N-MULTISIX®

REAGENT STRIPS FOR URINANALYSIS

DIRECTIONS:
Must be followed exactly.

1. Dip test areas of strip in FRESH, *well-mixed*, uncentrifuged urine. Remove immediately.

2. While removing, run the edge of the strip against the rim of the urine container to remove excess urine. Hold the strip in a horizontal position to prevent possible mixing of chemicals from adjacent reagent areas and/or soiling of hands with urine.

3. Compare test areas closely to corresponding Color Charts at times specified.

PLEASE READ PACKAGE INSERT BEFORE USE.

Ames Division MILES

Ames Division, Miles Laboratories, Inc.
P.O. Box 70, Elkhart, Indiana 46515

©1979 Miles Laboratories, Inc.
3109   R7119   55M

UROBILINOGEN	45 sec.	**NORMAL** 0.1 1	2	**Ehrlich units/dl urine** 4	8	12	
NITRITE	40 sec.	NEGATIVE		POSITIVE (any degree of uniform pink color)			
BLOOD	25 sec.	NEGATIVE	NON-HEMOLYZED TRACE / HEMOLYZED TRACE	SMALL +	MODERATE ++	LARGE +++	
BILIRUBIN	20 sec.	NEGATIVE		SMALL +	MODERATE ++	LARGE +++	
KETONE	15 sec.	NEGATIVE		SMALL +	MODERATE ++	LARGE +++	
GLUCOSE	10 sec. qual / 30 sec. quan	g/dl NEGATIVE	1/10 TRACE	1/4 +	1/2 ++	1 +++	2 or more ++++
PROTEIN	TIME NOT CRITICAL MAY BE READ IMMEDIATELY	mg/dl NEGATIVE	TRACE	30 +	100 ++	300 +++	over 2000 ++++
pH HANDLE	NEAREST		5	6	7	8	9

Many simple tests can be done during an office visit to aid the physician in diagnosis. Urine may be analyzed with reagent strips for correct levels of not only glucose, but many other components. (Courtesy of Ames Division of Miles Laboratories, Inc.)

(The color reproductions on these pages are for illustrative purposes only and must not be used to analyze actual test results)

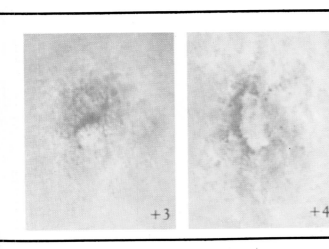

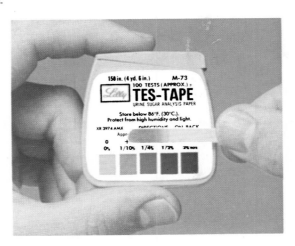

It is important for diabetics to have an immediate, accurate indication of urine sugar level. The patient can be counseled in the use of Tes-Tape®, as shown. (Courtesy of Eli Lilly and Company.)

THE
MEDICAL ASSISTANT:
ADMINISTRATIVE AND CLINICAL

MARY E. KINN, CPS, CMA-A

Assistant Professor, Health Technologies, Retired
Long Beach City College
Long Beach, California

Past President, American Association of Medical Assistants

Former Chairman, American Association of Medical Assistants Certifying Board

MARY ANN WOODS, RN, CMA, PhD

Professor, Health Sciences and the Arts Division, and
Director of Medical Assistant & Medical Records Programs,
Fresno City College, Fresno, California

Member of California Medical Assistants Association Certifying Board

Member of American Medical Writers Association

ELEANOR F. DERGE, RN, MS, CMA

Formerly Program Director, Medical Assisting Program, and
Instructor, Medical Assisting Program,
Madison Area Technical College, Madison, Wisconsin

SEVENTH EDITION

W.B. SAUNDERS COMPANY
A Division of Harcourt Brace & Company
PHILADELPHIA   LONDON   TORONTO   MONTREAL   SYDNEY   TOKYO

W.B. SAUNDERS COMPANY
A Division of Harcourt Brace & Company

The Curtis Center
Independence Square West
Philadelphia, Pennsylvania 19106

Library of Congress Cataloging-in-Publication Data

Kinn, Mary E.
    The medical assistant: administrative and clinical/Mary E.
Kinn, Mary Ann Woods, Eleanor F. Derge. — 7th ed.
        p. cm.
    Includes bibliographical references and index.
    ISBN 0–7216–4691–3
    1. Medical assistants.   I. Woods, Mary Ann.   II. Title.
    [DNLM: 1. Allied Health Personnel.   2. Medical Secretaries.   W 80
K55m 1993]
    R728.8.K493   1993
    610.73′7 — dc20
    DNLM/DLC   93-6719

The Medical Assistant: Administrative and Clinical, 7th Edition   ISBN 0–7216–4691–3

Printed in the United States of America

Last digit is the print number: 9   8   7   6   5

PREFACE

It is with pride and excitement that we have written this seventh edition of *The Medical Assistant: Administrative and Clinical.* Beginning with the refreshing new cover and ending with the last page of the glossary, you will find creative ideas and many interesting changes. Advances in the technology of equipment and educational methodology as well as an emphasis on new medical discoveries and procedures have made this edition a challenge to write and a joy to present.

This book is designed for use in the community college or vocational/technical school, by the medical office or clinic in-service, and in independent study programs. It can also aid the practicing medical assistant who wishes to upgrade a skill or needs a reference book.

Each chapter opens with a detailed outline. This is followed by a vocabulary list and competency objectives, which provide a road map for the chapter. These objectives have been carefully edited to ensure that every item in the current *DACUM Analysis of the Medical Assisting Profession* has been addressed and promotes the achievement of the basic entry-level skills. The chapter outline and competency objectives guide the instructor in preparing the material to be covered in the chapter and may also serve as a lecture outline for teaching the material. By previewing each chapter's outline and vocabulary, the student is mentally prepared to study that chapter's content.

Section 1, The Health Care Team (Chapters 1 to 7), addresses interactions of medical assistants with all health professionals and includes a brief history of medicine to provide background information on those events that have led to today's medical accomplishments, modern forms of medical practice, and current types of medical care. The cornerstones of medical ethics, from historical codes to the *AMA's Principles of Medical Ethics,* are discussed in some detail. The legal responsibilities and limitations of practicing medical assistants as well as those of physicians are included in Chapter 5, Medicine and the Law. A new chapter on personal communication (Chapter 6) guides the medical assistant in relations with his or her employer, colleagues, and patients. Section 1 concludes with situations that the medical assistant can expect when completing an externship and seeking employment.

Section 2, The Administrative Medical Assistant (Chapters 8 to 22), includes instruction in the areas generally described as "front-office," including appointment scheduling and patient reception, records management, fees and collections, accounting systems, computer applications, banking, and health and accident insurance. An entirely new chapter on dictation and transcription has been added to this edition. Section 2 concludes with extensive material on management responsibilities and the office environment.

Section 3, The Clinical Medical Assistant (Chapters 23 to 40), presents basic clinical medical assisting principles and procedures. The chapter sequence follows the logical progression of training of the medical assistant, from the basic to the advanced level of learning and competency. Each chapter is an entire learning package and serves as a "learning loop" that ties it both to the previous chapters and to those that follow. Added to every chapter are discussions of the medical assistant's responsibilities concerning patient education and legal and ethical matters as they specifically relate to the content of that chapter.

Highlights include a totally new chapter on Acquired Immune Deficiency Syndrome (AIDS), an updated chapter on nutrition, and reorganization of the chapters on surgery. In addition, three chapters have been devoted to examination techniques and procedures, starting with the generic examination, continuing with examination concerning the family unit, and concluding with types of specific specialty examination. The medical assistant's role in assessing the patient, which is specific to each type of examination, is described.

An extensive student review manual and an instructor's manual are also available; the review manual provides a variety of learning tools to aid the student in mastering and retaining the material discussed in the textbook, while the instructor's manual helps the teacher present the material in the text in the most effective manner possible.

We hope that the instructors, the students, and the practicing medical assistants who use this text will attain the sense of fulfillment and professional achievement that the medical assisting profession provides.

MARY E. KINN, CPS, CMA-A
MARY ANN WOODS, RN, CMA, PHD

ACKNOWLEDGMENTS

Over the 25 years that I have worked on *The Medical Assistant: Administrative and Clinical,* scores of individuals have contributed to its evolution. For this 7th edition, I acknowledge with great appreciation those who have directly assisted in bringing it to fruition:

Howard Langhans, Marketing Specialist of Credit Service Systems in Anaheim, CA, for his thorough review of Chapters 15 and 18, the verification of credit laws, and suggestions for improvement.

Mary Ray, office manager for Orthopedic Surgery, Orange, CA, for her assistance with the chapter on management responsibilities.

Experienced practicing medical assistant–members of the California Medical Assistants Association: Philomena Ten Eyck, CMA, CMT, and Judy Casto in San Diego, CA; June Miller, CMA-A, in Riverside, CA; Dee Ford, CMA-AC, in Laguna Hills, CA; and Rosalinda Salinas in Anaheim, CA, all of whom shared current materials and information.

Mark Farminger in Fresno, CA, for the unique artwork in the Student Manual.

Med-Index Publications in Salt Lake City, UT, for supplying current information on insurance coding and billing procedures.

Bibbero Systems in Petaluma, CA, and Colwell Systems, Inc. in Champaign, IL, for their continued support in providing sample forms for illustrating various administrative procedures.

The officers and members of the American Medical Writers Association, the American Association of Medical Assistants, and the California Medical Assistants Association for the privilege of membership, for the sharing of their friendship and accumulated knowledge, and for fostering the challenge of excellence.

Most of all, I thank Mary Ann Woods, RN, CMA, PhD, for sharing her wealth of experience and knowledge, for her effervescent good nature, and for being up when I was down.

MARY E. KINN, CPS, CMA-A

Many people gave of their time and energy to assist me in preparing this edition. I'm grateful to the editorial and production staffs at W.B. Saunders Co., who kept the project on track, and to the members of their Art Department, who worked meticulously on the many illustrations.

Thanks are also due to members of the medical profession who read and offered expert advice on many of the chapters. Their suggestions helped shape the manuscript into its final form.

I acknowledge with great appreciation:

Kathleen Thompson, RN (AORN), surgical nurse at Clovis Community Hospital, Clovis, CA, for her thorough review and assistance in rewriting the chapters on surgery.

Craig C. Stepp, MT (ASCP), medical technologist for Sierra Community Hospital, Fresno, CA, for his hours of assistance in evaluating and rewriting the chapters on laboratory techniques and procedures.

Emma Pelham, RN for helping to set up the procedures for the photographer.

Dr. Michael Maruyama, Physician's Plaza, Clovis, CA, for the use of his office, examination rooms, and equipment, which made the procedure photographs meaningful.

To my husband Bob, for spending countless hours proofreading, researching data, and xeroxing manuscript.

To all the medical assistant and medical records students at Fresno City College, Fresno, CA, who gave up their Saturdays to help with the photography.

To Mary Kinn, who became my mentor, my confidant, and, most of all, my friend, a deeply heartfelt "thank you," for without her love and talent, none of this would have been possible.

MARY ANN WOODS, RN, CMA, PhD

BRIEF CONTENTS

Detailed Contents

SECTION III
THE CLINICAL MEDICAL ASSISTANT

THE
MEDICAL ASSISTANT:
ADMINISTRATIVE AND CLINICAL

SECTION 1
THE HEALTH CARE TEAM

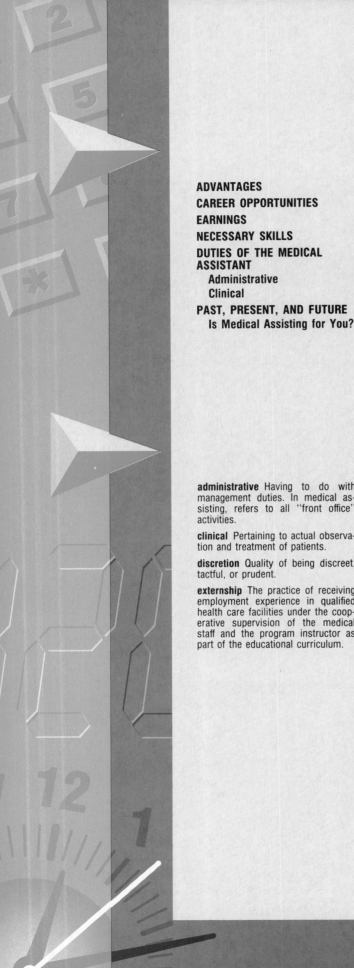

CHAPTER OUTLINE

ADVANTAGES

CAREER OPPORTUNITIES

EARNINGS

NECESSARY SKILLS

DUTIES OF THE MEDICAL
ASSISTANT
  Administrative
  Clinical

PAST, PRESENT, AND FUTURE
  Is Medical Assisting for You?

FIRST IMPRESSIONS
  Professional Appearance

TRAINING
  Getting Started
  Initial Job Training
  Continuing Education

PROFESSIONAL
ORGANIZATIONS
  American Association of
  Medical Assistants (AAMA)

Registered Medical Assistant
Program of the American
Medical Technologists (RMA/
AMT)

American Association for
Medical Transcription (AAMT)

Professional Secretaries
International (PSI)

VOCABULARY

administrative Having to do with management duties. In medical assisting, refers to all ''front office'' activities.

clinical Pertaining to actual observation and treatment of patients.

discretion Quality of being discreet, tactful, or prudent.

externship The practice of receiving employment experience in qualified health care facilities under the cooperative supervision of the medical staff and the program instructor as part of the educational curriculum.

freestanding emergency center An emergency facility not associated with a hospital.

group practice The provision of services by a group of at least three practitioners.

health maintenance organization (HMO) An organization that provides comprehensive health care to an enrolled group for a fixed periodic payment.

jargon The technical vocabulary of a special group.

mandatory In the nature of a mandate or command; obligatory.

regional Pertaining to a region or territory; local.

rural Pertaining to the country, as distinguished from a city or town.

solo private practice One physician practicing alone.

technical Pertaining to the practical or procedural details of a trade or profession.

urban Characteristic of or pertaining to a city or town.

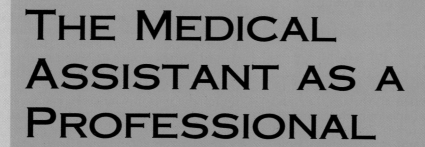

THE MEDICAL ASSISTANT AS A PROFESSIONAL

LEARNING OBJECTIVES

Upon successful completion of this chapter you should be able to:

1. Identify at least 10 career opportunities that are available to the trained medical assistant.

2. List five personality traits that are beneficial to the successful medical assistant.

3. Identify at least five skill areas in which the medical assistant should be proficient.

4. Differentiate between administrative and clinical responsibilities of the medical assistant.

5. Briefly describe the programs that are available for training medical assistants and list their required courses.

6. Name three professional organizations that provide educational opportunities and certification examinations to medical assistants.

A career as a medical assistant is challenging and offers variety, job satisfaction, opportunity for service, fair financial reward, and possibility for advancement. It is open to both men and women.

ADVANTAGES

The trained medical assistant is equipped with a flexible, adaptable career. The skills acquired by the medical assistant can be carried all through life, and employment is readily available anywhere in the world that medicine is practiced. Although medical assisting holds many opportunities for young people, it is one career that usually does not have a **mandatory** retirement age. Many medical assistants are still employed far beyond the usual retirement age because physicians realize the value of experienced, mature employees.

CAREER OPPORTUNITIES

The delivery of health care has changed dramatically in the last two decades. Increasing health care costs have created a trend away from hospital-based treatment toward the delivery of care in physicians' offices and in outpatient centers. Although doctors have employed assistants in their practices for many years, computerization and technologic advances have created more opportunities for qualified medical assistants and increased their responsibilities; as a result, the need for those trained in this profession has grown.

As the requirements that medical assistants must fulfill have become more clearly defined, the quality of their training has improved and become more accessible. Medical assisting is recognized as an important allied health profession. Employment opportunities in allied health are abundant, extremely varied, and increasing every day because of the growing concern about the availability of health protection for every individual in the United States. More medical assistants are employed by practicing physicians than any other type of allied health care personnel.

As a medical assistant, your work can be **administrative, clinical,** or **technical.** You can be a receptionist in a hospital or physician's office, a transcriptionist, insurance specialist, financial secretary, billing and collection specialist, a clinical assistant involved in patient care, or an emergency technician, to name just a few. You may choose to work for a physician in **solo private practice,** for a medical partnership or **group practice,** a **health maintenance organization (HMO),** a hospital, or a **freestanding emergency center.** The physician(s) may be either in general practice or engaged in a specialty such as surgery, internal medicine, dermatology, obstetrics, pediatrics, psychiatry, or radiology.

There are career opportunities in public health facilities, hospitals, laboratories, medical schools, research institutions and universities as well as in voluntary health agencies and medical firms of all kinds. There are also opportunities for work with such federal agencies as the Department of Veterans Affairs, the United States Health Service, and Armed Forces clinics or hospitals.

Although appropriate training equips you for work in a variety of settings, this text is designed primarily for the person who seeks employment in a medical office or who is already employed as a medical assistant.

Ideally, you should have both administrative and clinical training, even though you may have a personal preference for one or the other. The physician's staff should be able to handle all responsibilities of the office except those requiring the services of a physician or other licensed personnel. Where there are several assistants, each should be able and willing to substitute in an emergency for any of the others. Few physicians in private practice attempt to get along without at least one assistant. The great majority have at least two, and many have five or more.

EARNINGS

What kind of earnings can the medical assistant expect? As in any other career field, there are **regional** differences. There is usually some difference between earnings in **rural** and in **urban** areas. However, as a medical assistant, you can generally expect a satisfactory return on your investment in training, experience, and skill. Physicians have come to realize that a good medical assistant is worth a good salary. Many have learned through bitter experience that "bargain" help is often the most expensive.

The job turnover among medical assistants is surprisingly low. This fact may indicate that medical assistants derive a high degree of satisfaction from their work. Many instances have been reported of medical assistants who were hired when a physician started practice and remained until the physician's retirement.

NECESSARY SKILLS

Every profession or trade has its special vocabulary or **jargon;** the language of medicine must be understood by every allied health professional. The medical assistant must have a basic knowledge of law and ethics as they relate to the medical profession. Additionally, to qualify for administrative duties, the medical assistant must have good handwriting, be a proficient typist, and have good language, communication, and mathematics skills. Knowledge of shorthand is helpful, but in most medical facilities, electronic dictation and word processing are the current trend. Some training in records management is desirable for both the administrative and clinical assistants as are skills in human relations and personal communications. All medical assistants should be trained in cardiopulmonary resuscitation (CPR) and emergency first aid. The clinical medical assistant must be skilled in certain patient care arts and must have the necessary training to perform common medical tests. The laws governing which medical tests a clinical assistant may perform, however, vary from state to state.

DUTIES OF THE MEDICAL ASSISTANT

The duties of the medical assistant vary from one facility to the next, since the schedule must be geared to the type of practice and the working habits of the individual physician. In the office with only one employee, the medical assistant's time is divided between administrative and clinical duties. In the multiple-employee office, the positions tend to be more specialized.

Administrative Duties

A medical assistant's duties are similar to those of any administrative assistant to a top executive, but they have specific medical aspects. They include:

- answering telephones
- scheduling appointments
- interviewing and instructing new patients
- screening nonpatient visitors and salespersons
- explaining the doctor's fees to patients
- opening and sorting mail
- answering routine correspondence
- pulling patient charts for scheduled appointments
- filing reports and correspondence
- making arrangements for patient admission to a hospital and instructing the patient regarding admission
- making financial arrangements with patients
- completing insurance claim forms
- maintaining financial records and files
- preparing and mailing statements
- preparing checks for the doctor's signature
- maintaining a file of paid and unpaid invoices
- preparing and maintaining employees' payroll records (or submitting payroll information to an outside accountant)

Sometimes you may act as an informal editorial assistant to the doctor by helping in the preparation of manuscripts or speeches or by clipping articles from professional journals and assisting with the maintenance of the doctor's personal medical library.

Clinical Duties

Clinical duties are also varied. In general, the medical assistant:

- helps patients prepare for examinations and other office procedures
- takes the medical history
- assists the doctor when requested to do so
- cleans and sterilizes instruments and equipment
- instructs patients regarding preparation for x-ray and laboratory examinations
- keeps the supply cabinets well stocked

You may also collect specimens from patients and either send them to a laboratory or perform certain diagnostic tests for which you have been trained. You may also perform electrocardiography and, depending on state laws, assist in radiography. You may take and record a patient's temperature, pulse rate, respiratory characteristics, blood pressure, height, and weight. You may also prepare treatment or surgical trays and assist with patient treatments or surgery. You may occasionally be called upon to administer emergency first aid.

PAST, PRESENT, AND FUTURE

The first medical assistant was probably a neighbor of a physician who was called to help when an extra pair of hands was needed. As the practice of medicine became more complicated, some physicians hired registered nurses to assist in their office practices. When recordkeeping, data reporting, and an increasing number of business details began to be burdensome, the physician realized a need for an assistant with business training. Slowly, training programs that focused on both administrative and clinical skills began to appear in community and junior colleges. Medical assistant organizations on county and state levels were established. A national organization for medical assistants was formed in 1957, and a few years later, national certification for medical assistants became possible. In recent years, legislation regarding the scope of practice of medical assistants has been enacted in some states. Whether to enter the field of medical assisting is a big decision. Medical assisting is more than just a job — it is a career requiring dedication, integrity, and a commitment to continuing education.

IS MEDICAL ASSISTING FOR YOU?

- Do you have a friendly and pleasant disposition?
- Are you considerate, respectful, and kind?
- Can you view a situation through the eyes of others?

The services performed by a medical assistant are extremely personal. For this reason, the manner in which these services are performed can actually affect the health and welfare of a patient.

- Are you attentive to details?
- Are you accurate and dependable?
- Can you remain calm and accept responsibility during an emergency?

You may be called upon to assume charge of the office when the doctor is out. The doctor must depend on the medical assistant's good judgment when he or she is left alone.

Discretion and concern for the patient are very important. Many patients have chosen other physicians because of a seeming lack of concern on the part of medical assistants. The patient who feels comfortable with the medical assistant will probably feel comfortable with the doctor.

FIRST IMPRESSIONS

Appearances and first impressions can mean a great deal in any situation. This is especially true in the health care provider's establishment, where an atmosphere of cleanliness and order must prevail. The impression that the patients receive from the medical assistant often colors their impressions of the doctor and of the care they expect.

Professional Appearance

Health and Grooming

A well-groomed assistant in professional attire has a good psychologic effect on patients. The essentials of a professional appearance are good health, good grooming, and appropriate dress.

Good health means getting adequate sleep, eating balanced meals, and getting sufficient exercise to keep fit. Medical assistants need to maintain a sensible and healthful lifestyle that includes regular checkups of their own physical condition. A radiantly healthy office staff promotes the best possible public relations image for the physician.

Good grooming is little more than attention to the details of personal appearance. Personal cleanliness, which includes taking a daily bath or shower, using a deodorant, and practicing good oral hygiene, is vital. The female medical assistant's makeup should be carefully selected and applied. Harsh or exaggerated makeup is out of place in the professional office. Subtle eye makeup and clear or natural shades of nail polish may enhance the assistant's appearance. Both male and female medical assistants should be sure that their hair is clean, neatly styled, and off the collar.

Attire

Appropriate dress for the medical assistant is usually a uniform. The uniform not only gives a professional look but also identifies the assistant as a member of the health care team. Synthetic fabrics and fashionable styling make it possible for the medical assistant's uniform to be both practical and attractive.

Women have a choice of pantsuits that are available in white or a variety of colors, perhaps with a blouse or shirt in a contrasting color; alternatively, they may select a two-piece dress uniform (in white or a color) or an attractively styled traditional white uniform. Men usually wear white slacks with a white or light-colored shirt, jacket, or pullover top. A laboratory coat may be worn over casual "street" clothes by men or women if this is within the facility's dress code. Today's easycare fabrics make it unthinkable to wear a uniform more than one day without laundering. Even spills and spots that occur during the course of the working day can usually be rinsed out immediately.

The shoes the assistant wears should be appropriate for a uniform and be spotless and comfortable. White shoes must be kept white by daily cleaning. Remember that if you wear a laced shoe, shoestrings also need cleaning.

In some offices, the physician prefers that the medical assistant not wear a uniform. Some psychiatrists and some pediatricians, for example, feel that the clinical appearance of a uniform can have an adverse effect on patients. Nevertheless, the medical assistant who does not wear a uniform should follow the dictates of good taste and propriety in choosing a professional wardrobe. The garments worn while on duty must be comfortable, becoming, allow easy movement, and still look fresh at the end of a busy day.

Whatever uniform style the assistant chooses, it should be personally becoming and worn over appropriate undergarments. It should not have ornamentation. When wearing a uniform, jewelry should be limited to an engagement ring, wedding band, and professional pin. If there is more than one assistant in the office, name pins worn by all members of the staff can help patients to identify each one by name.

TRAINING

Getting Started

Medical assistants who were already employed in the field were among the first to recognize the need for more trained personnel in doctors' offices. Through the work in chapters of the American Association of Medical Assistants (AAMA) and aided by local medical societies, they have been instrumental in rapidly accelerating the development, refinement, and accessibility of such training. Formal training is essential for today's medical assistant.

Many community colleges and private vocational schools offer courses in medical assisting. Upon satisfactory completion of a course, the student receives a certificate, diploma, or, in the case of some community colleges, an associate degree. In the community college, the course of training takes from 10 months to 2 years to complete. Students are usually admitted only once or twice per year. Private schools more frequently have ongoing enrollment, and many courses are completed in 7 months.

The curriculum includes all or most of the following:

anatomy and physiology

medical terminology

medical law and ethics

psychology

oral and written communications

administrative procedures, such as typewriting and transcription

financial recordkeeping

insurance billing

medical records management

clinical procedures, such as preparation, assisting, and follow-up of patients for medical examinations

first aid

principles of CPR

pharmaceutical principles and administering medications

specimen collection and processing

basic office diagnostic procedures

Effective training also includes an **externship** of at least several weeks to provide practical experience in physicians' offices, accredited hospitals, or other health care facilities.

Initial Job Training

The physician, probably more than any other employer, tends to expect employees to perform independently, with little or no direct supervision. Conversely, the success of the physician's practice is highly dependent on teamwork of the staff members:

"The quantitative and qualitative acceptance of the team approach to health care is reflected in the changing ratio of physicians to other health professionals and in the increasing involvement of organizations representing allied health professionals. In the early 60s, the ratio was eight allied health professionals to one physician; by the late 60s, the ratio was twelve to one; and in the late 70s, the ratio was estimated at twenty to one." (American Medical Association, *Allied Health Education Directory,* 1990)

As a new employee, you should be told exactly what duties you are responsible for fulfilling. You may be asked to read the description of your job as it appears in an office procedure manual and then discuss it with the physician or your supervisor. If no one offers direction, you should ask for it. Poor performance reviews are too often the result of an employee never having been told what was expected of him or her.

You will bring many intangibles to your job that are not found in your job description. Courtesy toward others and a capacity for teamwork are necessary personal attributes. A positive attitude, enthusiasm, initiative, and dedication are also important assets. Respond to your initial training by showing that you are responsible and can be depended on. After you are thoroughly acquainted with your own job, you will probably want to learn what other employees are doing so that you can offer them assistance when needed. In this way, you become a full member of the health care team. Remember that you always learn by doing.

Continuing Education

Education does not end with the completion of formal training. The amount of medical knowledge gained since the beginning of medical history is now said to double every 5 years. The practicing medical assistant must keep current with the rapid changes within the profession. Most physicians appreciate the medical assistant who asks questions about unfamiliar conditions or procedures.

Much can be learned by reading or at least briefly reviewing the medical literature that arrives in the daily mail or the articles that appear in newspapers, news magazines, and specialized newsletters. The medical assistant who wishes to advance is an active member of a professional organization, has an inquisitive mind, and attends available professional seminars and workshops.

PROFESSIONAL ORGANIZATIONS

American Association of Medical Assistants (AAMA)

The AAMA was formally organized in 1956 as a federation of several state associations that had been functioning independently. In 1991, the AAMA had affiliated societies in 42 states and the District of Columbia, with national headquarters in Chicago, Illinois.

The AAMA has been the force behind establishing a national certifying program for medical assistants, the accrediting of medical assisting training programs in community colleges and private schools, and setting minimum standards for the entry-level medical assistant. AAMA members have the opportunity to attend local, state, and regional meetings, where they can participate in workshops, learn of educational advances in their field, hear prominent speakers, and establish a networking system with other medical assistants. The Association publishes a bimonthly journal, *The Professional Medical Assistant (PMA)*. Members may wear the AAMA insignia (Fig. 1–1).

Since 1963, the AAMA has offered a certifying examination, with successful completion leading to a certificate and recognition as a Certified Medical Assistant (CMA). The National Board of Medical Examiners participates in the construction and administration of the examination. The examination is given in January and June of each year at designated centers throughout the United States. Certification is available to students or graduates of programs accredited by the Committee on Allied Health Education and Accreditation (CAHEA), medical assisting instructors, and experienced medical assistants. Applicants need not be members of AAMA. Since 1988, revalidation every 5 years has been mandatory and can be accomplished through continuing education units (CEUs) or reexamination. The Certified Medical Assistant is permitted to wear the CMA pin (Fig. 1–2).

Registered Medical Assistants of the American Medical Technologists, RMA(AMT)

In the early 1970s, the American Medical Technologists (AMT) a national certifying body for laboratory personnel since 1939, began offering an examination for medical assistants. The solid success of this project brought about the formulation of the Registered Medical Assistant (RMA) Program within AMT in 1976. Since that time, the RMAs

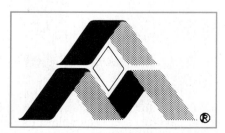

FIGURE 1–1. Insignia of the American Association of Medical Assistants. (Courtesy of the American Association of Medical Assistants, Chicago, IL.)

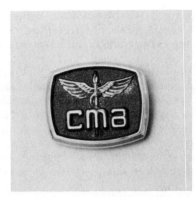

FIGURE 1–2. Pin worn by the Certified Medical Assistant. (Courtesy of the American Association of Medical Assistants, Chicago, IL.)

have earned great respect in their own right. They have played an active role in public relations and professional recognition, protective legislation, improvements in training programs, and the provision of continuing education materials and opportunities.

The RMA certification examination is given in March, June, and November of each year throughout the United States and as needed at schools accredited by the Accrediting Bureau of Health Education Schools (ABHES). Applicants must be graduates of a medical assisting course accredited by ABHES, a regional accrediting commission, or other acceptable agency or must meet certain experience requirements. All RMA members of the AMT Registry are certified medical assistants by examination and are entitled to wear the RMA insignia (Fig. 1–3). RMA national headquarters is located in Park Ridge, Illinois.

There are benefits to being a member of a medical assisting organization (see chart).

BENEFITS FROM MEMBERSHIP IN A MEDICAL ASSISTING ORGANIZATION
Both AAMA and RMA (AMT) offer opportunities for:
● Participation at local, state, and national levels
● Continuing education events with CEUs being recorded and reported, and a revalidation program
● Group insurance programs
● A professional journal

There are independent unaffiliated medical assistant organizations in some states that offer professional participation at the local and state level.

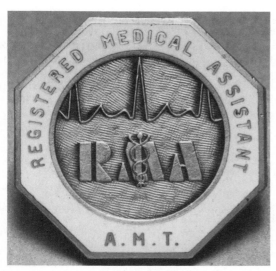

FIGURE 1–3. Pin worn by the Registered Medical Assistant. (Courtesy of the RMA/American Medical Technologists, Park Ridge, IL.)

American Association for Medical Transcription (AAMT)

Many medical offices employ medical word specialists as medical transcriptionists; such professionals will find membership in AAMT valuable. The Association was incorporated in 1978 with headquarters in Modesto, California. Certification by experience was available through December 1983. A certification examination has been offered since 1981, and since January 1, 1984, the only route to certification has been by successful completion of this examination (Fig. 1–4). Certification is voluntary; once achieved, it must be maintained through continuing education. AAMT publishes a professional journal four times per year and a newsletter six times per year. It offers an outstanding education program and holds an annual national convention.

Professional Secretaries International (PSI)

The administrative medical assistant may profit from membership in PSI. Formerly known as The

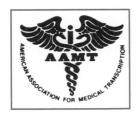

FIGURE 1–4. Insignia of American Association for Medical Transcription. (Courtesy of American Association for Medical Transcription, Modesto, CA.)

National Secretaries Association (International), PSI was founded in 1942 and is headquartered in Kansas City, Missouri. Through its Institute for Certifying Secretaries, PSI sponsors the Certified Professional Secretary (CPS) Examination, which covers behavioral science in business, business law, economics and management, accounting, office administration and communication, and office technology. The rating of CPS is obtained by meeting educational and work experience requirements and by passing the six-part, two-day examination (Fig. 1–5). The organization publishes *The Secretary* magazine nine times per year, holds an international convention each July, and sponsors Collegiate Secretaries International and the Future Secretaries Association in colleges and high schools, respectively.

By joining a professional organization and participating in the activities it affords, you can grow personally and professionally and keep abreast of current trends. Participation in a recognized professional organization indicates to an employer that you are serious about your career and are an asset to his or her practice. The rewards are limitless.

SUMMARY

In this first chapter, you have learned about the advantages of becoming a trained medical assistant and about some of the many career opportunities available. The necessary skills that you must develop were emphasized, and you are now aware of the general knowledge that you must acquire in order to function successfully in the medical arena.

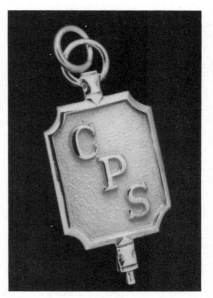

FIGURE 1–5. Pin worn by the Certified Professional Secretary. (Courtesy of Professional Secretaries International.)

However, skills alone do not bring success to the aspiring medical assistant. For this reason, personality traits and professional appearance have been emphasized in this introductory chapter. You have also learned the importance of getting the right start when entering new employment and the necessity for continuing education. An understanding of some of the history of the development of medical assisting as a career will help you to find your own niche in this rapidly changing profession. As your career develops, you will probably choose to affiliate with one of the professional organizations mentioned in this chapter.

Although this first chapter is an introduction to your training as a medical assistant and precedes the presentation of performance skills, it is recommended that you review it immediately prior to interviewing for a position in this fascinating field of health care.

 ## LEARNING ACHIEVEMENTS

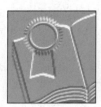

Are you able to:

1. Identify at least 10 career opportunities that are available to the trained medical assistant?
2. List five personality traits that are beneficial to the successful medical assistant?
3. Identify at least five skill areas in which the medical assistant should be proficient?

4. Differentiate between administrative and clinical responsibilities of the medical assistant?
5. Briefly describe the programs that are available for training medical assistants and list their required courses?
6. Name three professional organizations that provide educational opportunities and certification examinations to medical assistants?

REFERENCES AND READINGS

American Medical Association: *Allied Health Education Directory,* 11th ed., Chicago, The Association, 1990.
Gettys, R. C., and Zasa, R. J.: *Medical Group Practice Management,* Cambridge, MA, Ballinger Publishing Co., 1977.

PROFESSIONAL ORGANIZATIONS

American Association of Medical Assistants, 20 North Wacker, Suite 1575, Chicago, IL 60606.
American Association for Medical Transcription, P.O. Box 576187. Modesto, CA 95357.
Professional Secretaries International, 10502 N.W. Ambassador Drive, P.O. Box 20404, Kansas City, MO 64195–0404.
Registered Medical Assistant (AMT) 710 Higgins Road, Park Ridge, IL 60068.

CHAPTER TWO

——

A BRIEF HISTORY OF MEDICINE

CHAPTER OUTLINE

MEDICAL LANGUAGE AND MYTHOLOGY

MEDICINE IN ANCIENT TIMES

PIONEERS IN MODERN MEDICINE

WOMEN IN MEDICINE

MODERN MIRACLES

LOOKING AHEAD

LEARNING ACHIEVEMENTS

VOCABULARY

anesthesia Natural or artificially induced absence or loss of feeling or sensation.

anthrax An acute infectious disease caused by a bacillus. Humans contract the disease from contact with animal hair, hides, or waste matter.

aphonia Loss of the ability to speak.

aphrodisiacs Drugs that cause sexual arousal.

attenuated Made thin or weaker.

auscultation The act of listening for sounds within the body.

bacteria Single-celled microscopic organisms.

cervical vertebrae The upper seven bones of the spinal column; the skeleton of the neck.

chemotherapy The treatment of disease using chemical agents.

cholera An acute, infectious, bacillus-caused disease involving the entire small bowel. *Chicken cholera* Cholera that affects chickens.

contamination The act of soiling, staining, or polluting; especially the introduction of infectious materials or germs that produce disease.

cyanosis A bluish discoloration of the skin.

dialysis Separating out from the blood the harmful waste products of the body that are normally excreted in the urine.

dissection The process of cutting apart or separating tissues for anatomic study.

embryology The science or study of the development of living organisms during the embryonic stage.

fallopian tubes The tubes that carry the ovum from the ovary to the uterus; the oviducts.

hemiplegia Paralysis of one side of the body.

histologist One who specializes in the study of the minute structure, composition, and function of the tissues.

immunology A science that deals with the phenomena and causes of immunity and immune responses.

innovation Act of introducing something new or novel.

invulnerable Incapable of being injured or harmed.

ligation The process of tying up something to close it, usually a blood vessel, during surgery. The ties are called *ligatures*.

microorganism An organism of microscopic or ultramicroscopic size.

millennia Thousands of years (*mille* = thousand).

mons veneris The rounded, elevated area overlying the symphysis pubis that is covered with hair after puberty.

mysticism The experience of seeming to have direct communication with God or ultimate reality.

mythology A branch of knowledge that deals with the interpretation of myths.

neophyte A beginner.

oviducts The pair of tubes in the female that carry the egg from the ovary to the uterus; fallopian tubes.

pandemic Affecting the majority of the people in a country or a number of countries.

pathologic Altered or caused by disease.

percussion The act of striking a part of the body with short, sharp blows as an aid in diagnosing the condition of the underlying parts by the sound obtained.

perfusion The passing of a fluid through spaces.

phagocytosis The engulfing of microorganisms, other cells, and foreign particles by phagocytes.

placenta The vascular structure that develops within the uterus during pregnancy and through which a fetus receives nourishment.

protozoa Primitive animal organisms, each of which consists of a single cell.

puerperal fever The fever that accompanies an infection of the birth canal following delivery of a child; childbed fever.

purulent Consisting of or containing pus.

pustule A raised pus-filled area or sac.

putrefaction Decomposition of animal matter that results in a foul smell.

rabies An acute infectious disease of the nervous system caused by a virus, usually communicated to humans through animal bite.

rete mucosum The innermost layer of the epidermis (*rete* = network of nerves or vessels).

spermatozoa Mature male germ cells.

stethoscope An instrument for listening to sounds within the body.

swine erysipelas A contagious disease affecting young swine in Europe.

syphilitic chancre The primary sore of syphilis.

vagina The canal in the female that extends from the vulva to the cervix.

virulent Exceedingly pathogenic, noxious, or deadly.

vivisection Operation or cutting on a living animal for research purposes.

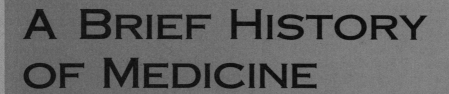

A BRIEF HISTORY OF MEDICINE

LEARNING OBJECTIVES

Upon successful completion of this chapter you should be able to:

1. Identify:

   The Greek physician who was revered as the "God of Medicine";

   The early physician who gave medicine a scientific basis;

   The man who first observed bacteria and protozoa through a microscope;

   The physician who pioneered the use of the microscope in the study of plants and animals;

   The 18th century surgeon who was given the title "Founder of Scientific Surgery";

   The physician who discovered the smallpox vaccine and identified the relationship between cowpox and smallpox;

   The physician who discovered the importance of percussion in diagnosis and the physician who developed the stethoscope;

   The physician who first diagnosed puerperal fever.

2. List four diseases to which Louis Pasteur devoted many years of study.

3. Identify at least four women who played important roles in the fields of nursing and medicine.

4. Name the individuals who were responsible for the discovery of:

x-ray therapy	penicillin
insulin	polio vaccine

Modern medicine reflects its history in the names given to anatomic and physiologic phenomena, medications, diseases, instruments, and specialties. Even the latest medical discoveries often have names drawn from the ancients. It is impossible to live in the world of medicine and to talk its language without being constantly touched by this fascinating past. The rich cultural heritage of medicine is interesting to study and to draw upon, but it is also a process filled with hardships and disappointments that were pushed aside by determined men and women who wanted to pursue their dreams and goals. It can be inspiring to think of these pioneers and realize that we too are part of the heritage of caring and discovery that continues to improve health care throughout the world.

MEDICAL LANGUAGE AND MYTHOLOGY

It may seem strange for modern medicine to borrow so liberally from ancient **mythology** and to use so actively the classical language that most civilizations abandoned centuries ago. Yet today's medicine uses words whose origins stem from the romance and fantasy of this long "dead" world. Anatomy, especially, seems to reach back to the dawn of history and, although some terms today are erroneous when translated literally (because the ancients did not correctly understand body functions), many early anatomic terms have reached modern times almost unchanged.

Greek and Roman mythology have contributed a major portion of our medical terms, but we have also borrowed liberally from Arabic, Anglo-Saxon, and German sources, with a heavy dash of the Bible added. Here are a few of the many examples from the classical past: the anatomic name for the first **cervical vertebra** upon which the head rests is aptly named Atlas, for the famous Greek Titan, who, according to mythology, was condemned by Zeus to bear the heavens on his shoulders. The tendon of Achilles reminds us of the story of the youth whose mother held him by the heel and dipped him into the river Styx to make him **invulnerable.** This particular tendon was not immersed, and later, a mortal wound was inflicted in Achilles' heel. The dubious honors given in medicine to Venus, the Roman Goddess of Love, are paid to her not so much as the goddess of love but of lust. She has a portion of the female anatomy, the **mons veneris,** dedicated to her memory. Venereal diseases are also named after her. Aphrodite, the Greek Goddess of Love and Beauty, gave her name to the sex arousing drugs known as **aphrodisiacs.**

Aesculapius, the son of Apollo, was revered as the God of Medicine. The early Greeks worshiped the healing powers of Aesculapius and built temples in his honor, where patients were treated by trained priests. His daughters were Hygeia, Goddess of Health, and Panacea, Goddess of All Healing and Restorer of Health. These two names are prominent in our language today.

MEDICINE IN ANCIENT TIMES

Though religion and myth were the basis of care for the sick for **millennia,** there is evidence of drugs, surgery, and other treatments based on theories about the body from as early as 5000 to 2000 BC. In the well-developed societies of the Egyptians, Babylonians, and Assyrians, certain men acted as physicians and used their scant knowledge to try to treat illness and injury.

Around 1205 BC, Moses incorporated rules of health into the Hebrew religion. He was thus the first advocate of preventive medicine and could even be called the first "public health officer." Moses knew that some animal diseases may be passed on to man and that **contamination** may linger on unclean dishes. Thus, it became a religious law that no one was permitted to eat animals that were not freshly slaughtered or to eat or drink from dirty dishes, lest they become defiled and lose their souls.

Hippocrates (460–377 BC) is the most famous of the ancient Greek physicians and is known as the "Father of Medicine." He did much to separate medicine from **mysticism** and gave it a scientific basis. He is best remembered for the "Hippocratic Oath" (see Chapter 4) exacted from his pupils. This oath has been administered to physicians for more than 2000 years. Hippocrates' astute clinical descriptions of diseases and his voluminous writings on epidemics, fevers, epilepsy, fractures, and instruments were studied for centuries. He believed that the body tends to heal itself and that it is the physician's responsibility to help nature. In his time, very little was known about anatomy, physiology, and pathology, and there was no knowledge of chemistry. In spite of these handicaps, many of his classifications of diseases and his descriptions of symptoms are being used today.

Many Greek physicians practiced, studied, and taught in Rome in the time after Hippocrates. One was Galen (131–201 AD), who came to Rome in 162 AD and became known as the "Prince of Physicians" (Fig. 2–1). Galen is said to have written 500 treatises on medicine. He wrote an excellent summary of anatomy as it was known at that time, but his work was faulty and inaccurate, for it was based largely on the **dissection** of apes and swine. He is considered to be the father of experimental physiology and the first experimental neurologist. He was the first to describe the cranial nerves and the sympathetic nervous system, and he made the first experimental sections of the spinal cord, producing **hemiplegia.** Galen also produced **aphonia** by cutting the recurrent laryngeal nerve, and he gave the first valid explanation of the mechanism of respiration.

The profound influence of the writings of Hippoc-

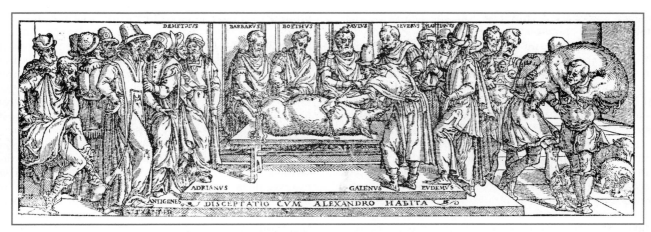

FIGURE 2–1. Galen. (Courtesy of the National Library of Medicine.)

rates and Galen on the course of medicine gives praise to these great thinkers, but their unquestioned authority actually had a negative effect on the progress of science throughout the "Dark Ages." Their theories and descriptions were held to as law, so **innovation** was rarely attempted. Experimenters were scoffed at by their contemporaries. Later, the Christian religion taught people to care for the sick and encouraged the establishment of institutions where the sick could find help. This provided an opportunity for physicians to observe, analyze, and discuss the progress of a variety of patients. The establishment of universities led more to a study of theories of disease rather than to observation of the sick. It was not until the 16th century that Andreas Vesalius (1514–1564) began to correct some of Galen's errors (Fig. 2–2).

Vesalius, a Belgian anatomist, is known as the

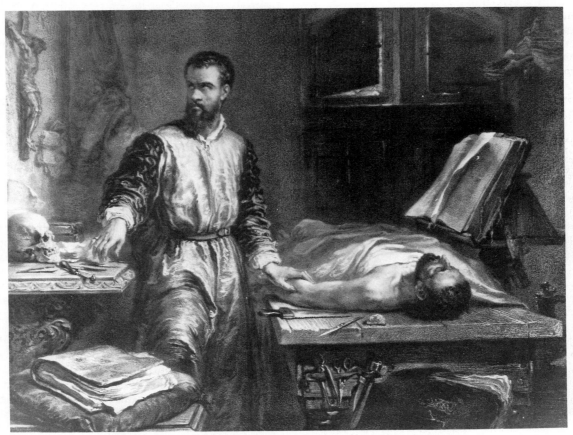

FIGURE 2–2. Andreas Vesalius. (Courtesy of the National Library of Medicine.)

"Father of Modern Anatomy." At the age of 29, he published his great *De Corporis Humani Fabrica,* in which he described the structure of the human body. This work marked a turning point by breaking with the past and throwing overboard the Galen tradition. Vesalius introduced many new anatomic terms, but because of his radical approach he was subjected to some persecution from his colleagues, his teachers, and his pupils. Despite his great contributions to the science of anatomy, his name is not used to identify any important anatomic structures. A student of Vesalius, Gabriele Fallopius, was also an accurate and detailed dissector who described and named many parts of the anatomy. He gave his own name to the **oviducts,** known as the **fallopian tubes.** He also gave the **vagina** and the **placenta** their present names.

In 1628, William Harvey (1578–1657) made his pronouncement—based on experimental **vivisection, ligation,** and **perfusion** as well as brilliant reasoning—that the heart acts as a muscular force-pump in propelling the blood along, and that the blood's motion is continual and continuous and in a cycle or circle (Fig. 2–3). The work of this English physician was not fully recognized until 1827, when the full importance of his work was substantiated. Harvey's writings were recognized in Germany before the English permitted their publication at home. Modern England now considers Harvey to be its "medical Shakespeare."

Great advances in medicine were somewhat stilled for a century or so, but the unseen world of **microorganisms** was opened as Anton van Leeuwenhoek (1632–1723), a Dutch linen draper and haberdasher by trade, pursued his hobby of grinding lenses. He ground over 400 lenses during his lifetime, most of which were very small—some no larger than a pinhead—and usually mounted between two thin brass plates that were riveted together. In grinding lenses Leeuwenhoek discovered how to use a simple biconvex lens to magnify the minute world of organisms and structures that had never been seen before. Leeuwenhoek was the first man ever to observe **bacteria** and **protozoa** through a lens. His accurate interpretations of what he saw led to the sciences of bacteriology and protozoology. He described for the first time the **spermatozoa** from insects, dogs, and man. He studied the structure of the optic lens, striations in muscles, and the mouthparts of insects. Leeuwenhoek extended Marcello Malpighi's demonstration in 1660 of the blood capillaries by giving (in 1684) the first accurate description of red blood cells. From 1673 until 1723, he communicated by means of informal letters most of his discoveries to the Royal Society of England, to which he was elected as a fellow in 1680.

The greatest of the microscopists was Marcello Malpighi (1628–1694), who was born near Bologna, Italy, entered the University of Bologna in 1646, and in 1653 was granted doctorates in both medicine and philosophy. Malpighi pioneered the use of the microscope in the study of plants and animals, after which microscopic anatomy became a prerequisite for advances in physiology, **embryology,** and practical medicine. He may be regarded as the first **histologist.** In 1661, he identified and described the pulmonary and capillary network connecting the small arteries with small veins, one of the most important discoveries in the history of science. When Malpighi found that the blood passed through the capillaries, it meant that Harvey was right—that blood was not transformed into flesh in the periphery, as the ancients had thought. Malpighi continued to pursue his studies with the microscope while teaching and practicing medicine. He identified the taste buds and described the minute structure of the brain and optic nerve. He was the first to see the red blood cells and to attribute the color of blood to them. He discovered the **rete mucosum** or Malpighian layer of the skin. His work on the structure of the liver, spleen, and kidney is recalled today when we speak of the Malpighian bodies of the kidney and spleen, Malpighi's pyramids (pyramides renales) and Malpighi's vesicles (alveoli pulmonis).

A few years after Leeuwenhoek's death, the famous English surgeon and anatomist John Hunter (1728–1793) was born (Fig. 2–4). Hunter has been given the title "Founder of Scientific Surgery" because his surgical procedures were soundly based on **pathologic** evidence. He was the first to classify teeth in a scientific manner. In 1778, he introduced artificial feeding by means of a flexible tube passed into the stomach. His description of the **syphilitic chancre** is classic, and the lesion is sometimes called the "Hunterian chancre." In an unsuccessful

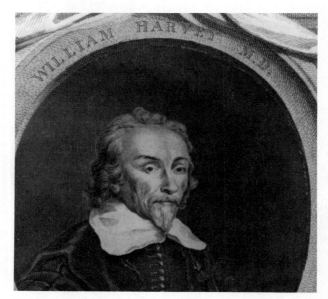

FIGURE 2–3. William Harvey. (Courtesy of the National Library of Medicine.)

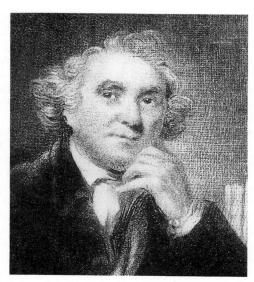

FIGURE 2-4. John Hunter. (Courtesy of the National Library of Medicine.)

attempt to differentiate gonorrhea from syphilis, Hunter inoculated himself with what he thought was gonorrhea, but instead acquired syphilis. His great collection of anatomic and animal specimens formed the basis for the museum of the Royal College of Surgeons. He was also a member of the Royal Society of Medicine and the Royal Academy of Surgery in Paris. Hunter wrote many papers on anatomy and physiology; he was a brilliant lecturer and teacher. Among his many students was one who would become famous and well loved: Edward Jenner.

PIONEERS IN MODERN MEDICINE

Edward Jenner (1749–1823) was a country physician in Dorsetshire, England (Fig. 2–5). He is listed among the immortals of preventive medicine for his discovery of the smallpox vaccine. The story goes that one day, while Jenner was serving as an apprentice in the office of Daniel Ludlow, a dairy maid was being given treatment. Smallpox was mentioned, and she said, "I cannot take that disease, for I have had cowpox." Smallpox at that time was the deadliest of **pandemics.** Jenner observed that farmers and dairy maids who once had cowpox never contracted smallpox. Later, as a practicing physician, Jenner continued investigating the relationship between cowpox and smallpox, to the extent that other medical society members became bored by him and threatened to expel him from their ranks.

On May 14, 1796, Dr. Jenner took some **purulent** matter from a **pustule** on the hand of Sarah Nelmes, a dairy maid, and inserted it through two small superficial incisions into the arm of James Phipps, a healthy 8-year-old boy. This was the first vaccination. Later, on July 1, a **virulent** dose of smallpox matter was given to young Phipps in the same arm. It had no effect: Phipps had been vaccinated and was safe from the dreaded disease. Edward Jenner's method of vaccination spread throughout the world. The results of his methods and experiments were published in 1798. He called this method of protection "vaccination" because the Latin word *vacca* means cow. Cowpox was called "vaccinia." Pasteur applied the term "vaccine" to suspensions of dead bacteria or **attenuated** bacteria. This term has come to be used in reference to other immunizing antigens not derived from cows.

Victor Robinson, in *Pathfinders in Medicine,* said of Dr. Jenner, "He died where an intellectual man should die — in his library. The village which gave him birth received his illustrious ashes. When his worn-out body was laid to rest, it would not be surprising if some humble woman, whose child he had saved from smallpox, imagined that Edward Jenner had gone to heaven — to vaccinate the angels."

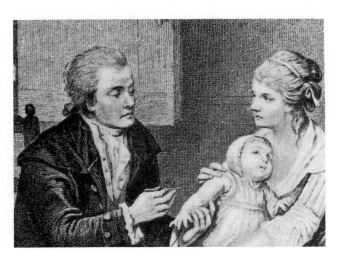

FIGURE 2-5. Edward Jenner. (Courtesy of the National Library of Medicine.)

Percussion and **auscultation** have been the very basics of physical examination for many years. But no physician had a real understanding of what went on inside the body until anatomists had paved the way for an Austrian physician, Leopold Auenbrugger (1722–1809), who developed the use of percussion in diagnosis, and a French physician, René Laënnec (1781–1826), who developed the **stethoscope.** Auenbrugger became physician-in-chief to the Hospital of the Holy Trinity at Vienna in 1751, and it was there that he tested his discovery, which afterward made him famous but which was generally ignored and scorned by his contemporaries. Laënnec invented the stethoscope in 1819, but at first it was only a cylinder of paper in his hands. His book concerning the stethoscope was readily accepted and translated into many languages. It is said to be the most important treatise in diseases of the thoracic organs ever written.

The first American treatise on psychiatry, *Medical Inquiries and Observations upon the Diseases of the Mind,* published in 1812, was written by Benjamin Rush (1745–1813), a member of the Continental Congress in 1776 and a signer of the Declaration of Independence.

In the early 1800s, there were several men who are remembered for their fight against **puerperal fever** and for their concern for women's health. Puerperal fever, an infectious disease of childbirth, is also known as puerperal sepsis or childbed fever. This term is from puerpera, denoting a woman in childbed, from the Latin *puer,* a child, and *pario,* to bring forth. The word "puerperium" now designates the period from delivery to the time the uterus returns to normal size.

The best known of these men is the Hungarian physician Ignaz Philipp Semmelweis (1818–1865). History has called him the "Savior of Mothers." His fight against puerperal fever is a sad story of hardships and resistance, especially from his instructor in Vienna, Professor Klein. Semmelweis noted the terrible results of puerperal fever in lying-in hospitals and observed that it occurred with special frequency in cases delivered by medical students who came directly from the autopsy or dissecting room. Semmelweis directed that in his wards the students were to wash and disinfect their hands with a solution of chloride of lime after leaving the dissection room and before going to the wards to examine a woman and deliver her child. This brought about a marked reduction of cases of childbed fever on his ward, but violent opposition was given by the hospital's medical men, and especially by Dr. Klein. As his theories were proven correct, Semmelweis began to feel the horror of the deaths that had been caused in the past by doctors themselves.

At the age of 47 years, Semmelweis died, ironically from the very infection he had fought, which was brought on by a cut in his finger while he was doing an autopsy. A monument to Semmelweis in Budapest is given great care, and it has been said that if people had been as tender to the man as they are to his statue, his career would have been happier.

Surely Semmelweis' death was a matter of tragic timing, for his grave had hardly been closed when the causes of this deadly disease were beginning to be understood as a result of the works of two great men, Louis Pasteur and Joseph Lister.

Louis Pasteur (1822–1895), a Frenchman, did brilliant work as a chemist, but his studies in bacteriology made him one of the most famous men in medical history and earned him the title of "Father of Bacteriology" (Fig. 2–6). He has also sometimes been honored with the name "Father of Preventive Medicine." His skills and studies reached far beyond the outermost boundaries of the knowledge of the time. He pursued everything with the fire of genius. His adventures included studying the difficulties in the fermentation of wine. He saved the most important industry of France at that time from disaster by a process now called pasteurization. By this process of supplying enough heat to destroy microorganisms, wine was prevented from turning into vinegar. This made great improvements in spirit and malt liquors. The French people called on Pasteur again to help the ailing silkworm industry. The silkworm epidemic in the south of France had reached such proportions that whole plantations were ruined. Pasteur devoted 5 years to the conquest of the two diseases that infected the silkworm. His work was interrupted only when he was stricken with hemiplegia. But after a long, difficult recovery when his mind was always fully active, he continued his work with a stiff hand and a limping foot.

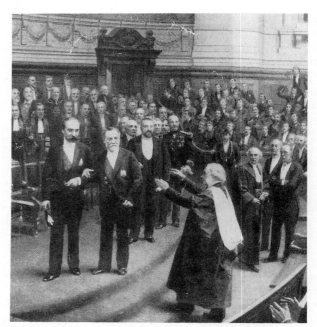

FIGURE 2–6. Louis Pasteur. (Courtesy of the National Library of Medicine.)

With the conviction that the "infinitely small" world of bacteria held the key to the secrets of contagious diseases, he again left chemistry, this time to become a medical man. Many renowned scientists denied the germ theory of disease and devoted themselves to degrading Pasteur. In the midst of all this "controversy" he became involved in the prevention of **anthrax,** which threatened the health of the cattle and sheep of France as well as of the world. Pasteur's name was also honored for work on many other diseases, such as **rabies,** chicken cholera, and **swine erysipelas.**

Pasteur died in 1895, with his family at his bedside. His last words were said to be, "There is still a great deal to do."

Joseph Lister (1827–1912) was to revolutionize surgery through the application of Pasteur's discoveries. He saw the similarity between the infections that were taking place in postsurgical wounds and the processes of **putrefaction,** which Pasteur had proved were caused by microorganisms. Before this time, surgeons accepted infection in surgical wounds as inevitable. Lister reasoned that microorganisms must be the cause of infection and must, therefore, be kept out of wounds. Lister's own colleagues were quite indifferent to his theories, since they felt infections were God-given and natural. Lister had once seen pain quelled by the administration of an anesthetic, and pain had been thought to be God-given and inevitable also. He developed antiseptic methods by using carbolic acid for sterilization. By spraying the room with a fine mist of the acid, by soaking the instruments and ligatures, and by washing his hands in carbolic solutions, Lister proved his theory. He is honored with the title of "Father of Sterile Surgery."

Pasteur and Joseph Lister met at the Sorbonne after years of great mutual admiration. The meeting was filled with emotion, and Robinson, in *Pathfinders in Medicine,* has said that "a new star should have appeared in the heavens to commemorate the event. Only a small percentage of the human race entertains any adequate realization of how much we really owe to the combined labors of Louis Pasteur and Joseph Lister."

The name Robert Koch (1843–1910) is familiar to all bacteriologists, for the first law learned as a **neophyte** in this microscopic world is Koch's Postulates, which state rules that must be followed before an organism can be accepted as the causative agent in a given disease.

Robert Koch was a German physician who truly earned great honors in bacteriology and public health. He gave the bacteriology laboratory many of its "tools," such as the culture-plate method for isolation of bacteria. He discovered the cause of **cholera** and demonstrated its transmission by food and water. This discovery completely transformed health departments and proved the importance of bacteriology. It also established a place of great respect for Koch in the scientific world. A great disappointment in Koch's career was his failure to find a cure for tuberculosis. In this attempt, however, he isolated tuberculin, the substance produced by tubercle bacteria. Its use as a diagnostic aid proved to be of immense value to modern medicine.

Koch's work took him throughout the world. He traveled to America, Africa, Bombay, Italy, and anywhere nations sought his help in ridding themselves of feared diseases. He was investigating anthrax at the same time as Pasteur, but the ill-concealed animosity between the two men prevented any cooperative effort.

In 1885, the University of Berlin created the Chair of Hygiene and Bacteriology in his honor. He became the Nobel Laureate in 1905.

While Robert Koch's brilliant career was nearing an end because of advanced age and illnesses, the work of Paul Ehrlich (1854–1915) was reaching its zenith (Fig. 2–7). Ehrlich had been greatly honored when Koch had invited him to work in his laboratory. Koch had known Ehrlich well, since he had been a distinguished student of his and had already made a place for himself in scientific circles.

Ehrlich was a German physician, and one of the pioneers in the fields of bacteriology, **immunology,** and especially **chemotherapy,** a fairly new science. He was only 28 years old when he wrote his first paper on typhoid, but his greatest gift to mankind was to be called his "magic bullet," or "606," and was designed to fight the terrible disease, syphilis. Only 3 years before, Bordet and Wasserman had identified the organism and devised a test that would smoke it out of hiding. With the offending germ identified, Ehrlich set out to find a chemical that would destroy the organism but not harm the germ's host, the human body. The search was long and tedious, and history tells us it was the 606th

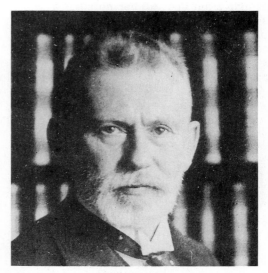

FIGURE 2–7. Paul Ehrlich. (Courtesy of the National Library of Medicine.)

drug that Ehrlich tried that finally did the healing. He called the drug "salvarsan" because he felt it offered mankind salvation from this disease. This also was the beginning of the practice of injecting chemicals into the body to destroy a specific organism.

Later, in 1912, Ehrlich discovered a less toxic drug, called neosalvarsan, to replace the original 606. The new drug bore the number 914. In 1908, Ehrlich shared the Nobel prize with Eli Metchnikoff, who is remembered for his theory of **phagocytosis** and immunology.

WOMEN IN MEDICINE

Much time is spent with honoring great men in medical history, but women have also played important roles, which during those times was not an easy thing to do. Two famous women, in particular, are Florence Nightingale (1820–1910) and Clara Barton (1821–1912). You may notice that their careers overlap almost to the year.

Florence Nightingale has been honored and known far and wide as "The Lady with the Lamp" and is immortalized as the founder of nursing (Fig. 2–8). She was of noble birth, and somewhat late in life she sought nurse's training in both England and Europe. By the time of the Crimean War in 1854, she already had a reputation for her work in hospital organization. She was invited by the Secretary of War to visit the Crimea to correct the terrible conditions that existed in caring for the wounded. She created the Women's Nursing Service at Scutari and Balaklava. The doctors at Scutari regarded Florence Nightingale as a troublesome female intruder and treated her and her nurses quite shabbily. Only a crisis that brought thousands of wounded and sick soldiers to army hospitals persuaded the doctors to accept help from her and her nurses.

Miss Nightingale ruled her nurses with an iron hand. Aside from the practical work she did, it was she who insisted the nursing profession get public recognition and that nursing require special training and experience. From donated funds she organized a school of nursing that bears her name. The modern conception of nursing is based largely on the foundations she laid.

The American counterpart to Florence Nightingale is Clara Barton (Fig. 2–9). She was a nurse and philanthropist whose work during the American Civil War led her to recognize that very poor records, if any at all, were kept in Washington to aid in the search for missing men wounded or killed in combat. This led to the formation of the Bureau of Records. Clara Barton's fame spread as a result of her organization and recruitment of supplies for the wounded. In 1870, she observed the work of the Red Cross in the Franco-Prussian War, and in 1881, she organized a Red Cross Committee in Washington, forming the American Red Cross, of which she served as the first president from 1881 to 1904.

Elizabeth Blackwell (1821–1910) was the first woman in the United States to receive the Doctor of Medicine degree from a medical school. Blackwell's family immigrated to New York from England in 1832. Young Elizabeth began her medical education by reading medical books and later on had private instruction. Medical schools in New York and Pennsylvania refused her applications for formal study, but finally, in 1847, she was accepted at the Geneva (New York) Medical College. Ten years later, when Blackwell was practicing medicine in New York City, she established the New York Infirmary, a hospital staffed by women. In 1869, Dr. Blackwell returned to her native England and became professor of gynecology (1875–1907) at the London School of Medicine for Women, of which she was a founder.

Another great contribution to medical care was made by Lillian Wald (1867–1940), a social worker

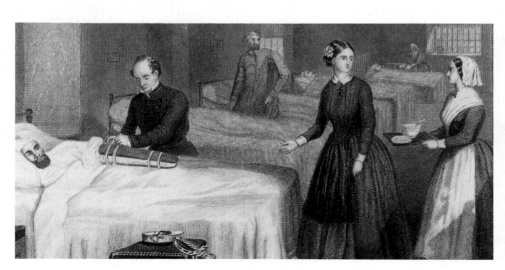

FIGURE 2-8. Florence Nightingale. (Courtesy of the National Library of Medicine.)

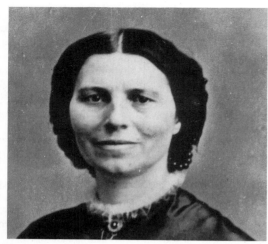

FIGURE 2-9. Clara Barton. (Courtesy of the National Library of Medicine.)

and nurse who founded the internationally known Henry Street Settlement at 265 Henry Street, New York City. Wald operated a visiting nurse service from this establishment. When one of her nurses was assigned to the city's public schools in 1902, the New York City municipal board of health established the world's first public school nursing system.

MODERN MIRACLES

Anyone who has ever been spared the pain of surgery through the sleep of an anesthetic can give thanks to the memory of two dentists, Dr. Horace Wells and Dr. William T. G. Morton, and a physician, Dr. Crawford Williamson Long. There has been considerable controversy as to whom should be given final credit for the actual discovery of **anesthesia,** but it now seems to be established that Dr. Long (1815–1878) was the first to employ ether as an anesthetic agent. Early in 1842, after lectures on chemistry, a group of students would have a social gathering and inhale ether as a form of amusement. At one of these so-called "ether frolics," Dr. Long observed that people under the influence of ether did not seem to feel pain. After considerable thought, Dr. Long decided to use ether for a surgical operation. On March 30, 1842, he removed a tumor from the neck of James M. Venable after placing him under the influence of ether. Long did not report this operation or his discovery until 1848. Wells reported his discovery in 1844, and Morton his in 1846, when he extracted a tooth after the patient had been given ether; he also used ether at Massachusetts General Hospital for a surgical procedure.

Surgery undoubtedly owes most to Wilhelm Konrad Roentgen (1845–1922), who discovered the x-ray in 1895. Roentgen was awarded the Nobel prize in Physics in 1901. Although he called his ray the x-ray, science has honored him by calling it the roentgen ray.

In 1900, Walter Reed, U.S. Army pathologist and bacteriologist, proved that yellow fever is transmitted by the bite of a mosquito; in 1901, action by U.S. military engineers in Cuba freed Havana from the disease by eliminating the mosquitoes.

Anyone who has had an x-ray or has received radium therapy should know the long struggle of Marie and Pierre Curie leading to the discovery of radium in 1898. Diabetics should be grateful to Frederick Banting, the Canadian physician who discovered insulin in 1922. Children born with **cyanosis** due to a malformed heart (tetralogy of Fallot) owe thanks to Helen B. Taussig, M.D., of Baltimore, Maryland, who, together with Alfred Blalock, M.D. (1899–1964), developed the lifesaving operation for so-called "blue babies." While the Blalock-Taussig procedure, first performed in 1944 at Johns Hopkins University Hospital, may seem simple today, 40 years ago it was revolutionary and led to a major change of direction in the treatment of heart disease.

In 1928, Sir Alexander Fleming (1881–1955), a British bacteriologist, discovered penicillin. While working with staphylococcal bacteria, Fleming noticed a bacteria-free circle around a mold growth that was contaminating a culture of the staphylococci. Upon investigation, he found a substance in the mold that prevented growth of bacteria even when the substance was diluted 800 times. He called it penicillin. Fleming shared the 1945 Nobel prize for Physiology or Medicine with Ernst Boris Chain and Howard Walter Florey for further discoveries related to penicillin.

The vaccines developed by Jonas Edward Salk and Albert Sabin in the 1950s almost eradicated polio, once the killer or crippler of thousands in the United States. The work of Dr. Christiaan Barnard in the 1960s inspired transplantation of hearts and other organs.

William Worrall Mayo, who immigrated to the United States from England in 1845, was the founder, in 1863, of the surgical practice in Rochester, Minnesota, that evolved into today's Mayo Clinic. Mayo's two sons, William James Mayo and Charles Horace Mayo, both became doctors and carried on the work begun by their father. A third-generation Mayo, Charles William Mayo (born in 1899), son of Charles Horace, also became a skilled surgeon and a member of the Mayo Clinic board of governors. The clinic is world renowned and is associated with the University of Minnesota. By the 1980s, the staff included more than 800 physicians and over 7000 support staff. Thousands of physicians have received some or all of their residency training at the Mayo Clinic and the Mayo Foundation connected with it.

And history continues. Bypass surgery has made thousands of hearts more functional. Organ trans-

TABLE 2–1. MILESTONES IN THE HISTORY OF MEDICINE

Dates	Person	Achievement	Dates	Person	Achievement
1205 BC	Moses (First "Public Health Officer")	Incorporated rules of health into the Hebrew religion	1749–1823	Edward Jenner	Discovered smallpox vaccine
460–377 BC	Hippocrates (Father of Medicine)	Gave scientific basis to medicine Hippocratic Oath	1781–1826	René Laënnec	Invented the stethoscope
131–201 AD	Galen (Father of Experimental Physiology)	First to describe cranial nerves and sympathetic system	1818–1865	Ignaz Philipp Semmelweis (Savior of Mothers)	Developed theory of childbed (puerperal) fever
1514–1564	Andreas Vesalius (Belgian anatomist; Father of Modern Anatomy)	Corrected some of Galen's errors Published *De Corporis Humani Fabrica* describing structure of human body	1820–1910	Florence Nightingale (Lady with the Lamp)	Founder of nursing
			1821–1912	Clara Barton	Founder of American Red Cross
1578–1657	William Harvey	Described pumping action of heart and circulation of the blood	1821–1910	Elizabeth Blackwell	First woman in United States to receive Doctor of Medicine degree from a medical school
1628–1694	Marcello Malpighi (First histologist)	Pioneered microscopic anatomy Identified the taste buds; described minute structures of brain and optic nerve	1822–1895	Louis Pasteur (Father of Bacteriology)	Developed germ theory of disease and destruction of microorganisms through use of heat
1632–1723	Anton van Leeuwenhoek	Discovered lens magnification First to observe bacteria and protozoa through a lens Made first accurate description of red blood cells	1827–1912	Joseph Lister	Applied Pasteur's theories and developed sterile techniques in surgery
			1843–1910	Robert Koch	Bacteriologist who developed culture-plate method for isolation of bacteria Set down Koch's postulates
1722–1809	Leopold Auenbrugger	Developed the use of percussion in diagnosis	1845–1922	Wilhelm Konrad Roentgen	Discovered x-ray in 1895
1728–1793	John Hunter (Founder of Scientific Surgery)	Introduced artificial feeding by insertion of flexible tube into stomach Made classic description of syphilitic chancre (Hunterian chancre)	1854–1915	Paul Ehrlich	Began the use of injecting chemicals into the body to destroy a specific organism Developed drug used to fight syphilis
1745–1813	Benjamin Rush	Published first American treatise on psychiatry in 1812	1867–1940	Lillian Wald	New York City nurse who operated a visiting nurse service and helped establish the world's first public school nursing system

plants are becoming almost commonplace. Great advances have been made in the treatment of cancer —who will find a real breakthrough? **Dialysis** machines allow people with nonfunctional kidneys, who would have died a few decades ago, to lead relatively normal lives. Countless unnamed people are engaged in research or are implementing new developments. Let us not forget those who are involved in organizing public health services and have thus contributed to bettering the availability and distribution of health care.

It is tremendously exciting simply to be open to such advancements and to be aware of their potential. The supportive role of medical assisting is very important in maintaining the quality of medical service and in making today a strong foundation for the progress of tomorrow.

LOOKING AHEAD

Learning the history of the development of modern medicine is not necessary in order to perform your duties as a medical assistant, just as a study of the genealogy of your family is not necessary for you to live a full life. However, both of these pursuits add interest and a uniqueness to the quality of your life. If you have been enlightened by this brief history of medicine, further study of medical history will add an extra dimension to your study of medical assisting.

Volumes could be—and have been—written about the medical miracles of the last 50 years. The nature of this text does not permit the exploration of every one of these miracles. You will undoubtedly be witness to many more discoveries in the course of your career. Perhaps you will contribute some miracles of your own.

► LEARNING ACHIEVEMENTS

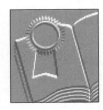

Are you able to:

1. Name the Greek physician who was revered as the "God of Medicine" and his two daughters whose names are common in today's language?
2. Explain how the term *vaccine* got its name?
3. Recall the reason that John Hunter was given the title "Founder of Scientific Surgery"?
4. State which physician named many parts of the anatomy, including the oviducts, vagina, and placenta?
5. Recall the name of the physician who discovered the use of percussion in diagnosis?
6. Explain what is meant by the term *puerperal fever?*
7. Name the chemist whose discovery led to the ability to destroy microorganisms?
8. Name the person who:
    Founded the American Red Cross?
    Was responsible for the formation of the National Bureau of Records?
9. Name the person responsible for the discovery of:
    X-ray therapy?
    Insulin?
    Penicillin?
    Polio vaccine?
10. Name the physician who developed the stethoscope?

REFERENCES AND READINGS

Bordley, J., III, and Harvey, A. M.: *Two Centuries of American Medicine,* Philadelphia, W. B. Saunders Co., 1976.
Garrison, F. H.: *History of Medicine,* 4th ed. (reprint), Philadelphia, W. B. Saunders Co., 1929.
Marks, G., and Beatty, W. K.: *The Story of Medicine in America,* New York, Scribners, 1974.
Robinson, V.: *Pathfinders in Medicine,* New York, Medical Life Press, 1929.
Smith, W. D.: *The Hippocratic Tradition,* New York, Cornell University Press, 1979.
Thorwald, J.: *The Century of the Surgeon,* London, Thames & Hudson, 1957.

CHAPTER OUTLINE

VOCABULARY

accelerating Causing to act or move faster.

concurrent Operating or occurring at the same time.

dissemination The act of broadcasting or spreading over a considerable area.

endorsement Sanction or approval.

isolation The act of placing alone, apart from others.

liability State or quality of being liable; that for which one is liable, such as debts.

prudent Capable of directing or conducting oneself wisely and judiciously.

quackery Pretense of medical skill.

reciprocity An obligation under which something is done or given by each of two to the other.

statutory body A part of the legislative branch of a government.

substantiated Having been established as true by proof or competent evidence; verified.

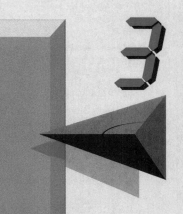

MEDICAL PRACTICE

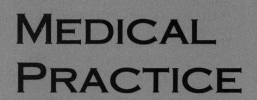

LEARNING OBJECTIVES

Upon successful completion of this chapter, you should be able to:

1. Define the terms listed in the Vocabulary.

2. Name the medical school that was the most famous in the world at the end of the 19th century.

3. Name a 20th century educator who played a major role in the development of medical education in the United States.

4. State at least two reasons for great changes in the 20th century delivery of medical care.

5. State the purpose of medical practice acts and how they are established.

6. List the three methods by which licensure may be granted.

7. State the three general categories of cause for revocation or suspension of license.

8. Name and briefly describe three forms of medical practice.

9. Name four types of medical care delivery.

10. Identify at least 10 allied health occupations that might be represented in a physician's office.

EARLY DEVELOPMENT OF MEDICAL EDUCATION

In our brief review of the history of medicine in Chapter 2, we found that in early times medical knowledge developed slowly, often in **isolation,** and that **dissemination** of knowledge was poor. Before the advent of printing, there was very little exchange of scientific knowledge and ideas, and scientists were not well informed about the works of others.

In the middle of the 15th century, Johann Gutenberg's invention of movable type and adaptation of a certain kind of press for printing marked a turning point in history. Gutenberg's invention resulted in a relatively fast way to produce multiple identical copies of any single text. Printing rapidly replaced the laborious method of scribes, who had to copy manuscripts by hand. The greater availability of books enlarged the number of literate people throughout Europe. In turn, ever greater refinements in the printing press were developed to meet the growing demand for books.

Another development of great importance to science that occurred in the 17th century was the establishment in Europe of academies or societies consisting of small groups of men who met to discuss subjects of mutual interest. The academies provided freedom of expression which, together with the stimulus of exchanging ideas, contributed significantly to the development of scientific thought. One of the earliest of these academies was the Royal Society of London, an organization formed in 1662 by the incorporation of several smaller groups under one royal charter.

A significant aspect of these societies was their publications, such as the Royal Society of London's *Philosophical Transactions.* Marcello Malpighi and Anton van Leeuwenhoek (mentioned in Chapter 2) both were invited to join the Royal Society and contributed works to *Philosophical Transactions.*

As the development of communications improved, society also became more complex, and the need for regulation became greater. The passage of the Medical Act of 1858 in Great Britain was considered one of the most important events in British medicine. It established a **statutory body,** the General Medical Council, which controlled admission to the medical register and had great power over medical education and examinations.

In the United States, medical education was greatly influenced by the example set in 1893 by the Johns Hopkins University Medical School in Baltimore. It admitted only college graduates with a year's training in the natural sciences. Its clinical work was superior because the school was supplemented by the Johns Hopkins Hospital, which had been created expressly for teaching and research by members of the medical faculty. The first four professors at Johns Hopkins were Sir William Osler, professor of medicine; William H. Welch, chief of pathology; Howard A. Kelley, chief of gynecology and obstetrics; and William D. Halsted, chief of surgery. Together, these four men transformed the organization and curriculum of clinical teaching and made Johns Hopkins the most famous medical school in the world.

Abraham Flexner (1866–1959), an educator, also played a major role in the development of medical education in the United States. After publishing an appraisal of educational institutions in the United States in 1908, Flexner received a Carnegie Foundation commission to study the quality of medical colleges in the United States and Canada. The Flexner report, published in 1910, rated 155 schools according to the quality of instruction and facilities available to the students. The publication of this report resulted in the closure of many low-ranking schools and the upgrading of many others.

By the mid-20th century, medical practice was experiencing many changes. Rapid developments in medical science encouraged more specialization. The **accelerating** cost of maintaining an office was becoming prohibitive for a solo practitioner, especially the new graduate. Medical insurance for the patient was the rule rather than the exception. More and more government programs, with their accompanying regulations, were developing, and the management of a medical practice required more and better-trained personnel.

All of these developments brought many changes in the delivery of medical care. It is estimated that by the year 2000, 50 per cent of the U.S. population will be receiving their medical care in prepaid comprehensive care facilities. Although there are still many solo practitioners in medicine, the trend is toward multiple-practitioner practices.

MEDICAL PRACTICE ACTS

Medical practice acts are established by *statute* in each of the 50 states. They define what is included in the practice of medicine within that state and govern the methods and requirements of licensure and the grounds for suspension or revocation of license.

Medical practice acts existed as early as in colonial days. However, these acts were later repealed, and in the mid-19th century practically none of the states had laws governing the practice of medicine. As might be expected, there was a rapid decline in professional standards. The general welfare of the people was endangered by medical **quackery** and inadequate care; by the beginning of the 20th century, medical practice acts were again in effect in every state.

LICENSURE AND REGISTRATION

Licensure

A Doctor of Medicine degree (M.D.) is conferred upon graduation from medical school. Some graduates may not wish to actually engage in the practice of medicine; their interests may lie in research or administration or even in the practice of law with a special interest in medical **liability.** In such cases, it is not necessary for them to be licensed. However, before a doctor of medicine can engage in the practice of medicine, he or she must be licensed. **Physicians in the Armed Forces, Public Health Service, or Veterans Administration facilities need not be licensed in the state where they are employed.** The license to practice medicine is granted by a state board, frequently known as the Board of Medical Examiners or Board of Registration.

Licensure may be by any one of the following:

- Examination
- Endorsement —*exam*
- Reciprocity

Examination

All states require medical doctors to pass a written examination for initial licensure. All licensing jurisdictions in the United States (except Puerto Rico), use the Federation Licensing Examination (FLEX) as the official medical licensing examination. Puerto Rico endorses scores from both the National Board of Medical Examiners (NBME) and FLEX for licensing purposes.

To be eligible for NBME certification, an individual must fulfill all of the following prerequisites:

- Have received the M.D. degree from a medical school in the United States or Canada that is accredited by the Liaison Committee on Medical Education (LCME) at the time the M.D. degree was granted.
- Have passed Parts I, II, and III of the NBME examination.
- Have completed, with a satisfactory record, one full year of an accredited residency.

Endorsement

Most graduates of medical schools in the United States have been licensed by **endorsement** of their National Board certificate. Those graduates who have not been licensed by endorsement are required to pass a state board examination (usually the FLEX). In all states, graduates of foreign medical schools seeking licensure by endorsement must meet the same requirements as graduates of medical schools in the United States, in addition to various other qualifying factors.

Reciprocity

Some states grant a license to practice medicine by **reciprocity;** that is, they endorse a license held in another state or jurisdiction. If an applicant is certificated by the National Board of Medical Examiners, he or she may be granted a license by endorsement in all licensing jurisdictions except Louisiana, Texas, and the Virgin Islands.

New Single Licensing Examination

The Federation of State Medical Boards and the National Board of Medical Examiners agreed in 1990 to establish a single licensing examination for graduates of accredited medical schools. The new examination, entitled the United States Medical Licensing Examination (USMLE), was to be gradually phased in starting in 1992.

Registration and Re-Registration

After a license is granted, periodic re-registration is necessary. A physician can be **concurrently** registered in more than one state. The issuing body notifies the physician when re-registration is due; however, not all states do this at the same time of the year. **Periodic re-registration is necessary annually or biennially.**

The medical assistant can aid the physician by being aware of when the registration fees are due, thus preventing a possible lapsing of the registration. Pennsylvania is the only jurisdiction that does not require a re-registration fee. The other states charge fees ranging from $15 to $200. Many states require proof of continuing education in addition to payment of a registration fee.

Continuing education units (CEUs) are granted to physicians for attending approved seminars, lectures, and scientific meetings, as well as formal courses in accredited colleges and universities. Fifty hours a year is the average requirement for license renewal. The medical assistant may be expected to help the physician make arrangements for completing the required units for license renewal.

Revocation or Suspension

Under certain conditions, the license to practice medicine may be revoked or suspended. Grounds for revocation or suspension of medical license generally fall within three categories:

- Conviction of a crime
- Unprofessional conduct
- Personal or professional incapacity

Conviction of a crime may include felonies such as murder, rape, larceny, narcotics violations, and others. *Unprofessional conduct* is a failure to uphold the ethical standards of the medical profession. Betrayal of patient confidences, giving or receiving rebates, and excessive use of narcotics or alcohol are examples. *Personal or professional incapacity* is more difficult to label or prove. For instance, advanced age or an injury may reduce the apparent capacity of some physicians. Certain illnesses can affect the memory or judgment necessary to practice medicine.

FORMS OF MEDICAL PRACTICE

Sole Proprietorship

Sole proprietorship is commonly referred to as "solo practice." A sole proprietor is an individual who holds exclusive right and title to all aspects of the medical practice. The sole proprietor may employ other physicians to participate in the practice. The employed physician would be entitled to any employee fringe benefits, but the owner would not be so entitled. Additionally, the owner would be potentially liable for all of the acts of his professional employees. Solo practice is steadily declining. In 1984 it was estimated that solo practices were diminishing by 20,000 a year.

In 1991, about one third of the nation's 566,000 nonfederal physicians practiced in groups, compared with one tenth in 1965. The average group has grown from 6.3 physicians in 1969 to 11.5 in 1992. About 15% of all group physicians practice in groups of three to four. One third of all group physicians practice in groups with 100 or more doctors.*

Associate Practice

Often, two or more physicians agree to share office space and employees but conduct their practices as sole proprietors. They have an agreement among themselves as to the manner in which the practice is to operate.

Group Practice

The governing bodies of the American Medical Association, the American Group Practice Association, and the Medical Group Management Association have formally adopted the following definition of medical group practice:

> Medical Group Practice is the provision of health care services by a group of at least three licensed physician-practitioners, engaged full-time in a formally organized and legally recognized entity; sharing the group's income and expenses in a systematic manner; and sharing facilities, equipment, common records, and personnel, involved in both patient care and business management.

An association of 3 to 7 physicians is considered a small group; 8 to 30 physicians, a medium group; and more than 30 physicians a large group.

---

* From American Medical News, September 7, 1992.

A small or medium-sized group might be a single-specialty group with all the physicians engaged in the same specialty. Family practice and anesthesia services are two common examples. A large group would more likely be a multispecialty practice. Group practice may take the legal form of a partnership or a corporation.

Partnership

When two or more physicians elect to associate in the practice of medicine, they may draw up a partnership agreement. While it is not necessary that the agreement be in writing, no **prudent** person would enter into such an arrangement without a written agreement prepared with the aid of a competent attorney. The agreement should show all the rights, obligations, and responsibilities of each partner. One of the major disadvantages of partnership is the liability of each for the acts and conduct of one another unless otherwise specified in the partnership agreement.

Professional Corporation

A corporation may be defined as an artificial entity having a legal and business status that is independent of its shareholders or employees. Corporations are regulated by state statutes, so their requirements vary. However, they do have many similarities. The physician shareholders are employees of the corporation. Even one physician in solo practice can incorporate. There are income and tax advantages to all employees of the corporation. Usually, an attractive fringe benefit package is offered to the employees, which might include pension and profit-sharing plans, medical expense reimbursement, life insurance, disability income insurance, and employee death benefit. Fringe benefits to the corporate employee are separate from salary—that is, they are tax deductible to the corporation and not taxable to the employee. Professional employees of a corporation are liable only for their own acts. Another advantage of the corporate entity is the continuous life of the corporation.

In an unincorporated solo practice, the practice dies with the owner, and in a partnership practice, the death or discontinuance of practice of a partner necessitates a new agreement. A corporation, however, is an entity unto itself and does not end with a change in shareholders.

TYPES OF MEDICAL CARE DELIVERY

General and Family Practice

The physician who does not specialize or limit his or her practice is said to be in general practice. Family or general practice encompasses the care of all members of the family regardless of age or sex and covers a vast range of medical problems. This allows for continuity of care for the individual and for integration of care for the family as a whole.

Prepaid Comprehensive Care through Health Maintenance Organizations (HMOs)

An HMO is an organization that provides for comprehensive health care to an enrolled group for a fixed periodic payment. HMOs are not an entirely new concept. The Ross-Loos Medical Group of Los Angeles has operated a prepaid group practice since early 1929. For many years, however, organized medicine resisted all arrangements for compensation except on a basis of fee-for-service.

In the early 1970s, the federal government, which bears a great percentage of the costs of medical care, took action to contain the potential abuses of overtreatment and overutilization of health care services. The enactment of Public Law 93-222, the HMO Assistance Act, in December 1973, created Title XIII of the Public Health Service Act. Title XIII is intended to encourage and promote the growth of HMOs with the intent of cost containment. As the name implies, the HMO concept stresses the maintenance of health and preventive medicine. Members of HMOs are more inclined to see their physician before major and more costly problems arise because their contract provides for comprehensive care. Employers who provide health care benefits to employees are required to offer federally qualified HMOs as an option.

Specialty Practice

Many physicians have a special interest in a particular branch of medical practice and eventually direct their efforts to becoming expert in their chosen field. Physicians who decide to limit their practice to a specialized field will have to spend an additional 3 to 6 years in a residency program after completion of internship and will probably seek certification by one of the specialty boards.

Preventive Medicine and Public Health

The practice of medicine does not always involve patient care. The community is the public health physician's patient. All branches of medicine are committed to preventive medicine, and the public health physician complements the efforts of the private physician. The United States Public Health Service and the World Health Organization are both concerned with preventive medicine. The American Board of Preventive Medicine requires completion of 2 years of approved residency, 1 year of study in a School of Public Health, and 3 years of full-time experience in public health work before a candidate is eligible for certification examinations.

General preventive medicine is concerned with the relation of environment to health and with special concern for the health requirements of population groups.

Public Health is a special field of preventive medicine embodying the use of medical and administrative methods to prevent disease and improve general health through community efforts in areas such as sanitation and education.

Occupational medicine, another branch of preventive medicine, is concerned with the medical problems and practices related to occupation and especially to employment in industry.

AMERICAN BOARD OF MEDICAL SPECIALTIES

Presently, there are 23 specialty boards under the umbrella of the American Board of Medical Specialties. These specialty boards assist in improving the quality of medical education by elevating the standards of graduate medical education and approving facilities for specialty training. The primary function of each approved specialty board is to evaluate the qualifications of candidates in its field who apply voluntarily for examination and to certify as diplomates those who are qualified.

To accomplish this function, specialty boards determine if candidates have received adequate preparation in accordance with established educational standards; they provide comprehensive examinations to such candidates; and they issue certificates to those physicians who have satisfied the requirements. Those physicians who are Board-certified are known as diplomates of a specific specialty board—for example, Fredrick B. Mears, M.D., Diplomate of the American Board of Surgery.

A listing of the 23 specialty boards is found in Table 3–1. The American Board of Medical Specialties is located at One American Plaza, Suite 805, Evanston, Illinois, 60201. It regularly publishes a directory listing all physicians certified as diplomates by the specialty boards, including biographic sketches detailing their educational qualifications. Many physicians consult the directory in making referrals.

AMERICAN COLLEGE OF SURGEONS

The American College of Surgeons may also confer a degree on an applicant from a surgical specialty. The applicant is required to have completed a course of postgraduate training equivalent to "Board requirements" and to have submitted 50 detailed, **substantiated** case reports of varied surgical proce-

TABLE 3–1. APPROVED SPECIALTY BOARDS OF THE UNITED STATES

American Board of Allergy and Immunology
American Board of Anesthesiology
American Board of Colon and Rectal Surgery
American Board of Dermatology
American Board of Emergency Medicine
American Board of Family Practice
American Board of Internal Medicine
American Board of Neurological Surgery
American Board of Nuclear Medicine
American Board of Obstetrics and Gynecology
American Board of Ophthalmology
American Board of Orthopaedic Surgery
American Board of Otolaryngology
American Board of Pathology
American Board of Pediatrics
American Board of Physical Medicine and Rehabilitation
American Board of Plastic Surgery
American Board of Preventive Medicine
American Board of Psychiatry and Neurology
American Board of Radiology
American Board of Surgery
American Board of Thoracic Surgery
American Board of Urology

dures in which the applicant has been the chief surgeon during the last 3 years of practice prior to application. Successful applicants are identified as a Fellow of the American College of Surgeons (FACS).

AMERICAN COLLEGE OF PHYSICIANS

The American College of Physicians issues a similar fellowship degree (FACP) to applicants who have completed approved postgraduate training and who have exhibited special interest and competence in one of the nonsurgical specialties.

SPECIALTIES OF MEDICINE

Aerospace Medicine

Aerospace medicine is the specialty concerned with the physiologic, pathologic, and psychologic problems encountered by humans in space. At present, this field is mostly confined to the space agencies of the federal government.

Allergy & Immunology

An allergy is an abnormal reaction to substances that are harmless to most people. Substances that frequently bother the allergic person include pollens from grass, weeds, and trees, molds, house and other dusts, dog and cat danders, certain foods and medications, and the stings of insects.

There are many kinds of medicines and treatments that can help relieve the allergic symptoms, but it is essential first to identify the cause. The allergist is specially trained to diagnose and treat allergy problems with a high degree of accuracy and success.

The American Board of Allergy and Immunology is a Conjoint Board of the American Board of Internal Medicine and the American Board of Pediatrics. To become an allergist, the pediatrician or internist must take several years of additional specialty training and pass another certifying examination.

Anesthesiology

An anesthesiologist is a physician who administers local and general anesthesia, usually to prepare and maintain a patient for surgery, and in some cases for relief of pain. An anesthesiologist monitors the surgical patient through the surgical process until stable consciousness returns postoperatively.

Dermatology

Dermatologists are medical doctors who have extensive specialized training in the medical and surgical treatment of disorders of the skin, hair, and nails.

Because of specific training, the dermatologist is able to determine the best treatment approach to skin disorders. This approach may involve the use of medicines, both internal and external, or it may involve skin surgery. In addition to common dermatologic procedures such as removal of moles, warts, cysts, benign tumors, and skin cancers, many dermatologists are also trained in certain surgical and cosmetic procedures. These include skin grafts and flaps, hair transplants, dermabrasion, and collagen implants.

Emergency Medicine

The emergency medicine specialist is a physician who specializes in the immediate recognition and treatment of acute illnesses and injuries. These specialists may also be involved in the administration, teaching, and research of systems designed to help patients seeking emergency care. Qualifications for this specialty include a formal emergency medicine residency training or experience and continuing medical education.

Traditionally, specialists in emergency medicine provide 24-hour coverage of emergency departments in acute care hospitals, making emergency care available at all times. These specialists also provide the authority and license under which paramedic prehospital care is provided.

Family Practice

Family or general practice encompasses the care of all members of the family regardless of age or sex and covers a vast range of medical problems. This allows for continuity of care for the individual and integration of care for the family as a whole.

Internal Medicine

Internal medicine is the specialty concerned with the complete nonsurgical care of the adult. Internists are experts in the medical diagnosis and treatment of adult disorders as well as in the areas of health maintenance and wellness. General internists are responsible for a broad range of adult medical problems. There are multiple subspecialties within internal medicine, including allergy, cardiology, endocrinology, gastroenterology, gerontology, hematology, infectious disease, nephrology, oncology, pulmonary diseases, and rheumatology.

Neurology

Neurology is concerned with the nonsurgical management of neurologic disease. Generally, the neurologist manages infectious, metabolic, degenerative, and systemic involvement of the nervous system.

Nuclear Medicine

Nuclear medicine is a specialty field in which radioactive substances are used for the diagnosis and treatment of disease.

Obstetrics & Gynecology

Obstetrics is the specialty involved in the care and management of women during pregnancy, labor, delivery, and the puerperium. Gynecology is the specialty devoted to the medical and surgical treatment of diseases of women, especially those of the reproductive organs and functions.

Ophthalmology

Ophthalmology involves the diagnosis and treatment of eye and vision disorders, utilizing surgery and other corrective techniques.

Otolaryngology

Otolaryngology is professionally known today as Otolaryngology/Head and Neck Surgery. The specialty is broadly based, encompassing medical and surgical treatment of ear, nose, and throat disorders, allergy therapy, facial cosmetic and reconstructive surgery, and tumor problems in the head and neck. Otolaryngology is advancing in the fields of microsurgery and laser surgery.

Pathology

Pathology is the science that deals with the causes, mechanisms of development, and effects of disease. The pathologist seeks to determine the actual nature of disease—not just the physical symptoms or how it feels to the patient, but what the disease is from a biologic standpoint; that is, what visible or measurable changes it produces in the cells, fluids, and life processes of the entire body.

The practice of pathology is divided into two major areas, Anatomic Pathology and Clinical Pathology, and these areas are further subdivided into more numerous subspecialties. The function of the anatomic pathologist is to render a diagnosis on the basis of examination of a tissue specimen and to determine as precisely as possible the extent of the disease. The clinical pathologist is in charge of the medical laboratory, in which a wide variety of diagnostic studies are performed. Forensic pathology is a subspecialty dealing with various aspects of medicine and the law.

Pediatrics

Caring for the health of children from birth to adolescence is the unique purpose of pediatrics, the medical specialty that continually strives to prevent and treat all aspects of childhood diseases. The extent of the pediatrician's interest and responsibilities spans such areas as infectious diseases, newborn care, hospital care of children, environmental hazards, school health problems, nutrition, accident prevention, children with handicaps, drugs, allergy, cardiology, and pediatric pharmacology. The pediatric specialist is able to handle the problems of acutely ill children as well as to provide guidance to parents regarding the development and preventive care of children who are well.

The neonatologist deals with the diseases and abnormalities of the newborn.

Physical Medicine and Rehabilitation

Physical Medicine and Rehabilitation is concerned with the diagnosis and treatment of disorders and disabilities of the neuromuscular system. A physician in this specialty is called a physiatrist. He or she uses the physical elements such as heat, cold, water, electricity, and exercise to help restore physical function and independence.

Preventive Medicine

Preventive Medicine is concerned with preventing the occurrence of both mental and physical illness and disability. Analysis of present health services and planning for future medical needs are part of Preventive Medicine, as are Occupational Medicine and Public Health.

Psychiatry

A psychiatrist is a physician whose specialty is the diagnosis and treatment of persons with mental, emotional, or behavioral disorders. The psychiatrist is qualified to conduct psychotherapy and to prescribe medications when necessary. This allows the psychiatrist to comprehensively treat complex interactions of biologic, psychologic and social factors that affect patients.

Radiology

Radiology is a specialty in which x-rays (roentgen rays) are used for diagnosis and treatment of disease. A diagnostic radiologist specializes in using x-rays, ultrasound, nuclear medicine, computed tomography (CT), and magnetic resonance imaging (MRI) for detection of abnormalities throughout the body. Therapeutic radiology involves the use of ionizing radiation in the treatment of cancer and other tumors.

Surgery

Surgery is the correction of deformities, defects, diseases, or injured parts of the body by means of operative treatment. By making an incision into body tissue or by passing instruments through the skin, the diseased or injured tissues or organs can be corrected, modified, removed, or replaced. The various specializations contained within the broad field of surgery are listed below:

GENERAL SURGERY. General Surgery may include all aspects of surgery other than those included under special groups. Many general surgeons restrict their practice to surgery of abdominal conditions, traumatic situations, or tumor conditions. However, there is no restriction on the general surgeon's scope of activities, and many general surgeons take on additional fields as their training, interest, and capabilities dictate.

COLON AND RECTAL SURGERY. Colon and Rectal Surgery is a surgical subspecialty that concentrates on surgical treatment of the lower intestinal tract, which includes the colon and rectum.

NEUROSURGERY. A neurosurgeon specializes in the diagnosis and surgical treatment of the nervous system (the brain, spinal cord, and nerves) and the surrounding bony structures.

ORTHOPEDIC SURGERY. Orthopedic Surgery is that branch of medicine that deals with the treatment of maladies of the musculoskeletal system.

It not only involves treatment of musculoskeletal injuries but also deals with congenital deformities and acquired deformities, including spinal curvatures and arthritis. Orthopedic techniques are also used to treat sports injuries, more successfully now than ever with the advent of arthroscopic techniques to maximize rehabilitation.

Although orthopedics is a branch of surgery, many conditions are actually treated without surgery, including most fractures and muscle and tendon infirmities.

ORAL SURGERY. Oral Surgery is that branch of dentistry dealing with the extraction of teeth and the treatment of fractures of the jaws and adjacent facial bones as well as with other surgical procedures on the jaws, oral tissues, and adjacent tissues

TABLE 3–2. LIST OF ALLIED HEALTH PROFESSIONS FOR WHICH THE AMA HAS COLLABORATED IN ESTABLISHING ACCREDITATION OF EDUCATIONAL PROGRAMS

Abbreviation	Professional Title
AA	Anesthesiologist's Assistant
CVT	Cardiovascular Technologist
CYTO	Cytotechnologist
DMS	Diagnostic Medical Sonographer
EMT-P	Emergency Medical Technician-Paramedic
ENDT	Electroneurodiagnostic Technologist
HT	Histologic Technician/Technologist
MA	Medical Assistant
MI	Medical Illustrator
MLT-AD	Medical Laboratory Technician (Associate Degree)
MLT-C	Medical Laboratory Technician (Certificate)
MRA	Medical Record Administrator
MRT	Medical Record Technician
MT	Medical Technologist
NMT	Nuclear Medicine Technologist
OMT	Ophthalmic Medical Technician/Technologist
OT	Occupational Therapist
PA	Physician's Assistant
PERF	Perfusionist
RAD	Radiographer
RADTT	Radiation Therapy Technologist
REST	Respiratory Therapist
RESTT	Respiratory Therapy Technician
SA	Surgeon's Assistant
SBBT	Specialist in Blood Bank Technology
ST	Surgical Technologist

TABLE 3-3. MEMBERS OF THE HEALTH CARE TEAM

Occupation	Education Requirements	Employment
Anesthesiologist's Assistant (AA)	*Prerequisite:* Baccalaureate degree with strong science major *Training program:* 2 years	Works under direction of licensed and qualified anesthesiologist; assists in preoperative tasks; assists in administering anesthetics
Cardiovascular Technologist (CVT)	*Training program:* 1-4 years	Provides recovery room care and diagnostic examinations under direction of physician
Cytotechnologist (CYTO)	*Prerequisite:* Strong background in basic chemistry and biologic sciences *Training program:* varies but at least 1 year	Works with pathologist to detect changes in body cells, particularly those related to cancer; prepares cellular samples for study; examines samples to assist in diagnosis
Diagnostic Medical Sonographer (DMS)	*Prerequisite:* High school diploma or equivalent *Training program:* 1-4 years	Uses diagnostic ultrasound under supervision of a physician
Emergency Medical Technician-Paramedic (EMT-P)	*Prerequisite:* Evidence of certification as EMT-ambulance and a high school diploma or equivalent *Training program:* 600-1000 hours	Works under direction of physician, often through radio communication; trained to recognize, assess, and manage emergency care
Electroneurodiagnostic Technologist (ENDT)	*Training program:* 1 year or more	Works in neurology departments of hospitals or private offices; records and studies electric activity of the brain
EKG (ECG) Technician	*Training program:* Provided in most medical assisting programs	Works in offices of general practitioners; performs electrocardiograms
Histologic Technician (HT) and Histotechnologist	*Training program:* Varies; the Histotechnologist has more training than the Histologic Technician	May work in hospitals or private offices; prepares sections of body tissue for examination by physician
Medical Laboratory Technician (MLT)	*Training program:* Varies; requires at least 1 year of professional/clinical education	Usually works in a hospital, but might work in a physician's office; performs routine, uncomplicated procedures in hematology, serology, blood banking, urinalysis, microbiology, and clinical chemistry
Medical Technologist (MT)	*Training program:* At least 1 year of processional/clinical education	Usually works in a hospital, but might work in a physician's office or clinic; develops data on blood, tissues, and fluids in the body for the detection, diagnosis, and treatment of disease
Medical Record Administrator (MRA)	*Training program:* Baccalaureate degree	Manages medical records and reports in a hospital
Medical Record Technician (MRT)	*Training program:* Usually 2 years; may receive associate degree	Works as technical assistant to MRA; compiles, analyzes, and prepares health information needed by patients and health facilities
Nuclear Medicine Technologist (NMT)	*Prerequisite:* High school diploma or equivalent *Training program:* 1 year	Performs tasks that complement the performance of nuclear medicine physician and that involve patient care, technical skills, and administration
Ophthalmic Medical Technician and Ophthalmic Medical Technologist (OMT)	*Prerequisite:* High school diploma *Training program:* 1 year for technician; 2 years for technologist	Assists ophthalmologist in wide range of activities, including taking medical history, administering diagnostic tests, assisting in surgery, and testing ocular functions
Occupational Therapist (OT)	*Training program:* 4-year program leading to baccalaureate degree	Works in hospitals, schools, and public agencies; provides services to individuals whose ability to perform normal functions is impaired
Physical Therapist (PT)	*Training program:* Baccalaureate degree	Works in hospitals, nursing homes, rehabilitation centers, and schools for crippled children; concerned with restoration of function and prevention of disability following disease or injury of muscles, nerves, joints and bones or after loss of body part; treats patients with exercise, heat, cold, water, electricity, ultrasound, and massage
Physician's Assistant (PA) and Surgeon's Assistant (SA)	*Training program:* State laws govern qualifications and job descriptions; most states require 2 years of study plus work experience	PA most often works with family physician or internist; takes patient history; performs physical examinations; diagnoses and monitors patient care; performs therapeutic procedures; counsels patients; SA may additionally perform pre- and postoperative care
Radiographer (RAD)	*Prerequisite:* High school diploma *Training program:* 2-4 years	Works under direct supervision of physician in hospital or private office.
Radiation Therapy Technologist (RADTT)	*Training program:* 1-4 years	Administers radiation therapy services under supervision of a radiation oncologist; observes patient under treatment; maintains records of treatment and progress
Respiratory Therapist (REST) and Respiratory Therapy Technician (RESTT)	*Prerequisite:* High school diploma or equivalent *Training program:* For REST, usually 2 years; RESTT may be qualified after 1-year program	Both may be employed in hospitals, nursing care facilities, clinics, doctors' offices, or emergency oxygen services; administers general respiratory care
Surgical Technologist (ST)	*Training program:* Can vary in length from 9-24 months	Works in hospital operating room or in surgeon's private office
Certified Medical Transcriptionist	*Prerequisite:* Must have above average typing and word processing skills, an understanding of human anatomy and physiology, and a knowledge of medical terminology used in medical records, medical and surgical procedures, and laboratory tests	Transcribes medical dictation; employed in hospitals, clinics, and medical research and teaching centers, private offices; sometimes works as independent contractor

TABLE 3–3. MEMBERS OF THE HEALTH CARE TEAM Continued

Occupation	Education Requirements	Employment
Translator	*Prerequisite:* Must be competent in speaking and understanding one or more languages other than English	Employed as a patient advocate for non-English speaking patients
Licensed Practical Nurse (LPN) or Licensed Vocational Nurse (LVN)	*Training program:* Scope of practice and training determined by each state	Works under direction of physician in hospital or in physician's office; the scope of practice and protocols are determined by each state
Registered Nurse (RN)	*Training program:* 2 or 3 years of training or 4-year baccalaureate program	May practice in hospital, physician's office, schools, or employment services or independently; scope of practice determined by state in which individual is licensed
Nurse Practitioner (NP)	*Prerequisite:* Must be Registered Nurse *Training program:* Additional year or more required	May work alone or with physician

to treat or correct disease and other abnormal conditions.

PLASTIC SURGERY. Plastic Surgery includes the operative repair of defects by graft, tissue transfer, or cosmetic alteration of tissue. A plastic surgeon specializes in burns, congenital defects, and hand and extremity reconstruction as well as in the treatment of skin wounds and lesions and the performance of aesthetic surgery of the face and body contouring.

THORACIC (CARDIOVASCULAR) SURGERY. Thoracic or Cardiovascular Surgery is a surgical subspecialty concerned with the operative treatment of the chest and chest wall, lungs, and respiratory passages. Specialists in this field are involved with heart surgery, including both valvular and coronary heart surgery.

Urology

Urology is a medical specialty concerned with the treatment of diseases and disorders of the urinary tract of men, women, and children as well as of the male genitalia.

SUPPORT PERSONNEL

In the complex delivery of 20th century medical care, the physician is the maestro, but for every practicing physician there are many behind-the-scenes support personnel. As the delivery of medical care has become more fragmented, the close relationship that used to exist between family physician and patient has diminished, and the specialist often enters the picture as a complete stranger. The med-

ical assistant is the professional who can bridge this gap. Familiarity with the training and scope of practice of other allied health occupations can help the medical assistant in this role.

For more than 50 years, the American Medical Association (AMA) has been involved in the setting of standards and the accreditation of allied health education programs. In 1935, the training of the occupational therapist was the first in allied health education to be accredited by the AMA. By 1989, the AMA Council on Medical Education was accrediting the training of 26 allied health professions (Table 3–2). The medical assisting program was accredited in 1969.

Table 3–3 defines various members of the health-care team and their functions.

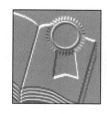 ▶ **LEARNING ACHIEVEMENTS**

Are you able to:

1. Define the terms listed in the Vocabulary of this chapter?
2. Discuss the circumstances that brought Johns Hopkins University the reputation as the world's most famous medical school?
3. Explain how the Flexner report affected the practice of medicine?
4. Name the most rapidly expanding type of medical practice today?
5. State the purpose of medical practice acts and how they are established?
6. List the three methods by which licensure may be granted to physicians?
7. State three general categories of cause for revocation or suspension of a physician's license?

8. Explain the difference between *associate* practice and *partnership* practice?
9. Name four types of medical care delivery?
10. Compare the responsibilities of a medical assistant with those of other allied health occupations?

REFERENCES AND READINGS

American Medical Association: *Allied Health Education Directory,* 19th ed., Chicago, The Association, 1991.

American Medical Association: *U. S. Medical Licensure Statistics and Current Licensure Requirements,* Chicago, The Association, 1992.

Manning, F. F.: *Medical Group Practice Management,* Cambridge, Massachusetts, Ballinger Publishing Co., 1977.

Orange County Medical Association: *Reference Guide to Medical Resources,* Orange, California, The Association, 1991.

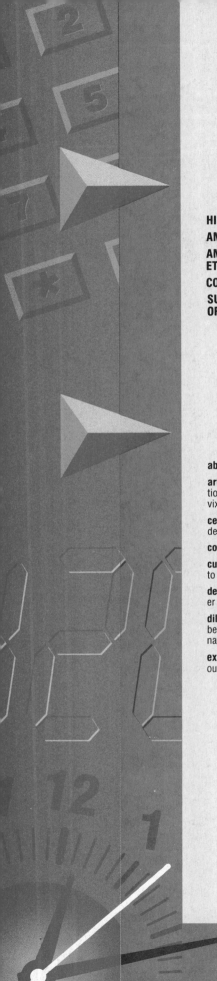

CHAPTER OUTLINE

HISTORICAL CODES

AMA CODE OF ETHICS

AMA PRINCIPLES OF MEDICAL ETHICS

COUNCIL OPINIONS

SUMMARY OF CURRENT OPINIONS OF THE COUNCIL
  1.00 Introduction

2.00 Social Policy Issues

3.00 Interprofessional Relations

4.00 Hospital Relations

5.00 Confidentiality, Advertising, and Communications Media Relations

6.00 Fees and Charges

7.00 Physician's Records

8.00 Practice Matters

9.00 Professional Rights and Responsibilities

ETHICS FOR THE MEDICAL ASSISTANT

SUMMARY

LEARNING ACHIEVEMENTS

VOCABULARY

abet To encourage or support.

artificial insemination The introduction of semen into the vagina or cervix by artificial means.

censure The act of blaming or condemning sternly.

compulsory Obligatory; enforced.

culminate To reach a decisive point; to bring to a head.

deceptive Misleading; having the power to deceive.

dilemma A situation involving choice between equally unsatisfactory alternatives.

expulsion Act of expelling or forcing out.

fee splitting Sharing a fee with another physician, laboratory, or drug company not based on services performed.

genetics The branch of biology dealing with heredity and variation among related organisms.

ghost surgery A situation in which a patient has consented to have surgery done by one surgeon, but without the patient's knowledge or consent, the surgery is actually performed by another surgeon.

preamble An introductory portion; a preface.

precept A practical rule guiding behavior or technique.

public domain The realm embracing property rights that belong to the community at large and that are subject to appropriation by anyone.

resident A graduate and licensed physician receiving training in a specialty in a hospital.

revocation The act of annulling by recalling or taking back.

surrogate A substitute; someone appointed to act in the place of another.

suspension The act of interrupting or discontinuing temporarily, but with an expectation or purpose of resumption.

technologic Relating to the application of scientific knowledge or methods.

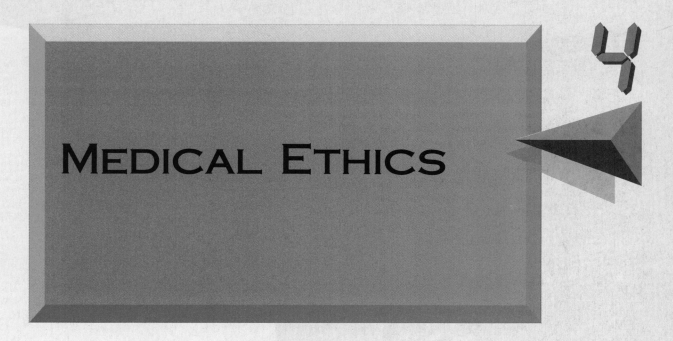

MEDICAL ETHICS

4

LEARNING OBJECTIVES

Upon successful completion of this chapter, you should be able to:

1. Define the terms listed in the Vocabulary.

2. Differentiate between the terms *ethics* and *etiquette*.

3. Identify the earliest written code of ethical conduct for medical practice.

4. Name the ancient Greek oath that remains an inspiration to physicians today.

5. Identify a code that was an example for the AMA Principles of Medical Ethics.

6. State a significant reason for the 1980 revision of the AMA Principles.

7. State the maximum penalty that a medical society can impose upon a member for unethical conduct.

8. Discuss what and to whom information about a patient may be released.

9. Discuss the application of ethics in dealing with fees and charges.

10. Compare the provisions of the AAMA Code of Ethics with those of the AMA Principles.

Ethics concerns the thoughts, judgments, and actions on issues that have the greater implications of moral "right" and "wrong." A "morally right" attitude is usually understood to be directed toward an ideal form of human character or action, which should **culminate** in the highest good for humanity. From the desire to achieve this good comes the sense of moral duty and a system of interpersonal moral obligations.

Medical etiquette should not be confused with medical ethics. *Etiquette* deals with courtesy, customs, and manners; *ethics* concerns itself with the underlying philosophies in the ideal relationships of humans. These relationships are often formally set forth in social contracts and codes.

HISTORICAL CODES

Ethics—judgments of right and wrong—have always been a concern of human beings. It is not surprising that for centuries the medical profession has set for itself a rigid standard of ethical conduct toward patients and colleagues. The earliest written code of ethical conduct for medical practice was conceived around 2250 BC by the Babylonians and was called the Code of Hammurabi. It went into much detail regarding the conduct expected of a physician, even prescribing the fees that could be charged. Probably because of its length and detail, it did not survive the ages.

About 400 BC, Hippocrates, the Greek physician known as the Father of Medicine, developed a brief statement of principles that has come down through history and remains an inspiration to the physician of today. The Oath of Hippocrates has been administered to medical graduates in many European universities for centuries.

THE OATH OF HIPPOCRATES

I swear by Apollo, the physician, and Aesculapius, and Health, and Allheal, and all the gods and goddesses, that, according to my ability and judgment, I will keep this oath and stipulation, to reckon him who taught me this art equally dear to me as my parents, to share my substance with him and relieve his necessities if required; to regard his offspring as on the same footing with my own brothers, and to teach them this art if they should wish to learn it, without fee or stipulation, and that by precept, lecture, and every other mode of instruction, I will impart a knowledge of the art to my own sons and to those of my teachers, and to disciples bound by a stipulation and oath, according to the law of medicine, but to none other.

I will follow that method of treatment which, according to my ability and judgment, I consider for the benefit of my patients, and abstain from whatever is deleterious and mischievous. I will give no deadly medicine to anyone if asked, nor suggest any such counsel; furthermore, I will not give to a woman an instrument to produce abortion.

With purity and holiness, I will pass my life and practice my art. I will not cut a person who is suffering with a stone, but will leave this to be done by practitioners of this work. Into whatever houses I enter I will go into them for the benefit of the sick and will abstain from every voluntary act of mischief and corruption; and further from the seduction of females or males, bond or free.

Whatever, in connection with my professional practice, or not in connection with it, I may see or hear in the lives of men which ought not to be spoken abroad, I will not divulge, as reckoning that all such should be kept secret.

While I continue to keep this oath unviolated, may it be granted to me to enjoy life and the practice of the art, respected by all men at all times, but should I trespass and violate this oath, may the reverse be my lot.

The most significant contribution to ethical history subsequent to Hippocrates was made by Thomas Percival, a physician, philosopher, and writer from Manchester, England. In 1803, he published his Code of Medical Ethics. Percival's personality, his interest in sociologic matters, and his close association with the Manchester Infirmary led to the preparation of a "scheme of professional conduct relative to hospitals and other charities," from which he drafted the code that bears his name.

In 1846, as the American Medical Association (AMA) was organized in New York City, medical education and medical ethics were being considered from a national point of view. At the first AMA annual meeting in Philadelphia in 1847, a Code of Ethics was formulated and adopted. It specifically acknowledged Percival's Code as its basic example and became a part of the fundamental standards of the AMA and of its component parts.

EVOLUTION OF MODERN CODE OF MEDICAL ETHICS

2250 BC	Code of Hammurabi
400 BC	Oath of Hippocrates
1803 AD	Percival's Code of Medical Ethics
1980 AD	AMA Principles of Medical Ethics (latest revision)

AMA CODE OF ETHICS

The AMA's Code of Ethics has three components:

- Principles of Medical Ethics
- Current Opinions of the Council on Ethical and Judicial Affairs
- Reports of the Council on Ethical and Judicial Affairs

The Principles comprise seven broad precepts that set the basis of ethical conduct for physicians. The Current Opinions address specific ethical issues, and the Reports are detailed accounts of the considerations that guided the Council in arriving at their opinions of the issues involved.

AMA Principles of Medical Ethics

The AMA Principles of Medical Ethics have been revised on several occasions to keep them consistent with the times, but there has never been a change in their moral intent or overall idealism. Major revisions were made in 1903, 1912, and 1947. In 1957, the AMA Principles of Medical Ethics were condensed to a preamble and 10 sections, a major change in format from the 1847 code. The 1980 revision of the code, which contains a **preamble** and only seven sections, was done "to clarify and update the language, to eliminate reference to gender, and to seek a proper and reasonable balance between professional standards and contemporary legal standards in our changing society." (See Principles of Medical Ethics.)

AMA PRINCIPLES OF MEDICAL ETHICS

PREAMBLE

The medical profession has long subscribed to a body of ethical statements developed primarily for the benefit of the patient. As a member of this profession, a physician must recognize responsibility not only to patients, but also to society, to other health professionals, and to self. The following Principles adopted by the American Medical Association are not laws, but standards of conduct which define the essentials of honorable behavior for the physician.

I. A physician shall be dedicated to providing competent medical service with compassion and respect for human dignity.

II. A physician shall deal honestly with patients and colleagues, and strive to expose those physicians deficient in character or competence, or who engage in fraud or deception.

III. A physician shall respect the law and also recognize a responsibility to seek changes in those requirements which are contrary to the best interests of the patient.

IV. A physician shall respect the rights of patients, of colleagues, and of other health professionals, and shall safeguard patient confidences within the constraints of the law.

V. A physician shall continue to study, apply and advance scientific knowledge, make relevant information available to patients, colleagues and the public, obtain consultation, and use the talents of other health professionals when indicated.

VI. A physician shall, in the provision of appropriate patient care except in emergencies, be free to choose whom to serve, with whom to associate, and the environment in which to provide medical services.

VII. A physician shall recognize a responsibility to participate in activities contributing to an improved community.

(From Code of Medical Ethics, Current Opinions of the Council on Ethical and Judicial Affairs of the American Medical Association, Copyright 1992, American Medical Association)

As stated in the Preamble, these Principles are not laws but standards. Laws vary from state to state and from community to community, but ethical standards are universal. Ethical standards are never less than the standards required by law; frequently they are greater. Violation of the ethical standards of an association or society may result in **censure, expulsion,** or **suspension** of membership. Expulsion from membership is the maximum penalty that a medical society may impose upon a physician. Violation of a law followed by conviction may result in punishment by fine, imprisonment, or **revocation** of license.

The Council on Ethical and Judicial Affairs of the AMA consists of nine active members of the AMA, including one Resident Physician member and one Medical Student member, and is charged with interpreting the Principles as adopted by the House of Delegates of the AMA. The Council periodically publishes a compilation of its interpretations, opinions, and statements. Some of the interpretations of the Principles set forth in the *Current Opinions of the Council on Ethical and Judicial Affairs of the AMA, 1989,* are discussed later in this chapter. Although the code and the interpretations are directed specifically toward physicians, the medical assistant, as a member of the medical team, must be familiar with these principles and cooperate with the physician in practicing within their concepts.

Council Opinions

The opinions of the Council elaborate and expand the **precepts** in the Principles of Medical Ethics. They are continually updated to encompass developing situations, and they reflect the changing challenges and responsibilities of medicine.

For a fuller appreciation of the ethical issues in medicine, the medical assistant should obtain a copy of the *Current Opinions of the Council* for complete study (Write to: Order Department, OP 122/9, American Medical Association, P.O. Box 10946, Chicago, IL 60610).

Current Opinions, 1989, is presented in nine parts; only a brief summary of these parts appears in the following section.

SUMMARY OF CURRENT OPINIONS OF THE COUNCIL

1.00 Introduction

The introduction explains the terminology used and the relationship between law and ethics. If a physician violates ethical standards involving a breach of *moral* duty or principle, the maximum penalty that the medical society can impose is expulsion. If there is alleged *criminal* conduct relating to the practice of medicine, the medical society is obligated to report it to the appropriate governmental body or state board.

2.00 Social Policy Issues

ABORTION. The physician is not prohibited by ethical considerations from performing a lawful abortion in accordance with good medical practice.

ABUSE. The discovery that a patient is abusing a child or a parent creates a difficult situation for the doctor's office. The law requires that such abuse be reported. If the physician does not report such abuse in accordance with the law, an added ethical violation is created that may result in continued abuse to the victim.

ALLOCATION OF HEALTH RESOURCES. Society must sometimes decide who will receive care when it is not possible to accommodate all who need it. In the case of organ transplantation, for example, there may be several who need the transplant and only one available donor. Who shall be the recipient?

Kidney dialysis is another situation where the demand is greater than the supply. This creates a conflict with the physician expected to participate in the decision. The Council opinion is that priority should be given to persons who are most likely to be treated successfully or derive long-term benefit.

ARTIFICIAL INSEMINATION. Artificial insemination requires the informed consent of the woman receiving the artificial insemination and the consent of her husband. In the case of artificial insemination by a donor, the physician is ethically responsible for complete screening of the donor for any defects that may affect the fetus. The identity of the donor is not revealed to the recipient or the resulting child.

CAPITAL PUNISHMENT. The physician, being a member of a profession dedicated to preserving life, should not participate in a legally authorized execution, but may certify the death.

CLINICAL INVESTIGATION. Without clinical investigation, there could be no new drugs or procedures. However, all such investigation must follow a competently designed systematic program with due concern for the welfare, safety, and comfort of patients. The physician-patient relationship does exist in clinical investigation, and whenever treatment of the patient is involved, voluntary written consent must be obtained from the patient or the patient's legally authorized representative. Additional restrictions apply when the subject is a minor or a mentally incompetent adult. When participating in the clinical investigation of new drugs and procedures, physicians should show the same concern for the welfare and safety of the person involved as would prevail if the person were a private patient.

COST. Technologic developments add to the ethical **dilemmas** facing the physician. New expensive treatments are available, and the physician must balance the advantages of these treatments to the patient against their sometimes exorbitant costs.

GENETIC COUNSELING. Genetic counseling and organ transplantation may require personal and ethical decisions concerning the quality of the life that is to be saved.

ORGAN DONATION. The physician should encourage the donation of organs when it is appropriate. However, it is considered unethical to participate in proceedings in which the donor receives payment, except for reimbursement of expenses directly incurred in the removal of the donated organ.

The rights of both the donor and the recipient must be equally protected. In a case involving the transplantation of a vital, single organ, the death of the donor must be determined by a physician other than the recipient's physician.

QUALITY OF LIFE. Physicians must sometimes decide the fate of a person whose future is dim, such as a deformed newborn or a person of advanced age with many physical problems. The first thought may be the burden to be borne by the family or by society in caring for this person. Ethically, the physician's primary consideration must be what is best for the patient.

SURROGATE MOTHERS. Although **surrogate** motherhood is no longer an isolated entity, many cases are reaching the courts for various reasons. For example, the surrogate may claim bonding to the child and refuse to give it up; the surrogate may decide to have an abortion; or a defective child may be borne and neither the surrogate nor the adoptive parents wish to accept custody. The Council does not favor surrogate motherhood as a reproductive alternative for a couple who would otherwise be unable to parent a child because of the many associated concerns.

WITHHOLDING OR WITHDRAWING LIFE-PROLONGING MEDICAL TREATMENT. A physician is committed to *saving life* and *relieving suffering.* Sometimes these two goals are incompatible, and a choice between them must be made. If at all possible, the patient may make this decision. Often, the patient makes his wishes known to a responsible relative or other representative in the event that he or she becomes incapacitated. Patients who live in a state that has "living will" statutes may have some choice if such a will has been established. The living will is a document that states the wishes of that person in the event of a terminal illness. Usually, it is done to prohibit heroic measures being taken in a situation in which the patient would be unable or incompetent to make a decision himself or herself. In the absence of preplanning, the physician must act in the best interest of the patient. If it has been determined beyond a doubt that the patient is permanently unconscious, it is not unethical to cut off life-prolonging treatment.

3.00 Interprofessional Relations

The interprofessional relations of the physician are mostly governed by ethics; however, some legal restrictions do exist. There are state laws that prohibit a physician from aiding and **abetting** an unlicensed person in the practice of medicine or from aiding and abetting a person with a limited license in the provision of services beyond the scope of that license.

The Council addresses the relations of the physician with respect to nurses and specialists, sports medicine and optometry, and involvement with teaching as well as to the referral of patients to other physicians.

If a nurse recognizes or suspects that there is something wrong in a physician's orders, it is the nurse's obligation to report this to the physician. The medical assistant also has this obligation, even if it means risking the displeasure of the physician.

Physicians often refer a patient to another physician for diagnosis or treatment when it is beneficial to the patient. The physician should make these referrals only when he is confident that the patient will receive competent treatment.

In the absence of legal restrictions, a physician is free to choose whom to serve. However, even though the physician may limit his practice, he cannot choose to neglect a patient already in his care.

The sports physician must keep in mind that his professional responsibility at a sporting event is to protect the health and safety of the participants, with his judgment being governed only by medical considerations.

An ophthalmologist may employ an optometrist as ancillary personnel to assist him or her, provided that the optometrist is identified to patients as an optometrist. If the physician does not employ an optometrist, he or she may send a patient to a qualified optometrist for optometric services. Of course, the physician would be ethically remiss if, before doing so, he or she did not ensure that there was an absence of any medical reason for his patient's complaint; the physician would be equally remiss if he or she referred a patient without having made a medical evaluation of the patient's condition.

4.00 Hospital Relations

Most practicing physicians have staff privileges at one or more hospitals. Guidelines for the physician-hospital relationship are developed in this section and include the following:

- It is considered unethical for a physician to charge a separate fee for the routine, nonmedical services performed in admitting a patient to a hospital.
- The physician may ethically bill a patient for services rendered the patient by a **resident** under the physician's personal observation, direction, and supervision, if the physician assumes responsibility for the services.
- The granting of hospital privileges should be based on the training, competence, and experience of the applicant.
- **Compulsory** assessments should not be a condition of granting medical staff membership or privileges.

5.00 Confidentiality, Advertising, and Communications Media Relations

There are no restrictions on advertising by physicians except those that can be specifically justified to protect the public from **deceptive** practices. Standards regarding advertising and publicity have been liberalized over the years, but any advertisement or publicity must be true and not misleading. Testimonials of patients, for instance, should not be used in advertising, as they are difficult, if not impossible, to verify or measure by objective standards. The physician can safely include information on educational background, fees, available credit, and any other nondeceptive information, but statements regarding the quality of medical services are highly subjective and difficult to verify.

HMOs routinely seek members through advertising. Physicians who practice in such prepaid plans must abide by the same principles of ethics as do other physicians. Any deceptive advertising — for example, any that would be misleading to patients or prospective subscribers — is unethical.

Although information regarding some patients, such as celebrities and politicians, may be considered "news," the physician may not discuss a patient's condition with the press without authorization from the patient or the patient's lawful representative. The physician may release only authorized information or that which is public knowledge.

Certain news is a part of the public record. News in this category is known as news in the **public domain** and includes births, deaths, accidents, and police cases.

A statement may be made that the patient was injured by a knife but not that the injury was a result of an assault or accident or that it was self-inflicted. You cannot assert that an action was a suicide or an attempted suicide, nor whether intoxication or drug addiction was involved.

The medical assistant must be aware that only the physician is authorized to release information, and under no circumstances should the medical assistant violate the confidential nature of the physician–patient relationship.

One item of particular interest to the medical assistant is what information may be disclosed by the physician's office to the representatives of insurance companies. It is important to remember at all times that the history, diagnosis, prognosis, and other information acquired during the physician–patient relationship may be disclosed to an insurance company representative *only* if the patient or the patient's lawful representative has consented to the disclosure. You should not even certify that the individual was under the physician's care without the patient's permission. The same restriction applies to discussions with the patient's lawyer.

A physician may testify in court or before a workers' compensation board in any personal injury or related case. In the case of a pre-employment physical examination, although no physician–patient relationship exists, the physician is still bound to the rule of confidentiality; if the physician treats a patient, then the physician–patient relationship is established.

The expanding use of computer technology permits the accumulation and storage of an unlimited amount of medical information. With the use of computers in the physician's office and the employment of computer service organizations, confidentiality becomes more difficult. Detailed guidelines are included in the *Current Opinions.* and are reproduced in Chapter 8, p. 105.

6.00 Fees and Charges

It is unethical for a physician to charge or collect an illegal or excessive fee. Illegal charges may occur through ignorance of the law when billing for treatment of Medicaid or Medicare patients. It is a medical assistant's responsibility to keep informed on current regulations and see that they are scrupulously followed.

FEE SPLITTING. If a physician accepts payment from another physician solely for the referral of a patient, both are guilty of an unethical practice called **fee splitting.** Fee splitting, whether with another physician, a clinic or laboratory, or a drug company, is unethical. The division of practice income among members of a group in joint practice or partnership is determined by the members of the group and is *not* fee splitting.

Lawyers often accept cases on a *contingency* basis, that is, the fee is contingent upon a successful outcome. A physician's fee is always based on the value of the service provided to the patient. Providing care for a fee based upon the success of the outcome would be considered unethical.

INSURANCE FORMS. An attending physician should expect to complete one insurance claim form for the patient without charge. Multiple or complex forms for the same patient may warrant a charge if this is in conformity with local custom.

INTEREST AND FINANCE CHARGES. It is entirely appropriate to request that payment be made at the time of treatment, particularly if there has been a past history of late payments. If the patient is notified in advance, it is also proper to add interest or other reasonable charges to delinquent accounts. Advance notice can be accomplished by posting a notice in the reception office or by notations on the billing statements. A more effective approach is the use of a Patient Information Folder that includes billing information; such a folder is provided for every new patient on the initial visit. Federal laws and regulations applicable to the imposition of interest charges are discussed in Chapter 15, Professional Fees and Credit.

7.00 Physician's Records

Notes made by the physician during the course of treating a patient are made for the physician's own use and are considered to be the physician's personal property. They are sometimes used to provide a summary of the patient's treatment to another physician or person at the request of the patient. Original records should never be released except on the physician's retirement or sale of a medical practice.

In some states, a patient is authorized by law to have access to his or her medical records. Health care professionals should familiarize themselves with the laws in their own states. Of primary concern regarding all records is the authorization of the patient before releasing any information, unless the release is required by law.

RECORDS OF PHYSICIANS ON RETIREMENT OR DEATH. There are many reasons that a patient might need access to his health records after a physician retires or dies. The records might be necessary for employment, insurance, litigation, or other reasons. When a physician retires or dies, the patients should be notified and encouraged to find a new physician and to authorize the transfer of their records. Records that are not forwarded to another physician should be retained by a custodian of the records in compliance with any legal requirements.

SALE OF A MEDICAL PRACTICE. A physician who retires or the estate of a deceased physician may wish to sell the practice. This sale usually includes the option of taking over the care of the patients who are served by the practice. In such cases, each patient is notified that the practice is being transferred to another physician and that this physician will have custody of the patient's records until such time as the patient may request that the records be sent to another physician.

8.00 Practice Matters

APPOINTMENT CHARGES. May a physician charge for an appointment that is missed or one that was not canceled within a stated time? Yes, but *only* if the patient has been fully advised in advance that such a charge will be made. Discretion should be used, however, in applying such a charge.

CONSULTATION. When a physician refers a patient to a consultant, the referring physician should provide the consultant with the patient's history and any other pertinent information in advance of the consultation. The consultant, in turn, should advise the referring physician of his or her findings and recommendations. On the other hand, if the patient seeks a second opinion from a physician of his own choice, that physician is not obligated to report to the patient's regular physician.

DRUGS AND DEVICES: PRESCRIBING. A physician may ethically own or operate a pharmacy or dispense drugs only if such ownership or activity does not result in exploitation of patients. Patients should enjoy the same freedom of choice in deciding who will fill a prescription as they have in choosing a physician. A prescription is an essential part of a patient's medical record, and the patient is entitled to a copy.

HEALTH FACILITY OWNERSHIP BY A PHYSICIAN. A physician may ethically own or have a financial interest in a for-profit hospital or other health care facility such as a freestanding clinic. However, before admitting or referring a patient to that facility, the physician has an ethical obligation to disclose such ownership to the patient. Additionally, the patient's welfare must not be jeopardized by the physician's financial interest; this could happen if the physician unnecessarily hospitalizes or prolongs the patient's stay in the health care facility.

INFORMED CONSENT. The patient's right of self-decision can be effectively exercised only if the patient possesses enough information to make an intelligent choice. (Informed consent is discussed in more detail in Chapter 5.)

GHOST SURGERY. The substitution of another surgeon without the patient's consent is called **ghost surgery.** The patient has a right to choose his own physician or surgeon, and to make a substitution without consulting the patient is deceitful and unethical.

9.00 Professional Rights and Responsibilities

The final section of *Current Opinions* addresses the following:

Accreditation

Agreements restricting the practice of medicine

Civil rights and professional responsibility

Discipline

Due process

Free choice

Medical testimony

New medical procedures

Patents

Peer review

Physician impairment

Physician–patient relationship

Physicians and infectious diseases

ETHICS FOR THE MEDICAL ASSISTANT

The Code of Ethics of the American Association of Medical Assistants is a standard for all medical assistants to honor. The Code is patterned after the AMA Principles and is adapted to the professional medical assistant who accepts this discipline as a responsibility of trust. (See Code of Ethics.)

A. render service with full respect for the dignity of humanity;

B. respect confidential information obtained through employment unless legally authorized or required by responsible performance of duty to divulge such information;

C. uphold the honor and high principles of the profession and accept its disciplines;

D. seek to continually improve the knowledge and skills of medical assistants for the benefit of patients and professional colleagues;

E. participate in additional service activities aimed toward improving the health and well-being of the community.

CREED

I believe in the principles and purposes of the profession of medical assisting.

I endeavor to be more effective.

I aspire to render greater service.

I protect the confidence entrusted to me.

I am dedicated to the care and well-being of all patients.

I am loyal to my physician-employer.

I am true to the ethics of my profession.

I am strengthened by compassion, courage and faith.

(Reprinted with permission of the American Association of Medical Assistants, Chicago, IL.)

CODE OF ETHICS

The Code of Ethics of AAMA shall set forth principles of ethical and moral conduct as they relate to the medical profession and the particular practice of medical assisting.

Members of AAMA dedicated to the conscientious pursuit of their profession, and thus desiring to merit the high regard of the entire medical profession and the respect of the general public which they serve, do pledge themselves to strive always to:

The Patient's Bill of Rights developed and approved by the American Hospital Association in 1973 should also be the credo of the practicing medical assistant. (See American Hospital Association: A Patient's Bill of Rights.)

AMERICAN HOSPITAL ASSOCIATION: A PATIENT'S BILL OF RIGHTS

The American Hospital Association presents a Patient's Bill of Rights with the expectation that observance of these rights will contribute to more effective patient care and greater satisfaction for the patient, his physician, and the hospital organization. Further, the Association presents these rights in the expectation that they will be supported by the hospital on behalf of its patients, as an integral part of the healing process. It is recognized that a personal relationship between the physician and the patient is essential for the provision of proper medical care. The traditional physician–patient relationship takes on a new dimension when care is rendered within an organizational structure. Legal precedent has established that the institution itself also has a responsibility to the patient. It is in recognition of these factors that these rights are affirmed.

1. The patient has the right to considerate and respectful care.

2. The patient has the right to obtain from his physician complete current information concerning his diagnosis, treatment, and prognosis in terms the patient can be reasonably expected to understand. When it is not medically advisable to give such information to the patient, the information should be made available to an appropriate person in his behalf. He has the right to know, by name, the physician responsible for coordinating his care.

3. The patient has the right to receive from his physician information necessary to give informed consent prior to the start of any procedure and/or treatment. Except in emergencies, such information for informed consent should include but not necessarily be limited to the specific procedure and/or treatment, the medically significant risks involved, and the probable duration of incapacitation. Where medically significant alternatives for care or treatment exist, or when the patient requests information concerning medical alternatives, the patient has the right to such information. The patient also has the right to know the name of the person responsible for the procedures and/or treatment.

4. The patient has the right to refuse treatment to the extent permitted by law and to be informed of the medical consequences of his action.

5. The patient has the right to every consideration of his privacy concerning his own medical care program. Case discussion, consultation, examination, and treatment are confidential and should be conducted discreetly. Those not directly involved in his care must have the permission of the patient to be present.

6. The patient has the right to expect that all communications and records pertaining to his care should be treated as confidential.

7. The patient has the right to expect that within its capacity a hospital must make reasonable response to the request of a patient for services. The hospital must provide evaluation, service, and/or referral as indicated by the urgency of the case. When medically permissible, a patient may be transferred to another facility only after he has received complete information and explanation concerning the needs for and alternatives to such a transfer. The institution to which the patient is to be transferred must first have accepted the patient for transfer.

8. The patient has the right to obtain information as to any relationship of his hospital to other health care and educational institutions insofar as his care is concerned. The patient has the right to obtain information as to the existence of any professional relationships among individuals, by name, who are treating him.

9. The patient has the right to be advised if the hospital proposes to engage in or perform human experimentation affecting his care or treatment. The patient has the right to refuse to participate in such research projects.

10. The patient has the right to expect reasonable continuity of care. He has the right to know in advance what appointment times and physicians are available and where. The patient has the right to expect that the hospital will provide a mechanism whereby he is informed by his physician or a delegate of the physician of the patient's continuing health care requirements following discharge.

11. The patient has the right to examine and receive an explanation of his bill regardless of source of payment.

12. The patient has the right to know what hospital rules and regulations apply to his conduct as a patient.

No catalog of rights can guarantee for the patient the kind of treatment he has a right to expect. A hospital has many functions to perform, including the prevention and treatment of disease, the education of both health professionals and patients, and the conduct of clinical research. All these activities must be conducted with an overriding concern for the patient, and, above all, the recognition of his dignity as a human being. Success in achieving this recognition assures success in the defense of the rights of the patient.

The prime objective of the medical profession is to render service to humanity, and this must be the medical assistant's first concern. The importance of respecting the confidentiality of information learned from or about patients in the course of employment cannot be overemphasized. It is not right to reveal patient confidences to *anyone* — this includes your family, your spouse, your best friend, your beautician, and other medical assistants. The medical assistant must avoid even mentioning the names of patients, for sometimes the doctor's specialty reveals the patient's reason for consultation.

Never discuss one patient's case with another patient; if you are asked questions by a curious patient, change the subject. When patients ask questions of a medical nature about their own case, they should be referred to the doctor for information. Patients may sometimes ask for your advice on personal matters, and you should avoid such involvements. Patients tend to identify your remarks as being those of the doctor. By staying silent in all instances, you are protecting the physician, yourself, and the patient. Confidential papers, case histories, and even the appointment book should be kept out of sight of curious eyes to protect the patient as well as the doctor and office staff.

The medical assistant has an obligation to keep abreast of developments that affect the practice of medicine and care of the patients. Membership in a professional organization provides access to continuing education for improvement of knowledge and skills.

On rare occasions, a medical assistant is faced with a situation in which the physician-employer's conduct appears to violate established ethical standards. Before making any judgments, the medical assistant must be absolutely sure of all the facts and circumstances. If there has in fact been a history of unethical conduct, the medical assistant must then make some decisions. Is it wise to remain under these circumstances or would it be better to seek other employment? This is a difficult decision, particularly if the relationship and employment conditions have been satisfactory and congenial. Will a decision to remain adversely affect future opportunities for employment with another physician?

A medical assistant is not obliged to report questionable actions of the physician or to attempt to change the practice. However, an ethical medical assistant does not wish to participate in the continuance of known substandard practices that may be harmful to patients or that are unlawful.

SUMMARY

In this chapter's treatment of medical ethics, we have discussed the evolution of the codes and the application of ethical principles to the practice of medicine. The medical assistant is bound to ethical practices as are all health care providers. Specifically, the medical assistant must be aware that:

- the primary objective of the medical profession is to render service to humanity
- it is important for the medical assistant to keep informed and to follow current regulations
- *only* the physician is authorized to release information about a patient
- it is unethical for the medical assistant to discuss a patient's case with anyone

▶ LEARNING ACHIEVEMENTS

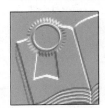

After completing this chapter, are you able to:

1. Define the terms listed in the Vocabulary of this chapter?
2. Explain how *etiquette* differs from *ethics?*
3. Briefly explain how the Code of Hammurabi differed from the modern Principles of Medical Ethics?
4. Name the oath that has been administered to medical graduates for centuries?
5. Recall the significant contribution to ethics made by Thomas Percival?
6. State the significance of the 1980 revision of the AMA Principles?
7. Summarize the manner in which a medical society might penalize a member for unethical conduct?
8. Discuss what and to whom information about a patient may be released?
9. Apply the Principles of Medical Ethics in dealing with fees and charges?
10. Compare the provisions of the AAMA Code of Ethics with those of the AMA Principles?

REFERENCES AND READINGS

American Medical Association: *Current Opinions of the Council on Ethical and Judicial Affairs,* Chicago, The Association, 1989.

Flight, M. R.: *Law, Liability, and Ethics for Medical Office Personnel,* Albany, NY, Delmar Publishers, Inc., 1988.

Lewis, M. A., and Warden, C. D.: *Law and Ethics in the Medical Office,* 2nd ed., Philadelphia, F. A. Davis Co., 1988.

CHAPTER FIVE

—

MEDICINE AND THE LAW

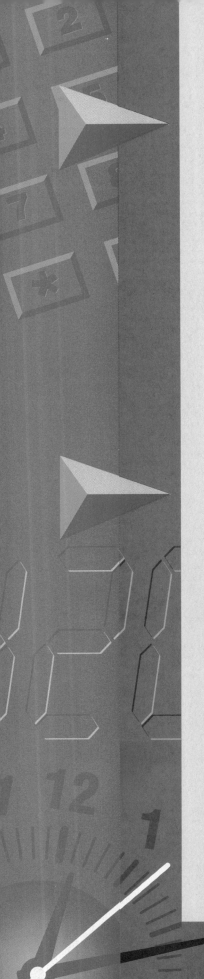

CHAPTER OUTLINE

VOCABULARY

administer To instill a drug into the body of a patient.

administrative law Regulations set forth by government agencies.

arbitration The hearing and determination of a cause in controversy by a person or persons either chosen by the parties involved or appointed under statutory authority.

arbitrator A neutral person chosen to settle differences between two parties in controversy.

assault An intentional, unlawful *attempt* of bodily injury to another by force.

battery A willful and unlawful use of force or violence upon the person of another.

communicable Capable of being transmitted from one person to another.

compensatory damages General or special damages without specific monetary value.

contagious Transmitted readily from one person to another by direct or indirect contact.

contract law Enforceable promises.

dispense The giving of drugs, in some type of bottle, box, or other container, to the patient. (Under the

Controlled Substances Act of 1970, the definition of "dispense" includes the administering of Controlled Substances.)

emancipated minor A person under legal age who is self-supporting and living apart from parents or a guardian.

exemplary Serving as a warning.

felony A crime of a graver nature than one designated as a misdemeanor. Generally, an offense punishable by imprisonment in a penitentiary.

infectious Capable of causing infection.

informed consent A consent in which there is understanding of what treatment is to be undertaken and of the risks involved, why it should be done, and alternative methods of treatment available and their attendant risks. The alternatives include the failure to treat and the attendant risk.

infraction Breaking the law.

litigation Contest in a court of justice for the purpose of enforcing a right.

malfeasance The doing of an act that is wholly wrongful and unlawful.

malpractice Professional misconduct, improper discharge of professional duties, or failure to meet the standard of care by a professional that results in harm to another.

misdemeanor A crime less serious than a felony.

misfeasance The improper performance of a lawful act.

nominal Existing in name only.

nonfeasance The failure to do something that should have been done.

perjured testimony Telling what is false when sworn to tell the truth.

prescribe To issue a prescription for the patient; to direct, designate, or order use of a remedy.

punitive Inflicting punishment.

tort An act that brings harm to a person or damage to property, caused negligently or intentionally.

treason A crime against the United States.

trespass To exceed the bounds of what is lawful, right, or just.

venereal Due to or propagated by sexual intercourse.

MEDICINE AND THE LAW

5

Upon successful completion of this chapter, you should be able to:

1. Define the terms listed in the Vocabulary.

2. Explain the difference between a *crime* and a *tort.*

3. Define a *contract* and explain its importance in a health care facility.

4. Explain the steps a physician must take for legal protection when terminating an established doctor-patient relationship.

5. Define *medical professional liability.*

6. List the four "Ds of Negligence" as published by the AMA.

7. Describe briefly what is meant by an *arbitration procedure* and identify at least three advantages from using this process.

8. List the six components of informed consent.

9. Explain the purpose of Good Samaritan Acts.

10. State two restrictions imposed on physicians by the Uniform Anatomical Gift Act.

Closely allied with medical ethics are certain medicolegal principles that must be considered in the daily operation of the physician's office. Law is the system by which society gives order to our lives. For our purposes, the law may be divided into two general categories: criminal law and civil law.

CRIMINAL LAW

Criminal law governs violations of the law that are punishable as offenses against the state or government. Such offenses involve the welfare and safety of the public as a whole rather than of one individual.

Classifications of Criminal Law

Criminal offenses are classified as:

- Treason
- Felony
- Misdemeanor
- Infraction

Treason is defined by the Constitution as a crime against the United States. **Felonies** are major crimes that include robbery, arson, issuing bad checks, forgery, and using the mail to defraud. Conviction may result in imprisonment for 1 year or more. **Misdemeanors** are lesser offenses that might result in imprisonment for from 6 months to 1 year. An example of a misdemeanor is possession of a hypodermic syringe or needle by an unauthorized person. **Infractions** are minor offenses that are often associated with traffic laws or drug violations; they usually result in a fine only.

CIVIL LAW

Civil law is concerned with the relations of individuals with other individuals, with corporations or other organizations, or with government agencies. Classifications of civil law that affect the practice of medicine are:

- Contract Law
- Tort Law
- Administrative Law

Contract law—governs enforceable promises. **Tort law**—governs acts, intentional or unintentional, that bring harm to a person or damage to property. **Administrative law**—involves regulations set forth by government agencies, for example, the Internal Revenue Service.

LAW OF CONTRACTS

A contract need not be formal to be binding. The law of contracts touches our lives in many ways practically every day, but usually we do not give it much thought. The physician–patient relationship is governed by the law of contracts, and as a medical assistant, you must be aware of what constitutes a contract.

A contract is an agreement creating an obligation. It may be written or oral, express, or implied. To be valid or enforceable, a contract must have the following four basic elements:

Manifestation of assent (an offer and an acceptance). The parties to the contract must understand and agree on the intent of the contract. The party making the offer is known as the *offeror,* and the party to whom the offer is made is the *offeree.*

Legal subject matter. An obligation that requires an illegal action is not an enforceable contract.

Legal capacity to contract. Both parties to the contract must be adults of sound mind.

Consideration. There must be an exchange of something of value.

If any of these four elements is missing, there is no contract.

The physician–patient relationship is generally held by the courts to be a contractual relationship that is the result of three steps:

1. The physician invites an offer by establishing availability.
2. The patient makes an offer by arriving for treatment.
3. The physician accepts the offer by undertaking treatment of the patient.

Prior to accepting the offer, the physician is under no obligation, and no contract exists. Once the physician has accepted the patient, however, an implied contract does exist that the physician (1) will treat the patient, using reasonable care, and (2) possesses the degree of knowledge, skill, and judgment that might be expected of another physician in the same locality and under similar circumstances. It is extremely important that no express promise of a cure be made, for this then becomes a part of the contract.

The patient's part of the agreement includes the liability for payment for services and a willingness to follow the advice of the doctor. Most physician–patient relationships are implied contracts. After the physician–patient relationship has been established, the physician is obligated to attend the patient as long as attention is required, unless a special arrangement is made.

Termination of Contract

The physician–patient relationship may be terminated by the physician or the patient.

Termination by Physician

Before withdrawing from the relationship, the physician may want to take into consideration the condition of the patient, the size of the community, and the availability of other physicians. When a physician does terminate the relationship, the patient must be given notice of the physician's intention to withdraw in order that the patient may secure another physician.

The physician may write a letter of withdrawal from the case to the patient, similar to the one shown in Figure 5–1. The letter should state that:

- professional care is being discontinued
- the physician will turn over the patient's records to another physician
- the patient should seek the attention of another physician as soon as possible

The letter should be sent by certified mail with a return receipt requested, and a copy of the letter should be placed in the patient's medical record. When the return receipt arrives, it should be attached to the copy of the letter and retained permanently.

In order to protect the physician against a lawsuit for abandonment, make certain that details of the circumstances under which the physician is withdrawing from the case are included in the patient's medical record.

Termination by Patient

In the event that the patient terminates the relationship, the termination of the contract and the circumstances surrounding it should be carefully documented in the physician's records. This may be accomplished by the physician's confirming the discharge by a certified mail letter similar to the one shown in Figure 5–2.

Statute of Frauds

In 1677, a statute was adopted in England aimed at reducing the evil of **perjured testimony** by providing that certain contracts could not be enforced if they depended upon the testimony of witnesses alone and were not evidenced in writing. The provisions of this English statute have been closely followed by statutes adopted in all the states of this country. Under the Statute of Frauds, some contracts, in order to be enforceable, must be in writing. One of these is the promise to pay the debts of another. Thus, if a third party, not otherwise legally responsible for the person's debts, agrees to pay a patient's medical bills, the agreement cannot be enforced unless it is in writing. Another contract that falls within the Statute of Frauds is one that cannot be completed within a year. If the physician entered into an agreement to perform a series of treatments for a given sum, and this series covered a time span of more than 1 year, it would have to be in writing to be enforceable.

MEDICAL PROFESSIONAL LIABILITY

Medical professional liability is governed by the *law of torts*. The term "medical professional liability" encompasses all possible civil liability that a

FIGURE 5–1. Letter of withdrawal from case.

Date

Dear (Patient):

I find it necessary to inform you that I am withdrawing from providing you medical care for the reason that _____

_____

As your condition requires medical attention, I suggest that you promptly place yourself under the care of another physician. If you do not know of other physicians, you may wish to contact the county medical society for a referral.

If you so desire, I shall be available to attend you for a reasonable time after you have received this letter, but in no event for more than 15 days.

When you have selected a new physician, I would be pleased to make available to him or her a copy of your medical chart or a summary of your treatment.

Very truly yours,

Date

Dear (Patient):

This will confirm our telephone conversation of today in which you discharged me from attending you as your physician in your present illness.

In my opinion, your condition requires continued medical treatment by a physician. If you have not already done so, I suggest that you employ another physician without delay.

At your request, I would be pleased to make available to him or her a summary of the diagnosis and the treatment you have received from me.

Very truly yours,

FIGURE 5-2. Letter to confirm discharge by patient.

physician can incur as a result of professional acts. It is preferred over the term "medical malpractice" because the latter carries some negative overtones. Medical professional liability is more easily prevented than defended.

Classifications

All medical professional liability claims fall into one of three classifications:

- Malfeasance
- Misfeasance
- Nonfeasance

Feasance simply means the "performance" or the doing of an act. Add the prefix *mal-* (meaning "bad"), and the result is **malfeasance**—the performance of an act that is wholly wrongful and unlawful. **Misfeasance** is the improper performance of some lawful act. Failing to perform an act that should have been done is **nonfeasance.** Any and all of these situations are considered *professional negligence.*

Negligence

When applied to the medical profession, negligence is called **malpractice.** Negligence is generally defined as the doing of some act that a reasonable and prudent physician would not do or the failure to do some act that such a person should or would do. The standard of prudent conduct is not defined by law but is left to the determination of a judge or jury.

A physician who performs an operation carelessly or contrary to accepted standards, performs an unnecessary operation, or fails to render care that should have been given may be found guilty of negligence or malpractice.

A medical assistant whose responsibilities are clearly set forth in a policy and procedure manual may be guilty of negligence through failure to carry out these responsibilities or to exercise reasonable and ordinary care in so doing. The medical assistant must also avoid rendering any care to a patient that might be construed as the practice of medicine.

Standard of Care

If a physician were to be held legally responsible for every unsuccessful result occurring in the treatment of a patient, no person would undertake the responsibility of practicing medicine. The courts hold that a physician must use reasonable care, attention, and diligence in the performance of professional services, follow his or her best judgment in treating patients, and possess and exercise the best skill and care that are commonly possessed and exercised by other reputable physicians in the same or a similar locality.

Physicians who represent themselves as specialists must meet the standards of practice of their specialty. Whether or not they have met these requirements in treating a particular patient is generally a matter for the court to decide on the basis of expert testimony provided by another physician. *Negligence is not presumed; it must be proved.*

Physicians are not required to possess extraordinary learning and skill, but they must keep abreast of medical developments and techniques, and they cannot experiment. They are also bound to advise their patients if they discover that the condition to be treated is one beyond their knowledge or technical skill.

Importance of the Physician–Patient Relationship

When injury results to a patient as a result of a physician's negligence, the patient can legally initiate a malpractice suit to recover financial damages. Experience has shown, however, that the incidence of malpractice claims is directly related to the personal relationship existing between the physician and the patient. Deterioration of the physician–patient relationship is a frequently demonstrated reason for a patient's initiating a malpractice suit, even though there was no real injury to the patient.

Medical Assistant's Role in Claims Prevention

The medical assistant also has an important role in claims prevention. For instance, a patient who is kept waiting for an inexcusably long time without explanation or reassurance has developed some feeling of hostility before ever seeing the physician. A few words from the medical assistant at the appropriate time may forestall hostility and promote understanding.

The medical assistant must be very careful in his or her choice of words when reassuring an apprehensive patient. Rather than saying, "I'm sure you will soon be entirely well," a gentle touch or a friendly smile will comfort the patient but be noncommittal. Any time a medical assistant has reason to believe that a patient is dissatisfied, it is the medical assistant's duty to pass along such information to the physician.

The Four Ds of Negligence

In a report by the Committee on Medicolegal Problems of the American Medical Association (AMA), it was stated that:

"To obtain a judgment against a physician for negligence, the patient must present evidence of what have been referred to as the "four Ds." He must show: (1) that the physician owed a *duty* to the patient, (2) that the physician was *derelict* and breached that duty by failing to act as the ordinary, competent physician in the same community would have acted under the same or similar circumstances, (3) that such failure or breach was the *direct cause* of the patient's injuries, and (4) that *damages* to the patient resulted therefrom."

DUTY. Duty exists when the physician–patient relationship has been established. That is, the patient has sought the assistance of the physician, and the physician has knowingly undertaken to provide the needed medical service.

DERELICT (NEGLECTFUL OF OBLIGATION). Proof of dereliction, or proof of negligence of an obligation, must be shown in obtaining a judgment for malpractice.

DIRECT CAUSE. There must be proof that the injury or death was directly caused by the physician's actions or failure to act and that it would not otherwise have occurred.

DAMAGES. There are three kinds of damages recognized by the law:

- Nominal
- Punitive or exemplary
- Compensatory or actual

Nominal (existing in name only) damages are a token compensation for the invasion of a legal right in which no actual injury was suffered. **Punitive** (inflicting punishment) or **exemplary** (serving as a warning) damages require allegations and proof of willful misconduct and are unusual in lawsuits against physicians. It is the compensatory or actual damages that are most frequently involved in professional liability cases. **Compensatory damages** may be general or special.

Compensatory or actual damages for injuries or losses that are the natural and necessary consequences of the physician's negligent act or omission are referred to as *general damages*. General damages include compensation for pain and suffering, for loss of a bodily member or faculty, for disfigurement, or for other similar direct losses or injuries. The fact of the losses must be proved—the monetary value need not be proved.

Special damages are those injuries or losses that are not a necessary consequence of the physician's negligent act or omission. These may include the costs of medical and hospital care, loss of earnings, cost of travel, and so forth. Both the fact of these injuries or losses and the monetary value must be proved.

The Committee on Professional Liability of the California Medical Association in 1971 called these same four elements the "ABCDs" of negligence in medical practice:

ABCDs OF NEGLIGENCE IN MEDICAL PRACTICE

A. Acceptance of a person as a patient

B. Breach of the physician's duty of skill or care

C. Causal connection between the breach by the physician and the damage to the patient

D. Damage of a foreseeable nature—that is, injury, pain, loss of earnings, and so on—that could reasonably have been foreseen to result

WHEN THE PHYSICIAN IS SUED

Malpractice suits are far from rare, and every physician faces the probability of being sued at least once during his or her career. When a suit is filed, the medical assistant may become involved in scheduling depositions or court appearances and in preparing materials for court.

Interrogatory

Before the trial, the physician may be requested to complete an *interrogatory*. An interrogatory is a list of general questions from another party to the lawsuit. Answers to the interrogatory must be provided within a specified time and must be answered under oath. Interrogatories are limited to parties named in the lawsuit.

Deposition

There may be a request for a *deposition*. A deposition is oral testimony taken from a party or witness to the litigation and is not limited to parties named in the lawsuit. A witness who is not a party to the lawsuit will be summoned by subpoena for the deposition. The deposition is usually taken in the attorney's office in the presence of a court reporter and must be taken under oath to tell the truth, just as in a court of law. The person giving the deposition is called the *deponent*. The transcribed deposition is sent to the deponent for review, and the deponent is at liberty to make any necessary changes or corrections. Only deponents who are not parties to the suit are compensated for their time.

Subpoena

A *subpoena* is a document issued by the court requiring the person to whom it is directed to be in court at a given time and place to testify as a witness in a lawsuit.

Subpoena Duces Tecum

A *subpoena duces tecum* is an order to provide records or documents of some sort and is usually addressed to the custodian of the records. This may be the medical assistant. The custodian of the records may expect to be compensated for the time spent in compiling the records and for photocopying charges. The fee must be demanded at the time the subpoena is served, or it is considered to be waived.

Some states have laws that permit patients to obtain a copy of their records upon request, although a photocopying charge may be made. It is never wise to release the original records.

ARBITRATION

Arbitration, the settlement of a dispute by a third party or parties that have been selected because of their familiarity with the practices involved, is common in modern business life. Arbitration is established by statute and is available to the medical profession in many states. Arbitration is an alternative method of resolving legal disputes between doctor and patient. Many physicians and lawyers see it as one way to help solve the malpractice crisis. Instead of taking the disagreement through the long and expensive process of court **litigation,** which may take as long as 7 or 8 years, the patient and the physician (or hospital) agree in advance to submit the dispute informally to a neutral person or persons.

An arbitration agreement is a contract and is subject to the judgment of the courts only as to the fairness of the agreement. The agreement is precisely worded by an attorney and should not be paraphrased when explaining it to a patient (Fig. 5–3). Signing the agreement is a voluntary act on the part of the patient, who has a period of grace in which to revoke the agreement if he or she later decides against it. Both the patient and the physician have the opportunity to agree on who will arbitrate the case, so that it does not favor one side over the other. By prior agreement, the **arbitrator**(s) may be appointed by or from the American Arbitration Association, which is a neutral, private, nonprofit association dedicated solely to the advancement of out-of-court remedies. Its panels of arbitrators are made up of persons from business, the professions, and public interest groups.

Advantages of Arbitration

- Less expensive
- Faster
- More confidential

After an informal hearing, the arbitrator(s) then renders a binding decision, based on very specific rules of arbitration, as to any award. Arbitration applies essentially the same rights and the same measure of damages as a court. Arbitration is fair, it is less expensive, it is faster, and it is more confidential than court litigation.

If an arbitration statute exists in your state, you should get details of the procedure from your state or local medical society. If a physician elects to implement the procedure, every member of the physician's staff should know the details of the agreement, how to sign patients up, and how to answer the patient's questions. The fairness with which the physician's personnel present the program to the patient and the willingness with which the personnel answer the patient's questions largely determine whether or not the court will uphold the arbitration agreement. Furthermore, when the physician's per-

Physician's Copy

PATIENT-PHYSICIAN ARBITRATION AGREEMENT

1. It is understood that any dispute as to medical malpractice, that is as to whether any medical services rendered under this contract were unnecessary or unauthorized or were improperly, negligently or incompetently rendered, will be determined by submission to arbitration as provided by California Law and not by a lawsuit or resort to court process except as California Law provides for judicial review of arbitration proceedings. Both parties to this contract, by entering into it, are giving up their constitutional right to have any such dispute decided in a court of law before a jury, and instead are accepting the use of arbitration.

2. I have read and understood Article 1 above and I voluntarily agree, for myself and all persons identified in Article 3 below, to submit to arbitration any and all claims involving persons bound by this Agreement whether those claims are brought in tort, contract or otherwise. This includes, but is not limited to, suits for personal injury, actions to collect debts, or any other kind of civil action.

3. I understand and agree that this Arbitration Agreement binds me and anyone else who may have a right to assert a claim on my behalf. I further understand and agree that if I sign this Agreement on behalf of some other person for whom I have responsibility (including my spouse or children, living or yet unborn) then, in addition to myself, such person(s) will also be bound, along with anyone else who may have a right to assert a claim on their behalf. I also understand and agree that this Agreement relates to claims against the physician and any consenting substitute physician, as well as his/her partnership, professional corporation, employees, partners, heirs, assigns or personal representatives. I also hereby consent to the intervention or joinder in the arbitration proceeding of all parties relevant to a full and complete settlement of any dispute arbitrated under this Agreement, as set forth in the Medical Arbitration Rules and/or CHA-CMA Rules for the Arbitration of Hospital and Medical Fee Disputes.

4. I agree to accept medical services from the undersigned physician and to pay therefor. I UNDERSTAND THAT I DO **NOT** HAVE TO SIGN THIS AGREEMENT TO RECEIVE THE PHYSICIAN'S SERVICES, AND THAT IF I DO SIGN THE AGREEMENT AND CHANGE MY MIND WITHIN 30 DAYS OF TODAY, THEN I MAY REVOKE THIS AGREEMENT BY GIVING WRITTEN NOTICE TO THE UNDERSIGNED PHYSICIAN WITHIN THAT TIME STATING THAT I WANT TO WITHDRAW FROM THIS ARBITRATION AGREEMENT. I further understand that after those 30 days, this Agreement may be changed or revoked only by a written revocation signed by both parties.

5. On behalf of myself and all others bound by this Agreement as set forth in Article 3, agreement is hereby given to be bound by the Medical Arbitration Rules of the California Hospital Association and California Medical Association and the CHA-CMA Rules for the Arbitration of Hospital and Medical Fee Disputes, as they may be amended from time to time, which are hereby incorporated into this Agreement.

6. I have read and understood the attached explanation of the Patient-Physician Arbitration Agreement and I have read and understood this Agreement, including the Rules. I understand and agree that this writing makes up the entire arbitration agreement between me and/or the person(s) on whose behalf I am signing and the undersigned physician and/or consenting substitute physicians.

NOTICE: BY SIGNING THIS CONTRACT YOU ARE AGREEING TO HAVE ANY ISSUE OF MEDICAL MALPRACTICE DECIDED BY NEUTRAL ARBITRATION AND YOU ARE GIVING UP YOUR RIGHT TO A JURY OR COURT TRIAL. SEE ARTICLE 1 OF THIS CONTRACT.

Dated: _____, 19___ _____
(Patient)

Physician's Agreement to Arbitrate

In consideration of the foregoing execution of this Patient-Physician Arbitration Agreement, I likewise agree to be bound by the terms set forth in this Agreement and in the Rules specified in Article 5 above.

Dated: _____, 19___ _____
(Physician)

_____   _____
(Name of partnership or   (Title—e.g., Partner, President, etc.)
professional corporation)

© California Medical Association, 1977, 1981

FIGURE 5–3. Arbitration agreement used in the state of California.

sonnel "speak for the physician," any representations made by the personnel could be held against the physician.

SECURING A PATIENT'S INFORMED CONSENT OR INFORMED REFUSAL

A physician must have consent to treat a patient even though this consent is usually implied by virtue of the patient's having come to that physician for treatment. This implied consent is sufficient for common or simple procedures that are generally understood to involve little risk. A blood screen, chest x-ray, or electrocardiogram are examples. When more complex procedures are anticipated, the physician must obtain the patient's **informed consent** for *each* procedure. A physician who fails to secure some formal expression of consent could be charged with **trespass** or **assault** and **battery.**

A number of states have passed specific AIDS laws that require the written informed consent of a patient before a test for the AIDS antibody may be performed by a health care facility, physician, or other health care provider.

Even in cases in which the treatment was not negligent, the physician can be sued for failing to obtain an informed consent. Under such circumstances, the physician must be prepared to prove in court that a full explanation was given to the patient before obtaining the patient's consent.

An informed consent implies an understanding of:

- What is to be done
- Why it should be done
- The risks involved
- Expected benefits of recommended treatment
- Alternative treatments, including the failure to treat
- The attendant risks of alternative treatment

The informed consent is not satisfied merely by having the patient sign a form. A discussion must occur during which the physician provides the patient or the patient's legal representative with enough information to decide whether or not to undergo the proposed therapy. After such a discussion, the patient either consents or refuses to consent to the proposed therapy and may be required to sign a consent form. In any event, the discussion should be fully documented in the patient's medical record. If a form is used, a copy of the signed form should also be included in the patient's record. Treatment may not exceed the scope of the consent.

Forms on which a patient can grant written consent for operations or other procedures are kept in most physicians' offices.

WHO MAY GIVE CONSENT?

If a mentally competent adult expressly indicates assent to a particular form of treatment, then consent has been obtained. If the act consented to is unlawful—for instance, an abortion in states where abortion is prohibited—the consent is invalid. The consent is also invalid if it is given by a person unauthorized to do so or if it is obtained by misrepresentation or fraud.

Emergencies

In an emergency, one may render aid or care to prevent loss of life or serious illness or injury. However, implied consent in this circumstance lasts only as long as the emergency, and formal consent must be obtained for follow-up procedures done after the emergency has passed.

Incompetent Adults

Adults who have been found by a court to be insane or incompetent usually cannot consent to medical treatment. Consent must be obtained from the guardian.

Minors

Generally, when the patient is a minor, consent for surgery or treatment must be obtained from a parent or guardian except in an emergency requiring immediate treatment. If the parents are legally separated or divorced, consent should be obtained from the parent who has legal custody. There are exceptions.

Treatment of **venereal** disease, drug abuse, alcohol dependency, or pregnancy usually do not require parental consent.

Emancipated Minors

Emancipation is defined by statute and varies from state to state. An **emancipated minor** is a person under the age of majority (usually 18 or 21 years) who is one or more of the following:

- married
- in the armed forces
- living separate and apart from parents or a legal guardian
- self-supporting

Some statutes include a minimum age for emancipation.

Unless a statute declares otherwise, a minor who has the right to consent to treatment is entitled to the protection of his or her confidences, even from parents.

> ### GOOD SAMARITAN ACTS
>
> The purpose of a Good Samaritan Act is to protect the physician from liability for any civil damages as a result of rendering emergency care.

Physicians are sometimes reluctant to fulfill an ethical obligation to render aid in an emergency to someone who is not their patient for fear they may later be charged with negligence or abandonment by a total stranger (Fig. 5–4). In 1959, California passed the first *Good Samaritan Act,* and today all 50 states have Good Samaritan statutes. Although there are minor variations in the state statutes, their purpose is to protect the physician from liability for any civil damages as a result of rendering emergency care to accident victims, provided that such care is given in good faith and with due care under the circumstances. In some states, the law applies to nurses and other health professionals as well as to physicians. There is no creation of a contract in giving emergency care.

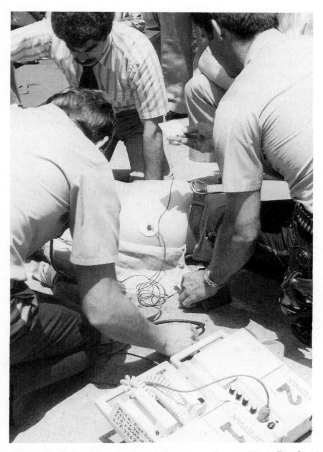

FIGURE 5–4. Physician treating at the scene of an accident. The Good Samaritan Act protects the physician from liability for any civil damages as a result of rendering emergency care. (From Henry, M., and Stapleton, E. R.: *EMT Prehospital Care,* Philadelphia, W.B. Saunders Co., 1991.)

UNIFORM ANATOMICAL GIFT ACT

The Uniform Anatomical Gift Act was approved by the National Conference of Commissioners on Uniform State Laws in 1968. Although many states had passed laws prior to this time that permitted living persons to make a gift of their body or portions of it after death, the laws were so different from state to state that arrangements for a donation in one state might not be recognized in another. All states have adopted the Uniform Anatomical Gift Act or similar legislation.

Essentially, the model law for donation states that:

- Any person of sound mind and 18 years of age or over may give all or any part of his body after death for research, transplantation, or placement in a tissue bank.
- A donor's valid statement of gift is paramount to the rights of others except where a state autopsy law may prevail.
- If a donor has not acted during his lifetime, his survivors, in a specified order of priority, may do so.
- Physicians who accept organs or tissues, relying in good faith on the documents, are protected from lawsuits. The physician attending at the time of death, if acquainted with the donor's wishes, may dispose of the body under the Uniform Anatomical Gift Act.
- The time of death must be determined by a physician who is not involved in the transplantation, and the attending physician cannot be a member of the transplant team.
- The donor may revoke the gift, or the gift may be rejected.

The most important clause permits the donation to be made by a will (without waiting for probate) or by other written or witnessed documents, such as a card designed to be carried on the person (Fig. 5–5). The Uniform Donor Card is considered a legal document in all 50 states.

The provisions of the Uniform Anatomical Gift Act are so designed that the offer is exercised only after death. Therefore, the donors should reveal their intentions to as many of their relatives and friends as possible and to their physician. Since the human body or its parts are not commodities in commerce, no money can be exchanged in making an anatomical donation.

LEGAL DISCLOSURES

The physician is charged with safeguarding patient confidences within the constraints of the law, but according to state laws, which vary somewhat throughout the nation, certain disclosures must be made.

UNIFORM DONOR CARD

OF _____

Print or type name of donor

In the hope that I may help others, I hereby make this anatomical gift, if medically acceptable, to take effect upon my death. The words and marks below indicate my desires.

I give: (a) _____ any needed organs or parts
(b) _____ only the following organs or parts

_____

Specify the organ(s) or part(s)

for the purposes of transplantation, therapy, medical research or education;

(c) _____ my body for anatomical study if needed.

Limitations or
special wishes, if any: _____

Signed by the donor and the following two witnesses in the presence of each other:

_____ _____
Signature of Donor   Date of Birth of Donor

_____ _____
Date Signed   City & State

_____ _____
Witness   Witness

This is a legal document under the Uniform Anatomical Gift Act or similar laws.

FIGURE 5–5. Uniform donor card.

Births and deaths must be reported. Births out of wedlock must be reported on special forms in some states; some require detailed information about still-births.

Physicians are required to report cases that may have been a result of violence, such as gunshot wounds, knifings, or poisonings. They also must report deaths from accidental or unexplained causes.

In some states, occupational diseases must be reported within 10 days or 2 weeks.

Venereal diseases are reportable in every state. All fifty states require that confirmed cases of AIDS be reported to state public health officials. In at least 13 states, a seropositive test result is also a reportable condition. Individuals are reported either by name or by patient identifiers.

Child abuse is now a leading cause of death among children under 5 years of age, and health professionals are required by law to report any suspected cases of child abuse. This should be done as soon as evidence is discovered. Suspected abuse of elderly persons often creates a dilemma for the physician and other health care personnel. The elderly person may deny the abuse in fear of further mistreatment if it is made known. The law requires that suspected cases of physical abuse to children, elderly persons, or any others at risk be reported to the authorities.

The physician must report any cases of **contagious, infectious,** or **communicable** diseases. Local health departments publish lists of diseases that are reportable as well as the method of reporting. Often, the report may be made by telephone. When reporting by mail, the appropriate forms, which are supplied by the health department, must be used. In many areas, the county health department issues regular bulletins that are sent to all physicians in the county. Check with the local authorities for specific procedures in your area.

Controlled Substances Act of 1970

On May 1, 1971, the Controlled Substances Act of 1970 became effective, replacing the former Narcotic Acts and the Drug Abuse Control Amendments. In October 1973, the regulatory agency became known as the Drug Enforcement Administration (DEA).

Registration

Prior to administering, prescribing, or dispensing any of the scheduled drugs, a physician is required to register with the Registration Branch, Drug Enforcement Administration, P.O. Box 28083, Central Station, Washington, D.C. 20005, or with the nearest regional office. Registration is renewable annually. If a physician administers or dispenses any of the drugs listed in the five Schedules at more than one office, he or she must register each office. Regulations regarding the writing, telephoning, and refilling of prescriptions vary according to which Schedule is involved.

Schedules

Under the Controlled Substances Act, drugs are categorized into Schedules I, II, III, IV, and V. Drugs in Schedule I have the highest potential for abuse, and those in Schedule V have the least potential.

Schedule I substances are those that have no accepted medical use in the United States and have a high potential for abuse. Examples include heroin and LSD. Only the physician who is involved in conducting research with such drugs is concerned with Schedule I substances.

Schedule II substances have a high abuse potential with severe psychic or physical dependence liability. They include certain narcotic, stimulant, and depressant drugs. Examples are opium, morphine, and codeine.

Schedule III substances have an abuse potential that is lesser than that of the first two schedules. They include compounds that contain limited quantities of certain narcotic drugs combined with nonnarcotic substances. Paregoric, Empirin Compound with Codeine, and Tylenol with Codeine are examples.

Schedule IV substances have still less potential for abuse. Phenobarbital, Diazepam (Valium), and Propoxyphene (Darvon) are examples.

Schedule V substances have less abuse potential than those in Schedule IV but still warrant control. They include preparations that contain moderate quantities of certain narcotics such as may be found in cough medicines and antidiarrheal products.

WRITTEN PRESCRIPTIONS. Any prescription for any drug classified in Schedule II requires an official prescription issued by the Department of Justice. Official preprinted triplicate prescription forms are obtained from the DEA. Separate prescription blanks must be used for each controlled substance prescribed.

The prescription must be prepared in triplicate, in ink or indelible pencil in the handwriting of the prescriber, and include the following information:

- Name and address of the person for whom the prescription is made
- Name and quantity of the controlled substance prescribed
- Directions for use
- Address, category of license, and federal controlled substance number of the prescriber

The pharmacist keeps the original of the prescription, endorses the triplicate copy, and sends the copy to the Department of Justice. The physician keeps the other copy for the office record.

Schedule III, IV, and V substances are subject to the following prescription requirements:

- The prescription must be signed and dated by the prescriber.
- It must contain the name and address of the person for whom the controlled substance is prescribed, the name and quantity of the substance, and the directions for its proper use.
- For all controlled substances classified in Schedule III, the signature, date, and information described above must be written in ink or indelible pencil in the handwriting of the prescriber.
- The prescription must contain the name, address, telephone number, category of professional license, and DEA registration number of the prescriber.

ORAL PRESCRIPTIONS. The physician may dispense any Schedule III, IV, or V controlled substance by an oral prescription, but the prescription must be put in writing by the pharmacist who fills it. With permission from the physician, any employee may orally transmit a prescription for controlled substances *only* in Schedules III, IV, or V, again with the prescription being put in writing by the dispensing pharmacist. An employee cannot, under any circumstances, orally transmit a prescription for a controlled substance classified in Schedule II.

NARCOTIC DRUGS. Physicians who **prescribe** or **administer** narcotic drugs in the course of professional practice are not required to keep records of those transactions. The physician who **dispenses** a narcotic drug to a patient is required to keep a record of such dispensing. The physician who expects to dispense Schedule II controlled drugs must obtain these drugs by the use of a triplicate order form supplied by the DEA. Federal law mandates that an inventory must be maintained and kept for 2 years. Some states require the inventory to be kept 3 years.

NON-NARCOTIC DRUGS. A physician who regularly engages in dispensing any of the non-narcotic drugs listed in the Schedules as a regular part of the professional practice and who charges for the drugs either separately or together with other professional services must keep records of all such drugs received and dispensed. The records must be kept for a period of 2 years and are subject to inspection by the DEA. If the physician only occasionally dispenses a non-narcotic controlled drug to a patient (such as a physician's sample), he or she is not required to maintain a record of such dispensing.

SECURITY. Stored controlled substances must be kept in a locked cabinet or safe. Any loss of controlled drugs by theft must be reported to the regional office of the DEA at the time the theft is discovered. The local police department should also be notified.

DISCONTINUANCE OF PRACTICE. A physician who discontinues medical practice must return his or her Registration Certificate and any unused order forms to the nearest office of the DEA. The regional DEA office will advise on the disposition of any controlled drugs still on hand.

LEGAL RESPONSIBILITIES OF THE MEDICAL ASSISTANT

Generally, the law holds that every person is liable for the consequences of his or her own negligence when another person is injured as a result. In some situations, this liability also extends to the employer. Physicians may be held responsible for the mistakes of those who work in their offices and sometimes must pay damages for the negligent acts of their employees.

Physicians are legally responsible for the acts of their employees when the employees are acting within the scope of their duties or employment. Physicians are also responsible for the acts of assistants who are not their own employees if they commit acts of negligence in the presence of the physician while under the physician's immediate supervision. For example, a nurse who is a hospital employee makes an error in a procedure while acting under a physician's direction. The court may determine that the nurse came so completely under the direction and supervision of the physician that the physician is liable for the nurse's negligence. This is known as the doctrine of *respondeat superior* (let the master answer). On the other hand, if a special nurse is employed by the patient, the physician is not usually held liable for negligent acts of the special nurse. When physicians practice as partners, they are liable not only for their own acts and those of their partner but also for the negligent acts of any agent or employee of the partnership. The medical assistant, while acting within the scope of the employment contract, is considered an agent of the employer.

A physician who properly writes a prescription is not liable for a pharmacist's negligence in compounding it, but may be liable in cases in which there is misunderstanding as to the ingredients when the prescription is ordered over the telephone.

Need for Extreme Care

Medical assistants who are guilty of negligence are liable for their own actions, but the injured party generally sues the physician because there is a better chance of collecting. However, even an assistant who has no money can still be liable for any negligent actions. This fact illustrates the continuing importance of exercising extreme care in performing all duties in the professional office. While working under pressure, there is always the danger of interchanging blood, serum, or medications or of mixing names or improperly preparing labels. Medication and treatment solutions should be labeled clearly and their expiration dates checked. Never proceed with administration of a medication or treatment without checking all details at least three times. It is an accepted rule that the medication label should be read three times: (1) when you remove the container from its storage place; (2) when you are preparing the medication; and (3) when you return the medication to the storage place.

Rechecking Equipment

One person in the office should be designated to make periodic safety checks of reception room and treatment room furniture and of the condition of instruments and supplies. Every person on the staff should be alert for potential hazards, such as slipping rugs, exposed telephone and light cords, highly waxed floors, and protruding objects, since patients who are harmed as a result of these conditions can sue for damages (Fig. 5–6).

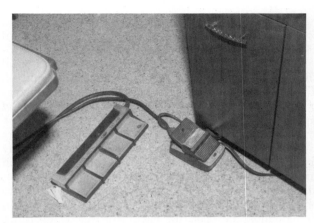

FIGURE 5–6. Example of a possible safety hazard.

Illegal Practice of Medicine

A physician studies many years to learn the profession before becoming licensed by the state to practice medicine. The medical assistant is not licensed to practice medicine and must never prescribe or try to diagnose a patient's ailment. This is the *illegal practice of medicine*. For this reason, it is not good policy for the medical assistant to discuss patients' complaints with them because patients tend to identify the medical assistant's remarks as being the opinion of the physician.

Instructions to Patients

Both the physician and the medical assistant must be thorough when giving instructions to patients. Written instructions should be provided whenever possible. A patient might forget oral instructions, resulting in drug-related injuries stemming from poor understanding of the proper use of the medications, their limitations, and their contraindications. The AMA has developed a Patient Medication Instruction program consisting of printed 5½″ × 8½″ sheets with information on over 80 common drug types.

Assisting at Patient Examinations

Except in an actual emergency, the physician should not examine a patient unless a third person is present. Allegations of sexual misconduct are made against physicians of all specialties. The charge of undue familiarity against a physician is very damaging. For this reason, the assistant generally stands by during examinations.

Emergency Aid

The question sometimes arises: Should the medical assistant give emergency care to a patient brought into the office during the physician's absence? In a medical emergency, the medical assistant, like any other layperson, may do whatever is reasonably necessary, provided the action taken is within that person's skill and competence. The physician should instruct the medical assistant regarding what course of action to take in such instances. The medical assistant must immediately get in touch with a physician to care for the patient once any emergency measures have been performed.

CLAIMS PREVENTION

The majority of patients never entertain the thought of taking legal action against their physicians, and the medical assistant should not develop an attitude of skepticism. The medical assistant can, however, play a role in claims prevention by following these suggestions:

- Give scrupulous attention to the needs of each patient.
- Avoid leaving patients alone (especially children and elderly patients).
- Avoid destructive and unethical criticism of the work of other physicians.
- Do not give out information either orally or in writing without the patient's consent.
- Verify the identity of anyone requesting information.
- Use discretion in telephone and office conversations.
- Be aware of your tone of voice and attitude during spoken communications.
- Communicate office policies and procedures to patients in advance of treatment whenever possible.
- Keep records that clearly show what was done and when it was done.
- Make no promises as to outcome of treatment.
- Record the facts if a patient discontinues treatment or fails to follow instructions.
- Avoid making any statement that might be construed as an admission of fault.
- Check the office equipment regularly to see that it is operating properly and safely.
- Make periodic safety inspections of furniture.
- Keep toxic substances out of reach of patients and clearly labeled.
- Keep drug samples and prescription pads out of sight.
- Never diagnose, prescribe, or offer a prognosis.
- Perform only those tasks that are within your scope of knowledge and training.
- Keep abreast of new procedures and technical advances in health care.

GLOSSARY OF LEGAL TERMS

agent A person authorized by another to act for him.

battery A willful and unlawful *use of force* or violence upon the person of another without his consent. A surgical operation is a technical "battery" regardless of its result and is excusable only where there is express or implied consent by the patient.

breach The breaking or violating of a law, right, or duty.

breach of duty In a general sense, any violation or omission of a legal or moral duty.

burden of proof The necessity or duty of affirmatively proving a fact or facts in dispute in a case at law.

civil law That division of municipal law that is concerned with the enforcement of civil rights as distinguished from criminal law.

common law Law derived from court decisions; law as established by a judge.

contributory negligence An act or omission amounting to lack of ordinary care on the part of the patient, which, concurring with defendant's negligence, is proximate cause of injury.

criminal case A suit instituted to punish an infraction of the criminal laws.

criminal law Law that deals with conduct offensive to society as a whole or to the state.

defamation Offense of injuring another's reputation by false and malicious statements.

defendant The person against whom relief or recovery is sought in an action or lawsuit.

deposition The testimony of a witness taken in writing, under oath, and before a judicial officer in answer to oral or written interrogatories.

emancipation A term principally used with reference to the emancipation of a minor child by its parents, which involves an entire surrender of the right to the care, custody, and earnings of such child, as well as a renunciation of parental duties.

ethics That branch of moral science that treats of the duties a member of a profession owes to the public, to his colleagues, and to his patient or client.

expert testimony Testimony given in relation to some scientific, technical, or professional matter by experts, that is, persons qualified to speak authoritatively by reason of their special training, skill, or familiarity with the subject.

feasance The doing of an act; a performance. *Malfeasance* The doing of an act that is wholly wrongful and unlawful; *misfeasance* The improper performance of some act that may lawfully be done; *nonfeasance* The omission of an act that a person ought to do.

grievance committee A committee established by a local medical society to hear and investigate the complaints of patients regarding professional care rendered by an attending physician or of allegedly excessive fees charged.

invasion of privacy The right of privacy is the right to be "left alone" to live in seclusion without being subjected to unwarranted or undesired publicity. Thus, without the knowledge and authorization of the patient, there should be no publication of his medical case record and no showing of a photograph or motion picture from which the identity of the patient is determinable.

judgment The official decision of a court of justice upon the respective rights and claims of the parties to an action or suit therein litigated and submitted to its determination.

judicial Relating to or connected with the administration of justice.

jurisprudence The science or philosophy of law.

liable Bound or obliged according to law or equity.

libel Defamatory words that are printed, written, or published that injure the character or reputation of another. See **slander.**

locum tenens "Holding the place." A deputy, substitute, or representative.

medical audit A study of the patient's medical record for the purpose of determining the quality of medical care the patient received.

negligence The omission to do something that a reasonable person, guided by those considerations that ordinarily regulate human affairs, would do or the doing of something that a reasonable and prudent person would not do.

non compos mentis Not sound of mind; insane. This is a very general term, embracing all varieties of mental derangement.

plaintiff The person who brings an action; the party who complains or sues in a personal action and is so named in the record.

proximate cause That which, in a natural and continuous sequence, unbroken by any efficient intervening cause, produces the injury, and without which the result would not have occurred.

prudence Carefulness, precaution, attentiveness, and good judgment, as applied to action or conduct.

qui facit per alium facit per se "He who acts through another acts himself."

quid pro quo Something for something.

res gestae "Things done." Res gestae is considered as an exception to the hearsay rule. In its operation, it renders acts and declarations that constitute a part of the things done and said admissible in evidence, even though they would otherwise come within the rule excluding hearsay evidence or self-serving declarations.

res ipsa loquitur "The thing speaks for itself."

res judicata A thing judicially acted upon or decided.

respondeat superior "Let the master answer." This maxim means that a master is liable in certain cases for the wrongful acts of his servant, and a principal for those of his agent.

rule of discovery Statute of limitations does not

begin to run until the patient knew or should have known of the injury.

slander Oral defamation; speaking falsely about another with resulting injury to his reputation. See **libel.**

statute An act of the legislature declaring, commanding, or prohibiting something. This word is used to designate the written law, in contradistinction to the unwritten law.

statute of limitations A legal limit on the time one has to file suit in civil matters, usually measured from the time of the wrong or from the time a reasonable person would have discovered the wrong.

statutory Relating to a statute; conforming to a statute.

subpoena A writ or order directed to a person and requiring his attendance at a particular time and place to testify. *Subpoena duces tecum* The writ may also require bringing any books, documents, or other things under his control that he is bound by law to produce in evidence.

suit An action or process in a civil court for the recovery of a right or claim. The term is seldom applied to a criminal prosecution.

suspend To discontinue temporarily, but with an expectation or purpose of resumption.

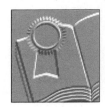

▶ LEARNING ACHIEVEMENTS

Are you able to:

1. Define the terms listed in the Vocabulary of this chapter?
2. Give the legal classifications of issuing a bad check and of the possession of a hypodermic syringe by an unauthorized person?
3. List the three components of a legal contract and explain how they apply to the physician–patient relationship?
4. Discuss the termination of the physician–patient relationship with an uncooperative patient, and what precautions apply?
5. State how the *law of torts* affects medical practice?
6. Explain the meaning of the four "Ds of Negligence"?
7. Compare the processes of *arbitration* and *litigation?*
8. Discuss the importance of *informed consent* and *informed refusal?*
9. State what law protects a person who renders first aid at the scene of an accident?
10. Discuss the purpose of the Uniform Anatomical Gift Act and the restrictions it imposes on physicians?

REFERENCES AND READINGS

American Medical Association: *Medicolegal Forms with Legal Analysis,* Chicago, The Association, 1991.

California Medical Association: *Arbitration for Physicians in Private Practice,* San Francisco, The Association, 1975.

California Medical Association: *Professional Liability,* San Francisco, The Association, 1971.

California Medical Association: *California Physician's Legal Handbook,* San Francisco, The Association, 1992.

Cowdrey, M. L.: *Basic Law for the Allied Health Profession,* Monterey, CA, Wadsworth Health Sciences Division, 1984.

Flight, M. R.: *Law, Liability, and Ethics for Medical Office Personnel,* Albany, NY, Delmar Publishers, Inc., 1988.

Hemelt, M. D., and Mackert, M. E.: *Dynamics of Law in Nursing and Health Care,* Reston, VA, Reston Publishing Co., 1979.

Hirsch, C. S., Morris, R. C., and Moritz, A. R.: *Handbook of Legal Medicine,* 5th ed., St. Louis, C. V. Mosby Co., 1979.

Lewis, M. A., and Warden, C. D.: *Law and Ethics in the Medical Office,* 2nd ed., Philadelphia, F. A. Davis Co., 1988.

Medical Insurance Exchange of California: *Malpractice Prevention Guide for California Medical Practices,* San Francisco, The Exchange, 1983.

State of California Department of Consumer Affairs, Board of Medical Quality Assurance: *Guidebook to Laws Governing the Practice of Medicine by Physicians and Surgeons,* 3rd ed., Sacramento, CA, State of California Department of Consumer Affairs, 1981.

5

CHAPTER OUTLINE

DEVELOPING YOUR PERSONAL COMMUNICATION SKILLS
- Attitudes

BODY LANGUAGE
- Nonverbal Communication

PATIENT COMMUNICATION
- Orienting Yourself to the Patient
- Listening

COMMUNICATION TECHNIQUES
- Silence
- Establishing Guidelines
- Give the Patient Broad Openings
- Reduce the Distance
- Acknowledgment

COMMUNICATION WITH YOUR COWORKERS
- Cooperation
- Dependability
- Politeness
- Patience

GETTING ALONG WITH YOUR SUPERVISOR/EMPLOYER-PHYSICIAN
- Establishing A Working Relationship
- The Physician

RECOGNIZING DISCRIMINATION
- Prejudice and Stereotyping
- Civil Rights Act
- Subtle Discrimination
- Confrontation or Walking Away
- Resistance with Patience

CULTURAL INFLUENCES

SEXUAL HARASSMENT

PATIENT EDUCATION

LEARNING ACHIEVEMENTS

VOCABULARY

acknowledgment Recognition given to a patient for contribution to the conversation.

anxiety A feeling of uneasiness, apprehension, or dread; fear of the unknown.

empathy Intellectual and emotional awareness of another person's thoughts, feelings, and behavior.

establishing guidelines Making statements regarding roles, purpose, and limitations for a particular interaction.

focusing Questions and statements used to help the patient develop an idea.

laissez faire Management style of "hands off" when dealing with employees.

listening An active process of receiving information and examining one's reaction to the messages received.

open-ended questions General questions that ask the patient to determine the direction the communication should take.

rapport A relationship of harmony and accord between the patient and the health care worker.

reducing distance Diminishing the physical space between the medical assistant and the patient.

reflecting Directing back to the patient his ideas, feelings, questions, or concerns.

restating Repeating to the patient what you believe is the main thought or idea expressed.

seeking clarification Asking for additional inputs to understand the message received.

seeking consensual validation Attempts to reach a mutual meaning for a specific word used in the conversation.

silence Periods of no verbal communication.

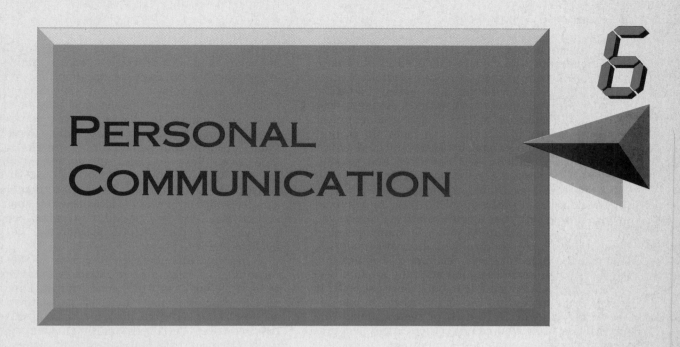

PERSONAL COMMUNICATION

LEARNING OBJECTIVES

COGNITIVE

Upon successful completion of this chapter, you should be able to:

1. Define the terms listed in the Vocabulary.

2. List four nonverbal communication tactics.

3. Elaborate on three skills for communication with co-workers.

4. List pros and cons of three management styles.

5. Discuss three patterns of listening.

6. Compare the three categories of verbal messages.

7. List and summarize five communication methods other than listening.

8. Differentiate between *prejudice* and *stereotyping.*

9. Discuss the Civil Rights Act and affirmative action.

10. Clarify sexual harassment.

PERFORMANCE

Upon successful completion of this chapter, you should be able to:

1. Display a better understanding of yourself.

2. Help a coworker recognize a correctable bad habit.

3. Interview someone in management and decide what their management style is.

4. Talk to a patient using therapeutic communication techniques.

Communication is a major requirement for success in any endeavor. Individuals employed in the health care profession are expected to have certain characteristics. A medical assistant must always be tactful and should know instinctively when speaking is wise and when listening is better. Effective communication is necessary to establish and maintain rapport among staff members and between staff and physician, staff and patient, and physician and patient. You are an important communication link.

As a medical assistant, you must perform your role not only as a professional but also as a human being. Throughout your medical assisting career, you will have the opportunity to touch many people's lives and to learn to display humanistic qualities. You will be able to foster feelings of compassion, fellowship, understanding, and empathy among individuals, physicians, staff members, and patients. It is important to develop the ability to relate one-on-one to the individuals in each of these groups. The medical assistant who can effectively apply communication skills is extremely important in today's medical office.

DEVELOPING YOUR PERSONAL COMMUNICATION SKILLS

Attitudes

It is important to understand yourself and to feel good about yourself. Confidence and self-esteem can affect your success, and feeling "down on yourself" can lead to failure. When you expect to fail, it is almost inevitable that you will. However, when you believe in yourself and expect to succeed, the likelihood of your success is greatly improved.

It is natural for human beings to be learning constantly. We gain knowledge by studying and by using our logical and critical thinking abilities. We develop skills by practice and careful repetition of behavior, and demonstration and coaching from others help us to improve our abilities. When an emotion accompanies an event time after time, it creates an attitude or feeling that may be very intense and difficult to change. No one can see your inner feelings, but those feelings have such a profound effect on your behavior that you are unable to hide them. Your attitudes are written in your behavior (Fig. 6–1).

Attitudes are infectious. Very often, how one person feels has a powerful influence on how others around feel. This is especially true when people are involved in a team effort, as you will be in the medical facility.

A negative attitude usually creeps up on us because it is so easy to be negative. It takes no effort to let a feeling of self-pity steal over us. Disappointments occur every day. It is easy to let them engulf us. Replacing negative thoughts with positive ones requires effort, but the effort is well spent. The way to combat negativity is to take the first steps toward a positive attitude:

- **Smile.** If you make the corners of your mouth turn up instead of down, it will be easier to think of something positive to say.
- **Say Something Pleasant.** Think of something positive, good-natured, or complimentary to say to others at every opportunity.
- **Use Positive Statements.** When you start to complain to a coworker, stop yourself and consider possibly altering your statement so that it will be more positive. For example, if you feel as if you want to say "Why can't you put things back where they belong?" instead try saying "Why don't I help you put things back where they belong?" You will be surprised at the way your relationships with people will improve.

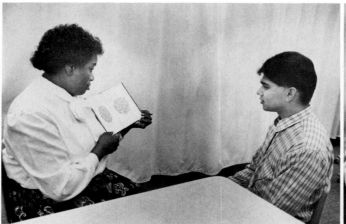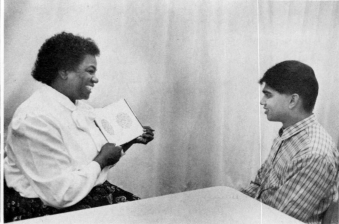

FIGURE 6–1. Look at these two individuals and think about the attitudes each conveys.

- **Change Problems into Opportunities.** When you see a problem in the office, use it as an opportunity to get other staff members to work together to find a solution. Use positive statements; they will generate positive replies.

Learn to share the sense of accomplishment gained from a job well done. This is important in maintaining a smooth-working office team. Sharing praise for your work, ideas, or plans may be difficult. Developing this kind of unselfishness is not easy. In our fiercely competitive society, most of us try to shine individually. We dislike sharing with others the honors that rightfully belong to us.

BODY LANGUAGE

When we think about communication, we most often think about talking. The fact is, we communicate more with our actions than we do with our words. Communication includes not only what you say but also how you say it. Do you smile or frown, or are you expressionless? Do you appear agitated or calm and relaxed? Do you appear really interested in what is being said or do you think about something else and not even listen? Communication is never one-way. There must be a receiver as well as a sender in any kind of discourse. Remember that it is as important to listen as it is to speak. The listener who maintains eye contact with the person with whom he or she is speaking communicates interest in what is being said.

Nonverbal Communication

You always communicate. You were communicating with your first cry at birth, and you have never stopped communicating since. You can stop communicating with words, but there are many modes of communication that do not use words. You use these modes whether you intend to or not; they include facial expression, the use of time, hand gestures, the position taken in a room, eye contact, posture, style of dress, loudness of voice, and touch.

Each of these modes and the many ways in which each can be used are potentially important in promoting relationships. Each can be used to communicate underlying feelings and motives between you and the people around you.

We are usually not aware of our own nonverbal signals and recognize only a small number of the signals sent by others. Our ability to help others increases greatly as we increase our own skills in interpreting nonverbal communication.

Nonverbal behaviors are habits; this means that they are automatic and that we are generally not aware of them. Try this experiment to demonstrate the strength of habits: Place your hands in front of you with palms together and clasp your hands with your fingers intertwined. Note how natural it feels. Notice which thumb is on top. Place the other

thumb on top and reposition the fingers so that they are again intertwined. This probably feels quite awkward. The way you did it the first time is the way you always do it. You have a habit of clasping your hands together in a certain way. If you clasped your hands in both ways with equal frequency, then each would feel equally natural. Changing habituated nonverbal patterns is a long and difficult process. Even so, if you find yourself using nonverbal behaviors that reduce your ability to be helpful to others, it may be worth the effort required to change them.

Since nonverbal behaviors are habits, it is difficult to deceive another person with words—your nonverbal gestures reveal your true feelings even though you seek to disguise those feelings with your own words. For example, if a person sits with hands clasped white knuckled, lips pinched tightly together, forehead wrinkled into a deep scowl and says to you, "Oh, things are fine, just fine. I'm cool. Not a care in the world," would you believe him or her? Of course not! When verbal and nonverbal messages are in contradiction, we usually believe the nonverbal message. Nonverbal channels are the primary means of expressing emotion.

Nonverbal messages may have different or even opposite meanings from one culture to the next. There are no truly universal meanings. For example, in our society, a simple up-and-down head nod means "yes," and a side-to-side shake means "no," but in Bulgaria and among the eskimos, these signals have the opposite meaning. As a medical assistant, you need to be aware of the nonverbal messages being sent by the persons with whom you interact, as well as of the nonverbal messages you are returning. Although you do not consciously control many of your nonverbal behaviors, you can become aware of them and work to control some of them. Table 6-1 summarizes some of the behaviors most frequently seen in the medical office.

TABLE 6-1. NONVERBAL COMMUNICATION

Message	Low-Level Behavior	High-Level Behavior
Empathy	Frown resulting from lack of understanding	Positive head nods; facial expressions that reflect the content of the conversation
Respect	Mumbling; patronizing tone of voice	Devoting one's full attention
Warmth	Apathy; fidgeting; signs indicating a desire to leave	Smiling; physical contact
Genuineness	Evasive eye contact	Congruence between verbal and nonverbal behavior
Self-disclosure	Bragging gestures; pointing to oneself	Gestures that minimize references to oneself
Confrontation	Pointing a finger or shaking one's fist; speaking in a loud tone of voice	Speaking in a natural tone of voice

PATIENT COMMUNICATION

Each person who enters your office needs to be greeted. Your job is to meet that need in a warm and caring manner. Make direct eye contact as soon as you can. Remember that as the medical assistant, you will be setting the tone for the entire visit. Courtesy helps to relax patients who are anxious about their visits and creates a caring **rapport** between you and them. Helping the patient to relax makes it easier to take the patient's history, since he or she is more willing to talk.

Orienting Yourself to the Patient

As the medical assistant, you observe the nonverbal behaviors of the patient. These observations can assist you in understanding the needs of the patient. "Helping" transactions demand your presence, that is, your "being with" the patient. In order to solve a problem, a working relationship needs to be established between you and the patient. This relationship will help you to gather the kind of data needed to clarify and define the problem. Your nonverbal behavior can have either a positive or negative influence on the patients. It can invite or encourage them to trust you, to open up, and to explore the significant dimensions of their problems, or it can promote their distrust and lead to a reluctance to reveal their thoughts to you. If you hear but do not truly listen, you will most likely miss data that are needed to clarify a situation.

Listening

Listening is the act of selectively discriminating among the available aural inputs within any given environment. It is a specific and important human behavior that is simple to grasp and easy to do, yet it is amazing how often people fail to listen to one another. Becoming a better listener requires energy, effort, and continual practice. Listening is more than merely hearing; we hear many things, but we listen to only a few. Listening is a combination of attention, hearing, understanding, and remembering. Effective listening involves all the senses. People want more than your physical presence when they communicate something to you; they want you to be fully attentive as well.

Three listening patterns are used in the medical facility: passive, active, and evaluative:

- **Passive** listening is simply "lending an ear." You do not need to offer a verbal response to the speaker; a nod or smile may be all that is necessary.
- **Active** listening involves direct communication. You need to offer *feedback,* ask questions, and be actively involved in the listening process.

- **Evaluative** listening is the most complex form of listening. You are asked to judge or evaluate and to provide an immediate response. This type of listening is required when answering the telephone in the medical office.

As you listen to patients communicate, you will understand that verbal messages can be organized into three categories:

- **Experiences** (what happens to patients). If a patient tells you that he gets a pain in his stomach every time he eats raw vegetables, he is discussing his problem in terms of an experience.
- **Behaviors** (what they do or fail to do). If the patient tells you that she cries for no reason at all, she is talking about her problem in terms of behavior.
- **Affect** (the feelings that have arisen from or are associated with either experiences or behaviors). If the patient tells you that he loses his temper every time he and his wife discuss finances, he is talking about affect.

Once you establish the category of the problem, you can become an active participant in the communication process. You will have a better understanding of what is really important to the care of the patient.

COMMUNICATION TECHNIQUES

There is no doubt that listening is the most effective communication technique available. However, other techniques can also be employed to enhance the communication process.

Silence

Patients very often find it impossible to put their thoughts into words. The medical assistant can use periods of **silence** to nonverbally communicate genuine interest to the patient. Short periods of silence often give the patient an opportunity to organize his or her thoughts. It is also a valuable opportunity for you to examine the nonverbal communication of the patient as well as your own. The appropriate use of silence has a great therapeutic value, but prolonged use may provoke the patient and produce feelings of **anxiety** in him or her.

Establishing Guidelines

Guidelines should be established at the beginning of the interaction. It is a basic courtesy to tell the patient if there is a time limit or a confidentiality limit to your interaction. Never make a promise to the patient that you know you cannot keep.

Give the Patient Broad Openings

Always remember that this initial time belongs to the patient. They are paying for your attention. Questions that you ask should emphasize the patient's needs. Examples of **open-ended questions** might be:

- "How have things been going?"
- "For what reasons did you come to the clinic today?"
- "Is there something special you would like to discuss with the doctor today?"
- "Why are we seeing you today?"

Continue to focus the conversation on the direction the patient desires. Use statements such as "And then what happened?" and "Yes, go on."

Reduce the Distance

Standing or sitting across the room or behind a desk gives the patient a negative nonverbal message of noninvolvement. Remember to **reduce the distance.** Your body style should reflect openness. Do not fold your hands over your chest or keep them in your pockets. Maintain eye contact; this gives the nonverbal message of involvement. "I want to get to know you," and "I want to hear what you have to say," are messages that can be communicated by removing physical distance (Fig. 6–2).

Acknowledgment

Acknowledgment is the recognition given to persons for their contribution to a communicative interaction. Without acknowledgment, communication often resembles a command. The communication techniques of **restating, reflecting, seeking clarification, seeking consensual validation,**

TABLE 6–2. THERAPEUTIC COMMUNICATION TECHNIQUES

Technique	Therapeutic Value
Acknowledgment	Emphasizes the importance of the patient in the communication process
Establishing guidelines	Helps patients to know what is expected of them
Focusing	Directs the conversation toward important topics
Listening	Communicates your interest in the patient
Open-ended comments	Helps patients to decide what is relevant and encourages them to continue discussion
Reducing distance	Communicates your involvement to the patient
Reflecting	Shows the patient the importance of his or her ideas and feelings
Restating	Lets the patient know how you interpreted the message that he or she communicated
Seeking clarification	Demonstrates your desire to understand what the patient is communicating
Silence	Communicates your acceptance of patient

and **focusing** acknowledge the patient's participation in the relationship (Table 6–2).

True communication can exist only when there is understanding among all parties. The communicator must be aware of possible language barriers. The worried patient may be a "nonlistener" because he or she has a high level of anxiety. When giving instructions to a patient, it may be necessary to ask him or her to repeat what you have said, that is, to verify understanding of the message. At other times, it may be wise to repeat or clarify to the patient what he or she has said or to restate the message if you think that the patient has failed to state clearly the intended thought or problem. Patience and courtesy are extremely important.

FIGURE 6–2. Reduce the distance. Eye contact gives the nonverbal message "I want to hear what you are saying."

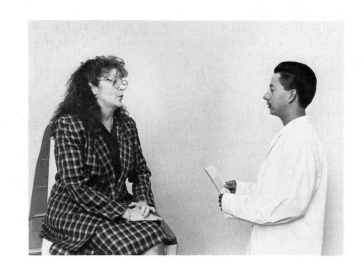

COMMUNICATION WITH YOUR COWORKERS

Medical assistants are hired because they have the specific skills and knowledge needed to get a job done. They are not hired because they have interests, personalities, or backgrounds that are in common with those of others in a medical practice. Establishing a good working team is not always an easy task. No two people are alike. Your coworkers may perceive things very differently than you do. Their habits, values, traits, and personalities may be different, and they may conflict with yours.

Patients are usually quite sensitive to the degree of harmony that exists in the medical facility, and it is important to their well-being that they be treated in a harmonious atmosphere. If personality problems exist among staff members, these problems should be openly discussed so that they can be resolved. If there are several staff members in your office, care must be taken to avoid constantly criticizing others and participating in office gossip.

Cooperation

Cooperation is the ability to work with others effectively. It requires your extending yourself to be helpful to others. You learn cooperation not by thinking of your immediate comfort but rather of the ultimate welfare of your medical facility and of your patients. Cooperation is actually an expression of self-interest and unselfishness. It demands that you adjust your immediate pleasure to benefit the interests of others.

As a medical assistant, you will be expected to cooperate often and in many ways. You will need to keep your work place and belongings neat and orderly, assume additional duties and responsibilities without complaint, work overtime when there is a need, and offer your services even when you are not obligated to do so. Refrain from expressing statements that are contrary to office policies. For example, if you are asked to help another employee, you would not respond with "That's not my job." Share ideas and listen when others are trying to help you. Work harmoniously with others to advance the interests of the medical facility.

Dependability

Teamwork is based on the ability of one worker to depend on another. Every person on the team is important and must complete his or her share of the workload if the team is to succeed. As you think of yourself as a team member, keep in mind that there are some rules that you need to be very aware of:

- Never take advantage of coworkers.
- Think before you speak.
- Never let your emotions take control over you.
- Don't make hasty judgments about others.

Politeness

Little phrases like "please," "thank you," "good morning," and "good night" are very powerful in the work environment. Comments of politeness let others know that you care about them and appreciate them. A simple "good morning" may minimize the impact of an unpleasant event that occurred earlier in the day and contribute to a cooperative working atmosphere.

Patience

Not everyone catches on to new ideas and routines at the same rate. It is important for you to remain calm when helping a coworker perform a new routine. Be patient when you are asked questions. A negative attitude may quickly lead to conflict and a negative work environment. Remember that someone took the time to teach you, so when the time comes for you to be the teacher, you should do the very best job you can.

Some people find contentment in gossiping, backstabbing, and petty quibbling. Such behavior is not only negative for those around you but is ultimately self-destructive for the initiator. Understand that working in an office is among the most stressful occupations. It offers the potential for the development of an environment that facilitates dehumanization and frustration. Remember that humor is one of the greatest relievers of stress. You might use it to resolve problems with a coworker or to relieve pent-up tension in your medical facility.

GETTING ALONG WITH YOUR SUPERVISOR/EMPLOYER-PHYSICIAN

Everyone has the same needs. Your *supervisor,* who may appear to you to be extremely successful, may feel completely unappreciated. It has been said that "the higher you climb on the ladder of success, the more lonely you may become." Like the rest of us, supervisors have personality quirks, strengths and weaknesses, good days and bad days, and hopes and fears. It is important that you learn to respond to your supervisor as a real person. You will find that you will get along better with your supervisor if you remain positive and accept and respect him or her as a unique human being.

Establishing A Working Relationship

As an individual, your supervisor has a definite style of managing people. By becoming acquainted with the various styles of management, you will be able to develop a good working relationship with him or her. The three basic styles of management are autocratic, democratic, and **laissez faire.** Each style has its own set of rules and characteristics.

THE AUTOCRATIC SUPERVISOR. An autocratic supervisor is a leader. This person dictates procedure, policy, and tasks. This individual tells you how to do a task and when to do it. An autocratic person may feel uncomfortable in delegating authority. He or she seldom accepts employees who have traits such as initiative, creativity, and assertiveness. When working for such a supervisor, be sure you follow directions and adhere strictly to the rules of the facility.

THE DEMOCRATIC SUPERVISOR. The democratic supervisor encourages participation in the management process. This individual exercises only a moderate degree of control over employees and seeks input from them. This person is sometimes referred to as a "born teacher": he or she always seems to have the time to explain policies and procedures to employees. If this is the type of supervisor you have, you are encouraged to see yourself as part of the management team; your ideas are requested and considered. In the office with a democratic supervisor, committees of staff members often make decisions and develop policy.

THE LAISSEZ FAIRE SUPERVISOR. The supervisor who follows the laissez faire management style exercises little or no control over his or her employees. This person provides only general guidance and allows the staff to work independently. In the facility with such a supervisor, initiative and creativity are encouraged. You have the freedom to complete your work using your best judgment and creative talents and relying on your past experiences. If you are assertive and creative and possess a degree of self-confidence, you will work well under this type of supervisor.

Remember your supervisor's style of management will not change. As the employee, you will have to learn to adapt to the style. When you discover which style of management best suits you, you should direct your efforts toward securing employment in a health care facility where the management style suits your style.

The Physician

Because of contrasts in educational levels and training, the medical assistant is often placed in a position that is subordinate to the physician's. Your physician may have a poor "bedside manner," not only in his or her interactions with patients but also with other staff members. You can offset educa-tional differences by using your human relations skills to improve interactions with the physician. Be patient. It may take time, but even the gruffest of doctors eventually responds to humanistic efforts. A compliment, some light-hearted humor, or reassurance can soften the heart of one who must continually withstand the emotional consequences of facing the eventual death of a terminally ill patient, attending to life-threatening emergencies, and dealing daily with the medical complaints of a full caseload of patients. Understandably, such a routine can harden even the most dedicated physician. Be sure not to let a doctor's complaints and frustrations affect you personally. Use your personal energy to break through barriers and to get in touch with the vulnerable human being inside the physician's coat.

RECOGNIZING DISCRIMINATION

Discrimination is a word used to describe unfair treatment of a particular person because of his or her race, sex, religious affiliation, or handicap. Discrimination is a behavior that is often based on an attitude. Such an attitude might be the belief that people of a particular race tend to be lazy. If you refuse to work with a person of a certain race or refuse to care for a person with a certain handicap, you are guilty of discrimination.

Prejudice and Stereotyping

Two other terms associated with discrimination are *prejudice* and *stereotyping.* To show prejudice is to prejudge. An opinion is based on prejudice if it has been formed without taking the time or trouble to judge in a fair manner. Prejudice results in the unfair treatment of others. If you have decided that people belonging to a particular minority race are stupid, incompetent, and lazy, you will likely prejudge all people you meet who belong to that race.

Whenever you judge others not as unique individuals but rather based on widely held beliefs about various groups, you are guilty of stereotyping. If you stereotype an individual, you "pigeonhole," or categorize, him or her. You attribute to that person characteristics that may be untrue, unfair, and undeserved.

The first step in coping with discrimination in the medical facility is to become aware of it. When prejudice becomes a part of your personality or when you learn to accept unfair treatment based on prejudice, you begin to experience a form of personal decay. Work becomes less satisfying, and conflict becomes a part of each day. You must learn to recognize and refuse to accept discrimination in the workplace. You must be sensitive to what is going on around you and must recognize your personal prejudices in order to change them. Prejudice and stereotyping are very difficult to overcome.

Civil Rights Act

The Civil Rights Act became law in 1964 and was amended in 1972. The amendment to the Act states that employers are not allowed to discriminate in any area of employment. These areas include race, color, national origin, religion, sex, family status, handicaps, and age. The agency responsible for enforcement of the amendment (Title VII) is the Equal Employment Opportunity Commission (EEOC).

Affirmative action is designed to correct the effect of past discrimination against minorities and women. Affirmative action programs must be implemented by organizations that receive federal funds or contract with the federal government and all its agencies, the public, and employers.

Subtle Discrimination

Discrimination that is not entirely defined by law may be just as harmful as the discrimination that is defined. This type of discrimination is often referred to as *subtle discrimination*. Subtle discrimination is not obvious and seldom expressed openly. It includes discrimination based on a person's appearance, values, or lifestyle or on some other personal factor.

Much of the discrimination that occurs in medical facilities falls into this category. Examples include discrimination against overweight people, divorced people, gay people, people receiving state assistance, and people with sexually transmitted diseases. Often, you may not even be aware that your words or actions reflect subtle discrimination against another.

For example, a heavyset medical assistant may not be hired by a particular facility because it might be believed that such a person will have a negative impact on the facility's "image." The facility may not have an image policy, but through tradition it has perhaps unknowingly favored slim and athletic-looking applicants.

When you are aware that discrimination and prejudice are present in the facility in which you work, there are several decisions that you can make. Keep in mind that prejudice and discrimination are destructive and can often be offset by developing tolerance and understanding for other individuals (Fig. 6–3). Tolerant people are those who are sure of themselves and are able to separate the important from the unimportant. A willingness to try to accept and understand others as they are goes a long way in helping you preserve a good rapport with patients and staff.

Confrontation or Walking Away

You may find yourself in situations in which you consider the costs of confrontation to be too high. For example, in the office where you work, you may be witness to discrimination that you cannot tolerate. You may feel that the least painful solution to free yourself from a situation is to walk away from the pressure, resign your position, or ask for a transfer. If you walk away, the discrimination or prejudice will not be brought to light, and the unfair practices will continue. Keep your own rights in mind and make the decision that is right for you.

Resistance with Patience

You usually can overcome prejudice with time and patience. Demonstrate through your own actions that you do not tolerate prejudice. Do your best to express to each patient your consideration and **empathy.** By clearly recognizing and confronting problems, you let your coworkers know that you are aware that the problems exist and that you are uncomfortable with them. Very often, maintaining such an attitude can help to correct a situation that has gone wrong.

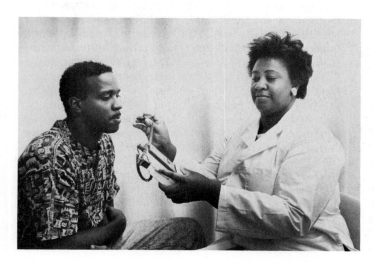

FIGURE 6–3. Do you sense any subtle discrimination in this picture?

CULTURAL INFLUENCES

Culture is the sum of traditions, practices, beliefs, and values developed by a group of people and passed on, most often through families, from generation to generation. Cultural factors determine which signs of behavior are perceived as normal or abnormal. Culture influences the behavior of the patient in illness and how he or she seeks health care.

Medical assistants should take an interest in the cultural subgroups that live in the area in which they are employed. Understanding how cultural influences work aids the health care team to care for each patient. The following are examples of cultural practices that can impact on a patient's care:

- The husband speaks for his wife. The wife does not speak to the physician.
- The hand motion signaling one to come or follow that is performed with the back of the hand facing the patient is used only when calling an animal.
- Direct eye contact shows no respect.
- Clothing is not removed without the presence of another female family member.
- Emotional crying and sobbing denote femininity.
- Going to the doctor is a sign of weakness.
- The female medical assistant never touches the male patient.
- Acquaintances are permitted to stand no less than 3 feet from the patient; only immediate family members are permitted to stand closer.

These are only a few examples. If you work in a practice that predominately serves a distinct ethnic group, discuss possible cultural differences with the physician and with influential people within the cultural group. Learning to understand cultural differences helps you to gain the confidence and respect of patients.

SEXUAL HARASSMENT

Sexual harassment in the workplace is defined as the conduct of one worker (employee or employer) that focuses on a coworker's sexual role at the expense of that individual's role as a worker. Sexual harassment may consist of objectionable looks or remarks or may go as far as physical assault. It can occur at any level of the hierarchy within the workplace.

The consequences of such abuse can result in a great deal of personal distress for the object of the harassment. A person may feel obligated to quit a job because of the harassment that he or she experiences, or he or she may even be fired for resisting another's advances.

The equal opportunity laws and civil rights agencies provide help for those who feel they are being sexually harassed. If you feel you are being harassed on the job, remember that you have the right to be free from such pressure and abuse. Inform the coworker that his or her behavior is unacceptable. Some forms of harassment (such as physical assault) are crimes. Do not hesitate to go to your local police department, EEOC office, or your local human rights agencies if you are a victim of such a crime.

PATIENT EDUCATION

As a member of the health care team, the medical assistant has the opportunity to perform a vital service for all the patients who enter the medical facility. Educating patients is well worth the time and effort and reflects favorably on the medical practice. As a health educator, the medical assistant can provide the patient with valuable information about medical care facilities and providers of medical services that he or she may need, such as information on laboratories, therapeutic facilities, and hospitals.

Patients experience anxiety when they do not understand why a procedure is necessary or how it will be accomplished. You can work with other members of the team to create an atmosphere that fosters patient confidence and trust. You should volunteer information regarding appointment schedules, billing, insurance services, telephone hours, office hours, and emergency coverage.

If patients feel uneasy about asking the physician questions, let them know that you are available to transmit their questions to the physician. You might suggest that they prepare a list of their questions before their appointments and that they give this list to the physician when they come to the office. By acting as the patient's advocate, the medical assistant helps to establish a positive rapport between the patient and the physician.

Medical information and new treatment methods are favorite topics for coverage by the news media. Patients often ask questions about medical news that they have heard. The medical assistant can help by alerting the physician to the patient's concerns or by encouraging the patient to speak to the physician directly. Information about fees for services, office policy, and Medicare should be readily available to patients.

The medical assistant is the representative of the physician and the facility to the general public. In this role, you can expect to have contact with outside physicians, staff members, salespersons, supply company representatives, and service representatives. Courtesy, patience, and effective communication skills help to promote a positive public image of the facility for which you work. Your mastery of these skills is an asset and enhances your value to your employer.

▶ ## LEARNING ACHIEVEMENTS

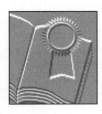

Upon completion of this chapter, can you in the time allowed by your evaluator:

1. Analyze a personal behavior skill that you want to improve?
2. Describe the importance of coworker cooperation?
3. Effectively restate, reflect, and focus on statements made by a patient during a patient interview?

REFERENCES AND READINGS

Eagan, G.: *The Skilled Helper,* 2nd ed., Belmont, California, Wadsworth Health Sciences, 1982.

Griffith, H. W.: *Instructions for Patients,* 4th ed., Philadelphia, W. B. Saunders Co., 1989.

King, M., Novik, L., and Citrenbaum, C.: *Irresistible Communication: Creative Skills for the Health Professional,* Philadelphia, W. B. Saunders Co., 1983.

Sundeen, S., Stuart, G., DeSalvo Rankin, E. A., and Cohen, S. A.: *Nurse–Client Interaction,* 4th ed., St. Louis, C. V. Mosby Co., 1989.

Wallace, H., and Masters, L.: *Personality Development for Work,* 6th ed., Cincinnati, South-Western Publishing Co., 1989.

CHAPTER SEVEN

——

EXTERNSHIP AND FINDING THE RIGHT POSITION

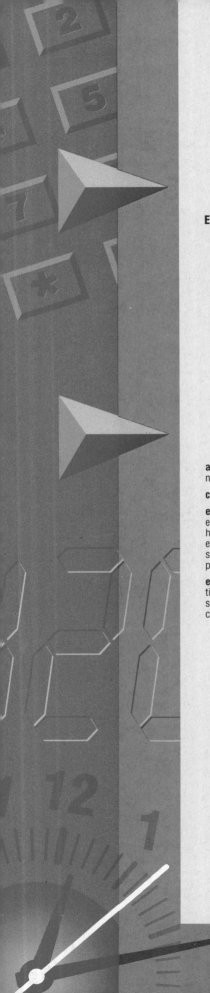

CHAPTER OUTLINE

VOCABULARY

avocational Pertaining to a subordinate occupation or a hobby.

chronologic In the order of time.

externship The practice of receiving employment experience in qualified health care facilities under the cooperative supervision of the medical staff and the program instructor as part of the educational curriculum.

extracurricular Relating to those activities that form part of the life of students but are not part of the courses of study.

format Shape, size, and general makeup of a publication, such as a resumé.

objective Something toward which effort is directed; an aim or end of action.

personal inventory A *complete* summary of pertinent information about oneself.

re-entry student One who has been away from formal education or employment for several years and who is now preparing to re-enter the workplace.

resumé A *selective* summary of one's education and employment record tailored to the position being sought.

seminar A group of students meeting regularly and informally with a professor to discuss ideas and problems.

EXTERNSHIP AND FINDING THE RIGHT POSITION

LEARNING OBJECTIVES

COGNITIVE

Upon successful completion of this chapter, you should be able to:

1. Define the terms listed in the Vocabulary.

2. Explain the essentials of an externship.

3. Briefly explain four responsibilities of the student during externship.

4. Describe the responsibilities of an externship office or agency.

5. Explain how a student will benefit from the externship experience.

6. List the three steps in applying for a position.

7. Identify the five essential parts of a personal inventory.

8. List seven basic items that should be included in every resumé.

9. Specify five items that must not be inserted in a resumé.

10. Cite five sources of leads for employment as a medical assistant.

11. List three avenues of evaluation that an interviewer may use in selecting an employee.

PERFORMANCE

Upon successful completion of this chapter, you should be able to perform the following activities:

1. Prepare a personal inventory.

2. Prepare two examples of a resumé.

3. Demonstrate a telephone request for an interview.

4. Write a letter in response to a newspaper help-wanted ad.

5. Compose a follow-up letter of thanks following an interview for a position.

EXTERNSHIP

As you progress in your training, you will be giving thought as to just how and where you will fit into the health care arena, and you will undoubtedly have acquired certain preferences.

One aid in defining and focusing your interests is an **externship** program that provides practical experience in a variety of qualified physicians' offices, accredited hospitals, or other health care facilities. Externship experience is included by most schools and colleges that have a complete curriculum for medical assistants. In those programs accredited by the Committee on Allied Health Education and Accreditation (CAHEA) in collaboration with AMA and AAMA, an externship is mandatory. A minimum of 160 hours is recommended.

What is Externship?

The externship phase of your training may also be known as *work experience* or *on-the-job training*

(Fig. 7–1). The physicians and health care facilities are serving as an extension of the college when they accept students for externship. You may be expected to carry malpractice insurance during the externship. You will probably be required to undergo a physical examination, chest x-ray, and appropriate serologic tests.

During the very important weeks of your externship, you will have an opportunity to apply your administrative and clinical skills under the supervision of a practicing medical assistant. Your supervisor and the physician(s) at the externship site will be evaluating your personal qualities as well as the skills you have learned in the classroom. These will include your:

- grooming
- poise
- integrity
- punctuality
- initiative
- relations with coworkers and patients
- reaction to criticism and direction

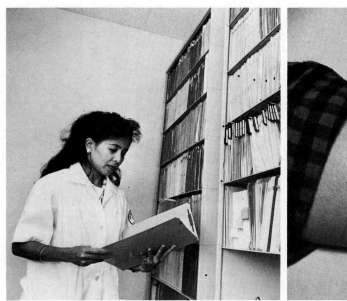
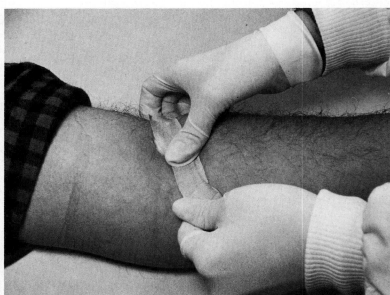

FIGURE 7–1. The medical assisting externship will include both administrative and clinical duties.

- respect for ethical standards
- consideration for others

They will be responsible for an ongoing evaluation of your performance, as directed by your instructor, and this evaluation will become a part of your student records.

Duration and Time of Externship

The duration of the externship and the time at which it is introduced into the program vary, depending on the school or college. Some schools have the student spend a day or two in a health facility near the beginning of the training to provide a frame of reference for later instruction. Some programs combine work experience with classroom instruction throughout the training period. The majority of schools prefer a concentrated period of externship near the conclusion of the classroom instruction.

Student Responsibilities

During your externship, both your appearance and actions must be professional. You will report to work at a specified time on specified days, just as if you were a regular employee, but you will not be paid by the training facility. You may spend all your externship in one facility, but it is usually preferable to rotate among several types of practice for a well-rounded experience. Do not be surprised if you are expected to apply and be interviewed for the position just as you will later on when you are seeking employment. This is valuable experience and should be welcomed.

You, as a student, should recognize that a health care agency that cooperates with your education is accepting a great responsibility. You will require continual supervision, and your questions must be answered. You must be aware of ethical and legal concerns and of the potential for a claim of medical malpractice. One large concern is that of patient privacy. You must reveal no information concerning a patient or the practice to persons outside the facility. Some agencies may ask you to sign an oath of privacy while in that facility.

Externship Sites

The school or college will designate a specific individual to be your externship coordinator, who will carefully choose and screen suitable training facilities. The supervising staff at the health care facility must agree to provide ample opportunity for you to practice your skills and to complete an evaluation of your performance. Quite often, the coordinator will seek out offices where former graduates of the program are employed. This ensures greater understanding and cooperation as well as the assurance

that work habits and procedures meet the standards promoted in the classroom. In rare instances, a student may feel that the training facility is taking advantage of a situation and simply using the student to perform menial tasks. If you do have such an experience, it should be reported to your instructor.

The value of the externship is enhanced when the training program includes a weekly **seminar** at which all the students serving externship and their instructor may share experiences, problems, and solutions.

Benefits from Externship

All three parties to the agreement—the school, the externship office or facility, and the trainee—benefit from the experience.

The school has a line of communication to the community and is better able to assess the needs and requirements of the public for which it is training prospective employees.

The externship agency benefits from the new ideas and methods that the trainee may introduce. If the facility is looking for additional help, this is an ideal way to evaluate the performance of a trainee without involvement in the hiring process.

You, the trainee, benefit most of all by exposure to practical experience in a variety of settings. This practical experience in the "real world" removes a great deal of the anxiety that you might otherwise have in a first employment situation. If you perform well during the externship you may be offered a permanent job with the facility where you trained, but you should not assume that this will happen. The externship facility may also be used as a reference when you are seeking a permanent position. When you know that you have performed well and have a comfortable relationship with the supervisory staff in the training facility, you may ask for a reference to be used later on when interviewing for employment.

FINDING THE RIGHT POSITION

After you have completed your classroom training and externship, the next step will be to find the right position. Your aptitudes and skills must be matched with the requirements of a physician or facility in need of an employee. Whether you are seeking your first position or are returning to the field after an absence of several years, or even if you are an experienced medical assistant preparing to change employers, the steps in applying for a position are essentially the same:

1. Preparing for the interview
2. Locating prospective employers
3. Interviewing

Looking for work is a job in itself. Establish a schedule and stick to it.

Preliminary Steps

Before seeking an interview, ask yourself some pertinent questions:

- What type of work do I really want?
- Where can I function best?
- Do I prefer clinical or administrative duty?
- What are my skills?
- Do I prefer to work in a small practice or in a large medical group?
- Would I enjoy the variety of a general practice or the concentration of a specialty practice?
- How important to me are salary, hours, and location?

In your externship experience, you may have formed some rather definite preferences, or you may feel absolutely certain of some things that would cause you to be dissatisfied.

Preparation for the Interview
Personal Inventory

It sometimes happens that your first position is so ideally suitable that you will accept and stay in it for the remainder of your working years. More likely, though, you will have to make several changes of employment during your lifetime.

A **personal inventory,** to which you will add as you gain additional experience and education, will prove invaluable to you later as well as now. The personal inventory is for your own information and reference. It will be a ready source of information in preparing and updating your **resumé.** The personal inventory is complete information about yourself; a resumé is selected information tailored to the position you are seeking.

1. Start with a page for biographic data: your name, birth date, Social Security number, address, and telephone number.

BIOGRAPHIC DATA
Name _____ Birth Date _____
Soc. Sec. No. _____
Address _____
Tel. No. _____

2. Prepare a separate page for your employment history. This is especially important for the **re-entry student.** Not all students enter vocational training directly out of high school or early in their employment careers. Many have spent intervening years as full-time homemakers or in other employment. The experience gained during these years

should be included in your personal inventory. It could be important in future situations. If you have never been employed but have done volunteer work requiring personal responsibility, list that here. The employment history should include dates of employment, name of employer, type of business, your position title, and major duties. Because this will be a continuing record that you will add to as you gain experience, it is prepared in **chronologic** order, starting with the first major job you held. When you use this information in a resumé, however, it will be listed in reverse chronologic order, beginning with the latest position.

EMPLOYMENT HISTORY
June ___ 19xx ___ to ___ June ___ 19xx Employer <u>Looking Good</u>
Month Year   Month Year
Type of Business ___ Women's clothing
Position Held ___ Part-time sales clerk
Major Duties: Assisting customers in their selections, registering sales, closing out register at end of day
Satisfactions: Enjoyed personal contacts / Learned to accept responsibility
Dissatisfactions: Not related to my goals

3. Next, record your educational data, beginning with high school. List the dates, the institution attended, and the year of graduation, plus the diploma or degree earned. Make note of the areas of study you enjoyed most and list special competencies, awards, or honors. As time goes by, it may be difficult to recall these details, and you never know what will be important to an employer in the future. Remember, you are starting a permanent record for your own information and as a handy reference tool when needed. As with the employment history, the educational data is listed here in chronologic order but will appear in reverse chronologic order in a resumé, starting with the highest degree or certificate.

EDUCATIONAL DATA		
Dates	Institution Attended	Year Graduated/Degree
19xx–19xx	Valley High School Ola Vista	19xx Diploma
19xx–19xx	Ola Vista Community College	19xx Associate in Science, Medical Assisting
Special Competencies:		
Typing Certificate (70 WPM)		
Limited X-ray permit, 19xx		
CPR Certificate, 19xx, renewed annually		
Fluency in Spanish		
Awards:		
Dean's List, all four semesters in college		

4. You may wish to include a page for your extracurricular interests and activities. List organization memberships and activities and any positions of leadership you held. Your volunteer activities might be included here if they are not in your employment record. Also include any significant hobbies.

EXTRACURRICULAR INTERESTS AND ACTIVITIES

Organization Memberships	Year	Personal Participation
Associated Women Students	19xx	Secretary 19xx–19xx
American Association of Medical Assistants	19xx	Student member Page, 19xx convention
Girl Scouts of the U.S.A.	19xx	Brownie group leader, 19xx

Hobbies
Oil painting, backpacking

5. Finally, have a page for your personal goals. What are your immediate goals? your long-term goals? What concessions are you willing to make in order to reach your goals?

PERSONAL GOALS

Date	Immediate Goals	Long-Term Goals
19xx	Medical assistant position, preferably in pediatric practice	Bachelor of Science in Business Administration Administrative position in large group practice or HMO

Resumé

The final and most important step in preparing for an interview is producing a resumé that will arouse the interest of a prospective employer.

If you do not feel confident in doing this yourself, get help. If you are a student in a 2-year college, there is probably a career center on campus where you can ask for assistance. There are also many guidebooks in the public library and in bookstores where you can find ideas galore. See the references at the end of this chapter.

PURPOSE OF THE RESUMÉ. The purpose of the resumé is to get an interview, not to get a job. Keep this in mind as you decide what to include. Using your personal inventory, select the information that applies to the position you have in mind. Choose an attractive format, and type the information on one sheet of paper with absolutely no errors or misspelled words (Figs. 7–2 and 7–3). Tinted paper will make the resumé more distinctive, but avoid using bright colors or arty headings. The resumé gives you an opportunity to display the qualifications that enhance your appeal to prospective employers. Omit anything that cannot help you or anything that would detract from your image. Once you are in the interview, you can clarify any item not entirely explained on the resumé.

WRITING THE RESUMÉ. There is no standard **format** for a resumé, but it should be typewritten on 8½″ × 11″ good-quality paper. It should be concise and honest and have a professional look.

Heading. At the top of your paper, place the necessary personal information: name, address, and telephone number. Display this prominently so that it stands apart and can be easily identified (it may be centered).

Objective. The modern trend is to omit reference to an **objective,** particularly if your qualifications are vocationally specific. If you do include an objective, avoid such words as "challenge" or "opportunity," as this focuses on what the applicant wants instead of showing understanding of what the employer wants and needs.

Education and Experience. If you are a recent graduate with little or no experience, list your education first and then your employment, if any. College graduates need not include high school backgrounds. If you have a good history of recent employment, make this the first item, followed by education. In both cases, start with your most recent position and list the rest in reverse chronologic order.

Professional Licenses. Include any professional licenses or certificates and list memberships in professional organizations.

Extracurricular Activities. List any **extracurricular** or **avocational** interests that would be applicable to the position sought.

References. State on your resumé that references will be furnished upon request. (Do not list names and addresses of references on the resumé.) Be prepared to furnish the names of at least three references at the time of your interview. These should have been typewritten on a separate page in the same style as your resumé. Don't forget to obtain permission from the persons you are listing before you provide their names.

Items to Exclude:

your photograph

names of spouse and/or children

reasons for terminating previous position

past salaries or present salary requirements

names and addresses of references

THERESA O'SULLIVAN, CMA

233 West Wentworth Street   San Diego, CA 92184   (619) 239-2345

EDUCATION

Associate in Science, Ola Vista Community College
June 1994   (Dean's List, four semesters)
Diploma, Valley High School, June 1992

CERTIFICATES

CPR certificate (renewed annually since 1992)
Certificate in Medical Assisting, Ola Vista Community College, 1993
Certified Medical Assistant, 1994, Certificate #0000

**SPECIAL
COMPETENCIES**

Speak Spanish fluently
Hold Limited X-ray Permit

EMPLOYMENT

Part-time Medical Assistant, June 1993 to June 1994
Duties included: preparing patients for examination in general practice office;
taking height, weight, and vital signs; answering the telephone and reception; and
appointment scheduling, four afternoons per week.

Part-time Salesperson, Baxters Department Store, June 1991 to June 1993
Duties included: assisting customers in making their selections; registering sales;
and closing out register at end of day.

**AVOCATIONAL
INTERESTS**

Student Member, American Association of Medical Assistants
Secretary, Associated Women Students OVCC

REFERENCES

Furnished upon request.

FIGURE 7–2. Sample chronologic resumé.

THERESA O'SULLIVAN, CMA

233 West Wentworth Street   San Diego, CA 92184   (619) 239-2345

STATEMENT OF EMPLOYMENT ASSETS
FOR A CAREER IN MEDICAL ASSISTING

GENERAL

Take pride in appearance
Display professionalism
Recognize and respond to verbal and nonverbal communication
Apply legal and ethical concepts of medical practice
Work as a team member
Speak Spanish fluently

ADMINISTRATIVE

Appointment scheduling, filing, pegboard and electronic billing systems, account collections, insurance billing, coding, recordkeeping, bank deposits and statement reconciliation, patient histories, medical terminology, machine transcription, word processing

CLINICAL

Understanding of anatomy and physiology, symptoms and diseases, collecting and handling laboratory specimens, procedures for assisting with physical examination, emergency first aid and CPR, injections, sterile techniques, ECG, inventory and supplies

REFERENCES

Furnished upon request.

FIGURE 7–3. Sample skills resumé.

PROCEDURE 7-1 PREPARING A RESUMÉ

GOAL To prepare a resumé of education and experience that will be informative to a prospective employer and create interest in arranging an interview for employment.

EQUIPMENT AND SUPPLIES

Summary of personal data
Quality stationery
Typewriter or computer

PROCEDURAL STEPS

1. Assemble all personal data necessary for resumé.

2. Arrange in reverse chronologic order.
   Purpose: To enable you to proceed in orderly fashion in preparing the resumé and to check accuracy of dates.

3. Typewrite heading that includes your name, address, and telephone number.
   Purpose: For easy identification by reader.

4. List highest education degree or diploma, including name of institution and year. Include high school if you are not a college graduate.
   Purpose: Training may be important to your employability.

5. List all work experience in reverse chronologic order.
   Purpose: To demonstrate transferable experiences toward future employment.

6. Include any professional licenses, certificates, and memberships in professional organizations.
   Purpose: Indicates employability and personal interest in profession.

7. List any extracurricular or avocational interests applicable to the position sought.

8. State that references will be furnished upon request.
   Purpose: Prospective employers may wish to verify your experience and character.
   Note: Obtain permission prior to listing anyone as a reference.

9. Review resumé for accuracy, completeness, and attractive format.

Locating Prospective Employers

If you are a student in an accredited school, your instructor or the school may be able to give you names of prospective employers. Other good sources for leads are the local medical society, other medical assistants, branches of the United States Employment Service, and state-operated employment offices. You may also wish to check the classified advertisements in your local newspaper (Fig. 7–4) or place your name with an employment agency. Private employment agencies generally charge a fee equivalent to 2 to 4 weeks' salary to successful applicants. This fee is sometimes paid by the employer after a probationary period.

The Interview

Requesting an Interview

If you are responding to an advertisement that lists a telephone number, *telephoning to request an interview* is preferable to writing a letter, but an unsolicited telephone call may be disruptive and destroy the opportunity for an interview. If no telephone number is included in the advertisement,

PROCEDURE 7-2   ANSWERING A HELP-WANTED ADVERTISEMENT

GOAL To write a letter in response to a newspaper advertisement that will relay your qualifications and generate interest in arranging an interview.

EQUIPMENT AND SUPPLIES

Recent newspaper with classified employment ads
Stationery
Typewriter or computer
Pen

PROCEDURAL STEPS

1. Review letter writing information in Chapter 12, Correspondence and Mail Processing.

2. Draft a letter to include:
   - Name of newspaper, date of publication, and title of position for which you are applying.
   Purpose: Employer may be running more than one advertisement.
   - Information about where you can be contacted.
   Purpose: To enable interested employer to reach you.

3. Express enthusiastic interest in the position offered, and state your qualifications.

4. Request a response to your letter by telephone or letter.
   Purpose: So that an interview can be arranged if position is still open and employer is interested in your qualifications.

5. End the letter with an expression of thanks for considering your request.
   Purpose: To demonstrate your knowledge of courtesy.

6. Review the letter for content and accuracy.
   Purpose: To make certain that you have included all essential information and that the letter is free of errors.

---

there will be an address listed (usually a box number) to which you may direct a letter requesting an interview.

LETTER IN RESPONSE TO ADVERTISEMENT. A *cover letter responding to an advertisement* should include:

- A reference to the advertisement, including name of newspaper, date of publication, and position title. The employer may be running more than one recruitment ad.
- An enthusiastic expression of interest in the position.
- A comparison of your own qualifications with those of the position to be filled.
- Information about where you can be contacted.
- A request for a response or interview.
- Thanks for considering your request.

UNSOLICITED INTERVIEW REQUEST. You may decide to canvas a number of medical facilities to determine whether there are openings for a medical assistant. Write a letter such as the one shown in Figure 7–5 and enclose your resume. Then follow up with a telephone call in about 1 week.

Day of the Interview

Your appearance is extremely important. Clothing should be conservative, neat, and well-pressed. Women should wear a dress or suit with a skirt. Slacks or pantsuits and open sandals are considered inappropriate for job interviews. Men should wear a suit and tie and appropriate dress shoes. The man or woman who is still actively in a student program

MEDICAL COMPUTER BILLING & INSURANCE
Mature, some bkkppg a must. Recent checkable refs. Xlnt benefits pkg. New Beverly Hills Ortho office.   310-000-0000

● **MEDICAL TRANSCRIBER** ●
Exp'd only for multi-specialty grp. to work in Beverly Hills or Sherman Oaks offic. F/T. Good sal/bnfts. Carla, 818/000-0000

MEDICAL Exper person for medical office, front or back. Brentwood 310/000-0000

Medical-PHLEBOTOMISTS NHL has many P/T opptys. See ad 3/15. 5601 Oberlin Dr,SD 92121

MEDICAL. Team Coordinator. See Sunday ad. Home Health Plus. 1-800-000-0000W.Cov.

MEDICAL ASSISTANT Full time. Experienced, for busy Bev.Hls. Derm. office.   310/000-0000

Medical Records Coder
See Sun 4/26 ad.
St. John's Hospital

FIGURE 7–4. Help wanted advertisements.

may wish to go to the interview in a fresh, clean uniform bearing the school insignia (Fig. 7–6).

Hair should be well-groomed and worn in a professional-looking style. Keep jewelry to a minimum and avoid heavy scents of perfume or antiperspirants. Women should be careful and conservative in applying makeup and should carry a modest purse that is not bulging with unnecessary items.

Take a critical look at yourself in the mirror before leaving home and again just before entering the prospective employer's office (see Interviewing Tips).

INTERVIEWING TIPS

● Arrive promptly for the interview. Under no circumstances should you be even so much as a minute late and then have to make a weak excuse.

● Go alone. You may want moral support, but you will be more relaxed if there is no one waiting for you.

● Enter the office confidently and without appearing rushed.

● Introduce yourself to the receptionist, then express appreciation when you are asked to be seated.

● If you must wait, try to relax, but avoid slouching in your chair.

● *Do not* smoke or chew gum.

When you prepared your resumé, you listed your job skills, your education, or both. The interviewer already knows how well you ought to be able to do the job. However, you will be judged in at least two other areas of evaluation:

● *What kind of coworker you will be.* Work in a health care facility requires team effort, and your ability to work in cooperation and coordination with others bears heavily on how well you will do your job, apart from how good your specific job skills may be.

● *What kind of employee you will be.* Dependability, trustworthiness, dedication, loyalty, and other personal characteristics are always important to an employer.

Employment Application

Completing an employment application is not standard procedure in smaller medical practices, but you should be prepared for this if asked (See Chapter 22, Management Responsibilities). Larger health agencies such as hospitals and HMOs will definitely ask you to fill out their application form.

Make notes in advance of your Social Security number, driver's license, and telephone numbers where you can be reached. Your resumé should have the information you will need regarding education and employment. Be prepared to furnish telephone numbers for previous employers if asked, and have available the names, addresses, and telephone numbers of three references who have given you their permission to list them.

The appearance and completeness of your filled-in application will be considered in your overall evaluation. By law, employers cannot require you to answer questions regarding your place of birth, ethnic origin or religious preference, or about your age, marital status, or number of children. If these questions are on the application, you may choose to leave them blank, but all allowable questions should be answered honestly and completely. Print your answers or write as plainly as possible. Having your own favorite pen with you may help.

During the Interview

When you are ushered into the interviewer's room, wait to be seated until you are invited to do so. Let the interviewer lead the conversation. Be prepared to answer such questions as "Tell me about yourself," and "Why do you want to work here?" One reason for an opening such as this is to provide a little time to relax and get acquainted. You might start out by reviewing your professional background and training and then progress to personal interests, hobbies, and so forth.

Remember that the interviewer will be observing your manners, poise, speech, alertness, and ability to give direct answers. A relaxed, friendly manner with good eye contact is important. You must look di-

THERESA O'SULLIVAN, CMA

233 West Wentworth Street   San Diego, CA 92184   (619) 239-2345

June 1, 19xx

Arthur M. Blackburn, M.D.
2200 Broadway
Anytown, US 98765

Dear Dr. Blackburn:

In a few weeks, I will complete my formal training in medical assisting with an Associate in Science Degree from Ola Vista Community College.

The medical assisting program at Ola Vista has included theory and practical application in both administrative and clinical skills. My six weeks supervised externship gave me additional practical experience in two specialty practices.

While studying at Ola Vista, I have also worked part-time for a busy physician in family practice, while maintaining a 3.5 grade point average. My experience as Dr. Madden's employee is outlined on the enclosed resume. I have enjoyed my work in Dr. Madden's office and am now seeking full-time employment.

If you will require a replacement or addition to your staff in the near future, may I be considered as an applicant? I will follow up with a telephone call within a week.

Sincerely yours,

Theresa O'Sullivan, CMA

Enc. Resume

FIGURE 7-5. Sample cover letter.

rectly at the person to whom you are speaking. Your sense of humor may be tested as well, and questions may be directed to you that will test your common sense and frankness. You can promote yourself honestly and graciously by showing that you enjoy others, are willing to work and accept responsibility, and that you have an open mind about the position and are willing to learn.

Recent legislation in fair employment practices has influenced hiring practices nationwide. Employers are restricted in the information that can be required on an application or asked in an interview. But while you may not be required to answer questions regarding your age, birthplace, marital status, and so forth, a prospective employer might appreciate your mentioning any such pertinent information

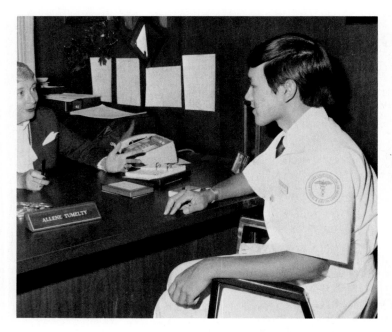

FIGURE 7–6. Student being interviewed for a job. (Courtesy of Southern California College of Medical and Dental Careers, Anaheim, CA. Photo by Don Santucci.)

THERESA O'SULLIVAN, CMA

233 West Wentworth Street   San Diego, CA 92184   (619) 239-2345

June 15, 19xx

Arthur M. Blackburn, M.D.
2200 Broadway
Anytown, US 98765

Dear Dr. Blackburn:

Thank you for taking the time to talk with me today about the medical assistant position in your office and for considering my qualifications for filling that position.

I would be pleased to accept your offer if you should decide that I meet your requirements.

Sincerely yours,

Theresa O'Sullivan, CMA

FIGURE 7–7. Thank-you letter following an interview.

in conversation. Remember your objective—to obtain a position.

At the end of the interview, if the interviewer has not mentioned hours and salary, you may properly inquire at this time. If you are not really interested in the position, do not bother to ask, but if the position sounds satisfactory and is one that you would like to accept, you may then ask if the interviewer wishes to discuss the salary. This should be enough of a lead, since it was probably an oversight on the interviewer's part. If the interviewer seems reluctant to discuss it, though, do not press the issue, as this may be an indication that your qualifications do not fit the position and there is no reason to pursue the interview further.

If you have been given a tour of the office, you may make some pleasant observations and comments, but do not be falsely overenthusiastic. When you are introduced to the staff, be gracious and friendly. Try to remember their names so that you can thank them later. Show enthusiasm, but do not overdo it because it may appear to others that you are "putting on an act."

Closing the Interview

The interviewer will usually take the initiative in closing the interview, perhaps by sliding back the chair and asking whether you have further questions. Do not show disappointment if the position is not offered to you at the time of the interview. There may be other applicants to see or the interviewer may wish to check your references before making a commitment. Express your thanks for the interview as you leave, and remember, too, to thank the receptionist and say a friendly goodbye.

Follow-up Activities

A brief, well-worded letter of thanks sent to the interviewer immediately after the interview could be crucial in deciding whether you will be hired. This is one of the most essential steps in the whole job-seeking process—and the one most overlooked by job-seekers. Simply write a brief note expressing appreciation for the interview and interest in the position (Fig. 7–7).

After a few days, you may call the office and ask if the position has been filled and tell them you are interested because you enjoyed your interview and the office. If the position is still open, ask whether you may inquire again in a few days. Be brief and thank the person with whom you are speaking.

If you do not get the job, ask yourself some pertinent questions:

- Did I look my best?
- Did I show enthusiasm for the job?
- Did I listen carefully during the interview?
- Did I say or do something I should not have?

Even if you are not hired, you should never feel that an interview is a waste of time. You learn from each experience, and with experience you are better able to promote your qualifications in future interviews.

If you are hired, ask the interviewer if you may borrow the policy and procedure manual to review before you report to work. If this is allowed, jot down items that you find important to remember in your own notebook.

On your first day of work, arrive promptly and eager for your new experience. And remember to bring your notebook!

► LEARNING ACHIEVEMENTS

Upon completion of this chapter, are you able to:

1. Define the terms listed in the Vocabulary?
2. Discuss the reasons for and essentials of externship?
3. Describe the responsibilities of the student and of the externship agency?
4. Discuss the benefits you will derive from the externship experience?
5. List the three steps in applying for a position?
6. Explain what a *personal inventory* is and identify its five essential parts?
7. List the seven basic items that should be *included* and five specific items that should be *omitted* from a resumé?
8. Cite several sources of leads for employment as a medical assistant?
9. Prepare a personal inventory and a resumé?
10. Write a letter in answer to a newspaper help-wanted ad and an appropriate letter of thanks following an interview for a position?

REFERENCES AND READINGS

Beatty, R. H.: *The Resume Kit,* New York, John Wiley & Sons, Inc., 1991.

Bolles, R. N.: *The Three Boxes of Life, and How to Get Out of Them,* Berkeley, CA, Ten Speed Press, 1983.

Bolles, R. N.: *What Color Is Your Parachute?* Berkeley, CA, Ten Speed Press, 1991.

Bostwick, B.: *Resume Writing,* New York, John Wiley & Sons, Inc., 1990.

Camden, T. M.: *How to Get a Job in the Boston Area (The Insider's Guide Series),* Chicago, IL, Surrey Books, 1992. (This is one of a series available for large cities in the U.S. and contains excellent information.)

Holtz, H.: *The Winning Resume: How to Sell Yourself,* Glenview, IL, Scott Foresman Professional Books, 1991.

Jackson, T.: *The Perfect Resume,* Garden City, NY, Anchor Press, 1990.

Lewis, A.: *How to Write Better Resumes,* Woodbury, NY, Barron's Educational Series, 1989.

Reed, J. [ed]. *Resumes That Get Jobs,* New York, Arco Publishing, Inc., 1990.

SECTION 2

THE ADMINISTRATIVE MEDICAL ASSISTANT

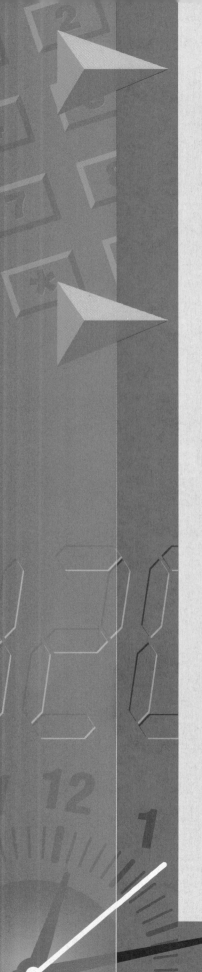

VOCABULARY

batch A collection of similar work that can be processed in one operation.

command An instruction telling the computer to do something with a program.

computer A machine that is designed to accept, store, process, and give out information.

CPU Central Processing Unit; the part of a computer system that processes information.

cursor A symbol appearing on the monitor that shows where the next character to be typed will appear.

daisy wheel A printing element of an electric typewriter or printer that consists of a disk with spokes bearing type.

database A collection of related files that serves as a foundation for retrieving information.

demographics Relating to the statistical characteristics of populations, such as births, marriages, mortality, and health.

directory A logical area on a disk within which programs and data are stored. Each directory functions similarly to a single floppy disk.

disk A flat, circular plate with a magnetic surface that is capable of storing computer programs. Some disks are flexible *(floppy disks)* and some are hard *(hard disks)*.

disk drive A device that loads a program or data stored on a disk into a computer.

dot matrix printer An impact printer that forms characters using patterns of dots.

electronic mail Communications transmitted via computer using a telephone modem.

file An orderly, self-contained collection of data that is stored on a permanent storage device such as a disk.

floppy disk (diskette) A thin disk (diskette) of magnetic material capable of storing a large amount of information. The floppy disk was developed to provide users of small computer systems with an inexpensive and convenient way of storing information.

format To magnetically create tracks on a disk where information will be stored; to initialize.

hard copy The readable paper copy or printout of information.

hardware Computer machinery.

I/O (input/output) *Input* is any information that is entered into and used by the computer; *output* is any information that is processed by the computer and transmitted to a monitor, printer, or other device.

main memory The section of the computer where information and instructions are stored.

microcomputer Desk-top computer, originally designed as a personal computer.

minicomputer Medium-size computer that has a larger storage capacity than a microcomputer and that can accommodate multilocation terminals.

modem An acronym for **MO**dulator **DEM**odulator; a device that enables data to be transmitted over telephone lines.

monitor A device used to display computer-generated information; a video screen; a CRT.

peripheral A device—such as a printer, disk drive, or mouse—that can be attached to a computer for input, output, or storage purposes.

printout The output from a printer; also called *hard copy*.

prompt A symbol used by some computers to indicate when the computer is ready to accept input.

random access memory (RAM) The computer's temporary memory; it stores data and programs that are input.

read-only memory (ROM) Memory that can be altered only by changing the physical structure of the computer chip. ROM chips are usually used to store information that is essential to the operation of the computer.

scanner An input device that converts printed matter into a computer-readable format.

software The programming necessary to direct the hardware of a computer system; computer programs.

stand-alone system Any complete computer system located within an office.

syntax error A computer system response to a mistake in instructions, such as a transposition of characters or an omission of a character or word.

telecommunications The science and technology of communication by transmission of information from one location to another via telephone, television, or telegraph.

tutorial Instruction on paper or disk intended to give practical information about using a specific computer program.

word processing (WP) A system used to process written communications through the use of modern equipment, greater employee specialization, and an increase in the application of standardized procedures.

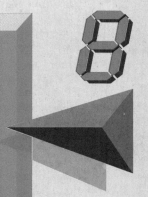

The Computer in Medical Practice

LEARNING OBJECTIVES

COGNITIVE

Upon successful completion of this chapter, you should be able to:

1. Define the terms listed in the Vocabulary.

2. Distinguish among the three types of computer systems.

3. Name three kinds of outside service bureaus.

4. Demonstrate the ability to use the elementary language of computers effectively.

5. Cite at least ten medical office functions that can be performed using a computer.

6. List three advantages of electronic processing of insurance claims.

7. List six ways that a computer can improve the medical assistant's working environment.

8. State the reason for the establishment of security guidelines for computerized data in the medical office.

PERFORMANCE

When given the necessary information and equipment, the student with hands-on computer experience should be able to perform the following activities:

1. Start the computer.

2. Load a program.

3. Format a disk.

4. Make a back-up copy of a document.

5. Generate a patient record.

6. Prepare a billing statement.

7. Complete a patient insurance form.

8. Personalize a computerized form letter.

9. Access, add, correct, and delete information on the computer.

10. Shut down the computer.

Less than 50 years ago, in 1946, the first electronic **computer** (ENIAC) was completed after 2½ years in the making. It weighed 30 tons, required a space of 15,000 square feet, and cost over one million dollars. Since that time, a computer explosion has taken place, brought about at first by the application of the transistor, then integrated circuits, and now silicon chips. A compact personal computer in the home and a desk-top monitor in the office are now commonplace.

The age of the computer has also arrived in the physician's office. For many years, the computer has been used in hospitals and large group practices, but the proliferation of software, the drop in cost of hardware, and the sharp increase in paperwork that must be done in the medical marketplace have brought computerization into private medical practices. The use of a computer in the physician's office is no longer a question of "if" but "when."

The development of computers, their programming, and internal operation is extremely compli-cated. Entire volumes have been written on the minute technical details of the computer. Fortunately, this technical knowledge is not necessary in order to use the computer, just as it is not necessary to be a mechanic in order to drive an automobile or to be an electrician in order to operate a light switch. But a knowledge of the functions that a computer can perform, how it influences our daily lives, and how it is used to perform tasks in the workplace has become a necessary part of the general education of all students. This chapter is intended to deal only with the use of the computer by the medical assistant as a tool in a medical facility.

BASIC COMPUTER LANGUAGE

The physical equipment of the computer is called **hardware. Software** is the programming necessary to direct the hardware of a computer system. **Peripherals** are devices that are connected to the

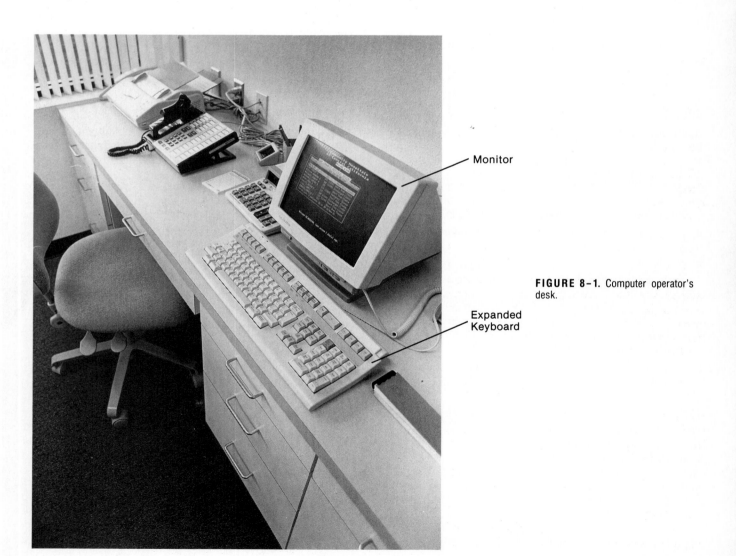

FIGURE 8-1. Computer operator's desk.

Monitor

Expanded Keyboard

computer but that are not part of the computer itself, for example, **disk drives** and printers. **Input** to the computer is accomplished via a keyboard or other input apparatus, such as a mouse or voice-activated input device. The computer keyboard looks very much like an ordinary typewriter keyboard but has a few extra keys; these are called *special function keys.* These are used to perform specific **word processing** or computer-related operations. Used alone, a special function key may create bold print, underline, indent, or call up a "HELP" screen, as well as other functions. Used in conjunction with the *Ctrl, Alt,* or *Shift* keys, function keys can produce other desired results, such as activate the printer, insert the current date into a document, retrieve a file, and move a designated block of text. **Output** is information processed by the **central processing unit (CPU)** and displayed on the **monitor** of the terminal, which resembles a television screen (Fig. 8–1).

TYPES OF COMPUTERS

Computers can be roughly divided into three types:

- Microcomputers
- Minicomputers
- Main-frame computers

Microcomputer

The **microcomputer** is a desk-top computer. Originally designed as a personal computer, today's microcomputer has many business applications and may be suitable for the small medical practice.

Minicomputer

More commonly found in health agencies, the **minicomputer** historically has had larger storage capacity and multilocation terminals. Both the microcomputer and the minicomputer can be installed in an average office environment without the need for special rooms or air conditioning.

Main-Frame Computer

Main-frame computers (or "main frames") are capable of manipulating and storing great amounts of information and are usually found in large facilities such as hospitals, clinics, and service bureaus. Because main-frame computers are susceptible to changing environmental conditions, they must be housed in temperature-controlled and humidity-controlled rooms.

Any complete computer system located within an office is known as a **stand-alone system.**

OUTSIDE SERVICE BUREAUS

Computer services are available to the office that does not have total in-house capabilities through service bureaus. Service bureaus have been providing computer services to the medical profession for more than 30 years. They provide three basic types of service:

- On-line time sharing
- On-line servicing
- Off-line batch system

On-line Time Sharing

With this type of service, the medical facility has its own terminal that is connected directly to the service bureau's main-frame computer. It shares access to the computer with other subscribers. The medical facility usually has its own printer. Access to the computer may not always be available when it is needed.

On-line Servicing

With on-line servicing, the medical facility has its own terminal through which it provides the service bureau with data via telephone lines. The service bureau then responds by producing reports, statements, or whatever has been contracted for in the service agreement. The medical facility may have its own printer for the preparation of reports.

Off-line Batch System

The medical facility that uses a **batch** system sends information daily, by mail or messenger, to a central location; at this location, the data is entered into a main-frame computer. The service bureau then prepares statements, insurance forms, and reports and returns them to the physician by mail or messenger. One of the major problems with this system is the time lag between the sending and the receiving of information; however, it is the simplest and the least expensive way to use a service bureau.

SYSTEM COMPONENTS

- *Hardware:* the electrical, electronic, and mechanical equipment (the computer and various peripherals, such as disk drives and printer)
- *Software:* the programming (instructions) that directs the hardware how to complete the desired task
- *Input and Output Devices:* the components that allow the computer to communicate with the operator or other computers

Hardware

CPU

The CPU is the most important piece of hardware. It is the "brain" of the computer. Although you cannot see it, within the CPU is the memory; it consists of electronic or magnetic cells, each of which contains information (Fig. 8–2).

Memory

There are two kinds of memory: **ROM, or read-only memory,** and **RAM, or random access memory.** ROM is internal memory that contains the entire operating system and a computer language. It is also known as **main memory.** With this permanent memory, much less information has to be transferred from a disk to start the computing process. The ROM cannot be overwritten and is not erased when the power is shut off. RAM can be thought of as the internal scratch pad of the computer. It contains the program instructions and the data that it is currently processing. This memory is normally erased automatically when the power is turned off.

Disk Drives

A disk drive is a device that holds, "reads," and records on a data storage disk. There are two kinds of disk drives: hard or rigid disk drives and floppy disk drives. In the classroom, you may use a computer that has two floppy disk drives. They are identified as "Drive A" and "Drive B." A hard disk is identified as "Drive C." Floppy disks may be 8 inches, 5.25 inches, or 3.5 inches in diameter.

If a computer has a hard disk drive, it still must have at least one floppy disk drive; this is because most software packages (programs) are purchased on floppy disks. The software is read by the floppy disk drive and entered onto the hard disk.

Information Storage

Information may be saved (stored) on a **disk** for future reference or printing. The amount of information that can be stored depends on the type of disk the system uses. Storage is achieved either on a hard disk or **floppy disks (diskettes),** or both. Floppy disks are frequently used for data storage on personal and small-business computer systems, and the size of the floppy disk needed depends on the type of computer being used. The hard disk is usually necessary in a medical practice. Hard disks store much more information than do floppy disks and make possible faster information access. They may be fixed or removable from the computer. Hard disks with various storage capacities are available.

Diskette Files

Before information can be stored on a diskette, the diskette must be initialized, or **formatted.** When correctly instructed, your computer formats the diskette by magnetically creating tracks (recording bands) on the diskette where information is to be stored. Diskettes that are preformatted are also available at slightly higher cost than nonformatted diskettes. After a diskette has been formatted, the disk operating system (DOS) can both read data from the diskette and "write" data onto the diskette. When information is stored only on diskettes, it is always wise to make back-up or duplicate diskettes in case the original diskettes are lost or damaged. Floppy diskettes are more easily damaged than are hard disks and must be carefully stored (always in a jacket) and filed for easy reference. For tips on the proper care of diskettes, see the Care of Diskettes chart.

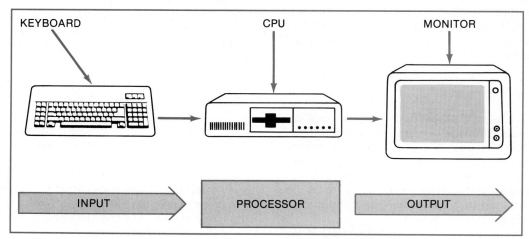

FIGURE 8–2. Components of a computer system.

CARE OF DISKETTES

- Avoid exposing the diskette to extremes of temperature.

- When the diskette is not in use, always return it to its storage envelope, where it will not collect dust.

- Avoid laying a diskette on top of the monitor because this could scramble information on the diskette.

- Keep your fingers off the surface of the diskette, especially around the window in the jacket. Body oils can permanently destroy data.

- Hold the diskette with your thumb on the label.

- Write or type on the label before attaching it to the diskette, if possible, or write with a soft felt tip pen. Never write with a ballpoint pen or pencil on a label that is on a diskette. Also, do not erase on a diskette label. All of these can cause impressions in the diskette, and the ink can run.

- Do not force a diskette into a disk drive or its storage envelope. If there is resistance, pull it out and try again. Bending or folding a diskette will render it useless.

- Store the diskettes vertically in dust-tight containers.

- Keep smoke, food, and drink away from the area of use.

Hard Disk Management

The hard disk is the filing cabinet of the computer. Thousands of files can be placed on a hard disk and retrieved with a few specific keystrokes.

A hard disk system usually comprises two or more rigid metal plates enclosed in a sealed case. It stores data by magnetic encoding similar to that when using a floppy disk or cassette tape. Hard disks provide much greater storage capacity than do floppy diskettes. The storage capacity of a 20-megabyte hard disk is about 56 times greater than that of one 360K floppy diskette. For efficiency in retrieving a given piece of information, a **directory** is established for each main topic; subdirectories can be set up within directories. Computer **files** are organized in much the same fashion as ordinary files that contain paper records (Fig. 8–3).

When a disk becomes overcrowded, more time is required for the system to retrieve a specific file. The hard disk needs to be purged of files that are outdated or no longer useful just as does any other filing system.

Monitors

The monitor, which looks like a television screen, is a device used to display computer-generated information. When using the usual medical office software, it is possible to type in a patient's name and have all the information concerning that patient appear on the screen. The monitor displays **prompts** (messages) to instruct the operator what to do. A blinking marker on the screen, called the **cursor,** indicates the position where the next information can be added or inserted.

Some monitors are black and white only but may be adjusted for screen brightness and contrast. Color monitors allow the operator to choose the background color that is most pleasing to the eye and easiest to read (see Fig. 8–2).

Printers

Documents appearing on the monitor may be directed to a printer to produce what is called a **hard**

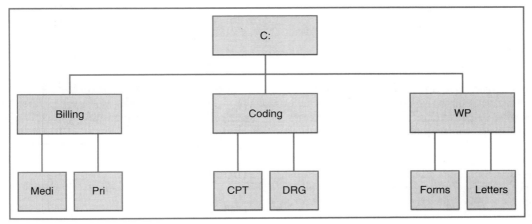

FIGURE 8–3. Schematic drawing of computer directories and subdirectories.

(paper) **copy** or **printout.** Some printers have built-in paperfeeders, whereas others require accessory feeders. The single-sheet or cut-sheet feeder is used for feeding single sheets of letterhead or other paper into the printer. Continuous forms, such as bills, insurance forms, and reports, require a *tractor feeder,* which feeds in the continuous sheets, aligns the paper, and automatically advances it as necessary. Four types of printers are commonly used with computers:

- dot matrix
- letter-quality or print wheel
- ink-jet
- laser

Many printers print bidirectionally (i.e., they print both from left to right and from right to left). Some are capable of both draft-quality and correspondence-quality printing.

DOT MATRIX PRINTERS. Dot matrix printers are the least expensive of the four types of printer and are very popular. They are used almost exclusively in the classroom. Dot matrix printers form the letters or shapes that they are directed to print by arranging patterns of dots on the paper. They operate more quickly than do letter-quality machines, but their print lacks the clarity generally desired for a professional look.

LETTER-QUALITY PRINTERS. Letter-quality printers may be either mechanical or electronic. The electronic letter-quality printer generally uses a print wheel, or **daisy wheel,** that is interchangeable for variations in print style or size. Many printers have 10-, 12-, and 15-pitch typing capability as well as proportional spacing capability.

INK-JET AND LASER PRINTERS. Ink-jet and laser printers are the latest generation of high-quality printers. They are very fast, the quality of the documents they produce is comparable with that of typeset documents, and they are now quite affordable. Unlike dot matrix or daisy-wheel printers, both of which print by striking the paper, the print wires, or a print hammer, the ink-jet and laser printers are nonimpact printers; that is, no mechanical device strikes the paper to produce the printed image. Ink-jet printers use an ink cartridge that feeds an array of nearly microscopic tubes, each of which has a heating element that is energized during the printing process. Ink-jet printers cost less than do laser printers, but the ink cartridges they use are fairly expensive, bringing their operating cost to about double that for laser printers. Laser printers use xerographic technology similar to that in photocopiers, so the laser printer is able to produce an almost limitless variety of type forms and sizes as well as complex graphics. One disadvantage of ink-jet and laser printers is that they are incapable of producing multiple copies with carbon sets or multicopy forms, such as many types of insurance forms.

Software and Its Capabilities

Software is the most important component of a computer system. Software—that is, the programs that a computer uses—is the "roadmap" for the computer. It contains instructions as to what the computer is to do with the data you input. Software can account for a major portion of the cost of a computer system.

Functions performed in the physician's office for which computer software has been designed include:

- Processing insurance claims
- Maintaining patient ledger
- Keeping medical records
- Billing and collections
- Accounting processes
- Database management
- Appointment scheduling
- Clinical research
- Electronic mailing
- Word processing

Processing Insurance Claims

Claims information can be sent from the physician's office directly to the computer of an insurance company using a **modem,** which transmits information over telephone lines. Electronic processing of insurance claims not only saves transit time but also provides immediate information as to whether a given claim will be accepted. Errors in coding or procedure are immediately evident, and such errors result in the rejection of the claim by the insurance company's computer. Corrections can then be made instantly using the computer.

The codes that are most commonly used for claims processing can be stored on the computer disk and retrieved when needed (Fig. 8–4).

Many insurance companies give preferential treatment to providers who file claims electronically (Fig. 8–5*A* and *B*).

In medical offices that do not file insurance claims for patients, a computer can generate a *superbill* for the patient to attach to his or her own insurance form. The superbill gives information about diagnosis and procedures that is needed to file a claim.

Patient Ledger

The **demographic** information about a patient (e.g., his or her name, address, telephone number, and insurance carrier) will appear on the patient's computerized ledger (Fig. 8–6). As services are rendered, all charges and payments are entered into the computer. This results in the availability of a current balance at all times.

Medical Records

Computer systems can store clinical information about patients using much less space and with

CHARGE RECORD

Code	✓	Description	Code	✓	Description	Code	✓	Description	Code	✓	Description
Physician Services			93000		ECG	**Chemistries**			**Microbiology O/L**		
		Comp. Extended Exam	99150		ECG Monitoring	82040		Albumin			Fungus Culture
90020		Comp. Exam New Pt.	93040		ECG Rhythm Strip (1 min.)	84075		Alk. Phos.			GC Culture
90020-52		Comp. Exam New Pt. Brief	93262		Holter Monitoring	84520		BUN			Stool O & P
90600		Office Consult Brief	94150		Peak Flow Rate	82310		Calcium			TBC Culture
90610		Office Consult Extended	93015		Treadmill ECG	80112		Chem. Panel 12			Urine Culture
90605		Office Consult Intermed.	**Hematology**			82465		Cholesterol			Urine Sens.
90040		Office Visit Brief	85024		CBC	82565		Creatinine			Viral Serologies (Specify)
90060		Office Visit Estab. Pt.	85170		Clot Retraction	82251		Direct Bilirubin			
90070		Office Visit Extended	85009		DIFF	84231		FSH & LH	**Serologies O/L**		
90010		Office Visit New Pt. Int.	82728		Ferritin	82977		GGTP			ANA
90050		Office Visit Limited	85014		HCT	82948		Glucometer			C-Reactive Prot.
90030		Office Visit Minimal	85018		HGB	82947		Glucose			Febrile Agglts.
90060-01		Office Visit-No Charge	85021		Indices	83036		Glycohemoglobin			Premarital & Rubella
90080		Re-Exam	85000		Ivy Bleeding Time	83718		HDL Cholesterol			RPR Premarital
90080-52		Re-Exam School	85580		Platelet Count	83720		LDL Cholesterol			RPR Routine
			85610		Protime	83735		Magnesium			Rubella Titer
90026-22		Subsp - Comp. Exam Extd.	85730		PTT	84100		Phosphorus			
90020-22		Subsp - Comp. Exam New	85041		RBC	84132		Potassium	**Serologies - Miscellaneous**		
90020-01		Subsp - Comp. Exam New Br.	85044		Retic Count	84450		SGOT	831		Heterophile / EBV
90010-22		Subsp - Int. Exam New Pt.	85048		WBC	84460		SGPT	86006		RA Factor
90600-22		Subsp - Off. Consult Br.	85651		Westergren Sed. Rate	84295		Sodium	86008		RA Quant.
90610-22		Subsp - Off. Consult Ext.				82250		Total Bilirubin	89205		Stool Hemoccult X3
90605-22		Subsp - Off. Consult Inter.				84155		Total Protein	89205-01		Stool Hemoccult X1
90050-22		Subsp - OV Brief	**Special Hematology O/L**			84475		Triglycerides	82997		UCG
90060-22		Subsp - OV Estab. Pt.			Blood Group & Type	84443		TSH	87205-03		10% KOH Prep.
90070-22		Subsp - OV Extended			B12	84250		T3 Resin			
90080-22		Subsp - Re-Exam			Cold Aggluts.	84251		T4R	**Hepatitis Testing O/L**		
40260		Anoscopy			Coombs, Direct	84550		Uric Acid			Anti Hav IGG
85100		Bone Marrow A/S			Coombs, Indirect	**Chemistries O/L**					Anti Hav IGM
85102		Bone Marrow Bx.			Folate			Acid Phosphatase			Anti HBC
99080		Chart Review			Haptoglobin			Aldolase			Anti HBE
96501		Chemo Inf. Drip Tech.			HGB Electrophor			Amylase Blood			Anti HBS
96500		Chemo Inf. Push Tech.			Serum Iron			NA, K, CL, CO2			HBE AG
69210		Ear Irrig.			Sickle Cell Prep.						HBS AG
90015		Int. Exam, Intermed.			TIBC	**Outside Miscellaneous**					Hepatitis Panel
99070		IV Injection						Chem. Panel			Panel With E
20610		Joint Aspir. Infus.						Lipoprotein EPG			
90749		Joint / Bursa Inj.	**Blood Assays O/L**			**Chemistries Complement O/L**			**Drug Levels**		
31505		Laryngoscopy			Alpha Fetoprotein			C'3			Alcohol
95834		Neurol Exam.			Anti DNA			C'4			Amitryptiline
90040		Pelvic			Anti - Thyroid Antibody			C'H50			Barbiturates
96450		Phlebotomy			Beta HCG			Complement Profile	82643		Digoxin
40240		Sigmoidoscopy			Calcitonin			CPK			Disopyramide
10000		Soft Tissue Aspir.			CEA			CPK Isoenzymes			Imipramine
90040-52		Suture Removal			Cortisol			Immunoglobulins (All)			Lithium
					C-Peptide			IGG			Phenytoin
Nursing Service & Supplies					Estradiol			IGM			Procainamide NAPA
95150		Antigen Inj.			Free Testosterone			IGA			Quinidine
90030-01		Blood Pressure			FSH			LDH			Salicylates
90030-02		Clean / Dress Wound			Insulin			LDH Isoenzymes	84420		Theophylline
86490		Cocci Skin Test			LH			Lead			
69210		Ear Irrig.			Parthormone			Lysozymes			
90724		Flu Vaccine			Prolactin			Mercury	**Cytologies O/L**		
90730		IM Med. Injection			Testosterone			SPEP			Pap Smear
90030-04		Injection, Instruct.			T3 RIA						Sputum Cytology X1
99070-03		IV Meds.									Sputum Cytology X3
86540		Mumps Skin Test	**Urines**			**Microbiology**					
90729		Other Immuniz.	82575		24 Hr. Creatinine Clear	85535		Bone Marrow Fe Stain	**Laboratory Tests / Outside Labs**		
90732		Pneumovax	81000		Urinalysis Multi 10SG	86235		Chlamydia	**Preparation of Specimens**		
86580		PPD Skin Test	84175		24 Hr. Urine Protein	87205-02		Gram Stain	99022-12		American
92551		Screening Audio	82335		Calcium	87060		Nose / Throat Culture	99026		Cab to Outside Lab
99070-03		Supplies	84550-01		Uric Acid	87070-02		Other Culture (Specify)	99022-06		Dianon
90703		Tet. Tox. / Diphth.				87205-01		Prostatic Wet Mount	99023		Home Collect by Tech.
92081-52		Vision Test	**Organ Related Panels**			87184		Sensitivities	99023-01		Lab Drawing
			80099		Bone Disease	87070		Sputum Culture	99022-05		MAAS
Laboratory Tests - In Office			80062		Coronary Risk	87082		Stat Strep Serology	99022-02		Nichols Lab
Cardiopulmonary			80065		Diabetic	87045		Stool Culture			
94010		AB (FVC & MVV)	80058		Hepatic	87205		Stool Smear WBC			
94060		ABC (+ / – Bronchodil)	80060		Hypertension	87086		Urine Colony Ct.			
94160		Breath FEVI & VC	825		Lipid	87081		Urine Culture			
71022		Chest Xray Oblique Only	80073		Renal	88150		Vaginal Wet Mount			
71020		Chest Xray PA & Lat.				87070-01		Wound Culture			
71010		Chest Xray PA Only									

07/22/57
3

COURTESY - BILL INS
429-27-7469
06/09/92

CHART COPY

FIGURE 8-4. Computer coding for an internal medicine practice.

FIGURE 8–5. *A*, Computer-generated Medicare bill.

greater security than can papers in a patient chart. Anyone who has worked in a medical office understands the problems that a "lost" patient chart can cause. The chart stored on the computer can be set up in such fashion that a printout of only the most important information can be reviewed by the physician at the time of the patient's visit; as a result, he or she does not have to thumb through an ever-growing stack of papers (Fig. 8–7). Reports from outside sources can be added to the computer record using a **scanner.**

DO NOT STAPLE IN BAR AREA

PROVIDER NAME AND ADDRESS

FASTEN HERE

2

1. CLAIM CONTROL NUMBER		F.I. USE ONLY
2. MEDI-CAL PROV. NO.	CHECK	
00G611450		
3. MEDICARE PROV. NO.	DIGIT	
W1202		
6. ZIP CODE		
92103		

PROFESSIONAL/SUPPLIER CLAIM FORM

AFFIX LABEL HERE

4. ☒ MEDI-CAL
5. ☐ MEDICARE

Elite Pica 7 (AREA) ◄ PROVIDER PHONE NO.

PLEASE TYPE ALL REQUIRED INFORMATION
Typewriter Alignment

Elite Pica

PATIENT'S COMPLETE NAME, AND ADDRESS
8

MEDICARE NUMBER	SEX M/F	WAS CONDITION RELATED TO EMPLOYMENT	DATE OF ONSET	TAR CONTROL NUMBER
9	10 F	11 N	12	13

MEDI-CAL I.D. NUMBER		DATE OF BIRTH	PATIENT ACCOUNT NUMBER
14 3760947328667 9	15	032832	16 15001

SERVICES RELATED TO HOSPITALIZATION FROM	THRU	EMER. CERT.	OTHER COV.	BILLING LIMIT	ATTACH-MENTS	D.M.E. CODE	MEDICARE STATUS
17	18	19	20	21	22	23	24 O

26 OTHER HEALTH INS. COV.-ENTER NAME OF POLICY HOLDER, PLAN NAME, ADDRESS AND POLICY NO. 25 PATIENT'S PHONE NUMBER (AREA)

NAME & ADDRESS OF FACILITY WHERE SERVICES WERE RENDERED (IF OTHER THAN HOME OR OFFICE)	FACILITY PROVIDER NO.
28 MERCY HOSPITAL	27 HSC30077F

29 OUTSIDE LAB 30 LABORATORY NAME AND ADDRESS

31 NAME OF REFERRING PROVIDER 32 REFERRING PROVIDER NUMBER

PRIMARY DIAGNOSIS DESCRIPTION
33 CONGESTIVE HEART FAILURE 34 PRIMARY ICD-9-CM 4280 35 SECONDARY DIAGNOSIS DESCRIPTION 36 SECONDARY ICD-9-CM

DESCRIPTION	BILLING PROVIDER CHARGE FOR OUTSIDE LAB SERVICES	DELETE	DATE OF SERVICE	PLACE OF SERVICE	FP/CHDP	RENDERING PROV. NO. IF OTHER THAN BILLING PROV.	PROCEDURE CODE	MOD	QUANTITY	SERVICE CHARGES
37 SUBSQNT HSP-MINOR CM	38	39 ☐1	40 040192	41 3	42	43 WG61145A	44 99232	45	1	46 5416
47	48	49 ☐2	50	51	52	53	54	55		56
57	58	59 ☐3	60	61	62	63	64	65		66
67	68	69 ☐4	70	71	72	73	74	75		76
77	78	79 ☐5	80	81	82	83	84	85		86
87	88	89 ☐6	90	91	92	93	94	95		96
97	98	99 ☐7	100	101	102	103	104	105		106
107	108	109 ☐8	110	111	112	113	114	115		116

REMARKS/EMERGENCY CERTIFICATION STATEMENT:

AEVS 9215650612

		117 BLOOD PINTS	BLOOD DEDUCT		TOTAL CHARGES
M E D I - C A L / F I U S E		118			119 5416
	120 MEDICARE DEDUCTIBLE	MEDICARE CO-INSURANCE 121			MEDICARE PAID 122
	123 MEDICARE DISALLOWED	PATIENT'S SHARE OF COST 124	OTHER COVERAGE 125		DEDUCTIONS 126
		DATE OF EOMB 127	DATE BILLED 128 060392		NET AMOUNT BILLED 129 5416
	130 ☐	131 ☐ 132 ☐	133 ☐	134	**M E D I C A R E** 135 TOTAL CHARGES
					136 AMOUNT PAID
					ANY UNPAID 137 BALANCE DUE

SIGNATURE REQUIRED FOR EMERGENCY CERTIFICATION DATE __/__/__

PATIENT'S OR AUTHORIZED PERSON'S SIGNATURE (READ BACK BEFORE SIGNING). I authorize the release of any Medical Information necessary to process this claim and request payments of Medicare Benefits either to myself or to the party who accepts assignment.
138 _____ SIGNED _____ DATE

This is to certify that the information contained above is true, accurate, and complete and that the provider has read, understands, and agrees to be bound by and comply with the statements and conditions contained on the back of this form.
139 _____ SIGNED _____ DATE
Signature of provider or person authorized by provider to bind provider by above signature to statements and conditions contained on this form.

140 ☒ I DO ACCEPT ASSIGNMENT
141 ☐ I DO NOT ACCEPT ASSIGNMENT

40-1C 4/91

SEE YOUR PROVIDER MANUAL FOR ASSISTANCE REGARDING THE COMPLETION OF THIS FORM.

FOR PROVIDER RECORDS ONLY

B

FIGURE 8–5 *Continued B*, Billing for a Medi-Cal (Medicaid) patient.

```
                                                              PAGE    1

                                            Tax ID
                                            95-2585978




                         June 10 , 1992

To:




Diagnosis:                        Patient  :
1 4659   UPPER RESPIRATORY INFECTI  Acct #   :
2 4959   ALLERGIC ALVEOLITIS & PNE  SS#      :
3 7856   LYMPHADENOPATHY            D.O.B.   :
                                    Phone    :
                                    Employer :
                                    Claim No.:
                                    Group    :


 #    Date  Dr Pl Svc     Description  Bil  Charge   Credit      Bal    Prev
 ------------------------------------------------------------------------------
 1.  052992           777  COURTESY ADJU B          -30.50      0.00    30.50
 2.  052992           742  DEBIT ADJUSTM B           97.50     30.50   -67.00
 3.  043092  INSURANCE BILLED     B/C PRUDE 0401-0430(  30.50)
 4.  043092  INSURANCE BILLED     RISK MANA 0401-0430(  30.50)
 5.  040692   9  1 8706000  NOSE\THROAT C *   30.50         -67.00   -97.50
 6.  093091           751  COURTESY DISC B          -97.50    -97.50    0.00
                                          2/11-2/14/91
 7.  053091           751  COURTESY DISC B         -253.75     0.00   253.75
                                          4/23/91
 8.  043091  INSURANCE BILLED     B/C PRUDEN 0401-0430 253.75
 9.  043091  INSURANCE BILLED     RISK MANAG 0401-0430 253.75
10.  042391   9  1 9902301  LABORATORY DR *    5.75        253.75   248.00
11.  042391   9  1 8444300  TSH           *   35.00        248.00   213.00
12.  042391   9  1 8425100  T4R           *   21.00        213.00   192.00
13.  042391   9  1 8425000  T3 RESIN      *   21.00        192.00   171.00
14.  042391   9  1 8429500  SODIUM        *    9.25        171.00   161.75
15.  042391   9  1 8413200  POTASSIUM     *    9.25        161.75   152.50
16.  042391   9  1 8371800  HDL CHOLESTER *   27.50        152.50   125.00
17.  042391   9  1 8011200  CHEM PANEL 12 *   42.50        125.00    82.50
18.  042391   9  1 8272800  FERRITIN,EIA  *   47.00         82.50    35.50
19.  042391   9  1 8565100  WESTERGREN SE *   13.50         35.50    22.00
20.  042391   9  1 8502400  CBC           *   22.00         22.00     0.00
21.  041991           751  COURTESY DISC B          -41.00     0.00    41.00
                                          BAL APPLD TO DED
22.  022891  INSURANCE BILLED     B/C PRUDEN 0201-0228  97.50
23.  022891  INSURANCE BILLED     RISK MANAG 0201-0228  97.50
24.  022191           751  COURTESY DISC B          -56.50    41.00    97.50
                                          D.O.S. 11/12/90
25.  021491   4  1 9006000  OFFICE VISIT- *   48.75         97.50    48.75
26.  021191   4  1 9006000  OFFICE VISIT- *   48.75         48.75     0.00
27.  013191           751  COURTESY DISC B          -56.50     0.00    56.50
                                          TO DEDUCTIBLE
```

FIGURE 8-6. Patient ledger.

```
                                                          PAGE    2
28.  112390  INSURANCE BILLED       AETNA LIFE 1001-1123    56.50
29.  111290  10  1 8720503  10% KOH PREP  *    10.50         56.50      46.00
30.  111290   6  1 9006000  OFFICE VISIT- *    46.00         46.00       0.00
31.  053190              751  COURTESY DISC B        -220.25  0.00     220.25
32.  022890  INSURANCE BILLED       AETNA LIFE 0201-0228   178.00
33.  020290   6  1 9902200  ALLIED CLINIC *     8.00        220.25     212.25
                                    \FERRITIN
34.  020290   6  1 8444300  TSH           *    33.00        212.25     179.25
35.  020290   6  1 8425100  T4R           *    19.75        179.25     159.50
36.  020290   6  1 8425000  T3 RESIN      *    19.75        159.50     139.75
37.  020290   6  1 8371800  HDL CHOLESTER *    26.00        139.75     113.75
38.  020290   6  1 8011200  CHEM PANEL 12 *    38.00        113.75      75.75
39.  020290   6  1 8565100  WESTERGREN SE *    12.75         75.75      63.00
40.  020290   6  1 8502400  CBC           *    20.75         63.00      42.25
41.  093089  INSURANCE BILLED       AETNA LIFE 0901-0930    42.25
42.  091989   3  1 8565100  WESTERGREN SE *    12.00         42.25      30.25
43.  091989   3  1 8503100  Not in ISAM   *    19.50         30.25      10.75
44.  091989   3  1 9902201  ALLIED SPECIM *    10.75         10.75       0.00
                                    /FER,IBC,SE IRON
45.  010089   3  1 9999900  BALANCE FORWA B     0.00          0.00       0.00
                                    COMPRESSED TO BALF

              Current    30-day    60-day    90-day    120 +     Balance
Bal Fwd Age:    0.00      0.00      0.00      0.00      0.00        0.00

Treatment Rendered by:
Referring Physician   : NO REFERRAL
Please Make Check Payable to:
```

FIGURE 8-6 *Continued*

Billing and Collections

At the appropriate time, the computer can print a patient's billing statement that shows detailed charges, payments, adjustments, and a balance (Fig. 8–8). Additionally, the computer can be programmed to age the accounts according to any criteria selected and to include this information on the billing statement. A series of collection letters can also be developed and personalized for individual patients as they are needed.

Accounting Processes

With the appropriate software, the computer can easily handle all accounting processes, including:

- Recording payables and receivables
- Computing the payroll
- Keeping track of bills to be paid
- Generating checks
- Producing a deposit slip for the bank
- Reconciling bank statements
- Preparing daily, monthly, and annual financial and statistical reports

Database Management

The amount and character of information that can be stored on a computer **database** about patients, procedures, diagnoses, and other topics are limitless. After the data is recorded on the disk, it can be sorted into any chosen order and retrieved as desired (Fig. 8–9).

Appointment Scheduling

The computer can replace the appointment book, but this is practical only in large practices and clinics. Software for appointment scheduling ranges from relatively simple programs that merely display available and scheduled times to sophisticated systems into which the operator may enter information such as the length and type of appointment required and day and time preferences of the patient; the computer then selects the best appointment time based on inputed information.

The computer can also be used to keep track of future appointments. For example, when a patient calls and inquires about an appointment, the system can search by his or her name to find the time and date. The computer can provide printouts of the daily schedule that include the patients' names and telephone numbers and the reason for their visiting. Multiple copies of these schedules can be made according to the needs of the practice.

A big advantage of computer scheduling is that more than one person can access the system at one time, and the information is available to all operators. In many facilities, employees still maintain an appointment book as a back-up to computer scheduling.

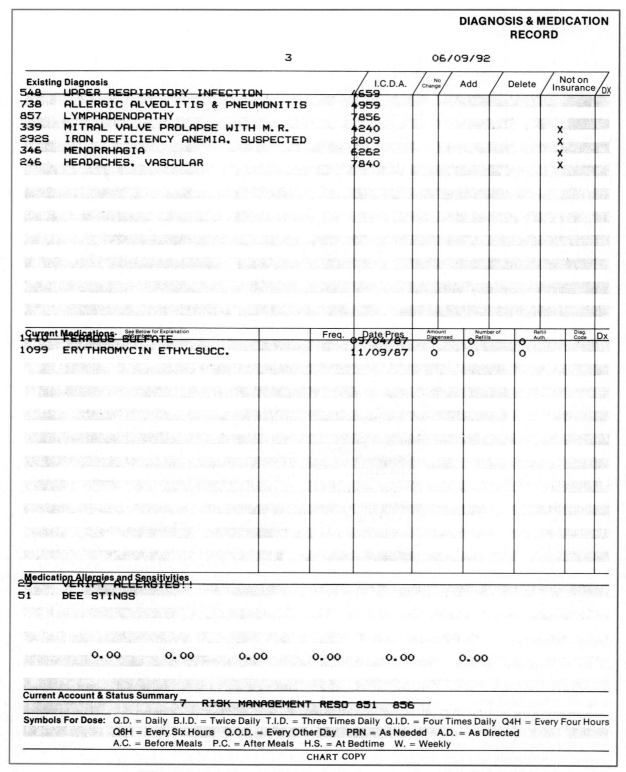

DIAGNOSIS & MEDICATION RECORD

3   06/09/92

Existing Diagnosis		I.C.D.A.	No Change	Add	Delete	Not on Insurance	DX
548	UPPER RESPIRATORY INFECTION	4659					
738	ALLERGIC ALVEOLITIS & PNEUMONITIS	4959					
857	LYMPHADENOPATHY	7856					
339	MITRAL VALVE PROLAPSE WITH M.R.	4240				X	
292S	IRON DEFICIENCY ANEMIA, SUSPECTED	2809				X	
346	MENORRHAGIA	6262				X	
246	HEADACHES, VASCULAR	7840				X	

Current Medications See Below for Explanation of Symbols		Freq.	Date Pres.	Amount Dispensed	Number of Refills	Refill Auth.	Diag. Code	Dx
1110	FERROUS SULFATE		09/04/87	0	0	0		
1099	ERYTHROMYCIN ETHYLSUCC.		11/09/87	0	0	0		

Medication Allergies and Sensitivities

29	VERIFY ALLERGIES!!
51	BEE STINGS

0.00   0.00   0.00   0.00   0.00   0.00

Current Account & Status Summary   7   RISK MANAGEMENT RESO 851   856

Symbols For Dose: Q.D. = Daily B.I.D. = Twice Daily T.I.D. = Three Times Daily Q.I.D. = Four Times Daily Q4H = Every Four Hours
Q6H = Every Six Hours Q.O.D. = Every Other Day PRN = As Needed A.D. = As Directed
A.C. = Before Meals P.C. = After Meals H.S. = At Bedtime W. = Weekly

CHART COPY

FIGURE 8-7. Diagnosis and medication record for an internal medicine practice.

Clinical Research

The physician who stores patient information in a database can develop research reports from this source. For example, if a study were being done on the results of a specific treatment, the physician could gather the needed information from the database.

Electronic Mail

Telecommunication (or **electronic mail**) software allows one computer to communicate with an-

Statement

Date	Diagnosis	*	RVS / CPT	Description	Doctor	Amount
05/27/92	4779	11	90060	OFFICE VISIT-EST.PT.	MM	51.00
05/27/92	4779	11	8502424	CBC	MM	23.00
05/27/92	4779	11	8565124	WESTERGREN SED RATE	MM	14.25
05/27/92	2724	11	8006224	CORONARY RISK PANEL	MM	51.00
05/27/92	2724	11	8005824	HEPATIC FUNCTION PANEL	MM	57.00
05/27/92	7851	11	8444324	TSH	MM	36.75
05/27/92	7851	11	36415	LABORATORY DRAWING	MM	6.00
053192			INSURANCE BILLED			
			FOR DATE RANGE 501--531 (FOR THE AMT. OF 239.00)			

Patient Name

Account Number	Statement Date
12992	5/31/92

Billed To

Return this portion with your payment in the envelope provided.
Make your check payable to:

IRS # 95-2585978

Check Number

Current Charges	Previously Billed Charges Now Past Due				Balance Due
	Over 30 Days	Over 60 Days	Over 90 Days	Over 120 days	
$239.00	$0.00	$0.00	$0.00	$0.00	$239.00

Balance Due	Amount Enclosed
$239.00	

Account Number
12992

Patient Name

Billed To:

Change of Address: Note Below

*Location Codes:
1. Inpatient Hospital
2. Outpatient Hospital
3. Office
4. Residence

Save this portion of your bill for Major Medical and Income Tax Purposes.

FIGURE 8-8. Patient bill.

other computer via telephone lines through the use of a modem. Letters and reports can travel along telephone lines to your computer, which can provide a printout in a manner not unlike that previously discussed concerning the electronic transmission of insurance claims.

Word Processing

Word Processing software is available for all desktop computers. A sophisticated software package with the capability to create footnotes, bibliographies, indexes, graphics, and so forth will appeal to the physician who does academic writing.

SECURITY GUIDELINES FOR COMPUTERIZED DATA

As we learned in an earlier chapter, the patient is entitled to utmost confidentiality with respect to his or her medical records and the release of any information of a personal nature. Since computer technology allows the accumulation and storage of a vast amount of data that may be accessible to a variety of individuals, it is imperative that guidelines be set up for the protection of that data. Security guidelines have been established by the Council on Ethical and Judicial Affairs of the American Medical Association and are included in the box entitled Security Guidelines for Computerized Data.

SECURITY GUIDELINES FOR COMPUTERIZED DATA

Guidelines on a computerized database:

1. Confidential medical information entered into the computerized database should be verified as to authenticity of source.

2. The patient and physician should be advised about the existence of computerized databases in which medical information concerning the patient is stored. Such information should be communicated to the physician and patient prior to the physician's release of the medical information. All individuals and organizations with some form of access to the computerized data bank, and the level of access permitted, should be specifically identified in advance.

3. The physician and patient should be notified of the distribution of all reports reflecting identifiable patient data prior to distribution of the reports by the computer facility. There should be approval by the physician and patient prior to the release of patient-identifiable clinical and administrative data to individuals or organizations external to the medical care environment, and such information should not be released without the ex-

```
DATE : 06/10/92 TIME : 08:37 AM                                    PAGE    1

LIST OF PATIENTS


                           R E G I S T R A T I O N
06/10/92
 1.CHART #:                        10.RESP PARTY:
 2.NAME    :                       11.ADDRESS    :
 3.ACCT #  :                       12.CITY/STATE:
 4.DR/PL #: 03/01                  13.ZIP        :
 5.SEX     : F                     14.RELATION   :
 6.MARITAL: M                      15.PHONE RES  :
 7.BIRTH  :   7/22/57              16.PHONE BUS  :
 8.REF DOC:    1  NO REFERRAL      17.EMPLOYER   :
 9.ACC DAY:   /  / 0               18.SSN        :
- - - - - - - - - - - - - - - I N S U R A N C E - - - - - - - - - - - - -
 20.CODE   : 851                   26.CODE       : 856   B/C PRUDENT BUYER
 21.PRIMARY: RISK MANAGEMENT RESO  27.SECONDARY :
 22.ID #   : 429-27-7469           28.ID #       :
 23.GROUP  : 664-626               29.GROUP      : 336631/101/3
 24.ASSN:1            25.STAT: 0   30.ASSN:0            31.STAT: 0
- - - - - - - - - - - - - - - - - - - - - - - - - - - - - - - - - - - - -
 32.NOTE 1: PARENTS     524-8240 34.RECALL DATE:08/18/88 36.RECALL TYPE:  0
 33.NOTE 2: SISTER     -524-6995 35.RECALL DONE:08/30/88 37.PAN:NEW INS 1/91
- - - - - - - - - - - - - - - - - - - - - - - - - - - - - - - - - - - - -
 38.ICD #1:4659    39.DESC:UPPER RESPIRATORY INFECTI  44.ADMITTED   :00/00/00
 40.ICD #2:4959    41.DESC:ALLERGIC ALVEOLITIS & PNE  45.DISCHARGED :00/00/00
 42.ICD #3:7856    43.DESC:LYMPHADENOPATHY            46.LAWYER     :   0


SECPAG - Extra Patient Information

 1. Pat Address :              10. Family Planning  :
 2.     Address :              11. Other Accident   :
 3.     City St :              12. Patient Employed  : Y
 4.         Zip :              13. Patient P/T Std.  :
 5. O.I. Emp/Sch:              14. Patient F/T Std.  :
 6. Time of Inj.:              15. Insured's Sex     : F
 7. Active/Ret. :              16. Other Ins. Sex    : M
 8. Date to Clinic   :         17. Insured's D.O.B.  : 07/22/57
 9. Discharge Date   :         18. Other Ins. D.O.B. : 10/21/45

19. Refered Out :              25. Auto Accident   :
20.     Contact :              26. Work Related    :
21.     Address :              27. Return Mod Work:
22.     City St :              28. Return Reg Work:
23.         Zip :              29. Claim #         :
24.       Phone :              30. Examiner        :

31. Extra Info 1:


              Change what # ( 0 for none ) :
```

FIGURE 8-9. Patient registration.

press permission of the physician and the patient.

4. The dissemination of confidential medical data should be limited to only those individuals or agencies with a bona fide use for the data. Release of confidential medical information from the database should be confined to the specific purpose for which the information is requested and limited to the specific time frame requested. All such organizations or individuals should be advised that authorized release of data to them does not authorize their further release of the data to additional individuals or organizations.

5. Procedures for adding to or changing data on the computerized database should indicate individuals authorized to make changes, time periods in which changes take place, and those individuals who will be informed about changes in the data from the medical records.

6. Procedures for purging the computerized database of archaic or inaccurate data should be established, and the patient and physician should be notified before and after the data has been purged. There should be no commingling of a physician's computerized patient records with those of other computer service bureau clients. In addition, procedures should be developed to protect against inadvertent mixing of individual reports or segments thereof.

7. The computerized medical database should be on-line to the computer terminal only when authorized computer programs requiring the medical data are being used. Individuals and organizations external to the clinical facility should not be provided on-line access to a computerized database containing identifiable data from medical records concerning patients.

8. Security:
   a. Stringent security procedures for entry into the immediate environment in which the computerized medical database is stored and/or processed or for otherwise having access to confidential medical information should be developed and strictly enforced so as to prevent access to the computer facility by unauthorized personnel. Personnel audit procedures should be developed to establish a record in the event of unauthorized disclosure of medical data. A roster of past and present service bureau personnel with specified levels of access to the medical database should be maintained. Specific administrative sanctions should exist to prevent employee breaches of confidentiality and security procedures.
   b. All terminated or former employees in the data processing environment should have no access to data from the medical records concerning patients.
   c. Involuntarily terminated employees in the data processing environment in which data from medical records concerning patients are processed should immediately upon termination be removed from the computerized medical data environment.
   d. Upon termination of computer service bureau services for a physician, those computer files maintained for the physician should be physically turned over to the physician or destroyed (erased). In the event of file erasure, the computer service bureau should verify in writing to the physician that the erasure has taken place.

From CURRENT OPINIONS, The Council on Ethical and Judicial Affairs of the American Medical Association, copyright 1989, American Medical Association.

APPLYING YOUR KNOWLEDGE

Even with some basic knowledge of computer components and of what computers can do, if you have had no "hands-on" experience with a computer, you may feel some initial fear—fear of the unknown, fear of machines, or fear of not being able to master the computer. You will soon overcome any such fears if you will remember that you really are smarter than the computer. All it can do is perform the tasks that you tell it to do. It cannot think. It cannot make decisions, and it will wait for your commands. What it can do is:

- relieve you of repetitive clerical tasks
- reduce errors
- speed up production
- recall information on command
- save time

- reduce paperwork
- allow more creative use of your time

As you begin your familiarization with the computer, you may key in some wrong information. As a result, the computer will become confused and will respond with a question mark or a comment such as:

- FILE NOT FOUND
- INVALID DRIVE SPECIFICATION
- **SYNTAX ERROR**

It will give you the opportunity and time to figure out the correct information and input it. If you are in doubt about what to do next, take a look at the screen. Most of the time it will indicate what to do next. If the answer is not readily available on the screen, check the list of **commands** and instructions in your manual. The answer should be there. Most programs have a **tutorial.** Refer to it frequently until you are thoroughly familiar with operation of the program.

You cannot break the computer simply by hitting the wrong keys. It is even unlikely that you will destroy records accidentally; a specific command is necessary. However, if you shut off the computer without saving the information on disk or tape you will lose what you have put in. By using a computer in the classroom, you will gain familiarity with computer operation and confidence that you can master it. Mastery can be accomplished only through practice.

The computer that you will actually encounter on the job is likely to be different from the one on which you will learn in the classroom. The programs and tasks performed may also be different, but you will be given training with that specific system, either by the vendor or by a member of the staff. It is important to keep an open mind while learning to operate any system.

With a knowledge of computer terms, the ability to follow step-by-step instructions, and a reasonable facility with a typewriter keyboard, you should have no problem with learning and using any computer system. In fact, many computer users consider them their best friends. You probably will, too.

ASSISTING WITH THE SELECTION OF A COMPUTER SYSTEM

The medical assistant who is already in the employ of a physician when the decision is made to invest in a computer system may be asked to participate in the selection of the system. The first step is to determine just what the computer can do for the practice and whether the practice really needs a computer. Types of computers, system components, and software capabilities have already been discussed in this chapter.

The goal is to get a computer system that will do everything you want it to do, offer options for expanded future use, and not cost more than you either need or want to spend.

Choosing a Vendor

After determining what you want the computer to do, the next important step is choosing a vendor. It is best to deal with an established vendor who has a reputation for reliability and who will be available for training, service, and help. Ask how many medical systems they have installed and the name of users who can be contacted for references. The success of the computer application may depend a great deal on the selection of the vendor, who will advise on the environmental requirements for temperature control, ventilation, power source, and so forth. The vendor's representative should be knowledgeable about medical practice and be able to advise what software can best perform the functions that you need and to help you select compatible hardware. He or she will understand your need for adequate instruction and continuing support after the system is installed. Ask how this support will be provided and what it will cost. How many experienced support personnel are available or on call? Satisfaction is usually greatest when the complete system is purchased from one vendor.

Desirable Hardware Features

There are certain physical features to look for that will assure the user's comfort:

- A tilt and swivel screen that can be adjusted to individual comfort when several persons will be using the terminal
- Adjustable screen brightness/contrast
- Easy-access disk drives
- A keyboard that is separate from the unit
- A separate numerical keypad for accounting entries
- Keys that are not over- or under-responsive

Choosing Software

Available software has a wide range of capabilities. Programs also require various degrees of training to attain proficiency in their use. Software is sometimes referred to as being "user-friendly," meaning that it is relatively easy to learn and use. User-friendly may also mean that the performable functions are limited, possibly too limited for a medical practice. In choosing software, it is important to consider the requirements of the practice first and to make arrangements for whatever training is necessary to operate the system.

Training

After a well-chosen system is in operation, its ultimate success will depend largely on the people who operate it. Formal training sessions are the best way to introduce new users to the system, and each person on the staff who will be operating the computer should receive this formal training. In the learning sessions, the new operators should practice their skills, using data similar in form and content to the actual data that will be processed by the system. Along with the formal training, the vendor should supply good operating manuals and a telephone number to call when difficulties arise that the operator cannot solve.

Computers are here to stay. Let's use and enjoy them.

ADDITIONAL COMPUTER TERMS

back-up Duplicate of a file that is made to protect information.

BASIC An acronym for **B**eginner's **A**ll-purpose **S**ymbolic **I**nstruction **C**ode; a computer language used in most microcomputers.

bit A binary digit; the smallest unit of data in a computer.

boot Starting up a computer.

buffer Temporary storage for data in a computer's memory.

bug Any mistake in a computer program.

byte A unit made up of 8 bits; a byte is roughly equal to one character on the computer keyboard.

CAI An acronym for Computer-Assisted Instruction.

catalog A list of files on the storage media.

chip Integrated circuit chip (ICC); a very tiny wafer of silicon containing thousands of integrated circuits.

CPI Characters per inch; a term used to measure type spacing.

CPS Characters per second; a term used to measure printer speed.

crash A breakdown resulting from software or hardware malfunction.

CRT **C**athode **R**ay **T**ube; the computer monitor.

DOS **D**isk **O**perating **S**ystem; a program that manages the operation of the computer.

font The size and style of type.

graphics Nontext designs and patterns displayed as output.

initialize To prepare a diskette to receive data.

K In electronics, K is short for *kilo*, a prefix meaning *one thousand;* for example, 64K = 64,000 bytes.

loading Storing information in the main memory.

memory Data held in storage in the computer.

menu The list of commands in a program available to the user.

mouse An input device that is separate from the keyboard.

nanosecond One billionth of a second; it is used to measure computer speed.

password A confidential code word or number that must be entered into a computer before the user can access a program or other data.

PC Personal computer.

plotter An output device that draws pictures and graphs on paper.

program A sequence of instructions written in computer language that is designed to cause the computer to carry out a given task.

scroll To move through information on a computer display, either vertically or horizontally, to view information otherwise excluded.

source document A document from which selected data is entered into the computer system.

spreadsheet An automated ledger sheet.

terminal An I/O device that has a keyboard for input and either a video screen or a printer for output.

text Refers to numbers, letters, or keyboard symbols (as opposed to graphics).

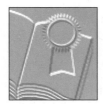

► LEARNING ACHIEVEMENTS

Are you able to:

1. Define the terms listed in the Vocabulary of this chapter?
2. Explain the meaning of the terms *computer hardware* and *software,* and give some examples of each?
3. Explain the need for *function keys* and how to implement their use?
4. Name the two kinds of computer memory and explain the difference?
5. List 10 or more medical office functions that can be performed using a computer?
6. State the reason that a laser printer is not the best printer to use in processing insurance claims?
7. Explain the statement: "Software is the most important component of a computer system"?
8. Discuss the necessity for security guidelines for computerized data in a medical facility?
9. Give a brief description of a computer service bureau?
10. List six ways in which a computer can improve the medical assistant's daily work?

REFERENCES AND READINGS

Diehl, M. O., and Fordney, M. T.: *Medical Typing and Transcribing,* 3rd ed., Philadelphia, W. B. Saunders Co., 1991.

Gylys, B. A.: *Computer Applications for the Medical Office,* Philadelphia, F. A. Davis Co., 1991.

Humphrey, D., and Sigler, K.: *The Modern Medical Office,* Cincinnati, South-Western Publishing Co., 1986.

Stwertka, E., and Stwertka, A.: *Computers in Medicine,* New York, Franklin Watts, Inc., 1984.

Tolos, P. C., and Moody, D.: *How to Choose the Right Computer for Your Medical Practice,* Santa Rosa, CA, Burgess Communications, 1986.

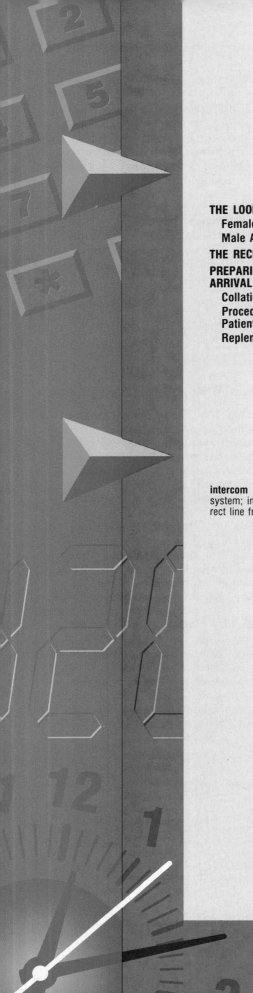

CHAPTER OUTLINE

VOCABULARY

intercom An intercommunication system; in a telephone system, a direct line from one station to another.

oral hygiene Proper care of the mouth and teeth for the maintenance of health and prevention of disease, characterized by clean teeth and absence of unpleasant breath.

phonetic Having to do with the pronunciation or transcription of speech sounds.

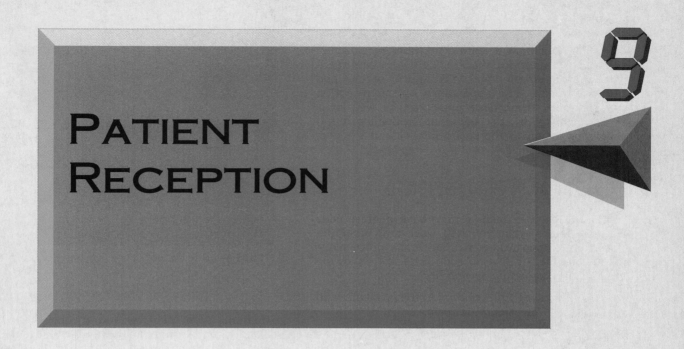

PATIENT RECEPTION

LEARNING OBJECTIVES

COGNITIVE

Upon successful completion of this chapter, you should be able to:

1. Define the words listed in the Vocabulary.

2. Describe the look of a professional.

3. List six considerations in keeping a reception room comfortable for patients.

4. Briefly discuss seven steps in collating patient charts for a day's appointments.

5. State two reasons for checking supplies at the beginning of each day.

6. Identify and discuss the importance of the three components of greeting an arriving patient.

7. Instruct a new patient about providing personal data for the records and completing a registration form.

8. List three actions a medical assistant might take to reduce stress caused by a delayed schedule.

9. Discuss ways a medical assistant might help a physically impaired, uncomfortable, or ill patient.

10. Suggest a way to successfully handle an angry patient.

PERFORMANCE

Upon successful completion of this chapter, you should be able to perform the following activities:

1. Demonstrate how the medical assistant maintains a professional appearance.

2. Follow correct procedure of collating and reviewing patient charts for the day's appointments.

3. Supervise completion of a new patient's registration form.

A first impression is a lasting impression. Nowhere is this more important than in the health care facility, where the environment must appear orderly and faultlessly clean. The appearance of the reception room and the front desk personnel as well as a cordial greeting by the personnel influence a patient's perception of the entire facility and the care he or she will receive.

THE LOOK OF A PROFESSIONAL

Your health care facility may have a dress code that determines what you will wear and other details of your appearance outlined in its office manual. If your facility has no such code, the following guidelines are generally acceptable:

- Appear ready to work in a fresh, clean, and pressed professional uniform.
- Clean and polish your shoes daily.
- Wear your name pin on the right side of your uniform where it can be easily read and wear your professional pin on the left collar.
- Use an unscented deodorant daily and pay particular attention to **oral hygiene.**
- Style your hair so that it is up and off your collar.
- Trim your nails and polish them as appropriate.

Female Assistants

- Wear full-length, neutral shade, run-free hosiery.
- Apply makeup conservatively and use no cologne or perfume.

Male Assistants

- Wear socks that are compatible with your shoes and uniform.
- Your face should be clean-shaven; if you have a mustache or beard, it should be clean and neatly trimmed.

THE RECEPTION ROOM

Take an objective look around the reception room periodically. Could it use a little brightening or freshening up? Try to look at it as if you were seeing it for the first time. The reception room is just that—a place to receive patients. It should be planned for the patient's comfort, made as attractive and cheerful as possible, and kept clean and uncluttered.

Fresh harmonious colors and cleanliness are the basis of an attractive room. Add comfortable furniture that is adequate to accommodate the peak load

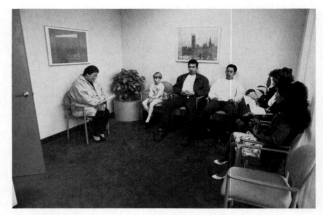

FIGURE 9-1. A comfortable, tasteful reception room.

of patients seen each day and arrange it in conversational groups. Individual chairs are usually best. People sometimes prefer to stand rather than sit next to a stranger on a sofa. Provide good lighting, ventilation, and a regulated temperature for additional comfort, and you have the essentials of an attractive reception room that tells the patient you care. A place to hang coats, rainwear, and umbrellas helps reduce reception room clutter (Fig. 9-1).

Most physicians' offices are well supplied with recent magazines in washable plastic covers. Patients seem to enjoy looking at pictures rather than something that requires concentrated reading. Pictorial travel books and magazines with short items of popular interest are favorites. The reception room, incidentally, is not the place for the physician's professional journals.

Some doctors place a writing desk and writing paper in the room for the convenience of patients; some play restful music over a concealed speaker. Even such additions as a television set, a lighted aquarium, or an educational display of some sort will enhance the attractiveness and individuality of the front door to the doctor's practice.

In pediatric practices, a children's corner, equipped with small-scale furniture and some playthings, is a good idea. It helps keep youngsters occupied who might otherwise get into mischief. Toys should be easily cleanable; plastic washable ones are especially good. Be scrupulously careful that the toy has no sharp corners that could injure a child and that it has no small parts that could be swallowed. Also, in selecting toys, make sure that they will not stimulate the child toward noisy activity. And no rubber balls, for obvious reasons!

It may be necessary to engage a professional designer to suggest reception room improvements that will add to the patient's comfort and enjoyment. The medical assistant is at least partly responsible for the appearance of the reception room by making sure that the room remains neat and orderly throughout the day. A quick check at intervals dur-

---

ADDED ATTRACTIONS FOR RECEPTION AREA

- Plants (fresh or artificial; if artificial arrangements are used, make sure they are dusted or cleaned regularly)
- Pictures
- Travel posters
- Bulletin board displays
- Recent general interest magazines
- Pictorial travel books
- Aquarium (built-in for safety)
- Safe toys for children's corner

---

ing the day and a minute or two devoted to putting the room in order help keep it looking its best.

If the medical assistant's desk is in the reception room or in open view of the patients, it should be free of clutter. In particular, patients' charts or financial cards should not be in sight. Personal articles, coffee cups, and ashtrays should not be on the receptionist's desk (Fig. 9–2).

PREPARING FOR PATIENT ARRIVAL

Advance preparation makes the day go more smoothly and contributes toward a more relaxed atmosphere for all concerned.

Collating Patient Charts

At the beginning of each day, review the appointment list to refresh your memory of the patients' names and any special notations. See that a duplicate of the appointment list is on the physician's desk. Pull the charts for the day, checking the patient's name on your list for accuracy. Occasionally, several patients may have the same or similar names. Double check to make certain you have the right chart.

Review each chart to make certain that any recently received information, such as laboratory reports and x-ray readings, has been correctly entered and that each chart is current. Arrange the charts sequentially in the order the patients are scheduled to be seen. You may be expected to place the charts of all the patients to be seen that day on the physician's desk. It is more likely that the physician will prefer to receive a patient's chart just prior to seeing him or her.

Replenishing Supplies

Supplies at the reception desk need to be replenished regularly. Stationery, appointment cards,

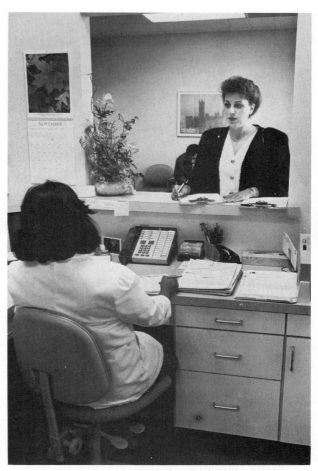

FIGURE 9–2. This reception desk is kept neat and orderly.

charge slips, sharpened pencils, and any items likely to be needed during the day should be on hand when the day begins.

In a multiple-employee practice, a clinical assistant has the responsibility of checking clinical supplies. However, in a small practice there may be only one assistant in charge. Before patients start arriving, everything should be ready for the day so that the doctor and medical assistant can give undivided attention to the patients' needs.

Check all rooms to make certain that:

- Everything is clean
- Cabinets are well-stocked
- Patients will receive complete attention

GREETING THE PATIENT

Every patient has the right to expect courteous treatment in the physician's office. No matter what the patient's economic or social status, each indi-

PROCEDURE 9-1   COLLATING PATIENT CHARTS

GOAL To collate patient charts for daily appointment schedule and have them ready for the physician before patients' arrival.

EQUIPMENT AND SUPPLIES

Appointment schedule for current date   Patient files
Clerical supplies (pen, tape, stapler,
   etc.)

PROCEDURAL STEPS

1. Review the appointment schedule.
2. Identify full name of each scheduled patient.
3. Pull patients' charts from files, checking each patient's name on your list as each chart is pulled.
   Purpose: To determine that the correct charts have been pulled and that none have been omitted.
4. Review each chart.
   Purpose: To reaffirm that:
   - All information has been correctly entered.
   - Any previously ordered tests have been performed.
   - The results have been entered on the chart.
5. Annotate the appointment list with any special concerns.
   Purpose: To alert the physician regarding matters that should be checked or discussed with the patient.
6. Arrange all charts sequentially according to each patient's appointment.
7. Place the charts in the appropriate examination room or other specified location.

---

vidual who enters the reception room should receive a cordial, friendly greeting.

- Using the personal touch in receiving patients is important. Cultivate the habit of greeting each patient immediately in a friendly, self-assured manner. Establish eye contact, smile, and introduce yourself to the new patient, giving your name and job title: "Good morning, I'm Elizabeth, Dr. Wade's medical assistant."
- Greet the established patient by name. Learn how to pronounce each patient's name correctly, as incorrect pronunciations may offend and irritate some people. If the name is unusual, write the **phonetic** spelling on the history for reference.
- Try to remember the patients' names and something personal about each one. Jot down key words on the patient's chart that will provide reminders for future conversations. Most patients appreciate the interest of the doctor and the staff in their families, hobbies, and work.

Ideally, the medical assistant's desk is placed for a clear view of all visitors who come into the office. If there is only one medical assistant, it is sometimes impossible for each new caller to be welcomed personally. In this situation, some announcement system must be worked out. The patient who enters an empty reception room does not know whether to sit down or to try to announce his presence in some way. Sometimes a register is placed in the reception room with a sign above it reading: "Please sign the register when you arrive. Doctor will see you shortly." This is a makeshift arrangement and should be avoided, since patient confidentiality is violated when others can read the register.

REGISTRATION FORMS: PERSONAL HISTORY

A patient coming in for a first visit requires certain introductory procedures. Most physicians use a patient information form of some kind to gather subjective information about the patient. The medical assistant may complete the form while interviewing the new patient or have the patient complete the form upon arrival for the first appointment. The form may be attached to a clipboard and handed to the patient with instructions to complete all parts of the form, with assurance that the assistant is ready and willing to answer any questions.

The patient's name and date of birth should appear prominently at the top of the form, followed by the name of the responsible person and pertinent information in logical order as follows:

- Patient's name and date of birth
- Responsible person's name
    Relationship to patient
    Address and telephone number
    Name, address, and telephone number of employer
    Occupation
    Social Security number
    Driver's license number
- Responsible person's spouse's name (in some community property states, both spouses are equally responsible)
    Include same information as for responsible person
- Nearest relative not living with patient and his or her relationship
- Source of referral, if any

Since the registration form is also, in effect, an application for credit, its content and form is subject to regulations of the Equal Credit Opportunity Act of 1975. Under this act, if you ask for marital status, only the terms married, unmarried, and separated may be used. Terms such as divorced or widowed are not permitted (Fig. 9–3).

When the completed form is returned to the medical assistant, it should be checked carefully to be certain that all the necessary information has been included.

The personal and medical history and the patient's family history may be obtained by asking the patient to complete a questionnaire; the physician can augment this information during the patient interview. The more experienced medical assistant may be expected to interview the patient for the patient's personal and medical history, family history, and chief complaint. This is a very specialized

procedure, and the interviewer will most likely be specifically trained for the individual practice.

CONSIDERATION FOR PATIENTS' TIME

Once the preliminaries have been completed, the patient will expect to see the doctor at the appointed time. The medical assistant should get the patient in to see the doctor as near the appointment time as possible or explain to the patient why he or she must wait. It is your responsibility as the medical assistant to convey both your own and the doctor's concern if there will be a delay. Consideration for the patient's time is extremely important.

Most experts agree that in a well-managed, busy office there are seldom more than three to five patients in the reception room. "Too long a wait in the doctor's office" is one of the most frequently heard criticisms of the medical profession. The patient who complains about medical fees or care may in actuality be complaining about the long wait or discourteous service.

A crowded waiting room is not always an indication of a doctor's popularity. It may simply mean that the doctor or the assistant is inefficient in scheduling patients.

Business people, for example, who are in the habit of making the most of their time, are particularly displeased at what may appear to them to be inefficient scheduling of appointments. Any delay of longer than 15 minutes should be explained to the person waiting.

When a prolonged wait is unavoidable, and this has been explained to the patient, the medical assistant may be able to help the patients pass the time by suggesting a particularly good story or article in a magazine to a patient who wants to read or by chatting briefly with a restless patient. It should, however, be the patient's decision as to whether or not to talk. Select conversation subjects that interest the patient—hobbies, family, business, profession, or recreational interests—and avoid discussions that include religion, politics, or the patient's health. A patient is favorably impressed with an assistant who is well versed on such subjects as health insurance, new medical discoveries, local health agencies, and other topics pertaining to medical care that patients may raise during conversation. Printed literature to answer patients' questions on these subjects is usually available from medical organizations. Active members of medical assistants' groups keep well informed by attending local meetings regularly.

Some personal attention, such as offering a drink of water, a cup of coffee, or a new magazine, sometimes calms a patient who is becoming visibly irritated at waiting.

Many patients are fearful and tense, but the medical assistant can often put them in a better frame

Today's Date _____

PATIENT INFORMATION SHEET

Patient's
Name _____
           First   Middle   Last

Date of Birth ___/___/___
    Mo Day Year

Responsible
Person's Name _____
         First   Middle   Last   Relationship

Address _____
    Number   Street   City   State   Zip   Area / Phone

Employer _____ Department or Occupation _____

Address _____
    Number   Street   City   State   Zip   Area / Phone

Social
Security Number _____ Driver's License Number _____

Spouse of
Resp. Person _____
         First   Middle   Last   Area / Phone

Employer _____ Department or Occupation _____

Address _____
    Number   Street   City   State   Zip   Area / Phone

Social
Security Number _____ Driver's License Number _____

Nearest relative
(not living with you) _____
                       Relationship

Address _____
    Number   Street   City   State   Zip   Area / Phone

Patient referred
to this office by _____

AUTHORIZATION TO PAY BENEFITS TO PHYSICIAN: I hereby authorize payment of any insurance benefits covering these medical charges directly to the physician/surgeon.
Signature of the Insured _____ Date _____

AUTHORIZATION TO RELEASE INFORMATION: I hereby authorize the physician/surgeon to release any medical information to my insurance company.
Responsible person's signature _____ Date _____

STATEMENT OF FINANCIAL RESPONSIBILITY: I, _____, do hereby agree to pay all medical charges incurred by the above listed patient. I further understand that these charges are my responsibility regardless of insurance coverage. Responsible person's signature _____

FIGURE 9–3. Patient information sheet and credit application. (Courtesy of Credit Service Systems, Anaheim, CA.)

of mind merely with a friendly smile and a show of concern.

The medical assistant can help keep the appointment schedule operating smoothly by immediately tidying each examination room and moving the next patient in so that the doctor need have no idle moments waiting for a patient to be prepared. Try not to place a patient in an examining room just to clear out the reception area. It is especially inconsiderate to keep the patient waiting after being gowned,

PROCEDURE 9-2 REGISTERING A NEW PATIENT

GOAL To complete registration form for a new patient, obtaining adequate information for credit and insurance claims.

EQUIPMENT AND SUPPLIES

Registration form
Clerical supplies (pen, clipboard)

Private conference area

PROCEDURAL STEPS

1. Determine whether the patient is new.

2. Obtain and record the necessary information:
   - Full name, birth date, name of spouse (if married)
   - Home address, telephone number (include ZIP code and area code)
   - Occupation, name of employer, business address, telephone number
   - Social Security number and driver's license number, if any
   - Name of referring physician, if any
   - Name and address of person responsible for payment
   - Method of payment
   - Health insurance information
   - Name of primary carrier
   - Type of coverage
   - Group policy number
   - Subscriber number
   - Assignment of benefits, if required

   Purpose: This information is necessary for credit and insurance claims.

3. Review the entire form.
   Purpose: To be certain that information is complete and legible.

---

draped, and positioned on the examining table. A magazine rack on the wall of the treatment room is a welcome addition in some offices.

ESCORTING AND INSTRUCTING THE PATIENT

Sometimes we become so accustomed to our own surroundings that we forget that the stranger may be confused or disoriented by all the hallways, doors, and rooms. Do take time to personally escort the patient to the appropriate examination or treatment room. This is usually the responsibility of the clinical medical assistant. If the patient is to disrobe, explain what garments, if any, can be left on, whether shoes are to be removed, that they must remove jewelry if an x-ray is to be taken, and so forth. If a gown is to be worn, specify whether the opening should be in front or back, and tell the patients where they can hang their clothes if this is not obvious. All instructions must be clear. Do not assume that patients will know what you want if you have not told them.

Be equally clear when the examination has been completed: "You can get dressed now and return to the consultation room," or "After you are dressed, please stop by the desk to make your next appointment."

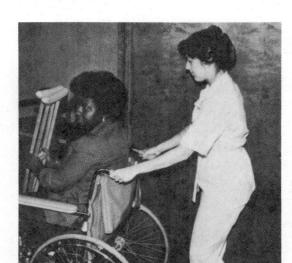

FIGURE 9-4. The medical assistant helps a disabled patient. (Courtesy of Ferris State College, Big Rapids, MI.)

ASSISTING THE DISABLED PATIENT

Some patients will be physically impaired, some will be very ill, and some will be severely uncomfortable.

Observe the patient's appearance and behavior. Is the patient pale or drawn looking? Do the eyes or voice reflect pain or discomfort? Find out how the patient is feeling before you suggest that he or she be seated to wait for the doctor. The patient may need to lie down in a cool room or perhaps should be seen as an emergency. The patient in a wheelchair or walker or using crutches may need a bit of personal attention. Some patients may need help in disrobing even when a disability is not obvious. Ask if you can be of assistance. The medical assistant must use good judgment in helping disabled patients, perhaps even bypassing some of the usual routines (Fig. 9–4).

HANDLING PATIENTS' COMPLAINTS

Even under the best of conditions, there will at times be complaints from patients. Remember that the practice of medicine is a personal service for individual personalities, and the medical assistant must cultivate the skill of listening. Each patient is a very important person, and any complaint should be taken seriously. Try to resolve the matter if it is within your realm of responsibility. Otherwise, assure the patient of your concern and explain that

you will try to find a solution. Then be sure to carry through.

PROBLEM SITUATIONS

The Talker

There are certain problem patients in any professional office. The talker, for example, takes up far more of the doctor's time than is justified. An alert medical assistant can usually spot this tendency during the initial interview. The patient's history can be checked with a symbol to alert the doctor. A prearranged agreement to contact the doctor on the **intercom** at the end of the appointment time, with the message that the next patient has arrived, gives the doctor an opportunity to conclude the interview. Once you have learned which patients take extra time, you can book them for the end of the day or simply allow more time for them.

Children

Children sometimes present special management problems. It is often advisable for young patients to go into the treatment room without the parent. This, of course, should be at the discretion of the physician.

While this practice of separating children from their parents to treat their needs is not always feasible, it sometimes can be applied with great success. In some offices, a token of the doctor's friendship, such as a trinket or toy, is given to the child at the completion of the visit.

The Angry Patient

Every medical assistant at some time is confronted with an angry patient. The anger may be simply a reflection of the patient's pain or fear of what the doctor may discover on the examination. It is usually best to let such patients talk out their anger. A calm attitude on the part of the medical assistant, with a few remarks interjected in a low voice, will often quiet the patient. Under no circumstances should the assistant return the anger or become argumentative.

The Patient's Relatives

A patient will sometimes be accompanied by a relative or well-meaning friend who may become restless while waiting for the patient and attempt to discuss the patient's illness. The medical assistant should sidestep any discussion of a patient's medical care, except by direction of the physician. Also avoid a too casual attitude, such as, "I'm sure there's nothing to worry about." A show of moderate concern and offering reassurance that "the patient is in good hands" usually takes care of the situation.

FRIENDLY FAREWELLS

A medical assistant should be ready to take charge of the patient as soon as the visit with the physician has been completed by assisting the patient in dressing, if necessary, and by making sure that any questions that the patient may have are answered. In a small practice, this may be the responsibility of the administrative medical assistant. If the patient has nontechnical questions that the assistant can capably answer, the assistant should answer them clearly and note this on the patient's chart. Some patient questions can be answered only by the physician; in such a case, the assistant can offer to get answers for the patient.

The assistant can help convey the impression of friendliness by terminating the patient's visit cordially. If the patient is returning for another visit, the medical assistant can say something like "We'll see you next week." If it is the patient's last visit, a pleasant "I certainly hope you'll be feeling fine from now on" is appropriate. The assistant may want to tell a patient on his (or her) last visit that he has been a fine patient and that it has been a pleasure to serve him. Whatever words of goodbye are chosen, all patients should leave the doctor's office feeling that they have received top-quality care and were treated with friendliness and courtesy.

▶ LEARNING ACHIEVEMENTS

Are you able to:

1. Define the terms in the Vocabulary of this chapter?
2. Maintain a professional appearance and understand its importance?
3. Make suggestions other than those mentioned in this chapter for keeping a reception room comfortable?
4. List and discuss the importance of the seven steps in collating charts for patient appointments?
5. Explain why the medical assistant should review the chart of an established patient who is scheduled for appointment?
6. Explain why it is important to check supplies at the beginning of each day?
7. State the acceptable limit of appointment delays, and discuss how the medical assistant can have a positive effect on the patient who must wait beyond the appointed time?
8. List at least 10 items that should be completed on a patient registration form?

REFERENCES AND READINGS

American Medical Association: *Winning Ways with Patients,* Chicago, The Association, 1979.
Conomikes Associates, Inc.: *Patient Flow Management,* 1991.

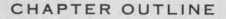

CHAPTER OUTLINE

APPOINTMENT SCHEDULING
 Open Office Hours
 Scheduled Appointments
 Flexible Office Hours
THE APPOINTMENT BOOK
 Selection
  Basic Features of
   Appointment Book
  Additional Considerations
 Advance Preparation
GUIDELINES FOR SCHEDULING
 Patient Need
 Doctor's Preferences and
 Habits
 Available Facilities
 Appointment Time Pattern
 Same-Day Service
TIME MANAGEMENT
 Wave Scheduling
 Procedure 10–1: Preparing
 and Maintaining the
 Appointment Book
 Modified Wave Scheduling
 Double Booking
 Grouping Procedures
 Advance Booking

**DETAILS OF ARRANGING
APPOINTMENTS**
 In Person
 Appointment Cards and
 Reminders
 Appointments by Telephone
 Appointments for New
 Patients
 Procedure 10–2: Scheduling
 a New Patient
 Special Problems
 Rescheduling an Appointment
**EXCEPTIONS TO APPOINTMENT
SYSTEM**
 Emergency Patients
 Acutely Ill Patients
 Physician Referrals
FAILED APPOINTMENTS
 Reasons for Failed
 Appointments
 No-Show Policy
 Charging for Failed
 Appointments
 Recording the Failed
 Appointment

**HANDLING CANCELLATIONS
AND DELAYS**
 When the Patient Cancels
 When the Doctor Is Delayed
 When the Doctor Is Called
 Out on Emergencies
 When the Doctor Is Ill or Is
 Called Out of Town
**SCHEDULING OUTSIDE
APPOINTMENTS**
 Surgeries
 House Calls
 Outside Appointments for
 Patients
 Procedure 10–3: Scheduling
 Outpatient Diagnostic Tests
**PATIENTS WITHOUT
APPOINTMENTS**
OTHER CALLERS
 Physicians
 Pharmaceutical
 Representatives
 Salespersons
 Miscellaneous
LEARNING ACHIEVEMENTS

VOCABULARY

deviation A noticeable or marked departure from accepted norms of behavior.

disruption A breaking down or upset.

integral Essential; being an indispensable part of a whole.

interaction A two-way communication.

intermittent Coming and going at intervals; not continuous.

matrix Something in which something else originates, develops, takes shape, or is contained; a base upon which to build.

no-show A person who fails to keep an appointment without giving advance notice of such failure.

prerogative An exclusive and unquestionable right belonging to a person or body of persons.

proficient Competent as a result of training and practice.

socioeconomic Relating to a combination of social and economic factors.

stat report An immediate report (from the Latin *statim*, meaning "at once").

tickler (file) A chronologic file used as a reminder that something must be taken care of on a certain date.

APPOINTMENT SCHEDULING AND TIME MANAGEMENT

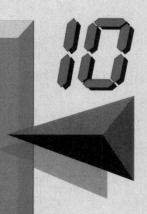

LEARNING OBJECTIVES

COGNITIVE
Upon successful completion of this chapter, you should be able to:

1. Define the terms listed in the Vocabulary.

2. Describe four important features of an appointment book.

3. List and explain the three basic guidelines to follow in scheduling appointments.

4. Identify and discuss the advantages of wave scheduling.

5. Cite three common situations that would require adjusting the appointment schedule.

6. Describe how you would determine whether a request for an appointment is an emergency.

7. State the reason for recording a failed appointment on the patient's chart.

8. Discuss the handling of cancellations and delays brought about by office situations.

9. List at least six points of information that will be necessary in scheduling surgery with a hospital.

10. State four items of information that must be available before arranging an outside laboratory appointment for a patient.

PERFORMANCE
Upon successful completion of this chapter, you should be able to perform the following activities:

1. Select an appropriate appointment book to suit a given type of practice.

2. Demonstrate the advance preparation that must be done before using a new appointment book.

3. Schedule patients according to the urgency of their complaints and the anticipated treatment time.

4. Rearrange the schedule in the event that the physician's arrival is delayed.

5. Explain the physician's unavailability to patients in the reception room.

6. Arrange a referral appointment for a patient.

7. Schedule a patient for a diagnostic test as indicated by the physician.

8. Schedule a surgery with the hospital, notifying all the persons and departments concerned.

9. Instruct a patient regarding preadmission requirements, hospital stay, and insurance information needed.

10. Arrange for a patient's admission to a hospital as ordered by the physician.

APPOINTMENT SCHEDULING

Appointment scheduling is the process that determines which patients will be seen by the physician, how soon they will be seen, and how much time will be allotted to each patient based on his or her complaint and the physician's availability. A vital step in efficient time management is to realize that there will always be unforeseen interruptions and delays. Most providers of medical care find that efficient scheduling of appointments is one of the most important factors in the success of the practice. However, some providers do no scheduling. They conduct their practices with open office hours.

Open Office Hours

With open office hours, the facility is open at given hours of the day or evening, and the patients are probably "scheduled" by the physician's or the medical assistant's saying something such as, "Come back in a couple of weeks." At a convenient time, the patients come in to see the doctor, knowing in advance that they will be seen in their order of arrival. Physicians who use this method say that it eliminates the annoyance of broken appointments and of the office "running late." The open office hours method has been referred to as "tidal wave scheduling."

Few doctors' offices in metropolitan areas have open office hours—no scheduled appointments—but this system is common in some rural areas, where the way of life is governed not so much by the clock as by the sun and the seasons. Another type of practice that has open hours is the growing number of emergency centers, many of which are open on a 24-hour basis. Although they are frequently called "emergicenters," they may in reality deal with many general practice types of cases.

There can be many disadvantages to open office hours:

- The office may be crowded when the doctor arrives, resulting in extremely long waits for some patients.
- There is the danger of rushing some patients through without giving them full attention.
- It is also possible that few or none will arrive before afternoon, and both doctor and staff will have to stay late to see everyone.
- Without planning, the facilities as well as the staff can be overburdened.

Scheduled Appointments

Studies have shown that physicians are able to see more patients with less pressure when they schedule appointments.

If appointments are made by telephone, that first telephone **interaction** creates the patient's impres-

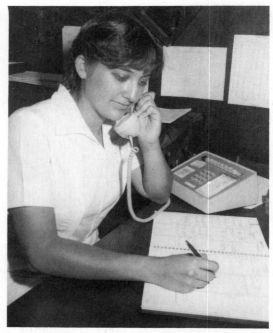

FIGURE 10-1. Medical assistant scheduling an appointment. (Courtesy of Southern California College of Medical and Dental Careers. Photo by Dan Santucci.)

sion of the medical facilities. Unfortunately, the skill required for the scheduling of appointments is often not fully appreciated by the physician, and this responsibility may be delegated to the least qualified medical assistant. But while the skill and attitude of the assistant who manages the appointment schedule is very important, the ultimate success of the system lies in the cooperation of the physician(s).

Efficient scheduling requires an understanding of the following:

- the practice
- the personality and habits of the physician(s)
- a close estimate of the time needed for each patient

Planning appointments realistically and seeing that the physician starts on time and sticks to the schedule will please the patients, bring economic gain to the physician, and assure a more regular schedule for both the medical assistant and the physician (Fig. 10-1).

Flexible Office Hours

Most scheduling practices are carryovers from the days when expectant mothers or families with young children relied on one wage-earner—the father. Today, families commonly have two working parents. Many health care providers, especially family physicians, pediatricians, obstetricians, gynecologists, and ophthalmologists, are turning to extended day and flexible office hours. Staff hours are affected by these changes. For example, on 1 day per week, office hours might begin at 7 AM and end at 3 PM; on a second day, office hours might be from noon to 8 PM; and on the remaining days, the traditional 9 AM to 5 PM schedule is maintained. In this manner, a variety of options are made available to patients. Flexible scheduling is most easily accomplished in group practices or partnerships.

THE APPOINTMENT BOOK
Selection

Office suppliers and stationers carry a variety of appointment book styles. One of the standard preprinted styles will be satisfactory for a physician who is just starting a practice, but as the practice develops, the physician may find the preprinted books too restrictive. When this happens, it is time to look for an appointment book that more closely suits the practice, or, failing this, to personally design one. In either case, there are certain basic features to consider.

Basic Features of Appointment Book
- Size conforms to the desk space available
- Large enough to accommodate the practice
- Opens flat for easy writing and reference
- Allows space for writing when, who, and why

Additional Considerations
- Pages that show an entire week at a glance
- Color coding, with a special color for each day of the week
- Multiple columns corresponding with the number of doctors in a group practice
- Division into time units suitable to the practice

Many professional stationers furnish planning kits and work with you to develop what is best for the practice. Some of these resources are listed at the end of the chapter (Fig. 10–2).

Advance Preparation

Having chosen an appropriate book, some advance preparation should be done. This is sometimes called "establishing the **matrix**." Block off, in pencil, those periods when the doctor is routinely not available to see patients (days off, holidays, hospital rounds, lunch, meetings, and so forth). In the space where you would ordinarily write the patient's name, write a memo showing the reason for blocking off these spaces. Always try to account for every time period in each day.

If the physician keeps you informed of social or family engagements, also make a note of these as a reminder.

GUIDELINES FOR SCHEDULING

The scheduling system must be individualized to each specific practice. The following guidelines are general and can be applied to any practice:
- Patient need
- Doctor's preferences and habits
- Available facilities

Patient Need

A major general consideration in determining office hours and appointment times is the **socioeconomic** status of the area being served—Is it agricultural? a retirement community? industrial? Who are the patients? Are evening and Saturday appointments essential for some?

More specifically, time must be allotted to patients on the basis of each one's particular needs. This can be assessed by asking patients such questions as:
- What is the purpose of the visit?
- What is the age of the patient? (A teenager will probably not require as much time as an older patient.)
- Will the patient require the doctor's time for the entire visit, or will another member of the staff be performing part or all of the service?
- Is the patient a young mother who prefers to schedule her appointments during the school hours?
- Is the patient a day-worker who cannot take time off?
- Is the patient a child whose parents are both working during the day?

Doctor's Preferences and Habits

Some doctors become restless if the reception room is not packed with waiting patients; others worry if one patient is kept waiting. All these personal preferences and habits become an **integral** part of the scheduling process. The preferences of the doctors in your facility must be considered before a schedule can be established.
- Is the doctor methodical and careful about being in the office when patient appointments are scheduled to begin? Some doctors are habitually late.
- Does the doctor move easily from one patient to the next? Some require a "break" time between patients.

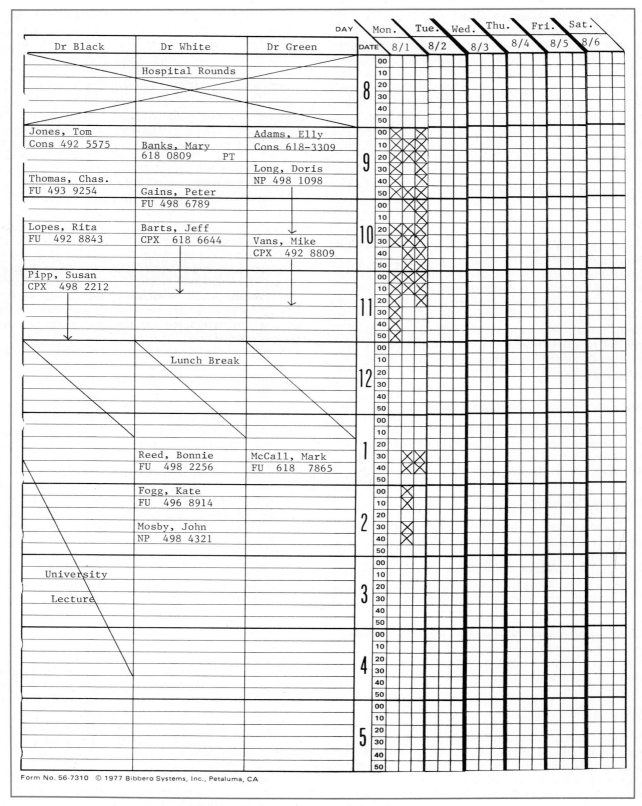

FIGURE 10–2. Sample appointment book page for three physicians.

- Would the physician rather see fewer patients and spend more time with each one? If so, this must be taken into account in the scheduling process.

Keep in mind that the physician cannot spend every moment of the day with patients. There are telephone calls to receive, reports to examine and dictate, meetings to attend, mail to answer, and many other business items that require the physician's attention. The experienced staff can handle many but not all of these tasks.

Available Facilities

There's no point in getting a patient into the office at a time when no facilities are available for the services needed. For instance, suppose that in a two-physician office there is only one room that can be used for minor surgery. You would not schedule two patients requiring minor surgery for the same time block even though both doctors could be available. If there is only one electrocardiograph, you would not book two ECGs at the same time. As you become **proficient** in scheduling, you should be able to pair patients' needs with the available facilities.

Appointment Time Pattern

The physician who has been practicing for years knows how much time is needed for the various kinds of office visits: complete physical, presurgery workup, well-child visit, eye examination, and so forth. The physician is the one who should decide how long a visit should be, and an estimated time schedule should be at the appointment desk. Since the doctor's timing does change through the years, an annual review of the time schedule should be made to accommodate these changes as well as changes in the patient profile.

It may be that a time pattern has never been determined. The medical assistant can do the preliminary work on this through an informal practice analysis, noting the arrival time, treatment or conference time, departure time, and service performed (Fig. 10–3). After a few weeks, a definite time pattern should be distinguishable for each type of service. When possible, smooth out the schedule by having some long and some short appointments and go over the schedule with the doctor at the beginning of each day.

APPOINTMENT TIME ANALYSIS

NAME	ARRIVED	BEGIN TREATMENT	END TREATMENT	SERVICE CODE

SUMMARY

SERVICE	AVERAGE WAITING TIME	AVERAGE TREATMENT TIME

FIGURE 10–3. Sample form for determining appointment pattern.

Same-Day Service

Ideally, the scheduling system should provide for same-day service for acutely ill patients, for emergencies, and for seeing all scheduled patients on time. New patients are sometimes treated as emergencies. Calls for appointments may be categorized as *emergencies, urgent,* or *routine.* Emergencies may include emotional crises as well as the more obvious physical problems, and patients having emergencies generally should be seen the same day. The physician should define what is to be considered urgent as well as the time frame for scheduling urgent appointments (probably within 1 to 4 days).

Every doctor's schedule should have at least one, or preferably two, appointment slots open each day. These slots are usually referred to as "buffer time." Family practitioners may want to leave as much as 25% of their time open for emergencies and work-in patients. Many doctors find that reserving one time slot at the end of the morning and one at the end of the afternoon works well and causes the least **disruption** of a schedule.

Time studies have shown that in the average medical practice, Mondays and Fridays are the most hectic days of the week. Patients may have waited the whole weekend to call for an appointment and expect to be seen immediately on Monday. Similarly, toward the end of the week, small problems that could magnify if left unattended over the weekend may prompt emotional emergencies on Friday. Hence, incorporating more empty slots on these 2 days can be worthwhile.

TIME MANAGEMENT

Wave Scheduling

Many scheduling systems lack flexibility. Wave scheduling is an attempt to correlate a time schedule with the variables brought about by patients who need more time or less time than planned for, by a patient who arrives late, and by other unavoidable **deviations** from the schedule, such as the patient who fails to keep an appointment **(no-show)** and unscheduled (work-in) patients. In wave scheduling, an attempt is made to start and finish each hour on time.

What happens when all patients are assigned the same length of time? With a patient scheduled every 20 minutes the schedule might look like this:

> 10:00 Alicia Barker
> 10:20 Colleen Davies
> 10:40 Edna Farber
>
> 11:00 Gertrude Havens
> 11:20 Irene Jackson
> 11:40 Katherine Lambert

Mrs. Barker, the first patient, arrives at 10:15. The physician has already lost 15 minutes. The patient needs 25 minutes instead of the allotted 20 minutes. Mrs. Davis, the second patient, also arrived at 10:15, 5 minutes early for her appointment, but is kept waiting until 10:40, the time that Mrs. Farber, the third patient, was to have been seen. Mrs. Farber is on time but will also be kept waiting. Fortunately, Mrs. Davis actually needs only 10 minutes, so Mrs. Farber can be seen at 10:50, but if she requires the allotted 20 minutes, Mrs. Havens, the fourth patient, will also have to wait, and so on throughout the day.

Wave scheduling assumes that the actual time needed will average out. If the average time is 20 minutes per patient, three patients will be scheduled for each hour and be seen in order of arrival. Thus, one person's late arrival will not disrupt the entire schedule. The appointment schedule would then look like this:

> 10:00 Alicia Barker
> Colleen Davis
> Edna Farber
>
> 11:00 Gertrude Havens
> Irene Jackson
> Katherine Lambert

Given the circumstances illustrated above, Mrs. Davis would have arrived first (5 minutes early), Mrs. Farber would be next (on time), and Mrs. Barker would be third (15 minutes late). All could have been seen within the hour, with no delay affecting the patients scheduled for the next hour.

Modified Wave Scheduling

There are several ways of modifying the wave schedule. One method is to have two patients scheduled to come in at 10:00 and the third at 10:30, with this hourly cycle repeated throughout the day. Another application is to have patients scheduled to arrive at given intervals during the first half of the hour, and none scheduled to arrive during the second half of the hour.

Double Booking

Booking two patients to come in at the same time, both of whom are to be seen by the doctor, is poor practice. Of course, if each is expected to take only 5 minutes or so, there is no harm in telling both to come at 2:00 and in reserving a 15-minute period for the two. This is an application of wave scheduling. However, if each patient requires 15 minutes, two will require 30 minutes; this should be reflected in the schedule. It is not considered double booking if a patient comes to the office to receive a treatment or injection from the medical assistant.

PROCEDURE 10-1   PREPARING AND MAINTAINING THE APPOINTMENT BOOK

GOAL To establish the matrix of the appointment page, arrange appointments for 1 day, and enter information according to office policy.

EQUIPMENT AND SUPPLIES

Page from appointment book
Office policy for office hours, and
   doctor's availability

Clerical supplies
Calendar
Description of patients to be scheduled

PROCEDURAL STEPS

1. Determine the hours that the physician will not be available.
   Purpose: So that those hours can be blocked out on the appointment page.

2. Establish the matrix of the appointment page for the day.
   Purpose: To leave available only those time slots that can be used for patient appointments.

3. Identify each patient's complaint.
   Purpose: You must have this information in order to allot time and space for the appointment.

4. Consult guidelines to determine the length of time necessary for each patient.

5. Allot appointment time according to the complaint and facilities available.

6. Enter information in the appointment book.
   Note: A telephone number must follow the patient's name. If the patient is new, add the letters N.P. (new patient) after his or her name.

7. Allow buffer time in the morning and afternoon.
   Purpose: To allow the physician and staff a short rest period and catch-up time.

Grouping Procedures

Another method of time management that appeals to some practitioners is the grouping of procedures; for example:

- An internist might reserve all morning appointments for complete physicals.
- A surgeon whose practice depends on referrals might reserve 1 day per week or specific hours on each day for referrals.
- A pediatrician might have well-baby hours.

By experimenting with different groupings, you will eventually find what works best for the practice at which you work. In applying a grouping system of appointments, the medical assistant may find it helpful to lightly color-code those sections of the appointment book being reserved for special procedures.

Advance Booking

When booking appointments weeks or months ahead, make it a policy to leave some open time during each day's schedule. Then, if a patient calls with a special problem that is not an immediate emergency, you will be able to book the patient for at least a brief visit. The busy doctor will always be able to fill these open slots, and the patients will appreciate being able to see their doctor within a reasonable time when the circumstances warrant it.

Some authorities recommend that appointments not be scheduled more than 3 months in advance.

If possible, set time aside in the morning and afternoon for a "breather," or work break. Even 15 or 20 minutes will give the doctor an opportunity to return calls from patients, verify prescription calls, or answer questions you may have that were not an emergency.

DETAILS OF ARRANGING APPOINTMENTS

Many return appointments are arranged while a patient is in the office. The patient's first appointment, though, will probably be made by telephone. Pleasantness on the part of the medical assistant who sets up the appointment is extremely important, whether he or she makes the appointment face-to-face or by telephone.

In Person

The physician will probably ask the patient to stop at the desk and make another appointment before leaving the office. While you reach for your pencil and the appointment book, look at the patient and say something such as, "Will next Thursday, the 8th, at 10:00 AM be satisfactory?" Avoid asking the question, "When would you like to come in?" Chances are that this will only initiate a debate, and the patient may finally decide on a time that you do not have available. Write the patient's name and telephone number in the book and give the patient a completed appointment card (after you have double-checked the date and time against the information in your book), along with your best smile. Give the patient any necessary instructions.

Appointment Cards and Reminders

Most offices use cards to remind patients of scheduled appointments, as well as to eliminate misunderstandings about dates and times (Fig. 10–4).

Make a habit of reaching for an appointment card while writing an entry in the appointment book. After you have written the date and time on the appointment card, double-check with the book to see that the entries agree. Patients who have made appointments in advance may be sent a reminder card or notified by telephone near the time of the appointment.

A patient who is due for an appointment but has not yet arranged a date and time may be sent a recall reminder. A simple way of handling this is to have a supply of postal cards on hand; while the patients are still in the office, have them write their name and address on a card. Then place it in a file box under the date it is to be mailed.

Appointments by Telephone

It is as important for the medical assistant to express pleasantness and a desire to be helpful when using the telephone as it is when meeting patients face to face. This is particularly essential in the arranging of appointments, since it is often the manner in which the booking is made rather than the convenience of the appointment time that makes a lasting impression.

Study the principles of telephone technique as set forth in the next chapter, Telephone Techniques. Be especially considerate if you must refuse an appointment for the time requested. Explain why and offer a substitute time and date. It should also be determined whether the patient has been in before and whether any necessary insurance information has been obtained. Comply with the patient's desires as much as possible and do not show impatience if a patient is not understanding of the problems involved in scheduling appointments. Most people do appreciate the need for a well-managed office and are willing to cooperate. End the conversation pleasantly with something like this: "Thank you for calling, Mrs. Albright. Dr. Wright will see you next Wednesday, the 28th, at 2:30. Goodbye." This little courtesy adds to the patient's feeling of esteem and additionally reinforces the time of the appointment. While you are saying this, you should be rechecking your appointment page to be certain you have written it in the right time slot on the right day.

Appointments for New Patients

Arranging the first appointment for a new patient requires a bit more time and attention to detail. Carefully check the correct spelling of the patient's name by repeating it or spelling it back. Obtain the address, the daytime telephone number where the patient can be reached, the patient's birth date, and the name of the referring doctor or individual. If possible, determine the nature of the visit so that the proper amount of time can be allotted in the appointment book. Financial arrangements should be made at the time of the first visit.

If the appointment is several days away, mail to the patient a Patient Information brochure (see Chapter 22, Management Responsibilities), a registration form, and a "welcome" letter. The brochure should provide advance information to the patient about the nature of the practice, introduce the doctor(s), and explain appointment policies and financial arrangements.

If another physician has referred the patient, the medical assistant may need to call the referring physician's office and obtain additional information before the patient's appointment. This information should be typed and given to the doctor in advance of the patient's arrival.

Affix this reminder to your calendar.

M__________________

HAS AN APPOINTMENT WITH

PARK AVENUE PROFESSIONAL GROUP
2100 WEST PARK AVENUE
CHAMPAIGN, ILLINOIS 61820
Telephone

APPOINTMENT
DR. ____________
Day ____________
Date ____________
Time ____________

ON _____ / _____ / _____ AM PM

THIS TIME IS RESERVED EXCLUSIVELY FOR YOU. 24 HOURS NOTICE IS APPRECIATED IF YOU ARE UNABLE TO KEEP YOUR APPOINTMENT.

ADMIT ONE

RESERVED SEATING

FOR __________________

DAY DATE TIME
24 HOUR NOTICE NECESSARY FOR CANCELLATION.

PARK AVENUE PROFESSIONAL GROUP
2100 WEST PARK AVENUE
CHAMPAIGN, ILLINOIS 61820
TELEPHONE

ADMIT ONE

M__________________

HAS AN APPOINTMENT WITH

PARK AVENUE PROFESSIONAL GROUP
2100 WEST PARK AVENUE
SUITE 1135
CHAMPAIGN, ILLINOIS 61820
TELEPHONE

FOR

MON. __________ AT______
TUES. __________ AT______
WED. __________ AT______
THURS. __________ AT______
FRI. __________ AT______
SAT. __________ AT______

IF UNABLE TO KEEP THIS APPOINTMENT KINDLY GIVE 24 HOURS NOTICE

M__________________

HAS AN APPOINTMENT ON

☐ MON. ☐ TUES. ☐ WED. ☐ THUR. ☐ FRI. ☐ SAT.

DATE____________ AT________ A.M. P.M.

LEONARD S. TAYLOR, M.D.

2100 WEST PARK AVENUE
CHAMPAIGN, ILLINOIS 61820
TELEPHONE

IF UNABLE TO KEEP APPOINTMENT KINDLY GIVE 24 HOURS NOTICE.

FIGURE 10–4. Examples of appointment cards. (Courtesy of Colwell Systems, Inc., Champaign, IL.)

Special Problems

Probably every doctor has a few patients who are habitually late for appointments. This seems to be a problem for which no cure has yet been found; consequently, you must find a way of booking such patients as the last appointments of the day. Then, if closing time arrives before a patient does, you need feel no obligation to wait. Some medical assistants simply tell the patient to come in one-half hour earlier than the time they actually write in the book. The point to remember is that you must learn to work around this patient, with the realization that in all likelihood he or she is not going to change.

When a former patient returns after a lengthy absence, the medical assistant should recheck his or her address, telephone number, insurance, and employment information and enter any changes on the patient's chart. If the appointment is made by telephone, be sure to ask for the patient's daytime telephone number. You may need to place a call to the

PROCEDURE 10-2   SCHEDULING A NEW PATIENT

GOAL   To schedule a new patient for a first office visit.

EQUIPMENT AND SUPPLIES

Appointment book
Scheduling guidelines

Appointment card
Telephone

PROCEDURAL STEPS

1. Obtain the patient's full name, birthdate, address, and telephone number.
   Note: Verify the spelling of the name.

2. Determine whether the patient was referred by another physician.
   Purpose: You may need to request additional information from the referring physician, and your physician will want to send a consultation report.

3. Determine the patient's chief complaint and when the first symptoms occurred.
   Purpose: To assist in determining the length of time needed for the appointment and the degree of urgency.

4. Search the appointment book for the first suitable appointment time and an alternate time.

5. Offer the patient a choice of these dates and times.
   Purpose: Patients are better satisfied if they are given a choice.

6. Enter the mutually agreeable time in the appointment book followed by the patient's telephone number.
   Note: Indicate that the patient is new by adding the letters "N.P."

7. If new patients are expected to pay at the time of the visit, explain this financial arrangement when the appointment is made.
   Purpose: The patient will be aware of the payment policy and can come prepared to pay at the time of the visit.

8. Offer travel directions for reaching the office as well as parking instructions.
   Purpose: To relieve any anxiety about being able to find the medical facility.

9. Repeat the day, date, and time of the appointment before saying goodbye to the patient.
   Purpose: To verify that the patient understands the date and time of the appointment.

patient, and you cannot safely assume that the number has not changed. You should also inquire into the nature of the current complaint.

Write legibly when making entries in the appointment book. Check off the patients' names as they arrive. Note any appointment failures or cancellations in ink on the appointment schedule.

Always write the patient's name in full, last name first, together with the reason for the appointment

immediately. DO NOT TRUST THE INFORMATION TO MEMORY! Be sure to cross off sufficient time for the appointment. It is a good idea to write the patient's daytime telephone number after every entry in the appointment book. You may have to cancel or rearrange that day's schedule in a hurry, and many precious minutes can be saved if you do not have to look up each patient's telephone number.

Rescheduling an Appointment

Sometimes changes must be made in the appointment schedule. For instance, the patient who has a 3:00 PM appointment next Monday calls and asks to have this changed to 1 week later. You find an opening at 3:00 PM on the following Monday and write in the patient's name, but in your haste you fail to cross out the first appointment. Someone else looking at the appointment book (or possibly even yourself a couple of days later) will either expect the patient on both days or be unable to determine which day is correct. Avoid this embarrassing situation by making it a habit to cross out the first appointment before writing in the new one.

You may have a patient who requires a series of appointments, for example, at weekly intervals. Try to set up the appointments on the same day of each week at the same time of day, if possible. This considerably reduces the risk of a forgotten appointment. A calendar that shows the dates several months in advance at a glance is useful to have on or near the appointment desk.

At the end of each day, prepare a typewritten list or computer printout of the next day's appointment schedule that shows each patient's name, appointment time, and reason for visiting. This list should be made available to the physician and any other members of the staff who have contact with patients. If changes occur during the day, be sure to correct the daily schedule sheet as well as your appointment book.

EXCEPTIONS TO APPOINTMENT SYSTEM

With even the best of appointment systems, certain situations require an immediate adjustment in the schedule. Some examples are discussed in the following paragraphs.

Emergency Patients

If someone telephones to report an emergency that can be taken care of in the office, the medical assistant should not hesitate to have the patient come immediately. In making such determinations, however, there must be some office protocol or previous understanding with the doctor concerning what kinds of emergencies will be seen in the office, the criteria for determining whether a particular case *is* an emergency, and what procedures the medical assistant should follow. Try to have a list of questions to ask the caller appropriate to the situation. For instance:

- Is there bleeding?
- Where is the blood coming from?
- What is the patient's temperature?

- Are there chills?
- Is there nausea or vomiting?
- If there is pain, is it steady or **intermittent?**
- Is the pain severe? sharp? dull?
- How long have the symptoms been present?

Acutely Ill Patients

Patients cannot always give advance notice of when they will need a doctor. There is sometimes a very fine line between an emergency patient and the acutely ill patient, but the latter should be seen as soon as possible. At the very least, let the physician decide whether the patient should be seen immediately or whether an appointment should be made for another day. (For example, a patient may report having had flu symptoms for several days, and now has an elevated temperature. The doctor will probably want more information before deciding whether the patient should be seen immediately or whether some other course of action is appropriate.) The 15- to 20-minute breather time you saved in the middle of the morning and the afternoon may rescue your schedule.

Physician Referrals

If another physician telephones and requests that a patient be seen by your doctor today, this is another exception you will have to make. Most physicians recognize the importance of keeping a schedule and will not be inconsiderate in this respect.

FAILED APPOINTMENTS
Reasons for Failed Appointments

Why do patients fail to keep appointments? Some patients are simply forgetful. If you detect this tendency in a patient, form the habit of telephoning a reminder the day before the appointment or send a postcard timed to arrive a day or two in advance of the appointment. If your office consistently runs behind schedule, with patients being kept waiting for more than 20 to 30 minutes, the patient whose own time is well-planned may simply elect not to run the risk of losing so much valuable time. Perhaps you gave a patient an appointment at a time that really was not agreeable to him. Or a patient who has been pressed for payment may stay away because of being unable to pay on that day. It is very important that you determine the reason for failed appointments and do what you can to remedy the situations. Telephone the patient to be sure there was no misunderstanding. If the patient's health is such that medical treatment must continue, write a letter explaining this to the patient. Send the letter by certified mail with return receipt requested and keep this letter in the chart for legal protection.

No-Show Policy

Some patients may not realize the importance of keeping their appointments. A busy practice must have a very specific policy on appointment no-shows and enforce it effectively. Michael Silver, Practice Management Consultant of Williamsville, New York, made these suggestions in *Physician's Management*, October 1978:

> The first time a patient fails to show, note the fact on the medical record or ledger card. The second time this happens, you'll have a warning, and if the patient is more than a half-hour late, call his or her home. The third time a patient fails to show without good reason, I suggest dropping the patient by using the customary methods that avoid legal problems.
>
> Incidentally, a patient with a major appointment—physical exams, counseling or the like—should be reminded by phone 24 to 48 hours before the appointment.

Charging for Failed Appointments

Legally, a patient may be charged for failing to keep an uncanceled appointment, if the patient was informed in advance about this policy and if it can be shown that this time was not used for another patient. However, few doctors attempt to collect for such occasions. The risk of poor public relations is too great; it generally results in a lost patient. Some other way must be found to handle failed appointments if they become a problem.

Recording the Failed Appointment

Whenever a patient fails to keep an appointment, a notation should be made in the patient's chart as well as in the appointment book. If the patient is seriously ill, the doctor should also be told about the failure. This may be a legal consideration at some later date. In some cases, it may be necessary for the doctor or the medical assistant to call and remind the patient that an unkept appointment may have serious effects on the patient's health.

HANDLING CANCELLATIONS AND DELAYS

When the Patient Cancels

It is inevitable that some cancellations will occur. If you keep a list of patients with advance appointments who would like to come in sooner, get busy on the telephone and try to get one of them in to fill the available time. By placing a colored dot alongside their names in the appointment book, these patients can be easily identified.

When the Doctor Is Delayed

There are days when the doctor is delayed in reaching the office. If you have advance notice of the delay, you can start calling those patients with early appointments and suggest they come later. If some have already arrived before you learn of the delay, you will have to explain that an emergency has prevented the doctor from getting in. Show concern for the patient, but avoid being overly apologetic, which might imply some degree of guilt. Most patients realize that a doctor has certain priorities, and that the patient who is able to be in the office may be inconvenienced but it is not a life-or-death matter. If this kind of situation occurs frequently, though, you may have to devise a different scheduling system.

When the Doctor Is Called Out on Emergencies

Physicians are conscious of their responsibilities for responding to medical emergencies, and most patients will be sympathetic to such occurrences if the medical assistant takes the time to explain what has happened. You may say something like, "Dr. Wright has been called away to answer an emergency. She asked me to tell you she is very sorry to keep you waiting. There will be at least a 1-hour delay."

Ask the patient, "Do you wish to wait? If it is inconvenient, I'll be glad to give you an appointment on another day. Or perhaps you'd like to have some coffee or do some shopping and return in an hour."

As quickly as possible, call the patients who are scheduled for a later hour. In many offices, especially those of obstetricians, surgeons, and general practitioners, it is sometimes necessary to cancel a whole day's appointments. For this reason, it is particularly important that you have the daytime telephone number of each patient available so that you can cancel the appointment and make a new one without delay. If it is at all possible, cancel appointments *before* the patient arrives in the office to find that the doctor is not in.

When the Doctor Is Ill or Is Called Out of Town

Physicians do get ill, too, and the patients who are scheduled to be seen during the course of the doctor's expected recovery period must be informed of this. They need not be told the nature of the illness. When the physician is called out of town for personal or professional reasons, the appointments will have to be canceled or rescheduled. It is customary to provide the patient with the name of another physician, or possibly a choice of several, who will take care of the doctor's patients during such absences. For security reasons, it is best to merely state that the doctor is unavailable. Stating over the phone that the doctor is out of town could lead to attempted burglary or other unauthorized intrusion of the premises.

SCHEDULING OUTSIDE APPOINTMENTS

There are other appointments that the medical assistant will make and that will appear on the appointment book, such as scheduled surgery at a hospital, consultations at a hospital or at another physician's office, and house calls at extended care facilities or in the home. The doctor must have time to get from one place to another, so allowance must be made for traveling time when arranging these appointments.

Surgeries

You may be responsible for scheduling surgeries. In scheduling with most hospitals, you should call the secretary in surgery first when your doctor plans an operation. Give the surgical secretary:

- The preferred date and time
- The type of surgery to be performed
- The approximate time required

After the date and hour have been established, give:

- The patient's full name
- Sex
- Age
- Telephone number

Then explain any special requests the doctor may have, such as the amount of blood to have available. Be sure you have all this information at hand before placing the call.

It may also be your responsibility to arrange for an assistant surgeon, the anesthesiologist, and the bed reservation.

Some hospitals request that the patient complete a preadmittance form so that all records can be processed before the patient is admitted. In such cases it may be the medical assistant's responsibility to see that this is done. These are general guidelines only, as procedures will vary in different areas and different hospitals.

House Calls

If the physician regularly makes house calls or sees patients in convalescent homes, you will probably set aside a special block of time for this on your appointment schedule. In arranging such appointments, be sure to get all the pertinent details:

- Name and address of patient
- Telephone number
- Best way to reach the home
- Nearest cross street
- Name of person making the request

Again, traveling time must be allowed for. Many physicians never make house calls, believing that the patient can best be examined and treated in the medical facility or in a hospital.

Outside Appointments for Patients

The medical assistant is often requested to arrange laboratory or x-ray appointments for patients. Before calling the laboratory or x-ray facility, you need to know:

- The exact procedure required
- Whether expediency is a factor
- Whether a **stat report** is necessary
- The patient's availability

With this information before you, you can set up the appointment with confidence. When you inform the patient of the time and place for the appointment, you can also relay any special instructions that may be necessary. Then note these arrangements on the patient's chart, and place a follow-up reminder on your **tickler** or desk calendar.

PATIENTS WITHOUT APPOINTMENTS

What will you do about "walk-in" patients, that is, those who arrive without an appointment? There must be a policy agreed upon by the doctor and then carried out by the medical assistant.

The patient who requires immediate attention will most likely be fitted into the schedule somehow. If the patient does not need immediate care, a brief visit with the doctor and a scheduled appointment at a later time may be the answer. Or you may simply have to turn down the request.

The medical assistant should always make it clear, even when sending patients without appointments in to see the doctor, that the office runs on an appointment basis. You might say, for example: "The doctor will be able to see you today, but we would appreciate it very much if you would make an appointment for your next visit." Or, "The doctor can see you now and I'm sorry you had to wait so long. Perhaps it would be possible for you to make an appointment the next time."

Try to convey the message that appointments save not only the doctor's time but the patient's time as well. Emphasize that the doctor is able to give them full attention and more time if an advance appointment is made.

PROCEDURE 10-3   SCHEDULING OUTPATIENT DIAGNOSTIC TESTS

GOAL To schedule patient for outpatient diagnostic test ordered by physician within the time frame needed by physician, confirm with the patient, and issue all required instructions.

EQUIPMENT AND SUPPLIES

Diagnostic test order from physician
Name, address, and telephone number
   of diagnostic facility

Patient chart
Test preparation instructions
Telephone

PROCEDURAL STEPS

1. Obtain an oral or written order from the physician for the exact procedure to be performed and the time frame for results.
   Purpose: The urgency of the test results affects the time and date of the appointment needed.

2. Determine the patient's availability.
   Purpose: To be sure that the patient will be able to comply with the arrangements for the test.

3. Telephone diagnostic facility:
   - Order the specific test needed.
   - Establish the date and time.
   - Give the name, age, address, and telephone number of the patient.
   - Determine any special instructions for the patient.
   - Notify the facility of any urgency for test results.

4. Notify the patient of arrangements, including:
   - Name, address, and telephone number of the diagnostic facility.
   - Date and time to report for the test.
   - Instructions concerning preparation for the test (eating restrictions, fluids, medications, enemas, and so forth).
   - Ask the patient to repeat the instructions.
   Purpose: To be certain that the patient understands the preparation necessary and the importance of keeping the appointment. If time permits, issue written instructions to the patient.

5. Note arrangements on the patient's chart.
   Purpose: To ensure follow-up on diagnosis and/or treatment.

6. Place reminder on a tickler or desk calendar.
   Purpose: To check whether the appointment was kept and report was received from the testing facility.

OTHER CALLERS

It is important to remember that there will be a wide range of other unscheduled callers with whom the doctor will need to meet.

Physicians

Another physician calling at your doctor's office should be ushered in to see the doctor as soon as possible regardless of the appointment schedule. If the doctor is seeing a patient, explain the situation and, if possible, take the visiting physician into a private room to wait. Then notify your doctor as soon as possible. The visits of other physicians are usually brief and do not appreciably affect your schedule.

Pharmaceutical Representatives

Also known as "detail persons," representatives from leading pharmaceutical houses are frequent visitors to physicians' offices and are generally welcomed when the schedule permits. They are well-trained and bring valuable information on new drugs to the physician. The medical assistant is often expected to screen such visitors and turn away those whose products would not be used in that practice. If you do not know the representative or the pharmaceutical company, ask for a business card, then check with the doctor, who will then decide whether or not to see the caller.

If the doctor is in a specialty practice or wishes to confer with only selected pharmaceutical company representatives, the medical assistant and the doctor can prepare a list of the representatives who will be seen by the doctor. Then, when a detail person calls, the medical assistant can deal with the caller confidently.

The medical assistant can say whether or not the doctor will be available that day and give an estimate of the waiting time or suggest a later time at which to return. The caller can then make a decision regarding whether to wait or return later. The pharmaceutical representative is usually quite understanding and cooperative and is willing to wait patiently a long while for just a brief visit with the doctor. The medical assistant should in turn treat the representative with courtesy, showing as much cooperation as possible. In some cases, the representative will just leave literature or materials for the doctor with the medical assistant. The detail person who is not on the calling list for a particular doctor will also appreciate the saving in time by knowing this. Most representatives say they would rather be told outright if the doctor does not wish to see them than to be given some evasive reply.

Salespersons

Salespersons from medical, surgical, and office supply houses call regularly at physicians' offices. Sometimes they want to see the doctor, but the medical assistant who is in charge of ordering supplies usually is able to handle these calls personally.

Unsolicited salespersons sometimes present a problem in the professional office. If the physician does not wish to see such callers, the medical assistant must firmly but tactfully send them away. You can suggest that they leave their literature and cards for the doctors to study and say that the doctor will contact them if further information is desired. Persistent callers who ignore a polite "No" can be discouraged by the suggestion that perhaps they would like to schedule an appointment, at the doctor's customary fee.

Miscellaneous

From time to time, other callers appear in the doctor's office. Some are civic leaders seeking the doctor's aid in community projects. Others may be church leaders, insurance representatives, solicitors for fund drives, and so forth. Most physicians inform their medical assistants of their general policy in regard to seeing such callers. Civic leaders should be treated with courtesy and consideration when they telephone or come into the office. Most doctors feel a responsibility to take an active part in community affairs, but no one can participate in all activities. Sometimes the responsibility for accepting or refusing such community appointments is delegated to the medical assistant. In this event, you must use discretion and exercise great tact and courtesy. Turning away community leaders with a blunt refusal does not create good medical public relations. If it is necessary to refuse such requests, be sure to explain that the doctor is already participating in such community projects as, for example, the Boy Scouts, Girl Scouts, Kiwanis, and the Health Council (naming specific activities or organizations), and cannot accept additional responsibilities at this time. The rules regarding tact, courtesy, and consideration apply to every caller in a physician's office.

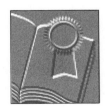

► **LEARNING ACHIEVEMENTS**

Are you able to:

1. Define the words in the Vocabulary of this chapter?
2. Describe what to look for in selecting an appointment book?
3. Prepare a new appointment page for scheduling patients?

4. Explain the reason for recording a failed appointment in the patient's chart?
5. Schedule a patient for a diagnostic test in an outside laboratory?
6. List and explain the three basic guidelines to consider in scheduling appointments?
7. Rearrange the day's schedule in the event the physician is late or unable to be present?
8. Determine whether a patient's situation is (a) an emergency, (b) urgent, or (c) delayable?
9. Identify the one single question that should not be asked when setting up a patient's appointment?
10. List at least six points of information that are necessary in scheduling surgery with a hospital?

REFERENCES AND READINGS

American Medical Association: *The Business Side of Medical Practice,* Chicago, 1989.
American Medical Association: *Winning Ways with Patients,* Chicago, The Association, 1981.
Conomikes Associates, Inc.: *Medical Office Management Institute,* 1991.
Manning, F. F. [ed]: *Medical Group Practice Management,* Cambridge, MA, Ballinger Publishing Co., 1977.

RESOURCES

Colwell Company, 275 Kenyon Road, Champaign, IL 61820.
Patient Care Systems, 16 Thorndal Circle, Darien, CT 06820.
VISIrecord Systems, 160 Gold Star Boulevard, Worcester, MA 01606.
Bibbero Systems, Inc., 1300 N. McDowell Boulevard, Petaluma, CA 94954.

CHAPTER ELEVEN

———

TELEPHONE TECHNIQUES

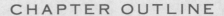

CHAPTER OUTLINE

VOCABULARY

clarity The state of being clear; lucid

diction Choice of words to express ideas, especially with regard to correctness, clearness, or effectiveness.

enunciation The act of pronouncing words distinctly.

monitor To listen to a matter transmitted by telephone as a third party.

noncommittal Not revealing any specific attitude or opinion.

pitch The vibratory frequency of a tone or sound.

pronunciation The act or manner of pronouncing words.

screen The act of determining to whom a telephone call is to be directed.

transmitter The part of a telephone into which one speaks.

WATS Wide Area Telephone Service

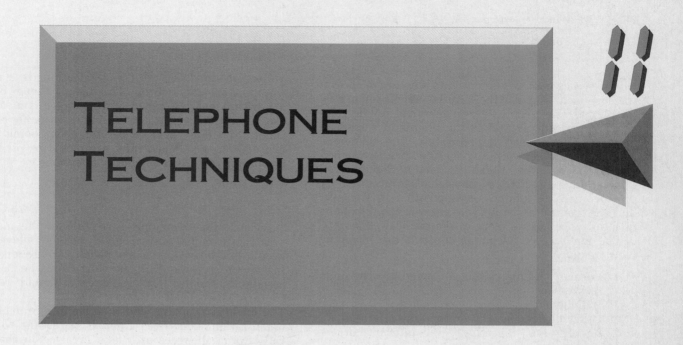

TELEPHONE TECHNIQUES

LEARNING OBJECTIVES

COGNITIVE

Upon successful completion of this chapter, you should be able to:

1. Define the terms listed in the Vocabulary.

2. Discuss the importance of telephone communications.

3. List ways by which the medical assistant can develop a pleasing telephone personality.

4. Cite seven items to be included in taking a complete telephone message.

5. Identify ten kinds of telephone calls that the medical assistant should be able to handle successfully.

6. Identify six kinds of telephone calls that will need to be referred to the physician for response.

7. Explain what is involved in monitoring telephone calls.

8. Discuss the useful information that may be found in a telephone directory in addition to telephone numbers.

9. Explain what is meant by *preplanning a call*.

10. Explain the ways in which an operator-answered telephone answering service can benefit a medical practice.

PERFORMANCE

Upon successful completion of this chapter, you should be able to perform the following role-play activities:

1. Demonstrate the appropriate method of placing and receiving telephone calls.

2. Using a multiple-line telephone, demonstrate the correct handling of two incoming calls, one of which must be transferred to another person.

3. Correctly record a telephone message from a laboratory facility reporting test results on a patient.

4. Respond to a call from a pharmacist regarding a request for a prescription refill, demonstrating appropriate precautions and completing necessary documentation.

5. Using a list of local social service agencies, respond to telephone calls for emergency treatment (at a poison or burn center) and for nonemergency services (at a facility for crippled children or a cancer-screening center).

6. Check a telephone answering device for recorded messages, and prepare and distribute message slips.

7. Call an operator-answered exchange to report on-call information for out-of-office messages.

GENERAL GUIDELINES

Ninety per cent of the patients who are seen in a medical facility make their initial appointments by telephone. The telephone is a powerful public relations instrument as well as the lifeline of a medical practice. When used appropriately, the telephone can help build a beginning medical practice; when used inappropriately, it can do much to destroy even a flourishing practice. A physician's office without one or more telephones is impossible to imagine, and the medical assistant who regards the telephone as a nuisance has no place in the medical office.

The majority of telephone contacts are incoming calls from:

- Former patients calling for appointments or to seek advice
- Individuals reporting emergencies
- Other physicians who are making referrals
- Laboratories reporting vital information regarding a patient
- New patients making a first contact

It is important to remember that although we put a great deal of emphasis upon rules for speaking, we often neglect the importance of good listening. The same attention should be given a telephone conversation that would be given a face-to-face conversation. Concentration is not always easy; it must be practiced. Effective listening is vital to the medical assistant.

Your Telephone Personality

When you receive a telephone call from a stranger, you probably try to visualize that person and form some opinion of his or her personality (e.g., he or she is a mature adult, is somewhat worried, thinks quickly, is fairly well educated, and so forth). The caller responds to you in the same way. To the caller, your voice is your entire personality. The caller cannot see you, your smile, or your facial expression. The caller's total impression of you and of the office is formed from your voice. What image do you create with your telephone personality?

- Is your voice warm and friendly?
- Does it sound confident?
- Is your conversation courteous and tactful?

Every caller should be made to feel that you have time to attend to his or her wishes. A small mirror, placed near the telephone, will remind you to smile. Smiling helps to relax your facial muscles and improves your tone of voice. If you are rushed when you pick up the telephone, wait a few seconds until you are able to answer graciously without seeming breathless or impatient.

Confidentiality

Keep in mind that all communications in a medical office are confidential. This means that if others are within hearing range of your voice, you are to use discretion when mentioning the name of the caller. You must also be careful about being overheard when you repeat any symptoms or other information you are receiving by telephone.

Personal Calls

Because the telephone is so vital to the medical practice, personal calls should not be allowed to keep a line busy. Physicians usually are understanding about occasional urgent calls from the medical assistant's family, but casual calls should be discouraged.

A medical assistant who is active in a professional organization sometimes finds it necessary to take calls from colleagues or others involved in the profession. Although these communications are not considered entirely personal, they too should be kept to a minimum. The doctor's telephone lines should be clear to receive the doctor's professional calls.

Holding the Telephone Handset Correctly

You may have developed some very casual personal habits when using the telephone that will need correction in the professional office. How do you hold the telephone handset? Is it placed so that your voice is relayed distinctly and accurately?

Practice holding the handset around the middle, with the mouthpiece about 1 inch from your lips and directly in front of your teeth. Never hold it under your chin. You can check the proper distance by taking your first two fingers and passing them through sideways in the space between your lips and the mouthpiece. If your fingers just squeeze through, your lips are the correct distance from the telephone and your voice will go over the line as close to its natural tone as possible.

Speak directly into the telephone immediately after removing it from its cradle. If you turn to face a window or another part of the room, make sure the telephone **transmitter** moves too, otherwise your voice will be lost.

Developing a Pleasing Telephone Voice

What are the qualities of a good telephone voice? How do you cultivate good voice quality? Here are some general tips:

- *Stay Alert.* Give the impression you are wide awake and alert and interested in the person who is calling. Let the caller know that he or she has your full attention.

- *Be Pleasant.* Build a pleasant, friendly image for you and your office. Be the "voice with a smile."
- *Talk Naturally and Be Yourself.* Use your own words and expressions. Avoid repetition of mechanical words or phrases. Do not use slang. Avoid the use of professional jargon.
- *Speak Distinctly.* Clear, distinct **pronunciation** and **enunciation** are vital. Move the lips, tongue, and jaw freely. Talk directly into the transmitter. Never answer the telephone when you are eating, drinking, or chewing gum.
- *Be Expressive.* A well-modulated voice carries best. Use a normal tone of voice, neither too loud nor too soft. Talk at a moderate rate, neither too quickly nor too slowly. Vary your tone. It will bring out the meaning of sentences and add color and vitality to what you say.

How Is Your Diction?

Everyone should have the experience of hearing his or her own voice; it reveals immediately the importance of careful **diction.** Try putting your voice on tape and listening to a playback. Each word and each sound must be given individual attention in order to achieve **clarity.** Slurring your words or dropping your voice too much at the end of a sentence can place a strain on your listener (see Guides to Good Diction chart).

GUIDES TO GOOD DICTION		
NUMERAL OR LETTER	**SOUNDED AS**	**PRINCIPAL SOUNDS**
0	oh	Round and long O
1	wun	Strong W and N
2	too	Strong T and long OO
3	th-r-ee	A single roll of the R and long EE
4	fo-er	Strong F, long O, and strong final R
5	fi-iv	I changing from long to short, strong V
6	siks	Strong S and KS
7	sev-en	Strong S and V, well-sounded EN
8	ate	Long A and strong T
9	ni-en	Strong N, long I, well-sounded EN
10	ten	Strong T and N
J	jay	Strong J and long AY
R	ahr	Strong R
M	em	Short E and strong M
W	dubble-yoo	Full value given to every syllable
F	ef	Short E and strong F

Do not overaccentuate; it causes you to sound artificial. Use a friendly natural style. Few words need to be spelled over the telephone if a person speaks slowly and clearly. Below are key words you can use when it is necessary to verify letters in spelling back over the telephone:

A as in Adams	J as in John	S as in Samuel
B as in Boston	K as in Katie	T as in Thomas
C as in Charles	L as in Lewis	U as in Utah
D as in David	M as in Mary	V as in Victor
E as in Edward	N as in Nellie	W as in William
F as in Frank	O as in Oliver	X as in X-ray
G as in George	P as in Peter	Y as in Young
H as in Henry	Q as in Queen	Z as in Zebra
I as in Ida	R as in Robert	

Try to avoid the habit of dropping "ers," "uhs," and long pauses into your conversation. Also, remember that it is seldom necessary to raise the **pitch** of your voice in order to be heard. If you have trouble being understood on the telephone you probably are:

- speaking too quickly
- enunciating poorly
- failing to speak into the transmitter

INCOMING TELEPHONE CALLS

You will be receiving many calls during the course of a single day. Each one deserves your most competent attention. See Office Telephone Rules for a summary of effective telephone rules to follow. Carefully review Pitfalls to Avoid to help you sidestep problems with telephone communications.

OFFICE TELEPHONE RULES
• Answer promptly.
• Visualize the person to whom you are talking.
• Hold the instrument correctly.

- Develop a pleasing telephone voice.
- Identify your office and yourself.
- Identify the caller.
- Offer assistance.
- Screen incoming calls.
- Minimize waiting time.
- Identify the caller when transferring a call.
- When answering a second call, identify the caller, then return to the first call.
- End each call pleasantly and graciously.

PITFALLS TO AVOID

- Having too few telephone lines. On request, the telephone company will do a traffic survey to determine how many busy signals are occurring and advise you as to whether you need additional lines. If collections and insurance processing require extensive use of the telephone, a special line just for this purpose may be advisable.
- Having too few assistants to handle the existing lines. One assistant can handle two incoming lines, but three lines are probably too many for one person. Another assistant should be assigned to pick up the phone after a specified number of rings.
- Wasting time looking up frequently called numbers. Keep these in a personal directory where they can be quickly and easily located.
- Incoming or outgoing personal calls by employees, except in emergencies. Most doctors have an unlisted private line to take care of their own personal and priority calls.
- Using the telephone to give travel directions to new patients (except for short notice appointments). This information should be included in a Patient Information Sheet or Folder sent to every new patient.
- Taking extensive patient histories over the telephone when this can be done more efficiently at the time of the patient visit.

- Diagnosing or giving medical advice without authorization from the physician.
- Releasing patient information without authorization.

Answering Promptly

Whenever possible, answer the telephone on the first ring, and always by the third ring. If you are unable to complete the conversation when you first answer the telephone, say, "Will you please hold for one moment? I will be right with you." Then wait for the caller to respond. It could be an emergency. Avoid such responses as, "Just a minute" or "Doctor's office, hold please." Tell the caller that you are placing the call "on hold." When you return, thank the caller for waiting.

Personalizing the Call

Try to use the caller's name three times during the conversation. Use other courtesy expressions, such as "thank you," "please," and "you're welcome," as often as possible.

Identifying the Office and Yourself

Your response to an incoming call should be to first identify the office and then yourself. Numerous telephone greetings can be used. You will probably wish to discuss which are best with the doctor or office manager. Your response might be something like this:

"Dr. Black's office—Miss Anderson."

If the doctor's surname is fairly common in your area, you may wish to use his or her given name to further clarify identification, saying:

"Dr. Sherman Black's office—Miss Anderson."

If there are two doctors in the office, both names should be included in the identification. Say:

"Drs. Smith and Taylor," or
"Drs. Taylor and Smith's office."

Some names do not blend smoothly; you should modify the identification so that it is easy to say and easy to understand.

Keep in mind the reason for using the doctor's name. You are telling the caller that the correct number has been reached. If callers frequently ask you to repeat, you need to analyze the failure to communicate and modify your response in some way.

Some authorities suggest preceding the identification with the words, "This is . . ." by saying:

"This is Dr. Black's office."

theorizing that the first two words are probably lost on the listener, who only begins to hear you when you have reached ". . . Dr. Black's office."

Answering an office telephone merely by repeating the telephone number or saying "Hello" is unsatisfactory. The caller will invariably ask, "Is this Dr. Black's office?" Rarely can a person immediately recall the number that he or she has just dialed. Time is wasted, the caller is psychologically rebuffed, and you have lost another opportunity to create a favorable impression of your office.

The use of salutations in telephone identifications is optional. Sometimes the addition of "Good morning" or "Good afternoon" to the identification is awkward. A rising inflection or a questioning tone in your voice indicates interest and a willingness to assist and eliminates the need for an additional greeting.

When you have decided upon the greeting to be used, practice it until you can say it easily and smoothly without having to think about what you are saying.

Identifying the Caller

If the caller does not identify himself or herself, you should ask to whom you are speaking. Repeat the caller's name by using it in the conversation as soon as possible; if other patients are within the range of your voice, remember that the caller's privacy should be respected.

Offering Assistance

You can offer assistance both by the tone of your voice and by what you say.

"May I help you?" or "How may I help you?"

will open the conversation and assure the caller that you are both willing and capable of being of service.

Screening Incoming Calls

Most doctors expect the medical assistant to **screen** all telephone calls. Good judgment in deciding whether to put a call through to the doctor comes with experience.

Do put through calls from other physicians at once. If your doctor is busy and cannot possibly come to the telephone, explain this briefly and politely, then say that you will ask the doctor to return the call as soon as possible.

Many callers ask, "Is the doctor in?" Avoid answering this question with a simple "Yes" or "No" or by responding with the question, "Who is calling,

please?" If the doctor is not in, say so *before* asking the identity of the caller. Otherwise, you create the impression that the doctor is simply not willing to talk with this person.

If the doctor is away from the office, the rule of offering assistance still holds. You can say:

"No, I am sorry, Dr. Black is not in. May I take a message?" or
"No, I am sorry, but Dr. Black will be at the hospital most of the morning. May I ask the doctor to return your call after 12 o'clock?"

Do not under any circumstances offer a medical judgment. Only the doctor can do that.

If the doctor is in and is available to speak on the telephone, a typical response would be:

"Yes, Dr. Black is in; may I say who is calling, please?"

If your doctor prefers to keep telephone calls to a minimum, you might say,

"Yes, Dr. Black is here, but I am not sure whether she is free to come to the phone. May I say who is calling, please?"

By answering in this way, the doctor is not committed to taking the call.

The doctor who is with a patient probably will not wish to be disturbed for a routine call. In this case, you might say:

"Yes, Dr. Black is in, but he is with a patient right now. May I help you?" or
"Yes, Dr. Black is in, but she is with a patient right now. Is there anything you would like me to ask her?"

Try to guard against being overprotective. A patient has a right to talk with the doctor, but unless it is an emergency, the patient is probably willing to do so at the doctor's convenience. Don't let it be said of your doctor, "He's a good doctor, but you can never talk to him." The medical assistant who answers the telephone should act as a screen, not a block.

Find out exactly how calls are to be handled when the doctor is out of the office and under what circumstances you can interrupt when the doctor is in the office. Be firm in your commitment to those preferences and cultivate a reputation for being helpful and reliable. You will save the doctor many interruptions if patients develop confidence in your ability to help them and have faith in your promise to take their messages and deliver them properly.

Minimizing Waiting Time

When a call cannot be put through immediately, ask:

"Will you wait, or shall I call you back when the doctor is free?"

If the caller elects to wait, remember that waiting with a silent telephone can be irritating. The waiting time, no matter how brief, always seems long. Let no more than 1 minute pass without breaking in with some reassuring comment, for instance:

"I'm sorry, Dr. Black is still busy."

If the wait is longer than expected, the caller may wish to reconsider and call back at another time or have the call returned, but he or she needs to communicate this to you. By going back on the line at frequent intervals, you give the caller an opportunity to express such concerns. In fact, you may ask the caller if he or she wishes to continue waiting. Say something like,

"I'm sorry to keep you waiting so long, Mr. Hughes. Would you prefer to have me return your call when Dr. Black is free?"

Try to give the caller some estimate of when he or she may expect the return call. In any event, irritation can be lessened by your consideration in saying:

"Thank you for waiting, Mr. Hughes."

When it is necessary for you to leave the telephone to obtain information, ask the caller:

"Will you please wait while I get the information?"

and then wait for a reply. When you return to the telephone, thank the caller for waiting.

If it will take longer than a few seconds to get the information, give some estimate of the time required and offer to call back. When a patient calls and asks a question that requires his or her chart, it may be best to take a message and call back.

Transferring a Call

Always identify the caller when transferring a call to the doctor. Any person who refuses to give a name should not be put through unless your doctor instructs you to do otherwise.

When the caller is a patient, the doctor will probably want the patient's chart at hand during the conversation. If there is no concern about others hearing your conversation, you can announce the caller's name on the intercom and tell the doctor you will bring the chart. If there are others within hearing range, you might simply take the chart to the doctor and say,

"Dr. Black, this party is waiting on the telephone to speak with you."

In this way, the patient's right to privacy is protected.

Answering a Second Call

If your office has several incoming lines or more than one telephone, it will sometimes be necessary for you to interrupt a conversation to answer another call. It is courteous to:

1. Excuse yourself by saying, "Pardon me just a moment, the other line is ringing."
2. Answer the second call, determine who is calling, and ask that person to hold while you complete the first call. Do not make the mistake of continuing with this call while the first one waits.
3. Return to your first call as soon as possible, and apologize briefly for the interruption.

Think of what you would do if there were a face-to-face conversation. You would not allow a second person to just interrupt a conversation and then ignore the one you were speaking with first.

If the second call is an emergency, you can still take a moment to return to the first line and alert the caller that you will have to keep him or her waiting or call back.

Never answer a call by saying,

"Hold the line, please."

without first finding out who is calling. It could be an emergency. It takes only a moment to be courteous—this courtesy could save a life.

Ending a Call

When a caller's requests have been satisfied; do not encourage needless chatting or permit the call to monopolize your time unnecessarily. The telephone lines should be cleared for other calls.

End the call pleasantly. It is considered good telephone etiquette to allow the person who placed the call to hang up first. It is a gracious gesture to thank a person for calling. Always close the conversation with some form of goodbye; do not just hang up abruptly. Replace the telephone on the cradle as gently as if you were closing a door in the office.

TAKING A TELEPHONE MESSAGE

Be Prepared

Always have a pen or pencil in your hand and a message pad nearby when you answer the telephone. You may be answering several calls before you have an opportunity to relay a message or carry out a promise of action. Therefore, the *written* message is vital.

What kind of message pad will you use? Probably the most satisfactory is an ordinary spiral-bound stenographer's notebook. It is inexpensive, sturdy, well-proportioned, will lie flat on your desk, and can be filed for future reference if desired. Do not be guilty of using small scraps of paper for messages. They are too easily lost. Date the bottom of the first blank page in your notebook at the beginning of each day. You will then have a permanent record that can be referred to later if the need arises. If you will draw a half-inch column down one side of each page, you can use this area to check off each message as it is delivered or taken care of. This is a good reminder system for yourself.

Information Required

The minimum information you will need from each call includes:

- Name of the person called
- Name of the caller
- Caller's daytime telephone number
- Reason for the call
- Action to be taken
- Date and time of the call
- Your initials

Transmitting and Recording the Message

Messages that are to be transmitted to another person may be rewritten on individual slips and delivered or posted on a message board later. Message pads that provide for a carbon copy of each page are good insurance that no message will be forgotten. The nature of the message will determine whether

you must report it immediately. Fig. 11–1 illustrates a model message form that can be adapted to the practice by inserting the patient symptoms and requests you hear most often. The person who completes the call must sign and date it. It is also possible to get message forms with a self-adhesive back that can be placed permanently in the patient's case history (Fig. 11–2). If the call is from a patient and relates in any way to the medical history, or if any instructions were given or queries answered, this information should be placed in the patient's chart.

Taking Action

The message procedure is not complete until the necessary action has been taken. Notations on the memo pad should be carried over to the following day if they have not been attended to. Just place an X in front of the item and move it onto the next page. Sometimes a notation will be carried over for several days until action can be completed. Do not trust to memory messages unattended to from previous days; always carry them forward in writing.

Make brief notations of patients' reactions while you are talking to them on the telephone. The doctor does not require a character study, but it is

---

TELEPHONE MESSAGE LOG

Date: _____ Time: _____ Taken by: _____

Caller: _____ Patient: _____ Age: _____
Phone # Day: _____ Evening: _____
Address: _____

Complaint: _____ How long: _____
Pain? _____ Location: _____
Any treatment? _____
Temperature: _____

____ Cough   ____ Lab Results
____ Sore throat   ____ Rx Refill
____ Vomiting   ____ Appointment
____ Diarrhea   ____ Insurance
____ Bleeding   ____ Billing

____ Return Call   ____ Will call back

Message: _____
_____
_____

Action taken: _____ Date: _____ Signature: _____

FIGURE 11–1. Telephone message log.

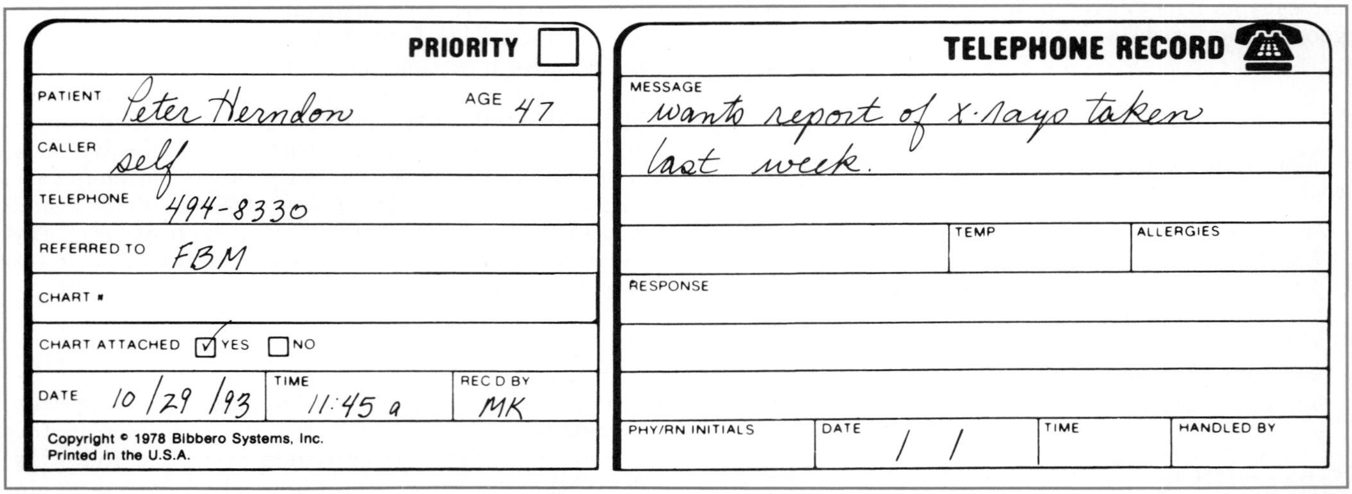
PRIORITY ☐

PATIENT Peter Herndon AGE 47

CALLER self

TELEPHONE 494-8330

REFERRED TO FBM

CHART #

CHART ATTACHED ☑ YES ☐ NO

DATE 10/29/93 TIME 11:45 a REC'D BY MK

Copyright © 1978 Bibbero Systems, Inc.
Printed in the U.S.A.

TELEPHONE RECORD

MESSAGE wants report of x-rays taken last week.

TEMP ALLERGIES

RESPONSE

PHY/RN INITIALS DATE / / TIME HANDLED BY

FIGURE 11–2. Message form with self-adhesive backing. (Courtesy of Bibbero Systems, Inc., Petaluma, CA.)

helpful to know when a patient appears fearful, apprehensive, or nervous. If a patient shows such symptoms, it may be wise to transfer the call to the doctor.

When your employer is talking to another physician in regard to a referral, you may sometimes be requested to take down a brief outline of the patient's case history by listening on the extension telephone. This information can be typed and placed on the doctor's desk just before the patient arrives in the office.

INCOMING CALLS THE MEDICAL ASSISTANT CAN HANDLE

One reason for having a medical assistant answer the incoming calls is to spare the physician unnecessary interruptions during visits with patients. Additionally, many calls relate to the administrative aspects of the office and can actually be better handled by the medical assistant. The doctor's policy regarding how calls are to be handled should be set forth in the office procedure manual. Figure 11–3 shows how the instruction page might be arranged in the manual. Listed below are some kinds of calls that can be handled by the medical assistant in most offices.

Appointments for New Patients

As mentioned in the chapter on scheduling appointments, the first appointment for a new patient requires more time and attention to detail. The medical assistant who is in charge of scheduling appointments should handle these calls. It is well to remember that you are in a sense "opening the door." The patient will form a first impression of the office, of you, and of the doctor from that first telephone contact. Follow all the prescribed rules of telephone courtesy in offering your friendly assistance.

Take the patient's full name, date of birth, complete address, daytime telephone number, name of the person who referred him or her, and the general type of examination required. This helps you to decide how much time to allot the patient on the appointment schedule. Your doctor also may ask you to give general instructions to patients seeking care for specific complaints; for example, to request the patient to bring in a urine specimen or to make certain that laboratory work is done prior to the appointment.

When you have recorded the necessary data, you may ask the patient, "Do you prefer morning or afternoon?" and then offer the first available date. Make certain the patient knows where the office is located and, if necessary, how to get there. If there are special parking conveniences, tell the patient. Ideally, transportation and parking instructions would be described in a Patient Information Folder to be mailed to the patient prior to a first visit, if time permits. Before hanging up, repeat the appointment date and time agreed upon and thank the person for calling.

Return Appointments

Usually it is necessary only to determine when the patient is expected to return and then to find a suitable time on the schedule. It is not necessary to

STANDARD PROCEDURE FOR TELEPHONE CALLS IN THE OFFICE OF

_____:

CALLS THE ASSISTANT CAN HANDLE:

Appointments for New Patients_____

Office Administration Problems_____

_____

_____

_____

_____

_____

_____

_____

CALLS TO BE PUT THROUGH IMMEDIATELY:

Calls from Other Physicians_____

Emergency Calls_____

_____

_____

CALLS TO BE REFERRED TO PHYSICIAN:

Unsatisfactory Progress Reports_____

Third Party Requests for Information_____

_____

_____

_____

_____

FIGURE 11-3. Page from procedure manual.

give extensive explanations about the location of the office and parking facilities. However, if it has been some time since the patient's last visit, it is advisable to ask whether the patient's address and telephone number remain the same. You may also wish to inquire whether the patient wants to see the doctor about a condition similar to the former one. A different complaint may require a longer or shorter visit than usual.

Inquiries About Bills

A patient may request to speak with the doctor about a recent bill. Ask the caller to "hold" for a moment while you pull the ledger. If you find nothing irregular on the ledger, you can return to the telephone and say,

"I have your account in front of me now. Perhaps I can answer your question."

Most likely, the caller will have some simple inquiry, such as "Is that my total bill?" "Has my insurance paid anything?" or "May I wait until next month to make a payment?" Not all patients realize that the medical assistant usually makes such decisions.

Inquiries About Fees

In some offices, the medical assistant is instructed *not to quote fees*. However, a caller who inquires,

"How much does Dr. Arnold charge for an examination?"

may not be pleased to hear

"That's impossible to say—it depends entirely on how extensive an examination is necessary."

The following response is equally **noncommittal** but far more satisfying to the caller:

"Mr. Barker, the fee usually varies with the nature of the problem. An uncomplicated physical examination without any laboratory tests or x-rays might run as low as $_____. On the other hand, the fee could be considerably higher if special tests are required."

If fees are regularly discussed on the telephone, write a suggested script in the policy manual. Do not be evasive. Have a schedule of fees available.

Requests for Insurance Assistance

Again, it is the medical assistant who is in a better position to answer inquiries about insurance. Often, patients find insurance claims very confusing and think they must answer questions with precise medical terminology. A simple statement to "just put it in your own words" may take care of this kind of inquiry. It is best to avoid interpreting insurance coverage by telephone.

Receiving X-ray and Laboratory Reports

Many physicians have x-ray and laboratory reports telephoned to their offices on the day the test is completed. The medical assistant can take these reports. Your task will be greatly simplified if you have blank forms on which you can just fill in the results; this eliminates the need to write the names of all the tests, particularly on laboratory reports. If it is impossible to get blank forms from the laboratory, you can type up your own and run it through the copy machine. By typing four or six to a page, the expense of duplication is cut considerably. They can then be cut to size. Save the original for future duplicating.

Satisfactory Progress Reports from Patients

Doctors sometimes ask a patient to "phone and let me know how you're feeling in a few days." The medical assistant can take such a call and relay the information to the doctor if the report is satisfactory. Assure the patient that you will inform the doctor about the call by saying, for example, "I'll relay this information as soon as the doctor arrives."

Routine Reports from Hospitals and Other Sources

There may be routine calls from the hospital and other sources reporting a patient's progress. If it is only a reporting procedure, take the message carefully, make sure that the doctor sees it, and then place it in the patient's history.

Office Administration Matters

Not all calls concern patients. There may be calls from the accountant or auditor or calls regarding banking procedures, office supplies, office maintenance, and so forth, all of which the medical assistant can either handle immediately or get the necessary information and call back.

Requests for Referrals

Doctors who are liked and respected by their patients are frequently asked for referrals to other specialists, for themselves or for friends. If the physician has furnished the medical assistant with a list of doctors for this purpose, these inquiries can usually be handled without referring them to the physician. The physician should always be told of such requests.

Prescription Refills

If the physician has placed a note on the patient's chart indicating that a prescription may be filled a certain number of times, the medical assistant can give an okay to the pharmacist after determining the number of times it has already been filled. This information should appear on the patient's chart, but it is always best to double-check. If there is any question, tell the pharmacist you will have to check with the doctor and call back.

CALLS THAT REQUIRE TRANSFER TO THE DOCTOR OR CALL BACK

Calls from Other Physicians

As stated earlier, calls from other physicians should be put through immediately. If it is impossible for the doctor to take the call at once, be sure to offer to call back as soon as possible.

Patients Who Will Not Reveal Symptoms

Occasionally, patients will call and wish to talk with the doctor about symptoms that they are reluctant to discuss with a medical assistant. Do not make the mistake of pressing for details. Even though you may not be embarrassed, patients have the right to privacy. Put these calls through or offer to have the doctor call back.

Unsatisfactory Progress Reports

If the patient reports that he or she "still is not feeling well" or that the "prescription the doctor gave me makes me feel sick," do not try to practice medicine by telling the patient "this is to be expected." Even if you think the doctor will say the same thing, the patient should hear it directly from the doctor for reassurance.

Requests for Test Results

When the physician orders special tests for the patient, the patient may be told to call the office in a couple of days for the results. Never assume that the patient will call for results. It is ultimately the responsibility of the physician to notify the patient of test results. Be sure the physician has seen the results and has given you permission to tell the patient before giving out any information. Particularly if the result is unfavorable, the physician should be the one to inform the patient and give further instructions. This call must be handled tactfully; otherwise, the patient may get the feeling that you are hiding something.

Some patients do not understand that the medical assistant does not have the privilege of giving out information without the permission of the physician. You might answer the inquiry like this: "The doctor has not seen the report yet; will you please call back after 2 o'clock? I will try to have the information for you then." Alternatively, you might offer to call the patient as soon as you have the necessary information.

Third-Party Requests for Information

If there is no legal requirement for disclosure of information, you must have the written permission of the patient before giving information to third-party callers. This includes insurance companies, attorneys, relatives, neighbors, employers, or any other third party.

Complaints About Care or Fees

You may be able to offer a satisfactory explanation to a patient who complains about the care he or she received or the fee charged. If a patient seems angry, you may say that it will take a few moments to pull the chart and offer to call back. This reassures the patient that someone is willing to talk about the problem and also gives the patient a chance to "cool off." However, if you are unable to appease the patient easily, the doctor would probably prefer to talk directly to the patient.

Call-Back System

The transfer of nonemergency calls as they occur may cause needless interruption in the physician's daily schedule. Some offices set aside a special time once or twice per day when the physician will accept or return calls—for instance, at the end of the morning office hours and again at the end of the afternoon. The person answering the telephone logs each caller's name, telephone number, and reason for calling. Patients' charts are pulled and given to the physician along with the log. When calls are handled in this manner, the physician is better prepared to answer questions and the caller is better assured of undivided attention to the call.

Unidentified Callers

Although it will happen rarely, you will sometimes encounter individuals who refuse to give you their name or business but are insistent upon speaking to the doctor. Such callers frequently are salespersons who are fully aware that if their identity is revealed they will never get the opportunity to speak to the doctor. Your own course in such instances is to say firmly, "Dr. Jones is very busy with a patient and has asked me to take all messages. If you will not give me a message, I suggest you write the doctor a letter and mark it 'personal.'"

Calls from Family and Friends

Every doctor receives a certain number of personal calls at the office from family and friends. As you become acquainted with the doctor's practice, you will soon know how to handle these calls. However, some persons abuse the telephone privilege. If a friend of the doctor calls too often and the doctor does not wish to take the calls, the medical assistant must deal with it. You can say, "Dr. Wilson is with a patient now and cannot be disturbed. We are booked rather heavily this afternoon, and you may have more time to talk with the doctor if you call at home this evening."

Angry Callers

No matter how efficient you are at the telephone or how well-liked your employer may be, sooner or later you will have an angry caller on the line. There may be a legitimate reason for the anger, or it may have resulted from a misunderstanding. It is a real challenge to handle such a call. You must:

- Avoid getting angry yourself
- Try to find out what the real problem is
- Provide the answers, if possible

If answers are not readily available, a friendly assurance that you will find the answer and call back will usually calm the angry feelings. Be sure to:

- Really listen while you let the caller talk
- Express interest and understanding
- Do not "pass the buck"
- Take careful notes
- Maintain your own poise
- Take the required action—even if it is to say that you will take the matter up with your employer as soon as possible and call back later.

Monitoring Calls

Occasionally you may be asked by your employer to **monitor** a telephone call. You will be expected to listen from an extension phone and take notes on the conversation. It is possible to record both sides of a telephone call by placing a tape recorder close to the telephone receiver. However, you should be aware that this is illegal unless the other person is told that the conversation is being recorded.

Requests for House Calls

Scheduling house calls was discussed briefly in Chapter 10. In response to a telephone request for a home visit, be sure to inquire as to the nature of the illness. Certain conditions are impossible to treat at home, and time will be saved if the patient is sent directly to the hospital, where the doctor can meet him or her. Alternatively, you might urge the patient to come to the office. You can point out that facilities for giving the best medical treatment are available there and that office visits are more economical. This also conserves the doctor's time.

Consult the doctor, if possible, before scheduling a house call. In most cases, you can explain to the patient that you will check with the doctor and call back immediately. If your doctor cannot make the house call, you should attempt to find other assistance for the patient. It is easier for you to call another physician than it is for the distraught patient. One of the most common complaints of patients about the medical profession is that patients are unable to get a doctor in an emergency. In communities that have paramedic teams, this is not such a problem.

Responding to Emergency Calls

The handling of telephone calls involving possible emergency situations was briefly discussed in Chapter 10. According to the American Medical Association's *The Business Side of Medical Practice:*

Many emergency calls are judgment calls on the part of the person answering in the medical practice. Good judgment only comes from proper training by the physician in what constitutes a real emergency in your type of practice and how such calls should be handled. If you are not immediately available, what should your staff do?

The person answering the telephone should first determine, "Is it urgent?" If the physician is in, the call should probably be transferred immediately. Some plan for the action to be taken when the physician is not present should be agreed upon (Fig. 11–4). It is estimated that fewer than 10% of medical assistants have such guidance.

The physician and medical assistant may also jointly develop typical questions to ask the caller in order to determine the validity and disposition of an emergency. For example:

- What are the chief symptoms?
- When did they start?
- Has this happened before?
- Are you alone?
- Do you have transportation?
- What is the telephone number where you can be reached?

Routine But Troublesome Calls

Many of the so-called "routine" calls coming into the physician's office will be difficult for a new medical assistant to handle (Fig. 11–5). Although no stock answer can be phrased for these calls, a gracious and prompt reply paves the way for a quicker handling of a call, since it tells the patient that you are capable, pleasant, and willing to offer assistance.

EMERGENCY CALL PROCEDURES

When the physician is not in the office, follow these emergency procedures:

Patient Complaint	Refer to Physician Below	Call RN	Call Paramedics	Have Patient	
				Go to Hospital	Come to Office
Severe bleeding					
Head injury					
Severe chest pain					
Broken bone					
Severe laceration					
Unconscious					
High fever					
Difficulty in breathing					

FIGURE 11–4. Form for instructions on emergency call procedures (when physician is not in office).

ASSISTANT'S GUIDE FOR HANDLING ROUTINE TELEPHONE CALLS	Refer immediately to physician	Physician will call back	Refer to clinical personnel: RN, CMA, PA	Other
New patient—ill and wants to talk to physician				
Established patient— wants to talk to physician				
Patient—request for lab results				
Family requesting patient information				
Patient or pharmacy— regarding Rx refill				
Another physician—wants to talk to physician				
Hospital—regarding a patient				
Insurance carrier or attorney requesting patient information				
Business calls for physician (attorney, accountant, broker)				
Professional society calls for physician				
Personal calls for physician (family, friends)				

FIGURE 11–5. The new assistant needs a guide for handling even routine calls.

The following are a few typical calls that any medical assistant might receive:

Appointment Changes

The Call: "I have an appointment with the doctor this morning and cannot keep it. May I come in this afternoon instead?"

The Answer: Even though this type of call throws the appointment book into confusion, showing irritation with the patient won't help the situation. Make a sincere effort to help the caller make a new appointment. Explain that appointments are made so that the doctor can give the very best care without rushing the patients and that consequently keeping appointments is to each patient's personal benefit.

Statements

The Call: "I received my statement this morning and I don't understand why it is so high."

The Answer: If billing matters are handled by another employee, tell the patient that you will transfer his or her call to the billing office. If you are responsible for billing, politely ask the patient to hold the line while you pull the financial card. When you return to the line, thank the patient for waiting and explain the charges carefully. If there is an error, apologize and say a corrected statement will be sent out at once. Thank the patient for calling. If patients are properly advised about charges at the time that services are rendered, the number of these calls will be considerably reduced.

Prescription Refill

The Call: "Last time I had an office call, the doctor gave me a prescription for some sleeping tablets. Please call the druggist and okay a refill."

The Answer: Remember that the medical assistant is not licensed to practice medicine. Ask the patient for the prescription number and date, the name, address, and telephone number of the pharmacy and obtain the patient's phone number. Explain that you will give the message to the doctor as soon as possible. Pull the patient's chart and have it ready with the message when the doctor comes in. If the doctor okays the refill, you may be asked to phone the pharmacy and the patient with the information.

Physician "Shopping"

The Call: "Does the doctor treat stomach trouble?"

The Answer: It depends upon the doctor's field of practice. Many people don't understand the various medical specialties, and this call may come from a person referred to the doctor by a friend who didn't explain that the doctor is a specialist. If your doctor is unable to handle the case, you may have to refer the patient to another doctor. Give the patient the names of at least three physicians, when possible; these should be only names that your employer has had you place on the referral list. Do not presume to make a diagnosis when a patient calls in with bizarre complaints; transfer the call to the doctor or take the caller's name and number and have the doctor return the call later.

Unauthorized Inquiry

The Call: "My next-door neighbor is a patient of the doctor's, and I am quite concerned about her. Could you tell me what is wrong with her?"

The Answer: Professional ethics is involved here. It is not the role of the medical assistant to give out any information about a patient's condition, except information that the physician has specifically okayed for "release." The caller in this case may be merely curious or may actually be a kindly neighbor who wishes to help a friend. Generally, refer such calls to the doctor. Your possible response might be, "I'm

PROCEDURE 11-1   ANSWERING THE TELEPHONE

GOAL To answer the telephone in a physician's office in a professional manner, respond to a request for action, and accurately record a message.

EQUIPMENT AND SUPPLIES

Telephone   Pen or pencil
Message pad   Appointment book

PROCEDURAL STEPS

1. Answer the telephone on first ring, speaking directly into the transmitter, with the mouthpiece positioned 1 inch from the mouth.
   Purpose: Answering promptly conveys interest in the caller. Proper positioning of the handset carries the voice best.

2. Speak distinctly with a pleasant tone and expression, at a moderate rate, and with sufficient volume for the calling party to understand every word.
   Purpose: Conveys interest in the caller and prevents a stressful response.

3. Identify the office and yourself.
   Purpose: The caller will know that the correct number has been reached and the identity of the staff member.

4. Verify the identity of the caller.
   Purpose: To confirm the origin of the call.

5. Provide the caller with the requested information or service, if possible.
   Purpose: The medical assistant can handle many calls and conserve time and energy of the physician or other staff members.

6. Take a message for further action, if required.
   Purpose: Not all calls can be responded to immediately.

7. Terminate the call in a pleasant manner and replace the receiver gently.
   Purpose: To promote good public relations.

---

unable to answer your question. Do you wish to speak to the doctor?" Very few of the merely curious will go this far.

TELEPHONE ANSWERING SERVICES

Because a physician's telephone is an all-important tool of the practice, it must be constantly "covered"—that is, there must be someone to answer it at all times—day and night, weekends and holidays. This presents no problem during weekdays, but nights and weekends require special attention. Most doctors subscribe to telephone answering services that provide around-the-clock coverage. Some telephone answering services are privately owned; others are owned and operated by the local medical society. Alternatively, the doctor may use an automatic answering device.

Operator-Answered Services

There are two types of operator-answered services.

Type 1

Doctor-subscribers leave messages with, or obtain patients' messages from, a service whose number appears in the local telephone directory in this way, "After _____ PM, call _____ [number]," or "If no answer, call _____ [number]." Such listings are placed immediately below the doctor's own telephone number in the directory. This form of service is somewhat inconvenient for the patient but is far better than no coverage at all.

Type 2

The answering service has a direct connection with the office telephone. When the telephone rings in the physician's office or at home, it also signals on the switchboard of the answering service. As long as the telephone is ringing, it will continue to signal at the answering service. If no one answers within a certain agreed-upon number of rings, the answering service operator takes the call. This method provides continuous telephone coverage.

Even during the day, such an answering service can function effectively. There may be times when you are assisting the doctor and it is impossible for you or anyone else to answer the telephone. Not answering the telephone is extremely poor policy, but if you have an agreement with the answering service (sometimes referred to as "the exchange"), its operators will accept calls for you in such situations. With this direct-wire answering method, the operator answers the telephone in your employer's name, as you would in the office, explaining "This is Dr. Wilson's exchange. May I take a message?"

The answering service will greatly appreciate your cooperation if you call them every day before leaving the office and tell them where the doctor will be during the evening or give them other special messages. Then, in the morning when you return to the office, call the exchange and ask for any messages they may have. Usually there will be messages from patients who called during the evening but whose calls were not urgent enough to merit an emergency call to the doctor. An exchange can act as a buffer for the physician and help eliminate too frequent, unnecessary calls during the night.

Here is how the system works: During the hours that the office is closed, the exchange will answer the doctor's office telephone, take a message, and relay it to the doctor. If it is urgent, the doctor will then return the call to the patient; if not, the exchange will call the patient and explain that the doctor will call first thing in the morning. Emergency calls, of course, are immediately put through by the exchange to the doctor.

Occasionally, it is a good idea to check up on your answering service by placing a few random calls at various hours. It may be that now and then the service does not answer the calls or the response may not meet your standards. The service may be enhanced by inviting the manager of the answering service in to see the office or by having the medical assistant go to the exchange facility to meet with the manager and staff. This personal contact frequently improves the rapport and quality of service you may expect.

Electronic Answering Devices

Some doctors use an answering device after office hours. Callers who dial the office number hear a recorded message either telling them how to reach the doctor (or a colleague who may be covering the practice) or inviting the caller to leave a message. The caller's message is recorded for later checking by the doctor or a staff member.

Most electronic answering devices are equipped with remote control to allow the subscriber to operate them from any Touch-Tone telephone. By using a personal code number, it is possible to:

- retrieve messages, including the times at which they were recorded
- reset the tape for future messages
- change the outgoing message when necessary

Voice Mail

Further sophistication of the answering machine has led to the development of what is called "voice mail." The call is answered by an automated operator that presents a list of options, such as "If you are calling about your account, push 'one'"; to change your address, push 'two'"; and so forth. The impersonal nature of voice mail does not lend itself to answering the telephone in a physician's office, but the medical assistant will encounter it frequently when placing outgoing calls.

ORGANIZING A PERSONAL TELEPHONE DIRECTORY

Organize your telephone numbers in an indexed 3 × 5 inch desktop file or a rotary file. Emergency numbers might be typed on a colored card or flagged with a color tab. Your personal directory of telephone numbers should include all the numbers that you call frequently, including:

- Specialists to whom your employer sometimes refers patients
- Professional facilities, such as hospitals, the Poison Control Center, pharmacies, ambulance companies, and laboratories
- Special duty nurses, along with their specialties and other pertinent information
- Administrative contacts, such as stationers, equipment dealers and repair services, laundry

and maintenance services, and surgical supply houses

- Personal numbers, such as the doctor's family, special friends, insurance agent, stockbroker, accountant, and lawyer.

OUTGOING CALLS

Preplanning the Call

Before placing a call, make certain you have the correct telephone number and the information you will need during the call at your fingertips.

If you are reporting a patient's history, have the complete record before you, including all the latest laboratory and x-ray reports.

If you are placing a call to order supplies, have the catalog in front of you, along with any previous order sheets or invoices. Also have a list of the items desired, the specifications for them, and any questions you may have regarding them.

Apply this rule to every call you make. The called party will be impressed with your competent organization, and you will save a great deal of time and prevent errors.

Placing the Call

Lift the receiver, listen for the dial tone, then start dialing your number. It sometimes happens that just as you pick up the telephone to place a call, an incoming call has reached your line but you lifted the receiver before the telephone had a chance to ring. If you start dialing without listening for the dial tone, you will not only fail to reach your number, you will have offended the ear of the party trying to reach you.

Touch-Tone telephones are rapidly replacing older models, but if your telephone has a rotary dial, use the index finger or a special dialing instrument for dialing your call. Do not use the eraser end of a pencil and do not let your finger remain in the dial openings on the return of the dial. It is the return of the dial that determines the number you reach, and if it is not allowed to return freely you may reach a wrong number.

Calling Etiquette

When placing a call to another doctor or to a patient at the doctor's request, your doctor should be ready to receive the call. Doctors, because of their busy schedules, sometimes are negligent in this respect.

> The telephone company's courtesy rule is that the person placing the call should be on the line and ready to speak when the called party answers.

If you are calling a patient to change an appointment, be ready to offer a new appointment time. Also, give the patient a logical reason for the inconvenience of having to change the original appointment. This change may cause considerable disruption of plans, and the patient is fully entitled to an explanation.

Remember that if your telephone is within hearing range of office patients, you should be careful when mentioning names or diagnoses.

By following these suggested techniques, you will be able to use the telephone wisely and efficiently. Correct use of the telephone is a skill and an art that can be developed only through actual practice. It is one of the most important skills that the medical assistant can possess.

Long Distance Service

Long distance calls are no longer reserved for special occasions. The calls are simple to place, inexpensive, and efficient. When information is needed in a hurry, it is much more expedient to telephone rather than wait for an exchange of letters.

Before placing a long distance call, have the correct number ready. This number often may be obtained from a letterhead or from other records. The telephone company also has a collection of major city telephone directories in every town. If you do not have the number, you may obtain directory assistance by dialing the area code of the party you are calling, then 555–1212. In some areas you must dial "1" before the area code.

It is important to keep in mind the different time zones when you are calling long distance (Fig. 11–6). The continental United States is divided into four standard time zones: Pacific, Mountain, Central, and Eastern. When it is 12:00 noon Pacific time, it is 3:00 PM Eastern time. If you are calling from San Francisco to New York, you will probably want to make the call no later than 2:00 PM if you are calling a business or professional office, because it will already be 5:00 PM on the East Coast.

Dialing Direct

By dialing your own long distance calls, you will pay the lowest rate and pay for only the minutes you talk (minimum 1 minute). Use direct dialing when you are willing to talk with anyone who answers the phone and you want the call charged to the number from which you are calling.

"800" WATS (Wide Area Telephone Service) Numbers

Many businesses and professional people have "800" **WATS** numbers to which long distance calls

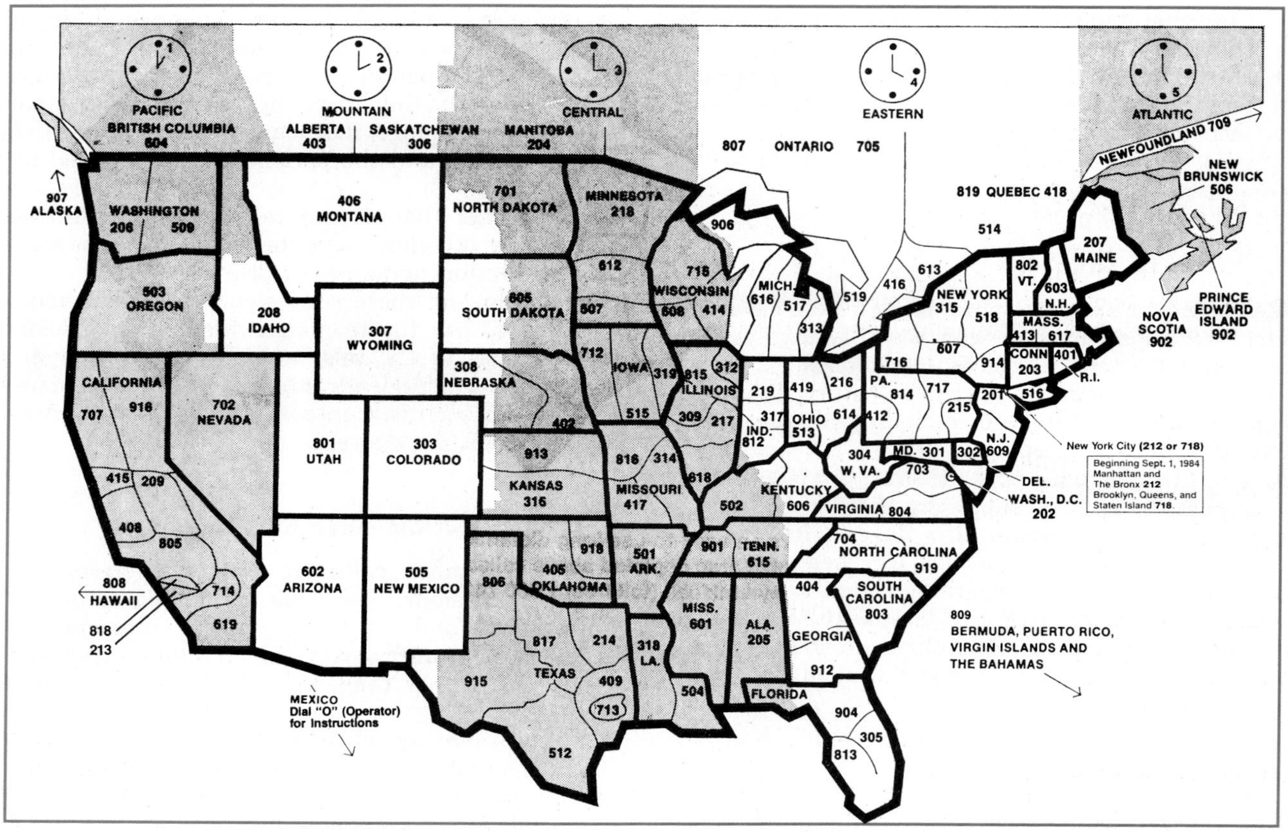

FIGURE 11-6. Time zones across the United States. (Courtesy of Bell Telephone.)

can be made without charge to the caller. To call an "800" number, dial 1 + 800 + the 7-digit telephone number. You can get the telephone numbers of those businesses and people who have 800 numbers by dialing 1 + 800 + 555–1212.

Operator-Assisted Calls

Operator-assisted calls include calls such as:

- Person-to-person
- Bill to a third number
- Collect
- Requests for time and charges
- Certain calls placed from hotels

There is a 1-minute initial period charge, and the rates are equal to the dial-direct rates plus a service charge.

International Service

International Direct Distance Dialing (IDDD) is available in many areas. International dialing codes are the same for all companies offering IDDD. De-

pending on your long distance company, additional numbers or codes may preface the international access, country, and city codes. IDDD is still not available in all areas. If it is available, you may place international station-to-station calls by dialing in sequence the:

1. International code 011
2. Country code
3. City code
4. Local telephone number
5. "#" button if your telephone is Touch-Tone

For example, to place a call to London you would dial:

International Access Code		Country Code		City Code
011	+	44	+	1

plus the local telephone number and "#" if Touch-Tone dialing. After dialing any international code, allow at least 45 seconds for the ringing to start.

Wrong Numbers

One slip in direct distance dialing can give you Los Angeles or New York instead of Dallas. If you reach a wrong number when dialing long distance, be sure to obtain the name of the city and state you have reached. By reporting this information promptly to the operator in your own city, you will not be charged for the call. If you are cut off before terminating your call, this too should be reported to the operator, who will either reconnect your call or make an adjustment of the charge.

Conference Calls

Conference telephone service is of great value to the medical profession in notifying and explaining to a family how a patient is progressing. It has exceptional value in family conferences, at which a quick decision by the entire family in regard to a patient's condition is required.

This service can connect from 3 to 14 points for a two-way conference in which each person can hear or talk to all others participating. Conference calls may be local or long distance calls. Charges are added for the number of places connected, mileage, and the length of the conversation.

To place a call, dial the operator and say you wish to make a conference call. Give the operator the names and telephone numbers of the people you want to connect. If prior arrangements are made with all parties, there is a better chance of reaching everyone at a given time.

TELEPHONE EQUIPMENT AND SERVICES

Number and Placement of Telephones

Familiarity with a multiple-line telephone is a must for the medical assistant. Few health care facilities can get along with just one telephone line. Two incoming lines along with a private outgoing line with a separate number for the physician's exclusive use is the minimum recommended.

One medical assistant can handle no more than two incoming lines, so the addition of more lines may also involve additional staffing. If there is a staff member assigned solely to dealing with insurance and billing, a separate line and listing in the telephone directory for this service may considerably lessen the load on the main incoming lines.

Telephones should be placed where they are accessible but private. Rather than placing telephones in the examining rooms, many practices have a wall telephone placed near a stand-up desk top outside the examining room. Some physicians place a telephone in the reception room for the convenience of patients and to prevent their asking to use the facility's phones.

Recent trends suggest a separate telephone line with a limited calling area for the convenience of patients who need to call out. This telephone should not be in the reception room but in an area available to patients upon request. It should be placed low enough for use by patients in wheelchairs. Wherever possible, telephones should be placed on the wall to conserve desk space.

Many physicians like to have a mobile phone for communication with their office or the hospital while they are traveling by car. Others carry a personal pager that is activated by the medical assistant or the answering service by calling a special number.

If patient care is spread over outlying calling areas, a **WATS** line for calling out and an "800" number for calling in may be practical.

Equipment Selection

There are many options to consider when selecting telephone equipment and services. The six-button key set with several incoming lines, an intercom line, and a hold button has been the standard business phone for decades. It is still being used in many offices. Lights within the buttons flash slowly for incoming calls and blink rapidly to remind of calls being held; a steady light indicates that the line is in use (Fig. 11–7).

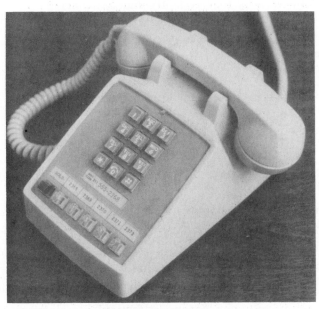

FIGURE 11–7. Key Set Touch-Tone. The Key Set features one "hold" button and five others for calling, signaling, or accessing other extensions. (Courtesy of AT&T.)

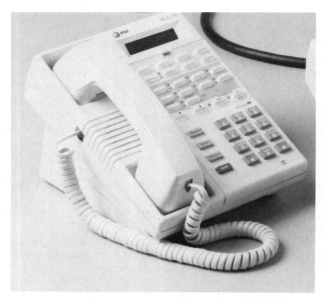

FIGURE 11–8. A two-line speaker phone. (Courtesy of AT&T.)

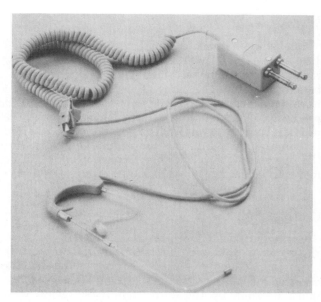

FIGURE 11–9. StarSet headset. (Courtesy of AT&T.)

A popular modern system is the two-line speaker phone that has distinctive ringing and flashing indicators that let you know which line is receiving a call. It also has other features, including:

- Last number redial
- Volume control on the receiver, ringer, and speaker
- Memory for frequently dialed numbers
- Intercom paging (Fig. 11–8)

Another available feature, "ring back on HOLD," allows the caller who dials a busy number to place it on hold. When the called line is free, the connection is completed and the caller is reminded.

Larger facilities tend to select small switchboard-type equipment. One system can start with as few as two lines and six extensions and expand to a maximum of 8 outside lines and 24 extensions.

Headsets

A popular headset is a very light plastic earphone and microphone combination that allows the wearer to move about the room and to have the hands free. One brand name is StarSet (Fig. 11–9). It was originally designed for the astronauts and weighs less than 1 ounce. It is worn behind the ear or clipped to the wearer's glasses. It can be equipped with a cord up to 10 feet in length for easy mobility. It also has an optional quick-disconnect feature that allows the user to separate the headset even during a call without breaking the connection.

Facsimile (FAX) Machines

The FAX machine is rapidly becoming standard equipment in the medical office. The FAX allows its user to send and receive copies of printed documents over telephone lines to other facilities that have FAX machines. It can be a great time and labor saver in conveying patient information from doctor to doctor or from doctor to hospital (Fig. 11–10).

USING THE TELEPHONE DIRECTORY

The primary purpose of the telephone directory, of course, is to provide lists of those who have telephones, their telephone numbers, and in most cases their addresses. In addition, the directory is an aid in checking the spelling of names and in locating certain types of businesses (through the yellow pages). Directories are usually organized in three sections:

- Introductory pages
- Alphabetic pages (white pages)
- Yellow pages

In metropolitan areas, the yellow pages appear in a separate volume.

The introductory pages are sometimes entirely overlooked by the subscribers. This section precedes the white alphabetic pages and provides basic information concerning the telephone services in the area, including:

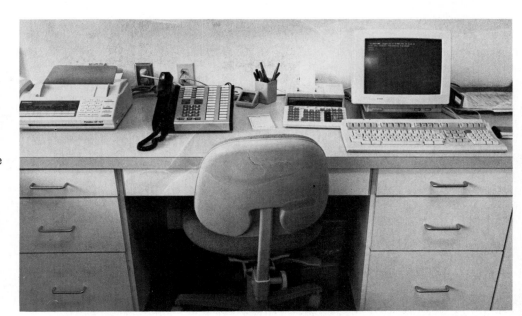

FIGURE 11-10. Facsimile machine on a receptionist's desk.

11

- Emergency services (fire, police, ambulance, and highway patrol)
- Service calls
- Dialing instructions for local and out-of-town calls
- Area codes for some cities

The introductory pages may also include:

- A survival guide
- Community service numbers
- Prefix locations
- Rates
- Long distance calling information
- International calling information
- Time zones
- Government listings

Some directories include ZIP Code maps for the local area. Take a few moments to familiarize yourself with your local directory; then use it frequently for getting information fast.

The white pages are an alphabetic listing of telephone subscribers with their telephone numbers and, in most cases, their addresses.

The yellow pages directory, sometimes published separately, contains listings for businesses arranged by the product or services they sell. Physicians are listed alphabetically, usually under the heading "Physicians and Surgeons," and have the option of another listing by type of practice.

In some areas, a Street Address Telephone Directory is published that lists street addresses, with the name and telephone number of the person or business at that address.

▶ LEARNING ACHIEVEMENTS

Are you able to:

1. Define the terms listed in the Vocabulary of this chapter?
2. Describe what is meant by a "good telephone personality"?
3. List five ways of improving your own telephone personality?
4. Demonstrate the five important steps in answering a professional telephone call?
5. List seven items of information that should be included in a complete telephone message?
6. Differentiate which telephone calls can be handled by a medical assistant and which should be referred to the physician?
7. Demonstrate the handling of two incoming calls on a multiple-line telephone system?
8. Take a call from a new patient who is calling for an appointment and record the six essential items of information?
9. Respond to a call from a patient about a problem with the billing statement?
10. Respond to a call involving a possible emergency situation?

REFERENCES AND READINGS

What Every Telephone User Should Know, General Telephone System.
Your Telephone Personality, Bell Telephone System.
Your Voice is You, Bell Telephone System.
The Business Side of Medical Practice, American Medical Association, 1989.

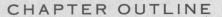

CHAPTER OUTLINE

VOCABULARY

academic degree A title conferred by a college, university, or professional school on completion of a program of study.

annotate To furnish with notes, which are usually critical or explanatory.

clarity The state of being clear or lucid.

concise Expressing much in brief form.

continuation page The second and following pages of a letter.

intrinsic Inward; indwelling.

portfolio A set of documents either bound in book form or loose in a folder.

CORRESPONDENCE AND MAIL PROCESSING

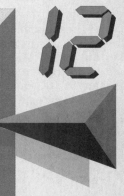

12

COGNITIVE

Upon successful completion of this chapter, you should be able to:

1. Define the terms listed in the Vocabulary.

2. Discuss the responsibility of the medical assistant with respect to office equipment.

3. Select stationery suitable for producing professional correspondence.

4. List the three basic sizes of letterhead stationery.

5. Name three types of essential references for the medical assistant's library.

6. State the five steps in getting ready to answer a letter.

7. Discuss the process of developing a correspondence portfolio.

8. Name four letter styles and discuss their differences.

9. List the four main parts of any business letter.

10. Explain how using ZIP Codes can save money for the mailer.

PERFORMANCE

Upon successful completion of this chapter, you should be able to perform the following activities:

1. Open, sort, and annotate incoming mail.

2. Prepare a response to an inquiry letter.

3. Compose original letters.

4. Address envelopes for optical scanning.

5. Fold outgoing mail for insertion into three styles of envelopes.

Correspondence and mail processing can consume the major part of the administrative medical assistant's day. Many physicians, when queried about the skills they most desire in an administrative assistant, have said, "Send me someone who can write a good letter." Or they may say, "My spelling is atrocious; I need help!" When a physician delegates to the medical assistant the responsibility of composing letters or reports that have the potential to reflect positively or negatively on the practice, he or she is expressing confidence in the assistant.

PUBLIC RELATIONS VALUE

Written communications offer the perfect opportunity for making a good impression on others, but they don't just happen. They require thought, preparation, skill, and a positive attitude. Written communications take many forms in the medical office. The medical assistant may be required to:

- Transcribe from machine or shorthand dictation
- Type consultation and surgical reports
- Compose original letters
- Reply to inquiries
- Respond to requests for information
- Write collection letters
- Order supplies
- Write instructions for patients
- Process a variety of other communications

Transcription is covered in Chapter 13. The other aspects of letter writing are discussed in this chapter.

Written communications should be *courteous* to the reader, *correct* in content, and **concise** without being curt.

Communication is an art as well as a skill. The ability to communicate effectively is extremely important to the medical assistant who is on the way "up the ladder."

EQUIPMENT AND SUPPLIES

In order to create a good impression with your letters, you must use good equipment and quality supplies.

Equipment

Whatever kind of equipment is available for your use, it is your responsibility to know how to use it to the best advantage and to keep it in good working condition. If the equipment manual is available, study it and keep it handy for reference when problems occur. Know how to maintain your equipment so that your best efforts always result in a quality appearance.

Supplies

The quality of paper unquestionably affects the reader's total impression of the communication. Your stationer or printer is qualified to advise on the selection of paper, which can range from all-sulfite (a wood pulp) to all-cotton fiber (sometimes called *rag*). Letterhead paper is usually on bond with a 25% or more cotton fiber content.

The weight of paper is described by a substance number. This number is based on the weight of a ream consisting of 500 sheets of 17 × 22 inch paper. The larger the number, the heavier the paper. If the ream weighs 24 pounds, the paper is referred to as "Sub 24" or "24-pound weight." Letterhead stationery and matching envelopes are usually 16-, 20-, or 24-pound weight.

Letterhead and Envelopes

There are three basic sizes of letterhead:

- Standard   8½ × 11 inches
- Monarch or Executive   7¼ × 10½ inches
- Baronial   5½ × 8½ inches

Standard letterhead is used for general business and professional correspondence. Some executives and professional persons also have letterheads in *Monarch* for informal business and social correspondence. *Baronial,* which is a half-sheet of Standard, is used for very short letters or memoranda. Each size letterhead should have its matching envelope (Table 12–1).

Continuation Pages

The second and continuing pages of a letter or report are typed on plain bond that matches the letterhead in weight and fiber content.

TABLE 12–1. LETTERHEAD

Type	Size	Uses
Standard	8½ × 11	General correspondence
Monarch or Executive	7¼ × 10½	Information, business, and social correspondence
Baronial	5½ × 8½	Very short letters or memoranda

Bond paper has a *felt* side and a *wire* side. Printing and typing is done on the felt side. Pick up a sheet of letterhead and hold it to the light; you will see a design or letters that can be read from the printed side. This design is called a *watermark* and is an indication of quality. The side from which you can read the watermark is the felt side of the paper and is the side on which typing should be done. Always have the watermark read across the page in the same direction as the typing.

Typewriter or Printer Ribbon

Most modern typewriters use correctable film ribbon that passes through the spool only one time. However, if your typewriter or printer uses a cotton or silk ribbon that becomes lighter with use, be sure to change the ribbon before the resulting type impression becomes too light.

YOUR PERSONAL TOOLS

Competent handling of written communications requires a basic knowledge of composition (i.e., sentence structure, spelling, and punctuation [see Chapter 13]). You will also need a personal reference library that includes an up-to-date standard dictionary, a medical dictionary, and a secretary's reference manual. Some suggestions are included in the reference list at the end of this chapter.

Spelling Aid

If you have difficulty with spelling (many people do), you may wish to keep a small looseleaf indexed notebook or card index of words that are troublesome. Whenever it is necessary to look up a word in the dictionary for spelling, record it in the notebook or card index where it can be more easily referred to.

Your physician or a medical assistant who is familiar with the practice might compile a basic list of frequently used medical terms and abbreviations as a reference for the trainee.

Table 12-2 lists 150 frequently misspelled or misused English words. Table 12-3 lists 100 frequently misspelled medical terms. Your list may be entirely different, depending on your capabilities and the branch of medicine in which you are involved.

COMPOSING TIPS

If your only experience in letter writing has been social correspondence, you will have a new set of rules to learn. Social letters tend to be long and chatty, "I" oriented, and do not necessarily follow any organized plan. Most business letters should be less than one page in length, "you" oriented, and

TABLE 12-2. 150 FREQUENTLY MISSPELLED OR MISUSED ENGLISH WORDS

absence	exceed	prevalent
accede	exhilaration	principal
accessible	existence	principle
accommodate	February	privilege
achieve	forty	procedure
affect	grammar	proceed
agglutinate	grievous	professor
all right	height	pronunciation
altogether	incidentally	psychiatry
analyses (pl.)	indispensable	psychology
analysis (s.)	inimitable	pursue
analyze	inoculate	questionnaire
anoint	insistent	rearrange
argument	irrelevant	recede
assistant	irresistible	receive
auxiliary	irritable	recommend
balloon	judgment	referring
believe	labeled	repetition
benefited	led	rheumatism
brochure	leisure	rhythmical
bulletin	license	ridiculous
category	liquefy	sacrilegious
changeable	maintenance	seize
clientele	maneuver	separate
committee	miscellaneous	siege
comparative	mischievous	similar
concede	misspell	sizable
conscientious	necessary	stationary
conscious	newsstand	stationery
coolly	noticeable	subpoena
corroborate	occasion	succeed
definitely	occurrence	suddenness
description	oscillate	superintendent
desirable	paid	supersede
despair	pamphlet	surprise
development	panicky	tariff
dilemma	parallel	technique
disappear	paralyze	thorough
disappoint	pastime	tranquility
disastrous	perseverance	transferred
discreet	persistent	truly
discrete	personal	tyrannize
discriminate	personnel	unnecessary
dissatisfaction	possession	until
dissipate	precede	vacillate
drunkenness	precedent	vacuum
ecstasy	predictable	vicious
effect	predominant	warrant
eligible	predominate	Wednesday
embarrass	prerogative	weird

carefully organized. This takes practice and preparation.

Getting Ready to Write

If you are asked to answer a letter, first organize your facts.

- Read carefully the letter you are to answer.
- Make note of or underline any questions asked or materials requested.
- Decide on the answers to the questions and verify your information. This is called **annotating.**

TABLE 12–3. FREQUENTLY MISSPELLED MEDICAL WORDS

abscess	homeostasis	peritoneum
additive	humerus	petit mal
aerosol	idiosyncrasy	pharynx
agglutination	ileum	pituitary
albumin	ilium	plantar
anastomosis	infarction	pleura
aneurysm	intussusception	pleurisy
anteflexion	ischemia	pneumonia
arrhythmia	ischium	polyp
bilirubin	larynx	prophylaxis
bronchial	leukemia	prostate
cachexia	malaise	prosthesis
calcaneus	malleus	pruritus
capillary	melena	psoriasis
cervical	mellitus	pyrexia
chromosome	menstruation	respiratory
cirrhosis	metastasis	rheumatic
clavicle	neurilemma	roentgenology
curettage	neuron	sagittal
cyanosis	occlusion	sciatica
defibrillator	optic chiasm	scirrhous
desiccate	oscilloscope	serous
ecchymosis	osseous	sessile
effusion	palliative	sphincter
epididymis	parasite	sphygmomanometer
epistaxis	parenteral	squamous
eustachian	parietal	staphylococcus
fissure	paroxysmal	suppuration
flexure	pemphigus	trochanter
glaucoma	percussion	venous
gonorrhea	perforation	wheal
graafian	pericardium	xiphoid
hemorrhage	perineum	
hemorrhoids	peristalsis	

• Draft a reply, using the tools you are most comfortable with (e.g., the typewriter, longhand, or shorthand).
• Rewrite for **clarity.**

Keep most of your sentences short. Put only one idea in each sentence. Eliminate the superfluous words. Be careful about using medical terms in correspondence with patients; use only language that the reader can understand.

Every person who writes letters develops his or her own personal style. Most physicians conform to a highly professional and formal style in their dictation.

The medical assistant who is given the responsibility of composing correspondence for the medical office should strive for the same degree of formality used by the physician. It would be inappropriate for the assistant to write in a breezy, informal style when acting as the representative of an employer who is strictly formal in his or her approach.

The principal thing to remember is that every letter produced in your office should project the image of the physician regardless of who composes or signs it.

Developing a Portfolio

Letter composition can be sped up by developing a **portfolio** of sample letters to suit the various situations that frequently arise. Suppose, for instance, you need to write to a patient to change an appointment. Compose the very best letter you can —one that is clear, concise, and courteous—and make an extra copy to place in your portfolio of letters. Alternatively, if you are using a computer, store the letter on a disk. Do this each time you write a new kind of letter. Soon you will be able to select a letter from your portfolio and change it slightly to suit the current situation. You will have your letters written in no time!

Watch for sample letters that appear from time to time in the doctor's business journals and clip them for your portfolio. Scan the textbooks and office manuals on the market or in your public library for additional help.

Other Written Forms of Communication

Written communications include more than letter writing. For example, consider telephone messages that you take. Are you sure that they are clearly stated and convey to the reader what you intend? You may need to mail a prescription to a patient, with instructions from the physician. Make sure that the patient is able to read and understand what you intend to communicate.

LETTER STYLES

A business letter is usually arranged in one of three styles: *block, modified block (standard),* or *modified block—indented.* A fourth style, called *simplified,* is occasionally used. The block and modified block (standard) styles are most commonly used in the physician's office.

Block letter style. All lines start flush with the left margin. This is considered most efficient but is less attractive on the page (Fig. 12–1).

Modified block letter style (standard). The date line, the complimentary closing, and the typewritten signature all begin at the center. All other lines begin at the left margin (Fig. 12–2).

Modified block with indented paragraphs. This is identical to the block style except that the first line of each paragraph is indented five spaces (Fig. 12–3).

Simplified letter style. All lines begin flush with the left margin. The salutation is replaced with an all-capital subject line on the third line below the inside address. The body of the letter begins on the third line below the subject line. The compli-

ELIZABETH BLACKWELL, M.D.
223 Orange Avenue, N.W.
Cottonwood, UT 84121

January 26, 19xx

Mr. Richard Fluege
3578 North Willow Avenue
Palm Beach, FL 33480

Dear Mr. Fluege:

Please send me full particulars on the
professional suites you expect to offer for
sale or rent in the Medical Arts Professional
Annex.

In about six months, I will be ready to open
my practice, and I am interested in locating
in Florida. My preference is a street-level
suite of approximately 2,000 square feet.

After I have had an opportunity to study the
information you send me, I will write or
telephone you if I have further questions.

Very truly yours,

Elizabeth Blackwell, M.D.

MK

FIGURE 12-1. Block letter style.

MEDICAL ARTS PROFESSIONAL ANNEX
3578 North Willow Avenue
Palm Beach FL 33480

January 29, 19xx

Elizabeth Blackwell, M.D.
223 Orange Avenue, N.W.
Cottonwood, UT 84121

Dear Doctor Blackwell:

We have two remaining street-level suites available for
occupancy about July 1. These are marked on pages 3
and 4 of the enclosed descriptive brochure. If either
of these suites appeals to you, we will be pleased to
customize it for your practice.

Please feel free to call me collect at the number on
the brochure for further discussion of your needs.

Sincerely yours,

Richard Fluege
Business Manager

RF:MK
Enclosure

FIGURE 12-2. Modified block letter style (standard).

12

WILLIAM OSLER, M.D.
1000 South West Street
Park Ridge, NJ 07656

January 26, 19xx

Robert Koch, M.D.
398 Main Street
Park Ridge, NJ 07656

Dear Doctor Koch:

<u>Mrs. Elaine Norris</u>

Thank you for referring your patient, Mrs. Elaine Norris, for consultation and care. She was examined in my office today.

FINDINGS: The patient complained of pain in the left lower quadrant and some abdominal tenderness. She had a temperature of 100.2 degrees.

RECOMMENDATIONS: The patient was placed on a soft, low-residue, bland diet, antibiotics, and bedrest for a few days. Upper and lower gastrointestinal X-rays will be performed next week.

TENTATIVE DIAGNOSIS: Diverticulitis of large bowel.

Mrs. Norris has been asked to return here for re-evaluation in about 10 days.

Sincerely yours,

William Osler, M.D.

WO:MK

FIGURE 12-3. Modified block letter style with indented paragraphs.

ROBERT KOCH, M.D.
398 Main Street
Park Ridge, NJ 07656

January 30, 19xx

William Osler, M.D.
1000 South West Street
Park Ridge, NJ 07656

ANNABELLE ANDERSON

You will be pleased to know, Bill, that Mrs.
Anderson is progressing nicely. Her wound is
healing. Her temperature has returned to
normal, and she is beginning to resume her
usual activities.

Mrs. Anderson has an appointment to return
here for one more visit next week. At that
time, I will ask her to return to you for any
further care.

ROBERT KOCH, M.D.

MK

FIGURE 12-4. Simplified letter style.

mentary closing is omitted. An all-capital typewritten signature is typed on the fifth line below the body of the letter (Fig. 12–4).

PUNCTUATION

Traditionally, the punctuation pattern is selected on the basis of letter style. Normal punctuation is always used *within the body* of a business letter. The other parts follow one of the following patterns:

Standard (mixed) punctuation. A colon is placed after the salutation, and a comma is placed after the complimentary closing. This is the punctuation pattern most commonly used. It is appropriate with the block or modified block letter styles.

Open punctuation. No punctuation is used at the end of any line outside the body of the letter unless that line ends with an abbreviation. This pattern is always used with the simplified letter style.

SPACING AND MARGINS

Generally speaking, a letter centered on a page is the most attractive. Accomplishing this requires experience, but a few guidelines with which to start are helpful:

Spacing. Business letters are almost always single-spaced. If a letter consists of only a few lines, you can double-space both the inside address and the message. In this case, you should indent the first line of each paragraph five spaces.

Top margin. Your first typed entry—the date—is usually placed on the third line below the letterhead or on line 15 if there is no letterhead. **Continuation pages** begin 1 inch from the top (line 7).

Side margin. On standard letterhead, the 6½-inch line is common and leaves 1-inch margins on each side. The appearance of a very short letter is improved by increasing the size of all margins.

Bottom margin. A 1-inch bottom margin is the minimum. This can be increased if the letter is to be carried over to a second page. Never use a second page to type only the complimentary closing and signature. Carry over a minimum of two lines of the body of the letter.

PARTS OF LETTERS

The parts of letters and their placement on a page has been fairly well standardized. There are four main parts of a letter:

- Heading
- Opening
- Body
- Closing

Heading

The heading includes the *letterhead* and the *date line*. The printed letterhead is usually centered at the top of the page and includes the name of the physician or group and the address. It may include the telephone number and the medical specialty (or specialties). In a group or corporate practice, the names of the physicians may also be listed. Occasionally, the heading also includes the name of an office manager.

The *date line* consists of the name of the month written in full, followed by the day and year. The date should not be abbreviated, nor should ordinal numbers (i.e., 1st, 2nd, and 3rd) be used following the name of the month.

Opening

The opening includes the inside address, the salutation, and the attention line (if there is one).

The *inside address* has two or more lines, starts flush with the left margin, and contains at least the name of the individual or firm to whom the letter is addressed and the mailing address.

When the letter is addressed to an individual, the name is preceded by a courtesy title, such as Dr., Mr., Mrs., Miss, or Ms. When addressing a letter to a physician, omit the courtesy title and type the physician's name followed by his or her **academic degree.** Do not use both a courtesy title and a degree that mean the same thing (e.g., Dr. Herbert H. Long, M.D.).

The *salutation* is the letter writer's introductory greeting to the person being addressed. It is typed flush with the left margin on the second line below the last line of the inside address. It is followed by a colon unless open punctuation is used. The words in the salutation vary depending on the degree of formality of the letter.

The *attention line,* if used, is placed on the second line below the inside address. If you know the name of the person for whom the letter is intended, use that person's name in the inside address and address him or her personally. If the letter is being directed to a division or department within a company, place that information on the line preceding the company name.

Body

The *body* of a letter includes the subject line, if one is used, and the message.

Frequently in medical office correspondence, the subject of a letter is a patient. The patient's name is used as the *subject line*. Because the subject line is considered to be a part of the body of the letter, it is typed on the second line below the salutation. It may start flush with the left margin or at the point of indentation of indented paragraphs, or it may be centered. The word "subject," followed by a colon, may be used or omitted entirely.

Begin typing the body of the letter (the message) on the second line below the subject line, or on the second line below the salutation if there is no subject line. The first line of each paragraph may be indented five spaces or may start flush with the left margin, depending on the letter style being used.

Closing

The closing includes the complimentary closing, the typewritten signature, the reference initials, and any special notations.

The *complimentary closing* is the writer's way of saying "goodbye." The words used are determined by the degree of formality in the salutation. For example, if the salutation is "Dear Herb:" the closing might be "Cordially" or "Sincerely yours." If the letter is addressed to a business, the complimentary closing generally used is "Very truly yours."

The complimentary closing is typed on the second line below the last line of the body of the letter and is followed by a comma unless open punctuation is used. Only the first word is capitalized.

The *typewritten signature* is a courtesy to the reader, especially if the name does not appear on the printed letterhead. Type the signature on the fourth line directly below the complimentary closing.

The *reference initials* identifying the typist are typed flush with the left margin on the second line below the typewritten signature. If the writer's name is included on the signature line, the writer's initials need not be included in the reference block unless desired. The writer's initials, if used, should precede the typist's initials and be separated by a colon or diagonal:

MEK   or   MMB:MEK   or   mmb/mek

Special Notations

Special notations are sometimes needed to indicate that enclosures are included with the letter or that copies of the letter are being distributed to others.

If the letter indicates an enclosure, type the word "Enclosure" or "Enc." on the first line below the reference initials. If there is more than one enclosure, specify the number (e.g., Enclosures 3).

If copies are to be sent to others, type this notation in the same manner as the enclosure notation or following it if both notations are needed. The copy notation is usually written as "cc:" or "xc:" followed by the name or names of those to whom a copy will be sent.

If the person to whom the letter is addressed is not to know that copies are being distributed to others, use the notation "bcc" for *blind carbon copy;* on all copies *except* the original, place this notation either in the upper left of the letter at the margin or below the last notation at the lower left margin.

Postscripts

Although a postscript may sometimes be used to express an afterthought, it is more often used to place emphasis on an idea or statement.

Begin the postscript on the second line below the last special notation. Follow the style of the letter, indenting the first line if paragraphs are indented in the body of the letter or at the margin if indentation was not used in the letter.

Continuation Page Heading

If the letter requires one or more continuation pages, the heading of the second and subsequent pages must contain three items of information:

- the name of the addressee
- the page number
- the date

There are three accepted forms for the heading (see Headings for Continuation Pages).

HEADINGS FOR CONTINUATION PAGES
Elizabeth Blackwell, M.D.   -2-   July 4, 19xx
William Osler, M.D. Page 2 July 4, 19xx
William S. Halsted, M.D. Page 2 July 4, 19xx Subject: Susan Barstow

The heading should begin on the 7th line from the top of the page; continuation of the body of the letter begins on the 10th line or the 3rd line below the heading.

SIGNING THE LETTER

Some physicians prefer to compose and sign all letters that leave their offices. The majority are more than pleased to delegate to a competent assistant the responsibility of composing and signing letters of a business nature.

Although not all authorities agree on the form to be followed, most recommend that a woman's typewritten signature include a title (Miss, Mrs., or Ms.) and that the title not be enclosed in parentheses. It is not necessary to include the courtesy title in the handwritten signature.

How will you know which letters to sign? In general, the physician signs all of the following:

- Letters that deal with medical advice to patients
- Letters to officers or committees of the medical society
- Referral and consultation reports to colleagues

- Medical reports to insurance companies
- Personal letters
- Any letters of a personal nature

The medical assistant usually signs letters concerning the following:

- Strictly routine or business matters, such as arranging or rescheduling appointments
- Ordering office supplies
- Notifying patients of surgery or hospital arrangements
- Collecting for delinquent accounts
- Letters of solicitation

PROCEDURE 12 - 1   COMPOSING BUSINESS CORRESPONDENCE

GOAL   To compose and type a letter ordering medical and office supplies using tabular placement of items and following the guidelines of a commonly used business letter style.

EQUIPMENT AND SUPPLIES

Typewriter or word processor
Draft paper
Letterhead paper
Pen or pencil

Want List of supplies needed
Medical and office supply catalog
Correcting tape, liquid, or eraser
  (optional)

PROCEDURAL STEPS

1. Locate items from Want List in the catalog.

2. Note the catalog number of each item, the unit price, size, and color, and any special information requirements.
   Explanation: Compare this information with the Want List to confirm the correctness of the order.

3. Prepare a draft of the letter by hand or typewriter, tabulating the items ordered.
   Purpose: To provide practice in composing a letter and the use of tabulation. (With sufficient experience, this step can be eliminated.)

4. Edit the draft carefully for correct information, grammar, spelling, and punctuation.

5. Insert letterhead in the typewriter.

6. Set line and margins for attractive placement of the letter.

7. Type the letter from the corrected draft.

8. Type your signature and identification initials.
   Explanation: The medical assistant signs letters ordering supplies.

9. Proofread the letter for composition errors and accuracy of the order.
   Purpose: Any necessary corrections are more easily accomplished while the paper is still in the typewriter.

10. Remove the completed letter and sign it.

PROCEDURE 12-2   WRITING INSTRUCTIONS

GOAL   To inform new patient of most desirable automobile route to doctor's office, including any known landmarks, and description of parking facilities at destination.

EQUIPMENT AND SUPPLIES

Local map
Name and address of patient
Typewriter or word processor
Draft paper
Pen or pencil

Bond paper
Envelope
Dictionary
Correcting tape, liquid, or eraser
   (optional)

PROCEDURAL STEPS

1. Locate the doctor's office on the map.

2. Locate the patient's address on the map.
   Purpose: To determine the most desirable route between these two points.

3. On draft paper, using a pencil or typewriter, compose directions, using street names and including any prominent intersections, right or left turns, landmarks just preceding the destination, and means of identifying the destination.
   Purpose: To create a mental picture of a route and directions that can be easily followed.

4. Read your copy for clarity and recheck with the map for accuracy.
   Purpose: Note the spelling of street names and check for the accuracy of direction turns.

5. Describe parking facilities and their utilization.
   Explanation: Include information about meters, validation, time limit, and so forth.

6. Describe route to doctor's office entrance from the parking facility.
   Purpose: To provide peace of mind to patients who feel apprehensive about traveling to an unfamiliar location.

7. Check the complete draft for clarity and detail.
   Purpose: It is very important that directions be accurate, clear, and complete.

8. Typewrite directions in narrative form on bond paper.

9. Proofread and correct any typographic errors.

10. Typewrite the patient's mailing address on an envelope using the format for optical scanning.

PREPARING THE OUTGOING MAIL

Addressing the Envelope

The United States Postal Service (USPS) is attempting to have all mail (in No. 10 and No. 6¾ envelopes) read, coded, sorted, and canceled automatically at regional sorting stations where mail can be processed at a rate of 30,000 letters per hour.

The success of automatic sorting depends on the cooperation of mailers in preparing envelopes in a format that can be read by automatic equipment. Key points are as follows:

- Use dark type on a light background; black on white is best.
- Do not use script or italic type; these cannot be read by an electronic scanner.
- Type all envelope addresses in block format and in the area on the envelope that the scanner is programmed to read.
- Capitalize everything in the address.

- Eliminate all punctuation in the address.
- Use the standard two-letter state code instead of the spelled out name of the state (Fig. 12–5).
- The last line of the address must contain the city, state code, and ZIP Code, and it must not exceed 27 characters in length. The characters should be distributed so that they will not exceed the following limits:

Allowance for city name	13
Space between city name and state code	1
Allowance for state code	2
Space between state code and ZIP Code	1
Space for basic ZIP Code	5
Space for hyphen and four additional characters	5
	27

If a city name contains more than 13 characters, you must use the approved code for that city as shown in the Abbreviations Section of the National Zip Code Directory.

The Postal Service provides three special sets of abbreviations: (1) state names; (2) long names of cities, towns, and places; and (3) names of streets and roads and general terms, such as University or Institute. By using these abbreviations, it is possible to limit the last line of any domestic address to 27 strokes. The next-to-last line in the address block should contain a street address or post office box number, as in the following examples:

```
MEDICAL ASSOCIATES INCORPORATED
4444 AVENIDA WILSHIRE
SAN CLEMENTE CA 92672-1500
```

```
HENRY B TURNER MD
P O BOX 845
JACKSONVILLE FL 32232-9950
```

Leave a bottom margin of at least ⅝ inch and left and right margins of at least 1 inch. Nothing should be written or printed below the address block or to the right of it.

TWO-LETTER ABBREVIATIONS

UNITED STATES AND TERRITORIES

Alabama	AL	Montana	MT
Alaska	AK	Nebraska	NE
Arizona	AZ	Nevada	NV
Arkansas	AR	New Hampshire	NH
California	CA	New Jersey	NJ
Canal Zone	CZ	New Mexico	NM
Colorado	CO	New York	NY
Connecticut	CT	North Carolina	NC
Delaware	DE	North Dakota	ND
District of Columbia	DC	Ohio	OH
Florida	FL	Oklahoma	OK
Georgia	GA	Oregon	OR
Guam	GU	Pennsylvania	PA
Hawaii	HI	Puerto Rico	PR
Idaho	ID	Rhode Island	RI
Illinois	IL	South Carolina	SC
Indiana	IN	South Dakota	SD
Iowa	IA	Tennessee	TN
Kansas	KS	Texas	TX
Kentucky	KY	Utah	UT
Louisiana	LA	Vermont	VT
Maine	ME	Virgin Islands	VI
Maryland	MD	Virginia	VA
Massachusetts	MA	Washington	WA
Michigan	MI	West Virginia	WV
Minnesota	MN	Wisconsin	WI
Mississippi	MS	Wyoming	WY
Missouri	MO		

CANADIAN PROVINCES AND TERRITORIES

Alberta	AB	Nova Scotia	NS
British Columbia	BC	Ontario	ON
Manitoba	MB	Prince Edward Island	PE
New Brunswick	NB	Quebec	PQ
Newfoundland	NF	Saskatchewan	SK
Northwest Territories	NT	Yukon Territory	YT

FIGURE 12–5. Two-letter abbreviations for states and territories should be used only with ZIP Codes in addresses.

The above regulations for addressing envelopes were developed mainly for volume mailers with computerized mailing lists. Some exceptions are acceptable to the Postal Service and its scanning equipment. For example, the traditional style of typing an address in lower case with initial capital letters is readable by the optical scanners. Also, if you cannot fit the ZIP Code on the line with the city and state, you can place it on the line immediately below.

Return Address

Always place a complete return address on your envelope. The USPS will not deliver mail without postage, and if you should forget to stamp the envelope or if the stamp should fall off and there is no return address, it will go to the dead letter office. There the postal employees will open the mail in an attempt to identify the sender.

If they find an address for the sender, they will return the mail in an official envelope with a notice of postage due. If they do not find an address for the sender, the mail is destroyed and you may never know what happened to it. At best, it causes a great delay.

Notations

Any notations on the envelope directed toward the addressee, such as "PERSONAL" or "CONFIDENTIAL," should be typed two lines below the return address and three spaces from the left edge of the envelope in all capitals.

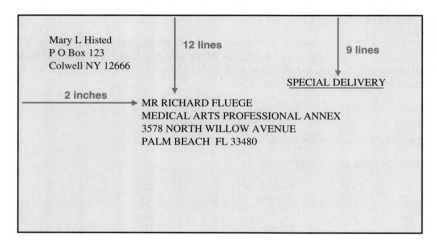

Placement of return address, mailing address, and mailing notation on 6 3/4 envelope

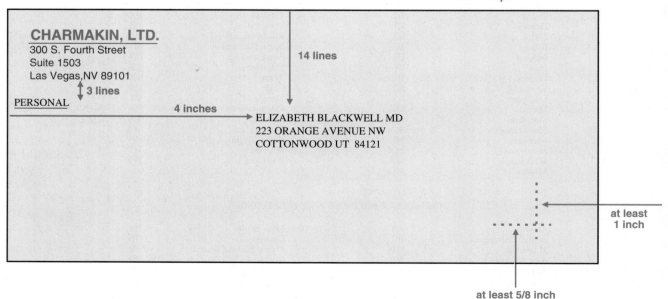

Placement of mailing address and Personal notation on No. 10 envelope

FIGURE 12-6. Addressing envelopes.

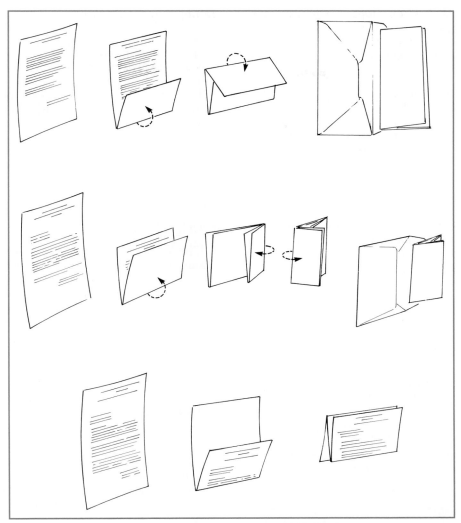

FIGURE 12–7. Correct methods of folding letters.

Any notations directed toward the postal service, such as "SPECIAL DELIVERY" or "CERTIFIED MAIL," should be typed in all capital letters in the upper right corner of the envelope immediately below the stamp area. If an address contains an attention line, it should be typed as the second line of the address (Fig. 12–6).

Folding and Inserting Letters

Standard ways of folding and inserting letters are used so that the letter fits properly into the envelope and so that it can be easily removed without damage (Fig. 12–7).

Number 10 envelope. For a standard-size letter, bring the bottom third of the letter up and make a crease. Fold the top of the letter down to within about ⅜ inch of the creased edge and make a second crease. The second crease goes into the envelope first.

Number 6¾ envelope. For a standard-size letter, bring the bottom edge up to within about ⅜ inch of the top edge and make a crease. Then, folding from the right edge, make a fold a little less than one third of the width of the sheet and crease it. Folding from the left edge, bring the edge to within about ⅜ inch of the previous crease. Insert the left creased edge into the envelope first.

Window envelope. To fold a letter for insertion into a window envelope, bring the bottom third of the letter up and make a crease, then fold the top of the letter back to the crease you made before. (The inside address should now be facing you.) This method is often followed for mailing statements.

Sealing and Stamping Hints

Here's a suggestion for speeding up the sealing of a number of envelopes; at statement time, for example, many envelopes go into the mail at once:

- Fan out unsealed envelopes, address side down, in groups of 6 to 10.
- Draw a damp sponge over the flaps and, starting with the lower piece, turn down the flaps and seal each one.

Do not use too much moisture, as this may cause the glue to spread and several envelopes to stick together.

A similar process simplifies stamping several letters at one time if you are not using a postage meter. If possible, purchase your stamps by the roll.

- Tear off about ten stamps from the roll.
- Fanfold the stamps on the perforations so that they separate easily.
- Fan the envelopes address side up.
- Wet a strip of stamps with the sponge and, starting at one end of the fanned envelopes, attach the stamp at the end of the strip, tear it off, and proceed to the next envelope.

MAILING PROCEDURES

Cost-saving Procedures

ZIP Codes

The ZIP Code is a very important part of an address, just as the area code is a very important part of a telephone number. ZIP Codes start with the number 0 on the East Coast and gradually increase to number 9 on the West Coast and Hawaii.

The 5-digit ZIP Code was introduced in 1961. The first three digits identify a major city or distribution point, and all five digits identify an individual post office, zone of a city, or other delivery unit.

The USPS has recently introduced the 9-digit ZIP Code, consisting of the original five digits followed by a hyphen and four additional digits that further identify the addressee's street location. The USPS claims that the ZIP-plus-4, when used with the automated letter-sorting machinery, can eliminate 20 mail handling steps and result in considerable savings. This saving is passed on to large mailers on mailings of 250 or more pieces of mail that have typewritten addresses in machine-readable format along with the 9-digit ZIP Code.

Presorting

Large mailers can get a discount on postage for presorting their mail. A discounted presort rate is charged on each piece that is part of a group of 10 or more pieces sorted to the same 5-digit code or a group of 50 or more pieces sorted to the same first 3-digit ZIP Code (Information Guide on Presorted First Class Mail, Publication 61).

Using Correct Postage

Although mailing fees are still one of our better bargains, the mailing costs for even a small office are a sizable item in the annual budget, and carelessness can cause them to soar.

If your office does not have a postage meter that dispenses postage exactly, then be sure that you are not putting too many stamps on your outgoing mail. Use an accurate postage scale and remember that only the first ounce requires the base rate; additional ounces are at a lower rate.

Getting Faster Mail Service

Postage Meter

The postage meter is the most efficient way of stamping the mail in a large business office (Fig. 12–8). It can print postage onto adhesive strips that are then placed onto the envelopes or packages, or it can print the postage directly onto an envelope.

Metered mail does not have to be canceled or postmarked when it reaches the post office. This means that it can move on to its destination faster. Meters vary in size and capabilities. Consult your office equipment dealer for your own needs.

Mailing Practices

Mailing early in the day is appreciated by your local post office. For large mailings, local letters should be separated from out-of-town letters. Letters or packages that need to be rushed should be taken directly to the post office for mailing. Others can be placed in street boxes or your own building's mail chute for pickup. Packages should always be taken to a post office.

Place a letter tray on your desk or some other convenient place so that you can keep all outgoing mail together until you are able to send it on its way.

CLASSIFICATIONS OF MAIL

Mail is classified according to type, weight, and destination. The ounce and pound are the units of measurement. The types of mail commonly handled in a medical office are:

Express Mail Next Day Service. Express Mail is available 7 days per week, 365 days per year for mailable items up to 70 pounds in weight and 108 inches in combined length and *girth*. Service features include:

- noon delivery between major business markets
- merchandise and document reconstruction insurance
- Express Mail shipping containers
- shipment receipt

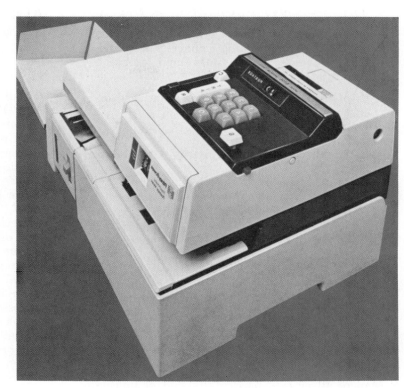

FIGURE 12-8. Example of one type of postage meter-mailing machine. (Courtesy of Pitney Bowes Company.)

12

- optional return receipt service
- optional COD service
- waiver of signature option
- collection boxes
- optional pickup service

First Class mail. This includes sealed or unsealed handwritten or typed material, such as letters, postal cards, postcards, and business reply mail. Postage for letters weighing 11 ounces or less is based on weight, in 1-ounce increments.

Envelopes larger than the standard No. 10 business envelope should have the green diamond border to expedite First Class delivery.

Priority Mail. First Class mail weighing over 11 ounces is classified as Priority Mail, and the postage is calculated on the basis of weight and destination, with the maximum weight being 70 pounds.

Second Class mail. This includes newspapers and periodical publications. Regular and preferred Second Class rates are available only to newspapers and periodicals that have been authorized to receive Second Class mail privileges.

Copies mailed by the public are charged at the applicable Express Mail, Priority Mail, or single piece First, Third, or Fourth Class rate.

Third Class mail. Third Class mail includes such items as catalogs, circulars, books, photographs, and other printed matter. Pieces should be sealed or secured so that they can be handled by machine but must be clearly marked with the words "Third Class."

Fourth Class mail. This consists of merchandise, books, printed matter, and so forth that are not included in the First or Second Class and that weigh 16 ounces or more but do not exceed 70 pounds. There are size limitations on Fourth Class mail; check with your post office regarding regulations on very large parcels. Rates are determined on the basis of weight and destination. Such mail may be sealed or unsealed.

SIZE STANDARDS FOR DOMESTIC MAIL

Minimum mail sizes. All mail must be at least 0.007 inch thick, and mail that is ¼ inch or less in thickness must be:

- At least 3½ inches in height and at least 5 inches long
- Rectangular in shape

Nonstandard mail. It is important to use an envelope of the correct size. For each piece of nonstandard mail, the USPS assesses a surcharge in addition to the applicable postage and fees. Envelope sizes were standardized when the Postal Service began sorting mail by machine. The following material is considered nonstandard mail: First Class mail (except Presort First Class and carrier route First Class) weighing 1 ounce or less, and all single-piece rate Third Class mail weighing 1 ounce or less if:

1. Any of the following dimensions are exceeded:
   Length — 11½ inches
   Height — 6½ inches
   Thickness — ¼ inch
2. The length divided by the height is not between 1.3 and 2.5.

SPECIAL SERVICES FOR DOMESTIC MAIL

Insurance

Insurance for coverage against loss or damage is available for all classes of mail in amounts up to $500.

Registry

Mail of all classes, particularly that of unusually high value, can be additionally protected by registering it. Evidence of its delivery may be requested by the sender. Registering a piece of mail also helps to trace delivery, if necessary.

When sending a registered letter, it is necessary to go to the post office and fill in the required forms. All articles to be registered must be thoroughly sealed with USPS approved tape (do not use cellophane tape) and have postage paid at First Class rates.

Upon receipt of the item, the recipient is required to sign a form that acknowledges delivery. A registered letter may be released to the person to whom it is addressed or to his or her agent. For an additional fee, a personal receipt may be requested. This assures that the letter will be released only to the individual to whom it is addressed. Such pieces bear the label "To Addressee Only."

Registered mail is accounted for by number from the time of mailing until delivery and is transported separately from other mail under a special lock. In case of loss or damage, the customer may be reimbursed up to $10,000, provided that the value of the registered article has been declared at the time of mailing and that the appropriate fee has been paid.

Postal Money Orders

Postal money orders are a convenient way of mailing money, especially for the individual who does not have a personal checking account. Postal money orders may be purchased in amounts as high as $700. If a sum greater than $700 is needed, additional money orders must be purchased in amounts of $700 or less.

Special Delivery

Mail of any class that has been marked "SPECIAL DELIVERY" is charged at the Special Delivery rate. Such pieces may be regular First or Second Class mail, registered, insured, or COD (Collect on Delivery) pieces. Special Delivery instruction generally does not speed up the normal travel time between two cities but does assure immediate delivery of the item when it arrives at the designated post office.

Special Delivery stamps may be purchased at the post office. Alternatively, the equivalent value in regular stamps may be affixed to the envelope, which should always be clearly marked "Special Delivery." Use Special Delivery when you need delivery of an item the same day as it is received at the addressee's post office (including weekend delivery that is not available with regular mail). Do *not* use Special Delivery for mail addressed to a Post Office Box or military installation. A fee based on the weight of the item is required in addition to the required postage.

Special Handling

For a small additional fee, Third and Fourth Class mail in this category receives the fastest handling and ground transportation practicable (about the same as that for First Class mail). This fee does not include insurance or Special Delivery at the destination, but Special Delivery, if desired, is available at an added cost. If a parcel is sent by Priority Mail, Special Handling is of no additional advantage because it is already traveling at the greatest possible speed. Fees are in addition to required postage and are determined according to weight.

Certified Mail

Any piece of mail without **intrinsic** value and on which postage is paid at the First Class rate will be accepted as Certified Mail. Such items as contracts, deeds, mortgages, bank books, checks, passports, insurance policies, money orders, and birth certificates that are not themselves valuable but that would be difficult to duplicate if lost should be certified. Certified Mail is also often used as an aid in collections.

Regular postage in addition to a Certified fee must be affixed. For an additional fee, a receipt verifying delivery can be requested. Certified Mail can be sent Special Delivery if the prescribed Special Delivery fees are paid. A record of delivery of Certified Mail is kept for 2 years at the post office of delivery; however, no record is kept at the post office of origin. Furthermore, this type of mail does not provide insurance coverage.

The medical assistant should keep a supply of Certified Mail forms and return receipts on hand (Figs. 12–9 and 12–10). These may be obtained at any post office. Full instructions are included on the forms. Fees and postage may be paid using ordinary postage stamps, meter stamps, or permit imprint. Certified Mail can be mailed at any post office, station, or branch, or can be deposited in mail drops or in street letter boxes if you follow specific instructions.

Certificate of Mailing

If a sender needs proof of mailing but is not especially concerned with proof of receipt of an item, the most economical method is to obtain a Certificate of Mailing. Obtain this form at your post office and fill in the required information. Attach a stamp for the current fee and hand the form to the postal clerk along with the piece of mail. The clerk will postmark the receipt, initial it, and hand it back as acknowledgment of having received the piece of mail at the post office. This is sometimes used when mailing tax reports or other items that must be postmarked by a certain date.

P 758 351 390

RECEIPT FOR CERTIFIED MAIL

NO INSURANCE COVERAGE PROVIDED
NOT FOR INTERNATIONAL MAIL
(See Reverse)

Sent to W B SAUNDERS	
Street and No. INDEPENDENCE SQ WEST	
P.O., State and ZIP Code PHILADELPHIA PA 19105	
Postage	$
Certified Fee	
Special Delivery Fee	
Restricted Delivery Fee	
Return Receipt showing to whom and Date Delivered	
Return Receipt showing to whom, Date, and Address of Delivery	
TOTAL Postage and Fees	$
Postmark or Date	

PS Form 3800, June 1985

Fold at line over top of envelope to the right of the return address

CERTIFIED

P 758 351 390

MAIL

FIGURE 12–9. Receipt for Certified Mail. Attach at top of envelope to the right of return address.

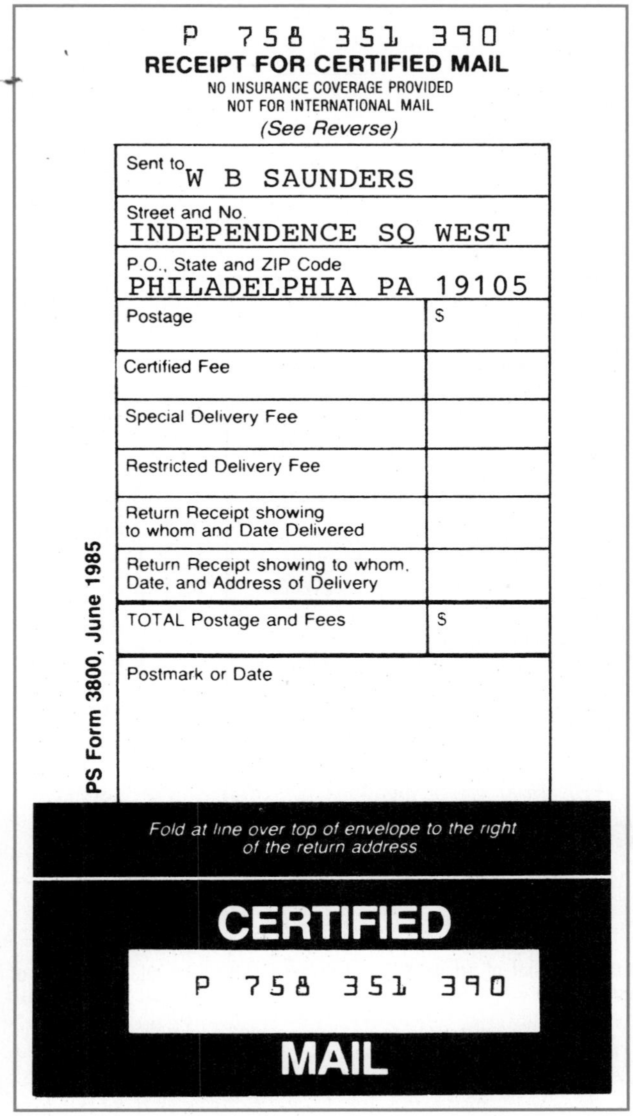

INTERNATIONAL MAIL

Letters to distant points of the globe are in almost all cases sent by air and can be expected to reach their destination within a very few days. The rates for international mail are based on increments of one-half ounce. A table of rates can be obtained from your post office. If you wish to supply a foreign correspondent with reply postage, international reply coupons may be purchased at the post office and sent to other countries.

PRIVATE MAIL SERVICES

Not all mail is delivered by the USPS. Many private services pick up and deliver mail overnight. Among these are Federal Express, United Parcel Service, Emery, and Purolator; all of these services are highly advertised and competitive. All large cities and many smaller communities have centralized points where packages can be dropped off for the service of the sender's choice. Pickup service is also available in many communities.

ELECTRONIC MAIL

Computer-to-computer communications systems are available for transmitting messages and documents. CompuServe, MCI Mail, Federal Express Corporation's ZapMail, and Western Union's Easy-Line are examples of providers of these services. The transmitting and receiving computers may be located on the user's own premises or on the service provider's premises. The messages and documents may be received electronically or on paper.

E-COM (Electronic computer-originated mail) service permits mailers to send computer-generated messages by electronic means at designated serving post offices. Messages are submitted in electronic form to one or more serving post offices, where they are transformed into printed letters, inserted into special marked envelopes, and delivered as First Class mail.

The facsimile (FAX) machine is emerging as standard equipment in medical offices and is discussed further in Chapter 11.

REMOVE TO EXPOSE ADHESIVE

UNITED STATES POSTAL SERVICE

OFFICIAL BUSINESS

SENDER INSTRUCTIONS

Print your name, address and ZIP Code in the space below.

- **Complete items 1, 2, 3, and 4 on the reverse.**
- **Attach to front of article if space permits, otherwise affix to back of article.**
- **Endorse article "Return Receipt Requested" adjacent to number.**

U.S.MAIL

PENALTY FOR PRIVATE USE, $300

REMOVE TO EXPOSE ADHESIVE

RETURN TO ➡

Print Sender's name, address, and ZIP Code in the space below.

KENNETH B MERETTI MD
483 SOUTH AUGUSTA STREET
MARINELAND CA 90000

Address Side

Is your RETURN ADDRESS completed on the reverse side?

● **SENDER:** Complete items 1 and 2 when additional services are desired, and complete items 3 and 4.
Put your address in the "RETURN TO" Space on the reverse side. Failure to do this will prevent this card from being returned to you. The return receipt fee will provide you the name of the person delivered to and the date of delivery. For additional fees the following services are available. Consult postmaster for fees and check box(es) for additional service(s) requested.
1. ☐ Show to whom delivered, date, and addressee's address. *(Extra charge)*
2. ☐ Restricted Delivery *(Extra charge)*

3. Article Addressed to: W B SAUNDERS INDEPENDENCE SQUARE WEST PHILADELPHIA PA 19106	4. Article Number P 758 351 390 Type of Service: ☐ Registered ☐ Insured XX Certified ☐ COD ☐ Express Mail ☐ Return Receipt for Merchandise Always obtain signature of addressee or agent and DATE DELIVERED.
5. Signature — Addressee X	8. Addressee's Address *(ONLY if requested and fee paid)*
6. Signature — Agent X	
7. Date of Delivery	

PS Form 3811, Apr. 1989 ★U.S.G.P.O. 1989-238-815 **DOMESTIC RETURN RECEIPT**

Thank you for using Return Receipt Service.

Information Side

FIGURE 12–10. Receipt for delivery of Certified, Registered, or Insured Mail. Attach to front of article if space permits. Otherwise, attach to back of article and endorse front of article with *"return receipt requested"* adjacent to the number.

HANDLING SPECIAL PROBLEMS

Forwarding Mail

First Class mail only may be forwarded from one address to another without payment of additional postage. Simply cross out the printed address and write in the address to which it should be delivered.

Obtaining Change of Address

If the mailer wants to know an addressee's new address, this service can be obtained from the post office by placing the words "Address Correction Requested" beneath the return address on the envelope. This can be handwritten, stamped, typewritten, or printed. The post office charges a postage-due fee for this service. For First Class mail, the post office will forward the piece of mail and return a card to the sender showing the forwarding address of the addressee. The card will have a postage due stamp on it for the amount of the required fee.

Recalling Mail

If you have dropped a letter in the mailbox and want it back, do not ask the mail collector to give it to you; he is not permitted to do this. Mail can be recalled, however, by making written application at the post office, together with an envelope addressed identically to the one being recalled. If your letter has already left the local post office, the postmaster, at the sender's expense, can telephone or telegraph the postmaster at the destination post office to return the letter.

Returned Mail

If a letter is returned to the sender after an attempt has been made to deliver it, it cannot be remailed without new postage. It is best simply to prepare a new envelope with the correct address, affix the proper postage, and remail.

Tracing Lost Mail

Receipts issued by the post office, whether for money orders, registered mail, certified mail, or insured mail, should be retained until receipt of the item has been acknowledged. If, after an adequate time elapses, no acknowledgment of receipt for such mailing arrives, notify the post office to trace the letter or package. Regular First Class mail is not easily traced, but the post office will make every attempt to find it for you. In tracing a lost letter or package, the post office requires that a special form be filled out; data from any original receipt should be written along with any other identifying information on this form.

INCOMING MAIL

Each day, a great variety of mail is received at the doctor's office and must be processed, including:

- General correspondence
- Payments for services
- Bills for office purchases
- Laboratory reports
- Hospital reports
- Medical society mailings
- Professional journals
- Promotional pieces and samples from pharmaceutical houses
- Advertisements
- Insurance claim forms to be completed

In large clinics and centers, the mail is opened by specially designated persons in some central department to speed up this daily task. But in the average professional office, the medical assistant opens the mail using the ordinary letter-opener method.

Mail Processing

Before opening any mail, the medical assistant should have an agreement with the physician as to what procedure to follow regarding incoming mail. In other words, what letters should be opened and what pieces does the doctor prefer to open personally? For instance, the physician may prefer to open any communications from an attorney or accountant, even when they are not marked "Personal." If there is any doubt in your mind in regard to opening a letter, the best rule to follow is, Don't! Treat your doctor's mail with the same consideration you expect others to exercise toward your own.

Before tackling the mail, assemble the equipment and supplies you will need:

- Letter opener
- Paper clips
- Stapler
- Transparent tape
- Date stamp

Sorting

Sort the mail according to importance and urgency:

1. Mailgrams or Special Delivery letters
2. Checks from patients
3. Doctor's personal mail
4. Ordinary First Class mail
5. Periodicals and newspapers
6. All other classes, including drug samples

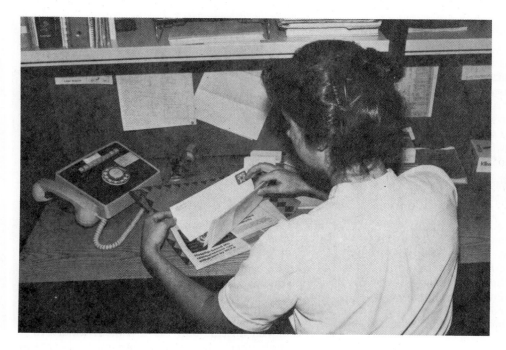

FIGURE 12–11. Medical assistant opening the mail. (Courtesy of Ferris State College, Big Rapids, MI.)

Opening

Even such a simple procedure as opening the day's mail can be done with more efficiency if a good system is followed (Fig. 12–11). Have a clear working space on your desk or counter, and proceed as follows:

1. Stack the envelopes so that they are all facing in the same direction.
2. Pick up the top one and tap the envelope so that when you open it you will not cut the contents.
3. Open all envelopes along the top edge for easiest removal of contents.
4. Remove the contents of each envelope and hold the envelope to the light to see that nothing remains inside.
5. Make a note of the postmark when this is important.
6. Discard the envelope after you have checked to see that there is a return address on the message contained inside. (Some offices make it a policy to attach the envelope to each piece of correspondence until it has received attention.)
7. Date stamp the letter and attach any enclosures.
8. If there is an enclosure notation at the bottom of the letter, check to be sure the enclosure was included. Should it be missing, indicate this on the notation by writing the word "no" and circling it. This may be as far as your employer will want you to proceed with handling the correspondence.

Annotating

If annotating the mail is within your duties, you can perform an additional service by reading each letter through, underlining the significant words and phrases and noting in the margin any action required. If it is a letter that needs no reply, you can code it for filing at this time. A nonprint pencil that does not photocopy may be used for the annotating, if desired.

When mail refers to previous correspondence, obtain this from the file and attach it. Or if a patient's chart is needed in replying to an inquiry, pull the chart and place it with the letter.

A specific place should be agreed upon for placing the opened and annotated mail. This will probably be some spot on the physician's desk. When you have completed the sorting, opening, and annotating of the mail, place those items that the doctor will wish to see in the established place, with the most important mail on top.

Personal mail, of course, is to remain unopened. Should you in error open a piece of personal mail addressed to your employer, fold and replace it inside the envelope, and write across the outside "Opened in error," followed by your initials. Use the same procedure with a piece of mail addressed to another office that may have been opened in error. In such a case, reseal the envelope with transparent tape and hand it to your carrier.

Responding to the Mail

In some offices, the doctor and the medical assistant go over the mail together. As you gain confidence, you will find that you can draft a reply to some inquiries. Most doctors are very pleased to delegate this responsibility, especially on matters that do not relate to patient care.

Letters of referral from other physicians should be carefully noted so that an answer may be sent after the doctor has seen the patient and can give a report. If considerable time may pass before such information can be sent, it is a courteous gesture to write a thank-you note to the referring physician advising that a detailed letter will follow. Some physicians send printed cards expressing thanks for referrals; others prefer to write thank-you letters to professional colleagues.

MAIL THE ASSISTANT CAN HANDLE

Cash Receipts

There will be some mail that the medical assistant can handle alone, for instance, payments from patients and insurance forms to be completed. All cash and checks should be separated and recorded immediately in the day's receipts.

Insurance Forms

Insurance forms for completion should be put in a predetermined place for handling at the appropriate time. If there is an insurance clerk or other individual who processes the claims, they should be passed along to that person immediately.

Drug Samples

Sample drugs and related literature may be in the mail. Determine from the physician what types of literature and samples should be saved. Most physicians keep pertinent new samples in their desks, along with the accompanying literature for immediate reference. Other drug samples are categorically stored. Drugs should never be tossed into the trash. (See Chapter 21.)

VACATION MAIL

When the doctor is away from the office, it is generally the responsibility of the medical assistant to handle all mail. In this event, all pieces should be studied carefully. The medical assistant can then make a decision in regard to handling each piece on the basis of the following questions:

- Is this important enough that I should phone or fax the doctor?
- Shall I forward this for immediate attention?
- Shall I answer this myself or send a brief note to the correspondent explaining that there will be a slight delay because the doctor is out of the office?
- Can this wait for attention until the doctor returns without appearing negligent?

If you are unable to contact the physician or to forward important mail, always answer the sender immediately, explaining the delay and requesting cooperation. Most offices have some kind of copy machine as part of the office equipment. Instead of forwarding an original piece of mail and risking possible loss, make a copy for forwarding. Then, if the physician wishes you to answer the letter, notations can be made on the copy and returned to you without defacing the original letter.

If your employer is traveling from place to place, the envelope on each communication should be numbered consecutively. Doing this enables the doctor to easily determine whether any mail has been lost or delayed. By keeping your own record of each piece of mail sent out, with its corresponding number, anything that might be lost can be identified and remailed if necessary.

Correspondence not requiring immediate action but that the medical assistant is unable to answer until the doctor returns should be placed in a special folder on the doctor's desk, marked "Requires Attention." Mail the medical assistant can answer but that requires the doctor's approval before mailing, should be put into another special folder, marked "For Approval." When the doctor returns, these letters can be rapidly checked and signed.

Any letters marked "Personal" that you hesitate to open and are unable to forward may be acknowledged to the return address on the envelope. The brief acknowledgment should state that the doctor is out of town for a certain length of time and will attend to the letter immediately upon returning. Your acknowledgment should also offer your help in any way possible in the meantime.

Discard any mail that you are sure the doctor would not wish to see. Some promotional literature falls into this category. (Make certain, however, that mailings from professional organizations, whether they are First, Second, Third, or Fourth Class, are saved.)

There may be rare periods when the entire office is closed. In such cases, the local post office should be notified to forward all First Class mail to an address supplied by the doctor, if possible. Your postal carrier cannot accept an oral request to leave the mail with the person next door for a few days. A formal request must be made. If forwarding is out of the question, place a request with the post office to hold the mail until a specified date when someone will again be on duty. Never leave mail unattended to gather outside a mailbox or clutter up a doorway in a hall. Even mail slots may become filled or magazines may become stuck in them, causing important mail to pile up outside the slot. Far too much money and mail of a confidential nature is sent to doctors' offices to take chances on mail theft or destruction.

Systematizing your routine for processing all incoming and outgoing mail can put you in control of the paper blizzard!

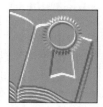

▶ LEARNING ACHIEVEMENTS

Are you able to:

1. Explain the terms listed in the Vocabulary of this chapter?
2. Discuss your responsibility with respect to the office equipment used in your employment?
3. Select professional quality stationery?
4. Identify three basic sizes of letterhead stationery and envelopes?
5. Select references for your professional library?
6. Use the five procedural steps to answer a professional inquiry letter?
7. Develop a correspondence portfolio?
8. Describe how your appropriate use of ZIP Codes could save money for your employer?
9. Generate a letter using the four main parts and their subdivisions for each of the four letter styles?
10. Address envelopes using the guidelines for optical scanning?
11. Correctly fold a letter and insert it into an envelope?

REFERENCES AND READINGS

Jennings, L. M.: *Secretarial and Administrative Procedures,* 3rd ed., Englewood Cliffs, NJ, Prentice-Hall, Inc., 1989.

Kutie, R., and Rhodes, J.: *Secretarial Procedures for the Electronic Office,* 2nd ed., New York, John Wiley & Sons, Inc., 1985.

Sabin, W.: *The Gregg Reference Manual,* 6th ed., New York, Gregg Division/McGraw-Hill, 1991.

Schwager, E.: *Medical English Usage and Abusage,* Phoenix, AZ, The Oryx Press, 1991.

Shertzer, M.: *The Elements of Grammar,* New York, Macmillan Publishing Company, 1986.

Strunk, W., Jr., and White, E. B.: *The Elements of Style,* 3rd ed., New York, Macmillan Publishing Company, 1979.

The Postal Manual, Superintendent of Documents, US Government Printing Office, Washington, DC.

Tilton, Rita S., et al.: *Secretarial Procedures and Administration,* 9th ed., Cincinnati, South-Western Publishing Co., 1987.

CHAPTER THIRTEEN

—

DICTATION AND TRANSCRIPTION

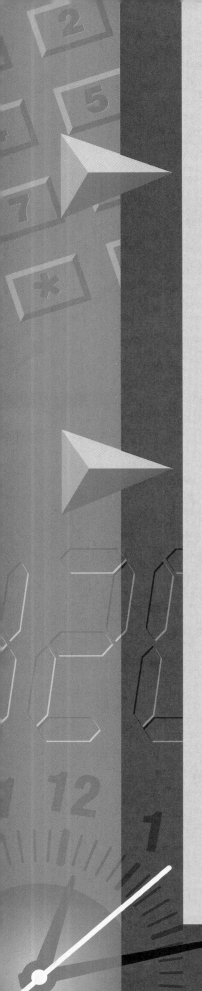

CHAPTER OUTLINE

VOCABULARY

alignment The state of being in the correct relative position.

cassette A magnetic tape wound on two reels and encased in a plastic or metal container. *microcassette* A very small cassette tape that may be used in a hand-held dictating unit.

consultation report A report of the findings of the consulting physician to be sent to the referring physician.

daisy wheel A printing element made of plastic or metal used on some typewriters and impact printers. It derives its name from its shape, which is like that of a daisy.

dictation The process of recording the spoken word onto a storage medium from which a printed copy will be produced.

discharge summary The final (progress) note for a hospital patient that contains the patient's admitting and discharge diagnoses, any surgeries performed, the patient's course while hospitalized, and his or her condition upon discharge.

editing The process of examining text to determine accuracy and clarity.

font A set of printing type that is of one size and style.

HCFA Health Care Financing Administration; the authority that administers Medicare

HCPCS Acronym for HCFA's Common Procedure Coding System, used in determining Medicare fees.

history and physical The record of a patient's present illness, past medical and surgical history, family history, and a review of the patient's present condition by body systems.

ICD-9-CM International Classification of Diseases, 9th Revision, Clinical Modification.

indicator strip A charted strip that is inserted into the dictation unit and on which the dictator marks the beginning and end point of each document and any corrections to be made.

keyboarding The process of entering characters into the memory of a word processor.

operation record A report dictated immediately following surgery that contains the pre- and postoperative diagnoses, the procedure performed, the anesthesia administered, the names of the patient, surgeon, assistant surgeon (if any), and the anesthetist, the beginning and end time of the surgery, and the patient's condition upon leaving the operating room. This becomes a permanent part of the patient's chart.

pathology report The report dictated by the pathologist following any surgery that involves removal of tissue in the hospital. The report contains a description of the tissue removed (gross and microscopic) as well as the diagnosis and is signed by the pathologist. It becomes a permanent part of the patient's chart.

progress notes Records of patient visits, telephone calls, progress, and treatment that are inserted into the patient's chart.

proofreading Checking a document for spelling, sentence structure, punctuation, capitalization, style, and format.

radiology reports Radiology reports are dictated in the radiology department of a hospital or imaging center and include reports of x-rays and other imaging procedures.

subscript A symbol or number written immediately below another character.

superscript A symbol or number written immediately above another character.

transcription Listening to recorded dictation and translating it into written form.

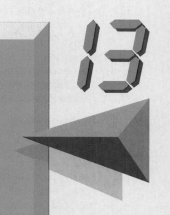

DICTATION AND TRANSCRIPTION

LEARNING OBJECTIVES

COGNITIVE

Upon successful completion of this chapter, you should be able to:

1. Define the terms listed in the Vocabulary.

2. List six basic educational requirements for the medical transcriptionist.

3. Name two primary requisites for the independently practicing transcriptionist.

4. List the three stages of activity in the machine transcription process.

5. List five functional features of a typical transcribing unit.

6. State the principal differences between a *dedicated word processor* and a *computer.*

7. Name three kinds of frequently dictated reports in the average physician's office.

PERFORMANCE

Upon successful completion of this chapter, and given the necessary equipment, you should be able to perform the following activities:

1. Estimate the length of a finished document prior to transcribing it.

2. Make any necessary corrections in keyboarding before removing the document from the machine.

3. Proofread and edit a transcribed document.

4. Correctly utilize basic rules of capitalization.

5. Follow the rules for word division.

6. Determine when to use figures for numbers.

7. Correctly format common medical reports.

A medical transcriptionist is a highly skilled professional whose educational background is similar in some respects to that of the administrative medical assistant. The medical transcriptionist must have the following skills and qualities:

- Above-average typing and word processing skills
- An understanding of human anatomy and physiology and of the pathologic conditions that affect the human body
- Knowledge of medical terminology used in medical records, medical and surgical procedures, and laboratory tests
- Knowledge of the names and correct spelling of surgical instruments and currently used drugs
- Superior command of grammar, sentence structure and style, spelling, and **editing** and **proofreading** skills
- Ability to use a medical dictionary and other standard reference materials

The professional medical transcriptionist may practice independently and may affiliate with the American Association for Medical Transcription and become certified (see Chapter 3). The independent transcriptionist will find that accuracy and speed are primary requisites. Income depends on the transcriptionist's productivity, which may be measured by the number of pages, characters, or lines typed. The person who intends to do transcribing exclusively would do well to take a special course in transcription techniques.

The medical transcriptionist in the physician's office is a part of the health care team. The smooth operation of the office may depend on the timely and accurate performance of assigned responsibilities, such as record documentation and the preparation of special reports.

The administrative medical assistant may find that transcribing **dictation** is one of his or her job requirements. Transcribing may be from handwritten notes, such as those in shorthand, or from machine dictation.

MACHINE TRANSCRIPTION PROCESS

Three stages of activity are involved in the process of dictation and transcription:

- Dictating into a dictation unit
- Listening to what has been dictated
- **Keyboarding** the dictated text to a printed document using correct format and required punctuation.

Equipment
Dictation Unit

The dictation unit is used by the physician to record matter to be typed. Dictation units vary in design and capabilities.

The desktop dictation unit is common in an office setting. This may be a combination unit used for both dictation and transcription. Alternatively, a machine used for dictation only may remain at the physician's desk; a separate **transcription** unit, including headphones and a foot pedal, remains at the transcriptionist's station.

A lightweight portable hand-held dictation unit may be used for times when the physician (dictator) wishes to dictate while traveling or attending meetings away from the office.

Physicians in a larger setting may install transcribing equipment that they can access by telephone wherever they may be. Many hospitals have this arrangement.

All produce a recording that the transcriptionist listens to while keyboarding the text.

Transcriber Unit

The unit operated by the transcriptionist may use magnetic tapes, **cassettes,** or disks. A desk-top unit using mini-, micro-, or standard cassettes is typical in the physician's office (Fig. 13–1).

There are many types and manufacturers of transcribing equipment, but most units contain certain standard features. Before using any equipment, you should study the manufacturer's instruction manual. Most transcription units have a minimum of the following features:

- A stop and start control, back up feature, and fast forward
- A speed control

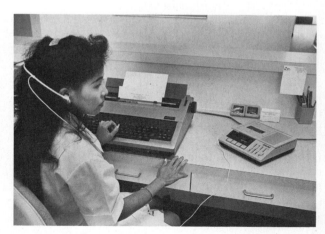

FIGURE 13–1. Transcriptionist using electronic typewriter and desk-top transcribing unit.

- A volume control
- A tone control
- An indicator for locating special instructions and determining the length of a document

Stop and start control A foot pedal allows the transcriptionist to start, stop, back up, or fast forward the unit. He or she may wish to stop the unit while catching up with the typing, back up to replay a portion that was not understood, pause to insert additional matter from another source, or stop to check spelling. Most have an optional adjustment so that a slight rewind of the tape occurs when the machine is stopped and restarted. This prevents the loss of any dictated material in the process.

Speed control The speed control feature can be used to slow down the recording of a fast dictator or speed up that of a slow dictator to match the speed of the transcriptionist.

Volume control The volume control in the headset can be adjusted to suit each unit of transcription. The headset also serves as a sound barrier by shutting out extraneous office sounds and preserving the confidentiality of the dictation.

Tone control The tone control feature allows the transcriptionist to increase or decrease the bass or treble to the pitch most understandable and pleasing to the ear.

Indicator strip For a long time, dictating and transcribing machines have had **indicator strips** that could be inserted into the machine to allow the dictator to mark the point at which each item begins and ends and where corrections, if any, are needed. These strips are then attached to the transcribing machine to aid the typist. All too often, the dictator refuses or neglects to use these indicators. When this happens, the transcriptionist should courteously remind the dictator of the importance of using this device.

Instead of an indicator strip, the machine may have a display window or cue-tone indexing capability that provides this same information. All of these features assist the transcriptionist in planning his or her transcribing duties.

The beginning transcriptionist tends to listen to a few words, stop the machine, type those words, and then restart the transcriber unit. Through practice, the transcriptionist learns to coordinate keyboarding activity with listening skills and "listen ahead," thereby retaining in memory more and more of the dictated material so that it becomes unnecessary to stop and start the machine for this purpose.

Keyboarding Unit

The most important piece of equipment for the transcriptionist is the typewriter or computer on which the printed text will be produced. Many improvements have occurred within the last few years.

The manual typewriter is now virtually a museum piece. The electric typewriter appears to be on its way out as well, having been replaced by the electronic typewriter. The machines of choice in the modern office are:

- The electronic typewriter, with or without memory
- The dedicated word processor (display text editor)
- The desk-top computer with word processing software

ELECTRONIC TYPEWRITER. The electronic typewriter improves upon the features of the electric typewriter by having the ability to automatically perform many tasks that save time and produce a more pleasing result. It is sometimes referred to as the *intelligent typewriter.* Instead of noisy "keys," it has a single element, which is most likely a **daisy wheel.** With a daisy wheel, the typist may choose from among many kinds of type styles and sizes by simply removing one wheel and substituting the one of choice. Automatic features, such as number **alignment,** automatic centering, underlining, indenting, caps lock, and carrier return, are accomplished with the stroke of a key. Most have the capability of storing a limited amount of text and may have a display screen and spell check capability.

DEDICATED WORD PROCESSOR. The term *word processing* was coined by IBM in the 1960s to describe its innovative Magnetic Tape Selectric Typewriter (MT/ST). The MT/ST was costly and met with some resistance because it required special training. Word processors today are much simpler. The word processor is a computer that is especially designed to perform one function only — word processing. It is more expensive than the electronic typewriter, but in situations that require a great amount of word processing, it is a good investment.

COMPUTER. A desk-top computer with word processing software is a third type of keyboarding equipment (Fig. 13–2). The principal difference between it and the dedicated word processor is that other tasks can be performed on the computer.

The person who uses a word processor can throw away the eraser and correcting fluid because the entire text can be edited on the monitor, any necessary corrections or changes made, and a perfect copy obtained before any printing is done.

- Revisions can be made easily without retyping a whole document.
- Blocks of text can be moved from one section of the document to another with just a few keystrokes. Even whole sections of text can be inserted into a document easily and quickly.

13

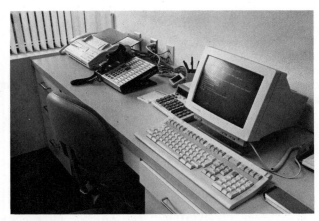

FIGURE 13-2. A desk-top computer can be used with word processing software for transcribing dictation.

- Paragraphs or statements that are used frequently in letters or reports can be saved as *macros* and with a stroke or two on the keyboard can be retrieved and inserted in the appropriate place without retyping.

Most word processing programs can instruct the printer to print in boldface or in alternate type **fonts.** Some can create **subscripts** and **superscripts.** A *spell check* feature can proofread a lengthy document in minutes with complete accuracy. One disadvantage of the spell checker is that it can determine only whether a word is spelled correctly. If an incorrect word that is correctly spelled is typed, the checker will not pick it up (for example, the use of "ilium" in place of "ileum"). With the text stored in memory or on a diskette, additional editing can be done and a corrected copy printed out almost effortlessly at any future time.

PROCEDURE 13-1   TRANSCRIBING A MACHINE-DICTATED LETTER USING A TYPEWRITER

GOAL   To transcribe a machine-dictated letter into a mailable document without error or detectable corrections, using a typewriter.

EQUIPMENT AND SUPPLIES

Transcribing machine	Letterhead paper
Typewriter	Correcting supplies
Draft paper	Reference manual

PROCEDURAL STEPS

1. Assemble supplies.
2. Turn on the transcription equipment.
3. Set *line* for double spacing.
   Purpose: To allow room for making changes or corrections.
4. Type a draft of the letter.
5. Edit the draft for spelling, insertions, and sentence structure.
6. Note any necessary corrections.
7. Set *line* and *margins* for attractive placement of the letter.
8. Retype the letter on letterhead paper.
9. Proofread the letter for content and errors before removing it from the typewriter.

PROCEDURE 13-2   TRANSCRIBING A MACHINE-DICTATED LETTER USING A COMPUTER OR WORD PROCESSOR

GOAL To transcribe a machine-dictated letter into a mailable document without error or detectable corrections, using a computer or word processor.

EQUIPMENT AND SUPPLIES

Transcribing machine
Word processor or computer with
    appropriate software

Stationery
Reference manual

PROCEDURAL STEPS

1. Assemble supplies.
2. Set up the format for selected letter style.
3. Keyboard the text while listening to the dictated letter.
4. Edit the letter on the monitor.
   Purpose: The letter should be in mailable form before printing.
5. Execute a spell check.
6. Direct the letter to the printer.

13

PREPARATION OF REPORTS

The scope of a transcriptionist's duties is determined by each specific employer. In most instances, the preparation of medical reports is a large part of the professional assignment. The reports most frequently dictated in the physician's office are:

- History and physical
- Progress notes
- Consultation reports
- Correspondence

History and Physical

The **history and physical** (H & P) may be dictated as the basis for the new patient's chart. When a patient is to be admitted to a hospital for surgery, the surgeon may dictate an H & P prior to admitting the patient, and this becomes a part of the patient's hospital chart. No universal standard form exists for the H & P, but Figure 13-3 is a typical example.

Many sections of this report have a standard response that occurs over and over, depending on the patient's complaint and condition. These responses can be stored in memory and used as needed with one or two strokes of the keyboard.

Progress Notes

The physician who sees many patients during a day does not have time to handwrite **progress notes** on the medical chart after each patient is seen. More than likely, the physician will either dictate notes in the presence of the patient or immediately after the visit. The transcriptionist will then prepare these notes as an addition to the chart (Fig. 13-4).

By using continuous pages of pressure-sensitive paper, a great deal of time and motion can be saved. The paper is inserted only once and is later separated for the appropriate charts. Some papers have interval perforations that expedite the separation of entries. When typing these progress notes, space is left at the end for the physician's signature. The

HISTORY AND PHYSICAL EXAMINATION

CHIEF COMPLAINT: Severe pain, left hip area, duration for the past couple of years.

PRESENT ILLNESS: The patient in 1940 was involved in a severe auto accident, at which time he sustained injury to his back and leg as well as to his right shoulder and left hip. He subsequently had back surgery performed as well as a fusion, which was performed at St. Francis Hospital in Yourtown. The patient, however, has had continued sciatica and has been seen by Dr. Thomas Brown. Appropriate studies have been done. It was felt that there is nothing from the neurosurgical standpoint which could be of benefit to his left leg sciatic type pain.

In June 1990, the patient underwent insertion of a total right shoulder because of severe progressive degenerative osteoarthritis of the right shoulder. He has done quite well with that, has improved his range of motion, and has minimal to no pain. The patient, however, has had progressive pain about his left hip that has not responded to anti-inflammatory medications. X-rays reveal a progressive degenerative osteoarthritis with cystic formation.

FORMER SURGERIES:
1. Removal of right kidney in 8/85.
2. Former back surgeries in the 1940s.
3. Right total shoulder in 7/90.

SERIOUS ILLNESSES: None.

MEDICATIONS: Occasional Darvocet for pain.

HABITS: Patient does not smoke.

REVIEW OF SYSTEMS:

HEENT: Patient denies any recent URIs or chronic sore throat.
CV: Patient denies history of chest pain or heart disease.
GI: Patient denies nausea, vomiting, diarrhea.
GU: Patient denies dysuria or frequency.
Musculoskeletal: See Present Illness.
Hem: Patient denies any bleeding tendencies.

VITAL SIGNS: Blood pressure 132/72.

GENERAL APPEARANCE: Patient appears to be in good health for his stated age.

HEENT: PERRL. Funduscopic examination within normal limits. Ears are clear, mouth negative.

NECK: Supple. Thyroid is not enlarged.

LYMPHADENOPATHY: None.

HEART: Regular rate, no murmurs. Patient has good bilateral carotid pulsations.

FIGURE 13-3. History and physical examination report (indented style).

Page 2

HISTORY AND PHYSICAL EXAMINATION

PHYSICAL EXAMINATION:

ABDOMEN: Soft, no abnormal masses.

GENITALIA: Normal male.

RECTAL: Prostate is somewhat firm; however, there are no changes
                     from exam in 1989.

EXTREMITIES: Patient has 0 internal rotation of the left hip. He has ab-
                     duction approximately 10 degrees, flexion marked pain
                     about 70 degrees. Patient has a very mild left hip flexion
                     contracture.

IMPRESSION: 1. Severe degenerative osteoarthritis, left hip.
                     2. Postoperative right total shoulder replacement.
                     3. Residual sciatica, left leg.

                     _____

                              xxxx, M.D.

13

FIGURE 13-3 *Continued*

1. Brought back to ofc. regarding wart, left dorsal hand, of about 6 mo duration.
   EXAM: 5-mm diameter raised, round, sharply marginated, gray-pink, finely papillomatous
            and keratotic lesion, left dorsal hand.
   IMP: Verruca vulgaris.
   DISP: 1) Discussed treatment by electrosurgery vs. cryotherapy with father, including
               scarring with electrosurgery.
            2) Lesion removed by D & C under local anesth with Xyl. + Epi.
            3) Monsels, DSD, H_2O_2 t.i.d.
            4) See prn

2. Has been treating superficial multicentric BCCA, distal left mandible, with Efudex 5% cream
   b.i.d. for 3 wks. See inflammation with central erosion and peripheral crusting in involved
   area. Response appears appropriate.
   DISP: 1) Cont Efudex 5% cream b.i.d.   2) See in 3 wks.

3. Pt. points out very small, quiescent-appearing actinic keratosis—inferior right lateral arm
   × 1 and proximal left extensor forearm × 1. Discussed nature of lesions with pt. L N2 about 10
   sec. each. Re/ck p.r.n. persistence.

4. Pt. inquires about lesion, medial right leg. Possibly present since birth. No change in size
   or color over time. No tmt to date.
   EXAM: Inferior right medial leg: 17 × 15-mm diameter round, sharply marginated, macular,
            uniformly medium-brown lesion; a few terminal hairs penetrate surface of lesion.
   IMP: Benign pigmented macule.
   DISP: 1) Discussed benign appearance of lesion with pt.
            2) No tmt at this time.
            3) Re/ck prn change.

FIGURE 13–4. Progress notes.

notes should never be entered into the chart without the physician's approval and signature.

Consultation Reports

Physicians who act as consultants are expected to prepare a detailed report of their findings and recommendations and send it to the referring physicians. The **consultation report** is dictated by the consulting physician to be transcribed within the office or by an independent transcriptionist if outside services are used. The consultation report is frequently quite long, and promptness in preparation is important (Fig. 13–5).

Other Reports

Other reports that usually are generated outside the office but which become a part of the patient's chart include:

- Operation records (Fig. 13–6)
- Pathology reports (Fig. 13–7)
- Radiology reports (Fig. 13–8)
- Discharge summaries (Fig. 13–9)

OTHER APPLICATIONS

The office that regularly sends out identical letters, such as recall notices or collection letters, will find word processing very helpful. Form letters can be stored in memory and personalized as needed.

The physician who does academic writing will want a program that can create footnotes, bibliographies, indexes, and so forth.

TRANSCRIBING: THE PROCESS

In most cases, the transcriptionist aims for finished copy and takes certain preliminary steps toward this goal. You should:

1. Estimate the length of the finished document by first checking the indicator slip or electronic cuing. By doing this, you can decide what margins and spacing to use to produce the desired end product.
2. Look for any special instructions or corrections from the dictator.
3. Try to "listen ahead" so that you can sense the meaning of a sentence and determine the punctuation necessary (some dictators include the punctuation marks).
4. If you are keyboarding an entire document before printing, you may be able to go back and change punctuation, paragraphing, and so forth, but if you are typing directly on paper, it is more important to keyboard correctly the first time.

5. Before removing a page from the typewriter or before printing out the document, check the page for any errors.

ABBREVIATIONS

If transcribing for a hospital, use only abbreviations approved by the hospital for which the reports are intended. The Joint Commission on Accreditation of Healthcare Organizations (JCAHO) requires that any abbreviations or symbols used in its medical records be from a list approved by that specific hospital. Progress notes done in the physician's office are less formal, and the physician's personally approved abbreviations are used to conserve space.

PROOFREADING AND EDITING

As a final step, the finished printed page should be checked twice—once for typing accuracy and once to be sure that the text makes sense. *Never* present material for signature unless it makes sense to you and is free of errors.

Proofreading is the process in which you determine whether the copy is exactly what was intended by the dictator and that all words are correctly interpreted and accurately spelled. Be especially careful to watch for sound-alike words, such as site/cite, ilium/ileum, right/write, and anti-/ante- (Table 13–1). Proofreading usually includes checking for sentence structure, correct punctuation, capitalization, style, and format. Watch for repeated words, substitutions that might change the meaning, the transposition of numbers, and inconsistencies of any kind.

Since you do not have another document against which you can compare the one you are working on, it is your responsibility to make any necessary corrections or, if you are unsure, to mark any questionable area for checking by the dictator. A reliable office worker's reference manual can be your guide in these matters.

Editing is the process of questioning the transcribed material for accuracy and clarity. Medical reports generally do not require extensive editing, but as you check for typing accuracy, you should also check the clarity of the text. In making corrections, be careful not to change the meaning. Always check with the dictator when making any changes in what was said.

SOME BASIC RULES

The following basic rules on capitalization, word division, forming plurals, and writing numbers can serve as a ready reference and are worth memorizing. For further assistance, always consult a reference manual.

December 10, 1997

Thomas Brown, M.D.
234 Maine Avenue
Yourtown, USA

Dear Dr. Brown:

Re: Rebecca Bloom

Rebecca Bloom is a 79-year-old, right-handed lady with known asthma who was seen in neurological consultation for progressive weakness in her legs.

She has had a prior neurological consultation, which suggested motor neuron disease. A muscle biopsy was consistent with neurogenic atrophy, and an EMG revealed positive sharp waves and fibrillation potentials in the quadriceps bilaterally and, to a lesser degree, in the distal groups of both legs below the knees. EMG of the upper extremities was normal.

Chemistry studies were unremarkable.

She denies any exposure to heavy metals or other neurotoxins. She has noted weakness in her legs for the past two years, initially above the knees, left greater than right. The problem has been slowly progressive, but she does not experience any weakness below the knees. She feels that her arms are strong, and she has experienced no difficulty with speech, swallowing, or eye movements. She has lost approximately 20 pounds in the last two years, which she attributes to nausea and poor dentures. She denies any significant muscle wasting or muscle twitching in the thigh muscles. She notes that her feet feel ''abnormal,'' but she does not describe true numbness or tingling. Bowel/bladder function is intact. She has had a vertebral compression fracture due to osteoporosis because of her chronic prednisone therapy for asthma.

Her past medical history is significant for right hip surgery; ectopic pregnancy; status post bladder repair; history of asthma-COPD; status post muscle biopsy; history of mild enlargement of her heart with a valvular dysfunction.

Her medications include prednisone, 7.5 mg q.d. for several years; Brethine; Theo-Dur, 150 mg p.o. b.i.d.; Lanoxin, 0.125 mg p.o. every day; supplemental folic acid; daily Coumadin therapy; Premarin; vitamin D, 50,000 units two times per week; as well as an Alupent Inhalor and Intal; Dyazide, 1 p.o. q.d.

Allergies: None known.

The patient denies tobacco or ethanol use. In the past six months, she has required the use of a cane to ambulate.

On physical exam, she is a well-developed, well-nourished female in no acute distress. She is oriented x three with an intact mental status exam. Speech is normal. Blood pressure is 120/80. Neck is supple. Carotids are 2+ bilaterally without bruits over the carotids or the supraclavicular region. Spine is nontender to percussion. HEENT: Normocephalic; atraumatic. Chest is clear to auscultation. Heart has a regular rate and rhythm; S1 and S2 without murmur. Cranial nerves: Olfactory sense is intact. Right disc is sharp with an intraocular lens present; left disc is nonvisible secondary to the presence of a cataract. The right pupil is greater than

FIGURE 13-5. Consultation report in full block letter style.

the left pupil by 0.5 mm; both are round and reactive to light. Visual fields are full. Extraocular movements are intact without nystagmus. Corneal reflexes are intact bilaterally, and there is normal facial symmetry and expression. Hearing is intact bilaterally, and the uvula is midline and upgoing. Sternocleidomastoid function is symmetric, and the tongue is midline.

Motor exam displays strength to be intact in the upper extremities bilaterally. The lower extremities display 3–4/5 strength in the iliopsoas and quadriceps bilaterally. There is trace weakness in the adductors and abductors, as well as hip extensors bilaterally. There is trace weakness of the hamstrings. There is no notable atrophy or fasciculation. The patient is unable to squat and has difficulty arising from a chair. Strength in the musculature distal to the knees is intact. There are no notable fasciculations. Thigh diameter is 33 mm on the right and 34 mm on the left, and the calves are both 30 mm in diameter. Sensory exam displays diminished vibratory and pinprick response in the feet, with position and soft touch intact. Finger-to-nose and heel-to-shin are intact. Fine motor movements and rapid alternating hand movements are normal. Deep tendon reflexes for the bicep, tricep, brachioradialis are 1–2+ bilaterally, with absent knee and ankle jerks; and the toes are downgoing. Gait and tandem are fair. Straight leg raise testing is unremarkable, as is bilateral hip rotation. Pedal pulses are 2+; the feet are cool in temperature, slightly erythematous, and swollen, with evidence of venous stasis.

Data Base: Nerve conduction studies of the lower extremities suggested a peripheral polyneuropathy, and an EMG of the upper extremities was normal. EMG of the left lower extremity revealed denervation to a greater extent in the left quadriceps and, to a minimal extent, in the left gastrocnemius. Some polyphasic small amplitude motor unit potentials were noted in the quadriceps that can be seen in myopathies.

Impression: Rebecca Bloom has evidence of proximal muscle weakness in her lower extremities with associated sensory deficits, including diminished vibratory and pinprick response in her feet and has been on chronic steroid therapy for her asthma-COPD. Her clinical picture, correlating with the electrical studies, suggests a peripheral polyneuropathy and possibly a proximal myopathy from chronic steroid use, rather than a motor neuron disorder, considering the lack of development of symptoms in the bulbar musculature or the upper extremities and the slow rate of progression.

Chemistry studies were unremarkable other than an elevated calcium of 11.3, and this will be further evaluated with the appropriate ionized calcium and PTH level.

I have recommended that we observe her over a period of time to document any evolution of her illness. I have referred her to physical therapy and pointed out that any reduction in her steroid use would be of value.

Further recommendations include a pelvic examination in view of the proximal muscle weakness in the lower extremities.

Her prior records will be reviewed, and the appropriate chemistry studies will be ordered.

Thank you for referring this pleasant lady for neurological evaluation.

Very truly yours,

FIGURE 13-5 *Continued*

REGIONAL MEDICAL CENTER
YOURTOWN, USA

REPORT OF OPERATION

DATE: 12/05/97

PREOPERATIVE DIAGNOSIS: MASS LEFT CALF

POSTOPERATIVE DIAGNOSIS: SAME, PROBABLY DEGENERATIVE MUSCLE
                               DISEASE LEFT CALF

PROCEDURE: OPEN BIOPSY LEFT CALF MUSCLE

SURGEON: XXXX, M.D.
ASST. SURGEON: XXXX, M.D.
ANESTHESIA: XXXX, M.D.   General endotracheal anesthesia

FINDINGS: Under general anesthetic, the patient's left lower extremity was prepped
and draped in the usual manner. The left leg was isolated in a sterile field, a well-
padded thigh tourniquet was inflated to 300 mm of mercury after elevating and exsan-
guinating the leg with an Esmarch bandage. Linear incision was made over the posterior medial aspect of the calf, and dissection was carried out through the skin and
subcutaneous tissue and superficial fascia. The gastrocnemius muscle was opened
posteromedially. It was obvious that the muscle appeared to be rather firm and woody
in consistency with infiltrating lighter tissue consistent with fatty tissue
throughout the muscle fibers. The muscle fibers also appeared to be essentially
relatively avascular and did not contract with direct stimulation. Samples of tissue were sent for frozen section, which indicated both degenerative and reparative
process within the muscle without evidence of any tumor infiltration or evidence of
infection. The specimens were sent for permanent section. At this point, the wound
was thoroughly irrigated with normal saline solution containing Bacitracin and Neomycin. Previously, the wound was cultured, aerobic and anaerobically. The tourniquet was deflated at 10 minutes of tourniquet time. The wound was closed in layers
with 0 and 2-0 Dexon followed by closure of the skin with subcuticular 4-0 Dexon
followed by Steri-Strips and dry sterile compression dressings. The patient tolerated the procedure well; she was awakened from the anesthetic and went to the recovery room in good condition. EBL less than 20 cc.

                                   _____ M.D.

NAME: XXXX
HOSPITAL NO: XXXX
ROOM NO: OP
ATTENDING: XXXX, M.D.

MEK

FIGURE 13-6. Operation report.

REGIONAL MEDICAL CENTER
PATHOLOGY REPORT

Name: _____   Pathology No.: _____

Hospital No.: _ Sex: _____ Age: _____ Room No.: _____ Date Received: _____

Physicians: _____

Preoperative Diagnosis: _____ Mass of left calf _____

Postoperative Diagnosis: _____ Pending _____

Procedure: _____ Open biopsy, left calf muscle _____

Specimens: (1) _____ Left calf mass—f/s _____

              (2) _____ Left calf mass—f/s _____

              (3) _____ Left calf mass _____

GROSS:

1. The specimen consists of 3 irregularly shaped fragments of dark maroon-brown muscle tissue measuring in aggregate $1.5 \times 1 \times 0.3$ cm. No discrete lesions are identified. A minimal amount of adipose tissue is present in the largest fragment. The entire specimen is submitted for frozen section diagnosis.

FROZEN SECTION DIAGNOSIS: Benign muscle tissue showing degenerative and regenerative changes.

After frozen section, the tissue submitted is resubmitted and labeled F/S.

2. The specimen consists of 2 fragments of maroon-brown muscle tissue measuring in aggregate $1 \times 0.7 \times 3$ cm. One of the fragments is submitted for frozen section diagnosis.

FROZEN SECTION DIAGNOSIS: Benign muscle tissue showing degenerative and regenerative changes.

After frozen section, the tissue submitted is resubmitted and labeled F/S.

3. Received is a wedge of grossly recognizable muscle tissue, brown-tan, and measuring $2.1 \times 1.2 \times 0.8$ cm in size. On sectioning, this is moderately firm and focally only slightly discolored. All processed.

MICROSCOPIC:

Sections from all three parts show skeletal muscle. There is variable fiber morphology ranging from severely atrophic to markedly hypertrophic. There are abnormal numbers of central nucleoli, and some muscle fibers are vacuolated. In the interstitium there is fatty infiltration but no significant inflammatory infiltrate. No vasculitis is noted.

DIAGNOSIS:

NONSPECIFIC DEGENERATIVE AND HYPERTROPHIC CHANGES CONSISTENT WITH SEQUELA OF PREVIOUS TRAUMATIC INJURY, LEFT LEG MUSCLE BIOPSY.

NOTE: The morphology is somewhat similar to a muscular dystrophy, but the clinical presentation is incompatible. Denervation myopathy could account for some of the features seen. An inflammatory myopathy such as polymyositis is excluded based on the hypertrophic fibers present.

_____
Pathologist

MEK

FIGURE 13-7. Pathology report.

RADIOLOGY MEDICAL GROUP, INC.

Name: _____ Age: _____ X-ray No.: _____

Doctor: _____ Date: _____

DOUBLE-CONTRAST ARTHROGRAM OF THE RIGHT KNEE:

Double-contrast arthrography of the right knee was performed under local anesthesia following intra-articular injection of Conray contrast medium and air.

Multiple views of the medial meniscus in various degrees of internal and external rotation demonstrate a faintly outlined vertically directed linear tear involving primarily the posterior horn and mid segment of the medial meniscus.

The lateral meniscus is intact with no evidence of tear or disruption. Overhead views show normal smooth synovial lining and articular surfaces. No popliteal cyst is demonstrated.

OPINION:

Faintly outlined vertically directed linear tear involving primarily the posterior horn and mid segment of the medial meniscus.

Normal lateral meniscus.

MEK

_____

Radiologist

FIGURE 13-8. Radiology report.

Hospital No.: _____

Patient Name: _____

Physician: _____

Date of Discharge: _____

YOURTOWN HOSPITAL

DISCHARGE SUMMARY

DATE OF ADMISSION: 12/15/97

DATE OF DISCHARGE: 12/18/97

ADMITTING DIAGNOSIS: 1. TEAR OF THE RIGHT ROTATOR CUFF

PRINCIPAL DIAGNOSIS: 1. TEAR OF THE RIGHT ROTATOR CUFF
2. HYPERTENSION
3. ALLERGIC REACTION

OPERATION:

BRIEF HISTORY: Patient came in for an elective surgery on the right rotator cuff. He had injured his shoulder while playing football and because of continuing pain, an ultrasound vasogram was performed, which revealed a tear of the right rotator cuff.

HOSPITAL COURSE: Approximately 24 hours following surgery, the patient was hooked up to a patient-controlled anesthesia with intravenous morphine and also receiving 1 g Ancef every eight hours. Patient developed rather severe itching and subsequent facial flush and mild rash. Both medications were discontinued. It is unknown which medication was the cause of his apparent allergic reaction.

Patient also had a very mild hypertension upon admission. During his admission, at times, blood pressure was as high as 190/116, and he ran a rather consistently elevated blood pressure for systolic and diastolic. Dr. Tom Brown was called in consultation because of both the allergic reaction and the hypertension, and initial studies were started concerning the hypertension. Patient was placed on Benadryl and responded rather appropriately to this treatment as far as allergic reaction was concerned.

DISPOSITION: Patient was discharged home in a sling and strap. He is to remain in this until I see him in approximately two weeks. He will also be followed up with Dr. Tom Brown concerning his hypertension in approximately two weeks, when all studies have been completed.

MEK

_____
Signature

FIGURE 13-9. Discharge summary.

TABLE 13–1. SOUND-ALIKE WORDS

addiction	diaphysis	menorrhea
adduction	diastasis	menorrhagia
abduction	diathesis	metrorrhagia
alveolus	epigastric	mucous
alveus	epispastic	mucus
alvus	embolus	nephrosis
amenorrhea	thrombus	neurosis
dysmenorrhea	endemic	palpation
antidiarrheic	epidemic	palpitation
antidiuretic	pandemic	paratenon
antiseptic	facial	peritenon
aseptic	fascial	precardiac
asepsis	foci	pericardium
arteritis	fossae	perineal
arthritis	gavage	peroneal
aural	lavage	perineum
oral	hypertension	peritoneum
bradycardia	hypotension	perivascular
tachycardia	hypocalcemia	perivesical
callus	hypokalemia	stasis
callous	ileum	staxis
carbuncle	ilium	sycosis
caruncle	infection	psychosis
furuncle	infestation	tenia
carpus	insulin	tinea
corpus	inulin	trachelotomy
chronic	keratosis	tracheotomy
chromic	ketosis	ureter
contusion	larynx	urethra
concussion	pharynx	vesical
convulsion	lymphangitis	vesicle
corneal	lymphadenitis	xerosis
cranial	macro	cirrhosis
cocci	micro	serosa
coxa	mastitis	
cystostomy	mastoiditis	
cystotomy		
cystoscopy		

Capitalization

- Capitalize the first word of:

  every sentence

  an expression used as a sentence

  each item in a list or outline

  the salutation and the complimentary closing of a letter

- Capitalize the official name of a particular person, place, or thing, for example:

  Andrew Jackson

  New York City

  the World Trade Center

- Capitalize a common noun when it is part of a proper name:

  "Give the paper to Professor Mary Woods."
  BUT: "Give the paper to the professor."

"The parade traveled along Madison Avenue."
BUT: "The parade traveled along the avenue."

Word Division

Avoid excessive division of words at the end of a line. Word divisions clutter a page and may even confuse a reader. Basic rules of word division include:

- Dividing words only between syllables
- Never dividing a one-syllable word
- Never setting off a one-letter syllable at the end or beginning of a word
- Never dividing abbreviations or contractions
- Never dividing a word unless you can leave a syllable of at least three characters (including the hyphen) on the upper line and carry a syllable of at least three characters (may include a punctuation mark) to the next line

Plurals

Some basic rules for forming plurals are:

- Plurals of nouns are usually formed by adding *s* or *es* to the singular form
- Plurals of abbreviations are formed by adding *s* (e.g., ECGs and CVAs); some use an apostrophe before the *s*, but this is unnecessary and losing popularity
- Medical terms: Many medical terms have Latin roots; the plural of a Latin noun is determined by its gender (masculine, feminine, or neuter):

	Singular	Plural
Nouns ending in	a	ae
Nouns ending in	is	es
Nouns ending in	um	a
Nouns ending in	us	i
Nouns ending in	ix, ex	ces

Numbers

Spell out numbers from 1 to 10. Use figures for numbers greater than 10 except at the beginning of a sentence.

- Use only figures (including 1–10) in tables and statistical matter and in expressing dates, money, clock time, and percentages.
- Express related numbers the same way
- Express measurements in figures
- Always use figures with AM and PM
- Do not use zeros with on-the-hour time (e.g. 9 AM, *not* 9:00 AM)
- Always write decimals in figures, without commas in the decimal part of the number
- Write percentages in figures and spell out *per cent* (e.g., 10 per cent)

- When typing figures in columns, Arabic numbers (e.g., 1, 2, and 3) are aligned on the right, decimal amounts (e.g., 1.23) are aligned on the decimal, and Roman numerals (e.g., I, II, and III) are aligned on the left

REFERENCE MATERIALS

The transcriptionist should have readily available reliable references.

Office worker's reference manual. A good reference manual can serve as a ready source of information when you are transcribing. In it, you will find in-depth information on punctuation, capitalization, writing numbers, the use of abbreviations, and plurals and possessives as well as spelling guides. It is also a source of information on typing manuscripts, reports, and bibliographies as well as other information that you may use only occasionally.

English language dictionary. Keep a good dictionary near your desk for those times when you are unsure of your spelling or of the meaning of a word (especially one that sounds like another).

Medical dictionary. Not all medical dictionaries have the same arrangement of entries. No matter which one you have available, you will soon become accustomed to finding what you need. In one popular dictionary, terms consisting of two words are primarily defined under the second word—usually the noun. For example, to find *acetic acid,* you would look under the noun *acid,* and then for the subheading *acetic;* to find *splenic vein,* you would first find the noun *vein,* and then the subentry *splenic. Syndrome* is a main entry; the dozens of kinds of syndromes are shown as subentries. Other examples are *tests, disease, culture,* and *method.* Just remember that whenever you must find a two-word entry, you will probably find it under the second word.

A specialized dictionary is available for almost every medical specialty. The transcriptionist in a specialty practice will find it worthwhile to invest in a reference for that specialty.

Physicians' Desk Reference (PDR). An unknown drug is difficult to spell, and the spelling must be verified by the transcriptionist. A drug may have three types of names: chemical, generic, and trade. The *chemical name* of a drug represents its exact formula, the *generic name* is the common name of the chemical or drug, and the *trade name* is the name by which a manufacturer identifies the drug.

The *PDR* is the reference of choice for checking the names and spelling of drugs. It is published each year, and during the year supplements are published to keep the reference up-to-date. The *PDR* contains seven different color-coded indexes:

- Alphabetical by Manufacturer
- Alphabetical by Brand Name
- Product (Drug) Category
- Generic and Chemical Name
- Product Identification
- Product Information
- Diagnostic Information

If your dictation contains an unfamiliar drug name, you should first look in the Alphabetical Index for the proper spelling. If this search is unsuccessful, try the Generic and Chemical Name Index. In typing the names of drugs, it is important to know whether it is a brand name or a generic name. For instance, *aspirin,* is a generic name, whereas *Bufferin* is a brand name. The first letter of a brand name is capitalized. Generic names are not capitalized. In addition to being helpful as a source for the spelling and capitalization of drug names, the *PDR* contains a vast amount of information about drugs and their specific uses.

Names of over-the-counter (OTC) drugs can be found in the *Physicians' Desk Reference for Nonprescription Drugs,* issued annually by the same publisher.

Standard abbreviations. As mentioned earlier in this chapter, except for the physician's own records, any abbreviations used in transcription should be standard and not subject to interpretation. Many good books are available for checking abbreviations and should be consulted when the meaning of an abbreviation is in doubt.

Coding books. If your transcription involves procedural or diagnostic coding, you should have copies of the most recent CPT (Current Procedural Terminology), **HCPCS,** and the **ICD-9-CM** in your reference library.

13

▶ LEARNING ACHIEVEMENTS

Are you able to:

1. Define the terms listed in the Vocabulary of this chapter?
2. Identify six basic educational requirements for the medical transcriptionist?
3. Discuss the special importance of speed and accuracy for the independently practicing transcriptionist?
4. List and briefly describe the three stages of activity in the machine transcription process?
5. Name and briefly describe five basic functional features of a typical transcribing unit?
6. Name and briefly describe three kinds of frequently dictated reports in the average physician's office?

7. List the basic contents of hospital reports that become a part of the patient's medical history?
8. Correctly type numbers in a dictated report?
9. Align figures in a column?
10. Correctly format common medical reports?

READINGS AND REFERENCES

Diehl, M. O., and Fordney, M. T.: *Medical Typing and Transcribing: Techniques and Procedures,* 3rd ed., Philadelphia, W. B. Saunders Co., 1991.

Fordney, M. T., and Diehl, M. O.: *Medical Transcription Guide: Do's and Don'ts,* Philadelphia, W. B. Saunders Co., 1990.

Logan, C. L., and Rice, M. K.: *Logan's Medical and Scientific Abbreviations,* Philadelphia, J. B. Lippincott Co., 1987.

Morrow, N. L.: *Being a Medical Transcriptionist,* Englewood Cliffs, NJ, Brady Books, A Division of Prentice Hall Press, Simon & Schuster, Inc., 1992.

Sabin, W. A.: *The Gregg Reference Manual,* 6th ed., Lake Forest, IL, Gregg/McGraw-Hill, 1991.

Schwager, E.: *Medical English Usage and Abusage,* Phoenix, AZ, The Oryx Press, 1991.

Schertzer, M.: *The Elements of Grammar,* New York, Macmillan Publishing Company, 1986.

Steen, E. B.: *Medical Abbreviations,* 5th ed., Philadelphia, W. B. Saunders Co., 1984.

Strunk, W., Jr., and White, E. B.: *The Elements of Style,* 3rd ed., New York, Macmillan Publishing Company, 1979.

Tessier, C. and Pitman, S. C.: *Style Guide for Medical Transcription,* Modesto, CA, American Association for Medical Transcription, 1985.

CHAPTER FOURTEEN

——

MEDICAL RECORDS MANAGEMENT

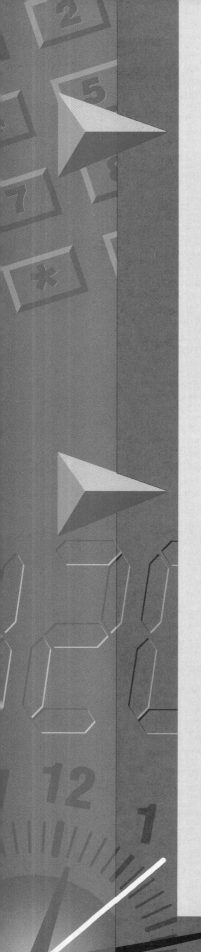

CHAPTER OUTLINE

VOCABULARY

alphabetic filing Any system that arranges names or topics according to the sequence of letters in the alphabet.

alphanumeric Systems made up of combinations of letters and numbers.

caption A heading, title, or subtitle under which records are filed.

chronologic order In the order of time.

continuity The quality or state of being continuous.

correlation The act or process of correlating; mutual relation.

cross-reference A notation in a file that indicates that a record is stored elsewhere and that gives the reference.

demographic Relating to the statistical characteristics of populations, such as births, marriages, mortality, health, and so forth.

direct filing system A filing system in which materials can be located without consulting an intermediary source of reference.

filing system A plan for organizing records so that they can be found when needed.

litigation Contest in a court of justice for the purpose of enforcing a right.

microfilming Photographing records in reduced size on film.

numeric filing Filing records, correspondence, or cards by number.

OUTfolder A folder used to provide space for the temporary filing of materials.

OUTguide A heavy guide that is used to replace a folder that has been temporarily removed from the filing space

pejorative Having negative connotations; a depreciatory word.

POMR Problem Oriented Medical Record.

retention schedule A listing of dates until which records are to be kept. The listing is determined based on statutes of limitations, tax regulations, and other factors.

sequential Succeeding or following in order or as a result.

shelf filing A system that uses open shelves (rather than cabinets) for storing records.

statute of limitations The time limit within which an action may legally be brought upon a contract.

subject filing Arranging records alphabetically by names of topics or things rather than by names of individuals.

tab The projection on a file folder or guide on which the caption is written.

tickler A chronologic file used as a reminder that something must be taken care of on a certain date.

transfer Removing inactive records from the active files.

unit Each part of a name that is used in indexing.

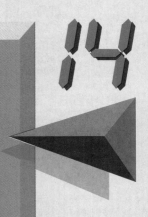

MEDICAL RECORDS MANAGEMENT

LEARNING OBJECTIVES

COGNITIVE

Upon successful completion of this chapter, you should be able to:

1. Define the terms listed in the Vocabulary.

2. State three important reasons for keeping good medical records.

3. Illustrate the meaning of subjective and objective information in a medical history.

4. List four categories each of subjective and objective information contained in a complete case history.

5. List the 15 items of personal data needed on a patient history.

6. Explain the basic differences between the traditional and the problem-oriented medical record (POMR), and three advantages of the POMR.

7. Discuss changing an entry in the medical record and the importance of following correct procedure.

8. List and describe the three classifications of patient files.

9. List and discuss the basic equipment and supplies in a filing system.

10. Describe the seven sequential steps in filing a document.

11. List and discuss application of the four basic filing systems.

12. Explain how color coding of files can be advantageous in a medical facility.

PERFORMANCE

Upon successful completion of this chapter, you should be able to perform the following activities:

1. Initiate a medical record for a new patient.

2. Add reports and correspondence into the patient's file in the correct manner and sequence.

3. Make a correction in a patient's chart in a manner affording legal protection.

4. Typewrite a list of names in indexing order and arrange them alphabetically for filing.

5. Arrange a group of patient numbers in filing sequence for a terminal digit filing system.

6. Using the color key in this chapter, state the tab color to be used for a given list of names.

Records management is not just a fancy name for storing information. Management of medical records includes not only assembling the medical record for each patient but also having an efficient system for the filing, retrieval, transferring, protection, retention, storage, and destruction of these records.

Some of the objectives of good records management are:

- Saving space
- Reducing filing equipment expenditures
- Reducing the creation of unnecessary records
- Faster retrieval of information
- Reducing misfiles
- Compliance with legal safeguards
- Protection of confidentiality
- Saving the physician's and the patients' time

Complete and accurate records are essential to a well-managed medical practice. They provide a continuous story of a patient's progress from the first visit to the last. The treatment and therapy prescribed are noted, along with regular reports on the patient's condition. When a patient is discharged, the degree of improvement is placed upon the record.

REASONS FOR MEDICAL RECORDS

There are three important reasons for carefully recording medical information:

1. **To Provide the Best Medical Care.** The doctor examines the patient and enters the findings on the patient's medical record. These findings are the clues to diagnosis. The doctor may order many types of tests to confirm or augment the clinical findings. As the reports of these tests come in, the findings fall into place like the pieces of a jigsaw puzzle. Now, with the confirmation data to support the diagnosis, the physician can prescribe treatment and form an opinion about the patient's chances of recovery, assured that every resource has been used to arrive at a correct judgment.

   Keeping good medical records helps a physician provide **continuity** in a patient's medical care. Earlier illnesses and difficulties that appear on the patient's record may supply the key to current medical problems. For example, the information on the record that the patient was treated for rheumatic fever as a child can be extremely important in determining the course of treatment the doctor prescribes for that patient when an illness develops a number of years later.

2. **To Supply Statistical Information.** Medical records may be used to evaluate the effectiveness of certain kinds of treatment or to determine the incidence of a given disease. **Correlation** of such statistical information may result in a new outlook on some phases of medicine and can lead

to revised techniques and treatments. The statistical data from medical records also are valuable in the preparation of scientific papers, books, and lectures.

3. **To Provide Legal Protection.** Sometimes a physician must produce case histories and medical records in court. For example, a patient may wish to substantiate claims made to an insurance company for damages resulting from an accident in which he or she was injured and required medical treatment. A patient may involve a physician in **litigation.** The physician's records can be a help or a hindrance, depending on the care with which they are kept.

CONTENT OF RECORD

For adequate legal protection, the patient record should include the following:

- Patient's medical history
- Results of examinations
- Records of treatment
- Copies of laboratory reports
- Notations of all instructions given
- Copies of all prescriptions and notes on refill authorizations
- Documentation of informed consent when applicable
- Any correspondence that relates to the patient's diagnosis or treatment
- Any other pertinent data

Specific quotes of comments made by the patient about symptoms or reasons for consulting the doctor are particularly helpful if there should ever be litigation. The doctor should also record what was told to the patient.

When a patient fails to follow instructions or refuses recommended treatment, a letter to this effect should be sent to the patient by certified mail, and a copy retained in the medical record. A similar type of letter should be sent if the patient leaves the doctor's care or if the doctor feels it is necessary to withdraw from the case.

ITEMS TO EXCLUDE FROM RECORDS

Some entries should not be made in the record. For instance:

1. Reports from consulting physicians should not be placed in the record until they have been carefully reviewed to ensure that the overall diagnostic and treatment plan is consistent or that any inconsistencies have been identified and justified. If the report contains confidential data from another source, release of such data without authorization can lead to legal difficulties.

2. Transferred records from the patient's previous physicians should never be added to the patient's new record until the physician has reviewed them. The same advice would apply to records received from any outside source (e.g., hospital emergency departments or freestanding urgent care clinics).

3. **Pejorative** or flippant comments should never be entered in the record. For example, one doctor might enter only one note in the record after seeing a patient who tended toward hypochondria: "Same verse, same refrain," or "New verse, same refrain." This comment would reflect negatively on the doctor in court. In some states, patients or their representatives have the legal right to a copy of their medical records.

STYLE AND FORM OF RECORDS

A record is any form of recorded information. It may be on:

- Paper
- Film
- A magnetic medium, such as computer tapes or disks

If a record is to be useful, it must be easily retrievable, orderly, complete, and understandable by anyone who needs to use it. To be helpful, it must be completely accurate. To be good, it must be brief.

Coding of information on records is sometimes a helpful shortcut, but any coding system used should be a standard one that can be understood by anyone who needs to consult the chart. If the coding does vary somewhat from the standard, an explanation of the code should be prepared and placed in the front of the files for immediate reference (Table 14–1).

The style and form selected by a physician for recording case histories depend partly on the nature of the practice. General practitioners and some specialists keep very detailed records. A specialist who sees patients only on a consultant basis, or a specialist who is likely to see a patient only once, such as a dermatologist, a radiologist, or an anesthesiologist, need not keep complex records.

The nature of the patient's complaint is also a factor in determining just how detailed a record should be. If a patient comes into a physician's office to have a foreign body removed from an eye or to have some minor injury such as a cut finger treated, a detailed past medical history or family history is unnecessary. In contrast, the patient who is being treated for cardiac, hypertensive, or diabetic symptoms requires a complete examination and a detailed history.

In some medical offices where detailed histories are not required, a simple patient registration slip (Fig. 14–1) can be used to record personal data, and a plain sheet of paper used to record the complaint and treatment given. In the great majority of offices,

TABLE 14–1. ABBREVIATIONS COMMONLY USED IN PATIENT HISTORY AND PHYSICAL EXAMINATION

Abbreviation	Meaning
A & W	Alive and well
CC	Chief complaint
CNS	Central nervous system
CR	Cardiorespiratory
CV	Cardiovascular
Dx	Diagnosis
FH	Family history
GI	Gastrointestinal
GU	Genitourinary
GYN	Gynecology
HEENT	Head, ears, eyes, nose, throat
MM	Mucous membrane
PH	Past history
PI	Present illness
prn	As necessary (pro re nata)
ROS/SR	Review of systems/Systems review
TPR	Temperature, pulse, respirations
UCHD	Usual childhood diseases
VS	Vital signs
w/d	Well developed
w/n	Well nourished
WNL	Within normal limits

14

```
                 REGISTRATION SLIP

PLEASE PRINT              DATE  April 20, 1992

NAME  Morris, Samuel Albert

ADDRESS  3810 Commonwealth Avenue

CITY  Los Angeles, CA           ZIP CODE  90056

Telephone 213 862 9917    Birth Date 04-05-40   Sex  M

 □ Single   ☒ Married   □ Widowed   □ Divorced

Occupation  Merchant          Phone 213 462 8122

Employed by  Morris Appliances (self)

Employer's address 5400 Hollywood Blvd, LA 90036
Name of Spouse
or Parent  Louise Marie

Occupation  Office Manager     Phone 213 462 8122

Employed by  Morris Appliances

Employer's address  (see above)

Referred by  Frank Gentry, M.D.
                          Soc. Sec.
INSURANCE:                 Number  012 34 5678

Medical Insurance Cert. No.  WD 4305

Company  Occidental

Hospital Insurance Cert. No. _____

Company _____

Other Health Insurance _____

FORM NO. 3320. COLWELL CO., CHAMPAIGN. ILL.
```

FIGURE 14–1. Patient registration slip. (Courtesy of Colwell Systems, a division of Deluxe Corporation.)

however, a more complete record and an individual folder for each patient is preferable.

The physician who uses just a plain sheet of paper for the patient record generally develops an outline that serves as a guide to taking down the information required for a history. The physician then dictates the history, and the medical assistant types it according to an established format and places it in the patient's folder after having it read and initialed by the physician. In every medical arena, you will find certain technical terms being used frequently in the doctor's reports. The medical assistant who types the reports should become familiar with the correct spelling and meaning of the medical terms. Because of the close similarity in the sound and spelling of some medical terms, it is wise to also check the definition to be sure the word fits the context in which it is used.

For the physician who wishes to use a more structured format, there are many different types of forms available from professional stationers: forms for general practice, obstetrics, surgery, pediatrics, internal medicine, or any other of the established specialties. Some physicians design their own forms to suit their particular practice and have them printed to order. Companies that specialize in medical forms sometimes provide a planning kit for the physician to use. Local printers, too, often can be very helpful with form design. The record may be **sequential,** or it may be separated into "problems," as described later, in the section on the problem-oriented medical record. Regardless of the form used, the case history will contain certain basic information.

CONTENTS OF THE COMPLETE CASE HISTORY

Recordkeeping in the hospital medical records department is deemed important enough that it is entrusted only to specially trained individuals. The position of medical record administrator requires a baccalaureate degree; a medical record technician requires an associate degree with specialization in the specifics of cataloging and recordkeeping in the hospital medical records department. The medical assistant in a doctor's office does not need such extensive training but must be familiar with the basic essentials of recordkeeping.

The medical case history is the most important record in a doctor's office. For completeness, each patient's record should contain:

Subjective Information Provided by the Patient

- Routine personal data about the patient
- Patient's personal and medical history
- Patient's family history
- Patient's complaint (in the patient's own words) and date of onset

Objective Information Provided by the Doctor

- Physical examination and findings; laboratory and x-ray reports
- Diagnosis and prognosis
- Treatment prescribed and progress noted
- Condition at time of termination of treatment

If these entries are completed, the case history will stand the test of time. No branch of medicine is exempt from the necessity of keeping records. Records aid the physician in the practice of medicine, as well as provide legal protection.

Subjective Information
Routine Personal Data About the Patient

The patient's case history begins with routine personal data, which the patient usually supplies on the first visit. The basic facts needed are:

- Patient's full name, spelled correctly
- If patient is a child, names of parents
- Patient's sex
- Date of birth
- Marital status
- Name of spouse, if married
- Number of children, if any
- Home address and telephone number
- Occupation
- Name of employer
- Business address and telephone number
- Employment information for spouse
- Health insurance information
- Source of referral
- Social Security number

Patient's Personal and Medical History

This portion of the medical record, which is often obtained by having the patient complete a questionnaire, provides information about any past illnesses or surgical operations that the patient may have had and includes data about injuries or physical defects, whether congenital or acquired. It also furnishes information about the patient's daily health habits.

Patient's Family History

The family history comprises the physical condition of the various members of the patient's family, any past illnesses or diseases that individual members may have suffered, and a record of the causes of death. This information is important, since a definite hereditary pattern is often present in the case of certain diseases.

Patient's Complaint

This is a concise account of the patient's symptoms, explained in the patient's own words. It should include the nature and duration of pain, if any, the time when the patient first noticed symptoms, the patient's opinion as to the possible causes for the difficulties, any remedies that the patient may have applied prior to seeing the doctor, and any other medical treatment received for the same condition in the past.

Objective Information

Objective findings, sometimes referred to as "signs," become evident from the physician's examination of the patient.

Physical Examination and Findings, and Laboratory and X-ray Reports

This section of the case history varies greatly with the specialty of the physician and the complaint of the patient. After the physician has examined the patient, the physical findings are recorded on the history. Results of other tests or requests for these tests are then recorded or, if they appear on separate sheets, attached to the history.

Diagnosis

The physician, on the basis of all evidence provided in the patient's past history, the physician's examination, and any supplementary tests, places the diagnosis of the patient's condition on the medical record. If there is some doubt, it may be termed "Provisional Diagnosis."

Treatment Prescribed and Progress Notes

The physician's suggested treatment is listed following the diagnosis. Generally, instructions to the patient to return for follow-up treatment in a specific period of time are noted here as well.

On each subsequent visit, the date must be entered on the chart, and information about the patient's condition and the results of treatment added to the history, on the basis of the physician's observations. Notations of all medications prescribed or instructions given, as well as the patient's own progress report, should be placed in the record. Any home visits are noted. If the patient is hospitalized, the name of the hospital, the reason for admission, and the dates of admission and discharge are recorded. Much of this information may be obtained from the hospital discharge summary.

Condition at Time of Termination of Treatment

When the treatment is terminated, the physician will record that information. For example:

August 18, 1993. Wound completely healed. Patient discharged.

PROBLEM-ORIENTED MEDICAL RECORD

The traditional patient record is "source-oriented"; that is, observations and data are catalogued according to their source—physician, laboratory, x-ray, nurse, technician—with no recording of a logical relationship between them. The problem-oriented medical record (POMR) is a radical departure from the traditional system of keeping patient records. It is sometimes referred to as the "Weed System" because it was originated by Lawrence L. Weed, M.D., a professor of medicine at the University of Vermont's College of Medicine. The POMR is a record of clinical practice that divides medical action into four bases:

- The *database* includes chief complaint, present illness, and patient profile and also a review of systems, physical examination, and laboratory reports.
- The *problem list* is a numbered and titled list of every problem the patient has that requires management or workup. This may include social and **demographic** troubles as well as strictly medical or surgical ones.
- The *treatment plan* includes management, additional workups needed, and therapy. Each plan is titled and numbered with respect to the problem.
- The *progress notes* include structured notes that are numbered to correspond with each problem number.

One company, which designed the Andrus/Clini-Rec Charting System, has developed a file folder for its recommended organization of patient data. The folder is preprinted on the front for age dating and easy access to basic information. With the calendar years printed on the cover, it is simple to keep track of when the patient was last seen. On the initial visit, the year, say 1990, is checked on the cover. If the patient appears again in 1992, and the year 1991 is not checked, you know immediately that more than a year has elapsed since the last visit (Fig. 14–2). The system has suggested dividers for lab reports, consultations, hospital reports, and x-ray and ECG reports (all scientific information) on the left side, and database and progress notes (communication and supervision) on the right side.

The chart is begun by obtaining a patient-completed database system record, which contains family and past medical history together with 135 carefully selected screening questions. It is so designed that the page that goes into the chart shows only the positive answers (Fig. 14–3). There are also questionnaires designed for screening problems in specialty practices.

The problem list is entered on the divider cover for lab reports. Special sections are provided for current major and chronic problems, and for inactive major or chronic problems. The divider cover

_____ CREDIT _____

Vol. No.: _____

Patient Name: _____

Patient Address: _____

City, State: _____

Patient Telephone: _____

Doctor: _____

PATIENT CLASSIFICATION

IND. ACCIDENT	MEDICAID	MEDICARE

ALLERGIC REACTIONS

DATE	SUBSTANCE	EFFECT

ORDER # 16-7100 CLINI-REC ® SHELF FOLDER
BIBBERO SYSTEMS, INC. PETALUMA, CA
TO ORDER CALL 800-BIBBERO(CA) or 800/358-8240(USA)

1991	
1992	
1993	
1994	
1995	
1996	
1997	
1998	
1999	
2000	
2001	
2002	
2003	
2004	
2005	
2006	
2007	
2008	
2009	
2010	
2011	

FIGURE 14-2. Andrus/Clini-Rec File Folder, preprinted on the front for age dating and easy access to basic information. (Courtesy of Bibbero Systems, Inc., Petaluma, CA.)

for progress notes is a chart for listing medications and other therapeutic modalities. Progress notes follow the SOAPing approach (Fig. 14–4):

S Subjective impressions
O Objective clinical evidence
A Assessment or diagnosis
P Plans for further studies, treatment, or management

The POMR has the advantage of imposing order and organization on the information added to a patient's medical record. The records are more easily reviewed, and the likelihood of overlooking a problem is greatly reduced. SOAPing essentially forces a rational approach to patient problems and assists in formulating a logical and orderly plan of patient care.

Whereas the POMR was practically unheard of before 1970, it has become increasingly popular and is especially advantageous in clinics, group practices, and hospitals, where more than one person must be able to find essential information in the chart.

OBTAINING THE HISTORY

The medical assistant usually secures the routine personal data. The personal and medical history and the patient's family history may be secured by asking the patient to complete a questionnaire, with the physician augmenting the information provided during the patient interview.

If the doctor delegates the taking of patients' histories to the medical assistant, care must be exercised to assure that the patient's answers are not heard by others in the reception room. If privacy is not possible, it is better to give the patient a form to fill out and then transfer this information to permanent records later. If convenient, it is time-saving to ask the patient questions and at the same time type

UESTIONNAIRE

27. Do you wear eyeglasses? . . . .
28. Do you wear contact lenses? . . . .
29. Has your vision changed in the last year? . . . .
30. How often do you have:
    a. Double vision? . . . .
    b. Blurry vision? . . . .
    c. Watery or itchy eyes? . . . .
31. Do you ever see colored rings around lights? . . . . . .
32. Do others tell you you have a hearing problem? . . . . .
33. Do you have trouble keeping your balance? . . . .
34. Do you have any discharge from your ears? . . . .
35. Do you ever feel dizzy or have motion sickness? . . . . .
36. Do you have any problems with your hearing? . . . . . .
37. Do you ever have ringing in your ears? . . . .

VISION/HEARING

	No	Yes	
			Wears eyeglasses
			Wears contacts
			Vision changed in last year

Rarely/Never	Occasionally	Frequently	
			Double vision
			Blurred vision
			Watery/itchy eyes
			Sees halos
			Hearing problem
			Loses balance
			Discharge from ears
			Dizzy/motion sickness

No___ Yes___ Hearing problems
No___ Yes___ Ringing in ears

NOSE/THROAT/RESPIRATORY

Rarely/Never	Occasionally	Frequently	
			Head colds
			Chest colds
			Runny nose
			Head congestion
			Sore/hoarse throat
			Coughing spells
			Sneezing spells
			Trouble breathing
			Nose bleeds
			Cough blood

No___ Yes___ Worked on a farm
No___ Yes___ Worked in a mine
No___ Yes___ Worked in a laundry/mill
No___ Yes___ Worked in high dust concentrations
No___ Yes___ Exposed to toxic chemicals
No___ Yes___ Exposed to radioactive materials
No___ Yes___ Exposed to asbestos

CARDIOVASCULAR

Rarely/Never	Occasionally	Frequently	
			Out of breath quickly when exercising
			Dizziness
			Fainted

CONFIDENTIAL

PART C – BODY SYSTEMS REVIEW

I. MEN: Please answ... skip to qu...
WOMEN: Pleas...

MEN ONLY

1. Have you h... prostate t...
2. Do you h... or with...
3. Have y... lesions o...
4. Have you ev... from your penis...
5. Do you ever have pain... or swelling in your testicles...
Check here if you wish to discuss any...

	Occasionally	Frequently
6. Is it sometimes hard to start your urine flow?
7. Is urination ever painful?
8. Do you have to urinate more than 5 times a day?
9. Do you get up at night to urinate?
10. Has your urine ever been bloody or dark colored?
11. Do you ever lose urine when you strain, laugh, cough or sneeze?
12. Do you ever lose urine during sleep?

WOMEN ONLY
Do you:

13. a. Have any menstrual problems?
    b. Feel rather tense just before your period?
    c. Have heavy menstrual bleeding?
    d. Have painful menstrual periods?
    e. Have any bleeding between periods?
    f. Have any unusual vaginal discharge or itching?
    g. Ever have tender breasts?
    h. Have any discharge from your nipples?
    i. Have any hot flashes?
14. How many times, if any, have you been pregnant?
15. How many children born alive?
16. Are you taking birth control pills? ... No___ Yes___
17. Do you examine your breasts for lumps every month? ... No___ Yes___
17a. What was the date of your last menstrual period? ... Date___

MEN & WOMEN
18. In the past year have you had any:
    a. Severe shoulder pain?
    b. Severe back pain?
    c. Muscle or joint stiffness or pain due to sports, exercise or injury?
    d. Pain or swelling in any joints not due to sports, exercise or injury?

19. Do you have dry skin or brittle fingernails? ... No___ Yes___
20. Do you bruise easily? ... No___ Yes___
21. Do you have any moles that have changed in color or in size? ... No___ Yes___
22. Do you have any other skin problems? ... No___ Yes___

23. In the last 3 months have you had:
    a. A fever that lasted more than one day? ... No___ Yes___
    b. Sores or cuts that were hard to heal? ... No___ Yes___
    c. Any cold sores (fever blisters)? ... No___ Yes___
    d. Any lumps in your neck, armpits or groin? ... No___ Yes___
    e. Do you ever have chills or sweat at night? ... No___ Yes___
24. Have you traveled out of the country in the last 2 years? ... No___ Yes, Traveled in: ___
25. Write in the dates for the shots you have had: Measles / Mumps / Polio — Smallpox / Tetanus / Typhoid
26. Have you had a tuberculin (TB) skin test? ... No___ Yes___ Date___
    If so, was it negative or positive? ... Neg___ Pos___

© 1979, 1983 Bibbero Systems International, Inc.   **PLEASE TURN THIS PAGE**   19-711-4 5/83

CONFIDENTIAL

Chart No. _____

ANDRUS/CLINI-REC® HEALTH HISTORY QUESTIONNAIRE

Identification Information   Today's Date _____

Name _____   Date of Birth _____

Occupation _____   Marital Status _____

PART A – PRESENT HEALTH HISTORY

I. CURRENT MEDICAL PROBLEMS
Please list the medical problems for which you came to see the doctor. About when did they begin?

Problems	Date Began

What concerns you most about these problems?

If you are being treated for any other illnesses or medical problems by another physician, please describe the problems and write the name of the physician or medical facility treating you.

Illness or Medical Problem	Physician or Medical Facility	City

II. MEDICATIONS
Please list all medications you are now taking, including those you buy without a doctor's prescription (such as aspirin, cold tablets or vitamin supplements)

III. ALLERGIES AND SENSITIVITIES
List anything that you are allergic to such as certain foods, medications, dust, chemicals, or soaps, household items, pollens, bee stings, etc., and indicate how each affects you.

Allergic To:	Effect	Allergic To:	Effect

IV. GENERAL HEALTH, ATTITUDE AND HABITS

How is your overall health now? .... Health now: Poor___ Fair___ Good___ Excellent___
How has it been most of your life? .... Health has been   Poor___ Fair___ Good___ Excellent___
In the past year:
  Has your appetite changed? .... Appetite: Decreased___ Increased___ Stayed same___
  Has your weight changed? .... Weight: Lost___ lbs. Gained___ lbs. No change___
  Are you thirsty much of the time? .... Thirsty: No___
  Has your overall 'pep' changed? .... Pep: Decreased___ Increased___ Stayed same___
Do you usually have trouble sleeping? ...... Trouble sleeping: No___ Yes___
How much do you exercise? .... Exercise: Little or none___ Less than I need___ All I need___
Do you smoke? .... Smokes: No___ Yes___ If yes, how many years?___
How many each day? Cigarettes___ Cigars___ Pipesfull___
Have you ever smoked? .... Smoked No___ Yes___ If yes, how many years?___
How many each day? Cigarettes___ Cigars___ Pipesfull___
Do you drink alcoholic beverages? .... Alcohol: No___ Yes___ I drink___ Beers___ Glasses of Wine___ Drinks of hard liquor - per day
Have you ever had a problem with alcohol? .. Prior alcohol: No___ Yes___
How much coffee or tea do you usually drink? .. Coffee/Tea: ___ cups of coffee or tea a day.
Do you regularly wear seatbelts? .... Seatbelts: No___ Yes___

DO YOU:	Rarely/Never	Occasionally	Frequently	DO YOU:	Rarely/Never	Occasionally	Frequently
Feel nervous?				Ever feel like committing suicide?			
Feel depressed?				Feel bored with your life?			
Find it hard to make decisions?				Use marijuana?			
Lose your temper?				Use "hard drugs"?			
Worry a lot?				Do you want to talk to the			
Tire easily?				doctor about a personal matter? No___ Yes___			
Have trouble relaxing?							
Have any sexual problems?							

Created and Developed by "Medical Economics" Professional Systems
Copyright © 1979, 1983 Bibbero Systems International, Inc.   STOCK NO. 19-711-4 5/83   Page 1

CONFIDENTIAL

14

FIGURE 14-3. Database self-administered general health history questionnaire. (Courtesy of Bibbero Systems, Inc., Petaluma, CA.)

OUTLINE FORMAT PROGRESS NOTES

Patient Name ___Fletcher, LeRoy___

Prob. No. or Letter	DATE	S Subjective	O Objective	A Assess	P Plans	Page _____
2	01/26/00	Patient complains of two days of severe high epigastric pain and burning, radiating through to the back. Pain accentuated after eating.				
			On examination there is extreme guarding and tenderness, high epigastric region. No rebound. Bowel sounds normal. BP 110/70			
				R/O gastric ulcer, pylorospasm.		
					To have upper gastrointestinal series. Start on Cimetidine 300 mg. q.i.d. Eliminate coffee, alcohol & aspirin. Return two days.	

Start each Progress Note (Subjective, Objective,   Assessment and Plans) at the appropriate   shaded column to create an outline form. Write
through the intervening columns to the right   margin of the page.

ANDRUS/CLINI-REC® PRIMARY CARE CHARTING SYSTEM FORM NO. 26-7115, ©1976 BIBBERO SYSTEMS, INC., PETALUMA, CA.

FIGURE 14-4. The SOAP Progress Note form. The four columns on the left indicate **S**ubjective impressions, **O**bjective clinical evidence, **A**ssessment or diagnosis, and **P**lans for further studies. (Courtesy of Bibbero Systems, Inc., Petaluma, CA.)

the answers directly on the record. This method offers an opportunity to become better acquainted with the patient as you complete the necessary records. In offices where lengthy questionnaires are to be completed by the new patient, the questionnaire is mailed to the patient with a request that it be completed and returned to the doctor's office prior to the appointment.

The patient's chief complaint may have been indicated to the medical assistant, but the physician will question the patient in more detail on this. The majority of doctors write their own entries on the chart in longhand. Others may dictate the material, either directly to the medical assistant or by using a recording device. If the material is dictated and typed, the physician should check each entry and then initial the entry to verify accuracy. Although the physician may find this is a bother, it should be encouraged. For a chart to be admissible as evidence in court, the person dictating or writing the entries should be able to attest that they were true and correct at the time they were written. The best indication of that is the physician's signature or initials on the typed entry.

MAKING ADDITIONS

As long as the patient is under the physician's care, the medical history is building. Each laboratory report, x-ray report, and progress note is added to the record, in **chronologic order,** with the latest information always on top. Although each item is important, the most recent is usually of greatest significance to the patient's care. Again, the physician should read and initial each of these reports before they are placed in the record.

Laboratory Reports

Different colors of paper are often used for reporting different procedures. For example, urinalysis report forms may be yellow, blood count forms pink, and so forth. Laboratory slips are usually smaller than the history form and should be placed on a standard 8½ × 11 inch sheet of colored paper. Type the patient's name in the upper righthand corner, and then, with transparent tape, fasten the first report even with the bottom of the page. The second laboratory report will be taped or glued in place on top of and about ½ inch above the first slip, allowing the date to show on the first report. By this method, called "shingling," the latest report always appears on top. When checking previous reports, it is necessary only to run your finger down the slips until you find the desired date; then flip up the slips above. Fifteen to twenty slips may be kept on one sheet by using this method, which is illustrated in Figure 14–5. Laboratory report carrier forms with adhesive strips may be purchased (Fig. 14–6).

X-ray Reports

X-ray reports are usually typed on standard letter-size stationery. X-ray reports are placed in the patient's history folder, with the most recent report on top. All x-ray reports may be stapled together or kept behind a special divider in the chart.

Progress Notes

Reports on the patient's progress are continually being added to the case history. Each visit of the patient should be entered on the chart, with the date preceding any notations about the call. The medical assistant can type or stamp the date on the chart when readying the charts for the patient's visits. Every instruction, prescription, or telephone call for advice should be entered with the correct date. If there are several persons handling and making entries on a patient's record, it is advisable to initial each entry. This aids in tracing entries about which there may be some question.

MAKING CORRECTIONS

Sometimes it is necessary to make corrections on medical records. Erasing and obliteration must be avoided. To correct a handwritten entry, follow these steps:

1. Draw a line through the error.
2. Insert the correction above or immediately following.
3. In the margin, write "correction" or "Corr.," your initials, and the date.

Errors made while typing are corrected in the usual way. An error discovered in a typed entry at a later date, however, is corrected in the same manner as described above for a handwritten entry.

KEEPING RECORDS CURRENT

One of the greatest dangers to good recordkeeping is procrastination. The record must be methodically kept current. It is the medical assistant's responsibility to see that this is done.

The case histories and reports may accumulate on the doctor's or the medical assistant's desk during the day. After the last patient has gone, check each history to make certain all necessary material has been recorded and that each entry is sufficiently clear for future understanding. Give the physician all extra reports, such as laboratory and x-ray reports, to read and initial so that they may be filed in the patient's case history folder.

While the doctor is reviewing these reports, you can pull the histories of any patients seen outside the office that day, as well as those of patients who

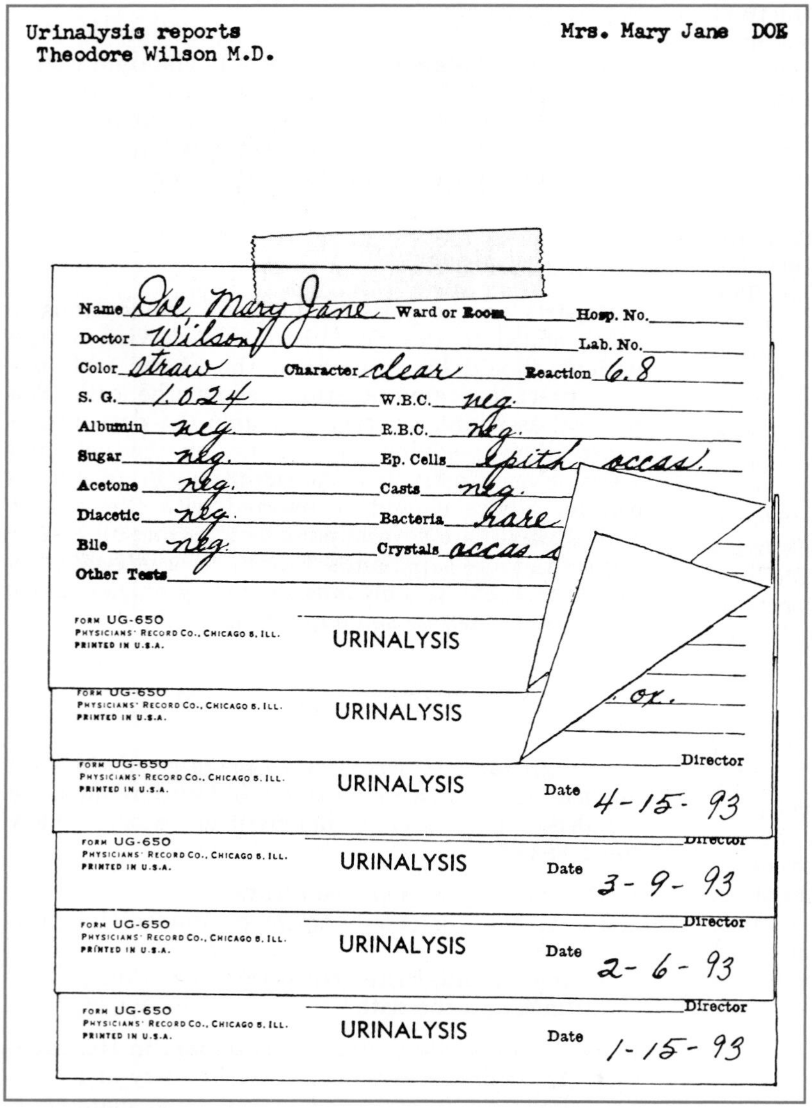

Urinalysis reports
Theodore Wilson M.D.

Mrs. Mary Jane DOE

Name Doe, Mary Jane Ward or Room ___ Hosp. No. ___
Doctor Wilson Lab. No. ___
Color straw Character clear Reaction 6.8
S. G. 1.024 W.B.C. neg.
Albumin neg. R.B.C. neg.
Sugar neg. Ep. Cells Epith. occas.
Acetone neg. Casts neg.
Diacetic neg. Bacteria rare
Bile neg. Crystals occas
Other Tests ___

FORM UG-650
PHYSICIANS' RECORD CO., CHICAGO 5, ILL.
PRINTED IN U.S.A.
URINALYSIS

FORM UG-650
PHYSICIANS' RECORD CO., CHICAGO 5, ILL.
PRINTED IN U.S.A.
URINALYSIS

FORM UG-650
PHYSICIANS' RECORD CO., CHICAGO 5, ILL.
PRINTED IN U.S.A.
URINALYSIS
Director
Date 4-15-93

FORM UG-650
PHYSICIANS' RECORD CO., CHICAGO 5, ILL.
PRINTED IN U.S.A.
URINALYSIS
Director
Date 3-9-93

FORM UG-650
PHYSICIANS' RECORD CO., CHICAGO 5, ILL.
PRINTED IN U.S.A.
URINALYSIS
Director
Date 2-6-93

FORM UG-650
PHYSICIANS' RECORD CO., CHICAGO 5, ILL.
PRINTED IN U.S.A.
URINALYSIS
Director
Date 1-15-93

FIGURE 14-5. Laboratory reports arranged chronologically on a page. (Courtesy of Physicians Record Company, Chicago, IL.)

have been given special instructions by telephone or for whom prescriptions were ordered. These entries are made in the same manner as for an office visit, but the type of call is explained in parentheses after the date. For example, here is what the history might include about a home visit to see a patient:

> May 23, 1993 (Res.) Routine PX. Temp 98.6. Chest clear. Cont. Rx. May now eat semi-bland diet.

When a patient telephones the doctor, the entry should be made on the patient's record, for example:

> June 26, 1994 (Tel.) To change Rx (Vit. B Comp) to one b.i.d. Force fluids. Feeling much better.

If tests are ordered for a patient, they should be charted in detail on the medical record:

> April 10, 1993. Consultation. Scheduled with Dr. Abbot for office consultation on April 26.
> Bilateral mammograms scheduled at SJH on April 17.

Prescriptions should be charted:

> April 25, 1993. Refill Tylenol c̄ Cod. #25.

A prescription pad, printed on no-smear, spot carbon paper, is available for a timesaving, write-it-once system. By placing the prescription blank over the patient's record, the prescription is automatically copied on the record as it is written (Fig. 14-7). Prescription carriers with adhesive strips are also available for the doctor who uses duplicate prescription blanks (Fig. 14-8).

The patient record should not leave the office. A Physician's Pocket Call Record, as shown in Figure 14-9, can be used for outside calls, and the information can be transferred to the chart in the office.

Also, at the end of the day, notations should be made of any unkept appointments or of refusals to cooperate with instructions.

After all records have been reviewed, they should

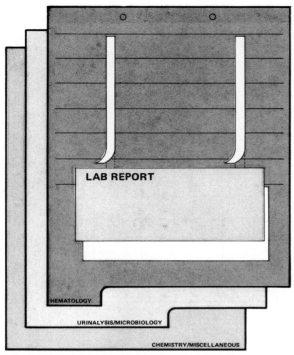

FIGURE 14-6. Quick-Stick color-coded lab carriers. Reports are affixed to proper carrier in chronological order by shingling from bottom of page to top. Remove zip tape from designated spot and press down on report. Be sure to indicate problem number on each report for future reference. (Courtesy of Bibbero Systems, Inc., Petaluma, CA.)

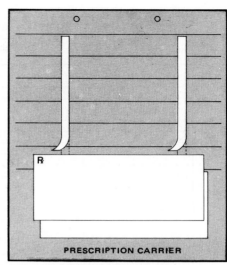

FIGURE 14-8. Quick-Stick Prescription Carrier for shingling copies of prescriptions in patient record. (Courtesy of Bibbero Systems, Inc., Petaluma, CA.)

14

FIGURE 14-7. Prescription pad for write-it-once system. (Courtesy of Bibbero Systems, Inc., Petaluma, CA.)

THOMAS A. SCOTT, M.D.
General Practice
135 SO. ELM STREET
SACRAMENTO, CALIFORNIA 94106
TELEPHONE: (916) 344-5550

CAL. LIC. #6099914
DEA #AK08888888

DATE *7/12/00*

PATIENT *John W. Bates*

ADDRESS *723 North Ave*
Crossville

	Rx Drug	Strength	Qty.	Rep.	Directions
1	*Esidrix*	*25 mgm*	*100*	*2x*	*1 tab p.c bid*
2.					
3.					
4.					

☐ Total Drugs

☐ Please label unless checked here

Strength is Mg. Units or %; Quantity is total amount to be dispensed. Rep. is number of refills.

Authority is given for dispensing by non proprietary name (generic equivalent) unless checked here. ☐

Thomas A. Scott M.D.
Thomas A. Scott, M.D.

FORM #25-8296

PHYSICIANS POCKET CALL RECORD			DATE _____			
NAME	ADDRESS OR REMARKS	SYMBOL	MONEY RECEIVED	HOME CHARGES	HOSPITAL CHARGES	
	Post these TOTALS to office book daily. ☞					

FIGURE 14–9. Physician's pocket call record for patient visits outside the office.

be placed in a file tray and locked away for the night, if there is insufficient time to file them the same day. Do not leave histories out in view at night, especially if the office has a night cleaning service.

On arrival the next morning, the medical assistant can index the histories for filing. Attach extra reports and information sheets; do not just drop them into the folders. It is best to attach them to the case histories with tape or rubber cement. When this is done, the records are ready for filing.

The doctor may prefer to dictate progress notes rather than write them in longhand. At appropriate moments during the day, everything is dictated: patient histories, physical examination findings, medications prescribed, follow-up findings, summaries of telephone conversations. At the end of the day the recorded information is handed to the medical assistant for transcribing onto the records.

A great deal of time may be saved in transcribing these notes by using a continuous roll or pages of self-adhesive strips (Fig. 14–10). When the transcription is completed, the doctor may wish to check the notes, underline important points, and initial each entry before returning the notes to the medical assistant for insertion in the charts. The use of self-adhesive strips saves removing the sheet from a chart that may be bound with metal fasteners, inserting the sheet into the typewriter, and putting the sheet back into the folder. It also simplifies the doctor's part in checking and initialing the notes, because only the transcribed material is handled, not the bulky charts.

TRANSFERRING FILES

Some system should be established for regular **transfer** of files. In most medical offices, records are filed according to three classifications:

- **Active files** are those of patients currently receiving treatment.
- **Inactive files** generally are those of patients whom the doctor has not seen for 6 months or longer. When such individuals return for care, their folders are replaced in the active file.
- **Closed files** are records of patients who have died, moved away, or otherwise terminated their relationship with the physician.

Charts for patients who are currently hospitalized may be kept in a special section for quick reference, then placed in the regular active file when the patient is discharged from the hospital.

In a surgical practice, there is frequently a specific date on which the patient is discharged from the doctor's care and the notation made on the chart, "Return prn." This record may be safely placed in the inactive file.

In a general practice office, the outside of the folder may be stamped with the date of the visit each time the patient is seen. It will then be a simple matter to determine when the chart should be transferred to the inactive status. In the parlance of filing, this is called the **perpetual transfer method.**

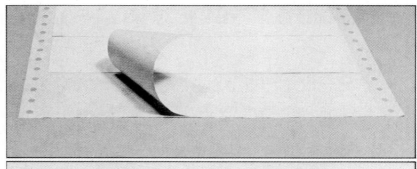

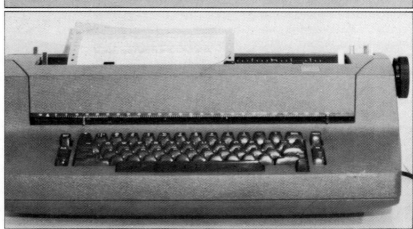

FIGURE 14–10. Adhesive transcription strips. Simply insert this continuous form of pressure-sensitive, adhesive-backed strips into the typewriter for easy dictation typing. Then peel off the strip and affix on Progress Notes or any other form. (Courtesy of Bibbero Systems, Inc., Petaluma, CA.)

14

RETAINING AND DESTROYING RECORDS

There is no standard rule to follow in establishing a records **retention schedule. Statutes of limitations** regarding professional liability litigation are a consideration in the retention of medical records. Tax regulations affect the retention of business records.

Case Histories

Space permitting, case histories are probably kept permanently or at least as long as the doctor is in practice. Then, if the patient is still living, the record may be made available to another doctor of the patient's own choosing. The record would not be given to the patient because of the possibility of misinterpretation.

Business Records

TAX RECORDS. Income tax returns are kept indefinitely; the last three returns are retained in a fireproof filing cabinet or safe; older returns are filed in dead storage.

INSURANCE POLICIES. Keep current policies in a fireproof cabinet or safe. When superseded by a new policy, throw away the old one *unless* a claim is pending. Professional liability policies are kept permanently.

CANCELED CHECKS. Keep in a fireproof file for 3 years, then indefinitely in dead storage.

RECEIPTS FOR BUSINESS EQUIPMENT. Keep until the item is fully depreciated.

GENERAL CORRESPONDENCE. Copies of correspondence should be reviewed periodically, as time permits, and any papers that are no longer of value destroyed. If the slightest doubt exists as to whether a paper should be destroyed, be sure to check with the doctor or retain the paper in the file.

MISCELLANEOUS. Many papers that are filed should instead be destroyed. Examples of these are letters of acknowledgement, announcements of meetings, duplicate copies, and letters of transmittal. Any document that is superseded by another in the file should be removed. For instance, when a new catalog is filed, destroy the old one; when a new fee schedule is received, destroy the old one. The Army has developed the technique of discarding papers to the highest level, and every document receives a date of destruction notation before it goes into the file.

PROTECTION OF RECORDS

Occasions may arise when records are temporarily out of the office. Some physicians release case histories to their colleagues, or an original record may be subpoenaed by the courts. In such instances an **OUTfolder** should be substituted in place of the regular folder and a notation made of the name, date, and to whom the record was released. Interim papers may be placed in the OUTfolder until the original is returned.

The sending out of original case histories should be avoided if possible. Instead, prepare a summary, or photocopy the materials needed for reference, and retain the original in the physician's office. Drawers and cabinets should be kept closed at all times when the office is unattended for further protection of the records.

STORAGE OF RECORDS

Large clinics and offices may find it advisable to **microfilm** records for storage. This permits storage of a considerable number of histories in a small space, saves time in searching, offers protection, and eliminates loss and misfiling. However, the cost is high, microfilm is hard to read for prolonged study, it is difficult to produce film in court, and if a patient returns, it is too small for refiling with the folders in the active file.

Some papers that should be kept but which need not be readily accessible may be placed in storage. Sturdy storage file boxes may be obtained from your stationery supply house. These boxes should be labeled to identify their contents in case it should be necessary to reclaim a file or refer to a record. The boxes are uniform in size and are available with a lift-off lid or in a drawer model. They can be kept in some out-of-the-way place or, if no room is available in the office, they can be placed with a storage company for a low monthly rental payment. If the latter is done, a record of the contents of each box should be kept in the office. When selecting a commercial records center, it is important to determine whether:

- It will retrieve items from a carton or only the entire carton
- The speed of retrieval is satisfactory
- It will deliver records (or must you pick them up?)
- It has an on-site work area available to the clients
- Fire protection and security is adequate
- The cost is reasonable

Thus far, the medical record itself has been emphasized. But this record must be filed so that it can be easily and quickly found when needed. This is sometimes the most neglected area of management practice. A **filing system** is only as good as the "findability" of everything in the files. A modern filing system should have three key components:

- A way to tell if the record is active or inactive from the outside of the jacket or folder, so that updating is continuous and easy
- Safeguards to prevent misfiling
- A filing technique that allows quick, accurate retrieval and refiling

FILING EQUIPMENT

The vertical four-drawer steel filing cabinet, used with manila folders with the patient's name on the **tab,** was the traditional system of choice for years. The most popular system today is color-coding on open shelves. There are also rotary, lateral, compactable, and automated files. Some records are kept in card or tray files.

Some of the considerations in selecting filing equipment are:

- Space availability
- Structural considerations
- Cost of space and equipment
- Size, type, and volume of records
- Confidentiality requirements
- Retrieval speed
- Fire protection

Regardless of the type or style of equipment, the best quality is always an economy.

Drawer files should be full-suspension; they should roll easily, close securely, and be equipped with a locking device. The best cabinets have a center trough at the bottom of each drawer with a rod for holding divider guides. Floor space of twice the depth of the drawer must be allowed so that the drawer can be pulled out to its full extent. A drawback of the vertical four-drawer files is that only one person can use a file cabinet at any given time. They are also slower because the drawer must be opened and closed each time a file is pulled or filed. They are relatively easy to move, but for safety reasons they should be bolted to the wall or to each other.

Shelf files should have doors to protect the contents. A popular type of shelf file has doors that slide back into the cabinet; the door from a lower shelf may be pulled out and used for work space. About 50% more material per square foot of floor space may be filed in shelf files as compared with the four-drawer file. Open shelf units hold files sideways and can go higher on the wall because there is no drawer to pull out. File retrieval is faster because several individuals can work simultaneously.

Open shelf units without doors are the most economical but offer little protection or confidentiality to the records. They are susceptible to water and fire damage. Shelf files are available in many attractive colors and can add a decorative note to the business office.

Special storage or shelf space should be provided for x-rays if many films are stored.

Rotary circular files can hold a large volume of records. They save space and clerical motion. The files revolve easily; some come with push-button controls. Several persons can work at one rotary file and use records at the same time. One disadvantage is that they afford less privacy and protection than files that can be closed and locked.

Lateral files are good for personal files and are especially attractive for the physician's private office. They use more wall space than the vertical file but do not extend out into the room so far. The folders are filed sideways in the lateral file, left to right, instead of front to back as in a vertical file. Some have a pull-out drawer, as the vertical file does; others have doors that slide into the cabinet, exposing the filing space.

The office with little space and a great volume of records might use *compactable files,* which are a variation of open shelf files. The files are mounted on tracks in the floor, and the units slide along the tracks so that access is gained to the needed records. They may be either automated or manual. One drawback is that not all records are available at the same time.

Automated files are very expensive initially and require more maintenance than do the other types of filing equipment. They will probably be found only in very large installations such as clinics or hospitals. These files bring the record to the operator instead of the operator going to the record. When the operator presses a button indicating the appropriate shelf, the shelf automatically moves into position in front of the operator for record retrieval. The automated or "power" file is fast and can store large amounts of records in a small amount of space. Only one person can use the unit at one time.

Almost every office has some occasion to use a *card file.* This may be for patient ledgers, a patient index, library index, index of surgical tray setups, telephone numbers, or numerous other records. A good-quality steel box or tray is a sound investment.

Special Items

Metal framework is available that can convert a regular drawer file into suspension-folder equipment. The assistant with a great deal of filing may wish to purchase a portable filing shelf that fits on the side of an opened drawer and can be moved from place to place as needed. A sorting file can be a great timesaver. A portable file cart for the temporary filing of unbilled insurance claims may be quite useful. Such a file cart may also be used for the preliminary sorting of charts to be refiled. This is sometimes called a "suspense file."

SUPPLIES

Divider guides. Each file drawer or shelf should be equipped with plenty of dividers or guides. Some authorities recommend one guide for approximately each inch and a half of material, or every 8 to 10 folders. Guides should be of good-quality pressboard. "Economy" guides will soon become bent and frayed and have to be replaced. Divider guides have a protruding tab, which may be either an integral part of the card or may be made of metal or plastic. The guides reduce the area of search and serve as supports for the folders. They are available in single, third, or fifth cut (one, three, or five different positions). The guide may have a projection at the bottom edge with a ring or hole through which a rod may go. This type of guide card is used in drawers that have a trough for the projection and a rod to hold the guides in place.

OUTguides. An OUTguide is a heavy guide that is used to replace a folder that has been temporarily removed. It should be of a distinctive color for quick detection. This makes refiling simpler and alerts the file clerk that a file is missing. Several colors may be used, each color designating the temporary location of the file. The OUTguide may have lines for recording information, or it may have a plastic pocket for inserting an information card.

Folders. Most records to be filed are placed in tabbed folders. The most commonly used is a general-purpose third-cut manila folder that may be expanded to ¾ inch. These are available with a double-thickness reinforced tab that will greatly lengthen the life of the folder. Folders kept in drawers have tabs at the top; those kept on shelves have tabs at the side.

There are many variations of folder styles obtainable for special purposes:

- *Classification folders* separate the papers in one file into six categories yet keep them all together.
- *OUTfolders* are used like the OUTguide and provide space for temporary filing of materials.
- The *vertical pocket,* which is heavier weight than the general purpose folder, has a front that folds down for easy access to contents and is available with up to 3½ inch expansion. These are used for bulky histories or correspondence.
- *Hanging or suspension folders* are made of heavy stock and hang on metal rods from side to side of a drawer. They can be used only with files equipped with suspension equipment.

- *Binder folders* have fasteners with which to bind papers within them. These offer some security for the papers but are time-consuming in filing the materials.

The number of papers that will fit in one folder depends on the thickness of the papers. Near the bottom edge of most folders are one or more score marks, which should be used as the contents of the folders expand. If folders are refolded at these score marks, the danger of their bending and sliding under other folders is reduced, and a neater file results. Papers should never protrude from the folder edges, and they should always be inserted with their tops to the left. When papers start to "ride up" in any folder, the folder is overloaded.

Labels. The label is a necessary "filing and finding" device. Use labels to identify each shelf, drawer, divider guide, and folder.

The label on the drawer or shelf identifies the nature of its contents. It should also indicate the range (alphabetic, numeric, or chronologic) of the material filed in that space. For example:

PATIENT HISTORIES (Active)
A – F

or

GENERAL CORRESPONDENCE
1994 – 1996

The label on the divider guide identifies the range of folder headings following that divider guide up to the next divider. For example:

Ba – Bo

The label on the folder identifies the content of that folder only. This may be the name of a patient, subject matter of correspondence, a business topic, or anything at all that needs to be filed. You will need to label a folder when a new patient is seen or existing folders are full, or when you need to transfer materials within the filing system.

Paper labels may be purchased in rolls of gummed tape or have adhesive backs that are peeled from a protective sheet. They are available in almost any size, shape, or color to meet the individual needs of any office. Visit your stationer and study the catalogs to find the best product for you.

A narrow label applied to the front of the folder tab is the easiest to use and is satisfactory for folders kept in a drawer file. Labels for shelf filing should be identifiable from both front and back. Always type the label before separating it from the roll or protective sheet. Type the **caption** on the label in indexing order (see Rules for Indexing, p. 223, and Table 14 – 2).

FILING PROCEDURES

Filing of all materials involves several steps. These steps are as follows:

Conditioning. Conditioning of papers involves removing all pins, brads, and paper clips; stapling related papers together; attaching clippings or items smaller than page size to a regular sheet of paper with rubber cement or tape; and mending damaged records.

TABLE 14–2. APPLICATION OF INDEXING RULES

Indexing Rule	Name	Unit 1	Unit 2	Unit 3
1	Robert F. Grinch	Grinch	Robert	F.
	R. Frank Grumman	Grumman	R.	Frank
2	J. Orville Smith	Smith	J.	Orville
	Jason O. Smith	Smith	Jason	O.
3	M. L. Saint-Vickery	Saintvickery	M.	L.
	Marie-Louise Taylor	Taylor	Marielouise	
4	Charles S. Anderson	Anderson	Charles	S.
	Anderson's Surgical Supply	Andersons	Surgical	Supply
5	Ah Hop Akee	Akee	Ah	Hop
6	Alice Delaney	Delaney	Alice	
	Chester K. DeLong	Delong	Chester	K.
7	Michael St. John	Saintjohn	Michael	
8	Helen M. Maag	Maag	Helen	M.
	Frederick Mabry	Mabry	Frederick	
	James E. MacDonald	Macdonald	James	E.
9	Mrs. John L. Doe (Mary Jones)	Doe	Mary	Jones (Mrs. John L.)
10	Prof. John J. Breck	Breck	John	J. (Prof.)
	Madame Sylvia	Madame	Sylvia	
	Sister Mary Catherine	Sister	Mary	Catherine
	Theodore Wilson, M.D.	Wilson	Theodore (M.D.)	
11	The Moore Clinic	Moore	Clinic (The)	
12	Lawrence W. Sloan, Sr.	Sloan	Lawrence	W. (1100 Main Street)
	Lawrence W. Sloan, Jr.	Sloan	Lawrence	W. (384 Turner Street)

Releasing. The term releasing simply means that some mark is placed on the paper indicating that it is now ready for filing. This will usually be either the medical assistant's initials or a FILE stamp placed in the upper left corner.

Indexing. Indexing means deciding where to file the letter or paper, and **coding** means placing some indication of this decision on the paper. This may be done by underlining the name or subject, if it appears on the paper, or writing in some conspicuous place the indexing subject or name. If there is more than one logical place to file the paper, the original is coded for the main location and a **cross-reference** sheet prepared, indicating this location and coded for the second location. Every paper placed in a patient's chart should have the name of the patient on it, usually in the upper right corner.

Sorting. Sorting is arranging the papers in filing sequence. Sort papers before going to the file cabinet or shelf. Do any necessary stapling of papers at your desk or filing table. Invest in a desk sorter with a series of dividers between which papers are placed in filing sequence. One general-purpose sorter has six means of classification: alphabetic sections, numbers 1 to 31, days of the week, months of the year, numbers in groups of five, and space on the tabs for special captions to be taped when desired. In the preliminary sorting, you place the papers in the appropriate division in the sorter. Then it is comparatively simple to arrange these groups into the proper sequence for filing.

Storing and Filing. In storing or filing papers in the folder, items should be placed face up, top edge to the left, with the most recent date to the front of the folder. Lift the folder an inch or two out of the drawer before inserting material, so that the sheets can drop down completely into the folder.

If you are refiling completed folders, arrange them in indexing order before going to the file cabinets.

Preventing Accidents

File drawers are heavy and can tip over, causing serious damage or injury unless reasonable care is observed. Open only one file drawer at a time and close it when the filing has been completed. A drawer left even slightly open can cause injury to a passerby.

Locating Misplaced Files

Unless files are promptly replaced after use, they may become lost. Papers may be misfiled, requiring a thorough search to find them. After you have made a methodical and complete search through the proper folder, there are several places you may look for a misplaced paper: in the folder in front of and behind the correct folder; between the folders; on the bottom of the file under all the folders; in a folder of a patient with a similar name; or in the sorter.

RULES FOR INDEXING

Indexing rules are fairly well standardized, based on current business practices. The Association of Records Managers and Administrators takes an active part in updating the rules. For the average physician's office, the following basic rules are all that is needed (see Table 14–2 for examples).

1. Last names of persons are considered first in filing; given name (first name), second; and middle name or initial, third. Compare the names from the first letter to the last. The first letter that is different in two names is the letter that determines the order of filing. Example:

   abE
   abI
   abX
   aCl
   acM
   aDa
   adE
   adI

2. Initials precede a name beginning with the same letter. This illustrates the librarian's rule, "Nothing comes before something." Example:

   Smith, J.
   Smith, Jason

3. Hyphenated names, whether first names, middle names, surnames of people, or business names, are considered to be one **unit.**

4. The apostrophe is disregarded in filing. Andersons' Surgical Supply is filed as Andersons Surgical Supply.

5. When you are indexing a foreign name and *cannot* distinguish the first and last name, you should index each part of the name in the order in which it is written:

   Cau Liu
   Talluri Devi

   If you *can* make the distinction, you should use the last name as the first indexing unit:

   Liu, Jason

6. Names with prefixes are filed in the usual alphabetic order. For example:

   DeLong is filed as Delong
   LaFrance is filed as Lafrance
   von Schmidt is filed as Vonschmidt

PROCEDURE 14-1   INITIATING A MEDICAL FILE FOR A NEW PATIENT

GOAL To initiate a medical file for a new patient that will contain all the personal data necessary for a complete record and any other information required by the agency.

EQUIPMENT AND SUPPLIES

Typewriter	ID card if using numeric system
Clerical supplies (pen, clipboard)	Cross-reference card
Information on agency's filing system	Financial card
Registration form	Routing slip
File folder	Private conference area
Label for folder	

PROCEDURAL STEPS

1. Determine that the patient is new to the agency.

2. Obtain and record the required personal data.
   Purpose: Complete information is necessary for credit and insurance claim processing.

3. Typewrite the information onto the patient history form.

4. Review the entire form.
   Purpose: To confirm that the information is complete and correct.

5. Select a label and folder for the record.
   Explanation: If color coding is used, a decision must be made regarding the appropriate color for the patient's name (see p. 226).

6. Type the caption on the label and apply to the folder.
   Explanation: Use patient's name for alphabetic filing or appropriate number for numeric filing.

7. For numeric filing system, prepare a cross-reference card and a patient ID card.
   Purpose: Numeric filing is an indirect system and requires a cross-reference to a patient's name for locating a chart. The patient will use the number of the ID card when arranging appointments or making inquiries.

8. Prepare the financial card, or place the patient's name in the computerized ledger.

9. Place the patient's history form and all other forms required by the agency into the prepared folder.

10. Clip a routing slip on the outside of the patient's folder.

---

7. Abbreviated names are indexed as if spelled in full. For example:

> St. John as Saintjohn
> Wm. as William
> Edw. as Edward
> Jas. as James

8. Mac and Mc are filed in their regular place in the alphabet:

> Maag
> Mabry
> MacDonald
> Machado
> MacHale
> Maville
> McAulay
> McWilliams
> Meacham

If your files contain a great many names beginning with Mac or Mc, you may, for convenience, wish to file them as a separate letter of the alphabet.

9. The name of a married woman is indexed by her legal name (her husband's surname, her given

name, and her middle name or maiden surname). For example:

Doe, Mary Jones (Mrs. John L.)
not
Doe, Mrs. John L.

10. Titles, when followed by a complete name, are disregarded in indexing:

Breckenridge, John J. (Prof.)

Titles without complete names are considered the first indexing unit:

Madame Sylvia
Sister Mary Catherine

Degrees are disregarded in filing but placed after the name, in parentheses:

Wilson, Theodore (MD)

11. Articles such as "The" or "A" are disregarded in indexing:

Moore Clinic (The)

12. Terms of seniority, such as Junior, Senior, or Second, are not considered in indexing. If two names are otherwise identical, the address is used to make the indexing decision (State, City, Street).

FILING SYSTEMS

There are four basic systems of filing:

- alphabetic by name
- numeric
- geographic
- subject

A fifth system, chronologic, is sometimes used. In the management of records in the physician's office, the medical assistant will probably be concerned with only three filing systems—alphabetic, numeric, and subject. Geographic filing is a specialized variation of alphabetic filing. The file is usually subdivided into a geographic hierarchy (country, state, county, city, and street), with each level alphabetized. Geographic filing is used in businesses that are interested in information by location rather than by name, such as sales organizations, mailing houses, or real estate firms. Chronologic filing refers to filing according to date and is used in a follow-up or tickler file, as described on page 228.

Alphabetic Filing

Alphabetic filing by name is the oldest, simplest, and most commonly used system. It is the system of choice for filing patient records in the majority of physicians' offices. If you can find a word in the dictionary or a name in the telephone directory, you already know some of the rules. Some people have difficulty remembering the sequence of letters in the alphabet. This can play havoc with alphabetic filing!

Alphabetic filing is traditional and simple to set up, requiring only a file cabinet or shelf, folders, and some divider guides. It is a **direct system** in that you need only know the name in order to find the desired file.

Alphabetic filing does have some drawbacks:

- You must know the correct spelling of the name
- As the number of files increases, more space is needed for each section of the alphabet. This requires periodic shifting of folders from drawer to drawer or shelf to shelf to allow for expansion.
- As the files expand, more time is required for filing or retrieving each folder because of the greater number of folders involved in the search. The time can be greatly reduced by color coding, which is discussed in detail later in this chapter.

Numeric Filing

Numeric filing is an indirect system, requiring the use of an alphabetic cross-reference in order to find a given file. Some people object to this added step and overlook the advantages. Management consultants differ in their recommendations; some recommend numeric filing only if there are more than 5,000 charts, more than 10,000 charts, or in some cases more than 15,000 charts. Others recommend nothing but numeric filing. This is an individual choice.

Some form of numeric filing combined with color and **shelf filing** is used by practically every clinic or hospital of any size. In numeric filing, each new patient is assigned a number, and an alphabetic cross-index card is prepared to identify the name. In a computerized office, the cross-index will probably be in the computer. It is possible to use the patient's ledger (financial) card as a cross-index by simply writing the patient's number at the top of the card. This does have one disadvantage in that ledger cards customarily are taken from the active file when the account is paid in full. The use of 3×5 cards attached to a Rolodex or Wheelodex system on the medical assistant's desk is usually more convenient and more efficient. Some clinics give each new patient an identification card bearing an assigned number, with instructions to give this number to the medical assistant each time the patient telephones or comes into the office.

Numeric filing allows unlimited expansion without periodic shifting of folders, and shelves are usually filled evenly. It provides additional confidentiality to the chart. The greatest advantage is the time saved in retrieving and refiling records quickly. One knows immediately that the number 978 falls between 977 and 979. By contrast, an alphabetic system, even with color coding, requires a longer search for the exact spot.

There are several types of numeric filing systems. In the *straight* or *consecutive* numeric system, patients are given consecutive numbers as they visit the practice. This is the simplest of the numeric systems and works well for files of up to 10,000 records. It is time consuming, and there is a greater chance for error when filing documents with five or more digits. Filing activity is greatest at the end of the numeric series.

In the *terminal digit system,* patients are also assigned consecutive numbers, but the digits in the number are usually separated into groups of twos or threes and are read in groups from right to left instead of from left to right. The records are filed "backward" in groups.

For example, all files ending in 00 are grouped together first, then those ending in 01, etc. Next the files are grouped by their middle digits so that the 00 22s come before the 01 22s. Finally the files are arranged by their first digits, so that 01 00 22 precedes 02 00 22. Example:

01 99 00
00 73 01
05 55 11
01 68 21
01 68 22
88 34 23
90 34 23

Middle digit filing begins with the middle digits, followed by the first digit and finally by the terminal digits.

Some practices use the last four digits of each patient's Social Security number to file patient records.

Numeric filing requires more training, but once the system is mastered, fewer errors occur than with alphabetic filing.

Subject Filing

Subject filing can be either alphabetic or **alphanumeric** (A 1-3, B 1-1, B 1-2, etc.) and is used for general correspondence. The main difficulty with subject filing is indexing, or classification—deciding where to file a document. Many papers require cross-referencing. All correspondence dealing with a particular subject is filed together. The papers within the folders are filed chronologically, the most recent on top. The subject headings are placed on the tabs of the folders and filed alphabetically.

Color Coding

When a color coding system is used, both filing and finding are easier, and misfiled folders are kept to a minimum. The use of color visually restricts the area of search for a specific record. A misfiled chart is easily spotted even from a distance of several feet. In color coding, a specific color is selected to identify each letter of the alphabet. The application of the principle may be through using colored folders, adhesive colored identification labels, or various combinations of these (Fig. 14–11). Any selection of colors may be used, and the division of the alphabet is determined by one's own needs. However, studies have shown that there is wide variation in the frequency with which different letters occur. The following division is one that has been used successfully; experience has proved that this breakdown results in almost equal representation of the five colors:

COLOR OF LABEL	LETTERS OF ALPHABET
Red	A B C D
Yellow	E F G H
Green	I J K L M N
Blue	O P Q
Purple	R S T U V W X Y Z

Alphabetic Color Coding

There are several ways of color coding files. One alphabetic system utilizes five different colored folders, with each color representing a segment of the alphabet. The *second* letter of the patient's last name determines the color, as in the following system:

Red Folder (second letters a, b, c, d)	Canfield
	Eberhart
	Ackerman
	Adams
Yellow Folder (second letters e, f, g, h)	Venable
	Effron
	Igawa
	Thill
Green Folder (second letters i, j, k, l, m, n)	Histed
	Bjork
	Akron
	Ullman
	Imhoff
	Anderson
Blue Folder (second letters o, p, q)	Gordon
	Epperley
	Aquino
	Greiner
Purple Folder (second letters r, s, t, u, v, w, x, y, z)	Osterberg
	Atherton
	Auer
	Uvena
	Owsley
	Oxford
	Nye
	Azzaro

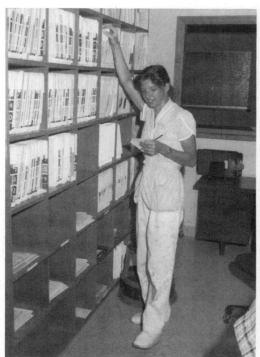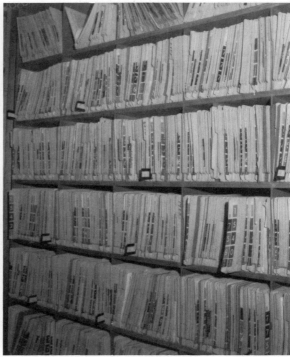

FIGURE 14–11. Color-coded numeric filing system. (Courtesy of Vista Medical Group, El Toro, CA. Photos by Dan Santucci.)

14

There are a number of ready-made systems available (e.g., Acme, Ames, Bibbero, Colwell, Remington Rand, TAB, VisiRecord). Self-adhesive colored letter blocks with either two or three letters in the specific colors are supplied in rolls. The color blocks with the appropriate letter are placed on the index tab of the folder, along with the patient's full name. The letters are in pairs so they can be seen from either side of the chart. Strong, easily differentiated colors are used, creating a band of color in the files that makes it easy to spot out-of-place folders.

Numeric Color Coding

Color coding is also used in numeric filing. Numbers 0 through 9 are each assigned a different color. In a terminal digit filing system, the colors for the last two numbers would be affixed to the tab. If the number 1 is red and 5 is yellow, all files with numbers ending in 15 form a red and yellow band. Usually a predetermined section of the number is color coded.

Other Color Coding Methods

There are many other ways to make color work for you. Small pressure-sensitive tabs in a variety of colors may be used to identify certain types of insured patients. For example, a patient on Medicaid may have a red tab over the edge of the folder; a Champus patient may be identified by a blue tab; a worker's compensation patient by a green tab, and

so forth. Matching tabs may be attached to the ledger cards. Research cases may be identified by a special color tab. In a partnership practice, it may be desirable to use a different color folder or label for each doctor's patients. Self-adhesive tabs are easily removed, less bulky than metal or plastic tabs, and not so likely to be inadvertently pulled from the record.

Color can be used to differentiate dates—one color for each month or year. Brightly colored labels on the outside of a patient chart can indicate certain health conditions, such as drug allergies.

The business records may also utilize color coding. Main divider guide headings may be of one color, subheadings in a second color, and subdivisions in a third color. (See Table 14–3 for an example of this type of arrangement.) A fourth color might be used for personal items. The use of color in the file is limited only by the imagination. One word of caution, though. Every person in the office who uses the files should know the key to the cod-

TABLE 14–3. COLOR CODING FOR BUSINESS RECORDS

Main Heading:	DISBURSEMENTS	Red label
Subheading:	Equipment	Blue label
Subdivisions:	Typewriter	Yellow label
	Copier	Yellow label
	Calculator	Yellow label

PROCEDURE 14-2   COLOR CODING PATIENT CHARTS

GOAL   To color code patient charts using the agency's established coding system to effectively facilitate filing and finding.

EQUIPMENT AND SUPPLIES

20 patient charts
Information on agency's coding system

20 file folders
Full range of color labels

PROCEDURAL STEPS

1. Assemble patient charts.

2. Arrange charts in indexing order.
   Purpose: When charts have been color coded, they will be in filing order.

3. Pick up the first chart and note the second letter of the patient's surname.
   Explanation: For purpose of this activity, the color coding system in the text will be used.

4. Choose a folder and/or caption label of the appropriate color.

5. Type patient's name on label in indexing order and apply to folder tab.
   Purpose: To identify sequence of folder in filing system.

6. Repeat steps 4 and 5 until all charts have been coded.

7. Check entire group for any isolated color.
   Purpose: If the order and color of the folders is correct, all charts of the same color within each letter of the alphabet will be grouped together.

---

ing, and the key should also be written in the agency's procedures manual.

ORGANIZATION OF FILES

Patient Records

It is very difficult for a physician to study a disorganized history. Some systematic method must be followed in placing the material in the patient folder. The content of the patient record has already been discussed. From the filing standpoint, it should be emphasized that when a patient record is not in actual use, there is only one place it should be — in the filing cabinet or shelf. Many precious hours can be lost in searching for misplaced or lost records that were carelessly left unfiled. The patient's full name, in indexing order, should be typed on a label and attached to the folder tab. The patient's full name should also be typed on each sheet within the folder. A strip of transparent tape can be placed on the label to prevent smudging if this is a problem.

Medical Correspondence

Correspondence pertaining to patients' medical records should be filed with the case history. Other medical correspondence should probably be filed in a subject file.

General Correspondence

The physician's office must be operated as a business as well as a professional service. There will be correspondence of a general nature pertaining to the operation of the office. In all likelihood, a special drawer or shelf is set aside for the general correspondence. The correspondence is indexed according to subject matter or names of correspondents. The guides in a subject file may appear in one, two, or three positions, depending on the number of headings, subheadings, and subdivisions. Examples are shown in Table 14–3.

Miscellaneous Folder

Papers that do not warrant an individual folder are placed in a miscellaneous folder. Within the folder, all papers relating to one subject, or with one correspondent, are kept together in chronologic order, the most recent on top, and then filed alphabetically with other miscellaneous material. Related materials may be stapled together. Never use paper clips for this purpose. When as many as five papers accumulate with one correspondent or subject, a separate folder should be prepared.

Business and Financial Records

The most active financial record is, of course, the ledger. In most offices, this will be a card or vertical tray file, and the accounts will be arranged alphabetically by name. There will be at least two divisions:

- active accounts
- paid accounts.

Special categories may be set up, for example:

- government-sponsored insurance

PROCEDURE 14-3 FILING SUPPLEMENTAL MATERIAL IN ESTABLISHED PATIENT HISTORIES

GOAL To add supplemental documents and progress notes to patient histories, observing standard steps in filing, while creating an orderly file that will facilitate ready reference to any item of information.

EQUIPMENT AND SUPPLIES

Assorted correspondence, diagnostic reports, and progress notes
Patient histories
Typewriter
Stapler

Mending tape
FILE stamp, or pen
Sorter

14

PROCEDURAL STEPS

1. Group all papers according to patients' names.
    Purpose: Some related papers may require stapling.

2. Remove any pins or paper clips.
    Purpose: Pins in file folders are hazardous; paper clips are bulky and may become inadvertently attached to other materials.

3. Mend any damaged or torn records.

4. Attach any small items to standard-size paper.
    Purpose: Small items are easily lost or misplaced in files.

5. Staple any related papers together.

6. Place your initials or FILE stamp in the upper left corner.
    Purpose: To indicate that the document is released for filing.

7. Code the document by underlining or writing the patient's name in the upper right corner.
    Purpose: To indicate where the document is to be filed.

8. Continue steps 2 through 7 until all documents have been conditioned, released, indexed, and coded.

9. Place all documents in the sorter in filing sequence.
    Explanation: Sorter can be taken to file cabinet or shelf for placing documents in patient folders.

- worker's compensation
- delinquent accounts
- collection accounts

Other business files include records of income and expense, financial statements, income and payroll tax records, canceled checks, and insurance policies. These papers may be filed chronologically.

Tickler or Follow-up File

The most frequently used follow-up method is that of a **tickler** file, so called because it "tickles" the memory that something needs to be done or followed up on a particular date. The tickler file is always a chronologic arrangement. In its simplest form, it consists of notations on the daily calendar. If information concerning a patient who has an appointment to come in is expected, such as an x-ray report or laboratory report, the medical assistant might make a note on the calendar or tickler file a day ahead to check on whether the report has arrived.

The tickler file is often a card file with 12 guides for the names of the months, and 31 guides printed with numbers 1 through 31 for the days of the month. The guide for the current month, followed by the 31 day guides, is placed at the front of the file. Notations of actions to be taken are placed behind the guides for specific days of the current month. Notations for future months are placed behind the guide for that month. In order to be effective, the tickler file must be checked the first thing each day. It is a useful reminder for recurring events, such as payments, meetings, and so forth. On the last day in each month, all the notations from behind the next month's guide are distributed behind the daily numbered guides, and the guide for the month just completed is placed at the back of the file.

Transitory or Temporary File

Many papers are kept longer than necessary because no provision is made for segregating those that have a limited usefulness. This situation is avoided by having a *transitory* or *temporary file*. For instance, if the medical assistant writes a letter requesting a reprint, the file copy is placed in the transitory folder. When the reprint is received, the file copy is destroyed. The transitory file is used for materials having no permanent value. The paper may be marked with a "T" and destroyed when the action involved is completed.

▶ LEARNING ACHIEVEMENTS

Are you able to:

1. Define the terms listed in the Vocabulary of this chapter?
2. State three important reasons for keeping good medical records?
3. Illustrate the meaning of *subjective* and *objective information,* and list four possible items in each category?
4. Create a patient history using 15 items of necessary personal data?
5. Explain the basic differences between the traditional and the *problem-oriented medical record (POMR)*?
6. State three advantages of the *POMR*?
7. Change an entry in a medical record?
8. Describe the three classifications of patient files?
9. Identify the basic equipment and supplies needed to set up a filing system?
10. Use the seven sequential steps to file a document?
11. Discuss applications of the four basic filing systems?
12. List three advantages of color coding files?
13. Correctly add reports and correspondence into a patient's file?
14. Arrange a group of patient numbers in filing sequence for a *terminal digit filing system*?
15. Type a list of names in indexing order and arrange them alphabetically for filing?

REFERENCES AND READINGS

Battista, M. E.: "Malpractice Risks of Documentation," Physicians' Management, February 1985, pp 232–258.

Chabner, D.-E.: *The Language of Medicine,* 4th ed., Philadelphia, W. B. Saunders Co., 1991.

Diamond, S. Z.: *Records Management: Policies, Practices, Technologies,* 2nd ed., New York, Anacom Book Division, American Management Association, 1991.

Jennings, L. M.: *Secretarial and Administrative Procedures,* 3rd ed., Englewood Cliffs, NJ, Prentice-Hall, 1989.

Johnson, M. M., and Kallaus, N. F.: *Records Management,* 4th ed., Cincinnati, South-Western Publishing Co., 1986.

Kinn, M. E.: *Medical Terminology Review Challenge,* Albany, NY, Delmar, 1987.

Krevolin, N.: *Filing and Records Management,* Englewood Cliffs, NJ, Prentice-Hall, 1986.

Sabin, W. A.: *The Gregg Reference Manual,* 6th ed., Westerville, OH, Glencoe Division Macmillan/McGraw-Hill, 1991.

Tilton, R. S., et al.: *Secretarial Procedures and Administration,* 9th ed., Cincinnati, South-Western Publishing Co., 1987.

CHAPTER FIFTEEN

—

PROFESSIONAL FEES AND CREDIT ARRANGEMENTS

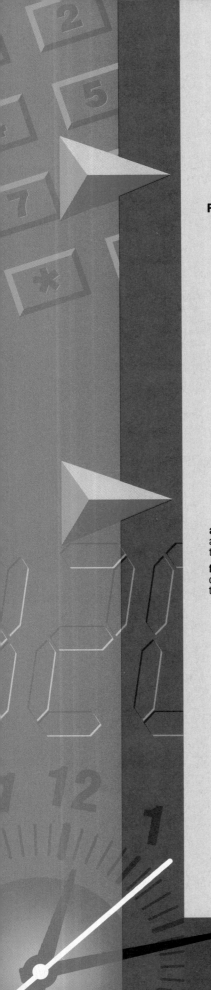

CHAPTER OUTLINE

VOCABULARY

assignment of benefits A statement authorizing the insurance company to pay benefits directly to physician.

fee profile A compilation of a physician's fees over a given period of time.

fiscal agent A financial representative.

medical indigent One who is able to take care of ordinary living expenses but who cannot afford medical care.

professional courtesy Reduction or absence of fee to professional associates.

third-party payor Someone other than the patient, spouse, or parent who is responsible for paying all or part of the patient's medical costs.

usual, customary, and reasonable (UCR) A formula for determining medical insurance benefits payable.

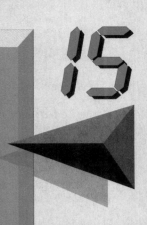

PROFESSIONAL FEES AND CREDIT ARRANGEMENTS

LEARNING OBJECTIVES

COGNITIVE

Upon successful completion of this chapter you should be able to:

1. Define the terms listed in the Vocabulary.

2. Name three values that are considered in determining professional fees.

3. Give an example of a usual and customary fee.

4. Explain how a physician's fee profile is determined.

5. List three reasons for giving patients an estimate slip.

6. Discuss the concept of professional courtesy in medical fees.

7. List four kinds of charges that should be avoided.

8. Explain what is meant by third-party liability.

9. Identify the three items of information that can be released in response to a request for credit information.

10. State three items that should be excluded in replying to a request for credit information.

PERFORMANCE

Upon successful completion of this chapter you should be able to perform the following activities:

1. Make financial arrangements with a patient requesting credit.

2. Prepare a Truth in Lending form.

3. Respond to patient's request for explanation of the physician's fee.

PROFESSIONAL FEES

While service to the patient is the primary concern of the medical profession, a physician must charge and collect a fee for such services in order to continue providing medical care. The practice of medicine is a business as well as a profession, and the details of conducting the business aspects are often the responsibility of the medical assistant. The physician determines what the fees are. The medical assistant usually bears the responsibility of informing the patient on financial matters, collecting the payment, and in some cases making arrangements for deferred payment.

How Fees Are Determined

Setting fees is no simple matter. The physician has three commodities to sell—time, judgment, and services. Yet the value of these commodities is never exactly the same to two different individuals. Medical care has little value except to the patient, and the value to the patient may not be consistent with the ability to pay. In every case, the physician must place an estimate upon the value of the services. This value may then be modified by other considerations.

Prevailing Rate in the Community

One of the bases for determining medical fees is the economic level of the community. Different communities reflect different living scales, and this situation is reflected in medical fees as well. Consequently, the prevailing rate in the community—the average composite fee—must be taken into consideration by each individual physician. Strangely enough, fees that are too low drive patients away just as quickly as do fees that are too high.

Usual and Customary Fee

Most insurance plans base their payments on what has become known as a usual and customary fee for a given procedure. Some include the word reasonable; that is, **usual, customary,** and **reasonable:**

Usual—The physician's *usual* fee for a given service is the fee that that individual physician most frequently charges for the service.

Customary—The *customary* fee is a range of the usual fees charged for that same service by physicians with similar training and experience practicing in the same geographic and socioeconomic area. There is now a growing tendency for fees to be determined by national trends rather than by local customs.

Reasonable—The term *reasonable* usually applies to a service or procedure that is exceptionally difficult or complicated, requiring extraordinary time or effort on the part of the physician.

It should be noted that under Medicare Part B, "customary" and "prevailing" correspond to "usual" and "customary" as defined here.

To illustrate, let us suppose that Dr. Wallace usually charges private patients $100 for a first office visit. The usual fees charged for a first visit by other doctors in the same community with similar training and experience range from $75 to $125. Dr. Wallace's fee of $100 is within the customary range and would therefore be paid by an insurance plan that pays on a usual and customary basis. If, on the other hand, the range of usual fees in the community is from $60 to $85, the insurance plan would allow only the maximum within the range, or $85, to Dr. Wallace.

Fee Setting by Third-Party Payors

The physician does not act alone in determining fees. Many **third-party payors** provide the physician with a predetermined fee schedule that they will approve for payment. Some require preapproval of the fee before service is rendered. A third-party payor may require precertification before it will pay for a specific service. Government programs such as Medicare and Medicaid (see Chapter 19) have strict guidelines regarding reimbursement for fees and the raising of fees.

Doctor's Fee Profile

The **fiscal agents** for government-sponsored insurance programs as well as some private plans keep a continuous record of the usual charges submitted for specific services by each individual doctor. By compiling and averaging these fees over a given period, usually a year, the doctor's **fee profile** is established. This fee profile is then used in determining the amount of third-party liability for services under the program. One of the objections voiced by doctors is the lag between the time of a private fee increase and the time it is reflected in payments by an insurance carrier. It may be as long as 2 to 3 years.

Insurance Allowance

In some individual cases, the physician may not wish to charge the patient in addition to what will be allowed by the patient's insurance. The full fee should be quoted to the patient and charged to the account, with the understanding that after the insurance allowance has been received, the balance will be discounted. If a smaller fee is quoted and charged, several problems may arise:

- The lower fee will alter the doctor's fee profile.
- If it should become necessary to bring suit for payment of the fee, only the reduced fee can be recovered.
- If the insurance allowance is paid on the basis of a certain percentage of the doctor's fee and a lower fee is charged, the insurance allowance will be correspondingly lower. Also, if the physician does this with many patients, the insurance company may take the position that the reduced fee is the doctor's usual fee and base its payments accordingly. It may even be considered fraudulent in some instances.

Advance Discussion of Fees

It is natural for the patient, particularly one new to the practice, to wonder, "How much is this going to cost?" However, some patients may be reluctant to voice this concern.

Responsibility to Discuss Fees

It is the responsibility of the doctor or the medical assistant to raise the discussion of fees if the patient does not do so. Be prepared to discuss fees with any patient who's interested, but don't assume you must do so with everyone. You might open the discussion of fees with something like this: "Mr. Willardson, do you have any questions about the costs of your operation? If you do, I'll be glad to review them." On the other hand, in this preliminary discussion of fees, the doctor must not sidestep the issue by saying "Don't worry about the bill, let's just get you well first." Avoid attempting to calm a worried patient about to undergo surgery by saying, "There's really nothing to it." The patient may later complain loudly about the bill because he misunderstood the complexity of the service.

Even in those cases where the doctor quotes a fee, the medical assistant often has the responsibility of explaining the doctor's fees to the patient. The medical assistant must know how fees are determined and why charges vary, as well as have a thorough knowledge of the physician's practice and policies in order to handle perplexing situations involving fees.

As your understanding of the practice increases, you can be something of a "salesperson" for the doctor's services by educating patients that money spent for medical care is an excellent investment in the future. It is a rare patient who understands the intricate procedures involved in diagnosis and treatment. Other points to emphasize are:

- The long years of training and study and the heavy expenses involved in securing a medical education
- That running a modern professional office is a costly process relying upon day-to-day income in return for services

Advance fee discussions help the patient to plan ahead for medical expenditures. Most patients want to pay their financial obligations but rightly insist upon an accurate estimate of those obligations before they contract for purchase of goods or services. When a doctor frankly discusses fees in advance with patients, even to the point of describing how a fee is established, misconceptions about overcharging and fee frictions are usually eliminated. One doctor wrote the American Medical Association that, with 95% of his patients, 3 minutes at the end of the visit spent in explaining the medical bill ensures financial success.

Because many physicians and patients are reluctant to broach the subject of fees, the American Medical Association sells, for a very modest price, an attractive wall plaque that encourages fee discussions, with this message:

> TO ALL MY PATIENTS—I INVITE YOU TO DISCUSS FRANKLY WITH ME ANY QUESTIONS REGARDING MY SERVICES OR MY FEES. THE BEST MEDICAL SERVICE IS BASED ON A FRIENDLY, MUTUAL UNDERSTANDING BETWEEN DOCTOR AND PATIENT.

This plaque should be placed in the physician's office, not in the reception room.

Explaining Additional Costs

Explanations of medical costs should extend beyond the doctor's own charges. For example, if a patient is to undergo surgery, the doctor should also explain the costs of the operation, the anesthetist's and radiologist's charges, the laboratory fees, and the approximate hospital bill. The importance of calling in another physician for consultation should be explained to patients when consultation becomes necessary. It should be made clear, in advance, that there will be a separate bill submitted by the consulting physician. Patients do not always understand that the consultation is for the benefit of the patient, not the physician.

Estimate Slips

Some physicians give patients an estimate of medical expenses before hospitalization (Fig. 15–1). A few medical societies cooperatively develop such estimate sheets with local hospitals. The American Medical Association includes an example of an estimate sheet in its publication, *The Business Side of Medical Practice.* Individual doctors occasionally

15

SURGICAL COST ESTIMATE

Name of Patient: _____ Date: _____

Procedure: _____

Your surgery has been scheduled at _____ Hospital on _____.

You should report to the Admitting Office between the hours of _____ (AM) (PM) and _____ (AM) (PM).

Although medical and hospital expenses are seldom welcomed, knowing in advance what expenses to expect and how to plan for them can lessen the burden. This estimate is prepared to assist you in budgeting your surgical costs.

PROFESSIONAL FEES

When you have major surgery, the surgical team includes the operating surgeon, the assistant surgeon, and the anesthetist. Each has an important part in your care, and each will render a separate statement for services. While each doctor will independently set his/her own fee, it is usually possible to estimate in advance an approximate range of fees. Assuming an uncomplicated course for your surgery, the charges are estimated as follows:

Operating Surgeon $ _____ to $ _____

Assistant Surgeon   _____ to   _____

Anesthetist   _____ to   _____

The assistant surgeon and the anesthetist usually base their fees on the operating time; consequently, if a surgical procedure turns out to be more complicated than was expected, their fees may be correspondingly increased.

The estimated duration of your hospital stay is _____ days at $ _____ per day for a (semi-private) (private) room. During your hospital stay there will be charges for laboratory tests, medications as required, and other services. It is impossible to estimate in advance what these charges will be; they will be itemized on your hospital bill. If you have health insurance, please take the appropriate forms and I.D. information with you on the day of your admittance.

PLEASE KEEP IN MIND THIS IS ONLY AN ESTIMATE

FIGURE 15–1. Form for surgical cost estimate.

---

work up their own estimate forms when a patient is embarking on long-term treatment. The doctor should, however, emphasize that it is an estimate only and that the actual cost may vary somewhat.

Estimate slips should be prepared in duplicate so that the patient may have a copy; the original is to be retained in the patient's file. Duplicate estimate slips may help to:

- Avoid your forgetting that a fee was quoted
- Eliminate the possibility of later misquoting the fee
- Simplify collection by preventing misunderstanding and confusion over charges.

Adjusting or Canceling Fees

Care for Those Who Cannot Pay

The medical profession has traditionally accepted the responsibility of providing medical care for indi-

viduals unable to pay for these services. In spite of the increased scope of government-sponsored care for the **medically indigent,** doctors still donate thousands of dollars' worth of such medical services each year.

In many instances, medical care of the indigent is available through social service agencies. The medical assistant should learn about any local organizations and agencies that can aid the patient in obtaining the necessary assistance. The doctor can provide only medical services. Other agencies must provide hospitalization, for example, or arrange for paying the costs of special therapy, rehabilitation, or medications. Unfortunately, there is still another segment of the population that consists of uninsured employees who are not eligible for public assistance, are not covered under a group policy, and cannot afford the high premiums for private medical insurance. Special attention must be given to helping these persons arrange to pay their medical bills.

PROCEDURE 15-1   EXPLAINING DOCTOR'S FEES

GOAL To explain the doctor's fees so that the patient understands his or her obligations and rights for privacy.

EQUIPMENT AND SUPPLIES

Patient's statement
Copy of physician's fee schedule

Quiet private area where the patient feels free to ask questions

PROCEDURAL STEPS

1. Determine that the patient has the correct bill.
   Purpose: To make certain it is this patient's bill and that the insurance numbers, the address, and the phone number are correct.

2. Examine the bill for possible errors.
   Purpose: To demonstrate that the patient's concerns are important and that you are willing to make any necessary adjustments.

3. Refer to the fee schedule for the services rendered.
   Purpose: To explain how physicians determine their fees. If an error has occurred, correct it immediately with a sincere apology.

4. Explain itemized billing:
   - Date of each service
   - Type of service rendered
   - Fee
   Purpose: To make certain that the patient realizes the number and extent of services rendered.

5. Display professional attitude toward the patient.
   Purpose: To reassure the patient that you have a thorough understanding of the fee schedule and show willingness to answer questions politely and completely.

6. Determine whether the patient has specific concerns that may hinder payment.
   Purpose: To provide an opportunity for making special arrangements if needed.

7. Make appropriate arrangements for a discussion between the physician and patient if further explanation is necessary for resolution of the problem.

If a doctor accepts a case for which a fee will not be paid, complete records must still be kept on the patient. The only deviation in procedure is that the financial record indicates no charge (n/c) in the debit column.

Fees in Hardship Cases

Sometimes a doctor is faced with the problem of deciding whether to reduce or cancel a fee in a hardship case. Before adjusting or canceling a fee,

the doctor or the medical assistant should encourage a frank discussion of the patient's financial situation. Find out whether the patient is entitled to an insurance settlement of some kind. Circumstances may qualify the patient for local or state public assistance programs. If so, the assistant may direct the patient to the appropriate agency.

If the circumstances of hardship are known before the services are rendered, thorough discussion of what the fee will be and how it will be paid should take place at that time. In most cases, it is far better to adjust a fee before rather than after treatment. The doctor may suggest that a medically indigent patient seek care at a county hospital with public assistance. A doctor should be free to choose his or her form of charity and not feel obligated to substantially reduce or cancel a fee when the circumstances are known in advance.

After the doctor and patient have agreed upon a fee, special circumstances may arise that create a hardship. If the doctor then agrees to reduce the fee, the patient should be told that the reduction will be effective only after the adjusted amount is paid in full. For instance, if a fee of $300 is reduced to $200, the full amount of the $300 charge should appear on the ledger and when $200 has been received, the remainder can be written off as an adjustment.

Pitfalls of Fee Adjustments

Great care should be taken in reducing the fee for care of a patient who dies. The doctor's sympathy is with the family in such instances, but the doctor's generosity in reducing a fee could be misinterpreted and result in a suit for malpractice.

If the doctor agrees to settle for a reduced fee in a situation in which the patient is disputing the fee, care should be taken to make certain the negotiations are "without prejudice." By taking this precaution, the doctor protects the right to collect the original sum should the patient refuse to pay the lowered fee. The offer of a discount, therefore, should be made in writing, with the insertion of the words "without prejudice," and a definite time limit for making payment stated. Make two copies of the agreement and have the signatures witnessed. Keep the original for the doctor and give a copy to the patient.

A fee should never be reduced on the basis of a poor result or as a means of obtaining payment to avoid the use of a collection agency. A reduction for these reasons degrades the doctor and the practice of medicine.

Professional Courtesy

Traditionally, doctors do not charge other doctors or their immediate dependents for medical care. Although the concept of **professional courtesy** is often attributed to Hippocrates, the foundations of professional courtesy today are actually derived from Thomas Percival's Code of 1803.

In some cases, the giving of professional courtesy represents the loss of a large amount of potential income. If there is a substantial outlay in the cost of materials, the professional colleague will probably wish to reimburse the physician for the materials used. Most doctors today subscribe to a health insurance plan. If the care they receive is covered by insurance, it is entirely ethical for the attending physician to accept the insurance benefits in payment for services.

If the services are frequent enough to involve a significant proportion of the doctor's professional time, or extend over a long period of time, the doctor may wish to charge on an adjusted basis.

If professional courtesy is offered, but the recipient insists upon paying, the physician need not hesitate on ethical grounds to accept a fee for services.

Professional courtesy is often extended beyond fellow physicians and their dependents. Most physicians treat their own medical assistants without charge and grant discounts to nurses and medical assistants not in their direct employ. Professional courtesy is sometimes extended to others in the health care field, for instance, pharmacists and dentists. There is a growing sentiment that professional courtesy has outlived its usefulness and should be abandoned.

Charges to Avoid

- Telephone calls
- Late payments
- Missed appointments
- First insurance forms

Telephone Calls

It is generally considered inadvisable to charge for telephone calls. Some physicians, especially pediatricians, find they must give considerable advice over the telephone. Many of these calls, however, are fairly routine to the office (although not to the worried mother or patient), and an able medical assistant can be trained to answer many of the questions, or a special time can be set aside for telephone calls.

Late Charges

Levying late charges on fees for professional services not paid within a prescribed time is usually not in the best interest of the public or the profession. However, the physician who has experienced problems with delinquent accounts may properly choose to request that payment be made at the time of treatment or add interest or other reasonable charges to delinquent accounts. The physician must comply with state and federal regulations applicable to the imposition of such charges (see Truth in Lending Act, p. 241).

Missed Appointments

Most physicians feel that charging for a missed appointment or for one not canceled 24 hours in advance, although not unethical if the patient is fully advised, is nevertheless not in the best interest of their patients or their practices.

First Insurance Forms

If the patient has multiple insurance forms to be completed, the physician is justified in making a charge but should be willing to complete the first standard form without charge.

CREDIT ARRANGEMENTS

Extending Credit

Whenever a service is rendered before payment is received, an extension of credit has been made. If payment is collected upon completion of the service, no problem exists. But if payment is deferred, credit arrangements are best made during the patient's initial visit. Successful collection of an account may depend upon the skill and tact with which the medical assistant conducts the first interview.

Federal law (Equal Credit Opportunity Act of 1977) bars discrimination in all areas of credit, with the purpose of ensuring that credit is made available fairly and impartially, and specifies "prohibited bases" under the law. The law prohibits discrimination against any applicant for credit

- because of race, color, religion, national origin, sex, marital status, or age
- because the applicant receives income from any public assistance program
- because he has exercised rights under consumer credit laws

Many medical assistants inform a patient telephoning for a first appointment that new patients are expected to pay cash for their first visit, at which time credit arrangements can be established if further care is needed. You can say, for example:

> "Mr. Barrington, your appointment is scheduled for 9:30 AM, Tuesday, September 25, with Dr. Newhouse. The usual charge for a first office visit is about XX dollars, and we ask that payment for a first visit be made at the time of service. If you wish to establish credit arrangements in case further care is needed, please plan to be here 15 minutes early so that the necessary papers can be completed."

This approach informs the patient in advance that he or she will be expected to complete a credit application.

Information from the Patient

Good records are essential to follow-up of collections. It is extremely important that the medical assistant get adequate information about the patient's ability to pay—on the first office visit, if possible. It is neither unprofessional nor time consuming to get full credit information from patients. The public is conditioned to supplying such information and respects a businesslike approach if it is done tactfully and without apology. Although a patient needing medical care is rarely turned away because of a credit risk, the information provided on the initial visit may alert the medical assistant to be cautious about allowing an account to fall in arrears.

Although the registration form the patient completes in the doctor's office is usually not as detailed as an application for credit in, for example, a department store, it must establish an information base, should future collection steps become necessary.

The medical assistant should check the completed form carefully, to make certain that nothing was overlooked. The new patient will view these questions as reasonable, but the established patient may resent such an inquiry. Consequently, it is important that the form be completed on the first visit.

Many printed forms are available on the market, but some physicians design their own to include specific information desired in their practices. Whatever form is used, it should include certain basic information and *not* ask for information that is disallowed under the 1975 Federal Equal Credit Opportunity Act. For instance, under the ECOA "marital status" can be requested only as *married, unmarried,* or *separated.* Terms such as *divorced, single,* or *widow/er* are illegal. *Age* is also forbidden, but *date of birth* is acceptable.

Patient's full name. The patient's first, middle, and last names, correctly spelled, should be at the top of the form.

Patient's birth date. With this information, the patient's age can be computed at any time.

Responsible person's full name. Relationship to the patient, his or her address, telephone number, social security number, and driver's license number should be included.

Responsible person's employer. Name, address, and telephone number of the employer and the responsible person's occupation or department.

Spouse of responsible person. Same information as for responsible person. (Community property laws in some states make each and both responsible.)

Nearest relative. Name, relationship to patient, address, and telephone number.

Referral. Name of physician or other person who referred the patient (see Fig. 9–3).

An individualized form can ask for further specific information appropriate for a particular practice. When a patient applies for credit:

- You *may not* ask the applicant's sex, race, color, religion, or national origin.
- You *may not* ask about birth control practices or plans to have children.

- You *may* collect this information when it is part of a medical history, but *not* when it is related to granting credit.

Under the Equal Credit Opportunity Act, once you agree to extend credit to one patient, you must offer the same arrangement to any other patient who requests it. You can refuse to do so only on the basis of ability or inability to pay. It is interesting that one way to avoid involvement with the credit laws is to accept bank credit cards.

Third-Party Liability

If financial responsibility is attributed to an individual other than the patient, spouse, or parent, be sure to obtain full name, address, employment data, and other credit information about that person. Also, contact the named individual for verification of the obligation. If a third-party payor's agreement to pay is contingent upon the patient's failure to pay, such an agreement must be in writing to be enforceable and must be made prior to treatment. Any agreement made after completion of treatment could be considered as a moral obligation only. The guarantee of a person to pay the account of another may be very simple. It may be typewritten or handwritten, stating:

I, the undersigned, do promise to pay for the medical services rendered by Theodore Wilson, MD, to my nephew, Robert L. Smith.
Date:
Signed:

or

I, the undersigned, promise to pay the medical bill of Robert L. Smith, if his mother, Mrs. Lydia Smith, does not pay by the 15th of July, 19xx.
Date:
Signed:

Accounts rendered to a spouse or child should always carry full data about the party responsible, which in most cases is the other spouse or the parent. Generally, a responsible spouse or parent pays the account without any follow-up collection procedures. In the case of a minor, it is generally held that the parent accompanying the child to the medical facility is responsible for paying. Any agreement between divorced or separated parents is solely between them and does not affect the obligation to the physician.

If you foresee legal difficulties in collecting an account in which divorce, legal guardianship, or the involvement of an emancipated minor complicates the matter, it is best to contact the physician's attorney for advice. The laws governing such matters vary according to each state. One reminder, however, is that you must always have the signature of the third party responsible for the debt if he or she is not otherwise obligated by law. An oral agreement is not binding.

Health Insurance Information

The initial interview is the best time to get full information on the patient's insurance coverage. The patient registration form usually provides a place for the name of the insurance company. Ask to see the patient's identification card and make a photocopy for your records. The card usually shows the name of the subscriber and the group and member number and often includes a service code indicating the patient's coverage. Also obtain information on any supplementary coverage—for instance, a plan in which the spouse is the subscriber and the patient is covered as a dependent. There may also be major medical or supplementary benefits to the patient's policy.

Assignment of Benefits

Many doctors ask the patient to execute an **assignment of insurance benefits** at this time. The assignment, authorizing the insurance company to pay benefits directly to the doctor, may be stamped on the insurance form or may be subsequently attached to a completed insurance form.

Consent for Release of Information

If a standard claim form is used or if the patient has brought along his own form, this is an appropriate time to have the patient sign the consent for release of the information that is necessary on most claims, so that the insurance form can be processed without delay as services are performed. Some states require a special form for release of information separate and apart from the insurance claim form itself. The medical assistant should check local regulations.

Installment Buying of Medical Services

Because installment buying is so much a part of our economic system today, the physician's office must be prepared to help patients budget for their medical care. Patients expect to use their credit resources and appreciate businesslike assistance in establishing a payment plan. The medical profession has too long suffered a poor collection record because of its fear of appearing "too commercial." The doctor should be ready to arrange credit when medical bills will be high or when a patient for some reason is unable to pay at the time of service. In general, fees for routine office calls and small medical bills should be kept on a pay-as-you-go basis.

Credit Cards

The acceptance of credit cards, sometimes called bank cards, has become commonplace in medical practice. Patients appreciate the convenience, and paying by credit card may help to improve collections. The signed credit card voucher is deposited to the doctor's bank account. The card company deducts a percentage (from 1% to 5% depending upon volume) for the collection service. The patient may pay the full amount when billed by the card company or may pay a portion and be charged interest on the balance.

Special Budget Plans

If a patient appears concerned about the ability to meet his financial obligations, the doctor or the medical assistant can suggest in a tactful way:

"Mr. Elwood, if you think you will have difficulty paying for your treatments at one time, we can work out some special arrangements."

This allows the patient to ask what sort of plan you have in mind, and the discussion progresses very easily into various payment plans. Generally, it is better to let the patient decide what arrangements are best rather than to suggest a plan. However, if the patient has no suggestion, the medical assistant can say:

"Mr. Elwood, would you be able to pay $50 each month until the account is paid in full?"

or

"Usually an account of this size can be settled in 3 to 4 months. Would you be able to pay $100 now, then $50 a month until the account is paid in full?"

When the amount of each installment has been agreed upon, it is then wise to establish definite dates on which the payments will be expected.

Truth in Lending Act

Regulation Z of the Truth in Lending Act, which is enforced by the Federal Trade Commission, requires that when there is a bilateral agreement between doctor and patient to accept payment in more than four installments, the doctor is required to provide disclosure of information regarding finance charges. Even if there are no finance charges involved, the form must be completed stating this fact. A copy of the form is retained by the doctor, and the original is given to the patient. Specific wording is required in the disclosure. The form in Figure 15–2 meets the requirements. Have the patient sign the agreement in your presence, as you must have proof of signing. The disclosure statement must be kept on file for 2 years. Although the disclosure statement is designed as protection for

LEONARD S. TAYLOR, M.D.
2100 WEST PARK AVENUE
CHAMPAIGN, ILLINOIS 61820

TELEPHONE 351-5400

FEDERAL TRUTH IN LENDING STATEMENT
For professional services rendered

Patient ___Joseph Brookhurst___

Address ___353 West Terry Lane___
___Birmingham, Alabama 35209___

Parent ___

1. Cash Price (fee for service)	$	1200.00
2. Cash Down Payment	$	200.00
3. Unpaid Balance of Cash Price	$	1000.00
4. Amount Financed	$	1000.00
5. FINANCE CHARGE	$	-0-
6. Finance Charge Expressed As Annual Percentage Rate		-0-
7. Total of Payments (4 plus 5)	$	1000.00
8. Deferred Payment Price (1 plus 5)	$	1200.00

"Total payment due" (7 above) is payable to ___Dr. Leonard S. Taylor___ at above office address in ___five___ monthly installments of $___200.00___ The first installment is payable on ___May 1___ 19__xx__, and each subsequent payment is due on the same day of each consecutive month until paid in full.

___4-15-19xx___   ___
Date   Signature of Patient; Parent if Patient is a Minor

FORM 9402 COLWELL SYSTEMS, INC. CHAMPAIGN, ILLINOIS

FIGURE 15–2. Disclosure statement. (Courtesy of Colwell Systems, a division of Deluxe Corporation.)

the debtor, it can be a good collection tool for the creditor.

It is recognized that physicians generally permit their patients to pay in installments, and as long as there is no specific agreement on the part of the physician for payment to be made in more than four installments, and no finance charge is made, the account is not subject to the regulation. If the patient chooses to pay in installments instead of the full amount, this is considered a unilateral action and the physician, in accepting such payments, probably would not be subject to the provisions of the regulation. The doctor's office, however, must be certain to bill for the full balance each time. If the statement is for only a partial payment, it then becomes a bilateral agreement and as such is subject to Regulation Z.

Helping patients budget their medical expenses is a rather new aspect of the business side of medical

PROCEDURE 15-2 MAKING CREDIT ARRANGEMENTS WITH A PATIENT

GOAL To assist the patient in paying for services by making mutually beneficial credit arrangements according to established office policy.

EQUIPMENT AND SUPPLIES

Patient's ledger
Calendar
Truth in Lending form
Assignment of Benefits form

Patient's insurance form
Typewriter
Private area for interview

PROCEDURAL STEPS

1. Answer thoroughly and kindly all questions about credit.

2. Inform the patient of office policy regarding credit:
   - Payment at the time of the first visit
   - Payment by bank card
   - Credit application
   Purpose: To ensure complete understanding of mutual responsibilities.

3. Have the patient complete the credit application.
   Purpose: To comply with office practices on the extension of credit.

4. Check the completed credit application.
   Purpose: To confirm that all necessary information is included.

5. Discuss with the patient the possible arrangements and ask the patient to decide which of those arrangements is most suitable.
   Purpose: Better compliance can be expected when the patient makes the choice.

6. Prepare the Truth in Lending form and have the patient sign it if the agreement requires more than four installments.
   Purpose: To comply with Regulation Z.

7. Have the patient execute an assignment of insurance benefits.
   Purpose: To comply with credit policy.

8. Make a copy of the patient's insurance ID and have the patient sign a consent for release of the information to insurance company.
   Purpose: Consent for the release of information is necessary on most insurance forms before a claim can be processed.

9. Keep credit information confidential.

practice. However, it is a real service to patients and demonstrates that the doctor and the office staff are sincerely anxious to help patients pay their own way. It may also prevent many collection problems.

Confidentiality

Obtaining Credit Information

Credit information is confidential. It should be guarded as carefully as a confidential medical history and should be disclosed to no one. When you ask for credit information from patients in the office, do so in a private area where others cannot overhear the conversation. A desk or table away from the reception area where a patient can sit in total privacy and complete a credit application is a great asset. Credit information is personal—it should be kept that way.

Credit Bureaus

Some doctors join a credit bureau, particularly in large cities where it is more difficult to gauge informally the patients' ability to pay. Credit bureaus gather credit information from many sources, pool it, and make it available to dues-paying bureau members. If you receive a request for credit information about one of your patients, it is permissible to furnish it because the debtor, by giving the doctor's name as a reference, has given implied consent; otherwise, the credit bureau would not have contacted you. According to the Fair Credit Practices Act Amendments of 1975, you can reply by giving ledger information only, including:

- When the account was opened
- How much the patient now owes
- The highest amount of the account at any time

You should avoid any reference to:

- character
- paying habits
- credit rating

Medical-Dental-Hospital Bureaus

The Medical-Dental-Hospital Bureaus of America (MDHBA), with headquarters in Chicago, is a na-tional organization of agencies serving physicians, dentists, and hospitals. It seeks to maintain the highest standards among its members and is committed to following the collection methods most acceptable to physicians. Doctors who use their collection services have access to credit information on accounts assigned by other clients. Member bureaus of the MDHBA frequently assist the medical assistant by sponsoring collection seminars as well as by providing speakers for medical assistant society meetings.

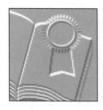 ▶ **LEARNING ACHIEVEMENTS**

Are you able to:

1. Define the terms listed in the Vocabulary of this chapter?
2. Name the three values that a physician considers in determining professional fees?
3. Give an example of a *usual and customary* fee?
4. Explain how a physician's fee profile is determined?
5. List three reasons for providing a patient with an estimate slip before starting treatment?
6. Discuss and give an example of *professional courtesy* in medical fees?
7. List the four kinds of charges that should be avoided?
8. Explain and give an example of what is meant by *third-party liability*?
9. State three items of information that *can* be released and three items that should be *excluded* in replying to a request for credit information?
10. Explain when and how to prepare a Truth in Lending form?

REFERENCES AND READINGS

American Medical Association: *The Business Side of Medical Practice,* Chicago, The Association, 1989.
Federal Reserve Board: *Equal Credit Opportunity Act,* October 28, 1975.
Manning, F. F.: *Medical Group Practice Management,* Cambridge, Ballinger Publishing Co., 1977.

15

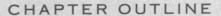

CHAPTER OUTLINE

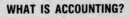

VOCABULARY

account A single financial record.

account balance The debit or credit balance remaining in the account.

accounting equation Assets = Liabilities + Proprietorship.

accounts payable Amounts charged and not paid.

accounts receivable Amounts owed to the doctor.

accounts receivable control A summary of unpaid accounts.

accounts receivable ledger The combined record of all patient accounts.

accounts receivable trial balance A method of determining that the journal and the ledger are in balance.

accrual basis of accounting Income is recorded when earned, and expenses are recorded when incurred.

adjustment column An account column, sometimes included to the left of the balance column, that is used for entering discounts.

balance column The account column on the far right that is used for recording the difference between the debit and credit columns.

balance sheet A financial statement for a specific date that shows the total assets, liabilities, and capital of the business.

bookkeeping The recording part of the accounting process.

cash basis of accounting Income is recorded when received, and expenses are recorded when paid.

cash flow statement A financial summary for a specific period that shows the beginning cash on hand, the cash income and disbursements during the period, and the amount of cash on hand at the end of the period.

cash payment journal A record of all cash paid out.

credit balance The amount of advance payment or overpayment on an account.

credit column The account column to the right of the debit column that is used for entering funds received.

daily journal The book in which all transactions are first recorded; the book of original entry, or general journal.

debit column The account column on the left that is used for entering charges.

disbursements Cash paid out.

disbursements journal Record of every amount paid out, the date paid, the check number, and the purpose of payment.

discount A subtraction from the patient's balance.

general journal The book of original entry in accounting.

in balance Total ending balances of patient ledgers equal total of accounts receivable control.

invoice A paper describing a purchase and the amount due.

packing slip An itemized list of objects in a package.

payables Amounts owed to others.

posting The act of transferring information from one record to another.

receipts Cash received.

receivables Amounts owing from others.

statement A request for payment.

statement of income and expense A summary of all income and expenses for a given period.

transaction The occurrence of a financial event or condition that must be recorded.

ACCOUNTING SYSTEMS

LEARNING OBJECTIVES

COGNITIVE

Upon successful completion of this chapter, you should be able to:

1. Define the terms listed in the Vocabulary.

2. List the two bases of accounting and explain their differences.

3. State the four kinds of information that the financial records of any business should show at all times.

4. Differentiate between a debit balance and a credit balance.

5. Describe and demonstrate the entry for a credit balance.

6. List six kinds of accounting records.

7. Compare the three most common accounting systems used in the professional office.

8. State the basic accounting equation.

9. Discuss the importance of a trial balance.

10. List and state the purpose of the five common periodic accounting summaries.

PERFORMANCE

Upon successful completion of this chapter, you should be able to perform the following activities:

1. Prepare a ledger account for a new patient.

2. Prepare a patient charge slip.

3. Journalize service charges and payments using a single-entry system.

4. Post the entries from the daily journal to patient ledger cards.

5. Prepare a daily posting proof.

6. Prepare a daily cash control proof.

7. Prepare a monthly trial balance.

8. Establish and maintain a petty cash fund.

9. Post service charges and payments using a pegboard.

A physician's business records are the key to good management practice. The medical assistant who can keep accurate financial records and who will conduct the nonmedical side of the practice in a businesslike fashion is genuinely needed and appreciated.

Financial records that are complete, correct, and current are essential for:

- Prompt billing and collection procedures
- Professional financial planning
- Accurate reporting of income to federal and state agencies

WHAT IS ACCOUNTING?

Accounting is the art or system of recording, classifying, and summarizing financial transactions.

Bookkeeping is mainly the recording part of the accounting process. The bookkeeping must be done daily and is the responsibility of the administrative medical assistant in a small practice. In a larger practice, the office manager or financial manager assumes this responsibility.

Account Bases

There are two bases for accounting: the **cash basis** and the **accrual basis** (Table 16–1). Expressed simply, this means that:

- charges for services are entered as income when payment is received
- expenses are recorded when they are paid

Most physicians use the cash basis of accounting. Merchants, on the other hand, generally use an accrual basis of accounting. On the accrual basis, income is considered earned when services have been performed or goods have been sold, even though payment may not have been received. Expenses are recognized and recorded when incurred, even though they have not been paid.

Financial Summaries

The financial records of any business should at all times show:

- How much was earned in a given period
- How much was collected

- How much is owed
- The distribution of expenses incurred

From the daily entries, the accountant can prepare monthly and annual summaries that provide a basis for comparing any given period with another similar period.

Periodic analyses of the financial records can result in improved business practices, better management of time, curtailment or elimination of unprofitable services, and better budgeting of expenses. With the appropriate software; these analyses can be accomplished using the computer.

BOOKKEEPING

Good Working Habits

A willingness to pay attention to detail, good organizational skills, and the ability to concentrate and maintain consistency in working patterns and procedures are all necessary qualifications for the person who has the responsibility of keeping financial records. The careful bookkeeper will:

- Use good penmanship
- Use the same pen style and ink consistently
- Keep columns of figures straight
- Write well-formed figures (a careless "9" may look like a "7"; an open "0" may resemble a "6")
- Carry decimal points correctly
- Check arithmetic carefully and not put blind faith in a calculator
- Not erase, write over, or blot out figures (if an error is made, a straight line should be drawn through the incorrect figure and the correct figure written above it)

Bookkeeping procedures are not difficult or complicated, but they do require concentration to avoid errors. There is no such thing as *almost* correct financial records. The books either balance or they do not balance. The bookkeeping is either right or wrong. This is not the place to be creative or take shortcuts.

The medical assistant should set aside a certain time each day for bookkeeping tasks, if possible. Do not attempt to work on financial records when you are busy attending patients or when there are other distractions.

Cardinal Rules of Bookkeeping

- Enter all charges and receipts immediately in the daily record or journal.

- Write a receipt in duplicate for any currency received. Writing receipts for checks is optional, but a consistent pattern should be followed.

TABLE 16–1. ACCOUNTING BASES

	Cash Basis	Accrual Basis
Income is recorded	When received	When service is performed or goods are sold
Expense is recorded	When paid	When incurred (even if not paid)

- Post all charges and receipts to the patient ledger daily.
- Endorse checks for deposit as soon as received.
- Deposit all receipts in the bank.
- Verify that the total of the deposit plus the amount on hand equals the total to be accounted for in the daily journal.
- Use a petty cash fund to pay for small unpredictable expenses. Pay all other expenses by check (a canceled check is the best proof of payment).
- Pay all bills before their due dates, after checking them for accuracy. Place date of payment and number of check on paid bills.

ACCOUNTING TERMINOLOGY

In order to understand and perform bookkeeping procedures, it is first necessary to learn some of the terminology of accounts.

A business **transaction** is the occurrence of an event or of a condition that must be recorded. For example:

- A service is performed for which a charge is made
- A patient makes a payment on account
- A piece of equipment is purchased
- The monthly rent is paid

Each is a transaction that must be recorded within the accounting system.

The **daily journal** is called the book of original entry because this is where all transactions are first recorded (Fig. 16–1).

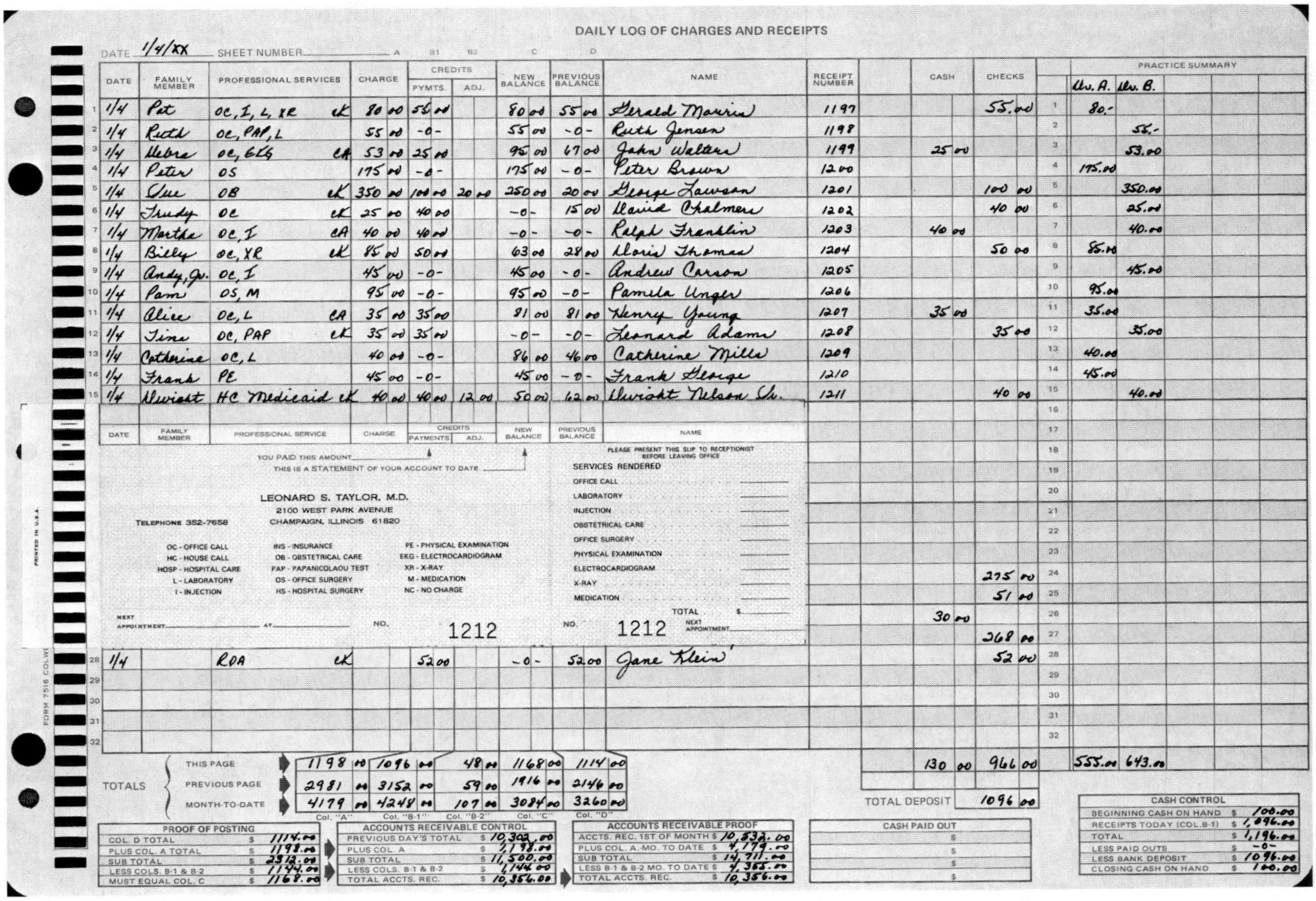

DAILY LOG OF CHARGES AND RECEIPTS

DATE 1/4/XX SHEET NUMBER

	DATE	FAMILY MEMBER	PROFESSIONAL SERVICES		CHARGE	CREDITS PYMTS.	CREDITS ADJ.	NEW BALANCE	PREVIOUS BALANCE	NAME	RECEIPT NUMBER	CASH	CHECKS		Dv. A.	Dv. B.
1	1/4	Pat	OC, I, L, XR	ck	80.00	55.00		80.00	55.00	Gerald Morris	1197		55.00	1	80.-	
2	1/4	Ruth	OC, PAP, L		55.00	-0-		55.00	-0-	Ruth Jensen	1198			2		55.-
3	1/4	Debra	OC, EKG	CA	53.00	25.00		95.00	67.00	John Walters	1199	25.00		3		53.00
4	1/4	Peter	OS		175.00	-0-		175.00	-0-	Peter Brown	1200			4	175.00	
5	1/4	Sue	OB	ck	350.00	100.00	20.00	250.00	20.00	George Lawson	1201		100.00	5		350.00
6	1/4	Trudy	OC	ck	25.00	40.00		-0-	15.00	David Chalmers	1202		40.00	6		25.00
7	1/4	Martha	OC, I	CA	40.00	40.00		-0-	-0-	Ralph Franklin	1203	40.00		7		40.00
8	1/4	Billy	OC, XR	ck	85.00	50.00		63.00	28.00	Doris Thomas	1204		50.00	8	85.00	
9	1/4	Andy, Jr.	OC, I		45.00	-0-		45.00	-0-	Andrew Carson	1205			9		45.00
10	1/4	Pam	OS, M		95.00	-0-		95.00	-0-	Pamela Unger	1206			10	95.00	
11	1/4	Alice	OC, L	CA	35.00	35.00		81.00	81.00	Henry Young	1207	35.00		11	35.00	
12	1/4	Tina	OC, PAP	ck	35.00	35.00		-0-	-0-	Leonard Adams	1208		35.00	12		35.00
13	1/4	Catherine	OC, L		40.00	-0-		86.00	46.00	Catherine Mills	1209			13	40.00	
14	1/4	Frank	PE		45.00	-0-		45.00	-0-	Frank George	1210			14	45.00	
15	1/4	Dwight	HC Medicaid	ck	40.00	40.00	12.00	50.00	62.00	Dwight Nelson Sr.	1211		40.00	15		40.00
24													275.00	24		
25													51.00	25		
26												30.00		26		
27													268.00	27		
28	1/4		RDA	ck	52.00			-0-	52.00	Jane Klein			52.00	28		

YOU PAID THIS AMOUNT
THIS IS A STATEMENT OF YOUR ACCOUNT TO DATE

LEONARD S. TAYLOR, M.D.
2100 WEST PARK AVENUE
CHAMPAIGN, ILLINOIS 61820
TELEPHONE 352-7658

OC - OFFICE CALL; HC - HOUSE CALL; HOSP - HOSPITAL CARE; L - LABORATORY; I - INJECTION; INS - INSURANCE; OB - OBSTETRICAL CARE; PAP - PAPANICOLAOU TEST; OS - OFFICE SURGERY; HS - HOSPITAL SURGERY; PE - PHYSICAL EXAMINATION; EKG - ELECTROCARDIOGRAM; XR - X-RAY; M - MEDICATION; NC - NO CHARGE

PLEASE PRESENT THIS SLIP TO RECEPTIONIST BEFORE LEAVING OFFICE
SERVICES RENDERED: OFFICE CALL, LABORATORY, INJECTION, OBSTETRICAL CARE, OFFICE SURGERY, PHYSICAL EXAMINATION, ELECTROCARDIOGRAM, X-RAY, MEDICATION, TOTAL $
NEXT APPOINTMENT AT
NO. 1212 NO. 1212

TOTALS	Col. "A"	Col. "B-1"	Col. "B-2"	Col. "C"	Col. "D"
THIS PAGE	1198.00	1096.00	48.00	1168.00	1114.00
PREVIOUS PAGE	2981.00	3152.00	59.00	1916.00	2146.00
MONTH-TO-DATE	4179.00	4248.00	107.00	3084.00	3260.00

Cash 130.00; Checks 966.00; Dv. A. 555.00; Dv. B. 643.00

TOTAL DEPOSIT 1096.00

PROOF OF POSTING	
COL. D TOTAL	$ 1114.00
PLUS COL. A TOTAL	$ 1198.00
SUB TOTAL	$ 2312.00
LESS COLS. B-1 & B-2	$ 1144.00
MUST EQUAL COL. C	$ 1168.00

ACCOUNTS RECEIVABLE CONTROL	
PREVIOUS DAY'S TOTAL	$ 10,302.00
PLUS COL. A	$ 1,198.00
SUB TOTAL	$ 11,500.00
LESS COLS. B-1 & B-2	$ 1,144.00
TOTAL ACCTS. REC.	$ 10,356.00

ACCOUNTS RECEIVABLE PROOF	
ACCTS. REC. 1ST OF MONTH	$ 10,532.00
PLUS COL. A.-MO. TO DATE	$ 4,179.00
SUB TOTAL	$ 14,711.00
LESS B-1 & B-2 MO. TO DATE	$ 4,355.00
TOTAL ACCTS. REC.	$ 10,356.00

CASH PAID OUT $ $ $ $

CASH CONTROL	
BEGINNING CASH ON HAND	$ 100.00
RECEIPTS TODAY (COL. B-1)	$ 1,096.00
TOTAL	$ 1,196.00
LESS PAID OUTS	$ -0-
LESS BANK DEPOSIT	$ 1096.00
CLOSING CASH ON HAND	$ 100.00

FORM 7516 COLWELL PRINTED IN U.S.A.

FIGURE 16–1. Sample day sheet for pegboard bookkeeping system, with deposit list of checks and optional business analysis summaries. (Courtesy of Colwell Systems, Inc., Champaign, IL.)

A patient's financial record is called an **account.** All of the patients' accounts together constitute the **accounts receivable ledger.**

Account cards vary in design, but all will have at least three columns for entering figures:

- The **debit** (abbreviation: Dr) column on the left is used for entering charges and is sometimes called the charge column.
- The **credit** (abbreviation: Cr) column to the right, sometimes headed "Paid," is used for entering payments received.
- The **balance** column on the far right is used for recording the difference between the debit and credit columns.
- An **adjustment** column is available in some systems and is used for entering professional discounts, write-offs, disallowances by insurance companies, and so forth (Fig. 16–2).

Posting means the transfer of information from one record to another. Transactions are posted from the journal to the ledger (this is accomplished in one writing in the pegboard system).

The **account balance** is normally a debit balance (charges exceed payments). A debit balance is entered by simply writing the correct figure in the balance column.

A **credit balance** exists when payments exceed charges; for instance, when a patient pays in advance. This is common in obstetric practices. To show a credit balance, record the figures in one of the following two ways:

- Write the credit balance on the card in regular ink and enclose the figure in parentheses or encircle it.
- Write the credit balance in red ink (this cannot be accomplished on the pegboard unless red carbon is inserted).
- **Discounts** are also credit entries and are entered in the adjustment column or, if there is no adjustment column, the discount is entered in the debit column in red ink or enclosed in parentheses. By making the entry this way, it is recognized as a subtraction from the charges. In totaling columns, any figure in red or in parentheses is always subtracted.
- **Receipts** are cash and checks taken in payment for professional services.
- **Receivables** are charges for which payment has not been received—amounts that are owing.
- **Disbursements** are cash amounts paid out.
- **Payables** are amounts owed to others but not yet paid.

KINDS OF ACCOUNTING RECORDS

General journal. The **general journal** (or daily journal) is the chronologic record of the practice —the financial diary. All information regarding services rendered, charges, and receipts is first recorded in the daily journal. It is important that every transaction be recorded.

In addition to professional services rendered in and out of the office, there may be income from other sources, such as rentals, royalties, interest, and so forth. Usually a special place is provided in the journal for such income. Any income that is not practice-related should be recorded separately from patient receipts.

Ledger. The **accounts receivable** ledger comprises all the patients' financial accounts on which there are balances. All charges and payments for professional services are posted to the ledger daily. The ledger then becomes a reliable source of information for answering all inquiries from patients about their accounts.

A separate account card or page is prepared for each patient (or each family) at the time of the first visit or service (Fig. 16–3). The heading of the account should include all information pertinent to collecting the account:

- Name and address of person responsible for payment
- Insurance identification
- Social Security number
- Home and business telephone numbers
- Name of employer
- Any special instructions for billing

Billing statements to the patient and the patient's insurance are prepared from the ledger.

Checkbook. All receipts are deposited in the checking account, and a record of the deposit is entered on the check stub. A copy of each deposit slip should be kept with the financial records. All bills are paid by check, and a record of the payment is entered on the check stub and in the disbursements section of the general journal (Fig. 16–4).

Disbursements journal. In simplified accounting systems, the **disbursements journal** usually consists of a section at the bottom of each daysheet and a check register page at the end of each month, plus monthly and annual summaries. It must show:

- Every amount paid out
- Date and check number
- Purpose of payment

Disbursements that are not practice-related should be recorded separately.

Petty cash record. A petty cash fund and voucher system should be established to take care of minor unpredictable expenditures such as:

- Postage due
- Parking fees
- Small contributions

BILLING NAME		NAMES OF OTHER FAMILY MEMBERS	
PATIENT S NAME			
RES PHONE	BUS PHONE		
OCCUPATION		RELATIVE OR FRIEND	
EMPLOYED BY		REFERRED BY	
INS INFORMATION			SOC SEC NUMBER
FORM NO. 40-8550		1976, BIBBERO SYSTEMS, INC., PETALUMA, CA.	

STATEMENT TO:

JANE L JONES
1211 EAST FIRST AVENUE
ANYWHERE US 10000

FIGURE 16-2. Account card/statement showing debit, credit, adjustment, and credit balance. (Courtesy of Bibbero Systems, Inc., Petaluma, CA.)

TEAR OFF AND RETURN UPPER PORTION WITH PAYMENT

19XX DATE	PROFESSIONAL SERVICE	FEE		PAYMENT		ADJUST-MENT		NEW BALANCE	
03/04	90010	125	00					125	00
04/20	90060-01	50	00	175	00			-0-	
04-21	4/20 VISIT, NO CHARGE					50	00	(50	00)
	DEBIT COLUMN ⟶								
	CREDIT COLUMN ⟶								
	ADJUSTMENT COLUMN ⟶								
	BALANCE COLUMN SHOWING CREDIT BALANCE ⟶								

16

NAME				CHARGE TO			
Johnson, Tom				self			

ADDRESS				ADDRESS			
2400 Main Street, Centerville, XX 10101				Dr. Maltby			

TELEPHONE		INSURANCE				REF. BY	
111-4545 Bus. 300-4365		Aetna Life		S.S.#000-00-0000			

DATE 1982	SERVICE	CHARGE	PAID	BALANCE	DATE	SERVICE	CHARGE	PAID	BALANCE
Feb 10	47600	800 –	–	800 –					
18	F. U.	–		800 –					
Apr 2	Insur paid		620 –	180 –					
25	Pers check		180 –	-0-					
May 13	F. U.	N/c		-0-					

NAME				CHARGE TO			
Dunn, Beatrice (Mrs Robert)				Robert Dunn			

ADDRESS				ADDRESS			
222 Center Street, Centerville, XX 10101							

TELEPHONE	INSURANCE				REF. BY	
714-5505	Mutual of Omaha (Robert Dunn Co. group) S.S.#213-00-7536				sister (M. Tucker)	

DATE 1982	SERVICE RENDERED	CHARGE	PAID	BALANCE
May 13	New patient exam 90020	60 –	60 –	-0-

NAME			
JONES, JANE LILLIAN (MRS ROBERT) SS # 000-00-0000			

ADDRESS			
1211 East First Avenue, Anywhere, USA 10000			

TELEPHONE			
443-7754 Not employed Mutual Ins			

DATE 1982	SERVICE RENDERED	CHARGE	PAID	BALANCE
3 4	Pre natal exam	30 –	100 –	70 –
4 20	"	20 –	100 –	150 –

FIGURE 16–3. Example of patient account cards. (Courtesy of Colwell Systems, Inc., Champaign, IL.)

In the average medical office, $25 to $50 is sufficient for the petty cash fund. If a larger sum is available, there is a tendency to pay too many bills out of petty cash.

When the check for this fund is exchanged at the bank for small bills and coins, the money is placed in a cashbox or drawer that can be locked or kept in the safe at night. One person only should be in charge of the petty cash fund. This person must be able to account for the full amount of the fund at any time.

Payroll record. The payroll record is an auxiliary disbursement record. A separate page or card for each employee, as well as a summary record, should be kept. This procedure is discussed in more detail in Chapter 22 as a management responsibility.

COMPARISON OF COMMON ACCOUNTING SYSTEMS

Success in accounting also requires a thorough understanding of the system and what it is expected to accomplish. There are many variations in accounting systems, from simple to complex, no one of which can meet the needs of every doctor. The basic principles are the same for all; only the system of recording varies.

The three most common systems found in the professional office are:

- Single-entry
- Double-entry
- Pegboard or write-it-once

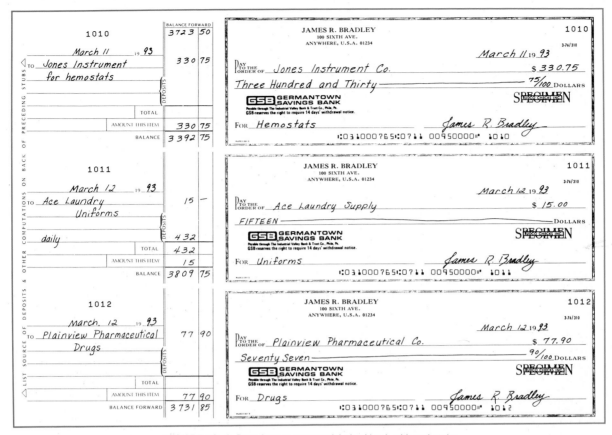

FIGURE 16–4. Page from a commercial checkbook with end stubs.

The recording process in all of these systems can be performed by hand or by computer; the choice usually depends on the volume.

An overview of the three systems is presented here (Table 16–2), followed later in the chapter by more detailed instruction for the pegboard system, which is currently the most widely used system in medical practices.

TABLE 16–2. ACCOUNTING SYSTEMS

	Advantages	Disadvantages
Single-entry	Inexpensive Requires little training Simple to use	Provides only simple summaries Errors difficult to locate No built-in controls
Double-entry	Provides comprehensive financial picture Built-in accuracy controls	Requires special training, more time, and greater skill
Pegboard	Generates all records with one writing Daily control on accounts receivable Daily record of bank deposits and cash on hand	Cost of supplies greater than single-entry system Some training required (usually included in medical assistant programs)

Single-Entry System

Single-entry accounting is inexpensive, simple to use, and requires very little training. It is the oldest and simplest of accounting systems and includes at least three basic records:

- A general journal, which may also be called a daily log, daybook, daysheet, daily journal, or charge journal (Fig. 16–5).
- A **cash payment journal,** which in its simplest form is a checkbook.
- An accounts receivable ledger, which is a record of the amounts owed by all the doctor's patients. The accounts receivable ledger may be a bound book, a loose-leaf binder, a card file, or loose pages in a ledger tray.

There may also be auxiliary records for petty cash and payroll records.

The records of charges and receipts are usually entered into a bound journal with a page for each day in the year, monthly summary pages, and an annual summary. Daily pages have columns for entering each transaction that show the patient's name, the service performed and the charge, any payments received, and the totals for charges and

October 20, 19xx

HOUR	NAME	SERVICE RENDERED	√	CHARGE	PAID
9:00	Brown, John	90030		30 00	
9:20	Sullivan, Bertha	90050		40 00	
9:40	James, Ella	P.O.Dressing		n/c	
10:00	Grover, Ellen	90030		30 00	30 00
10:20	Johnson, Tom	FU		n/c	
10:40	Taylor, Theo	90050		40 00	40 00
11:00	Sorenson, Betty	90730		30 00	
11:20	Boston, Stuart	81000		20 00	20 00
11:40	Daniger, Fred	90030		30 00	
12:00					
12:20					
12:40					
1:00	Marlow, Eva	FU		n/c	
1:20	Arnold, Anne	P.O.Dressing		n/c	
1:40	Tucker, Benjamin	90015		70 00	70 00
2:00					
2:20	Thompson, Dan	90015		70 00	70 00
2:40					
3:00	Dunn, Beatrice	90020		120 00	
3:20					
3:40					
4:00	Histed, J. B.	90000		50 00	
4:20	Roberts, Victor	90020		120 00	120 00
4:40					
5:00					

FIGURE 16–5. Page from a daily log used in single-entry bookkeeping. (Courtesy of Colwell Systems, Inc., Champaign, IL.)

receipts. The daily totals are entered on the monthly summary, and the monthly totals are carried forward to the annual summary.

The same bound book may also have space for recording cash payments, or the checkbook may be the only cash payment journal. Monthly and annual summaries would be done from the checkbook.

The accounts receivable ledger usually consists of an account card for each patient on which are entered the charges and payments from the general journal. The patients' statements are prepared from these cards (Fig. 16–6).

In a single-entry system, each entry is made separately:

1. The entry is recorded on the daily journal or log.
2. A patient receipt is written if payment was made.
3. The transaction is posted to the ledger.
4. A monthly statement is generated from the ledger.

Although the single-entry accounting system may satisfy the requirements for reporting to government agencies, it does have some drawbacks:

- errors are not easily detected
- there are no built-in controls
- periodic analyses are inadequate for financial planning

The single-entry system was at one time widely used in medical offices, but it is gradually being phased out in favor of more complete accounting systems.

Double-Entry System

Double-entry accounting is also inexpensive but requires a trained and experienced bookkeeper or the regular services of an accountant. In addition to the basic journals used in a single-entry system,

BILLING NAME		NAMES OF OTHER FAMILY MEMBERS	
AXELROD, FRANCIS			
PATIENT'S NAME		Wife: Alice	
Axelrod, Francis			
RES PHONE 399-7840 BUS PHONE 399-1846			
OCCUPATION Programmer		RELATIVE OR FRIEND	
EMPLOYED BY Topnotch Computers		REFERRED BY Dr. R. Burns	
INS INFORMATION Aetna Cas & Life		SOC. SEC. NUMBER 999 00 888	
FORM NO. MDP. 8550		1976 BIBBERO SYSTEMS, INC.-SAN FRANCISCO	

GEORGE D. GREEN, M.D.
JOHN F. WHITE, M.D.
Family Practice
100 MAIN STREET, SUITE 14
ANYTOWN, CALIFORNIA 90000
TELEPHONE: (999) 399-6000

STATEMENT TO:

FRANCIS AXELROD
1111 NORTH BROADWAY
SAN TOMAS XX 90000

TEAR OFF AND RETURN UPPER PORTION WITH PAYMENT

DATE	PROFESSIONAL SERVICE	FEE		PAYMENT	ADJUST-MENT	NEW BALANCE	
5/13/00	OFFICE CONSULT 90600	65	00			65	00

PROFESSIONAL SERVICE CODES:

1. OFFICE VISIT	9. COLLECTION OF LAB. SPEC.	17. SURGICAL
2. HOME VISIT	10. SPECIAL REPORTS	18. CASTS
3. HOSPITAL VISIT	11. OTHER SERVICES	19. LABORATORY
4. EMERGENCY ROOM	12. SPEC. DIAGNOSTIC SERVICES	20. X-RAY
5. CONSULTATION	13. SPEC. THERAPEUTIC SERV.	21. ALLERGY TEST.
6. IMMUNIZATION	14. EXTENDED CARE FACILITY	22. NO CHARGE
7. INJECTION	15. CUSTODIAL CARE	23. ADJUSTMENTS OR CORRECTIONS
8. DRUGS/SUPPLIES/MATERIALS	16. OBSTETRICAL CARE	24. TOTAL CARE

GEORGE D. GREEN, M.D.
CAL. LIC. # 6-2856

JOHN F. WHITE, M.D.
CAL. LIC. # G-5281

FIGURE 16-6. Combination account card/statement from accounts receivable ledger. (Courtesy of Bibbero Systems, Inc., Petaluma, CA.)

16

there may be numerous subsidiary journals. The system is based on the **accounting equation:**

Assets = Liabilities + Proprietorship (Capital)

Every transaction requires an entry on each side of the accounting equation, and the two sides must always be in balance. For this reason the system is called "double-entry." It is the most complete of the three systems.

Assets are the properties owned by a business, such as bank accounts, accounts receivable, buildings, equipment, and furniture. The rights to these assets are called *equities*. The equity of the owner is called *capital, proprietorship,* or *owner's equity*. The equities of the creditors (to whom money is owed) are called *liabilities*. The owner's equity (capital) is what remains of the value of the assets after the creditor's equities (liabilities) have been subtracted.

For example, if the doctor purchased equipment for $1,000, paid $250 down, and gave a promissory note for $750, the accounting equation would be:

$$\begin{array}{rl} \text{Assets } \$1,000 = & \text{Liabilities } \$\ \ 750 \\ & + \\ & \underline{\text{Capital} \qquad 250} \\ \overline{\$1,000} & \overline{\$1,000} \end{array}$$

The total value of the asset is $1,000. The owner's equity is $250 and the creditor's equity is $750. The accounting terms *capital, proprietorship, owner's equity,* and *net worth* are used interchangeably.

Few medical assistants are trained in accounting. If a double-entry system is used, it is usually set up by a practice management consultant or the accountant who does most of the actual bookwork and reports. The medical assistant in this instance generally maintains only the daily journal, from which the accountant takes the figures once a month.

The double-entry system provides a more comprehensive picture of the practice and its effect on the doctor's net worth. Errors show up readily and there are many built in accuracy controls, but because of the time and skill required, it is not frequently used in the small practice.

Pegboard or Write-It-Once System

The initial cost of materials for the pegboard system is slightly more than that for a single- or double-entry system but is still moderate. The system is simple to operate, and training is included in most medical assisting programs.

The system gets its name from the lightweight aluminum or masonite board with a row of pegs along the side or top that hold the forms in place. The accounting forms are perforated for alignment on the pegs. All of the forms used in any system must be compatible so that they may be aligned perfectly on the board.

The pegboard system generates all the necessary financial records for each transaction with one writing:

- Charge slip and receipt
- Ledger card
- Journal entry

It may also include a statement and a bank deposit slip.

The system provides current accounts receivable totals and a daily record of bank deposits and cash on hand, in addition to the record of income and expenses. The need for separate posting to patient accounts is eliminated, and the chance for error decreased. Pegboard accounting is the most widely used of the three systems in physicians' offices today.

USING THE PEGBOARD ACCOUNTING SYSTEM

The pegboard accounting system provides positive control over cash, collections, and receivables and ensures that every cent is accounted for and properly entered. It provides a record of every patient, every charge, and every payment. You have a daily recap of earnings—a running record of receivables and an audited summary of cash. The system requires a minimum of time. With one writing you can:

- Enter a transaction on the daysheet
- Give the patient a receipt for payment
- Bring the patient's account up to date
- Provide a current statement of account for the patient
- Give the patient a notation of the next appointment

All of these features communicate the "money message" to patients effectively and courteously and generate good financial records.

Materials Required

The pegboard may be of inexpensive masonite construction with pegs down the left side, or it may be a more sophisticated aluminum sliding board that allows flexible positioning of materials. The basic forms are:

- The journal daysheet
- The patient ledger
- The patient charge slip/receipt or superbill

All of the forms must be compatible and are available from medical office supply companies. They are customized to the practice, incorporating the usual services and procedure codes of the practice.

Preparing the Board

At the beginning of each day, place a new day-sheet on the accounting board. Some systems have a sheet of "clean carbon" attached to the daysheet; others use special carbon with holes for the pegs; some use NCR (no carbon required) paper. The carbon goes on top of the daysheet. Over the carbon, place the charge slip/receipt or superbill. The receipt has a carbonized writing line that should align with the first open writing line on the daysheet. If the slips are shingled, lay the entire bank of receipts over the pegs, with the top one aligned as mentioned. The remainder will be automatically in place. Receipts should be used in numeric order.

Pulling the Ledger Cards

If a great many patients are to be seen in one day, pulling the ledger cards for all the scheduled pa-tients at the beginning of the day will save time. Keep the cards in the order in which the patients are scheduled to be seen.

Entering and Posting Transactions

As each patient arrives, insert the patient's ledger card under the first receipt, aligning the first available writing line of the card with the carbonized strip on the receipt. Enter the receipt number and date, the account balance in the space labeled previous balance, and the patient's name. The information recorded on the receipt is automatically posted to the ledger and the daysheet (Fig. 16–7).

The charge slip is then detached and clipped to the patient chart to be routed to the doctor, who now has an opportunity to see how much the patient owes and can discuss the account in privacy, if desired.

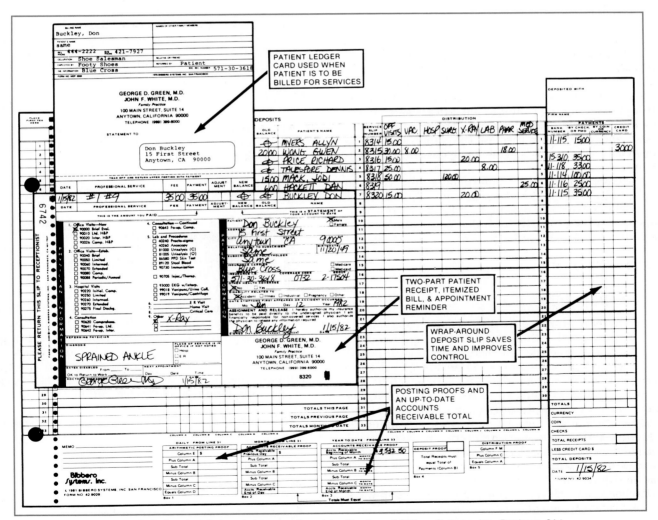

FIGURE 16–7. Sample daily log of charges and receipts. (Courtesy of Bibbero Systems, Inc., Petaluma, CA.)

After the service has been performed, the doctor enters the service on the charge slip and asks the patient or the nurse to return it to the medical assistant. The assistant then has an opportunity to ask the patient whether this is to be a charge or cash transaction before completing the posting.

Again, insert the ledger card under the proper receipt, checking the number that was previously entered to make sure you have the correct card. Record the service by procedure code, post the charge from the fee schedule, enter any payment made, and write in the current balance. If there is no balance, place a zero or straight line in the balance column. If another appointment is required, enter the date and time at the bottom of the receipt.

You have now posted the journal and the ledger and, if payment was made by the patient, automatically made a receipt. The service receipt is given to the patient; no other receipt is necessary. The ledger card is ready for refiling.

File the charge slips in numeric order for your internal audit. At the end of the month, the total of the charge slips should equal the total of the charges recorded on the daysheets for the month.

Recording Other Payments and Charges

Payments will be received in the mail and may be brought in by patients some time after a service was performed. These payments are entered on the daysheet and the ledger card in the same manner as previously explained. Payments by mail do not require a receipt.

The doctor may have daily charges for visits to patients in a hospital or convalescent facility. Enter these charges on the daysheet and ledger card only. Surgery fees are usually recorded as one entry that includes the surgery and aftercare.

End-of-Day Summarizing

At the end of the day, all columns must be totalled and proved. Although all bookkeeping is done in ink, it is a good idea to write the totals in pencil until they have been proved. If an error is discovered, you must correct the entry in which it occurred. Do not attempt to erase or write over the incorrect entry. Simply draw a line through it and make a new entry on the first open writing line. Remember that you must reinsert the ledger card for these corrections. Also, if the entry included a receipt for the patient, you must make a new receipt and notify the patient of the correction.

Pegboard accounting systems provide several ways for proving the arithmetic on the daysheet. Some examples are shown below.

```
POSTING PROOF FOR DAY

Old balance                          $_____
  Plus total charges                  _____
                     Subtotal    $_____
  Less payments received              _____
                     Subtotal    $_____
  Less adjustments                    _____
New balance                      *$_____
```
* This figure is carried forward to next page for "old balance."

```
CASH CONTROL PROOF

Cash on hand at beginning of day     $_____
  Cash received                       _____
                     Subtotal    $_____
  Less cash paid out                  _____
  Less bank deposit                   _____
Cash on hand at end of day       *$_____
```
* This figure is carried forward to next page for "cash on hand at beginning of day."

SPECIAL ACCOUNTING ENTRIES

The following special entries are necessary occasionally and may be used with pegboard or any other accounting system.

Adjustments

At times, it is necessary to enter a credit adjustment. Examples are:

- Professional discounts
- Insurance disallowances
- Write-offs

If the system has an adjustment column, enter them here. Otherwise, since the adjustment is actually a subtraction from the charge, enter it in the charge column with the figure enclosed in parentheses or circled, and an explanation of the entry in the description column. When the column of figures is totaled, this figure is *subtracted* rather than added. The learner has a tendency to ignore the circled figures. This is incorrect—they must be subtracted.

Credit Balances

A credit balance occurs when:

- A patient has paid in advance.
- There has been an overpayment

For example, an overpayment occurs if the patient made a partial payment and later the insurance allowance was more than the remaining balance. The difference between the total amount of money received and the amount owed must be entered in the balance column and enclosed with parentheses or circled. This indicates a credit balance.

In actuality, the credit balance is money owed to the patient. If the patient has paid in advance or wishes to leave the overpayment in the account in anticipation of future charges, care must be taken in figuring the balance on future transactions. Whereas normally a charge increases the balance, it will decrease a credit balance.

Refunds

If a patient wishes to have an overpayment refunded, write a check for the amount due and enter the transaction on the daysheet as follows:

1. Place the ledger card on the daysheet.
2. Enter an explanation in the description column.
3. Show the existing credit balance within parentheses or encircled.
4. Write the amount of the refund in the payment column in parentheses or encircled to show that it is a subtraction.
5. Show a zero balance.

NSF (Nonsufficient Funds) Checks

Sometimes a patient sends in a check without having sufficient funds to cover it; this check is later deposited to the physician's account. The bank will return the check to you marked NSF. You must now perform two accounting functions:

1. Deduct the amount from your checking account balance.
2. Add the amount back into the patient's account balance by:
   - Entering the amount in the paid column in parentheses
   - Increasing the balance by the same amount

A brief explanation of the transaction goes into the description column (Fig. 16–8).

One-Entry Cash Transactions

For the transient patient who has no ledger card and pays at the time of service, use a receipt as

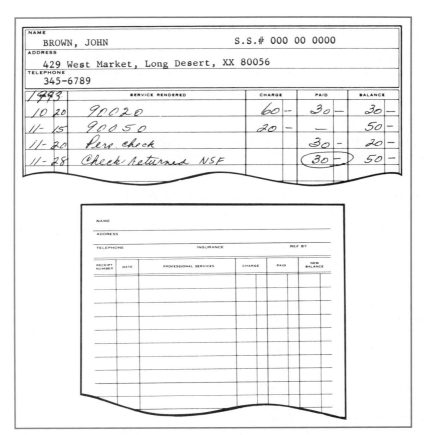

FIGURE 16–8. Entry for returned NSF checks.

PROCEDURE 16-1 POSTING SERVICE CHARGES AND PAYMENTS USING PEGBOARD SYSTEM

GOAL To post one day's charges and payments and complete daily accounting cycle using a pegboard.

EQUIPMENT AND SUPPLIES

Pegboard
Calculator
Pen
Daysheet

Carbon
Receipts
Ledger cards
Balances from previous day

PROCEDURAL STEPS

1. Prepare the board:
   - Place a new daysheet on the board.
   - Cover daysheet with carbon.
   - Place bank of receipts over the pegs aligning the top receipt with the first open writing line on the daysheet.

2. Carry forward balances from the previous day.
   Purpose: To keep all totals current.

3. Pull ledger cards for patients to be seen today.

4. Insert the ledger card under the first receipt, aligning the first available writing line of the card with the carbonized strip on the receipt.
   Purpose: To ensure that one writing will correctly post the entry to receipt, ledger, and daysheet.

5. Enter the patient's name, the date, receipt number, and any existing balance from the ledger card.

6. Detach the charge slip from the receipt and clip it to the patient's chart.
   Purpose: The doctor will indicate the service performed on the charge slip and return it to you.

7. Accept the returned charge slip at the end of the visit.

8. Enter the appropriate fee from the fee schedule.

9. Locate the receipt on the board with a number matching the charge slip.
   Purpose: To make certain it is the correct receipt.

10. Reinsert the patient's ledger card under the receipt.

11. Write the service code number and fee on the receipt.

12. Accept the patient's payment and record the amount of payment and new balance.
    Purpose: Brings patient's account up to date and provides current statement for patient.

13. Give the completed receipt to the patient.

14. Follow your agency's procedure for refiling the ledger card.

15. Repeat steps 4 to 14 for each service for the day.

16. Total all columns of the daysheet at the end of the day.
    Purpose: To determine total amount of charges, receipts and resulting balances for the day.

17. Write temporary totals in pencil.
    Purpose: To facilitate any necessary changes.

18. Complete proof of totals and enter totals in ink.

19. Enter figures for accounts receivable control.
    Purpose: To complete daily accounting cycle.

previously described. Enter the amount of the fee in the charge column and in the paid column, and a zero balance. This records the transaction on the journal page and provides a receipt for the patient. There is no need for a ledger card.

Collection Agency Payments

When a collection agency recovers an account for the physician, the agency deducts a commission, usually 40% to 50% of the amount recovered. For example, if the patient has a balance of $100 and pays it in full, the agency will send you $50. The patient now has a zero balance and you have only $50. To record this transaction on the ledger card and the daysheet you enter:

1. $100 in the previous balance
2. $50 in the cash received or paid column
3. $50 in the adjustment column
4. Zero in the new balance column

If there is no adjustment column, the $50 commission is entered in the charge column in parentheses ($50), so that the total charge business is reduced by this amount and the transaction is reflected correctly in the accounts receivable control.

ACCOUNTS RECEIVABLE CONTROL

The accounts receivable control is a daily summary of what remains unpaid on the accounts.

This is an integral part of the pegboard and double-entry systems but is a separate operation in single-entry accounting. A simple form such as the one illustrated in Figure 16–9 is useful. Using a separate page or card for each month, proceed as follows:

1. Total the unpaid balances from your entire ledger on the last day of the preceding month and enter this figure at the top of the card or page.
2. Total the charges and receipts at the end of each day and enter these figures in columns 1 and 2.
3. Determine the accounts receivable figure as follows:

   ■ If charges for the day are greater than the receipts, there is an increase in the accounts receivable. Enter this figure in column 4 and add it to the balance in column 6.
   ■ If receipts for the day are greater than the charges, there is a decrease in the accounts receivable. Enter this figure in column 5 and subtract it from the balance in column 6.

Note that the accounts receivable figure changes at the end of any day on which there is financial activity. The balance consists of the accounts receivable figure from the previous day, plus the charges for the day, minus the day's receipts and adjustments.

The total of the entire file of ledger card balances at the end of any given day should equal the accounts receivable balance shown for that day on the control form.

16

ACCOUNTS RECEIVABLE CONTROL

Month of _____December_____, 19___

Accounts receivable at end of last day of preceding month: ___$37,506___

Day	Value of Services Rendered	Received from Patients	Adjustments	+	−	Accounts Receivable Balance
1	785	1098			313	37,193
2	210	630			420	36,773
3	950	510	33	407		37,180
4						

FIGURE 16–9. Accounts receivable control for a single-entry bookkeeping system.

```
┌─────────────────────────────────────────┐
│        ACCOUNTS RECEIVABLE CONTROL        │
│                                           │
│   Total outstanding A/R balance           │
│     (from previous day)          $_____  │
│       Plus today's charges         _____ │
│                 Subtotal         $_____  │
│       Less today's payments        _____ │
│                 Subtotal         $_____  │
│       Less today's adjustments     _____ │
│   Balance outstanding           *$_____  │
└─────────────────────────────────────────┘
```

* This figure is carried forward to next page for "total outstanding A/R balance."

TRIAL BALANCE OF ACCOUNTS RECEIVABLE

A trial balance should be done once per month *after* all posting has been completed and *before* preparing the monthly statements.

The purpose of a trial balance is to disclose any discrepancies between the journal and the ledger. It does not prove the accuracy of the accounts.

For example, if a charge or payment were posted to the wrong account, or if the wrong amount were entered in the journal and then posted to the ledger, the totals would still "balance," but the accounts would not be accurate.

To begin, pull all the account cards that have a balance, enter each balance on the adding machine, and total the figures. This should equal the accounts receivable balance figure on your control.

If you have not kept a daily control, you must total all of the charges, all of the payments, and all of the adjustments for the month, and then do the computation illustrated below.

The end-of-month accounts receivable figure must agree with the figure arrived at by adding all the account card balances. The accounts are then said to be **in balance.** If the two totals do not agree, you must locate the error.

```
┌─────────────────────────────────────────┐
│  Accounts receivable at first of month  $_____ │
│    Plus total charges for month           _____ │
│               Subtotal          $_____ │
│  Less total payments for month            _____ │
│               Subtotal          $_____ │
│  Less total adjustments for month         _____ │
│  Accounts receivable at end of month    $_____ │
└─────────────────────────────────────────┘
```

Locating and Preventing Errors

After you have checked your tape and verified that you have not made an error in calculation, the first step in locating an error in your trial balance is to find the difference between the two totals. Then search the daily journal pages and the account cards for an entry of the identical amount. Check each one you find, to verify that it was posted correctly. Of course, there may be more than one error.

If there is only one error, and the amount of the error is divisible by 9, you may have transposed a figure. For example, if the difference is $81 (a number divisible by 9), you may find that you wrote $209 instead of $290. If the amount of the error is divisible by 2, you may have posted to the wrong column, reversing a debit and a credit.

A common error is made by entering the wrong amount in the "previous balance" column or in figuring the new balance. This kind of error will show up on the pegboard daily proof but could easily go undetected in the single-entry system.

Another common error is made by carrying forward a wrong total from one day to the next; for instance, carrying the beginning accounts receivable total rather than the ending accounts receivable total.

There is always a chance of sliding a number, that is, writing the first digit in the wrong column, such as writing 400 for 40, or 60 instead of 600.

Many bookkeepers avoid errors in the cents column by using a line (—) instead of writing two zeros when only even dollars are involved. For example, instead of writing $12.00, the bookkeeper will write $12.—. This eliminates the possibility of misreading zeros as other numbers. It also speeds the adding process when columns must be totaled.

If you are unable to locate any numeric error, there is the possibility that an account card was lost or overlooked, or was transferred as paid in full.

ACCOUNTS PAYABLE PROCEDURES

Invoices and Statements

When time purchases are made, that is, the item is not paid for at the time of purchase, the vendor usually includes a **packing slip** with delivery of the merchandise. A packing slip describes the items enclosed. The vendor may also enclose an **invoice.** An invoice describes the items and shows the amount due. Always check to verify that the items listed on the packing slip and invoice are included in the delivery.

Invoices should be placed in a special folder until paid. You may be making more than one purchase from the same vendor during the month. Some vendors request that payment be made from the invoice; others expect to send a statement later. A **statement** is a request for payment.

Paying for Purchases

At the time of payment, compare the statement with the invoice(s) to verify accuracy, fasten the

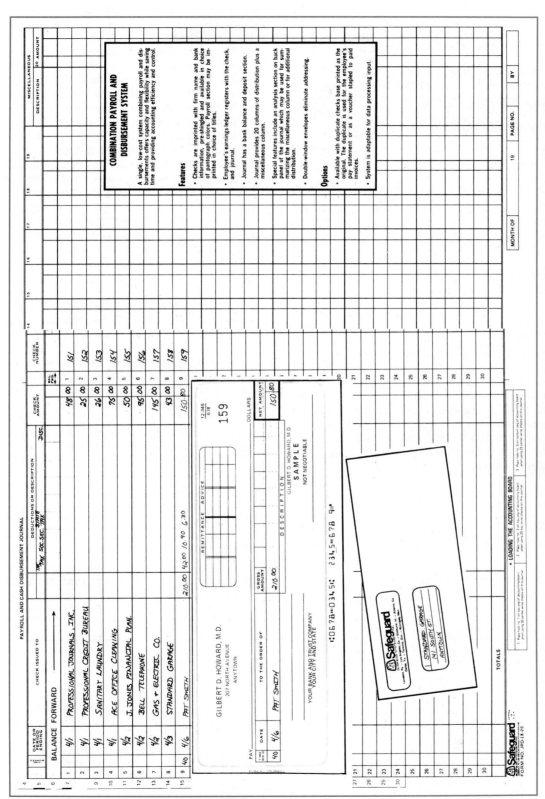

FIGURE 16-10. Payroll and cash disbursement journal showing payroll check that has been prepared for an employee and a window envelope for mailing a check. (Courtesy of Safeguard Business Systems, Atlanta, GA.)

16

statement and invoices together, write the date and check number on the statement, and place in the "paid" file.

Recording Disbursements

Both the pegboard and the single-entry accounting systems provide pages for recording disbursements. This is sometimes called a *check register* (Fig. 16–10). On these pages, disbursements are distributed to specific expense accounts such as:

- auto expense
- dues and meetings
- equipment
- insurance
- medical supplies
- office expenses
- printing, postage, and stationery
- rent and maintenance
- salaries
- taxes and licenses
- travel and entertainment
- utilities
- miscellaneous
- personal withdrawals

Each check should be entered on the disbursement page, showing the date, to whom the check was written, the number and amount of the check, and the payment allocated to one or more of the expense accounts. It is important to separate personal expenditures from business expenses. Business expenses are tax deductible and are considered in determining net income from the practice, but personal expenditures are not.

Recording Personal Expenditures

Some system must be established for transferring funds from the practice account to the physician's personal account. If the practice is incorporated, the physician is paid a salary. In the unincorporated practice, the transfer is usually accomplished through what is known in accounting terms as a *drawing account.*

The physician establishes a personal checking account and perhaps one or more savings accounts. Each month, or at any specified time, the medical assistant writes a check payable to the physician, which is then endorsed and deposited to the physician's personal account. In the disbursements journal, the amount of the check is posted in a special column headed "Personal" or "Drawing."

Although personal expenses are not deductible in determining net income from the practice, some qualify as personal deductions in computing personal income tax, so a careful accounting should be kept. Deductible expenses would include property taxes, interest paid out, contributions, and so forth.

Accounting for Petty Cash

The petty cash fund is a revolving fund. It does not change in amount except to increase or decrease the established fund. To establish the petty cash fund, a check is written payable to "Cash" or "Petty Cash" and entered in the disbursements journal under Miscellaneous. This is the only time the petty cash check is charged to Miscellaneous.

Each time the fund is replenished, the amount of the check is spread among the various accounts for which the money was used. This is determined from a record of expenditures such as that shown in Figure 16–11. The headings of the columns should correspond to headings in the disbursements journal to which they will be posted.

A pad of petty cash vouchers is kept in or near the box. For every disbursement from the fund, the petty cashier should either have a receipt or prepare a voucher similar to the one in Figure 16–12. The

No.	Date	Description	Amount	Office Expenses	Car	Misc.	Balance
	4-1	Fund established					50.00
1	4-2	Postage due	.46	.46			49.54
2	4-8	Parking fee	4.00		4.00		45.54
3	4-10	Delivery charge	2.32			2.32	43.22
4	4-25	Stationery supplies	5.47	5.47			37.75
		Total	12.25	5.93	4.00	2.32	
	5-1	Balance 37.75					
	ck #	376 12.25					
		50.00					

FIGURE 16–11. Petty cash record.

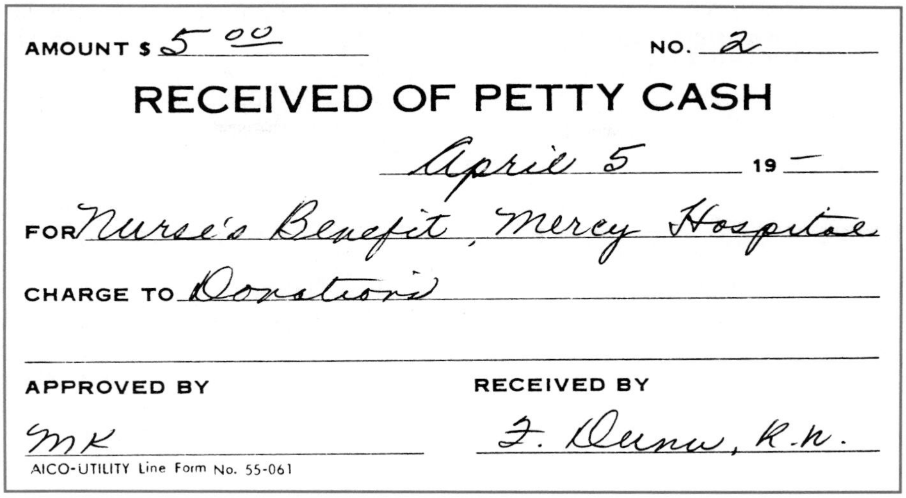
AMOUNT $ 5 00 NO. 2

RECEIVED OF PETTY CASH

April 5 19—

FOR Nurse's Benefit, Mercy Hospital

CHARGE TO Donations

APPROVED BY RECEIVED BY

MK F. Dunn, R.N.

AICO-UTILITY Line Form No. 55-061

FIGURE 16–12. Petty cash voucher.

total of the petty cash vouchers and receipts plus the amount of cash in the box must always equal the original amount of the fund.

Receipt and voucher total	$12.25
Cash on hand	37.75
Amount of fund	$50.00

Figure 16–11 shows that $50 was received into the fund on April 1. This is entered in the Description column and in the Balance column. On April 2, postage due was paid out, a voucher prepared, the number of the voucher and the amount of 46 cents entered, and a new balance brought down. On April 8, the doctor paid a parking fee. The amount of $4 was entered in the record, $4 taken from petty cash to reimburse the doctor, and the new balance of $45.54 brought down.

At the end of the month, or sooner if the fund is depleted, a check is written to "Cash" for replenishing the fund, but instead of being charged to Miscellaneous as previously, the amount of the check is divided among the various accounts affected. Our record shows that at the end of April, we have $37.75 remaining in the fund and need $12.25 to bring it back to $50.

When the check is written for $12.25, it is accounted for in the monthly distribution of expenditures by posting $5.93 as office expense, $4 as car expenses; and $2.32 as a miscellaneous expense. In this way, the expenditures from petty cash are charged to the actual accounts affected.

The accounted-for vouchers are clipped together and placed with paid invoices, the check for $12.25 is cashed, and the money is placed in the petty cash fund. The amount of the check is entered as being received into the fund, and the new balance of $50 is brought down.

Avoid the habit of borrowing from the petty cash fund. This admonition applies to the doctor as well as to the medical assistant. If the doctor requests cash from the fund, request a personal check or an office check in exchange for cash from the fund.

It is also poor policy to use the petty cash fund for making change. In facilities where patients frequently pay with currency, a separate change fund should be kept.

PERIODIC SUMMARIES

Financial summaries are compiled on monthly and annual bases. They may be prepared either by the medical assistant or by the accountant (or by computer). The common summary reports include:

- Statement of income and expense
- Cash flow statement
- Trial balance
- Accounts receivable trial balance and aging analysis
- Balance sheet

The **statement of income and expense** is also known as the profit and loss statement and covers a specific period. It lists all the income received and all expenses paid during the period. The total income is called "gross income" or "earnings." The income after deduction of all expenses is the "net income."

A **cash flow statement** starts with the amount of cash on hand at the beginning of the month (or for any specified period). It then lists the cash income and the cash disbursements made throughout the period and concludes with a statement of the amount of cash remaining on hand at the end of the period.

A **trial balance** is necessary in order to determine that the books are in balance. All of the columns on the disbursements journal must be totaled at the end of the month. The combined totals of all the expense columns must be equal to the total of

PROCEDURE 16-2   ACCOUNTING FOR PETTY CASH

GOAL To establish a petty cash fund, maintain an accurate record of expenditures for 1 month, and replenish the fund as necessary.

EQUIPMENT AND SUPPLIES

Form for petty cash fund
Pad of vouchers
Disbursement journal

Two checks
List of petty cash expenditures

PROCEDURAL STEPS

1. Determine the amount needed in the petty cash fund.

2. Write a check in the determined amount.
   Purpose: To establish a fund.

3. Record the beginning balance in the petty cash record.

4. Post the amount to miscellaneous on the disbursement record.
   Purpose: To account for original amount of fund.

5. Prepare a petty cash voucher for each amount withdrawn from the fund.
   Purpose: Voucher will be used for internal audit.

6. Record each voucher in the petty cash record and enter the new balance.
   Purpose: To record current balance and determine the need for replenishing the fund.

7. Write a check to replenish the fund as necessary.
   Note: The total of the vouchers plus the fund balance must equal the beginning amount.

8. Total the expense columns and post to the appropriate accounts in the disbursement record.
   Purpose: To record expenditures in the correct expense category.

9. Record the amount added to the fund.

10. Record the new balance in the petty cash fund.

---

the checks written. If the figures do not balance, it is necessary to recheck every entry until an error is found.

The **accounts receivable trial balance** is done prior to sending out the monthly statements. First, record the total of the accounts receivable ledger at the end of the previous month; then add the charges for the current month and subtract the adjustments and the payments received. The remainder should equal the total of the accounts receivable ledger at the end of the current month.

The **balance sheet,** also known as a statement of financial condition, shows the financial picture of the practice on a specific date. Often, it is done only on an annual basis. The balance sheet is set up using the accounting equation explained on page 254. The title of the statement had its origin in the equality of the elements—the balance between the sum of the assets and the sum of the liabilities and capital.

At the end of the accounting year, it is very simple to combine the monthly reports to compile the annual summaries. The annual summaries simplify the reporting of income for tax returns.

ACCOUNTING WITH THE AID OF THE COMPUTER

The office with an in-house computer and the appropriate software can accomplish all the described accounting operations and more in a fraction of the time required to do them manually. The role of the computer in the medical practice was discussed in Chapter 8. The office without a computer can still reap some of the benefits by using an outside computer service.

A computer service can relieve the office staff of the repetitive clerical procedures necessary in the recording of charges and in the preparation and mailing of statements and insurance forms. It can produce weekly and monthly financial reports that would be too time-consuming and perhaps beyond the capabilities of the staff to do manually.

One type of computer service is based on a telephone-linked terminal on a time-share basis with other users. Another is the batch type, in which the information is picked up at the office and taken to a computer center for processing. Whether to use computer services and the selection of what service to use are highly individualized decisions that require study and analysis of the practice. It is important to choose a service that will explain what can be expected from the computer and that will provide all the instruction and supervision necessary to ensure success in using it.

PAYROLL RECORDS

The office accounting system must include records of payroll, federal and state tax deductions, Social Security tax information, and quarterly and annual reports. These topics are discussed in Chapter 22, Management Responsibilities.

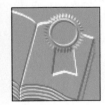

▶ **LEARNING ACHIEVEMENTS**

Are you able to:

1. Define the terms listed in the Vocabulary of this chapter?
2. Explain the differences between the two bases of accounting?
3. Cite the four kinds of information that the financial records of any business should show at all times?

4. Distinguish between a *credit balance* and a *debit balance*?
5. Complete a credit balance entry?
6. List six kinds of accounting records?
7. Name three accounting systems and list advantages and disadvantages of each?
8. State the basic accounting equation?
9. Discuss the importance of a trial balance?
10. Name five common periodic accounting summaries and their purpose?

Given the necessary information and materials, would you be able to:

1. Prepare the following items:
   Ledger account for a new patient
   Patient charge slip
   Daily posting proof
   Daily cash control proof
   Monthly trial balance
2. Journalize charges and payments in a single-entry system?
3. Post entries from the journal to the ledger?
4. Establish and maintain a petty cash fund?
5. Post service charges and payments using the pegboard system?

REFERENCES AND READINGS

Anthony, R. N., and Graham-Walker, R.: *Essentials of Accounting: A Reference Guide,* Menlo Park, CA, Addison-Wesley Publishing Co., Inc., 1985.

Colwell Systems: *One-Write Pegboard Bookkeeping System,* Champaign, IL, 1992.

Fess, P. E.: *Accounting Principles,* 6th ed., Cincinnati, South-Western Publishing Co., 1989.

Moscove, S. A.: *Accounting Fundamentals for Non-Accountants,* 2nd ed., Reston, VA, Reston Publishing Co., Inc., 1984.

16

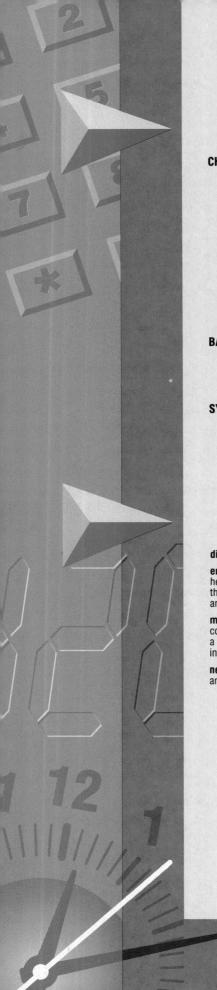

CHAPTER OUTLINE

VOCABULARY

disbursements Funds paid out.

endorser Person who signs his or her name on the back of a check for the purpose of transferring title to another person.

maker (of a check) Any individual, corporation, or legal party who signs a check or any type of negotiable instrument.

negotiable Legally transferable to another party.

payee Person named on a draft or check as the recipient of the amount shown.

payer Person who writes a check in favor of the payee.

power of attorney A legal statement in which a person authorizes another person to act as his or her attorney or agent. The authority may be limited to the handling of certain procedures. The person authorized to act as the agent is known as an *attorney in fact.*

reconciliation (of bank statement) The process of proving that the bank statement and the checkbook balance are in agreement.

teller A bank employee who is assigned the duty of waiting on the bank's customers.

third-party check A check written to the order of the person offering payment and unknown to the payee, who is a third party in the process.

17

BANKING SERVICES AND PROCEDURES

LEARNING OBJECTIVES

COGNITIVE

Upon successful completion of this chapter, you should be able to:

1. Define the terms listed in the Vocabulary.

2. State the four requirements of a negotiable instrument.

3. Discuss six advantages of using checks for the transfer of funds.

4. Explain why it is important to complete the check stub before writing a check.

5. State how you would handle mistakes made in preparing a check.

6. List and discuss eight precautions to observe in accepting checks.

7. State the purpose of a check endorsement.

8. Name and compare four kinds of endorsements.

9. Cite five reasons for depositing checks promptly.

10. Discuss the action necessary when a deposited check is returned.

PERFORMANCE

Upon successful completion of this chapter, you should be able to perform the following activities:

1. Prepare a bank deposit.

2. Correctly write a check.

3. Pay office bills by check.

4. Reconcile a bank statement with the checkbook balance.

Financial transactions in the professional office nearly always involve banking services and the use of checks. Therefore, the medical assistant must understand the responsibilities involved in accepting payments, in endorsing and depositing checks, in writing checks, and in regularly reconciling bank statements.

CHECKS

A check is a draft or an order upon a bank for the payment of a certain sum of money to a certain person therein named, or to the bearer, and is payable on demand. It is considered to be a negotiable instrument.

A **negotiable** instrument must:

- Be written and signed by a **maker**
- Contain a promise or order to pay a sum of money
- Be payable on demand or at a fixed future date
- Be payable to order or bearer

Types of Checks

You are probably already familiar with the standard personal check, but there are many additional types of checks in use in business transactions. You should be familiar with the following:

Bank draft. A check drawn by a bank against funds deposited to its account in another bank.

Cashier's check. A bank's own check drawn upon itself and signed by the bank cashier or other authorized official. It is also known as an officer's or treasurer's check. A cashier's check is obtained by paying the bank cashier the amount of the check, in cash or by personal check. Some banks charge a fee for this service. Cashier's checks are often issued to accommodate the savings account customer who does not maintain a checking account.

Certified check. This is the depositor's own check, upon the face of which the bank has placed the word "certified" or "accepted" with the date and a bank official's signature. Because the bank deducts the amount of the check from the depositor's account at the time it certifies the check, the bank can guarantee that the amount is available. A certified check, like a cashier's check, can be used when an ordinary personal check would not be acceptable. If not used, a certified check should be redeposited promptly, so that the funds previously set aside are credited back to the depositor's account.

Limited check. A check may be limited as to the amount written on it and as to the time during which it may be presented for payment. The limited check is often used for payroll or insurance checks.

Money order. Domestic money orders are sold by banks, some stores, and the United States Postal Service. The maximum face value varies according to the source. International money orders may be purchased for limited amounts, indicated in US dollars, for use in sending money abroad.

Traveler's check. Traveler's checks are designed for persons traveling where personal checks may not be accepted or for use in situations in which it is inadvisable to carry large amounts of cash. Traveler's checks are usually printed in denominations of $10, $20, $50, and $100, and sometimes $500 and $1,000. They require two signatures of the purchaser, one at the time of purchase and the other at the time of use. They are available at banks and some travel agencies.

Voucher check. A voucher check is one with a detachable voucher form. The voucher portion is used to itemize or specify the purpose for which the check is drawn. It is used for the convenience of the **payer** and shows discounts and various other itemizations. This portion of the check is removed before presenting the check for payment and provides a record for the **payee** (Fig. 17–1).

Warrant. A warrant is a check that is not considered to be negotiable but which can be evidence of a debt due because of certain services rendered, and the bearer is entitled to certain payment for this service. Government and civic agencies often issue such warrants. A claim draft on an insurance claim is a warrant issued by the insurance adjuster as evidence that the claim is valid. It authorizes the insurance company to pay the claim.

Advantages of Using Checks

Using checks for the transfer of funds has many advantages:

- Checks are both safe and convenient, particularly for making payments by mail.
- Expenditures are quickly calculated.
- Specific payments can be easily located from the check record.
- A stop-payment order can protect the payer from loss due to lost, stolen, or incorrectly drawn checks.
- Checks provide a permanent reliable record of disbursements for tax purposes.
- The deposit record provides a summary of receipts.
- Checking accounts protect the money while on deposit.

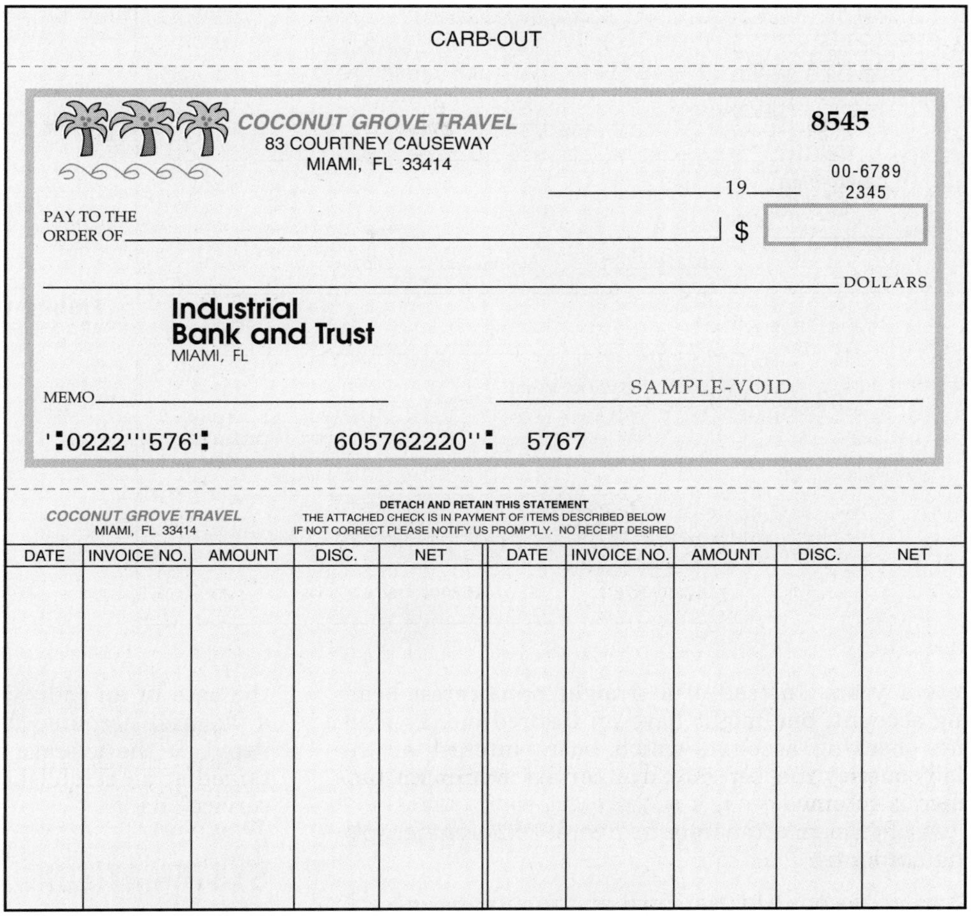

CARB-OUT

COCONUT GROVE TRAVEL
83 COURTNEY CAUSEWAY
MIAMI, FL 33414

8545

00-6789
2345

19____

PAY TO THE ORDER OF ____ $

____ DOLLARS

Industrial
Bank and Trust
MIAMI, FL

MEMO____

SAMPLE-VOID

⑆0222⑈576⑆ 605762220⑈ 5767

COCONUT GROVE TRAVEL
MIAMI, FL 33414

DETACH AND RETAIN THIS STATEMENT
THE ATTACHED CHECK IS IN PAYMENT OF ITEMS DESCRIBED BELOW
IF NOT CORRECT PLEASE NOTIFY US PROMPTLY. NO RECEIPT DESIRED

DATE	INVOICE NO.	AMOUNT	DISC.	NET	DATE	INVOICE NO.	AMOUNT	DISC.	NET

FIGURE 17–1. Page from bank order book showing sample voucher check.

17

ABA Number

The ABA number is part of a coding system originated by the American Bankers Association. It appears in the upper right area of a printed check. It is used as a simple way to identify the area where the bank upon which the check is written is located and the particular bank within the area. The code number is expressed as a fraction:

$$\frac{90\text{-}1822}{1222}$$

(Fig. 17–2). In the top part of the fraction, before the hyphen, the numbers 1 to 49 designate cities in which Federal Reserve banks are located or other key cities; the numbers from 50 to 99 refer to states or territories. The part of the number after the hyphen is a number issued to each bank for its own identification purposes. This whole ABA number is used in preparing deposit slips, to identify each check. The bottom part of the fraction includes the number of the Federal Reserve District in which the bank is located and other identifying information.

Magnetic Ink Character Recognition (MICR)

Characters and numbers printed in magnetic ink are found at the bottom of checks. They represent a common machine language, readable by machines as well as by humans. When a check is deposited, the amount of the check can also be printed in magnetic ink below the signature. MICR identification facilitates processing through a high-speed machine that reads the characters, sorts the checks, and does the bookkeeping.

BANK ACCOUNTS

Common Types of Accounts

Checking Accounts

By placing an amount of money on deposit in a bank, a depositor can set up a checking account. Simply stated, a checking account is a bank account against which checks can be written. Many variations in checking accounts have been developed in

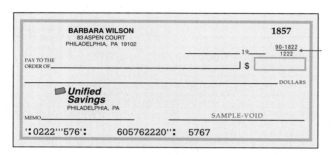

FIGURE 17-2. Sample checks. Arrows indicate ABA number.

recent years. Instead of a straight noninterest bearing account, one might have an insured money market checking account, which bears interest at the daily money market rate if a certain minimum balance is retained.

A physician often requires three different checking accounts:

- an account for personal and family expenses
- a separate checking account for office expenses
- a high-yield interest-bearing account for funds reserved for paying insurance premiums, property taxes, and other seasonal expenses

Savings Accounts

Money that is not needed for current expenses can be deposited in a savings account (Fig. 17-3). In most cases, savings accounts earn interest upon the amounts deposited; that is, the bank pays the depositor a certain percentage monthly or quarterly for the use of the money in the savings account.

The ordinary savings account draws interest at the lowest prevailing rate, has no minimum balance requirement, and no check-writing privileges.

An insured money market account requires a minimum balance, frequently $2500, draws interest at money market rates, and allows the writing of a specified number of checks (frequently three) per month. There may be a minimum amount for each transaction. Such checks are usually written for transfer of funds to a checking account.

Service Charges

In all types of accounts, the bank may charge a fee for services rendered in bookkeeping. Usually in the case of an individual account, it is a flat fee; in a business account, the fee is based on services rendered. If the average or minimum balance is maintained at an established level, the bank may forego a service charge.

SYSTEMATIZING BILL PAYING

A systematic plan should be established for the writing of checks and the paying of bills. Check writing usually is done on a specific day or days of each month. An exception sometimes arises when it is possible to realize a good discount if payment of a bill is made within a specified time, for instance 10 days. Such discounts usually are indicated at the bottom of invoices or billing statements.

When a check is written in payment of a statement or invoice, it is good practice to write on the invoice the number of the check and the date it was paid. Then, if any question arises about whether or when the bill was paid, you can readily locate the check stub.

The Business Checkbook

The checkbook most generally used in the professional office has three checks per page with a perforated stub at the left end of the check (Fig. 17-4). The checks may be in a bound soft cover or punched for a ring binder. The check and matching stubs are numbered in sequence and preprinted with the depositor's name and account number and any additional optional information such as address and telephone number. From 100 to 300 checks are usually ordered at one time, and the cost is charged against the account.

Statement of Account 14700 CT

014143759	R		1	12/20/91
Account Number	Type	Items	Page No.	Statement Date

001

Current Balance	Previous Statement Date	Previous Balance
2896.34	11/21/91	2886.59

ANSWERS TO YOUR BANKING QUESTIONS 24 HOURS A DAY,
7 DAYS A WEEK.   CALL ANSWERLINE TODAY

**** SUPER INSURED MONEY MARKET ACCOUNT ****

YOUR OPENING BALANCE OF: 2,886.59

NO   DEPOSITS LISTED TOTALING: .00

- - - - - - - - - - - - - - - OTHER   CREDITS   - - - - - - - - - - - - - - -
12-20 SUPER INSURED MONEY MKT. INT. PAID   9.75

1   CREDITS LISTED TOTALING: 9.75

NO   CHECKS LISTED TOTALING: .00

NO   DEBITS LISTED TOTALING: .00

EQUALS YOUR ENDING BALANCE OF: 2,896.34

DAILY ACCOUNT BALANCES
    DATE   BALANCE   DATE   BALANCE   DATE   BALANCE
    12-20   2896.34

- - - - - - - - - - - SUPER INSURED MONEY MARKET STATEMENT - - - - - - - - -

DATE	COLLECTED BALANCE	INTEREST RATES	DATE	COLLECTED BALANCE	INTEREST RATES
11-22	2,886.59	04.40	11-25	2,886.59	04.40
11-26	2,886.59	04.40	11-27	2,886.59	04.40
12-02	2,886.59	04.40	12-03	2,886.59	04.40
12-04	2,886.59	04.15	12-05	2,886.59	04.15
12-06	2,886.59	04.15	12-09	2,886.59	04.15
12-10	2,886.59	04.15	12-11	2,886.59	04.15
12-12	2,886.59	04.15	12-13	2,886.59	04.15
12-16	2,886.59	04.15	12-17	2,886.59	04.15
12-18	2,886.59	04.15	12-19	2,886.59	04.15
12-20	2,886.59	04.15			

********** CONTINUED ON NEXT PAGE **********

FIGURE 17-3. Example of Super Insured Money Market Account Statement. Limited check writing privilege.

17

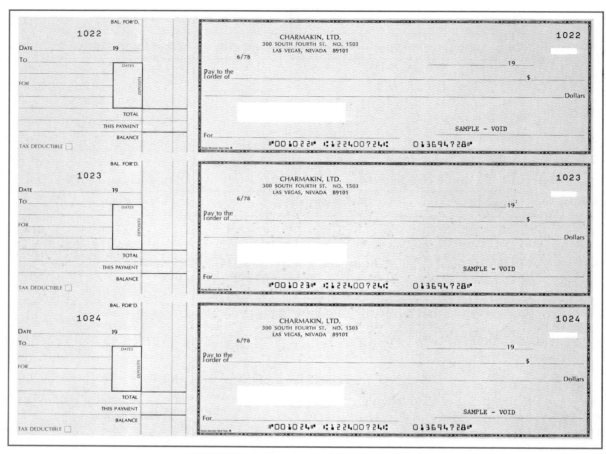

FIGURE 17-4. Example of business check with stub.

Numbered deposit slips are also supplied to the depositor.

Checkbook Stubs

The checkbook stub—the part that remains in the book after the check has been written and removed—is your own record of the checks written, date, amount, payee, and purpose. It is important that the stub be completed before the check. This prevents the possibility of writing a check and neglecting to complete the stub. If the stub is not completed and the check is sent out, you will have no record of the payee and the amount taken from the account until the canceled check is returned at a later date. Consequently, you will be unable to balance your account or determine the amount on hand until you receive those canceled checks.

Lost and Stolen Checks

If you lose any of your checks, report this to your bank promptly. The bank will place a warning on your account, and signatures on incoming checks will be carefully inspected to detect possible forgeries.

If you suspect that your checks have been stolen, first make a report to the police in the city or town where the theft took place. Then notify your bank and tell them the time, date, and place the police report was made. A warning will be placed on your account. In some cases, you may be asked to close your account and open a new one under a different number.

As long as you have reported your checks missing or stolen to the proper authorities, you usually will not be held responsible for losses due to forgery. The bank or merchant who accepts the forged checks will be charged for the loss. For this reason, anyone accepting a check from a person who is not known personally must be very careful about establishing the person's identity.

Writing Checks

The handling and writing of checks must be done with extreme care.

1. Before you write the check, fill out the stub or the place designated for recording your expenditures (Fig. 17-5). Include the date, name of payee, amount of check, the new balance to be

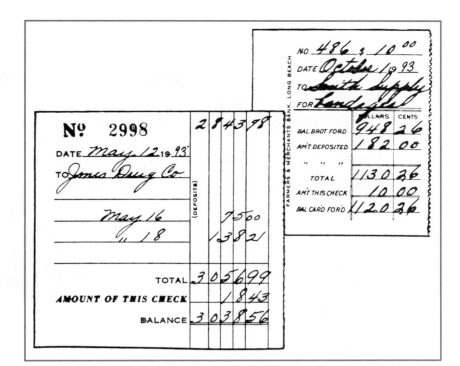

FIGURE 17–5. Methods of filling out check stubs.

carried forward, and usually the purpose of the check.

2. Both the check and the stub should be written in ink or typewritten. The typewritten check has a more professional look.

3. Date the check the day it is written (do not postdate).

4. Write the name of the payee after the printed words, "pay to the order of." Always try to write the name of the payee correctly. When paying bills, you will usually find a notation on the invoice stating "Make check payable to ____" with the necessary information following. Do not use abbreviations unless so instructed.

5. Leave no space before the name, and follow it with three dashes if there is space remaining.

6. Omit personal titles from the names of payees.

7. If a payee is receiving a check as an officer of an organization, the name of the office should follow the name. For example, "John F. Jones, Treasurer," or "Margaret F. Brown, President."

8. Double-check your figures to verify that the amount of the check is recorded correctly on the stub, in the box for the dollar ($) amount, and on the line where the amount is written in words.

9. Start writing at the extreme left of each space. Leave no blank spaces. Keep the cents notation close to the dollars figure to prevent alteration.

10. If necessary, a check can be written for less than one dollar, but be very careful to emphasize the amount. The figures by the $ sign may be circled to assure proper attention, as ($.65) or enclosed in parentheses, as $–(65¢). When writ-

ing out the amount of money, write "only sixty-five cents–". The word dollars should not be crossed out. Figures 17–6 and 17–7 show examples of correct and incorrect check writing.

Handling Corrections and Mistakes

Do not cross out, erase, or change any part of a check. Checks are printed on sensitized paper so that erasures are easily noticeable, and the bank has the right to refuse to pay on any check that has been altered.

If a mistake is made, write the word "VOID" on the stub and the check, but do not throw out or destroy the check. It should be filed with the canceled checks so that it is available for auditing purposes.

Writing "Cash" Checks

A cash check is a check made payable to cash or bearer. Such checks are completely negotiable. Since these checks are easily cashed without positive identification, it is poor policy to write cash checks unless they are to be cashed at the time they are written. Banks may require that the person receiving the cash endorse the check.

One-Write Check Writing

A one-write system of writing checks can save time and minimize errors in medical office **disbursements.** The office with a pegboard bookkeep-

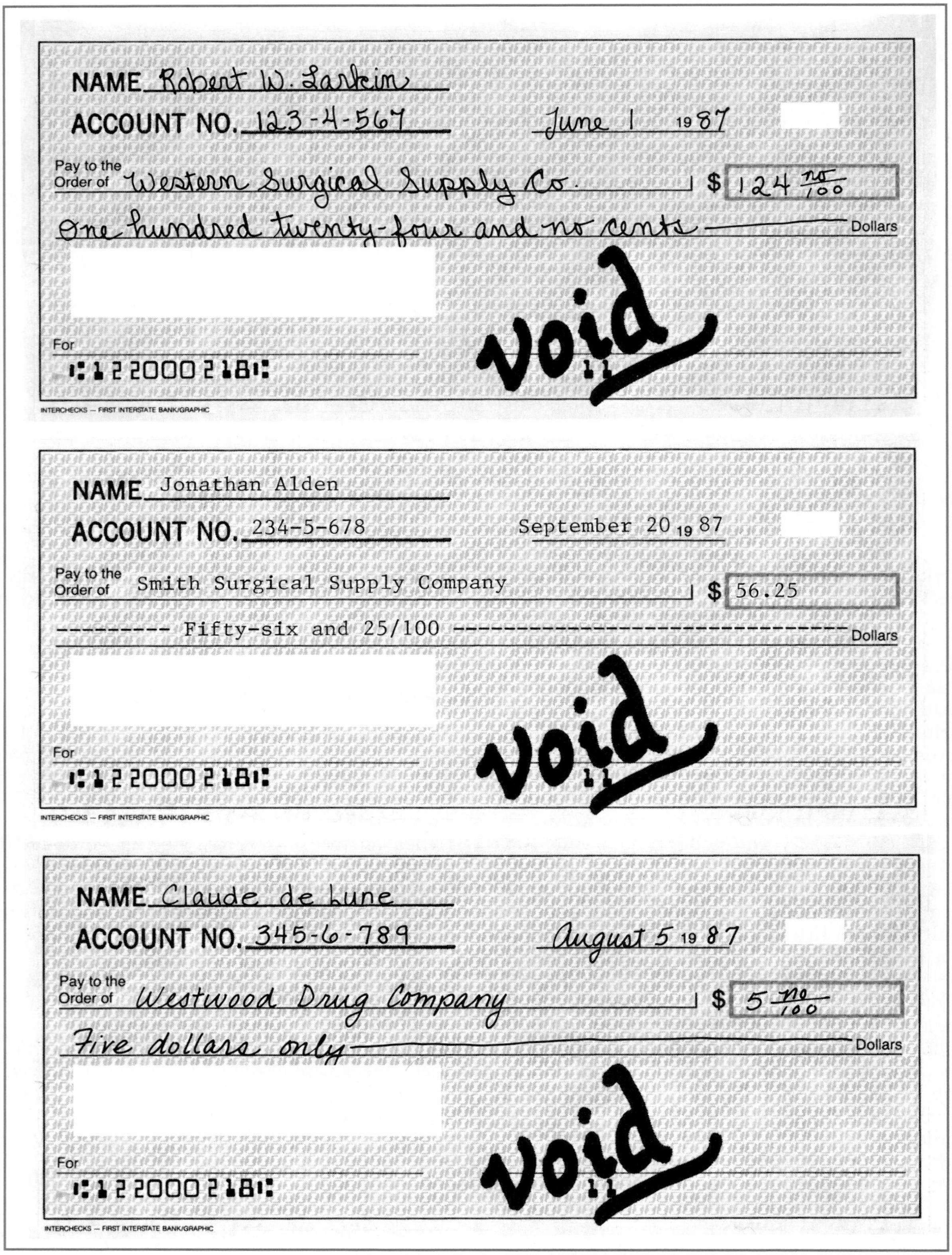
NAME Robert W. Larkin
ACCOUNT NO. 123-4-567 June 1 19 87
Pay to the Order of Western Surgical Supply Co. $ 124 no/100
One hundred twenty-four and no cents Dollars
For
⑆122000218⑆
void
INTERCHECKS — FIRST INTERSTATE BANK/GRAPHIC

NAME Jonathan Alden
ACCOUNT NO. 234-5-678 September 20 19 87
Pay to the Order of Smith Surgical Supply Company $ 56.25
--------- Fifty-six and 25/100 --------------------------------- Dollars
For
⑆122000218⑆
void
INTERCHECKS — FIRST INTERSTATE BANK/GRAPHIC

NAME Claude de Lune
ACCOUNT NO. 345-6-789 August 5 19 87
Pay to the Order of Westwood Drug Company $ 5 no/100
Five dollars only Dollars
For
⑆122000218⑆
void
INTERCHECKS — FIRST INTERSTATE BANK/GRAPHIC

FIGURE 17-6. Correct methods of writing checks.

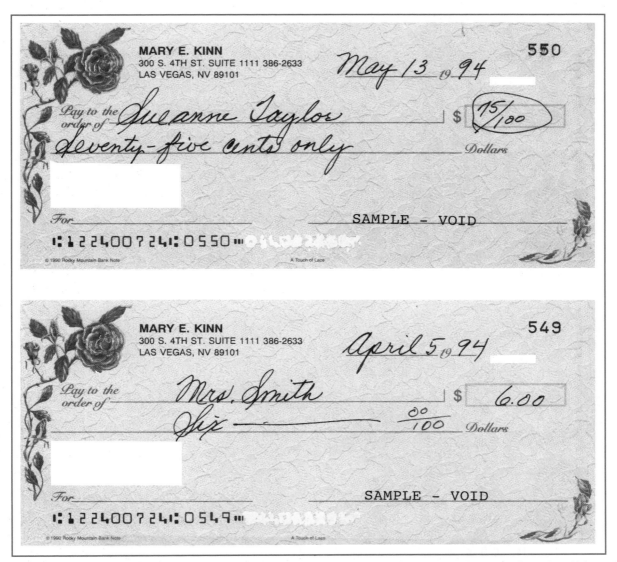

FIGURE 17-7. *Top,* Correct method of writing a check. *Bottom,* Incorrect method of writing a check: *1,* incomplete name; *2,* check could be made into $26 very easily; *3,* the "00" could be made into 88.

ing system (see Chapter 16) may wish to include one-write check writing. By using a combination check writing system, such as the one illustrated in Fig. 17–8, one check and one record of checks drawn handle both bill paying and payroll check writing.

When the check is written, a permanent record is created through the carbonized line of the check onto the record of checks drawn and the employee's payroll record, including a record of all deductions. Space is provided for the payee's address so that the check can be mailed in a window envelope. This not only saves time but ensures that the check goes to the right address. Suppliers of basic pegboard systems can also provide a check-writing system such as the one described.

Signing Checks

After all checks have been written, place them, along with the invoices or other verifying information, on the physician's desk for signature. In some facilities, the medical assistant who has charge of the financial matters is also allowed to sign the checks. This is accomplished by filing a **power of attorney** at the depositor's bank. The power of attorney may limit the check-signing authorization to a certain amount or to a limited time period.

Mailing Checks

When checks are sent through the mail, the check should not be visible through the envelope. Either place the check within a letter or fold it into a plain

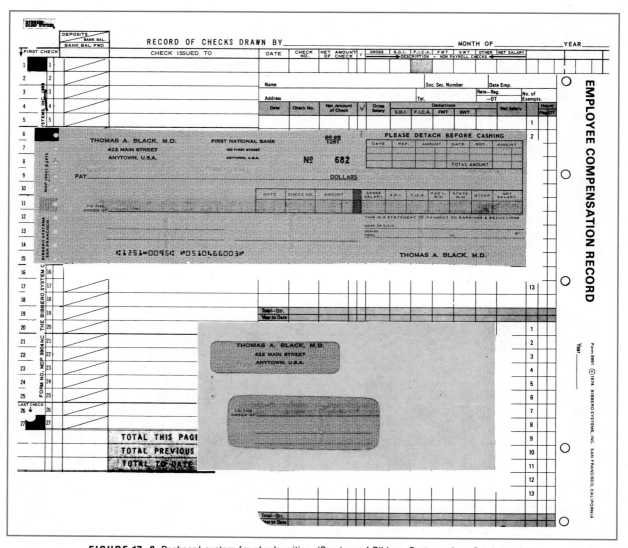

FIGURE 17-8. Pegboard system for check writing. (Courtesy of Bibbero Systems, Inc., Petaluma, CA.)

sheet of paper. Checks may be folded at the right end to conceal the amount of money written.

Make certain the envelopes are sealed before mailing, and mail all checks yourself as soon as possible after writing.

SPECIAL PROBLEMS WITH CHECKS

Special problems may arise when a check is written on nonexistent funds or when a payer wishes, for a legitimate reason, to prevent the payee from cashing a check.

Account Overdrawn or Overdraft

When a depositor draws a check for more than the amount on deposit in the account, the account becomes overdrawn. In most states, it is illegal to issue a check for more than the amount on deposit in the bank. Should this happen through error or oversight, the bank may refuse to honor the check and will return it to the bank that presented it for payment. Such a check is said to "bounce."

If the check is written by an established depositor, the bank may honor the check and notify the depositor that the account is overdrawn. If the bank thus pays or "covers" the check, it issues an overdraft on the depositor's account.

Stop-Payment Order

A depositor or maker of a check who wishes to rescind or stop payment of that check has the right to request the bank to stop payment on it. Stop-payment orders should be used only in emergencies. Reasons for stop-payment requests are:

- Loss of a check
- Disagreement about a purchase
- Disagreement about a payment

PAYMENT FROM PATIENTS

Acknowledging Payment in Full

If payment in full is to be recognized in regard to a given check, the statement "Payment in Full to Date" must appear on the back of the check, above the endorsement, not on the face of the check. Canceled checks are a receipt for the maker of the check, not for the payee.

Precautions in Accepting Checks

The medical assistant is frequently presented with checks in payment for the physician's services. In most cases, these are personal checks. The following guidelines should be observed:

- Scan the check carefully for the correct date, amount, and signature.
- Do not accept a check with corrections on it.
- If you do not know the person presenting a personal check, ask for identification and compare signatures.
- Accept an out-of-town check, government check, or payroll check only if you are well acquainted with the person presenting it and it does not exceed the amount of the payment.
- Acceptance of "third-party" checks is generally unwise. A **third-party check** is one made out to your patient by a party unknown to you. A check from the patient's health insurance carrier is an exception.
- When accepting a postal money order for payment, make certain it has only one endorsement. Postal money orders with more than two endorsements will not be honored.
- Do not accept a check marked "Payment in Full" unless it does pay the account in full up to and including the date on which it is received. If a check so marked is less than the amount due, you will be unable to collect the balance on the account once you have accepted and deposited such a check. It is illegal for you to scratch out the words "Payment in Full."
- Accepting checks written for more than the amount due is poor policy because, first, you will have to return cash for the difference between the amount of the check and the amount owed. If the check is not honored by the bank, your office will suffer the loss not only of the amount of the check but also of the amount returned in cash. Second, the canceled check could be used by the patient to indicate the amount paid on account.

ENDORSEMENT OF CHECKS

An endorsement is a signature plus any other writing on the back of a check by which the **endorser** transfers all rights in the check to another party. Endorsements are made in ink, with either pen or rubber stamp, on the back of the check across the left (or perforated) end.

Necessity for Endorsement

The Uniform Negotiable Instrument Act, applicable in all states, explains the need of an endorsement as follows:

> An instrument is negotiated when it is transferred from one person to another in such a manner as to pass title to another party. If payable to bearer, it is negotiated by delivery. If payable to order, it is negotiated by the endorsement of the holder completed by delivery.

The name of the last endorser of the check shows who last received the money. If a check is cashed for someone who did not endorse it and is returned for some reason, the bank will charge the check to the last endorser, not to the last person receiving the money. For this reason, it is not wise to cash a check made payable to another party without having the endorsement of the person who delivered the check to you for cashing.

Kinds of Endorsements

There are four principal kinds of endorsements. Blank and restrictive endorsements are the ones most commonly used.

Blank endorsement. The payee signs only his or her name. This makes the check payable to the bearer. It is the simplest and most common type of endorsement on personal checks but should be used only when the check is to be cashed or deposited immediately.

Restrictive endorsement. This specifies the purpose of the endorsement. You use a restrictive endorsement in preparing checks for deposit to the physician's checking account. An example is shown in Figure 17-9.

Special endorsement. This endorsement includes words specifying the person to whom the endorser makes the check payable. For instance, a check naming Helen Barker as payee may be endorsed to the physician by writing on the back of the check

Pay to the order of
Theodore F. Wilson, M.D.
Helen Barker

Pay to the Order of
Midwest National Bank
Main Branch
For Deposit Only
CARLOS MACAULEY
301-012697

FIGURE 17-9. Example of restrictive endorsement.

The check is still negotiable but requires Dr. Wilson's signature or endorsement.

Qualified endorsement. The effect of the endorsement is qualified by disclaiming or destroying any future liability of the endorser. Usually the words "Without Recourse" are written above by an attorney who accepts a check on behalf of a client but who has no personal claim in the transaction.

Endorsement Procedures

The medical assistant may use a blank endorsement when cashing a check to replenish the petty cash fund. This endorsement should be made only at the time of exchanging the check for cash.

As checks from patients and other sources arrive, they should be recorded on the ledger and immediately stamped with the restrictive endorsement "For Deposit Only." This is a safeguard against lost or stolen checks.

Any endorsement should agree exactly with the name on the face of the check. If the name of the payee is misspelled, it is usually necessary for the payee to endorse the check the way the name is spelled on the face, followed by the correctly spelled signature. The Uniform Commercial Code, Section 3-203, states:

> Where an instrument is made payable to a person under a misspelled name or one other than his own, he may endorse in that name or his own or both; but signature in both names may be required by a person paying or giving value for the instrument.

Most banks accept routine stamp endorsement that is restricted to "Deposit Only," if the customer is well known and maintains an established account.

Some insurance checks or drafts require a personal signature endorsement; a stamped endorsement is not acceptable. This will be stated on the back of the check. In such cases, ask the payee to endorse the check, then stamp immediately below the signature the restrictive endorsement "For Deposit Only."

MAKING DEPOSITS

Financial duties of the medical assistant include depositing checks and reconciling the bank statements with the checkbook.

Checks should be deposited promptly because:

- There is the possibility of a stop-payment order.
- The check may be lost, misplaced, or stolen.
- Delay may cause the check to be returned because of insufficient funds.
- The check may have a restricted time for cashing.
- It is a courtesy to the payer.

Preparing the Deposit

Deposit slips are itemized memoranda of cash or other funds that a depositor presents to the bank with the money to be credited to the account. All deposits must be accompanied by a deposit slip. A carbon or photocopy of the deposit slip should be kept on file.

There are several types of deposit slips, sometimes called *deposit tickets*. The commercial slip is used for the office checking account. The deposit slips are printed with the number of the account in magnetic ink characters to correspond with the checks. Preprinted deposit slips are ordered along with the checks.

Some write-it-once accounting systems include a deposit slip that the bank will accept as the itemization if it is attached to the customer's numbered deposit slip. The deposit slip should be prepared before you go to the bank, with the money organized and ready to present to the bank teller.

Payment on patient accounts is generally made by check, but some payments are made in currency (paper money). Each type of funds is recorded separately on the deposit slip. The currency is usually listed first. Organize the currency so that all of the bills are facing in the same direction—that is, the black side up and the portrait right side up. Place the larger bills on top, graduating down to the smallest ones.

The coin amount is listed next. Count the coins and place them in an envelope. If there is a large quantity of a certain coin, place it in rolls provided by the bank. The depositor should sign these rolls, since the rolled coins are usually not counted by the **teller.**

Checks are recorded individually by the ABA number. If the checks are arranged alphabetically by the names of the patient accounts, with these names included on your office copy of the deposit slip, you will have a ready reference of checks deposited should a question arise regarding a patient's payment. Follow this procedure:

1. List all checks on the back of the deposit slip (Fig. 17–10*A*).
2. Transfer the total to the front of the slip (Fig. 17–10*B*).
3. Enter the amount of the total deposit on the deposit slip stub (Fig. 17–10*C*).

Money orders, either postal, express, or others, are identified by "PO Money Order" or "Exp. MO." Remember that money orders cannot have more than two endorsements.

The deposit slip should be carefully totaled and the total entered in the checkbook. Any torn bills should be mended with transparent tape. Clip the currency together, and clip the checks in a separate packet. Then place the entire amount in a heavy envelope for taking to the bank. Deposit daily if possible.

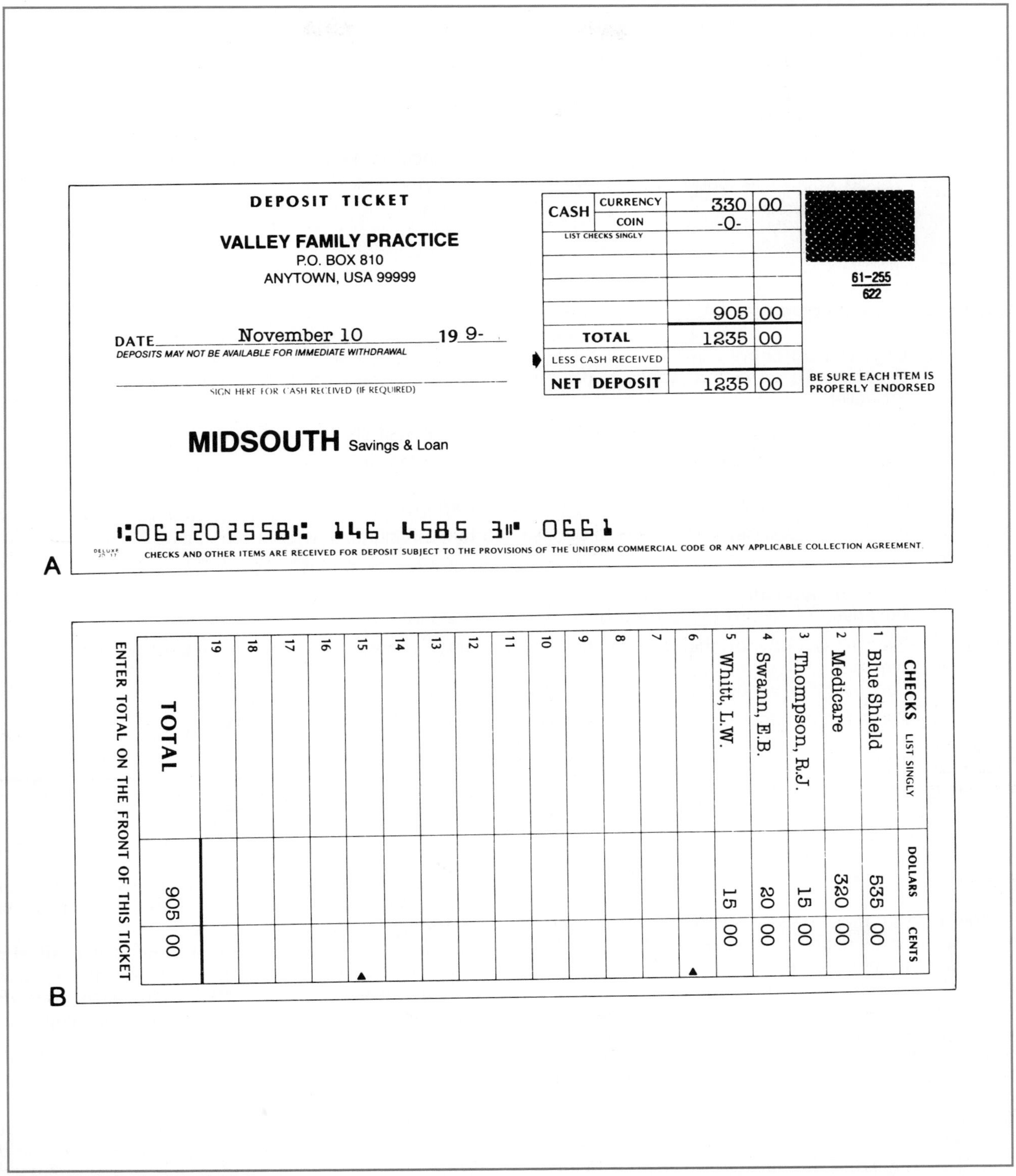

A

DEPOSIT TICKET

VALLEY FAMILY PRACTICE
P.O. BOX 810
ANYTOWN, USA 99999

DATE November 10 19 9-
DEPOSITS MAY NOT BE AVAILABLE FOR IMMEDIATE WITHDRAWAL

SIGN HERE FOR CASH RECEIVED (IF REQUIRED)

CASH	CURRENCY	330	00
	COIN	-0-	
LIST CHECKS SINGLY			
		905	00
TOTAL		1235	00
LESS CASH RECEIVED			
NET DEPOSIT		1235	00

61-255
622

BE SURE EACH ITEM IS PROPERLY ENDORSED

MIDSOUTH Savings & Loan

⑆0622025581⑆ 146 4585 3⑈ 0661

CHECKS AND OTHER ITEMS ARE RECEIVED FOR DEPOSIT SUBJECT TO THE PROVISIONS OF THE UNIFORM COMMERCIAL CODE OR ANY APPLICABLE COLLECTION AGREEMENT.

B

CHECKS LIST SINGLY	DOLLARS	CENTS
1 Blue Shield	535	00
2 Medicare	320	00
3 Thompson, R.J.	15	00
4 Swann, E.B.	20	00
5 Whitt, L.W.	15	00
6		
7		
8		
9		
10		
11		
12		
13		
14		
15		
16		
17		
18		
19		
TOTAL	905	00

ENTER TOTAL ON THE FRONT OF THIS TICKET

FIGURE 17-10. *A*, Back of deposit slip. *B*, Front of deposit slip. (From Lane, K.: Saunders Manual of Medical Assisting Practice. Philadelphia, W.B. Saunders Co., 1993, p. 103.)

PROCEDURE 17-1   PREPARING A BANK DEPOSIT

GOAL   To prepare a bank deposit for the day's receipts and complete appropriate office records related to the deposit.

EQUIPMENT AND SUPPLIES

Currency
Six checks for deposit
Deposit slip

Endorsement stamp (optional)
Typewriter
Envelope

PROCEDURAL STEPS

1. Organize currency.
   Purpose: To arrange currency in the best order for speedy and accurate presentation to the teller.

2. Total the currency and record the amount on the deposit slip.

3. Place restrictive endorsements on the checks, using an endorsement stamp or the typewriter.
   Purpose: To transfer title and protect checks from loss or theft.

4. List each check separately on the deposit slip by ABA number and its amount.

5. Total the amount of currency and checks and enter on the deposit slip.

6. Enter the amount of the deposit in the checkbook.
   Purpose: To record the current balance in the account.

7. Prepare a copy of the deposit slip for the office record, including the names of the payers.
   Purpose: For verification of checks deposited, if necessary.

8. Place the currency, checks, and deposit slip in an envelope for transporting to the bank.

Depositing by Mail

Depositing by mail saves time and is easily accomplished if the deposit consists of checks only. Banks usually supply their customers with special mailing deposit slips and envelopes upon request (Fig. 17–11). Some mailing deposit slips have an attached portion that the bank will stamp and return to the customer as a receipt. Others may provide the customer with a receipt card that is sent along with the deposit each time for the bank's notation. The mailer shown in Figure 17–11 has a peel-off receipt for your records. Mailed deposits are prepared in the same manner as are regular deposits, but certain precautions should be observed:

- Do not send cash or currency by mail. If this is absolutely necessary, then send it by registered mail.

- Use only a restrictive endorsement; use a deposit stamp or write the notation "For deposit only to the account of xxxx."

- If you have not obtained mailing deposit slips or your bank does not provide them, make duplicate slips and mail them with your deposit. Ask the bank to stamp one copy and return it to you as a receipt.

"Hold" on Account

Under certain circumstances, money that is deposited may not be immediately available for use. A "Hold for Uncollected Funds (UCF)" may be placed for the full amount of a check you deposit if it is:

- For a sizable amount
- Drawn on another bank or another branch of your bank

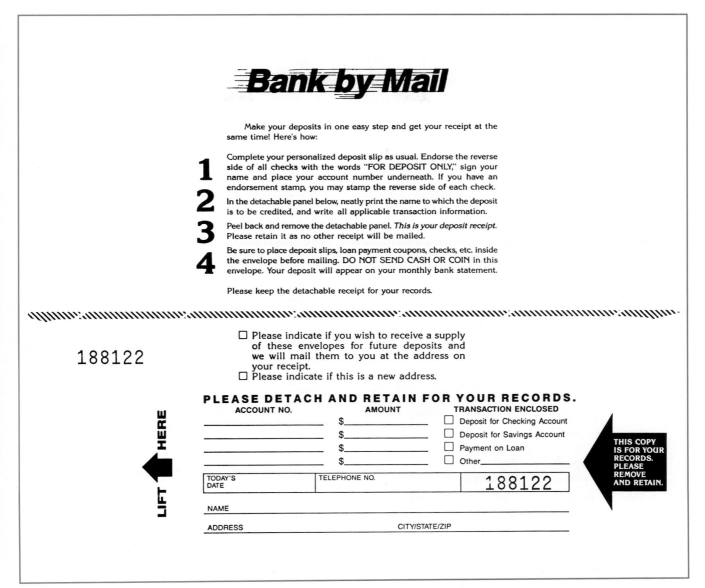

FIGURE 17–11. Example of bank-by-mail deposit envelope.

● Issued by a person or organization not known to the bank

The hold means that you cannot use the funds until the check has cleared (been processed and paid to your account).

You will be told if a hold has been placed on your account. The teller will note the hold in your deposit record by writing "UCF" and the number of days the hold will be in effect; this will appear next to the date of deposit. If the deposit was made by mail, you will be either telephoned or notified of the hold by return mail.

The hold will be for a specified number of business days and for the full amount of the check. After that time, you can begin to draw against the

funds. If for some reason the check does not clear, you will be notified.

Returned Checks

Occasionally, the bank may return a deposited check because of some irregularity such as a missing signature or missing endorsement. More often, it is because the payer has insufficient funds on deposit to cover the check.

If the check is stamped "NSF," indicating non-sufficient funds, do not delay in contacting the person who gave you the check. If you are unable to contact the maker of a bad check, waste no time in tracking down all leads, such as referrals, numbers

The Complete Statement®
DIRECT INQUIRIES TO (258)   (397) ACCT NO.   6
                                 (PER)   ITM028739   X

                                                                                  10
                                                                                  1 B

                                                           PAGE   1
                              THIS STATEMENT DATE   JANUARY 15, 1992
                              NEXT STATEMENT DATE   FEBRUARY 13, 1992

        WE MEAN BUSINESS... STAY LIQUID AND EARN SOLID INTEREST.
        OPEN A MARKET INTEREST ACCOUNT TODAY!

CHECKING ACCOUNT 253-5-21462   SUMMARY
    BALANCE FORWARD AS OF 12-13-91 . . . .   5,910.98
       TOTAL DEPOSITS/CREDITS. 2,888.64
       TOTAL CHECKS/DEBITS 787.87
       SERVICE CHARGES 00
    ENDING BALANCE 8,011.75
    MINIMUM BALANCE ON 01-13 . . . .   5,423.11
    AVERAGE BALANCE. 5,702.00

                        CHECKING ACCOUNT TRANSACTIONS
  CHECKS
  CHECK NO   DATE   AMOUNT   CHECK NO   DATE   AMOUNT   CHECK NO   DATE   AMOUNT
       131 12-26   100.00   378* 12-17   11.97   380 12-24   142.90
       376* 01-13   33.00   379 12-16   200.00   381 01-14   300.00
  DEPOSITS
  DATE   AMOUNT DATE   AMOUNT DATE   AMOUNT DATE   AMOUNT
  01-14   2,888.64

ONLY FIRST INTERSTATE BANK HAS THE EXTRA MILE SERVICE GUARANTEE.

A BALANCE PLUS CREDIT LINE TIED TO YOUR CHECKING HELPS PREVENT BOUNCED CHECKS.

LET US HELP YOU SAVE MONEY EASILY. OPEN AN AUTOMATIC SAVINGS PLAN TODAY!

Note: An asterisk (*) next to any check listed above means there has been a break in the numerical sequence of your checks.

Notice: Please see reverse side and any accompanying statement(s) for important information. Examine this statement carefully and report any irregularities promptly.

FIGURE 17–12. Example of regular checking account statement.

you obtained from credit cards, driver's license, and so forth. There are several places to which bad checks may be reported. Credit associations are often a great help when such a problem arises. Turn the account over to a qualified collection agency if you do not succeed in collecting on the account yourself within a short time.

If a check is returned to your office marked "No Account," and it is a check that you had deposited promptly, you have obviously been swindled. This check should be given to the police, the local Better Business Bureau, or your collection agency.

BANK STATEMENT

A statement is periodically sent by the bank to the customer; it shows the status of the customer's account on a given date. This statement indicates the beginning balance, deposits received, checks paid, bank charges, and ending balance at the time the statement is prepared (Fig. 17–12). The bank statement is usually accompanied by the customer's canceled checks.

Some banks are now microfilming canceled checks and storing the information in the bank's computer. The customer is asked for permission to use this procedure and has the privilege of requesting a copy of any check when needed. Bank statements are prepared at regular intervals, usually once per month. The bank statement is also known as a "bank reconciliation."

Reconciling the Bank Statement

The bank statement balance and the customer's checkbook balance will usually be different, except in a relatively inactive account. The two balances must be reconciled. The **reconciliation** discloses any errors that may exist in the checkbook or, on rare occasions, in the bank statement (Fig. 17–13). Most banks ask to be notified within 10 days of any error found in the statement. The bank statement should be reconciled as soon as it is received. You will usually find a form to follow in carrying out this procedure on the back of the bank statement.

The reconciliation procedure may be put in a formula, as shown below:

Bank statement balance	$_____
Less outstanding checks	$_____
Plus deposits not shown	$_____
CORRECTED BANK STATEMENT BALANCE	$_____
Checkbook balance	$_____
Less any bank charges	$_____
CORRECTED CHECKBOOK BALANCE	$_____

If these balances agree, you may stop here. If they do not agree, *subtract* the lesser from the greater; the difference will usually give you a clue to locating the error.

In searching for a possible error, ask yourself these questions:

- Did you forget to include one of the outstanding checks?
- Is your arithmetic correct?
- Did you fail to record a deposit or did you record it twice?
- Do all stubs and checks agree?
- Have you carried your figures forward correctly?
- Have you transposed a figure? (If the amount of your error is divisible by nine, you probably did.)
- Did your employer write a check without your knowledge?
- Did you fail to correct your checkbook balance at the time of the previous statement?

Many people find the reconciliation process confusing at first, but after a few times it becomes easier and fairly routine.

SAFE DEPOSIT BOX

Most commercial banks and many savings institutions have safe deposit boxes that may be rented by their customers. Safe deposit boxes provide protection for valuable papers and personal property for a moderate fee. They are obtainable in various sizes to suit the need of the customer. Chapter 14 (Medical Records Management) lists certain items that might be placed in a safe deposit box. The medical assistant may be asked to keep a perpetual inventory of the contents of the safe deposit box.

The box provides protection in several ways. The box itself is a metal container that is locked with two keys into a compartment in the bank's vault. One key is in the possession of the customer; the second key is held by the bank. The bank is very strict about giving access to the safe deposit boxes. The customer must register on a special form when requesting access to the box. After signatures have been compared, the customer is admitted to the vault, accompanied by a bank attendant. The attendant opens one lock with the bank key and opens the other lock with the customer's key. The box may then be removed and taken to a private room, or, if the customer merely wishes to place something in the box, this can be done and the box can be immediately replaced and locked.

The customer is given two identical keys upon renting the box. These must be guarded carefully because they cannot be duplicated, and the customer must return both keys to the bank when the box is relinquished. If a key is lost, the bank will charge a

17

BALANCING YOUR ACCOUNT

1. First, review this statement and mark off (✓) the corresponding entries in your account register.

2. **Add** to your register balance the amount of any deposits, interest credited, or other credits on this statement which you have not previously added.

3. **Subtract** from your register balance the amount of any checks or other charges recorded on this statement which you have not already subtracted. (For example, service charges, automated teller machine withdrawals, automatic loan or bill payments, transfers to other accounts, check printing charges, etc.)

4. List below all **outstanding** items (checks, automated teller machine withdrawals, automatic deductions, etc.) from your register that are not reflected on this statement and total them.

5. Using the Account Summary below, enter the ending balance as shown on the front of this statement.

6. Enter any deposits to your account after the statement date and add them to your ending balance.

7. Subtract the total amount of the outstanding items. The remaining balance should agree with your register balance. If it does not, use the check list at the bottom of this page to find the error.

**Outstanding Items Not
Charged On This Statement**

NO.	AMOUNT	NO.	AMOUNT
	$		$
	TOTAL $		

Account Summary

Ending Balance Shown
On This Statement $_____

ADD: Deposits Not
Credited On
This Statement
(if any) $_____

_____

_____

TOTAL $_____

SUBTRACT: Total
→ Outstanding Items $_____

BALANCE $_____

IF YOUR ACCOUNT DOES NOT BALANCE, PLEASE CHECK THE FOLLOWING:

_____ Have you checked all addition and subtraction in your register?

_____ Have you correctly entered all items in your register?

_____ Have you carried the correct balance forward from one register page to the other?

_____ Have you deducted all fees and charges?

_____ Have you added any interest credited to your register?

FIGURE 17–13. Reverse side of bank statement. Use for reconciling your checking account.

PROCEDURE 17-2   RECONCILING A BANK STATEMENT

GOAL   To reconcile a bank statement with the checking account.

EQUIPMENT AND SUPPLIES

Ending balance of previous statement
Current bank statement
Canceled checks for current month

Checkbook stubs
Calculator
Pen

PROCEDURAL STEPS

1. Compare the opening balance of the new statement with the closing balance of the previous statement.
   Purpose: To determine that the balances are in agreement.

2. Compare the canceled checks with the items on the statement.
   Purpose: To verify that they are your checks and that they are listed in the right amount.

3. Arrange the canceled checks in numeric order and compare with the checkbook stubs.

4. Place a checkmark (✓) on each stub for which a canceled check has been returned.
   Purpose: To locate any outstanding checks.

5. List and total the outstanding checks.

6. Subtract the total of the outstanding checks from the bank statement balance.
   Note: Do not include any certified checks as outstanding because their amount has already been deducted from the account.

7. Add to the total in Step 6 any deposits made but not included in the bank statement.
   Purpose: To correct the credits in the bank statement balance.

8. Total any bank charges that appear on the bank statement and subtract them from the checkbook balance. Such charges may include service charges, automatic withdrawals or payments, and NSF checks.
   Purpose: To correct the checkbook balance.

9. If the checkbook balance and the statement balance do not agree, repeat the process.

---

fee; if both keys are lost, the fee is considerably higher because the lock must be changed.

MEDICAL ASSISTANT'S POSITION OF TRUST

The medical assistant who manages the financial responsibilities of a medical practice is in a position of great trust. Conscientious and reliable attention to detail in this position can be a great source of job satisfaction and an attribute toward job security.

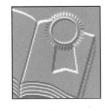

▶ **LEARNING ACHIEVEMENTS**

Are you able to:

1. Define the terms listed in the Vocabulary of this chapter?
2. Name the requirements of a negotiable instrument?
3. Discuss the advantages of using checks for the transfer of funds?
4. Show why the check stub should be completed before writing a check?
5. Show how you would correct any mistake made in preparing a check?

6. Discuss the precautions to observe in accepting checks?
7. Explain the purpose of check endorsements and compare the four kinds of endorsements?
8. List five reasons for depositing checks promptly?
9. Describe what you would do about a deposited check that is returned by the bank?
10. Correctly prepare a check?
11. Prepare a bank deposit?
12. Reconcile a bank statement?

REFERENCES AND READINGS

American Medical Association: *The Business Side of Medical Practice,* Chicago, The Association, 1989.

Brock, H., and Palma, C.: *Accounting Principles and Applications,* 6th ed., New York, McGraw-Hill Book Co., 1990.

Campbell, T.: *Principles of Accounting,* San Diego, Harcourt Brace Jovanovich, 1989.

Fess, P. E.: *Accounting Principles,* 6th ed., Cincinnati, South-Western Publishing Co., 1989.

CHAPTER EIGHTEEN

——

BILLING AND COLLECTING PROCEDURES

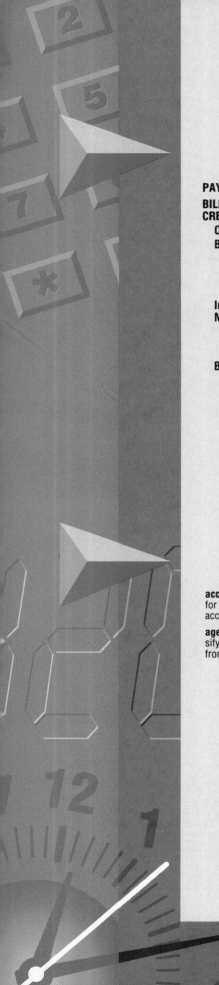

CHAPTER OUTLINE

PAYMENT AT TIME OF SERVICE

BILLING AFTER EXTENSION OF CREDIT

  Credit Policy

  Billing Methods

    Computerized Billing

    Microfilm Billing

    Copy Van or Centralized Photocopying

  Internal Billing by the Medical Assistant

    The Superbill

    Typewritten Statements

    Photocopied Statements

  Billing System

    Itemizing the First Statement

    Time and Frequency of Billing

    Once-a-Month Billing

    Cycle Billing

    Billing Third-Party Payers and Minors

Procedure 18–1: Preparing Monthly Billing Statements

PAYMENT COLLECTION

  Collection Goals

    Collection Ratio

    Accounts Receivable Ratio

  Importance of Collecting Delinquent Accounts

    Know When to Say No

    Why Patients Do Not Pay

  Aging Accounts Receivable

  Collection Techniques

    Telephone Collection

    Collection Letters

    Sample Letters

    Who Signs Collection Letters?

    Personal Interviews

  Procedure 18–2: Collecting Delinquent Accounts

  Special Collection Problems

    Tracing "Skips"

    Claims Against Estates

    Bankruptcy

  Statutes of Limitations

    Malpractice Statutes

    Collection Statutes

    Open Book Accounts

    Written Contracts

    Single-Entry Accounts

USING OUTSIDE COLLECTION ASSISTANCE

  Collecting Through the Court System

    Should We Sue?

    Small Claims Court

  Using a Collection Agency

    Selecting a Collection Agency

    Responsibilities to the Collection Agency

ACCOUNTS RECEIVABLE INSURANCE PROTECTION

LEARNING ACHIEVEMENTS

VOCABULARY

accounts receivable ratio A formula for measuring how fast outstanding accounts are being paid.

age analysis A procedure for classifying accounts receivable by age from the first date of billing.

collection ratio A formula for measuring the effectiveness of the billing system.

invasion of privacy Unauthorized disclosure of a person's private affairs.

statute of limitations The time limit within which an action may legally be brought upon a contract.

subsidize To aid or promote something (such as a private enterprise) with public money.

superbill A combination charge slip, statement, and insurance reporting form.

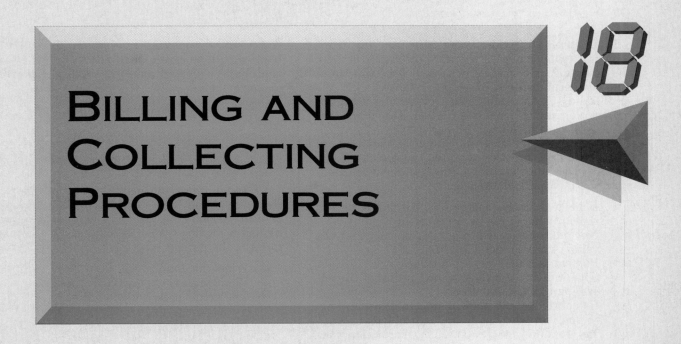

BILLING AND COLLECTING PROCEDURES

18

LEARNING OBJECTIVES

COGNITIVE
Upon successful completion of this chapter, you should be able to:

1. Define the terms listed in the Vocabulary.

2. Name the three ways by which payment for medical services is accomplished.

3. List nine items that should be addressed in developing a credit policy.

4. State three reasons for itemizing billing statements.

5. Describe cycle billing and its advantages.

6. Discuss the significance of determining the collection ratio and the accounts receivable ratio.

7. List the three most common reasons for patients' failure to pay accounts.

8. Discuss the do's and don'ts of telephone collection procedures.

9. Name five sources of information in tracing skips.

10. State the procedure to follow upon receiving notice of a debtor's bankruptcy.

11. List three advantages of using a small claims court for collecting delinquent accounts.

12. Discuss five appropriate follow-up actions after assigning accounts to a collection agency.

PERFORMANCE
Upon successful completion of this chapter, you should be able to perform the following activities:

1. Prepare patients' monthly statements.

2. Calculate a collection ratio and an accounts receivable ratio.

3. Prepare an age analysis of accounts receivable.

4. Initiate proceedings to collect delinquent accounts.

5. Demonstrate telephone collection techniques.

In Chapter 15 we discussed how fees are determined, the importance of advance discussion of fees, the adjusting or canceling of fees in hardship cases, and the legal aspects of credit arrangements. We also addressed the importance of getting adequate information on the first visit when it appears that an extension of credit will be necessary.

The collection of fees and financial management of the medical practice is often entrusted to the medical assistant. To be an effective financial manager, the medical assistant must:

- Believe that the doctor and the office have a right to charge for the services provided
- Not be embarrassed to ask for payment for the value of the service
- Possess tact and good judgment
- Give individual attention and personal consideration to each situation
- Be courteous and show a sincere desire to help the patient who has financial problems
- Try to find out the patient's reason for nonpayment when this occurs

The payment for medical services is accomplished in three ways:

- Payment at time of services
- Billing when extension of credit is necessary
- Using outside collection assistance

PAYMENT AT TIME OF SERVICE

Every practice in which there are patient visits should encourage time-of-service collection. This is especially important in an office-based primary care practice because many of the fees for these office visits are not covered by insurance and may be difficult to collect later. If patients get into the habit of paying their current charges before they leave the office, there are no further billing and bookkeeping expenses, and no risk that inflation will decrease the value of the account.

If patients are informed when making an appointment that payment is expected at the time of service, they are not surprised when you say at the end of the visit,

"Your charge for today is $xx. Will that be cash or check?"

Many patients are hesitant to ask about charges and are unsure whether to offer to pay or to wait until asked. You will make it easier for the patients by offering to accept their payments, since most people are prepared to pay small bills on a cash basis.

Even if a patient requests to be billed, you can say,

"The normal procedure is to pay at the time of service, but we can make an exception this time."

A patient who may have forgotten his or her checkbook should be given a self-addressed envelope with the charge slip and asked to send the payment in the next mail.

BILLING AFTER EXTENSION OF CREDIT

In some types of medical practice, particularly those involving large fees for surgery or long-term care, it becomes necessary to extend credit and establish a regular system of billing. This requires informing the patient of:

- What the charges will be
- What professional services these charges cover
- The credit policy of the office

Credit Policy

Many offices do not have a true credit policy; thus, each account continues to be evaluated individually. It is almost impossible to judge accounts objectively and equitably under such circumstances.

The doctor and the staff should think through their situation, decide what they expect of patients with respect to payments, and how they will inform the patient. Although there will always be exceptions to any rule, there must *be* a rule, which should be in writing and conveyed to the patient at the outset of the relationship.

Some medical practices prepare an information booklet that includes the payment policy. New patients are given a copy of the booklet. Any patient who needs special consideration can be counseled by the medical assistant.

Some of the issues to be addressed in the credit policy are:

- When payment is due from patients
- When the practice requires payment at time of service
- When or if assignment of insurance benefits is accepted
- Whether insurance forms will be completed by the office staff
- Billing procedures
- Collection protocol
- How long an account will be carried without payment
- Telephone collection protocol
- Sending accounts to a collection agency

The medical assistant who has the guidance and support of an established credit policy can perform with confidence in handling patient accounts.

Billing Methods

Computerized Billing

The medical office that "has gone on computer" for accounts receivable management will be completing statements and insurance forms by computer. These procedures are discussed in Chapter 8.

Microfilm Billing

Recommended by many management consultants, microfilm billing is particularly useful to offices with large volume billings. On a specified day of the month, a representative of the billing service brings portable camera equipment to the office and microfilms each ledger that has a balance due. This requires very little time, and the ledgers remain under the control of the office. The film is processed by the billing service, and a copy of the ledger is mailed to the patient. The mailing can include a self-addressed envelope for direct payment to the physician. An extra benefit of microfilming is that a duplicate set of ledger cards is generated, which would be useful in case of loss of the office records by fire or other causes.

Copy Van or Centralized Photocopying

In some areas, you may find a billing service with a copier mounted in a van that will call at the doctor's office once per month. The representative takes the ledger tray from the office to the van, runs the ledgers through a high-speed copier, and returns the ledgers to the doctor's office in a matter of minutes. The service can include inserting the copy in an envelope, stamping, and mailing. For the office without a photocopy machine, this may be the most inexpensive method of outside billing.

Internal Billing by the Medical Assistant

In a practice in which the number of accounts is not too great, the medical assistant handles the preparation and mailing of statements. This may be accomplished by:

- Superbill
- Typewritten statement
- Photocopied statement

The appearance of the statement carries a visual impact just as a letter does, so the statement heads should be carefully chosen and the typing clean and accurate. Statement heads usually are imprinted with the same information as the doctor's letterhead. They should be of good quality and large enough to allow itemization of charges. Envelopes should be imprinted with "Address Correction Re-

quested" under the return address to maintain up-to-date mailing lists. A self-addressed return envelope included with the bill encourages prompt payment. This is mainly for the convenience of patients who do not always have stationery available for sending a return payment or who are less likely to return a payment immediately if they must address an envelope.

The Superbill

The **superbill** is a combination charge slip, statement, and insurance reporting form. There are variations in styles, and they are usually personalized for the practice. Figure 18–1 is an example of a form used in an Ob-Gyn office. It has space for all the elements required in submitting medical insurance claims:

- Name and address of patient
- Name of insurance carrier
- Insurance identification number
- Brief description of each service by code number
- Fee for each service
- Place and date of service
- Diagnosis
- Doctor's name and address
- Doctor's signature

The superbill can be used as a charge slip for office treatments if the doctor checks the services performed at the completion of the visit and asks the patient to hand it to the medical assistant upon leaving. Either the doctor or the medical assistant may write in the amount of the fee. The doctor indicates at the bottom of the sheet when the patient should return, and the assistant can fill in the date and time. If a payment is made, it can be so indicated. Instructions to the patient for filing insurance claims are on the bottom left. The doctor's office keeps one copy; the patient is given the original and one copy for filing with the insurance company.

Statements must be correct and must include the patient's name and address as well as the balance owed. If statements are photocopied or microfilmed, special care must be taken with the ledger card because it will be duplicated in the billing process.

Typewritten Statements

The use of continuous form billing statements is a timesaver. The statements are printed in a roll with perforated edges for separation. The roll is fed into the typewriter for the first statement and remains until the last statement is typed, eliminating the time and energy necessary for inserting and removing each statement form from the typewriter.

18

UROLOGIC GYNECOLOGY
GENERAL GYNECOLOGY
OBSTETRICS

JERRY S. BENZL, M.D., F.A.C.O.G.

ID. #33-0306757

Nº 9411

☐ PRIVATE ☐ BLUE CROSS ☐ BLUE SHIELD ☐ IND. ☐ MEDICARE ☐ GOV'T. ☐ MEDI-CAL OR MEDICAID

PATIENT INFORMATION

| PATIENTS LAST NAME | FIRST | INITIAL | BIRTHDATE | SEX ☐ MALE ☐ FEMALE | TODAY'S DATE / / |

| ADDRESS | CITY | STATE | ZIP | RELATION TO SUBSCRIBER | REFERRING PHYSICIAN |

| SUBSCRIBER OR POLICY HOLDER | INSURANCE |

| ADDRESS | CITY | STATE | ZIP | INS. ID. | COVERAGE CODE | GROUP |

OTHER HEALTH COVERAGE?
☐ NO ☐ YES
IDENTIFY

DISABILITY RELATED TO: ☐ IND.
☐ ACCIDENT ☐ PREGNANCY
☐ OTHER

DATE SYMPTOMS APPEARED, INCEPTION OF PREGNANCY, OR ACCIDENT OCCURRED: /

ASSIGNMENT & RELEASE: I hereby assign my insurance benefits to be paid directly to the undersigned physician. I am financially responsible for non-covered services. I also authorize the physician to release any information required to process this claim.
SIGNED (Patient, or Parent, if Minor)
DATE:

		PROCEDURES	CPT-Mod	AMOUNT			PROCEDURES	CPT-Mod	AMOUNT			PROCEDURES	CPT-Mod	AMOUNT
		A. OFFICE VISITS				31	Post-Partum	59430			60	Urodynamic, Supplies	99070	
	1	New GYN, Limited	90010				**F. GYN PROCEDURES**					**I. UROLOGIC PROCEDURES**		
	2	New GYN, Intermed.	90015			32	Irrig. of Vagina	57150*			61	Urethral Dilation	53660	
	3	New GYN, Extensive	90017			33	Insert Pessary	57160*			62	Urethral Dilation, Repeat	53661	
	4	New GYN, Compreh.	90020			34	Pessary Supplies	99070			63	Bladder Instillation	51700	
	5	Return GYN, Minimal	90030			35	Colposcopy	57452			64	Periurethral Injection	53665	
	6	Return GYN, Brief	90040			36	Biopsy, Cervix	57500			65	Simple Catheterization	53670	
	7	Return GYN, Limited	90050			37	Biopsy, Vagina	57100			66	Manual Elect. Stimulation	97118	
	8	Return GYN, Intermed.	90060			38	Biopsy, Vulva	56600			67	Neuromuscular Reeducat.	97112	
	9	Return GYN, Extended	90070			39	Biopsy, Endometrium	58100				**J. LAB**		
	10	Return GYN, Compreh.	90080			40	BIOPSY, SKIN				68	Urine Analysis	81000	
	11	Return GYN, Post-Op	99024				0.5 cm.	11420			69	Urine Culture	87068	
		B. CONSULTATION					0.6 to 1.0 cm.	11421			70	Hematocrit	85015	
	12	GYN Consult., Limited	90600				1.1 to 2.0 cm.	11423			71	Hemogram	85021	
	13	GYN Consult., Intermed.	90605			41	Cryotherapy, Cervix	57511			72	Commercial - Lat.	87087	
	14	GYN Consult., Compreh.	90620			42	Destruct. Condyloma	56501			73	Wet Mount	87210	
	15	GYN Consult., Complex	90630			43	Diaphragm Fitting	57170			74	PG Test, Urine	86006	
	16	Second Opinion Surgery	90653			44	Diaphragm Supplies	99070			75	Antigen Test	86006	
		C. TELEPHONE CONSULTATION				45	IUD Insertion	58300			76			
	17	Telephone Consult., Simple	99013			46	IUD Supplies	99070			77	Cytopathology Smear	88155	
	18	Telephone Consult., Inter.	99014			47	IUD Removal	58301			78	Specimen Handling	99000	
	19	Telephone Consult., Comp.	99015				**G. CYSTOMETRICS**					**K. MISCELLANEOUS**		
		D. SPECIAL SERVICES				48	Cystourethroscopy	52000			79	Surgical Tray	99070	
	20	ER Service after Off. Hrs.	99064			49	Cystoureth., Supplies	99070			80	Therapeutic Injection	90782	
	21	ER Service during Off. Hrs.	99065			50	Cystoureth., Supplies, MC	A4550			81	Injection, Kenalog	J1870	
	22	Night Call Before 10 pm	99050			51	Cystometrogram	51725			82	Injection, Xylocaine	J3480	
	23	Night Call After 10 pm	99052			52	Electronic-Uroflow	51739			83	Injection, Estrogen	J2655	
	24	Sunday or Holiday Service	99054				**H. URODYNAMICS**				84	Injection, Progesterone	J2675	
	25	Office Non-Schedule	99058			53	UPP Studies	51772			85	Injection, Vit. B12	P4320	
		E. OB CARE				54	Cystometrogram, Complex	51726			86	Instillation, DMSO	J1212	
	26	Prenatal Dx, Consult.	90620			55	Electronic Uroflow, Compl.	51741			87	Booklets	99071	
	27	Initial OB, Normal	59400			56	EMG	51785			88	Special Reports	99080	
	28	Initial OB, High Risk	59400.22			57	Stimulus Evoked Response	51792						
	29	Return OB, Normal	59420			58	Voiding Pressure Studies	51795				**TODAY'S TOTAL FEE**		
	30	Return OB, High Risk	59420.22			59	Intra-Abd. Void Pressure	51797						

	DIAGNOSIS	CODE		DIAGNOSIS	CODE		DIAGNOSIS	CODE		DIAGNOSIS	CODE
	Abortion:			Breasts	216.5		Galactorrhea	676.6		Pregnancy Prenatal	V22
	Threatened	640.0		Vulva	221.2		Hemorrhoids	455.0		Pregnancy Postpartum	V24.2
	Incomplete	637.1		Breast Disorder (Mass)	611.72		Hypertension	401		Pyelonephritis	590.8
	Habitual	646.3		Bronchitis	491		Incontinence Of Urine	788.3		Rectocele	618.0
	Abnormal Urination	788.6		Carcinoma In Situ:			Interstitial Cystitis	595.1		Retention Of Urine	788.2
	Abnormal PAP Smear	795.0		Cervix	233.1		Irritable Colon	564.1		Stress Incontinence	625.6
	Adenomyosis	617.0		Uterus	233.2		Irregular Menstrual Cycle	626.4		Urethral Stricture	598
	Adnexal Mass	625.8		Female Genital Organs	233.3		Malignant Neoplasm:			Urethral Syndrome	597.81
	Amenorrhea	626.0		Cervical Dysplasia	622.1		Cervix	180.9		URI-Viral Syndrome	460
	Anemia	285.9		Cervicitis	616.0		Uterus	182.0		Uterine Leiomyoma	218
	Arthritis	716.9		Contraceptive Management	V25.0		Ovary	183.0		Uterine Prolapse:	
	Artificial Menopause	627.4		Cystocele	618.0		Vagina	184.0		Incomplete	618.2
	Asthma-Hayfever	493.0		Cystourethritis	595.0		Vulva	184.4		Complete	618.3
	Atrophic Vaginitis	627.3		Diabetes Mellitus	250.0		Menopausal Syndrome	627.2		Vaginal Disch.-Nonspecif.	623.5
	Bartholin Abscess	616.3		Thyroid Disorder	246.9		Menometrorrhagia	626.2		Vaginal Enterocele	618.6
	Benign Neoplasm:			Dysmenorrhea	625.3		Oligomenorrhea	626.1		Vaginal Prolapse	618.0
	Cervix	219.0		Dyspareunia	625.0		Obesity	278.0		Vaginal Vault Prolapse	
	Uterus	219.1		Dysuria	788.1		Ovarian Cyst	620.2		Post Hysterectomy	618.5
	Ovary	220		Ectopic Pregnancy	617.0		Pelvic Inflammatory Dis.	614.9		Vulvovaginitis:	
	Vagina	221.1		Endometriosis	617.9		Pelvic Peritoneal Adhesions	614.6		Non Specific	616.1
	Vulva	221.2		Enuresis-Unstable Bladder	788.3		Pigmented Nevus	216		Candida	112.1
	Benign Neoplasm Of Skin:			Frequency Of Urination	788.4		Polycystic Ovaries	256.4		Trichomonas	131.01
	Buttocks	216.5		Functional Disorder:			Postmenopausal Bleeding	627.1			
	Abdomen	216.5		Bladder Instability	596.5		Post-Op Wound Infection	998.5			

MISCELLANEOUS DIAGNOSIS

DOCTOR'S SIGNATURE

DATE:

SERVICES PERFORMED AT: ☐ Office ☐ E.R.
☐ Mission Comm. Med. Center ☐ Saddleback Women's Hosp.
27700 Medical Center Rd. 24451 Health Center Dr.
Mission Viejo, CA Laguna Hills, CA
☐ Hospital Calls at $_____ Per Visit
☐ Hospital Calls at $_____ Per Visit

ADMIT ___/___/___
DISCHARGE ___/___/___

RETURN VISIT INFORMATION
15 - 30 - 45 - 60
_____Days _____Weeks _____Months ☐ Will Call
Procedure:

ACCEPT ASSIGNMENT:
☐ YES
☐ NO

INSTRUCTIONS TO PATIENT FOR FILING INSURANCE CLAIMS
1. Complete patient information portion of this form.
2. Sign and date.
3. Mail this form directly to your insurance company with your own insurance company's form.
4. Patients with health care insurance please remember:
   A. Professional services are charged to the patient, and not to the insurance company.
   B. Insured patients are expected to take care of their fees as services are rendered.
   C. This office cannot accept responsibility for collecting your insurance claim or for negotiating a settlement on disputed claim.
   D. You are responsible for payment of your account.

TODAY'S FEE	
OLD BALANCE	
ADJUSTMENTS	
TOTAL DUE	
AMOUNT RECEIVED TODAY	
	☐ CASH ☐ CHECK ☐ C.C. ☐ K ☐ I.O. ☐ B
NEW BALANCE	

FIGURE 18-1. Example of a superbill.

Another timesaver is the multiple-copy statement. The Colwell Company calls its version "E-Z Statements." The E-Z Statement features three monthly statements plus one patient's ledger card in each set, all in NCR (no carbon required) paper.

Services and payments are posted during the month, and at billing time the top sheet is removed, folded, and mailed in a window envelope. If more than three mailings are required, a new set must be headed and the balance forwarded.

Photocopied Statements

Photocopy equipment is almost as standard as the typewriter in today's offices. The production of photocopied statements is a natural consequence. Coordinated ledger cards and copy paper are used, and a perfect statement is ready for mailing in minimum time. Extra care must be used in posting the ledgers, however. A black pen should be used in making entries on the ledger card. Other ink colors do not reproduce well. Writing must be clear and legible. There should be no personal notes made on the ledger cards unless it is something you wish conveyed to the patient. (It is possible to get pencils with nonreproducible lead if you feel this is necessary for making collection entries.) Usually, a window envelope is used for mailing, which means that the name and address on the ledger must be neat, correct, and in the right position for the window.

Billing System
Itemizing the First Statement

If the medical fee has been explained in advance, as discussed in Chapter 15, the monthly statement is merely a confirmation of what is owed, and there should be no misunderstanding. However, it is good business practice—and a courtesy to the patient—to itemize the charges. This is absolutely essential if the statement is to be used for billing the patient's insurance. Patients are entitled to an understanding of the doctor's statement for services (Fig. 18–2).

Itemizing statements is not difficult. The simplest method is merely to allow space on the original statement, below the "For Professional Services" line, on which to list the separate charges for office, house, or hospital calls, or for treatments or tests done in the doctor's office.

Many doctors have devised their own itemized charge slips; these are given to the patient when payment is made at the time of service, or later mailed in a combination statement-reply envelope. Use of such charge slips simplifies the itemization procedure, since filling out the slips is usually just a matter of checking the procedures listed. An itemized charge slip is shown in Figure 18–3.

Although the itemization of bills may seem an unnecessary waste of time, if you do itemize you will spend less time

- explaining services provided
- clearing up misunderstandings with patients
- following up on delinquent accounts

Time and Frequency of Billing

A regular system of rendering statements should be put into operation. Most people expect to receive statements from their creditors, and they plan their budgets around first-of-the-month bills received. Punctuality in billing encourages prompt payment.

Statements should be sent at least once each month. Some offices send bills immediately after treatment; others bill all patients on the same day each month. Mailing statements twice a month—

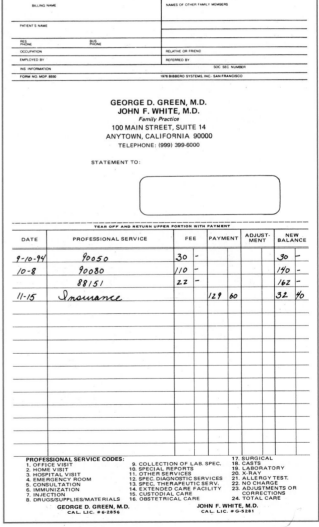

FIGURE 18-2. Example of an itemized statement.

RULINGS AND COLUMN HEADINGS TO MATCH YOUR CURRENT SYSTEM
PLEASE ENCLOSE SAMPLE FOR EXACT MATCH

1461

LYDIA R. THOMPSON, M.D.
Internal Medicine
2100 WEST PARK AVENUE
CHAMPAIGN, ILLINOIS 61820
Telephone: (217) 351-5400
Fax: (217) 351-5413

Tax I.D. # 123456
S.S. No. 000-00-0000
IL LIC. #00-00000

UPIN #E00000
MC #TA 000000
BCBS 123-45678-00

DATE _____
PATIENT _____
BIRTHDATE _____/_____/_____
SOCIAL SECURITY # _____
ADDRESS _____
_____
TELEPHONE _____

RESPONSIBLE PARTY _____
INSURANCE # _____
INSURED'S NAME _____

ASSIGNMENT AND RELEASE: I authorize my insurance benefits be paid directly to the physician. I am financially responsible for non-covered charges. I also authorize the physician to release any information required.

Signed _____

CPT	PROCEDURE	ICD-9 Ref. No.	FEE	CPT	PROCEDURE	ICD-9 Ref. No.	FEE	CPT	PROCEDURE	ICD-9 Ref. No.	FEE
	Office Visit - New Patient				*Office Procedures*				*Laboratory* (Cont.)		
☐ 90000	Brief Service		$	☐ 95115	Allergen, Single Injection		$	☐ 81000	Urinalysis, by Reagent Strips		$
☐ 90010	Limited Service		$	☐ 45330	Sigmoidoscopy, Flexible		$		Culture, Bacterial, Urine,		
☐ 90015	Int. Service		$	☐ 93015	Cardiovascular Stress Test		$	☐ 87086	Colony Count		$
☐ 90017	Extended Service		$	☐ 32000*	Thoracentesis		$	☐ 80070	Thyroid Panel		$
☐ 90020	Comprehensive Service		$	☐ 36600*	Arterial Puncture		$	☐ 84420	Theophylline		$
	Office Visit - Established Patient			☐ 86580	Tuberculosis, Intradermal		$	☐ 85048	Blood Count, WBC		$
☐ 90040	Brief Service		$	☐ 10060*	I & D Abscess		$		*X-Ray*		
☐ 90050	Limited Service		$	☐ 10120*	I & D Removal For. Bod. Subc.		$	☐ 71010	Chest, 1 View		$
☐ 90060	Int. Service		$	☐ 10160	Puncture Aspiration		$	☐ 71020	Chest, 2 Views		$
☐ 90070	Extended Service		$	☐ 58300*	Insertion IUD		$				
☐ 90080	Comprehensive Service		$	☐ 58301	Removal IUD		$				
	Consultations			☐ 69210	Cerumen Removal		$				
☐ 90600	Limited		$		*Laboratory*						
☐ 90605	Intermediate		$	☐ 36415*	Routine Venipuncture		$				
☐ 90610	Extended		$	☐ 86255	Fluorescent Antibody Screen		$				
☐ 90620	Comprehensive		$	☐ 85022	Hemogram (CBC), Manual		$		**TOTAL CHARGES** $		
☐ 90630	Complex		$		Differential		$				
	Confirm. Consultations			☐ 80050	General Panel		$				
☐ 90650	Limited		$	☐ 82643	Digoxin, RIA		$				
☐ 90651	Intermediate		$	☐ 82948	Glucose; Blood		$				
	Immunization Injection			☐ 82270	Blood; Occult, Feces		$				
☐ 90702	Diphtheria and Tetanus		$		Screening		$				
☐ 90724	Influenza Virus Vaccine		$	☐ 85014	Hematocrit		$		SIGNATURE OF PHYSICIAN Date		
☐ 90732	Pneumococcal Vaccine		$	☐ 86300	Heterophile Antibodies		$		PLACE OF SERVICE:		
☐ 90782	Therapeutic Injection		$	☐ 85580	Platelet Count		$		☐ Office ☐ Inpatient Hospital		
	Specify Material			☐ 84132	Potassium; Blood		$		☐ Skilled Nursing Facility ☐ Nursing Home		
☐ 90784	Therapeutic IV		$	☐ 85610	Prothrombin Time		$				
	Specify Material			☐ 84230	Quinidine, Blood		$		REFERRING MD:		
☐ J3420	Inj., B - 12		$	☐ 86592	Syphilis Test		$				
☐ J0290	Inj. Ampicillin, 500 mg.		$	☐ 87072	Culture, Commercial Kit		$				

(Watermark across center: IMPORTANT — THIS FORMAT IS ONLY A GUIDELINE TO AID YOU IN DESIGNING YOUR OWN SPECIALIZED FORM. PROCEDURES, CODES, AND LAYOUT CAN BE WHATEVER YOU NEED.)

DIAGNOSIS (ICD-9-CM): Correlate diagnosis to procedure by using the reference numbers listed below.

Ref. No.	DESCRIPTION	CODE	Ref. No.	DESCRIPTION	CODE	Ref. No.	DESCRIPTION	CODE	Ref. No.	DESCRIPTION	CODE
	Eye, Ears, Nose, & Throat		25.	Diverticulosis	562.10	50.			73.	COPD	496
1.	Allergic Rhinitis	477.0	26.	Gastritis, Acute	535.0		**Hematologic & Lymphatic**		74.	Emphysema	492.8
2.	Bronchiolitis, Acute	466.1	27.	G. I. Bleeding, Unspecified	578.9	51.	Anemia, NOS	285.9	75.	Influenza	487.1
3.	Conjunctivitis, Unspecified	372.30	28.	Hernia, Inguinal, NOS	550.90	52.	Anemia, Pernicious	281.0	76.	Pneumonitis	486
4.	Impacted Cerumen	380.4	29.	Irritable Bowel Syndrome	564.1	53.			77.	Upper Respir. Infection, Acute	465.9
5.	Laryngitis, Acute	464.0	30.	Rectal Bleeding	569.3		**Musculo - Skeletal**		78.		
6.	Pharyngitis, Acute	462	31.			54.	Arthritis, Rheumatoid	714.0		**Skin**	
7.	Sinusitis, Acute, NOS	461.9		**Metabolic**		55.	Bursitis	727.3	79.	Acne Vulgaris	706.1
8.	Tonsillitis, Acute	463	32.	Diabetes Mellitus, ID	250.01	56.	Ganglion Of Joint	727.41	80.	Dermatitis, Allergic	692.9
9.	Tonsillitis, Chronic	474.0	33.	Diabetes Mellitus, NID	250.00	57.	Osteoarthritis, Unspec. Site	715.90	81.	Herpes Simplex	054.9
10.			34.	Hypothyroidism, Primary	244.9	58.	Sprain, Ankle	845.00	82.	Herpes Zoster	053.9
	Symptoms		35.	Thyroid Disease, Unspecified	246.9	59.	Sprain, Muscle, Unspec. Site	848.9	83.	Hives / Urticaria	708.9
11.	Abdominal Pain	789.0	36.			60.			84.	Pilonidal Cyst	685.1
12.	Chest Pain	786.50		**Circulatory**			**Genito - Urinary / Breast**		85.	Skin Eruption, Rash	782.1
13.	Fever Of Undetermined Origin	780.6	37.	Angina, Unstable	411.1	61.	Abnormal Pap Smear	795.0	86.		
14.	Headache	784.0	38.	Arteriosclerosis	440.9	62.	Ovarian Cyst	620.2		**V-Codes**	
15.	Heart Murmur, Innocent	785.2	39.	Arrhythmia, NOS	427.9	63.	Pelvic Inflammatory Disease	614.9	87.	Family History Of Diabetes	V18.0
16.	Rash	782.1	40.	ASHD	414.0	64.	Postmenopausal Bleeding	627.1	88.	Gynecological Exam	V72.3
17.	Swollen Glands	785.6	41.	Chest Pain	786.50	65.	Premenstrual Tension	625.4	89.	Vaccination / Bacterial Dis.	V03.9
18.	Vertigo	780.4	42.	Edema	782.3	66.	Urinary Tract Infection	599.0	90.	Vaccination / Combination	V06.8
19.	Vomiting, Nausea	787.0	43.	Hypertension, Benign	401.1	67.	Vaginitis, Vulvitis, NOS	616.10	91.	Vaccination, Influenza	V04.8
	Gastro - Intestinal		44.	Hypertension, Malignant	401.0	68.			92.		
20.	Abdominal Pain	789.0	45.	Hypertension, W / O CHF	402.90		**Respiratory**				
21.	Cholelithiasis	574.20	46.	Leg Varicose Vein	454.9	69.	Asthma, Bron. w/Status Ast.	493.91			
22.	Constipation	564.0	47.	Mitral Valve Prolapse	424.0	70.	Asthma, Bron. w/o Status Ast.	493.90			
23.	Diarrhea	558.9	48.	Myocardial Infarction, Old	412	71.	Bronchitis, Acute	466.0			
24.	Diverticulitis	562.11	49.	Rheumatic Heart Disease, NOS	398.90	72.	Chest Pain	786.50			

FIGURE 18–3. An itemized charge slip. (Courtesy of Colwell Systems, Champaign, IL.)

for example, half of the accounts on the 10th and the remaining half on the 25th—is also a common practice.

According to the Fair Credit Billing Act of October 28, 1975, when a billing date for an account has been established, the date of mailing the state-ment must not vary more than 5 days without notification to the patient/debtor.

If there is a *balance due* or a *credit balance* of one dollar or more, the account must be billed every 30 days.

ONCE-A-MONTH BILLING. If a monthly pattern is followed, bills should leave your office in time to reach the patient no later than the last day of each month and preferably by the 25th of the month. Planning ahead for the preparation of statements can lighten the burden of once-a-month billing. The statement can be prepared at the time of service (or during slack periods), postdated, and mailed at the end of the month.

CYCLE BILLING. Many physicians prefer to use the cycle billing system, which calls for the billing of certain portions of the accounts receivable at given times during the month instead of preparing all statements at the end of each month. Cycle billing has been used for some time in large businesses such as department stores, banks, and oil companies. The system of cycle billing has become increasingly popular in the physician's office. Its many advantages include avoiding once-a-month peak workloads and stabilizing the cash flow. In a small office in which billing is done only once per month, the unexpected illness or absence of the medical assistant for any emergency can leave the doctor in a financial bind if the statements do not go out.

This is how the cycle billing system works: the accounts are separated into fairly equal divisions, the number of divisions depending on how many times you wish to do billing during a month. For example, if you expect to bill twice per month, divide the accounts into two equal sections; for weekly billing, divide into four groups; for daily billing, divide into 20 groups.

Small alphabetic groups can be combined to keep your divisions nearly equal in the number of statements to prepare on each billing day. If your files are color-coded, you may wish to use the same alphabetic breakdown in billing. Regardless of constant changes in the accounts themselves, the mailing dates for accounts in each section remain the same. A schedule for processing and mailing of accounts is thus established, and the load of work is apportioned throughout the entire month.

Cycle billing allows the medical assistant to continue all routine duties each day, handling the statements on a day-to-day or weekly schedule rather than in one intensive period at the end of the month. This means that whole days need not be sacrificed from other duties in order to get statements in the mail. By spacing the billing throughout the month, more time and consideration can be given to each statement, the itemization of bills is less burdensome, and the likelihood of error is decreased.

Patients generally accept the cycle billing system quickly, often with enthusiasm. However, if your office decides to change from a once-a-month billing system to a cycle billing system, patients should be notified in advance, and the new plan should be explained to them. To explain the new system to established patients, enclose a notice in each statement 2 months prior to the transfer, describing the plan and indicating the future dates on which each patient will receive the bill.

Before a doctor adopts the cycle billing system, particularly in a small community, several factors should be taken into consideration:

- What is the general income level of the community, and how and when does the average patient receive his pay?
- Do local companies pay employees at various times during the month, or are most paychecks handed out at the beginning of the month?
- Would cycle billing benefit patients as well as the overall operation of the office?

Billing Third-Party Payers and Minors

Collection problems may arise if the medical assistant fails to get the necessary insurance information, particularly Medicare and Medicaid information (see section on Credit Arrangement in Chapter 15).

In some instances, the insurance forms are not completed correctly, and the claim is denied because of minor infractions such as failing to name the responsible party or omitting Social Security information, the policy number, or the group number.

Time limits must also be observed in billing third-party payers. In cases of Medicare patients with a terminal illness, it may be best to accept assignment of benefits. If the doctor does not take assignment, sometimes the doctor will receive nothing, because the family is not obligated to pay and Medicare will not pay after a certain time or if the claim has not been correctly filed.

Bills for minors must be addressed to a parent or legal guardian. If a bill is addressed to a minor, the parent or parents could take the attitude that they are not responsible because they themselves never received the bill. If the parents are separated or divorced, the parent who brings the child in for treatment is responsible for payment. Whatever financial agreement exists between the parents is strictly their personal business and should not concern the medical office. The responsible parent should be so informed from the beginning. Minors cannot be held responsible for payment of a bill unless they are emancipated (see Chapter 5).

If an emancipated minor appears in the office and requests treatment and you can ascertain that the person is not living at home, the minor is responsible for the bill. It may be wise to make a determination either with the business manager or with the physician as to whether your office wishes to treat this emancipated minor.

18

PROCEDURE 18-1   PREPARING MONTHLY BILLING STATEMENTS

GOAL To process monthly statements and evaluate accounts for collection procedures in accordance with the agency's credit policy.

EQUIPMENT AND SUPPLIES

Typewriter   Agency's Credit Policy
Patient Accounts   Statement Forms

PROCEDURAL STEPS

1. Assemble all accounts that have outstanding balances.

2. Separate accounts that need special attention in accordance with the agency's credit policy.
   Explanation: Routine statements should be prepared first, after which special attention can be given to delinquent accounts.

3. Prepare routine statements, including:
   - Date the statement is prepared
   - Name and address of the person responsible for payment
   - Name of the patient if different from the person responsible for payment
   - Itemization of dates, services, and charges for the month
   - Any unpaid balance carried forward (may or may not be itemized, depending on office policy)

4. Determine the action to be taken on accounts separated in Step 2.

5. Make a note of the necessary action on the ledger card (telephone call, collection letter series, small claims court, or assignment to collection agency).
   Purpose: For guidance in executing an action and for later follow-up when necessary.

PAYMENT COLLECTION

Collection Goals

Management consultants for the medical profession say that if good financial practices are followed, the accounts receivable on a doctor's books should equal no more than 2 to 3 months' gross charges, but if the receivables start falling below the average of 1 month's total charges, perhaps the collection procedures are too stringent.

Evaluation of collections is based on the collection ratio and the accounts receivable ratio. The **collection ratio** measures the effectiveness of the billing system. The basic formula for figuring the collection ratio is:

$$\text{Collection Ratio} = \frac{\text{Total Collections}}{\text{Net Charges}}$$

A minimum of 6 to 12 months' data should be used in computing the collection ratio. Figure 18–4 illustrates how to calculate a collection ratio.

The **accounts receivable ratio** measures how fast outstanding accounts are being paid. The formula is:

$$\text{Accounts Receivable Ratio} = \frac{\text{Current Accounts Receivable Balance}}{\text{Average Gross Monthly Charges}}$$

Gross Charges		$125,000
Less:		
Courtesy discounts	$5,000	
Third party insurance allowance	6,000	
Other adjustments	1,000	
Total Adjustments		12,000
Net Charges		$113,000
Total Collections		110,000
Collection Ratio $\left(\dfrac{110,000}{113,000}\right)$		97%

FIGURE 18-4. Figuring the collection ratio.

A desirable accounts receivable ratio is less than 2 months. It is the medical assistant's responsibility to keep both the accounts receivable and collections within normal limits. Figure 18-5 is an example of how to calculate the accounts receivable ratio.

Importance of Collecting Delinquent Accounts

The reasons for pursuing collections go beyond the obvious one that a physician must be paid for services in order to pay expenses and continue to treat patients.

Failure to collect can result in the loss of a patient. A person who owes the doctor money and is not prodded gently into payment may stay away in embarrassment or may even change doctors.

Noncollection of medical bills may also imply guilt. A patient may infer that the doctor felt that the patient received inadequate or improper care, and a malpractice suit may result.

Nor is it fair to the paying patients to make no attempt to collect from nonpaying patients. Abandoning accounts without collection follow-up encourages nonpayers, and, as a result, the paying patients indirectly **subsidize** the cost of medical care for those who can pay but do not.

Most patients are honest; it is estimated that probably fewer than 4% never intend to pay. There may be a larger percentage who are financially "shipwrecked" and temporarily unable to pay. Also,

Annual Gross Charges	$125,000
Average Monthly Gross Charges $\left(\dfrac{125,000}{12}\right)$	10,417
Current Acc/Rec Balance	16,000
Acc/Rec Ratio $\left(\dfrac{16,000}{10,417}\right)$	1.54 months

FIGURE 18-5. Figuring the accounts receivable ratio.

a certain percentage of patients irresponsibly live beyond their incomes.

Figures 18-6 and 18-7 show notes that might be sent to patients in an effort to remind them of their financial obligations.

Know When to Say No

There must be some limit put on the time, effort, and expense invested in trying to collect an uncollectible account. Under some circumstances, it may be better simply to write off an unpaid account. An example of a letter that might be used to cancel the account and at the same time improve the image of the physician is shown in Figure 18-8.

Why Patients Do Not Pay

According to the American Medical Association, the three most common reasons for patients' failure to pay are:

- Negligence
- Inability to pay
- Unwillingness to pay

Aging Accounts Receivable

Aging is a term used for the procedure of classifying accounts receivable by age from the first date of billing. It should be done on a regular basis. Aging of accounts helps collection follow-up, since it enables the medical assistant to tell at a glance which accounts need attention in addition to a regular statement. Computer billing programs usually include this feature. With sufficient time, an age analysis may be accomplished manually (Fig. 18-9).

If the patient is billed on the day of service, the aging begins on that day; if the first billing is 30 days after service, the aging begins at 30 days. Some systems use a breakdown of Current, 30 days, 60 days, 90 days, and 90-plus days.

Looking at Figure 18-9, you see that:

- Patient A has a balance of $450. Unless regular payments are being made, this account may be heading toward a collection problem because $350 of the balance is over 3 months old.
- Patient B presents no problem because the entire balance is current.
- Patient C definitely is a potential problem even though the account is small. The entire balance is over 3 months old, and one fourth of it is over 6 months old.
- Patient D's account should never have been allowed to reach this stage of delinquency. If there had been a good collection policy established, it would not have.

The **age analysis** is simply a tool to show at a glance the status of each account. There is no need to do this every month if time is at a premium. If

If you are unable to pay your account this month, please telephone this office (776-4900) before ——————————— and let us know how you plan to take care of it.

Your balance due is $350.

FIGURE 18–6. Suggested note to patient for 60-day billing.

Every courtesy has been extended to you in arranging for payment of your long overdue account. Our auditor suggests that it no longer be carried on our books.

Unless we hear from you by ——————————, the account will be turned over to ——————————— for collection.

FIGURE 18–7. Suggested final letter to patient.

Date

Patient Name
Street Address
City, State ZIP Code

Dear Patient:

Your balance of $200 has been on our books for 23 months.

In view of the financial circumstances that make payment for these past services difficult for you, Dr. Johnson has instructed me to consider the debt cancelled. We will no longer bill you for it.

The doctor wants you to feel free to call on him for any future service you may require.

Sincerely yours,

Office Manager for
E. F. Johnson, M.D.

FIGURE 18–8. Example of a letter that cancels a fee.

ACCOUNTS RECEIVABLE AGE ANALYSIS

Dr _____

Address _____ Date _____

PATIENT'S NAME	TOTAL ACCOUNT RECEIVABLE	DISTRIBUTION OF ACCOUNTS RECEIVABLE BY AGE				REMARKS
		1-2-3 MONTHS	4-5-6 MONTHS	7-8-9-10-11-12 MONTHS	OVER 1 YEAR	
A	450.00	100.00	350.00			
B	50.00	50.00				
C	100.00		75.00	25.00		
D	200.00		10.00	150.00	40.00	
E	550.00		550.00			
F	42.50	42.50				
G	65.00	20.00	45.00			
H	325.00	325.00				

FIGURE 18-9. Form for accounts receivable age analysis.

you age the accounts quarterly, you will stay on top of the problem. Usually, a coding system with metal clip-on tabs or adhesive peel-off labels on the ledger cards is used in conjunction with the age analysis system.

For example, after two statements have been sent, a green tab is placed on the record, indicating that a courteous reminder was sent with the last statement.

The following month the green tab is replaced with a yellow tab, showing that a second payment request was sent in the form of a polite letter or printed request.

An orange tab is substituted the next month, indicating that the patient received a letter requesting prompt attention to the account.

Red tabs may be reserved for the accounts of patients who, as a last resort, have been notified of a specific time limit in which payment must be made, after which sterner measures will be taken. If you reach this stage in pursuing a particular account, make certain you record the date of the time limit on the patient's ledger.

The law requires that once you have made a statement in regard to a particular collection procedure, you must follow through or be liable for the consequences under the law (see Fair Debt Collection Practices Act 1977). If you say, for example, "I am going to turn your account over for collection unless it is paid within 10 days," then you must do so. If you state in a collection letter that you are going to take the debtor to small claims court if the account is not paid by a certain date, then you must do as you say. The intent of the law is to prevent the collector from making idle threats or harassing a debtor. A patient may sue for harassment if such idle threats are made.

> Fair Debt Collection Practices Act 1977 (Federal) states that the following conduct is a violation:
>
> Section 807 (5) The threat to take any action that cannot legally be taken or that is not intended to be taken.

Collection Techniques

Persuasive collection procedures include:

- Telephone calls
- Collection reminders and letters
- Personal interviews

Telephone Collection

A telephone call at the right time, in the right manner, is more effective than a collection letter (see General Rules to Follow in Telephone Collections). The personal contact of a telephone call will bring in more money than if a call is not made. In the absence of time to make calls, the collection letter is the next best avenue. If collections are a serious problem, it may pay to hire an extra person to do the telephoning. Written notification is a must, however, if it is a final demand for payment before collection or legal proceedings are started.

There are no hard and fast rules for pursuing collections by telephone (see Actions to Avoid). You must handle each case individually on the basis of your own acquaintance or experience with the person concerned.

18

GENERAL RULES TO FOLLOW IN TELEPHONE COLLECTIONS

1. Call the patient when you can do so in privacy.

2. Call between 8 AM and 9 PM

3. Determine the identity of the person with whom you are speaking. If you ask, "Is this Mrs. Noble?" and she answers "Yes," it could be the patient's mother-in-law or daughter-in-law, who is also "Mrs. Noble." Use the person's full name.

4. Be dignified and respectful in your attitude. You can be friendly and formal at the same time.

5. Ask the patient if it is a convenient time to talk with you. Unless you have the attention of the called party, there is little to be gained by continuing. If you are told that you have called at an inopportune time, ask for a specific time when you may call back, or get a promise for the patient to call you at a specified time.

6. After a brief greeting, state the purpose of your call. Make no apology for calling but state your reason in a friendly, businesslike way. You expect payment and are interested in helping the patient meet the financial obligation. "This is Alice, Dr. Brown's financial secretary. I'm calling about your account." A well-placed pause at this point in the call sometimes gets an immediate response from the debtor in regard to the non-payment.

7. Assume a positive attitude. For example, convey the impression that you know the patient intends to pay, and it is only a matter of working out some suitable arrangements.

8. Keep the conversation brief and to the point, and avoid threats of any kind.

9. Try to get a definite commitment— payment of a certain amount by a certain date.

10. Follow up on promises. This is best accomplished by a tickler file or a note on your calendar. If the payment does not arrive by the promised date, remind the patient with another call. If you fail to do this, your whole effort has been wasted.

ACTIONS TO AVOID WHEN CALLING TO COLLECT PAYMENT

1. Calling between 9 PM and 8 AM. To do so may be considered harassment.

2. Making repeated phone calls.

3. Calling at the debtor's place of work if you know that the employer prohibits personal calls.

4. If you do call the debtor at work and the person cannot take the call, you can leave a message asking to "call Mrs. Black at 727-9238" without revealing the nature of the call—that is, do *not* state that the call is from "Dr. Jones's office" or "Dr. Jones's medical assistant."

5. Losing your temper or showing hostility. An angry patient is a poor-paying patient. Insulted patients often do not pay at all.

Collection Letters

Some consultants believe that a printed collection letter or reminder enclosed with a statement is more effective than a personal letter. They believe that a patient may be embarrassed by a personal letter and feel that he or she has been singled out for attention. An impersonal printed message will probably encourage the patient to send a payment.

The printed form is a timesaver and is recommended if a lack of time is contributing to poor collection follow-up. Standard printed forms are readily available; you can also design your own (see Things to Avoid When Writing for Payment).

Letters that are friendly requests for an explanation of why payment has not been made are still effective in many cases. These letters should indicate that the doctor is sincerely interested in the patient and wants to help straighten out the financial obligations. The patient should be invited to visit the doctor's office to explain the reasons for nonpayment so that, if possible, special arrangements can be worked out. To give the patient an opportunity to save face, these letters can suggest that the patient may have overlooked previous statements.

Upon receipt of such a letter, most patients make some effort to explain their failure to make payment. If a patient really is having financial difficulties, the doctor may be able to get public assistance for him or her. Or, if it is a temporary financial embarrassment, the doctor and the patient may together be able to work out a satisfactory installment plan for payment.

The medical assistant often is given a free hand in designing collection patterns and composing collection letters. Many medical assistants compose a series of collection letters, using letters that they have found to be effective as models. Such a series usually includes at least five letters that range in varying degrees of forcefulness.

THINGS TO AVOID WHEN WRITING FOR PAYMENT

- Using the same collection letter for a patient with good paying habits as for one who is known to neglect financial obligations.
- Placing an overdue notice of any kind on a postcard or on the outside of an envelope. This is an **invasion of privacy.**

SAMPLE LETTERS. Following are some ideas for reminders and collection letters. These can serve as a guide for composing your own letters to suit the circumstances involved. Often, a gentle reminder brings good results:

SAMPLE REMINDER AND COLLECTION LETTERS

Your account has always been paid promptly in the past, so this must be an oversight. Please accept this note as a friendly reminder of your account due for $_____.

Since your care in this office in March, we have had no word from you in regard to how you are feeling or your account due.

If it is impossible for you to pay the full amount of $_____ at this time, please call this office before June 15 so that satisfactory arrangements can be worked out.

Medical bills are payable at the time of service unless special credit arrangements are made.

Please send your check in full or call this office before June 30.

If you have some question about your statement, we will be happy to answer it for you. If not, may we have a payment before the end of this month?

Unless some definite arrangement is made to reduce your balance of $_____, we can no longer carry your account on our books.

Delinquent accounts are turned over to our collection agency on the 25th of the month.

When a payment plan has been established, it can be reinforced by recognizing the first remittance with a letter of acknowledgment:

LETTER OF ACKNOWLEDGMENT

Thank you for the recent payment of $_____ on your account. We are glad to cooperate with you in this arrangement for clearing your account.

We will look for your next check at about the same time next month, and your final payment the following month.

When a payment schedule has been arranged by a telephone call, it can be confirmed by letter:

As agreed upon in our telephone conversation today, we will expect you to mail a payment of $50 on February 10; $50 on March 10; and the balance on April 10.

If some emergency should prevent your making one of these payments on time, please notify us immediately by telephone.

It is important to remember that you should:

- Individualize letters to suit the situation
- Design your early letters as mere reminders of debt
- Always imply that the patient has good intentions to pay, until lack of response over a period of time proves otherwise
- Send letters with a firmer tone only after you have sent one or two friendly reminders

Sometimes even the person with poor paying habits will pay the bill if treated with respect and consideration. See Figure 18–10 for a suggested collection program.

The medical assistant should never go beyond the authority granted by the physician in pursuing collections. If you have questions about special collection problems, always check with the doctor before proceeding. This is particularly important with patients whom you do not know personally—for example, patients the doctor has seen in the hospital or at home, and others for whom you have no credit history. It is difficult to say whether pressing collec-

GOAL	TIME	PROCEDURE
Inform patient of expected charges	Prior to or at time of service	Personal contact
Confirmation of charges	At time of service or next billing cycle	Billing statement
Reminder of charges or new balance	30 days after first billing	Billing statement with notation "Second Statement"
Determine whether there is a problem with payment or service	Prior to third billing	Telephone patient to arrange payment commitment
If previous step was unsuccessful or not completed	At 60 days	Third billing with note (see Fig. 18–6)
Ask for definite date and dollar amount of payment	Prior to fourth billing	Telephone patient; must have definite plan
Final notice 15 days before sending to collection	At 90 days	Fourth billing; send final notice (see Fig. 18–7) by Certified mail with return receipt requested
	At 105 days	Send to collector

FIGURE 18–10. A suggested collection program.

tions too hard loses more good will of patients than not pursuing collections diligently enough. The doctor and the medical assistant together should agree upon general collection policies as outlined earlier in this chapter, and then the policies should be followed. In all cases in which an account is assigned for collection, be sure that the doctor is aware of it.

WHO SIGNS COLLECTION LETTERS?. In most medical offices, the medical assistant signs them with the identification "Assistant to Dr. Brown" or "Financial Secretary" below the typewritten signature. Some physicians may wish to personally sign these communications, but generally the medical assistant who handles the accounts also signs the collection letters.

Personal Interviews

Personal interviews with patients can sometimes be more effective than a whole series of collection letters. By talking to a patient face to face, you can come to an understanding of the problem more quickly and reach an agreement about future payment plans.

Occasionally, a patient may undergo a long course of treatment and yet make no attempt to pay anything on account. Perhaps such a patient is only waiting for the doctor or the medical assistant to suggest that a payment be made. When there is advance knowledge that the patient will require extensive treatment, the matter of payment should be discussed early in the course of treatment, the credit policy explained, and some agreement reached as to a payment plan.

Since the fee for medical services is far more intangible than that on any commercial account, collection efforts must not be delayed too long. Any responsible, sincere patient will call or write the doctor's office after receiving a second statement and explain why payment has not been made, or ask for a payment plan.

If it becomes necessary to refer the account to a collector, a good agency should have a 35 to 40%

PROCEDURE 18-2   COLLECTING DELINQUENT ACCOUNTS

GOAL   To initiate proceedings to collect delinquent accounts.

EQUIPMENT AND SUPPLIES

Typewriter
Telephone
Delinquent accounts

Stationery
Collection letter series
Agency's credit policy

PROCEDURAL STEPS

1. Assemble the delinquent accounts.
2. Separate accounts according to the action required.
   Purpose: It is more efficient to process as a group all accounts requiring the same activity.
3. Make telephone calls to those so designated.
4. Record responses on the ledger cards.
   Purpose: For further action as necessary.
5. Review the accounts requiring collection letters.
6. Choose an appropriate letter from the collection series and individualize it for the account in question.
   Purpose: Form letters may be used as a guide, but should be individualized to suit the situation.
7. Typewrite the collection letter(s).
8. Make a notation of the action taken on the ledger card.
   Purpose: To avoid repetition of the same letter if further action is necessary.

18

recovery rate with an account that is assigned within 4 or 5 months. This may drop to 25% if the account is held only a few more months. If recovery by the agency is greater than 40%, it may indicate that the collection effort by the medical assistant needs to be intensified.

The value of medical accounts diminishes in direct proportion to the length of time that has elapsed since service was rendered. Do not fight the law of diminishing returns. All collection activity is costly. Know when to stop and call on the services of a professional agency.

Special Collection Problems

Tracing "Skips"

When a statement is returned marked "Moved—no forwarding address," you may consider this account as a "skip." This generally is accepted as an indication that the patient is attempting to avoid liability for debts. Some so-called skips are innocent errors. The person may have been careless in not leaving a forwarding address. Or the mistake may have occurred in the doctor's office; the wrong name or address may have been placed on the statement. However, immediate action should be taken in regard to returned statements. Do not wait until the next billing time to attempt to trace the debtor (see Suggestions for Tracing Skips).

The tracing of skips is a challenge to any medical assistant. A certified letter can be sent; by paying additional fees, you can request the Postal Service to obtain a receipt including the address where the letter was delivered. The certified letter may be sent in a plain envelope so that the patient will not refuse to accept the letter because of the letterhead.

If all your attempts fail, turn the account over to your collection agency without delay. Do not keep a skip account too long, since the trail may become so

SUGGESTIONS FOR TRACING SKIPS

1. Examine the patient's original office registration card.

2. Call the telephone number listed on the card. Occasionally a patient may move without leaving a forwarding address but will transfer the old telephone number. Or the new telephone number will be given when you call the old number.

3. If you are unable to contact the individual by telephone, make a few discreet calls to the references listed on the registration card to get leads.

4. Check the city directory to secure the name and telephone number of neighbors or the landlord, and contact these persons to secure information about the debtor's whereabouts.

5. Do not inform a third party that the person owes you money. Simply state that you are trying to locate or verify the location of the individual.

6. Check the debtor's place of employment for information. If the person is a specialist in his or her field of work, the local union or similar organizations may be contacted. Although they may not give you the person's current address, they will relay the message that you are seeking to contact him or her. Often, people will be stirred into paying a bill if they think that their employer may learn of their payment failure.

7. Do not communicate with a third party more than once. This is specifically forbidden by law (Public Law 95-109, Sec. 804) unless the third party requests the collector to do so.

cold as time elapses that even collection experts will be unable to follow it.

Claims Against Estates

A bill owed by a deceased patient may be handled a little differently than regular bills. Courtesy dictates that a bill not be sent during the initial period of bereavement, but do not delay more than 30 days. The person responsible for settling the affairs of the estate will be assembling outstanding accounts and will expect to receive the medical bills along with all others. Address the statement to:

Estate of (name of patient)
c/o (spouse or next of kin, if known)
Patient's last known address

Do not address the statement to a relative unless you have a signed agreement that that person will be responsible. If for some reason the statement cannot be addressed as suggested above — for instance, if the patient was in a convalescent home and you do not know the name of a relative — you may seek information from the county seat in the county in which the estate is being settled. A will is usually filed within 30 days of a death. A request to the Probate Department of the Superior Court, County Recorder's Office, will usually provide you with the name of the executor or administrator. The time limits for filing an estate claim are determined by the state in which the decedent resided.

After the name of the administrator or executor of the estate has been obtained, a duplicate itemized statement of the account should be sent to that person by certified mail, return receipt requested, so that you will know who received it. If no response is received in 10 days, you should contact the executor or the county clerk where the estate is being settled and obtain forms for filing claim against the estate. (Some states do not have special claim forms but will accept simple itemized statements.) This claim against the estate must be made within a certain length of time, varying from 2 to 36 months, depending on the state in which it is filed.

The executor of the estate will either accept or reject the claim and, if it is accepted, will send an acknowledgment of the debt. Payment is often delayed, owing to the legal complications in settling an estate, but if the claim has been accepted, you will receive your money in due time. If the claim is rejected and you have full justification for claiming the bill, you must file claim against the executor within a limited time, according to state laws. The time limit in such cases starts with the date on the letter of rejection that was sent you in response to your original claim.

Because states have different time limits and statutes in regard to such matters, it is advisable for the medical assistant to contact the doctor's attorney or the local court for the exact procedure to follow.

Bankruptcy

Bankruptcy laws were passed to secure equal distribution of the assets of an individual among the individual's creditors. Bankruptcy laws are federal and are applicable in all states. When you are notified that a patient has declared bankruptcy, you should no longer send statements or make any attempt to collect on the account from the patient.

Chapter VII bankruptcy is usually a "no asset" situation. Since the doctor's fee is an unsecured debt, there is little purpose in pursuing collection. Chapter XIII is known as "Adjustment of Debts of an Individual with Regular Income," according to the Revised Bankruptcy Act of October 1, 1979. Under Chapter XIII, the patient/debtor pays a fixed amount (agreed on by the court) to the trustee in bankruptcy. This is then passed on to the creditors. During this period, none of the creditors can attach the debtor's wages or otherwise attempt to collect the debt.

It is sometimes beneficial to file a claim under Chapter XIII because small payments will be made by the debtor under the supervision of the court over a period of 3 years.

Statutes of Limitations

A **statute of limitations** assigns a certain time after which rights cannot be enforced by action.

Malpractice Statutes

In many states, there are statutes of limitations in regard to malpractice lawsuits, which set a limit to the time during which malpractice actions can be filed. It is usually best to wait until this time has passed before pressing the account of a patient who may feel he is entitled to sue the doctor. However, this should not be made a blanket policy; each case should be judged on its own merit.

Collection Statutes

Statutes of limitations in regard to collections prescribe the time within which a legal collection suit may be rendered against a debtor; the term "outlaw" is sometimes used to refer to debts on which the time limit has passed. This legal time limit varies according to the state in which a doctor practices. Table 18–1 lists the time limits for collections in the various states. It should be noted that if the debtor moves out of state, either temporarily or permanently, the time spent out of state is not included in the time limit. Only the time during which the debtor resides within the state is included in the statute.

The time limit may vary according to the class of account. Generally, accounts may be placed in one of three classes:

- open book accounts
- written contracts
- single-entry accounts

OPEN BOOK ACCOUNTS. Open book accounts are accounts on the books that are open to charges made from time to time. The bill for each illness or treatment is computed separately, and the last date of entry—debit or credit—for that particular illness is the time designated by the statute of limitations for starting that specific debt. It is almost impossible to have a time limit on an account of a patient with a chronic condition, since there is no actual termination of the illness or treatment unless the patient changes physicians or dies. When legal time limits are set, they usually refer to these "open book accounts."

TABLE 18–1. STATUTE OF LIMITATIONS*

Location	Open Accounts (Years)	Contracts in Writing (Years)
Alabama	3	6
Alaska	6	6
Arizona	3	6
Arkansas	3	5
California	4	4
Colorado	6	6
Connecticut	6	6
Delaware	3	6
District of Columbia	3	3
Florida	4	5
Georgia	4	6
Hawaii	6	6
Idaho	4	5
Illinois	5	10
Indiana	6	10
Iowa	5	10
Kansas	3	5
Kentucky	5	15
Louisiana	3	10
Maine	6	6
Maryland	3	3
Massachusetts	6	6
Michigan	6	6
Minnesota	6	6
Mississippi	3	6
Missouri	5	10
Montana	5	8
Nebraska	4	5
Nevada	4	6
New Hampshire	6	6
New Jersey	6	6
New Mexico	4	6
New York	6	6
North Carolina	3	3
North Dakota	6	6
Ohio	6	15
Oklahoma	3	5
Oregon	6	6
Pennsylvania	6	6
Rhode Island	6	6
South Carolina	6	6
South Dakota	6	6
Tennessee	6	6
Texas	4	4
Utah	4	6
Vermont	6	6
Virginia	3	5
Washington	3	6
West Virginia	5	10
Wisconsin	6	6
Wyoming	8	10
Puerto Rico	15	—

* From Summary of Collection Laws published in the American Collectors Association, Inc., 1986 Membership Roster. (Reprinted with permission of American Collectors Association, Inc., Minneapolis, MN.)

WRITTEN CONTRACTS. Written contracts often have the same time limit as open book accounts, but in some states they have a longer time limit. The time limit on written contracts starts from the date due.

SINGLE-ENTRY ACCOUNTS. Single-entry accounts are accounts that have only one entry or charge. These accounts are usually short-lived and are for small amounts. Some states, such as California, place a shorter statute of limitations span on such accounts.

In many states, even though the legal time limit set by the statutes has passed, the account may be reopened and the date extended if you are able to obtain a written acknowledgment of the debt due. For instance, a letter from the patient stating "Yes, I know I owe you $150, but I do not intend paying Dr. Brown" is an acknowledgment of the debt. If this letter is signed and dated, keep it and contact your collector; on the basis of this letter, the collector can then proceed with collection. Also, a small payment on the account will extend the statute expiration date. Photocopy these small checks for proof of payment, should proof become necessary.

USING OUTSIDE COLLECTION ASSISTANCE

When you have done everything possible in your office to follow up on an outstanding account and have not received payment, the question arises as to what step to take next.

- Should the doctor sue for the amount?
- Should the account be turned over to a collection agency?
- Should the account be written off as a bad debt?

Before forcing an account, you must first consider the time element:

- Has the patient been given a fair chance to pay this bill?
- Have you sent statements regularly and used a systematic method of following the account?
- Ask yourself if there might be a misunderstanding in regard to the fee charged. Did you fully itemize the first statement? A large unexplained bill may frighten a patient into making no payments at all because the whole thing looks too big.

If you have used correct registration forms to secure advance credit information, you should know the financial abilities of the patient in regard to payment. However, illness may have caused a loss of salary and resulted in temporary inability to pay. A little investigation will reveal any such troubles.

Could the patient have been dissatisfied with the care received? For some unknown reason, a patient may feel that he or she was not treated correctly. Perhaps the patient expected a complete cure too soon. Only an explanation of the condition, prognosis, and care can enlighten such patients, and this is best handled by the doctor. If a bill is pressed too hard and the patient is dissatisfied for some reason, a malpractice suit may be filed by the patient to "get even."

Collecting Through the Court System
Should We Sue?

Will a doctor lose more good will by suing for a bill than by writing it off as a loss? One management official has related that, strangely enough, when a doctor-client sued two patients for large sums, the patients lost the cases, paid up, and were back in the office for treatment very shortly! However, most physicians feel it is unwise to resort to the court to collect medical bills unless there are extraordinary circumstances.

An account must be considered a 100% loss to you before legal proceedings are started. Remember that you should never threaten to instigate legal proceedings unless you are prepared to carry out the threat and have the doctor's consent to issue such a warning.

If your employer decides in favor of a lawsuit, investigate thoroughly before taking action. Litigation to collect a bill is generally in order in the following instances:

- When a patient can afford to pay without hardship.
- When the physician can produce office records that support the bill.
- When the physician can justify the size of the bill by comparison with fee practices in the community.
- When the patient's general condition after treatment is satisfactory.
- When the persuasive powers of an ethical collection agency have been exhausted, and the agency advises suing.
- When the patient can be given ample warning of the physician's intention to sue.
- When the defendant (whether a patient or a parent or legal guardian) is legally liable for the services rendered to the patient.
- When the defendant is not judgment-proof.*
- When the statute of limitations has ruled out any possible malpractice action.
- When the physician is not bubbling over with indignation and is not in a "he-can't-do-this-to-me" frame of mind.

The experienced practitioner establishes these 10 "whens" before plunging into costly litigation.

Small Claims Court

Many doctors' offices find the small claims court a satisfactory and inexpensive way to collect delinquent accounts. The law places a limit on the amount of the debt for which relief may be sought in the small claims court. Since this varies from state to state (from $300 to $5000) and in some

---

The Soldiers and Sailors Civil Relief Act (1940) protects the rights of servicemen and women on active duty.

instances even within a state, this limit should be checked locally before seeking recovery in this manner.

Parties to small claims actions may not be represented by an attorney at the trial, but may send another person to court in their behalf to produce records supporting the claim. Doctors often send their bookkeeper or medical assistant with records of unpaid accounts to show the judge.

In addition to the judgment for the amount owed, the plaintiff in small claims court may also recover the costs of the suit. This rarely exceeds $20. For a very small investment in time and money, the doctor who uses this method:

- Has saved the time of a regular court action
- Has had no attorney's fee to pay
- Has not sacrificed the commission charged by a collection agency

Remember, though, that the court has awarded only a judgment. You still must collect the money. Also, the only person in a small claims action who has the right of appeal is the defendant. An appeal by the defendant may have the judgment set aside. The plaintiff (doctor) cannot file an appeal in a small claims action; the decision of the court is final.

The forms for filing action and full instructions on the course to follow may be obtained from the clerk of the small claims court. The medical assistant who has never appeared in the court would probably be wise to attend once as a spectator only to preview the procedure and feel more at ease when appearing for the doctor.

A collection agency to which an account may have been assigned may not file or handle a small claims action. It must either sue in the regular municipal or justice court or attempt to collect the debt in some other way.

Using a Collection Agency

The medical assistant should try every means possible to collect accounts before they become delinquent. But as soon as the account is determined uncollectible through your office—that is, the patient has failed to respond to your final letter or has failed to fulfill a second promise on payment—send the account to the collector without delay. Skips should be assigned immediately.

Even though collection by an agency will mean sacrificing from 40 to 60% of the amount owed, further delay will only reduce the chances of recovery by the professional collector. If the agency finds that the case deserves special consideration, it will seek the physician's advice before proceeding further.

Selecting a Collection Agency

There are a number of agencies either owned and operated as an integral part of the county medical society or operated separately from the medical society but supervised by the medical profession. These bureaus provide specialized medical collection services.

Another type of collection agency is a division of the local credit association, recognized by the National Retail Credit Association. If the local credit association does not maintain a collection department, it will be able to recommend a reputable one. A nationally recognized credit association has considerable responsibility and a high standard to maintain. These factors act as monitors to its reliability.

The most common type of collection agency throughout the United States is the privately owned and operated agency. Many of these work with the local professional societies and strive to keep their work on a high ethical standard. Because a few bureaus are unethical and unscrupulous in their tac-

---

GUIDELINES FOR CHOOSING A COLLECTION AGENCY

- The best sources of referral for a collection agency are the doctor's colleagues, other doctors in the same specialty, and associates in the hospitals.

- For references of local agencies, you may check with the Medical-Dental-Hospital Bureaus of America, 111 East Wacker Drive, Chicago, IL 60601; the American Collectors Association, 4040 West 70th Street, Minneapolis, MN 55434; or the Associated Credit Bureaus of America, Collection Division, 6767 Southwest Freeway, Houston, TX 77074.

- Investigate the methods of collection used. Ask to see any letters, reminder notices, or follow-up literature used.

- Investigate to determine if the agency has contacts with other services to aid in the collection of out-of-town accounts.

- Find out the agency's collection ratio and the fees for various kinds of accounts assigned to them (large or small accounts, out-of-town accounts, skips). Its fees should be in line with the amount of effort expended to collect your accounts.

- The agency should rely heavily on a persuasive approach rather than being "suit-happy."

- Find out whether the agency will report cases deserving special consideration back to the physician's office.

- Generally speaking, one should not sign a contract.

tics, care should be taken to be sure that the one you choose is reliable and ethical (see Guidelines for Choosing a Collection Agency). For the sake of comparison, many health care facilities use two or three agencies.

Responsibilities to the Collection Agency

When the physician selects a reputable agency and decides to make use of its services, you must be prepared to provide the agency with all the necessary data to enable it to begin prompt collection procedures on overdue accounts. The agency should receive:

- Full name of the debtor
- Name of the spouse
- Last known address
- Full amount of the debt
- Date of the last entry on account (debit or credit)
- Occupation of the debtor
- Business address
- Any other pertinent data

After an account has been turned over to a collection agency, your office makes no further collection attempts. Once the agency has begun its work, follow these guidelines and procedures:

1. Send no more statements.
2. Mark the patient's ledger or stamp it so that you know it is now in the hands of the collector.
3. Refer the patient to the agency if he or she contacts you in regard to the account.
4. Promptly report any payments made directly to your office (a percentage of this payment is due the agency).
5. Call the agency if you obtain any information that will be of value in tracing or collecting the account.
6. Do not push the agency with frequent calls. The representatives of the agency will report to you regularly and keep you posted on collection progress.

ACCOUNTS RECEIVABLE INSURANCE PROTECTION

The potential income represented by the doctor's accounts receivable ledger is probably considerable, and the patient ledgers may be the only record the doctor has of what is owed. This potential income deserves insurance protection. The doctor's general insurance representative can obtain insurance protection for these records. Most insurance companies require that the ledgers be kept in a safe place, such as an insulated file cabinet. This is a good practice to follow in any case. They will also require that the accounts receivable balance be reported monthly, for

the cost of the insurance is usually based on the average balance during the year. The premium for this type of insurance is nominal. Anyone who has ever lost important records through fire or flood would say it is priceless.

In conclusion, we point out that to the best of our ability we have checked and verified all statements made in this chapter about collection law and legal procedures. However, laws do change, and it is recommended that you check with your local state regulations and laws to verify points pertinent to your special area. State law takes precedence over federal law if the state law is stronger. For a general textbook of this nature, it is impossible to check each of these state requirements to determine which are stronger and which would prevail over Federal Public Law 95-109.

▶ LEARNING ACHIEVEMENTS

Are you able to:

1. Define the terms listed in the Vocabulary of this chapter?
2. Name three ways in which payment for medical services might be made?
3. List nine items that should be considered in developing a credit policy?
4. State three reasons for itemizing billing statements?
5. Describe cycle billing and its advantages?
6. Calculate a collection ratio and an accounts receivable ratio and discuss their significance?
7. List the three most common reasons for patient failure to pay for services?
8. Discuss telephone collection procedures and actions that you should or should not take?
9. Name five sources of information to use in tracing skips?
10. Explain what you should do upon receiving notice of a debtor's declaration of bankruptcy?
11. Discuss the small claims court procedure for collecting delinquent accounts?
12. Describe what follow-up action you would take after assigning an account to a collection agency?
13. Given the necessary information, prepare an age analysis of accounts receivable?
14. Outline the sequence of events in a collection program?

REFERENCES AND READINGS

American Medical Association: *The Business Side of Medical Practice,* Chicago, The Association, 1989.
Fair Credit Billing Act, October 28, 1975.
Bankruptcy Act (Title 11, U.S. Code), October 1, 1979.

CHAPTER NINETEEN

—

HEALTH AND ACCIDENT INSURANCE

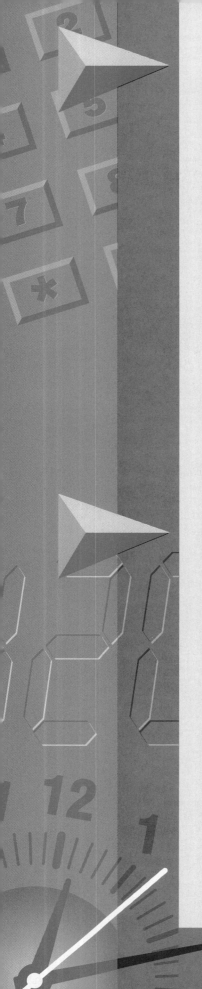

CHAPTER OUTLINE

VOCABULARY

assignment of insurance benefits A statement authorizing the insurance company to pay benefits directly to the physician.

beneficiary The person receiving the benefits of an insurance policy.

birthday rule The rule governing the hierarchy of coordination of benefits.

claim A demand to the insurer by the insured person for the payment of benefits under a policy.

coding Converting verbal descriptions of diseases, injuries, and procedures into numerical and alphanumerical designations.

coinsurance/copayment A policy provision by which both the insured person and the insurer share in a specified ratio of the expenses resulting from an illness or injury.

coordination of benefits (COB) The provision in an insurance contract that limits benefits to 100% of the cost.

crossover claim A claim for benefits under both Medicare and Medicaid.

deductible A statement in an insurance policy that the insuring company will pay the expenses incurred after the insured person has paid a specified amount.

disability The condition resulting from illness or injury that makes an individual unable to be employed.

established patient A patient who has received care from the physician within the last 3 years.

fee schedule A list of services or procedures indemnified by the insurance company and of the specific dollar amounts that will be paid for each service.

fringe benefit A benefit granted by an employer that involves a money cost but does not affect the basic wage rates of employees.

group policy A policy that covers a group—for example, all employees of one company—under a master contract.

indemnity A benefit paid by an insurer for a loss insured under a policy.

individual policy A policy usually held by a person who does not qualify for a group policy.

medical indigent One who is able to take care of ordinary living expenses but is unable to afford medical care.

member physician A physician who has agreed to accept the contracts of an insurer; this usually includes accepting the insurance benefits as payment in full.

new patient A patient who has not received any professional services from the physician in the past 3 years.

nonparticipating provider A physician who does not accept assignment under Medicare or the Blue Plans.

participating provider A physician who does accept assignment under Medicare or the Blue Plans.

pre-existing condition A physical condition of an insured person that existed prior to the issuance of the insurance policy.

premium The periodic payment required to keep a policy in force.

prepaid plan A plan that provides all covered services to a policyholder for payment of a monthly fee.

professional standards review organization (PSRO) A group of physicians working with the government to review cases for hospital admission and discharge under government guidelines; sometimes referred to as Peer Review.

rider A legal document that modifies the protection of a policy.

service benefit plan A plan that agrees to pay for certain surgical and medical services and that is not restricted to a fee schedule.

subscriber A person named as principal in an insurance contract.

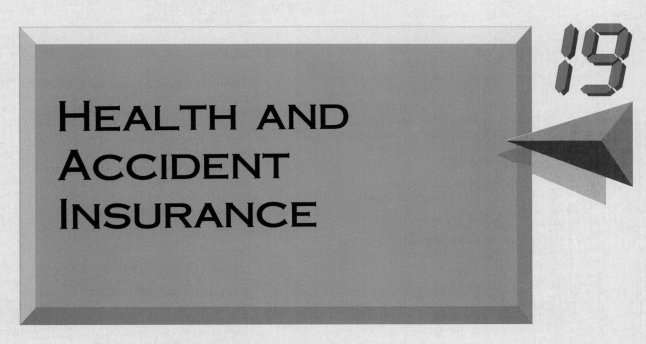

HEALTH AND ACCIDENT INSURANCE

LEARNING OBJECTIVES

COGNITIVE
Upon successful completion of this chapter, you should be able to:

1. Define the terms listed in the Vocabulary.
2. Cite three advantages of group insurance policies over individual policies.
3. Name seven major types of health insurance benefits.
4. State the meaning of the Birthday Law.
5. State the basic differences between *indemnity* and *service benefit* plans.
6. Identify four purposes of numerical diagnostic and procedural coding.
7. Name the principal coding systems that link the medical profession and the insurance system.
8. List 10 reasons for possible rejection of insurance claims.
9. State the maximum billing period for Medicare claims.
10. Explain why a patient's care under workers' compensation should be recorded separately from his or her care as a private patient.
11. List and briefly describe three types of managed care organizations.
12. List the five pieces of information in a patient's chart that are essential to assigning a case to a DRG.

PERFORMANCE
Upon successful completion of this chapter, you should be able to perform the following activities:

1. Identify and complete the appropriate insurance forms for patients covered by:
   a. Medicare
   b. CHAMPUS
   c. Workers' compensation
   d. Blue Cross and Blue Shield
2. Calculate the billing for patients whose insurance includes deductibles and coinsurance.

Health insurance is an important factor in the practice of medicine. As a medical assistant, you must understand insurance terminology, types of insurance coverage, the importance of obtaining consent for release of information, the effect of **assignment of insurance benefits,** and how to handle **claims.** You must also be able to communicate with patients about processing their insurance.

You may be expected to:

- Prepare insurance claim forms
- Maintain an insurance claims register
- Trace unpaid claims
- Evaluate claims rejection
- Report procedures to prepaid care plans
- Translate medical terminology into procedural and diagnostic codes

Fifty years ago, health insurance as we know it now was very uncommon. Today, most patients who come into a health care facility have some kind of health insurance coverage, either privately or through government-sponsored programs. Although the rapid growth of health insurance coverage is a recent phenomenon brought about by economic necessity, the concept of health insurance is not new.

BRIEF HISTORY OF HEALTH INSURANCE

The first company organized specifically to write health insurance was founded in 1847. The nation's earliest accident insurance company came into being in 1850 in response to public demand for coverage against frequent rail and steamboat accidents of the mid-19th century. By the turn of the 20th century, 47 American companies were issuing accident insurance.

In its early stages, the emphasis of health insurance was directed toward replacement of income rather than toward hospital or surgical benefits. The early insurance company policy protected the policyholder against loss of earned income due to a limited number of diseases, including typhus, typhoid, scarlet fever, smallpox, diphtheria, diabetes, and a few others. Emphasis on the income aspects of the insurance continued until 1929, the start of the Great Depression.

At this time, a group of school teachers banded together to form an arrangement with Baylor Hospital in Dallas, Texas, to provide themselves with hospital care on a prepayment basis. This was the origin of the Blue Cross service concept for provision of hospital care.

A further major change occurred during World War II. The freezing of industrial wages made the **fringe benefit** a significant element of collective bargaining. Group health insurance became a large part of the fringe benefit package.

PURPOSE OF HEALTH INSURANCE

Voluntary health insurance is designed primarily for those who can take care of the costs of routine illnesses but to whom a major illness may prove a real financial burden. Minor bills for preventive injections, routine office calls, and treatment of ailments of short duration such as colds should be considered a predictable expense in a family budget. Covering such items in an insurance program boosts administrative costs of the insurance plan out of proportion to the small benefits received.

Cost of Coverage

Few insurance policies pay all expenses resulting from accident or illness. The basic cost of health care coverage is an annual **premium** for which the insurer agrees to provide certain benefits. The real cost to the individual at the time of treatment includes:

- Deductibles
- Copayment
- Services not covered

The **deductible** is that portion of the bill that a **subscriber** must pay before insurance coverage is effective. The amount of the deductible is stated in the contract.

A **copayment** is a contribution the subscriber must make to cover some portion of each bill. This could be as low as $2 to $3 for each office visit or, more commonly, 20% of the total cost. Services not covered, such as eye examinations or dental care, are also a part of the total cost.

Coordination of Benefits

Coordination of benefits (COB) or nonduplication of benefits provisions are included in most group contracts. The purpose of COB provisions is to limit the benefits to 100% of the cost and to prevent duplication of benefits for the same service. Not all insurance plans have COB provisions. A plan that does not have COB provisions becomes the primary payer and pays benefits first. Laws establishing which payer is primary, including the Birthday Law, were enacted in January 1987 in many states.

In the case of an employed person who is eligible for Medicare benefits, the employer's plan is the primary carrier, and Medicare is the supplemental carrier.

In many families, both husband and wife are wage earners, and frequently, both are eligible for health insurance benefits through their own employment and their spouses'.

Coordination of benefits follows the rules of the plan that is the primary payer. If both plans have COB provisions:

- The policyholder's own plan is primary for that individual. An exception occurs if the policyholder is laid off or retired and not a Medicare recipient. In this case, the policyholder's plan pays second.
- The primary coverage for dependents of policyholders is determined by the **Birthday law.** The insurance plan of the policyholder whose birthday comes first in the calendar year (month and day, not year) provides primary coverage for each dependent.
- If neither of the above situations applies, the plan that has been in existence longer is the primary payer.

The primary plan for dependents of legally separated or divorced parents is more complicated.

- The Birthday rule is in effect if the parent who has custody of the dependent has *not* remarried. If the custodial parent *has* remarried, that parent's plan is primary for that dependent.
- If one parent has been decreed by the court as the responsible party, that parent's policy is primary. This is not always the parent with custody of the child.
- If one of the plans originated in a state that does not have the COB law, the plan that did originate in a state with a COB law will determine the order of benefits.

All of this emphasizes the need to determine whether there is a Birthday rule in your state.

AVAILABILITY OF HEALTH INSURANCE

Health insurance is available through **group policies, individual policies,** and subscription to **prepaid plans.** Many people are covered by government plans.

Group Policies

Insurance written under a group policy covers a group of people under a master contract, which is generally issued to an employer for the benefit of the employees. The individual employee may be given a certificate of insurance containing information regarding the master policy and indicating that the individual is covered under the policy. Professional associations also frequently offer group insurance as a benefit of membership.

Group coverage usually provides greater benefits at lower premiums, and a physical examination is seldom required for the enrollees. Every person in a group contract has identical coverage.

Individual Policies

Some individuals do not qualify for inclusion in a group policy, but most companies that write group insurance also offer individual policies. The applicant may be required to have a physical examination before acceptance and, if there is an unusual risk, may be denied insurance or may have to accept a **rider** or limitation on the policy. In any event, the individual premium will probably be greater and the benefits less than in a group policy.

Government Plans

In 1956, government became a major insurer with passage of Law 569, which authorized dependents of military personnel to receive treatment by civilian physicians at the expense of the government. We know this today as CHAMPUS (Civilian Health and Medical Program of the Uniformed Services).

Title XIX of Public Law 89-97, under the Social Security Amendments of 1965, provided for agreements with states for assistance from the federal government in providing health care for the **medically indigent** and is known as Medicaid.

Medicare under Social Security for the patient over 65 years of age went into effect on July 1, 1966. The law was expanded in 1973 to cover disabled persons under 65 years of age who had been receiving Social Security or railroad retirement checks for 2 or more years. This included disabled workers, persons who became incapacitated before age 22 years, disabled widows, and disabled dependent widowers.

The passage of the Health Maintenance Organization (HMO) Act in 1973 provided for federal aid to health insurance prepayment plans that met certain criteria. This brought about an accelerated growth of HMOs, which are organizations that provide for comprehensive health care to an enrolled group for a fixed periodic payment.

Title VI of the Social Security Amendments Act of 1983 contained the prospective payment system (PPS) for hospitals, which would begin the radical restructuring of the payment system to hospitals for Medicare inpatient services.

The resource-based relative value scale (RBRVS) reimbursement system put into effect in 1992 was the most fundamental change in the determination of physicians' fees under Medicare since the inception of Medicare in 1966.

The patient who is over 65 years of age probably is covered by Part B of Medicare under Social Security. The medically indigent patient may be eligible for Medicaid with or without Medicare. Dependents of military personnel are covered by CHAMPUS (Civilian Health and Medical Program of the Uniformed Services); surviving spouses and dependent children of veterans who died as a result of service-connected disabilities are covered by

19

CHAMPVA (Civilian Health and Medical Program of the Veterans Administration). Many wage earners are protected against the loss of wages and the cost of medical care resulting from occupational accident or disease through workers' compensation insurance.

All of these plans are dealt with in further detail later in this chapter.

TYPES OF INSURANCE BENEFITS

An insurance package is tailored to the needs of each individual or group policy, and the combinations of benefits are limitless. A policy may contain any one or any combination of the following kinds of benefits.

Hospitalization

Hospital coverage pays the cost of all or part of the insured person's hospital room and board and special hospital services. Hospital insurance policies frequently set a maximum amount payable per day and a maximum number of days of hospital care. Some insurance companies require that the hospital be an accredited or a licensed hospital. Most hospital plans exclude admission for diagnostic studies.

Surgical

Surgical coverage pays all or part of the surgeon's fee; some plans also pay for an assistant surgeon. Surgery includes any incision or excision, removal of foreign bodies, aspiration, suturing, and reduction of fractures. The surgery may be accomplished in the hospital, in a doctor's office, or elsewhere. The insurer frequently provides the subscriber with a surgical fee schedule that sets forth the amount payable for commonly performed procedures.

Basic Medical

Medical coverage pays all or part of the physician's fee for nonsurgical services, including hospital, home, and office visits, depending on the coverage. It may include provision for diagnostic laboratory, x-ray, and pathology fees. Many medical plans do not cover a routine physical examination when the patient does not have a specific complaint or illness.

Major Medical

Major medical insurance (formerly called *catastrophic coverage*) provides protection against especially heavy medical bills resulting from catastrophic or prolonged illnesses. It may be a supplement to basic medical coverage or a comprehensive integrated program providing both basic and major medical protection.

Disability (Loss of Income) Protection

Weekly or monthly cash benefits are provided to employed policyholders who become unable to work owing to an accident or illness. Many policies do not start payment until after a specified number of days or until a certain number of sick leave days have been used. Payment is made directly to the patient and is intended to replace loss of income resulting from illness. It is not intended for payment of specific medical bills.

Dental Care

Dental coverage is included in many fringe benefit packages. Some policies are based on a copayment and incentive program, with the company's copayment increasing each year until 100% coverage is reached.

Vision Care

Vision care insurance may include reimbursement for all or for a percentage of the cost for refraction, lenses, and frames.

Medicare Supplement

These are contracts insuring persons 65 years of age or older that supplement the coverage provided by Medicare.

Special Class Insurance

Applicants for health insurance who cannot qualify for a standard policy by reason of health may be issued special class insurance with limited coverage.

Special Risk Insurance

This insurance protects a person in the event of a certain type of accident, such as automobile or airplane crashes, or for certain diseases, such as tuberculosis or cancer. There is usually a maximum benefit.

Liability Insurance

There are many types of liability insurance, including automobile, business, and homeowners' policies. Liability policies often include benefits for medical expenses payable to individuals who are injured in the insured person's home or car, without regard to the insured person's actual legal liability for the accident.

Life Insurance

Life insurance policies sometimes provide monthly cash benefits if the policyholder becomes permanently and totally disabled. Sometimes, the proceeds from life insurance are used to meet the expenses of the insured person's last illness.

Overhead Insurance

A self-employed individual may carry overhead insurance that becomes effective during a period of illness or disability. Overhead insurance reimburses the insured person for specific fixed monthly expenses that are normal and customary in the operation and conduct of the person's business or office.

PAYMENT OF BENEFITS

Insurance benefits may be determined and paid in one of several ways:

- By indemnity schedules
- By service benefit plans
- By determination of the usual, customary, and reasonable fee
- By relative value studies

Indemnity Schedules

In **indemnity** plans, the insurer agrees to pay the subscriber a set amount of money for a given procedure or service. The insured person is given a schedule of indemnities **(fee schedule)** when the policy is purchased.

Indemnity plans do not agree to pay for the complete services rendered. Many times, there is a difference in the amount paid by the insurance company and the amount of the physician's fee. For example, the insurer may agree to pay up to $1000 for a specific operation, with no consideration for the time or complications of the surgery. If the physician charges $1200, the difference of $200 is the responsibility of the patient.

This type of plan takes the major expense out of medical bills and helps to keep the premiums down. The amount of the premium often determines the schedule of benefits. Indemnity benefits are usually paid to the person insured unless that person has authorized payment directly to the provider.

Service Benefit Plans

In **service benefit plans,** the insuring company agrees to pay for certain surgical or medical services without additional cost to the person insured. There is no set fee schedule.

In a service benefit plan, a surgery with complications would warrant a higher fee than an uncompli-

cated procedure. Premiums are sometimes higher for this type of coverage, but often payments are larger. Frequently, the payment for benefits is sent directly to the physician and is considered full payment for the services rendered.

Usual, Customary, and Reasonable Fee

Some insurance companies agree to pay on the basis of all or a percentage of the physician's usual, customary, and reasonable fee (see Chapter 15).

KINDS OF PLANS

Blue Cross and Blue Shield

In the early 1930s, hospitals introduced Blue Cross plans to provide coverage for hospital costs. Today, there are local Blue Cross plans operating in all states of the Union, the District of Columbia, Canada, Puerto Rico, and Jamaica.

In 1939, state medical societies in California and Michigan began sponsoring health plans to provide medical and surgical services; these became known as Blue Shield plans. Other states soon followed, and today Blue Shield is the largest medical prepayment system in the country.

Early in its development, Blue Shield was often known as "the doctor's plan." **Member physicians** agreed to bill Blue Shield for services to subscribers and abide by other prearranged procedures. Under many Blue Shield contracts, physicians accept Blue Shield's payment as payment in full for covered services. Blue Shield and its member physicians agree on methods of reimbursement in advance of the service performed.

In many plans, Blue Shield provides the medical and surgical coverage, and Blue Cross provides hospital coverage. However, in some areas, Blue Cross plans write medical and surgical insurance in addition to providing hospital coverage. Conversely, some Blue Shield plans offer hospital insurance as well as medical and surgical coverage.

Blue Cross benefits are normally paid to the provider of service. In some cases, a check issued jointly to the provider and the person insured is sent to the latter, who must then endorse and forward it to the provider.

Blue Shield makes direct payment to member physicians. For services of a nonmember physician, the payment is sent to the subscriber.

Blue Shield Reciprocity

Blue Shield reciprocity is an agreement among Blue Shield plans to provide benefits to subscribers who are away from home. It means the subscriber can receive benefits almost anywhere in the country.

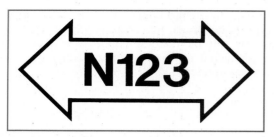

FIGURE 19-1. Blue Shield reciprocity symbol (From Fordney M: *Insurance Handbook for the Medical Office*, 3rd ed., Philadelphia, W.B. Saunders Co., 1989.)

The identification card of subscribers having reciprocity has a double-end red arrow symbol with an "N" followed by three digits (Fig. 19-1). When the reciprocity **beneficiary** receives covered care outside his or her own district, the physician bills the local Blue Shield plan using the local Blue Shield form. For those who do not have the double-end red arrow, the subscriber's home plan must be billed.

Foundations for Medical Care

A foundation for medical care is a management system for community health services. It takes the form of an organization created by local physicians through their medical society, and it concerns itself with the quality and cost of medical care. Under the foundation concept, the following procedure occurs:

- An insurance company sells and negotiates the policy. It collects the premiums, assumes all the risks, and reimburses the foundation for the cost of the claims office.
- The foundation sets policy standards; receives, processes, reviews, and pays claims to doctors; sets maximum fees based on current fees in the area; elects doctor-members yearly; and continually studies local medical-economic problems.
- Member doctors agree to accept foundation fees as full payment under foundation-approved policies.
- The local medical society legally controls the foundation and selects foundation trustees.
- The patient selects the doctor of his or her own choice; the patient or the patient's union or employer pays the premium directly to the insurance company.

Commercial Insurers

More than half of those covered by some form of health insurance are covered by private (commercial) insurance companies. Physicians and medical societies control neither the premiums paid nor the benefits received from such policies. Payment is normally made to the subscriber unless the subscriber has authorized that payment be made directly to the physician.

Government Plans
Medicare Under Social Security

There are two distinct parts (A and B) to the Medicare program.

PART A: HOSPITAL INSURANCE. Any person who is receiving monthly Social Security or railroad retirement checks is automatically enrolled for hospital insurance benefits and pays no premiums for this insurance. Part A is financed by special contributions paid by employed individuals as deductions from their salary, with matching contributions from their employers. These sums are collected along with regular Social Security contributions from wages and self-employment income earned during a person's working years.

There is a sizable deductible that the hospitalized patient must pay toward the hospital expenses.

PART B: MEDICAL INSURANCE. Those persons who are eligible for Part A are eligible for Part B, but must apply for this coverage and pay a monthly premium. Some federal employees and former federal employees who are not eligible for Social Security benefits and Part A may still enroll in Part B. Certain disabled persons under the age of 65 years are also eligible for Medicare (Fig. 19-2).

The patient with Medicare Part B has to meet an annual deductible before benefits become available, after which Medicare pays 80% of the covered benefits. The patient must pay the remaining 20% plus any amount not allowed by Medicare.

Many Medicare enrollees also carry private supplemental insurance that pays the deductible and the 20% copayment.

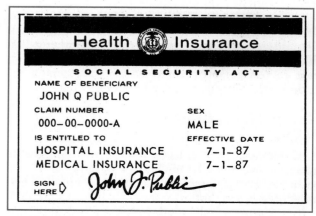

FIGURE 19-2. Identification card for a Medicare patient.

Medicaid

Title XIX of Public Law 89-97 under the Social Security Amendments of 1965 provides for agreements with states for assistance from the federal government in providing health care for the medically indigent. All states and the District of Columbia have Medicaid programs, but wide variations may exist among these programs.

The federal government provides basic funding to the state, after which the states individually elect whether to provide funds for extension of benefits. The state determines the type and extent of medical care that will be covered within the minimum requirements established by the federal government.

The physician may accept or decline to treat Medicaid patients. The physician who does accept Medicaid patients automatically agrees to accept Medicaid payment as payment in full for covered services. The patient *cannot* be billed for the difference between the Medicaid fee and the physician's normal fee. The patient *can* be billed for any services that are not covered by Medicaid.

Eligibility for benefits is determined by the respective states. Those who qualify include:

- Persons receiving welfare
- Persons who are medically needy, that is, they can provide for the expenses of daily living but are unable to afford medical care
- Recipients of Aid to Families with Dependent Children
- Persons who receive Supplemental Security Income (SSI)

A card or coupon showing proof of eligibility is usually issued to the beneficiary on a monthly basis. The dates of issuance vary, but the medical assistant must always check the patient's card or coupon to verify current coverage. Some nonemergency procedures require prior approval.

Medi/Medi

Some patients who qualify for Medicare are still unable to pay the portion for which they are responsible and may qualify for both Medicare and Medicaid. Medicare is the primary coverage, and any residual is paid by the Medicaid assistance program. Claims submitted for coverage under Medicare and Medicaid are sometimes referred to as **crossover claims.**

Military Medical Benefits

CHAMPUS. In 1956, the passage of Law 569 authorized dependents of military personnel to receive in-hospital treatment by civilian physicians at the expense of the government. This program was first called Medicare, but was later changed to CHAMPUS (Civilian Health and Medical Program of the Uniformed Services).

On September 30, 1966, the Military Medical Benefits Amendment Act of 1966 became law. This act added outpatient care benefits, including prescription drugs, to the in-hospital benefits previously allowed. The patient pays an out-of-pocket deductible (now $150, not to exceed $300 per family for claims after April 1, 1991) each fiscal year (October 1 to September 30), plus 20% of the balance for outpatient care. Families of active duty members pay at least $25 or a small fee for each day in a civilian hospital—whichever is greater.

Military retirees and their dependents as well as dependents of deceased members became eligible for outpatient benefits in January 1967, except that their copayment amount is 25% after the deductible.

In order to receive CHAMPUS benefits, eligible persons must be enrolled in the Defense Enrollment Eligibility Reporting System (DEERS), a computerized database that is used for verifying eligibility.

CHAMPVA. In 1973, a program similar to CHAMPUS was established for the spouses and dependent children of veterans suffering total, permanent, service-connected disabilities and for the surviving spouses and dependent children of veterans who have died as a result of service-connected disabilities. This is called CHAMPVA (Civilian Health and Medical Program of the Veterans Administration).

Eligibility is determined, and identification cards are issued, by the nearest Veterans Affairs medical center. The insured persons then are free to choose their own private physicians. Benefits and cost-sharing features are the same as those for CHAMPUS beneficiaries who are military retirees or their dependents, and dependents of deceased members of the military. Retirees, their families, and the families of service members who have died pay 25% of the cost of care in a civilian hospital.

Further information regarding these military medical benefit programs may be obtained by writing to OCHAMPUS, Aurora, CO 80045.

Workers' Compensation

All state legislatures have passed workers' compensation laws to protect wage earners against the loss of wages and the cost of medical care resulting from occupational accident or disease. State laws differ as to the classes of employees included and the benefits provided.

None of the states' workers' compensation laws cover all employees. However, if a patient says that he or she was injured in the workplace or is suffering from a work-associated illness, the medical assistant should check with the patient's employer to verify the insurance coverage.

Compensation benefits include medical care benefits, weekly income replacement benefits for temporary **disability,** permanent disability settlements, and survivor benefits where applicable. The provider of service (doctor, hospital, therapist, and so forth) accepts the workers' compensation payment as payment in full and does not bill the patient.

Time limitations are set forth for the prompt reporting of workers' compensation cases. The employee is obligated to promptly notify the employer; the employer in turn must notify the insurance company and must refer the employee to a source of medical care. In some states, the employer and the insurance company have the right to select the physician who will treat the patient. In essence, the purpose of workers' compensation laws is to provide prompt medical care to the injured or ill worker so that the person may be restored to health and return to full earning capacity in as short a time as possible.

Managed Care Organizations

- Health Maintenance Organization (HMO)
- Independent Practice Association (IPA)
- Preferred-Provider Organization (PPO)

HEALTH MAINTENANCE ORGANIZATION. The HMO is what first comes to mind when we speak of prepaid plans. An HMO plan agrees to provide specific services to every enrolled member for a prepaid fee. An HMO may be *closed-panel* or *open-panel*. A closed-panel HMO employs a staff of physicians and pays each one a salary. The HMO charges each patient a predetermined amount, which is usually negotiated through a group contract, and in addition may charge a small copayment for each visit. Public Law 93-222, the HMO Assistance Act, was enacted in 1973 to encourage and promote the growth of HMOs as a means of health care cost containment. Many Medicare recipients endorse their benefits over to an HMO for fully prepaid medical care. Employers who provide health care benefits to employees are required to offer federally qualified HMOs as an option.

INDEPENDENT PRACTICE ASSOCIATION. An IPA is a closed-panel HMO. Instead of maintaining its own staff and clinic buildings, the IPA contracts with independently practicing physicians who continue to practice in their own offices. The IPA may pay each doctor a set amount per patient in advance, or the fees charged for services to group members may be billed directly to the IPA rather than to the patient. Fees for services to nonmember patients are handled the same as any other fees for service.

PREFERRED-PROVIDER ORGANIZATION. The PPO preserves the fee-for-service concept that is desirable in the eyes of many physicians. An insurer, representing its clients, contracts with a group of providers (physicians) who agree on a predetermined list of charges for all services, including those for complex and unusual procedures. The care is not prepaid. Usually, there are deductibles of 20 to 25% of the predetermined charge that the patient pays; the insurer pays the balance.

A provider who joins a PPO does not need to alter the manner of providing care and continues to treat and bill the regular patients on a fee-for-service basis. When a patient covered under a PPO plan comes for treatment, the physician treats the patient and bills the PPO.

Life Insurance

When an individual whom the physician is treating or has treated in the past makes application for life insurance, the insuring company naturally wants to know the current state of the applicant's health and any significant past medical history.

In order to get an account of the applicant's current state of health, the insurance company authorizes one or more physicians in each community to perform physical examinations of prospective clients.

The insurance company's agent arranges the applicant's appointment for the physical examination and supplies the necessary forms for completion. The examining physician makes a report to the insurance company following the examination. The company may require that the forms be completed in the doctor's own handwriting. The physician is paid a stipulated fee by the insurance company upon receipt of the report.

For a summary of the applicant's past medical history, the agent asks the applicant to supply the names and addresses of any physicians consulted in the past. The company, in turn, requests reports from these physicians. Your physician may receive a request for such information concerning a current or previous patient. Before completing the form, make certain the applicant has signed an authorization for release of information.

The request form usually has a voucher check for a minimal fee attached. The physician may accept the proffered fee or, if it is inadequate, may bill the insurance company for "balance of fee." If the bill is reasonable, it is paid without question.

Disability Insurance

MANDATED. Several states require that employees be covered by nonindustrial disability (time loss) insurance. A small percentage (ranging from 0.3 to 1.2%) of the employee's salary may be deducted to cover the cost of this insurance. All regular employees, part- or full-time, are covered until they retire.

The weekly benefits are based on the employee's salary and calculated using a predetermined formula. There is a waiting period before benefits begin (usually 7 days) and a time limit ranging from 26 to 52 weeks for benefits to continue.

VOLUNTARY. In states that do not have mandated disability insurance, employees or groups may seek coverage from a commercial carrier.

CODING

In recent years, it has become necessary to identify diagnoses and services by code. Converting verbal descriptions of diseases, injuries, and procedures into numerical designations is the essence of **coding.** Numerical diagnostic and procedural coding was developed for a number of reasons:

- Tracking disease processes
- Classification of medical procedures
- Medical research
- Evaluation of hospital utilization

This transference of words to numbers also facilitated the use of computers in claims processing. Without the use of computers, it would be impossible to take care of the 60 to 65 thousand claims processed each day in an average mid-sized claims processing center.

Fee Schedules

Relative Value Scales (RVS)

The RVS was pioneered by the California Medical Association in 1956 to help physicians establish rational, relative fees, and other states soon followed suit. Hundreds of the most commonly performed procedures were compiled, assigned procedure numbers similar to those in the AMA's *Current Procedural Terminology,* and assigned a unit value. The assigned unit value represented the value of that procedure in relation to other procedures commonly performed. Although no monetary value was placed on the units, many insurance companies used the RVS to determine benefits by applying a conversion factor to the unit values. In 1978, the Federal Trade Commission interpreted the California RVS as a fee-setting instrument and prohibited its publication and distribution. The FTC was attempting to make medical practice more competitive by ruling against the setting of fees and by encouraging physicians to advertise.

Resource-Based Relative Value Scale (RBRVS)

We have now come "full circle" and are again practicing under a relative value scale nationally. The RBRVS is one of the outcomes of the Medicare Physician Payment Reform that was enacted in the Omnibus Budget Reconciliation Act of 1989 (OBRA 89). Since the beginning of Medicare, Part B of the program has paid physicians using a fee-for-service system based on "customary, prevailing, and reasonable" charges (CPR). The RBRVS, effective in 1992, has changed this. The RBRVS consists of three parts:

- Physician work
- Charge-based professional liability expenses
- Charge-based overhead

The *physician work* component includes the degree of effort invested by the physician in a particular service or procedure and the time it consumes. The *professional liability* and *overhead* components are computed by the Health Care Financing Administration (HCFA).

The fee schedule is designed to provide national uniform payments after being adjusted to reflect the differences in practice costs across geographic areas. The fee schedule includes a conversion factor (CF), which is a single national number applied to all services paid under the fee schedule.

Procedural Coding

Physicians' Current Procedural Terminology (CPT-4)

CPT-4 is a listing of descriptive terms and identifying codes that is used for reporting medical services and procedures performed by physicians. The purpose of the terminology is to provide a uniform language that accurately identifies medical, surgical, and diagnostic services and that can be used as an effective means for reliable, nationwide communication among physicians, patients, and third parties. CPT was developed initially in 1966 by the American Medical Association. There have been several revisions, and it is updated yearly.

CPT-4 is organized into six sections: Evaluation and Management (EM), Anesthesiology, Surgery, Radiology, Pathology and Laboratory, and Medicine. The EM section is new in the 1992 edition. EM identifies the location where the service was rendered (e.g., at an office or hospital), the category of patient (e.g., a **new patient** or an **established patient**), what service was performed, and the face-to-face time of the services.

An alphabetic index of procedures is located at the back of the CPT-4. Guidelines are found at the beginning of each section and explain items unique to that section that should be reviewed by the coder. Explanations as to the content of subsections, headings, and individual codes are found in the form of NOTES.

A number of specific code numbers have been designated for reporting unlisted procedures. Use of an unlisted code requires a special report. Two-digit modifiers may be attached to the five-digit code to indicate that the service or procedure has been altered. For example, "—50" indicates multiple or bilateral procedures, "—52" indicates reduced service,

"—62" indicates two surgeons, and "—80" indicates surgical assistant services.

HCPCS Coding System

Most Medicare carriers have converted to the Health Care Financing Administration Common Procedure Coding System (HCPCS). HCPCS, which is based on the current edition of the CPT, is a five-digit alphanumerical coding system that can accommodate the addition of modifiers. There are three levels of codes assigned and maintained by Medicare carriers:

- Level I codes include approximately 95 to 98% of all Medicare Part B procedural codes and comprise only CPT codes (excluding those for anesthesiology, which is currently designated by surgery codes).
- Level II codes are assigned by the Health Care Financing Administration (HCFA) and are consistent nationwide. These codes are for physician and nonphysician services not contained in the CPT system; they are alphanumerical, ranging from A0000 to V9999.
- Level III codes are assigned and maintained by each local fiscal intermediary. These codes represent services that are not included in the CPT system and are *not* common to all carriers. These codes range from W0000 to Z9999.

Diagnostic Coding

International Classification of Diseases, Ninth Revision, Clinical Modification (ICD-9-CM)

The International Classification of Diseases, Ninth Revision, Clinical Modification (ICD-9-CM) is published in three volumes:

Volume 1—*Diseases: Tabular (Numerical) Index*

Volume 2—*Diseases: Alphabetic List*

Volume 3—*Tabular List and Alphabetic Index of Procedures*

Volumes 1 and 2 are used in the physician's office to complete insurance claims. Volume 3 is used primarily in hospitals.

ICD-9 is used by health care providers in coding and reporting clinical information required for participation in Medicare and Medicaid programs and for statistical tabulation. Each single disease entity has been assigned a three-digit category. A fourth digit is added to provide specificity to the diagnosis regarding etiology, site, or manifestations. In certain cases, a fifth digit is added that, when permitted, is not optional.

Although diagnostic coding dates back to 17th-century England, and the first International Classification of Diseases (ICD) was published by the World Health Organization (WHO) in 1948, the

ICD-9 took on new significance in 1988 when Congress passed the Medicare Catastrophic Coverage Act. Since 1989, HCFA has mandated the use of ICD-9 codes on every Medicare Part B claim.

GUIDELINES FOR CLAIMS PROCESSING

Gathering Data and Materials

When the first appointment is made, the medical assistant should ask the patient for all insurance information:

- If the patient has an identification card, it should first be examined to determine that the coverage is current and then photocopied for the office record.
- If more than one insurance policy is involved, obtain the name, address, group, and policy number for each company.
- The information obtained for the patient record (see Chapter 14) is used for processing the insurance claim. Be certain that it is current.
- Obtain the name of the subscriber if it is someone other than the patient.
- Obtain a signed authorization form for releasing information if you are submitting the insurance claim for the patient.

Claim Forms

Universal Health Insurance Claim Form (HCFA-1500)

The Health Care Financing Administration Health Insurance Claim Form (HCFA-1500) has been designed to answer the needs of most health care insurers (Fig. 19–3). It is the basic form designed by HCFA for the Medicare and Medicaid claims of physicians and suppliers; however, it is not used to claim reimbursement for ambulance services. The HCFA-1500 has also been adopted by CHAMPUS and has received the approval of the American Medical Association Council on Medical Services.

Some commercial insurance companies do provide their own forms. When filing a claim with such a company, you can complete the HCFA-1500 form and attach it to the commercial form for submission to the insurance carrier.

Since many insurance carriers are using Optical Character Recognition (OCR) scanners to transfer the information on claim forms to their computers' memories, the original form printed in red must be used.

The Superbill

A private insurance carrier sometimes sends its own form to the patient. Rather than completing

APPROVED OMB-0938-0008

PLEASE
DO NOT
STAPLE
IN THIS
AREA

CARRIER

HEALTH INSURANCE CLAIM FORM

PICA | | | PICA

ALIGN BY TYPING AN X IN BOX

1. MEDICARE	MEDICAID	CHAMPUS	CHAMPVA	GROUP HEALTH PLAN	FECA BLK LUNG	OTHER	1a. INSURED'S I.D. NUMBER (FOR PROGRAM IN ITEM 1)
(Medicare #)	(Medicaid #)	(Sponsor's SSN)	(VA File #)	(SSN or ID)	(SSN)	(ID)	

2. PATIENT'S NAME (Last Name, First Name, Middle Initial)

3. PATIENT'S BIRTH DATE MM DD YY   SEX M F

4. INSURED'S NAME (Last Name, First Name, Middle Initial)

5. PATIENT'S ADDRESS (No., Street)

6. PATIENT RELATIONSHIP TO INSURED
Self   Spouse   Child   Other

7. INSURED'S ADDRESS (No., Street)

CITY   STATE

8. PATIENT STATUS
Single   Married   Other

CITY   STATE

ZIP CODE   TELEPHONE (Include Area Code) (   )

Employed   Full-Time Student   Part-Time Student

ZIP CODE   TELEPHONE (INCLUDE AREA CODE) (   )

9. OTHER INSURED'S NAME (Last Name, First Name, Middle Initial)

10. IS PATIENT'S CONDITION RELATED TO:

11. INSURED'S POLICY GROUP OR FECA NUMBER

a. OTHER INSURED'S POLICY OR GROUP NUMBER

a. EMPLOYMENT? (CURRENT OR PREVIOUS)
YES   NO

a. INSURED'S DATE OF BIRTH MM DD YY   SEX M F

b. OTHER INSURED'S DATE OF BIRTH MM DD YY   SEX M F

b. AUTO ACCIDENT?   PLACE (State)
YES   NO

b. EMPLOYER'S NAME OR SCHOOL NAME

c. EMPLOYER'S NAME OR SCHOOL NAME

c. OTHER ACCIDENT?
YES   NO

c. INSURANCE PLAN NAME OR PROGRAM NAME

d. INSURANCE PLAN NAME OR PROGRAM NAME

10d. RESERVED FOR LOCAL USE

d. IS THERE ANOTHER HEALTH BENEFIT PLAN?
YES   NO   *If yes*, return to and complete item 9 a-d.

READ BACK OF FORM BEFORE COMPLETING & SIGNING THIS FORM.

12. PATIENT'S OR AUTHORIZED PERSON'S SIGNATURE I authorize the release of any medical or other information necessary to process this claim. I also request payment of government benefits either to myself or to the party who accepts assignment below.

SIGNED _____ DATE _____

13. INSURED'S OR AUTHORIZED PERSON'S SIGNATURE I authorize payment of medical benefits to the undersigned physician or supplier for services described below.

SIGNED _____

14. DATE OF CURRENT: MM DD YY   ILLNESS (First symptom) OR INJURY (Accident) OR PREGNANCY(LMP)

15. IF PATIENT HAS HAD SAME OR SIMILAR ILLNESS. GIVE FIRST DATE MM DD YY

16. DATES PATIENT UNABLE TO WORK IN CURRENT OCCUPATION MM DD YY   MM DD YY
FROM   TO

17. NAME OF REFERRING PHYSICIAN OR OTHER SOURCE

17a. I.D. NUMBER OF REFERRING PHYSICIAN

18. HOSPITALIZATION DATES RELATED TO CURRENT SERVICES MM DD YY   MM DD YY
FROM   TO

19. RESERVED FOR LOCAL USE

20. OUTSIDE LAB?   YES   NO $ CHARGES

21. DIAGNOSIS OR NATURE OF ILLNESS OR INJURY. (RELATE ITEMS 1,2,3 OR 4 TO ITEM 24E BY LINE)

1. |___.___| 3. |___.___|

2. |___.___| 4. |___.___|

22. MEDICAID RESUBMISSION CODE   ORIGINAL REF. NO.

23. PRIOR AUTHORIZATION NUMBER

24. A DATE(S) OF SERVICE						B Place of Service	C Type of Service	D PROCEDURES, SERVICES, OR SUPPLIES (Explain Unusual Circumstances) CPT/HCPCS	MODIFIER	E DIAGNOSIS CODE	F $ CHARGES	G DAYS OR UNITS	H EPSDT Family Plan	I EMG	J COB	K RESERVED FOR LOCAL USE
From MM	DD	YY	To MM	DD	YY											
1															
2															
3															
4															
5															
6															

25. FEDERAL TAX I.D. NUMBER   SSN EIN

26. PATIENT'S ACCOUNT NO.

27. ACCEPT ASSIGNMENT? (For govt. claims, see back)   YES   NO

28. TOTAL CHARGE $

29. AMOUNT PAID $

30. BALANCE DUE $

31. SIGNATURE OF PHYSICIAN OR SUPPLIER INCLUDING DEGREES OR CREDENTIALS (I certify that the statements on the reverse apply to this bill and are made a part thereof.)

SIGNED _____ DATE _____

32. NAME AND ADDRESS OF FACILITY WHERE SERVICES WERE RENDERED (If other than home or office)

33. PHYSICIAN'S, SUPPLIER'S BILLING NAME, ADDRESS, ZIP CODE & PHONE #

PIN#   GRP#

PATIENT AND INSURED INFORMATION

PHYSICIAN OR SUPPLIER INFORMATION

(APPROVED BY AMA COUNCIL ON MEDICAL SERVICE 8/88)   ***PLEASE PRINT OR TYPE***

FORM HCFA-1500 (U2) (12-90)
FORM OWCP-1500   FORM RRB-1500

19

FIGURE 19-3. Health insurance claim form for patient signature.

this form, the office that uses the superbill discussed in Chapter 18 can simply attach a copy to the insurance form or give an extra copy to the patient if he or she is to submit the claim form. Make certain that the code descriptions on the superbill match those listed in the latest CPT code book.

Assignments

Some insurance companies honor requests for assignment of benefits to the physician. The medical assistant should request that the patient complete an Assignment of Benefits form (Fig. 19–4). This is an authorization to the insurance company to make payment of any benefits directly to the physician. It is the patient's responsibility to pay any balance that is not covered by the insurance.

All claims for government-sponsored insurance ask whether the physician will accept assignment. The physician must check either "Yes" or "No" in an appropriate box. Checking the "Yes" box means that the physician will accept the fee determination of the plan and that the insurance carrier will pay 80% of the fee directly to the physician. The patient is responsible for the remaining 20%.

Establishing a System

Keeping current with insurance information and changes is no small part of the medical assistant's responsibility. The procedure manual should be up-dated as changes occur (Fig. 19–5). Government programs are frequently modified, and these changes are reported in bulletins sent to all physicians. Read these bulletins carefully and save those that contain pertinent information.

Watch for workshops offered to medical assistants and physicians in your area and keep the information in a notebook or folder.

Keep a log of insurance claims as they are received and processed (Fig. 19–6). Date-stamp the forms as they are received and enter the information on the log. This log will enable you to determine immediately whether or not a claim form has been completed and mailed.

- If possible, set aside a definite time for completing insurance claims.
- Have a central location for all insurance forms.
- Have readily available the necessary manuals, code books, and other references needed.
- Create a master list of codes most often used by the practice, including 4th and 5th digits, if appropriate.
- Make it a practice to complete the forms as soon as possible after service is rendered.
- Use the superbill or HCFA-1500 form as often as possible.
- Complete the forms by category (all Blue Cross, all Medicare, and so forth).
- Set the tabulator stops on the typewriter for the form being completed. Make a note of these stops so they can be easily set up when completing the same kind of form again.

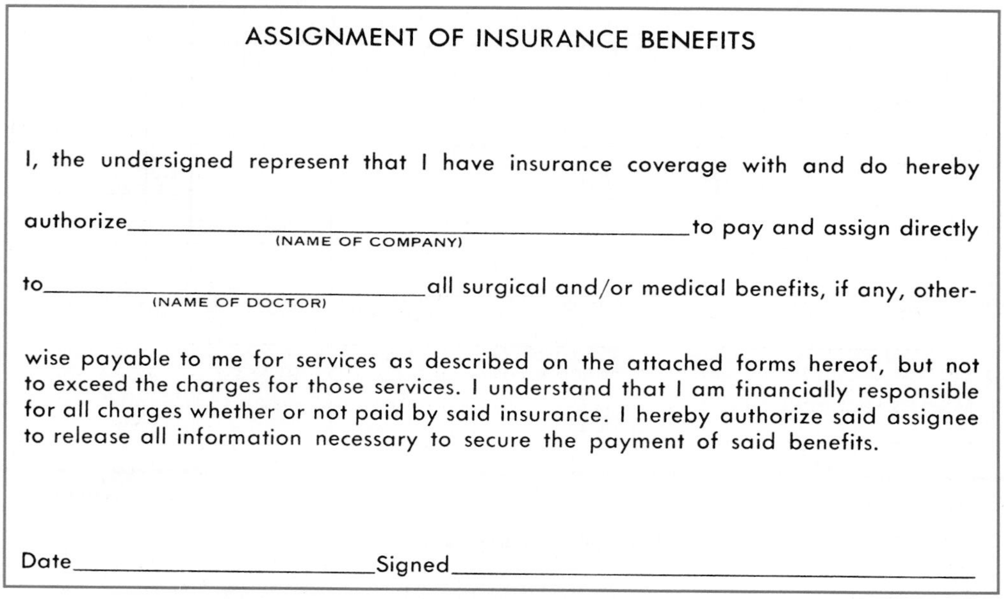

ASSIGNMENT OF INSURANCE BENEFITS

I, the undersigned represent that I have insurance coverage with and do hereby

authorize_____to pay and assign directly
(NAME OF COMPANY)

to_____all surgical and/or medical benefits, if any, other-
(NAME OF DOCTOR)

wise payable to me for services as described on the attached forms hereof, but not to exceed the charges for those services. I understand that I am financially responsible for all charges whether or not paid by said insurance. I hereby authorize said assignee to release all information necessary to secure the payment of said benefits.

Date_____Signed_____

FIGURE 19–4. Assignment of Benefits form.

INSURANCE CARRIER Name & Address	Department and Individual to Contact	POLICYHOLDER Indiv to Contact	Group or Policy Number	SPECIAL NOTES
BLUE SHIELD P O BOX 12345 Anytown, USA	Tom Jones Professional Relations 123-456-7890	Aerospace Industries Joan Crawford 123-888-3030	AI-89037	Tom Jones will speak to groups or give personal assistance in office
		Bell Burgers Nancy Donovan 123-465-2210	BB-3415Z	Scheduled Benefits
OCCIDENTAL P O BOX 42873 Anytown, USA	Cathy Redding Claims Dept. 213-440-3131	Town School Dist. Mary Embers 312-055-3210	Group No. 4414	Does not pay for assistant surgeon

FIGURE 19-5. A page from the procedure manual. Insurance problems can be diminished by knowing whom to contact at the insurance carrier and the policyholder.

Completing the Form

1. If you plan to mail the form directly to the insurance company, be sure that the patient has signed the Authorization to Release Information (Fig. 19-7).
2. Make sure Medicare patients sign an Extended Signature Authorization Form (Fig. 19-8).
3. Typewrite all claim forms and keep a photocopy of each.
4. Use accepted diagnostic and procedure codes, and be certain that the procedures are consistent with the diagnoses.
5. List all procedures performed, one procedure per line. Be specific. If a laceration is treated, give the location, length, and depth, the number of sutures required, and the duration of treatment involved. If a sterile surgical tray was used for office surgery, itemize and bill as a separate fee. If a treatment injection was given, state the injected material and the amount given.
6. Attach a copy of the x-ray report, hospital report, and/or consultant's report in complicated cases.
7. State the usual and customary fee on all claim forms, regardless of what payment is expected.
8. Never alter a claim as to services performed, date of service, or fees established.
9. If more than one visit per day was required, state the times of day so that the claims processor will know they were separate procedures.
10. Fill in all blanks. Type DNA (does not apply) or NA (not applicable) or simple dash lines (---) rather than leave an item blank. This is confirmation that the item was not overlooked.

INSURANCE CLAIM REGISTER

PATIENT	INSURANCE COMPANY	DATE FILED	AMOUNT BILLED	AMOUNT PAID	DIFFERENCE

FIGURE 19-6. Insurance log showing the date each claim is filed, the amount billed, the amount paid, and the difference that must be either discounted or billed to the patient.

```
RECORDS RELEASE                              DATE_____

TO_____
                        DOCTOR

_____
                        ADDRESS

I HEREBY AUTHORIZE AND REQUEST YOU TO RELEASE

TO_____
                        DOCTOR

_____
                        ADDRESS

THE COMPLETE MEDICAL RECORDS IN YOUR POSSESSION, CONCERNING MY ILLNESS

AND/OR TREATMENT DURING THE PERIOD FROM_____TO_____


                                 SIGNED_____
                                        (PATIENT OR NEAREST RELATIVE)

_____  RELATIONSHIP_____
        WITNESS

FORM 122 - EASTMAN, INC.
```

FIGURE 19–7. Authorization form for the release of medical information.

MEDICARE LIFETIME ASSIGNMENT

Name of Beneficiary: _____

Medicare Number: _____

I request that payment of authorized Medicare benefits be made to me or on my behalf to (physician/supplier name) for any services furnished me by that provider. I authorize any holder of medical information about me to release to the Health Care Financing Administration and its agents any information needed to determine benefits or the benefits payable for related services.

This authorization is in effect until I choose to revoke it.*

Signed: _____   Date: _____

  * If you are a patient in a hospital or skilled nursing facility, this authorization is in effect for the period of your confinement.

FIGURE 19–8. Patient's extended signature authorization for Medicare claims.

Electronic Claims Submission

The medical practice that is computerized probably uses the computer for processing electronic claims (E-claims). This may be handled in several ways—for example, by transmitting data via modem or by recording data on computer disk or tape and sending it to the payer or intermediary.

An obvious advantage of electronic billing is the amount of time saved with its use. The system interrupts the transmission of incomplete or incorrect data, giving the biller the opportunity for on the spot correction. You know immediately if the insurance company is accepting the claim.

Another advantage of electronic billing is that it speeds up the date of payment, which results in an increase in cash flow to the practice.

Electronic transfer of information is also advantageous to the payer. HCFA is a strong advocate and is said to give preference to the processors of E-claims.

Not all claims are suitable for electronic submission. For example, those claims that are complicated and require a cover letter or those that require some kind of attachment must be sent on hard copy (paper) in the mail.

Claim Rejection

If a claim form is not sufficiently detailed, complete, and accurate, it may be rejected by the insurance company. Some of the reasons for claim rejection are:

- Diagnosis is missing or incomplete.
- Diagnosis is not coded accurately.
- Diagnosis does not correspond with treatment.
- Charges are not itemized.
- Patient's group, member, or policy number is missing or incorrect.
- Patient's portion of the form is incomplete, or the patient's signature is missing.
- Patient's birth date is missing.
- Fee is not listed.
- Dates are incorrect or missing.
- Doctor's signature or address is missing.

BILLING REQUIREMENTS

Blue Plans

When a patient is covered under a Blue Plan, claims should be submitted as soon as possible after the service is provided. Many of the Blue Plans have adopted use of the HCFA-1500 form. Check with the local office or representative in your area.

Like Medicare, the Blue Plans have **participating** and **nonparticipating** arrangements with providers. Usually, the participating provider is paid directly for covered services and agrees not to bill the patient for any difference between the provider's fee and the allowed fee.

The Blue Plans have provider manuals that describe coverage and coding features of the Plan. These manuals are periodically revised. Contact your local representative if your manual might be outdated.

Medicare

Under Medicare, the physician may be a participating provider or a nonparticipating provider (sometimes referred to as *Par* and *Nonpar* providers). Both are required by law to file the HCFA-1500 insurance claim for all eligible patients. Many also file for a secondary carrier.

A participating provider accepts assignment on Medicare claims. The allowable payment comes directly to the physician and is accepted as payment in full. The patient is still responsible for the deductible and the 20% copayment.

A nonparticipating provider is not required to accept assignment. If such is the case, the patient is responsible for the balance after Medicare makes its payment. The allowable payment to the Nonpar provider is less than the payment to the Par provider.

The Nonpar provider who plans to perform elective surgery on a Medicare patient that costs $500 or more is subject to Medicare's $500 surgery rule (Fig. 19-9). The provider must prepare a financial statement showing the type of surgery to be performed, the estimated charge, the estimated payment from Medicare, and the patient's probable out-of-pocket expense. This statement must be signed by the patient. Give one photocopy to the patient and file another with the patient's chart.

Claims for Medicare must be filed by December 31st of the year following that in which the services were rendered. For example, care rendered in the year 1993 must be billed no later than December 31, 1994.

Medicaid

A physician is free to accept or to refuse to treat a patient under Medicaid. However, if the patient is accepted, requirements for rendering service and billing for services are strict and must be closely followed:

- The patient's identification card must be current. Some include labels that must be attached to the billing form.
- Prior authorization may be required for the service for which a form is completed. For an emergency situation, authorization may be secured by telephone but must be followed up with the appropriate form.

19

Dear Patient:

I do not plan to accept assignment for your surgery. The law requires that where assignment is not taken and the charge is $500 or more, the following information must be provided prior to your surgery. These estimates assume you have met the annual Part B Medicare deductible.

Type of surgery _____
Estimated Charge $_____
Estimated Medicare Payment $_____
Your Estimated Payment $_____
(This includes your Medicare co-insurance)

Physician's Signature _____

I have read and understand the above information.

X_____ _____
(Patient's Signature) (Date)

FIGURE 19–9. Nonpar provider's financial statement that is used to comply with Medicare's $500 surgery rule.

- There will be a time limit for billing after the termination of which the claim may be rejected.

It is important that the medical assistant check the local regulations and keep current on requirements.

Medi/Medi

The HCFA-1500 form is used, and the physician must always accept assignment. Failure to indicate acceptance of assignment will result in Medicare payment going to the patient and in rejection of the claim by Medicaid. A label from the patient's ID card or a photocopy of the current card may be required.

The claim form is first processed through Medicare and is then automatically forwarded to Medicaid. It is not necessary to prepare two claim forms.

CHAMPUS and CHAMPVA

Use Form HCFA-1500 for the covered portion of the fee. Bill the patient directly for the deductible and coinsurance portion. The claim must be filed no later than December 31st of the year following that in which services were provided.

Workers' Compensation

Records for the workers' compensation case (sometimes referred to as an "industrial case") should be kept separate from the physician's regular patient histories. If the patient who is seen for an industrial injury has previously been treated as a private patient, a new chart and ledger should be started that will be used only for the treatment rendered under conditions of the Workers' Compensation law.

The insurance carrier may request and is entitled to receive copies of all records pertaining to the industrial injury but not the records of a private patient. Information in the records of a private patient is privileged information and may be released only with the patient's consent. There could be a lawsuit or a hearing before a referee or Appeals Board for which records are subpoenaed. If separate records are kept, there is no question of privilege involved.

The physician who sees the injured or ill worker first will complete what may be called the Doctor's First Report of Work Injury within the time limit imposed by state regulations (Fig. 19–10). The medical assistant should make a minimum of five copies of this report. The insurance company usually requires at least two copies. One copy goes to the state regulatory body. The employer may get a copy, and one file copy should remain with the phy-

PROCEDURE 19-1   COMPLETING INSURANCE FORMS

GOAL To complete an insurance claim form for services to a Medicare patient for whom the physician accepts assignment.

EQUIPMENT AND SUPPLIES

Patient chart
Patient ledger

HCFA-1500 claim form
Typewriter or computer

PROCEDURAL STEPS

1. *Ask for patient's identification card.* **Purpose:** To determine whether the patient is insured under Medicare Part B.

2. Photocopy card and place the copy in the patient's file.

3. Have the patient sign an Extended Signature Authorization Form. **Purpose:** Grants lifetime signature authorization for the physician to submit assigned or unassigned claims on the beneficiary's behalf (must be canceled upon the patient's request).

4. Complete the following entries (blocks 1–33) on the HCFA-1500 form:

   1. Check the appropriate boxes for all types of health insurance coverage applicable to the claim.

   1a. Enter the insured person's identification number.

   2. Enter patient's full name.

   3. Enter six-digit birth date and sex.

   4. Enter word "same."

   5. Enter patient's permanent mailing address and telephone number (do not use P. O. Box for address).

   6. Enter patient's relationship to the insured person.

   7. Enter word "same."

   8. Check appropriate box for patient's marital status and whether he or she is employed or a student.

   9. Complete this block only if the patient has other coverage, such as (a) insurance primary to Medicare, (b) Medicare supplement policy, (c) Employer Retiree Coverage. Otherwise, type "NA" in this block.

   10. Check "yes" or "no."

   11. Complete only if the patient has other insurance.

   12. Reserve for the patient's signature.

   13. Reserve for the patient's signature if a Medicare supplement policy is indicated in block 9.

   14. Enter date of the current illness or injury.

   15. Leave blank.

   16. Leave blank.

   17. Name of referring and/or ordering physician.

   17a. Enter HCFA-assigned Unique Physician Identifier Number.

   18. Complete only when the medical service is related to hospitalization (enter admission and discharge dates).

   19. Enter the date the patient was last seen by the referring and/or ordering physician.

Continued

PROCEDURE 19 – 1   *Continued*

20. A "yes" check means that a lab test was performed outside the physician's office; a "no" check means that a test was performed by the billing physician. If "yes" is checked, block 32 must be completed.

21. Enter ICD-9-CM diagnosis codes in priority order.

22. Complete only for Medicaid.

23. Enter PRO prior authorization number, if any.

24a. Enter the month, day, and year for each service.

24b. Enter code for the place of service.

24c. Leave blank.

24d. Enter CPT/HCPCS codes with modifiers, if any.

24e. Enter diagnosis reference number from item 21.

24f. Enter charge for each listed service.

24g. Enter days or units.

24h. Leave blank.

24i. Check if service was rendered in an emergency room.

24j. Leave blank.

24k. Enter physician's PIN number.

25. Enter physician's Federal Tax Identification or Social Security number.

26. Enter patient's account number, if any.

27. Check "yes" or "no" for assignment of benefits.

28. Enter total charge for services. *Purpose:* No payment will be made unless the charge is entered on the form.

29. Enter the amount paid by the patient or other source.

30. Enter the balance due.

31. Reserve for the physician's signature.

32. See item 20.

33. Enter name, address, telephone number, PIN number, and group number of the provider who is billing for services.

---

sician's record. This report must be personally signed by the physician and should contain the following information:

- The history of the case as obtained from the patient, with notation of any **pre-existing condition** (injuries or diseases).
- The patient's symptoms and physical complaints.
- The complete physical findings, including laboratory and x-ray results.
- A tentative diagnosis.
- An estimate of the type and extent of the disability. In cases in which permanent disability has resulted, there should be a careful survey, and the extent of disability should be given in detail.

- Treatment indicated, including type, frequency, and duration. It may be necessary to attach a letter giving more detailed information to assist in making an evaluation of the case.
- Whenever possible, the date the patient may be able to return to work, if he or she has been totally disabled.

The insurance company may supply its own billing forms. Payment is usually made on the basis of a fee schedule. Any charges in excess of the fee schedule must be fully explained and documented.

In billing for the service, use the coding system specified in your state. Itemize the statement, including any drugs and dressings used.

STATE
COMPENSATION
INSURANCE
FUND

**DOCTOR'S FIRST REPORT OF
OCCUPATIONAL INJURY
OR ILLNESS
STATE OF CALIFORNIA**

Within 5 days of your initial examination, for every occupational injury or illness, send this report to **insurer or employer (only if self-insured).** Failure to file a timely doctor's report may result in assessment of a civil penalty. **In the case of diagnosed or suspected pesticide poisoning,** send one copy of this report directly to the Division of Labor Statistics and Research, P.O. Box 603, San Francisco CA 94101; and notify your local health officer by telephone within 24 hours and by sending a copy of this report within seven days. For a supply of this form, please call (415) 557-1924.

	PLEASE DO NOT USE THIS COLUMN
1. **INSURER NAME AND ADDRESS** STATE COMPENSATION INSURANCE FUND P.O. BOX 1316, SAN BERNARDINO, CA 92402-1316	
2. **EMPLOYER NAME**	Case No.
3. Address: No. and Street City Zip	Industry
4. Nature of business (e.g., food manufacturing, building construction, retailer of women's clothes)	County
5. **PATIENT NAME** (First name, middle initial, last name) 6. Sex ☐ Male ☐ Female 7. Date of Mo. Day Yr. Birth	Age
8. Address: No. and Street City Zip 9. Telephone number ( )	Hazard
10. Occupation (Specific job title) 11. Social Security Number - -	Disease
12. Injured at: No. and Street City County	Hospitalization
13. Date and hour of injury Mo. Day Yr. Hour or onset of illness _____ a.m. _____ p.m. 14. Date last worked Mo. Day Yr.	Occupation
15. Date and hour of first Mo. Day Yr. Hour examination or treatment _____ a.m. _____ p.m. 16. Have you (or your office) previously treated patient? ☐Yes ☐No	Return Date/Code

Patient please complete this portion, if able to do so. Otherwise, doctor please complete immediately. Inability or failure of a patient to complete this portion shall not affect his/her rights to workers' compensation under the California Labor Code.
17. **DESCRIBE HOW THE ACCIDENT OR EXPOSURE HAPPENED** (Give specific object, machinery or chemical. Use reverse side if more space is required.)

18. **SUBJECTIVE COMPLAINTS** (Describe fully. Use reverse side if more space is required.)

19. **OBJECTIVE FINDINGS** (Use reverse side if more space is required.)

A. Physical examination

B. X-ray and laboratory results (State if none or pending.)

20. **DIAGNOSIS** (If occupational illness, specify etiologic agent and duration of exposure.) Chemical or toxic compounds involved? ☐Yes ☐No

21. Are your findings and diagnosis consistent with patient's account of injury or onset of illness? ☐Yes ☐ No
If "no", please explain.

22. Is there any other current condition that will impede or delay patient's recovery? ☐Yes ☐No
If "yes", please explain.

23. **TREATMENT RENDERED** (Use reverse side if more space is required.)

If further treatment required, specify treatment.   Estimated duration

24. If hospitalized as inpatient, give hospital name and location.   Date admitted   Mo. Day Yr.   Estimated stay

25. **WORK STATUS**   Is patient able to perform usual work? ☐Yes ☐No
If "no", patient can return to: Mo. Day Yr.
Regular work _____
Modified work _____   Specify restrictions _____

Doctor's Signature _____   Date _____   CA License Number _____
Doctor Name and Degree (Please Type) _____   IRS Number _____
Address _____   Telephone Number (   ) _____

SCIF 3110 (REV. 7-89)

Incomplete information or delay in submitting this report may cause delay in benefits to your patient

FORM 5021 (Rev. 3)
1989

FIGURE 19–10. First report of occupational injury or illness.

In severe or prolonged cases, supplemental reports and billing should be sent to the insurance carrier at least once per month.

At the termination of treatment, a final report and bill are sent to the insurance carrier. Do not bill the patient.

HEALTH CARE AND COST CONTAINMENT

As mentioned earlier, since World War II, group insurance has become a significant fringe benefit in collective bargaining. It is believed by some that this has been a factor in increasing cost and overuse of medical care, because when the cost of care is borne by insurance, the patient loses awareness of the financial aspect. Attempts to meet the need for cost containment are being made by the medical profession, health insurance providers, and the federal government by modifying the delivery of medical care.

Fee-for-Service Payment

In the fee-for-service concept, the patient sees the doctor, receives care, and then gets a bill for the service. Insurance programs were first designed simply to pay those bills. The patient who had insurance paid an annual premium, and in return the insurance company paid at least a portion of the bills. Much of the fee-for-service care has been provided by Medicare, Medicaid, and the Blue Plans, but all of these plans are beginning to take steps toward cost containment and the identification of alternatives to fee-for-service insurance.

Peer Review Organizations (PROs)

Peer review organizations are an outgrowth of a 1972 amendment to the Social Security Act that brought about the formation of federal **professional standards review organizations (PSROs),** whose purposes were to monitor the validity of diagnoses and the quality of care and to evaluate the appropriateness of hospital admissions and discharges of patients covered by government-sponsored health insurance. The effectiveness of PSROs was continually debated, and the PSROs were gradually phased out.

In 1982, PROs were legislated as part of the Tax Equity and Fiscal Responsibility Act (TEFRA). The purpose of a PRO is identical to that of the PSROs. The primary difference is that the PROs are mostly limited to a single group within a state. PRO contracts are awarded by the Health Care Financing Administration to physician-based organizations within each state, and the mechanics of PROs vary slightly from state to state. In an attempt to control costs, an insurance carrier may require prior authorization from the PRO before a patient is hospitalized for elective medical or surgical care. If the patient's condition can be adequately and safely treated on an outpatient basis, payment for hospitalization will not be approved. It is important that the medical assistant be aware of the types of admission cases that require previous authorization and that the authorization be obtained prior to the admission date.

Prospective Payment System (PPS)

In April 1983, the Social Security Amendments Act of 1983 (Public Law 98-21) was signed into law. Title VI of this law contained the prospective payment system (PPS) for hospitals, which would begin the radical restructuring of the payment system to hospitals for Medicare inpatient services.

> As identified by the Health Care Financing Administration (HCFA), a major objective of the prospective payment system (PPS) is to establish the government as a "prudent buyer" of health care while maintaining beneficiaries' access to quality care. The "prudent buyer" objective is to be accomplished by paying Medicare providers a predetermined specific rate per discharge rather than on the basis of reasonable costs. Access to quality care is to be ensured through reviews by Peer Review Organizations of the validity of diagnoses, quality of care and appropriateness of admissions and discharges.[*]

If a hospital does not contract with a PRO, it is not eligible for payment from the Medicare program. The law provides authority to grant waivers from the PPS if a state has an approved hospital reimbursement control system. Additional criteria must be met by a state to receive approval and a waiver from the federal PPS.

Physician Prospective Payment System

Probability is high that HCFA will set up a PPS for physicians. Every claim form you file with Medicare or any other third-party payer becomes part of a permanent computerized record that may be used in the future as the basis of your physician's fee profile if the PPS is expanded to include reimbursement of physician charges. Your coding must be performed accurately and precisely if meaningful profiles are to be established. The two more likely approaches to a PPS for physicians are diagnosis-related groups (DRGs) (see the following section) and relative value scales (RVSs), discussed earlier in this chapter.

---

[*] *American Medical Association:* DRGs and the Prospective Payment System: A Guide for Physicians. *Chicago, The Association, 1984.*

Diagnosis-Related Groups (DRGs)

The DRG classification forms the basis for payment under the prospective payment system, as opposed to the traditional method of payment based on actual costs incurred in the provision of care. Payment to the hospital of a DRG amount generally constitutes payment in full for services rendered to Medicare patients.

The DRG system classifies patients on the basis of diagnosis and was developed by Yale researchers in the 1970s as a mechanism for utilization review. DRGs are derived from taking all possible diagnoses identified in the ICD-9-CM system, classifying them into 23 major diagnostic categories (MDCs) based on organ system, and further breaking them into 467 distinct groupings, each of which is said to be "medically meaningful."

In all, there are actually 470 DRGs. The first 467 are based on the principal diagnosis or procedure performed. Number 468 is assigned when the principal procedure performed does not conform with the principal diagnosis. Numbers 469 and 470 are codes that reflect coding errors and are automatically returned to the hospital for correction or verification. The principal diagnosis is the most critical factor in the assignment of DRGs. All diagnoses must reflect information contained in the patient's medical record.

In order to assign a case to a DRG, five pieces of information are necessary:

- The patient's principal diagnosis and up to four complications or comorbidities
- The treatment procedures performed
- The patient's age
- The patient's sex
- The patient's discharge status

PHYSICIAN'S RESPONSIBILITY. The major factor determining the assignment of a DRG is the physician's assessment of the principal diagnosis. It is the physician's responsibility to record the principal diagnosis as well as the other determining factors on a discharge face sheet. It is extremely important that the principal diagnosis, as stated by the physician, correspond to the various tests, procedures, and notes contained within the complete medical record.

Once the discharge face sheet has been completed by the physician, the chart is forwarded to the hospital's medical records department for review and coding. The codes contained in the ICD-9-CM are used for determining the DRG and, therefore, must be entered in the appropriate section of the discharge face sheet.

From the medical records department the information is forwarded to the financial office for completion of the bill to be submitted to the fiscal intermediary. The fiscal intermediary, through the use of a grouper computer program, determines the appropriate DRG and then calculates the payment to the hospital.

GLOSSARY OF PROSPECTIVE PAYMENT TERMS

Any discussion of the prospective payment system requires an acquaintance with the terminology involved.

capitation. A method of payment for health services in which an individual or institutional provider is paid a fixed, per capita amount for each person served without regard to the actual number or nature of services provided to each person.

comorbidity. A pre-existing condition that will, because of its presence with a specific principal diagnosis, cause an increase in length of stay by at least 1 day in approximately 75% of the cases.

complication. A condition that arises during the hospital stay that prolongs the length of stay by at least 1 day in approximately 75% of the cases.

diagnosis related groups (DRGs). A system developed by Yale University for classifying patients into groups that are clinically coherent and homogeneous with respect to resources used. There are 467 DRGs.

DRG creep. Inflating diagnoses to obtain a higher payment rate.

DRG weight. An index number that reflects the relative resource consumption associated with each DRG.

discharge face sheet (may also be called *discharge summary* or *discharge abstract*). A summary of the admission, prepared at the time of the patient's discharge from the hospital. Information contained on the discharge face sheet includes demographic information, source of payment, length of stay, principal diagnosis, secondary diagnoses or complications, procedures performed, services provided, and other information that may be relevant to a particular hospital.

grouper. Computer software program that is used by the fiscal intermediary in all cases to assign discharges to the appropriate DRGs using the following information abstracted from the inpatient bill: patient's age, sex, principal diagnosis, principal procedures performed, and discharge status.

ICD-9-CM (International Classification of Diseases, Ninth Revision, Clinical Modification). A system for classifying diseases and operations to facilitate collection of uniform and comparable health information.

major diagnostic category (MDC). An MDC is a broad clinical category that is differentiated from all others based on body system involvement and disease etiology. The 23 MDCs cover the complete range of diagnoses contained in the ICD-9-CM.

outliers (atypical cases). Cases involving an extremely long stay (day outlier) or extraordinarily high costs (cost outlier) when compared with most discharges classified in the same DRG.

peer review organization (PRO). An entity that is composed of a substantial number of licensed doctors of medicine and osteopathy engaged in the practice of medicine or surgery in the area, or an entity that has available to it the services of a sufficient number of physicians engaged in the practice of medicine or surgery, to assure the adequate peer review of the services provided by the various medical specialties and subspecialties.

principal diagnosis. That condition which after study is determined to be chiefly responsible for occasioning the admission of the patient to the hospital.

principal procedure. One that was performed for definitive treatment rather than for diagnostic or exploratory purposes, or one necessary to take care of a complication. It is that procedure most related to the principal diagnosis.

Prospective Payment Assessment Commission (Pro-PAC). A 15-member commission of independent experts with experience and expertise in the provision and financing of health care who are appointed to review and provide recommendations on: the annual inflation factor; DRG recalibration; and new and existing medical and surgical procedures and services.

sole community hospital (SCH). Those hospitals that, by reason of factors such as isolated location, weather conditions, travel conditions, or absence of other hospitals (as determined by the Secretary) are the sole source of inpatient hospital services reasonably available to individuals in a geographic area.

Tax Equity and Fiscal Responsibility Act (TEFRA). Signed into Federal law in 1982. Contains provisions for major changes in Medicare reimbursement.

uniform hospital discharge data set (UHDDS). A minimum data set required to be collected for each Medicare patient on discharge.

weight (DRG). An HCFA-derived figure intended to reflect the relative resource consumption of each DRG. The payment rate is multiplied by the appropriate DRG weight to determine the reimbursement amount for each patient.

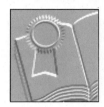

► LEARNING ACHIEVEMENTS

Are you able to:

1. Define the terms listed in the Vocabulary of this chapter?
2. Compare the attributes of group policies and individual policies?
3. Explain when the Birthday Law comes into effect?
4. State how eligibility for CHAMPUS benefits is determined?
5. Name the three components that establish the RBRVS?
6. Discuss the purposes for numerical diagnostic and procedural coding?
7. Explain under what circumstances DRG coding is used?
8. Discuss the difference between a *closed-panel* and an *open-panel* HMO?
9. Correctly prepare a Medicare claim form?
10. Correctly calculate a billing that includes a deductible and coinsurance?

REFERENCES AND READINGS

American Medical Association: *DRGs and the Prospective Payment System: A Guide for Physicians,* Chicago, The Association, 1984.

American Medical Association: *Physician's Current Procedural Terminology,* 4th ed., Chicago, The Association, 1992.

American Medical Association: *American Medical News,* a weekly newspaper.

Fordney, M.: *Insurance Handbook for the Medical Office,* 3rd ed., Philadelphia, W. B. Saunders Co., 1989.

Gosfield, A.G.: *RBRVS Special Report,* Salt Lake City, Med-Index Publications, 1991.

Med-Index: *HCPCS 1991–92,* 3rd ed., Salt Lake City, 1992.

Med-Index: *Reimbursement Strategies,* Salt Lake City, 1991.

CHAPTER TWENTY

———

EDITORIAL DUTIES AND MEETING AND TRAVEL ARRANGEMENTS

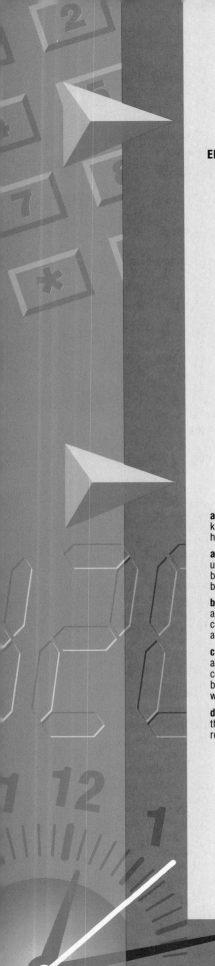

CHAPTER OUTLINE

VOCABULARY

abstract A written summary of the key points of a book, paper, or case history.

agenda A list of the specific items under each division of the order of business that is to be presented at a business meeting.

bibliography A list of the works that are referred to in a text or that were consulted by the author in producing a text.

colloquialism An expression that is acceptable and correct in ordinary conversation or informal speeches but unsuitable for formal speech or writing.

draft A preliminary outline or writing that the author expects to amend or revise.

footnote A comment placed at the bottom of a page that would be distracting if placed within the main text.

galley proof A printer's proof taken from composed type before page composition.

legend The heading or title of a figure.

manuscript A written or typewritten document, as distinguished from printed copy.

monograph A learned treatise on a small area of knowledge; a written account of a single thing or class of things.

order of business A list of the different divisions of business in the order in which each is to be addressed at a business meeting.

periodical A journal published with a fixed interval (greater than 1 day) between its issues or numbers.

prognosis Forecast of the course of a disease.

reprint A reproduction of printed matter.

summary A synopsis of the main points of a longer text.

treatise A systematic exposition or argument in writing.

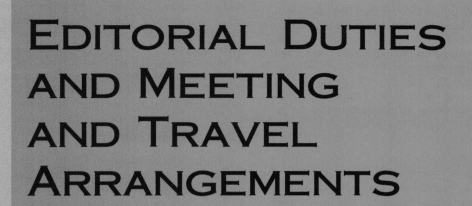
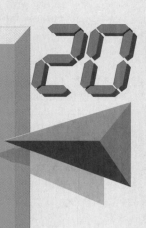

EDITORIAL DUTIES AND MEETING AND TRAVEL ARRANGEMENTS

LEARNING OBJECTIVES

COGNITIVE

After successful completion of this chapter, you should be able to:

1. Define the terms listed in the Vocabulary.

2. Originate and maintain a card catalog for a personal library.

3. Discuss the nature and importance of an abstract.

4. List the four items to include on a cross-reference card for a general reference file.

5. Name five items of information to include on a diagnostic file card.

6. Name the library classification system that uses decimal numbers.

7. Identify the classification system that uses a combination of letters of the alphabet and numerals.

8. Cite three indexes available in medical libraries for use in locating various periodical references.

9. Name two of the largest medical data bases for electronic retrieval of information.

10. List the seven items of information needed for each reference in a bibliography.

11. Briefly outline the general procedure for preparing a manuscript for publication in a periodical.

12. List the five items that should be included in the first paragraph of the minutes of a meeting.

PERFORMANCE

After successful completion of this chapter, you should be able to perform the following activities:

1. Type a speech in correct format and estimate the time necessary for delivery.

2. Prepare cards for an abstract file.

3. Set up a diagnostic file, including subject cards and the necessary subheadings to accommodate the patient charts.

4. Retype a manuscript that has been edited using proofreader's marks.

5. Make travel arrangements for a proposed trip.

6. Prepare a typewritten itinerary.

7. Make arrangements for a group meeting.

8. From a rough draft, type the minutes of a meeting in correct form, including the secretary's signature.

EDITORIAL DUTIES

The medical profession is unique in that the physician traditionally shares with others, through writing and speaking, the discoveries, information, and observations gained in practice, research, and private study. The medical assistant who becomes proficient in maintaining the physician's personal library and in assisting with the preparation of articles and speeches can be of immeasurable help in these endeavors.

The Physician's Library

The books that a physician acquires while in medical school are the nucleus of a personal library that will grow over the years. New books reflecting the changes in medicine and the physician's special interests are continually added (Fig. 20–1). The physician may accumulate a file of professional journals such as the *Journal of the American Medical Association* (JAMA), the journal of the state medical society, specialty journals, trade journals, and even informative material provided by pharmaceutical companies.

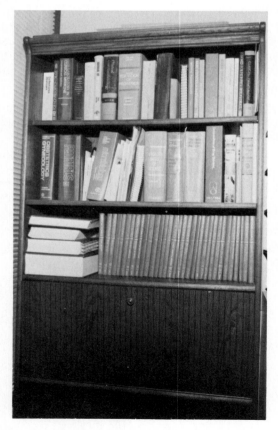

FIGURE 20–1. Typical basic library in physician's office. (Courtesy of Vista Medical Group, El Toro, CA. Photo by Dan Santucci.)

Journals should be bound at regular intervals, generally by volume, in order to preserve the individual copies. The medical assistant may be responsible for having the journals bound regularly and consistently. Most journals in the medical field publish indexes, annually, semiannually, or quarterly. The index should be bound with the journal pages. In most cities, the binding of **periodicals** can be done locally. The hospital librarian is a good source of information for locating a bookbinder.

Organizing the Library

While the physician's library may not be large, it must be systematically organized so that information is readily accessible.

In setting up or rearranging a small library, books should be classified by subject groupings that reflect medical specialties. Those dealing with related topics should be placed together.

Journals and periodicals are usually arranged alphabetically.

Card Catalog of Books

The books should be indexed in a card catalog or looseleaf binder. A 3 × 5 inch card file is practical for this purpose. Generally, three or more cards should be prepared for each book:

- Title card
- Subject card
- Author card(s)

Here's how to index a book in this manner, using the book you are reading as an example:

1. Prepare a title card with the heading "The Administrative Medical Assistant."
2. Prepare a subject card with the heading "Medical Assisting."
3. Prepare an author card (Fig. 20–2).
4. The three cards may then be filed alphabetically or, preferably, in a file divided into sections for title, subject, and author. With such a file and cross-reference system, any book can be located very quickly.

The computerized office undoubtedly stores this information on disk for ready retrieval.

Periodical File

One of the physician's greatest difficulties is keeping up with medical literature, particularly the articles appearing regularly in the periodicals. It is unlikely that the physician will want to maintain a complete index of all articles appearing in these periodicals, but most doctors want to keep track of those articles that are of particular interest. **Abstracts** are of great value in the continuing task of keeping abreast of scientific developments.

Administrative Medical Assistant, The, 3rd Edition

Mary E. Kinn
Philadelphia, W. B. Saunders Company, 1993

Textbook and reference covering all administrative
phases of medical assisting in the physician's office

TITLE CARD

Medical Assisting

The Administrative Medical Assistant, 3rd Edition,
Philadelphia, W. B. Saunders Company, 1993

Mary E. Kinn

SUBJECT CARD

Kinn, Mary E.

The Administrative Medical Assistant, 3rd Edition,
Philadelphia, W. B. Saunders Company, 1993

1. Medical Assisting

AUTHOR CARD

FIGURE 20–2. Title, subject, and author cards for referencing a book in
the personal library.

PREPARATION OF AN ABSTRACT. An abstract is a
kind of **summary** or epitome of a book, paper, or
case history. It is brief, indicates the nature of the
article, and summarizes the most important points
and conclusions. Abstracts prepared by professionals
are found in many medical journals as a service to
the individual physician.

Many physicians prepare abstracts of the articles
that they find of particular value, and in some offices, the medical assistant is trained to do abstract-
ing for the doctor. A medical assistant who can prepare a good abstract of an article can save the
doctor from reading 10 to 20 pages of the original
article and can help focus attention on information
of particular interest in the article.

Abstracts must clearly indicate the nature of the
information contained in the article. Each should
note:

- Any new procedures
- Results of studies and experiments
- Conclusions noted

The length and character of the article determine
the type and length of the abstract. In most scientific articles, the conclusions of the writer are sum-
marized at the end of the piece. This summary is of
great help in preparing an abstract.

The abstracts are typed on cards, with the text of
the abstract preceded by the following information:

- Title of the article
- Surname and initials of the author
- Name of the publication
- Volume
- Inclusive page numbers
- Month and year

The cards are then filed. If abstract cards are kept,
it is not necessary to clip and file the actual articles
separately. The journals in which they appear can
be kept in the usual alphabetic order.

Reprints

When physicians write articles or present papers
before scientific meetings, their work is often published in a periodical, and **reprints** of it are made
available to their colleagues. A portion of each doctor's library is usually composed of a collection of
such reprints. In some cases, the reprints come into
the office unsolicited, owing to the doctor's interest
in a particular person's writing in the past; in other
cases, the doctor may request the medical assistant
to write for a particular reprint. Sometimes, the
doctor may have a special postcard made up for
ordering reprints (Fig. 20–3).

Other physicians prefer to write personal letters
in which they compliment the author upon the excellence of the article and request copies of it for
their files. Reprints often present a filing problem in
the office because they are not of uniform size. This
problem can be solved by placing references to these
reprints in the library card file and storing the reprints in a separate drawer.

Other Reference Files

Physicians frequently need a variety of miscellaneous medical information in addition to book collections and periodicals and their indexes. For this
reason, they may accumulate a separate reference
file of valuable information. Often, this consists of
pages photocopied from journals or reference books.

ORGANIZATION OF REFERENCE FILES. The physician
and the medical assistant together may set up (1) a
subject index for filing the material and (2) a cross-

Please send me _____ copies of your article,
_____ (title) _____,

which appeared in _____ (publication)

_____ , 19 _____ .

_____ (Doctor's signature)

FIGURE 20–3. Typical card for ordering reprints.

reference card file for locating the material easily. Begin by tabbing file dividers with the main topics and folders with subheadings. When an article or item is photocopied, a card is made up with:

- The title of the article or chapter
- Its author
- The periodical or book in which it appeared
- The date of publication

The copy of the reference material is then filed in the appropriate folder and the card filed by subject for easy reference. As new developments occur, later articles may be filed and the outdated material discarded.

Diagnostic Files

Physicians often draw material for their writing and speaking from the case histories of their own patients. For this reason, many doctors like to set up diagnostic files so that they can quickly pull out information on, for example, the incidence of certain side effects among patients treated with a particular medication. The medical assistant must be familiar with medical terminology to maintain such a file.

ORGANIZATION OF THE DIAGNOSTIC FILE. The system used varies from office to office, but subject cards generally have:

- A main heading with the name of the disease or surgical procedure
- Subheadings for various aspects of the disease or procedure
- The patient's name, diagnosis, and type of treatment listed below

For example, one subject entry with subheadings might be:

BLOOD DISEASES
    Anemia
    Granulocytosis
    Hemophilia
    Leukemia
    Polycythemia
    Thalassemia
    Toxemia

Patient cards are headed with the patient's name and diagnosis, treatment, **prognosis,** and miscellaneous information below.

By keeping such a file, a physician can readily obtain the charts of all patients with a particular condition from the history files. This is particularly valuable to physicians who do a great deal of teaching, writing, or research. In the physician's office equipped with a computer, it is very easy to keep a detailed diagnostic file using these same principles.

Library for Patients

Many doctors keep a small library of educational information for patients. This library generally contains some books written in language that the average patient can understand as well as a number of pamphlets and reprints that the patient can take home. This might include information on such subjects as diabetes, heart disease, skin conditions, the danger signals of cancer, lung disease, first aid, and other subjects of interest to many patients. The specialist may have information dealing specifically with the doctor's specialty. A library service such as this saves the physician considerable time in repeating simple educational information and is generally welcomed by the patients.

Helping to Gather Information

The medical assistant who is employed by a doctor who teaches, writes, or lectures frequently may be called upon to assist with the preparation of papers. The duties might include:

- Making up a list of references for a talk or a paper for publication
- Doing actual research
- Preparing abstracts

Any medical assistant who is called upon to assume such responsibilities must know how to make the best use of the available library and reference facilities.

Using Library Facilities

Almost all doctors, even those practicing in rural areas, have access to medical libraries. The doctor who practices in a metropolitan area or near a medical center such as one affiliated with a university is particularly fortunate, since outstanding library facilities are readily at his or her disposal.

All general hospitals maintain medical libraries consisting of a basic collection of carefully selected, authoritative medical textbooks and reference works of the latest edition as well as files of current journals. The Medical Library Association sets standards for member libraries.

A physician usually has access to a county society library or can use the package library services of the state society. In addition, extension library facilities can be used to obtain information from special supplemental collections. The American Medical Association, for example, and some specialty societies, offer periodical lending services and package library services to their members.

The National Library of Medicine has established a system whereby doctors may get materials from a Regional Medical Library Program when information is not available locally. In those instances when the Regional Program cannot satisfy the need, the request is channeled to the National Library of Medicine.

All libraries systematically organize the books, periodicals, and other materials in a fairly uniform manner in order that the information can be easily located and is accessible. The medical assistant who finds it necessary to go to a library to do special work should seek out the librarian or an assistant and get an idea of what the library has to offer with respect to materials and their arrangement, privileges, rules, and regulations for use of the library. After a brief discussion, the trained medical librarian usually can suggest shortcuts that are of great help in locating references or doing research.

CARD CATALOG OF BOOKS. All books, **monographs, treatises,** handbooks, dictionaries, and encyclopedias contained in a library are indexed by author and subject and sometimes by title in the card catalog. This catalog is really an index of the book contents of the library. Cards are arranged alphabetically (with subject, author, and title cards alphabetized in one series) or are alphabetized within separate sections for subject, author, or title.

Although we still refer to it as the "card" catalog, in reality, the index is now frequently accessed via a computer terminal.

Classification Systems. There are a number of systems for classifying library books. In library procedure, classification means putting together materials on a given subject with related materials placed nearby. Medical libraries use various classification systems.

The Dewey decimal system, used not only in medical but in all types of libraries, is sometimes used for arranging medical library collections. This system uses decimal numbers to indicate specific subjects and arranges the book collection in numeric sequence for easy location. For example, "616" indicates "Pathology, Diseases, Treatment." Here's an example of how the Dewey decimal system works:

616.1	Diseases of the cardiovascular system
616.9	Communicable and other diseases
616.96	Parasitic diseases
616.99	Other general diseases
616.992	Neoplasms and neoplastic diseases

The Library of Congress classification system is also used. It consists of a number of separate, mutually exclusive classifications based on combination of letters of the alphabet and numerals:

QR:	Bacteriology
RD:	Surgery
RC 321-431:	Diseases of the nervous system

The National Library of Medicine classification system is replacing the Library of Congress system in many medical libraries.

There are other systems, such as the Boston Medical Library Classification, the Cunningham Classification, and the Barnard Classification, that are used by some medical libraries. A brief discussion with the librarian and a quick look at the card catalog will generally help acquaint you with the system used.

How the Card Catalog Can Help You Locate Books. No matter which system of classification is used, its main purpose is to help those who use the library to locate volumes quickly. The symbol for the particular book, whether it be a numeral, a letter, or a combination of numerals and letters, appears on the entry for the book in the card catalog. This symbol is called a classification mark. It also appears on the spine of the volume.

To locate a volume, check the classification mark on the card catalog entry, and if an open-shelf system is used, find that shelf in the library where corresponding symbols appear. If a closed-shelf system is used in the library, give the number of the book and its title to a librarian who will locate it for you.

PERIODICAL INDEXES. The bulk of current medical literature appears in medical journals, and some reference system for organizing and accessing the thousands of articles is necessary. The majority of journals publish their own indexes, one for each volume, sometimes with an annual index. If you know the name of the journal that published the article you are looking for, this is the fastest way to locate it. Otherwise, composite indexes may be consulted.

Clinical Medicine. The monthly *Index Medicus* and the annual *Cumulated Index Medicus,* published by the National Library of Medicine, include author and subject indexes for over 3000 periodicals. They are international in scope, representing foreign publications and languages as well as publications in English.

The monthly *Abridged Index Medicus* and the annual *Cumulated Abridged Index Medicus* are smaller versions of *Index Medicus* and *Cumulated Index Medicus,* and are limited to indexing 100 major periodicals in the medical field. These periodicals are readily available in the majority of medical libraries. The computer equivalent of both the *Index Medicus* and the *Abridged Index Medicus* is MEDLINE.

Nursing and Allied Health. The *Cumulative Index to Nursing & Allied Health Literature* is published by Glendale Adventist Medical Center.* This index is very comprehensive and is the only thorough source

---

* *1509 Wilson Terrace, Glendale, CA 91206*

for coverage of allied health. It is published bi-monthly with an annual cumulation. The computer equivalent is Nursing & Allied Health Index on Bibliographic Retrieval System (BRS) and Dialog.

The *International Nursing Index* is published quarterly, with an annual cumulation, by the *American Journal of Nursing*. The computer equivalent is MEDLINE.

Hospital and Health Care. *Hospital Literature Index* is published quarterly, with annual cumulations, by the American Hospital Association (AHA). The computer equivalent to *Hospital Index* is MEDLINE/Health file.

BIBLIOGRAPHY SEARCH. Information for **bibliographies** may be obtained by either a manual search through indexes or by a computer search.

For a manual search, you must look under the subject closest to the one on which you need information, then copy down all the information (author, title of journal, and complete bibliographic information, including volume number, pages, and date).

Most of the world's literature is now accessible through various vendors that provide computer access to specialized files. There are thousands of these databases. The major vendors in health care facilities are:

- National Library of Medicine
- Dialog Information Services, Inc.
- Bibliographic Retrieval System (BRS)
- Systems Development Corporation (SDC)

The National Library of Medicine is the least expensive of these four vendors.

ELECTRONIC RETRIEVAL OF INFORMATION. Two of the largest medical databases are MEDLINE and EMBASE, each of which includes citations and abstracts from thousands of publications.

MEDLINE is produced by the National Library of Medicine and covers materials from 1966 and later. *Index Medicus* is produced from this computer file.

EMBASE is produced by Excerpta Medica, and the *Excerpta Medica Index* is produced from this database. There is a great deal of overlap between the two databases, but EMBASE does include some literature not indexed in *Index Medicus.*

Computer access to MEDLINE is available in the majority of hospital libraries and is often provided as a free service to affiliates of the hospital. Many hospitals subscribe to at least one additional vendor (usually Dialog, BRS, or SDC's Orbit). With the aid of a computer, a researcher in a library can rapidly locate wanted information by using search terms such as topic, author, and publication. The computer search generates a bibliography of literature. The searcher must then locate a copy of the article. Some files provide abstracts that are available on-line. Articles not available from a local health care

library can usually be requested through that library as an interlibrary loan.

The individual physician or health care facility with a computer, a modem, telecommunications software, and a telephone line may subscribe to one or more information utilities. Some of the medically oriented utilities are:

- GTE Medical Information Network (MINET)
- BRS Colleague Medical
- DIALOG

Through GTE, access may be made to EMPIRES (Excerpta Medica Physician Information Retrieval and Education Service), the American Medical Association's clinical literature database that contains current and historical citations and abstracts from over 300 key medical journals.

The development of databases and electronic retrieval systems has provided an invaluable service to the medical profession by making possible easy access to references on an unlimited number of medical subjects. It is also possible for subscribers to read the complete text of books, journals, and other publications.

AMA/NET. The American Medical Association offers an on-line information service called AMA/Net free to its members. The user must have a computer terminal, telephone, and modem. The subscriber to this service has instant access to millions of published documents. MEDLINE and EMPIRES are two of the sources available through this service. AMA/Net also offers continuing medical education programs, several sources of medical news, and an electronic mail system.

OTHER REFERENCE SOURCES. There are a number of other specialized reference volumes that a medical librarian may use to locate literature. The Monthly Catalog of U.S. Government Publications, for example, contains certain medical listings and is sometimes valuable in research work. In securing biographic information about physicians or other professionals, it is often necessary to turn to such books as the *Directory of Medical Specialists, American Men of Science,* the *American Medical Directory,* or *Who's Who Among Physicians and Surgeons.* Encyclopedias such as *Encyclopedia Britannica* and the *Practical Medicine* series also are sometimes helpful in obtaining basic information.

CD-ROM. The computer has brought a world of information within reach of even the most isolated physician if he or she has a CD-ROM drive (Fig. 20–4). One small 5¼-inch compact disk can hold the equivalent of 250,000 typewritten pages, and a large choice of databases are available on CD. Frequent updates are available on many topics, and nearly instant retrieval of timely information is possible from numerous sources. For example, Core MEDLINE, *New England Journal of Medicine, The*

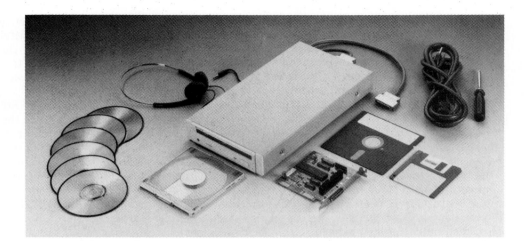

FIGURE 20-4. CD-ROM system. (Courtesy of Sony Corporation of America, San Jose, CA.)

Lancet, Yearbooks from Mosby, and *American Journal of Public Health* are just some of the resources that are available on CD. As an added benefit, some CD-ROM systems are able to play regular stereo CDs while you are working on the computer.

Preparing a Bibliography

Utilizing the various reference sources of the medical library, you can make up a bibliography or list of references on a specific topic with comparatively little difficulty. It does take time, since the list of references must be accurate. Many researchers recommend listing each reference separately on a card or in a small looseleaf notebook (Fig. 20-5). This simplifies the actual preparation of the formal bibliography that always accompanies any published medical paper. Take down the following information for each reference:

- Subject
- Author
- Title of book or article
- Publisher or periodical
- Volume
- Date of publication
- Page numbers

Sometimes card catalogs and other periodical references list brief summaries of the specific reference cited; this information is also helpful in research and should be noted.

Author	Subject
Title	Available at:
	Call No.
Publisher/Journal	Reference: Excellent, Good, Fair
Copyright Date Volume: Pages:	Illustrated:
Student's Name:	

(Summary, including problem, source of data, method, results, quotations, references.)

Summary:

FIGURE 20-5. Card for reporting bibliographic data.

Some libraries prepare medical bibliographies free of charge or for a small fee. Some also abstract or review literature, translate articles, and collect case reports. The library of the American College of Surgeons, for example, offers this service at a modest fee to its members. The American Medical Association also offers this service to its members.

Manuscript Preparation

In most cases, the medical assistant's tasks in connection with the preparation of a talk or a **manuscript** for publication are mainly mechanical; the doctor is responsible for the actual writing. However, since many physicians ask their medical assistants to serve in the capacity of editorial assistants and to smooth out and actually edit their copy before submitting it for publication, a basic understanding of the style, format, and characteristics of medical papers is helpful.

WRITING STYLE. Each medical journal has its own style for publishing papers. The individual hoping to publish in a specific journal should request a copy of the journal's guidelines for manuscripts in advance and then prepare the manuscript accordingly in order to minimize editorial changes. However, there are certain fairly uniform procedures to be followed in the preparation of a manuscript to be submitted for publication.

A good medical paper must present established new facts, modes, or practices; principles of value; results of suitable original research; or a review of facts on a subject from which the reader can draw a legitimate conclusion. The subject should be limited to a definite area or problem before writing is begun, and the purpose should be determined in advance.

The typical medical article begins with an introductory section outlining the nature of the material or problem to be covered, follows with actual discussion of the subject, and concludes with a summary in which conclusions are usually noted in numeric form. The format for case reports is somewhat similar. Case reports based on clinical information should be written clearly in smooth narrative style and should not read like a collection of telegraphic notes. There should be a clear presentation of the sequence of events. A brief abstract may appear at the beginning or end of any article. This summary should be rigidly condensed and should contain the deductions as well as clearly reflect the author's viewpoint. Only the actual conclusions reached should be numbered.

The writing in a scientific paper should be simple and straightforward. Excess words should be ruthlessly pared from the article. Grammatical construction must facilitate direct, clear expression. The paper should be well organized and proceed smoothly from beginning to end in a direct fashion.

Slang, **colloquialisms,** personal allusions, and reminiscences should generally be avoided in papers for publication, although they are often acceptable and add a friendly tone to a paper to be delivered in person before a medical meeting.

TYPING THE MANUSCRIPT. Many **drafts** of a paper may be made before the final copy. Using an electronic word processor or computer can greatly reduce the laborious retyping of manuscripts, but the author may still want a printout of each revision. Sometimes different colors of paper are used to distinguish between each draft. Double- or triple-space drafts to allow plenty of room for revisions by the author.

REVISING THE MANUSCRIPT. An important step in the preparation of any manuscript is a careful revision of copy. This is a duty sometimes delegated to the secretary or medical assistant. Revisions should be made with these specific objectives in mind:

- Organization
- Accuracy
- Content
- Conciseness
- Correct sentence and grammatic construction
- Clarity and smoothness

Check for correct spelling, using a medical dictionary as well as a standard dictionary.

PREPARING FINAL COPY. Use good-quality 8½″ × 11″ white paper. Type on one side of the paper only. Double-space the copy, allowing a margin of at least 1 inch at each side and at the bottom. Double-spacing provides space for the editor who receives the manuscript to make corrections or insert instructions for the printer. Unless otherwise instructed, number each page in the upper right-hand corner.

The original manuscript is submitted to the publisher, and the author should retain one or more copies. If the manuscript is on disk or tape, one printout is sufficient to retain in the file.

FOOTNOTES. When a paper is based on a study of the writing of others, it is necessary to acknowledge the sources used. In medical and scientific papers, **footnotes** usually provide exact references to sources of material. Forms of footnotes differ slightly, depending on the style of the particular periodical, but in general a footnote contains the following:

- Author's name
- Title of the work cited
- Facts of publication
- Exact page from which the citation was taken

The first time a book or article is mentioned in a footnote, all the information about publication should appear in the footnote; after that, references to the same source can be shortened to the author's last name and the page number cited. When a periodical is concerned, a later reference need contain only the author's name, the journal name, and the page number.

Detailed information about footnote preparation can be obtained from *The Chicago Manual of Style* or one of several published reference manuals for office workers.

FINAL BIBLIOGRAPHY. All scientific papers should carry a complete bibliography of source materials. List only those sources that directly pertain to the paper and that were used in its preparation. The form of bibliographies is fairly uniform.

A periodical listing includes:

- Author's name and initials
- Title of the article
- Name of the periodical
- Volume number
- Pages cited
- Date of publication

A book reference includes:

- Author's name and initials
- Title of the book
- Edition (only after the first edition)
- Place of publication
- Name of the publisher
- Year of publication

Bibliographies may be arranged alphabetically according to authors' names or numerically as the references appear in the text. Whatever form and punctuation are used should be consistent throughout the entire listing (Table 20–1).

ILLUSTRATIONS. All drawings, photographs, and other illustrative material submitted with a manuscript should be placed on separate sheets and keyed to the manuscript. In other words, illustrations should be numbered, and indications should be noted in the manuscript as to where each illustra-tion should be placed. Do not include such materials in the body of the manuscript. The explanation of the drawing or illustration should appear in a caption, or **legend.**

Glossy black and white photographs reproduce best. Captions for photos should be typed on separate sheets or may be attached with rubber cement below the photo. On the back of the photograph, the author's name and the number of the illustration should be penciled lightly. Do not use paper clips on photos. Credit lines should be given for copyrighted or commercial photos or illustrations. If x-ray films are submitted, make sure the prints are shiny; indicate on the back where they may be cropped, but leave localizing landmarks.

Charts and line drawings must be carefully prepared in order to achieve good reproduction. Such drawings preferably should be done with India or black ink on heavy white bond paper. Charts should be condensed and simplified as much as possible. Letters and identifying numerals can be placed on the face of the chart with the explanation in the legend below.

Tables should be typewritten on separate sheets in a uniform style; each table should be numbered consecutively and have a descriptive heading.

MAILING THE MANUSCRIPT. Generally, manuscripts should not be folded but should be mailed flat in a large envelope. Sometimes a paper of fewer than four pages can be folded twice and mailed in a regular business envelope, or a manuscript of four to eight pages can be folded once and mailed in a 6 × 9 inch envelope. A letter stating that the manuscript is being submitted for publication should be included. Photos and illustrations should be mailed flat, between sheets of protective cardboard.

PROOFREADING. A paper accepted for publication will be set in type, and proofs of the article will usually be returned by the editor to the author for checking. Since changes in a manuscript once it is set in type are costly, revisions should be limited to correction of errors and minor changes.

If possible, work as a team when checking **galley proofs,** with one person holding the proofs and the other person reading from the original copy. Check for typographic errors, omitted lines and words, and so forth. When correcting proofs, use a different-colored pencil from the one used by the proofreader on the publication. Corrections should be entered in the margins of the proof, next to the line with the error to be corrected. A knowledge of proofreader's marks is helpful (Fig. 20–6).

One corrected set of galley proofs should be returned to the editor, and one set of proofs should be retained by the author. If a second set of proofs is sent later, check the first corrected set against the second set to make sure all corrections have been made.

TABLE 20–1. ABBREVIATIONS USED IN MANUSCRIPT PREPARATION

Abbreviation	Meaning
cf.	compare
e.g.	for example
et al.	and other people
ibid.	in the same place
i.e.	that is
loc. cit.	in the place cited
op. cit.	in the work cited
sic	intentionally so written
q.v.	which see

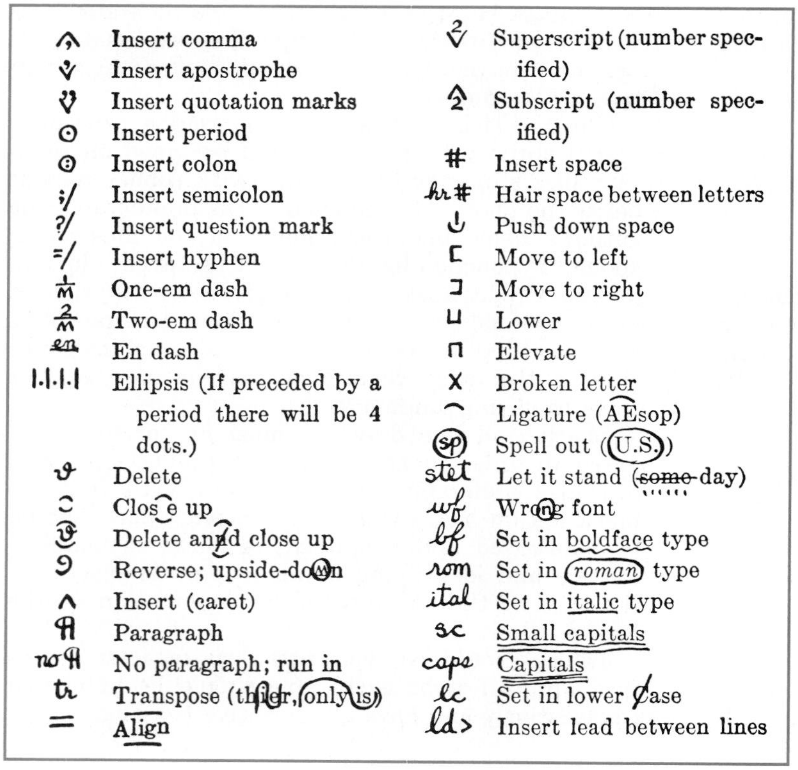

⌃	Insert comma	⌄	Superscript (number specified)
⌄	Insert apostrophe	⌃	Subscript (number specified)
⌄	Insert quotation marks	#	Insert space
⊙	Insert period	hr #	Hair space between letters
⊙	Insert colon	⌐	Push down space
;/	Insert semicolon	⊏	Move to left
?/	Insert question mark	⊐	Move to right
=/	Insert hyphen	⊔	Lower
1/M	One-em dash	⊓	Elevate
2/M	Two-em dash	X	Broken letter
en	En dash	⌒	Ligature (ÆEsop)
I.I.I.I	Ellipsis (If preceded by a period there will be 4 dots.)	ⓢⓟ	Spell out (U.S.)
		stet	Let it stand (some day)
ℰ	Delete	wf	Wrong font
⌣	Close up	bf	Set in boldface type
⌣℮	Delete and close up	rom	Set in roman type
9	Reverse; upside-down	ital	Set in italic type
∧	Insert (caret)	sc	Small capitals
¶	Paragraph	caps	Capitals
no ¶	No paragraph; run in	lc	Set in lower case
tr	Transpose (their only is)	ld >	Insert lead between lines
=	Align		

FIGURE 20–6. Proofreader's marks.

INDEXING. Often it is necessary to provide an index for a long paper or a book. An author and subject index can be made from page proofs. One system for indexing is to use slips of paper or 3 × 5 inch cards. Each index entry is listed on a separate card or slip; this simplifies alphabetizing under major headings later. The whole index can then be typed from the alphabetized cards. Manuscripts prepared by computer can be indexed quickly and accurately with the necessary software.

REPRINTS. At the time an article is set in type, the physician should order all reprints needed, since type is often destroyed after the original press run. Most doctors send copies of their articles to colleagues, to physicians who have evidenced an interest in their work, and to hospitals and teaching institutions with which they have had contact. They probably maintain a card file of names and addresses of those to whom they want to send reprints.

The medical assistant generally handles the ordering of the reprints, which may be as many as 500 copies or more. The order should be adequate to cover any future needs. Addresses in the card file should be checked from time to time in the *American Medical Directory* or by scanning membership and request lists. Some record of reprint mailing should be kept, and acknowledgments should be checked. A person who does not acknowledge two or three reprints should be taken off the mailing list.

An enclosure card, printed in advance, is sent by some authors with a copy of the reprint. Others prefer to enclose a short letter stating that the reprint is a complimentary copy.

SPEECHES. Not all papers are intended for publication. Some are prepared for presentation before medical and scientific meetings. Speeches should be typed and double-spaced; in some offices, a jumbo or magnatype machine is used so that the speech is easy to read. Special large-type elements, such as the IBM Orator, are available for single-element or daisy wheel typewriters.

At the bottom of each page, in the lower right-hand corner, type the first two or three words that appear at the beginning of the next page. The final draft of the paper should be carefully checked for typographic errors.

At large meetings, a speaker is usually allotted from 10 to 20 minutes to present a paper; at county society and small meetings, the speaker may have from 30 minutes to an hour for the presentation. Check in advance to find out exactly how much time will be allowed. The doctor or the medical assistant should time the speech. On the average, it takes about 2 minutes to read a page of copy on which there are about 200 to 250 words. If slides or

PROCEDURE 20-1   MAKING TRAVEL ARRANGEMENTS

GOAL   To make travel arrangements for the physician from his or her city of residence to Toronto, Canada.

EQUIPMENT AND SUPPLIES

Travel plan
Telephone
Telephone directory

Typewriter
Typing paper

PROCEDURAL STEPS

1. Verify the details of planned trip:
   - Desired date and time of departure
   - Desired date and time of return
   - Preferred mode of transportation
   - Number in the party
   - Preferred lodging and price range
2. Telephone the travel agency to arrange for transportation and lodging reservations.
3. Arrange for traveler's checks if desired.
4. Pick up tickets or arrange for their delivery.
5. Check tickets to confirm conformance with the travel plan.
   Purpose: To avoid any error due to misunderstanding and to verify compliance with requests.
6. Check to see if hotel reservations are confirmed.
7. Prepare an itinerary, including all the necessary information:
   - Date and time of departure
   - Flight numbers or identifying information of other modes of travel
   - Mode of transportation to hotel(s)
   - Name, address, and telephone number of hotel(s), with confirmation numbers if available
   - Date and time of return
8. Place one copy of the itinerary in the office file.
   Purpose: It may be necessary to contact the doctor or to forward mail.
9. Give several copies of the itinerary to the physician.
   Purpose: The physician may wish to have extra copies for family or friends.

20

other illustrations are planned, arrangements for showing this material must be made in advance and the necessary time allowed.

TRAVEL AND MEETING ARRANGEMENTS

Transportation and Hotel Arrangements

The medical assistant may be expected to make transportation and hotel arrangements for the doctor for out-of-town meetings. Although the doctor who is located in a metropolitan area probably uses a travel agent for most travel arrangements, the medical assistant may be responsible for working with the travel agent and preparing the detailed itinerary.

The medical assistant who does not deal with a travel agent may be expected to personally make the hotel and transportation arrangements. Keep a file of the telephone numbers of railroads, airlines, and buses, and descriptions and telephone numbers of hotels. Ask for the confirmation number of all hotel arrangements. The doctor who is a member of an auto club can use membership privileges to obtain names of good hotels and motels, road maps, and other important travel information.

Itinerary

When all arrangements are final, typewrite the itinerary. Keep one copy in the office file. Give the doctor the original and several copies for distribution to family members or other individuals. Since it is sometimes necessary to reach the doctor while traveling, it is important that the itinerary be carefully prepared, including locations and telephone numbers.

Meeting Calendar

A calendar of all meetings that the physician plans to attend should be kept by the medical assistant, with both the physician and the medical assistant retaining a copy. The calendar can be merely a sheet of paper but should include the following information for each event:

- Name of the meeting
- Date
- Place
- Time

Any changes or additions to the calendar should be made on both copies as notices are received. A reminder to the physician a few days in advance of each meeting is usually appreciated.

Meeting Responsibilities

The physician often accepts official responsibilities in his or her professional society or on the hospital board. The administrative medical assistant for this physician may be expected to assist in arranging meetings, preparing an agenda, and typing minutes of the meeting dictated by the physician.

The medical assistant who takes an active part in a professional society for medical assistants will have personal use for these skills as well.

Arranging a Meeting

You will need to have advance information of:

- The purpose of the meeting
- How many persons will be expected to attend
- Whether a meal is to be included
- The expected duration of the meeting
- The date, time, and place
- To whom notices are to be sent

Choosing the Location

Some groups meet regularly and use the same facility each time. In this case, it is necessary merely to confirm the date and time with the facility. If a meal is to be served, the menu, price, and approximate number expected to attend must be determined. If a new location is being used, you need to verify that:

- The space is adequate
- Any necessary electronic equipment is available
- Parking facilities are available if needed
- Lighting and ventilation are adequate
- Menus are available if a meal is to be included

Preparing the Notice of Meeting

Meeting notices are usually mailed to all members of the group. For a small committee meeting, the notice may be made by telephone. If there is to be a speaker, the name of the speaker and the topic is included in the meeting notice. The notice must include the date, time, and place of the meeting.

Preparing the Agenda

Organizations whose bylaws specify *Robert's Rules of Order, Newly Revised,* as the parliamentary au-

PROCEDURE 20-2   ARRANGING GROUP MEETINGS

GOAL To arrange a breakfast meeting for the physician's hospital committee.

EQUIPMENT AND SUPPLIES

Directory of committee members   Typewriter
Meeting plan   Post cards
Telephone

PROCEDURAL STEPS

1. Verify the proposed date and time for the meeting.

2. Gather details for meeting arrangements:
   - Purpose of the meeting
   - Expected attendance
   - Name of the speaker, if any, and the program topic
   - Expected duration of the meeting

3. Arrange for a meeting room based on the requirements.

4. Mail notice of the meeting to members and invited guests. Include:
   - Date
   - Time
   - Place
   - Name of the speaker and the topic
   - Cost, if any
   - Registration information

5. Arrange for any necessary equipment (e.g., microphone, projector, and screen).

6. Notify the meeting place of the number of reservations, if required.

7. Arrange for registration check-in.

8. Prepare the agenda.

9. Give the required number of copies of the agenda to physician.

20

thority and that have not adopted a special order of business use the following prescribed **order of business:**

1. Reading and approval of the minutes
2. Reports of officers, boards, and standing committees
3. Reports of special (select or ad hoc) committees
4. Special orders
5. Unfinished business and general orders
6. New business

The order of business lists the different divisions of business in the order in which each will be called for at business meetings.

An **agenda** is a list of the specific items under each division of the order of business that the officers or board plan to present at a meeting. The medical assistant who is expected to prepare the agenda should determine what topics are to be discussed, type them in the prescribed order, and duplicate enough copies for the meeting. For a large group, the program is usually printed. For the smaller group, photocopies are satisfactory.

Preparing the Minutes

The record of the proceedings of a meeting is called the *minutes*. The minutes contain mainly a record of what was done at the meeting, not what was said by the members.

The first paragraph of the minutes should contain the following information:

- The kind of meeting (regular, special, and so forth)
- The name of the association
- The date, time, and place of the meeting
- The fact that the regular chairman and secretary were present or, in their absence, the names of the persons who substituted for them
- Whether the minutes of the previous meeting were read and approved

The body of the minutes should contain a separate paragraph for each subject matter. It should include all main motions, including:

- The wording in which each motion was adopted or otherwise disposed of
- The disposition of the motion
- The name of the mover

The name of the seconder of the motion should not be entered in the minutes unless ordered by the assembly. The body of the minutes should also include any points of order and appeals, whether they were sustained or lost, and the reasons given by the chair for the ruling. The minutes may include the name and subject of a guest speaker, but no attempt should be made to summarize the speech.

The last paragraph should state the hour of adjournment.

The minutes should be signed by the secretary. In some organizations, the president also signs the minutes. The practice of including the words "Respectfully submitted" is obsolete and should not be used.

The medical assistant who might be expected to type the minutes of meetings should consult an authoritative book on the subject and prepare a model to follow in typing the minutes of each meeting so that every set of minutes will be in the same style.

▶ LEARNING ACHIEVEMENTS

Are you able to:

1. Define the terms listed in the Vocabulary of this chapter?
2. Develop and maintain a card catalog for a personal library?
3. Describe an abstract and its function?
4. Create a cross-reference card for a general reference file?
5. Prepare a diagnostic file card, including the five items of necessary information?
6. Specify the library classification system that uses decimal numbers?
7. State which classification system uses a combination of letters of the alphabet and numerals?
8. Cite three indexes available in medical libraries for use in locating various periodical references?
9. Name two of the largest medical databases for the electronic retrieval of information?
10. List the seven items of information needed for each reference in a bibliography?
11. Briefly describe the various steps in preparing a manuscript for publication in a periodical?
12. List the five items that should be included in the first paragraph of the minutes of a meeting?
13. Type a speech in correct format and estimate the time necessary for its delivery?
14. Prepare cards for an abstract file?
15. Set up a diagnostic file, including subject cards and the necessary subheadings to accommodate the patient charts?
16. Retype a manuscript that has been edited using proofreader's marks?
17. Make travel arrangements for a proposed trip?
18. Prepare a typewritten itinerary?
19. Make arrangements for a group meeting?
20. From a rough draft, type the minutes of a meeting in correct form, including the secretary's signature?

REFERENCES AND READINGS

Robert's Rules of Order, Newly Revised, Glenview, IL, Scott, Foresman and Co., 1990.

Strunk, W., Jr., and White, E. B.: *The Elements of Style,* 3rd ed., New York, Macmillan, 1979.

University of Chicago Press: *The Chicago Manual of Style,* 13th ed., Chicago, The Press, 1982.

Valancy, J.: Information at your fingertips: Tapping the resources, *Physician's Management,* April 1984, pp 29–32.

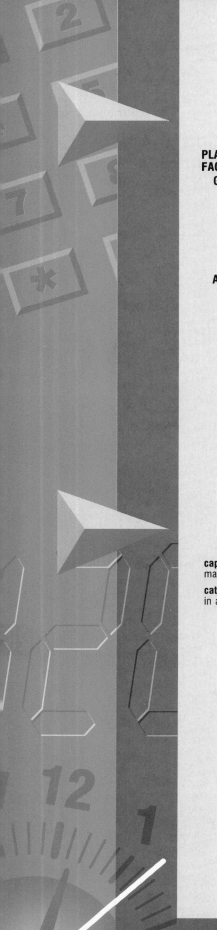

CHAPTER OUTLINE

PLANNING AND ORGANIZING FACILITIES
  General Environment
    Temperature
    Lighting
    Walls and Floor Coverings
    Traffic Control
    Sound Control
    Privacy
    Efficiency
  Area Utilization and Care
    Reception Area
    Administration Area
    Clinical Area
      Consultation Room
      Examination and Treatment
        Rooms
      Laboratory
      Recovery Room
    Lavatories
    Storage and Utility Rooms

MAINTENANCE
  Responsibilities of Staff
  Instructions to Maintenance Service
FURNITURE AND EQUIPMENT
  Acquisition
  Warranty Requirements
  Service
  Inventory
SUPPLIES
  Selecting Supplies and Suppliers
  Ordering Supplies
  Prevention of Waste
  Receiving and Storing
  Caring for Labels
  Drug Samples
  Procedure 21–1: Establishing and Maintaining a Supply Inventory and Ordering System

THE DOCTOR'S BAG
SAFETY AND SECURITY CONSIDERATIONS
  Detection of Hazards
  Drug Enforcement Administration (DEA) Regulations
  Smoke Alarms and Fire Extinguishers
  Fire Exits
  Contact with Security Systems
  Routine Office Security
LEARNING ACHIEVEMENTS

VOCABULARY

capital purchase The purchase of a major item of furniture or equipment.

categorically Pertaining to a division in any classification system.

caustics Substances that corrode or eat away tissues.

expendable Concerning supplies or equipment that is normally used up or consumed in service.

inventory A list of articles in stock, with the description and quantity of each.

reputable Honorable; having a good reputation.

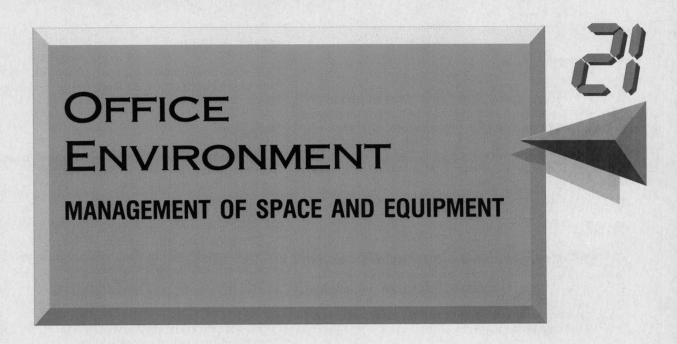

Office Environment

MANAGEMENT OF SPACE AND EQUIPMENT

21

LEARNING OBJECTIVES

COGNITIVE

Upon successful completion of this chapter, you should be able to:

1. Define the terms listed in the Vocabulary.
2. List seven items of concern in controlling the general environment of the medical facility.
3. Discuss the utilization of various areas of the medical facility.
4. Describe how the medical assistant would arrange for and supervise a maintenance service.
5. Explain the inventory process.
6. Explain the importance of the instructions and warranties accompanying new equipment purchases.
7. Cite precautions to be observed in storing poisons, narcotics, acids and caustics, and flammable items.
8. Discuss the procedure for storing supplies and drug samples.
9. List six possible safety hazards in a medical facility.
10. Discuss the importance of and procedures in routine office security.

PERFORMANCE

Upon successful completion of this chapter, you should be able to perform the following activities:

1. Write instructions for a maintenance service.
2. Set up an equipment inventory.
3. Organize and dispose of drug samples.
4. Establish and maintain a supply inventory and ordering system.

PLANNING AND ORGANIZING FACILITIES

The same principles of organization and planning that guide the business management of a medical office are essential in the organization and care of the facilities and supplies. A comfortable, attractive, clean environment lifts the spirits of patients and contributes to the efficiency and enthusiasm of the staff.

General Environment

Temperature

The ideal temperature for a reception room is about 74°F. Working areas can be somewhat cooler. There should be a constant exchange of air by means of open windows or air conditioning. However, you should guard against drafts, as people who are ill are very susceptible to chills.

Lighting

Working areas need to be well lighted. Fluorescent lights are usually preferable because their light is uniform and they do not give off heat. Lamps in the reception area can be decorative, but they are useful only if carefully chosen and properly placed. They should be at reading height; if they are too high they will shine into the eyes of others in the room. Lighting, furnishings, and comfort of the reception room are fully discussed in Chapter 9.

Walls and Floor Coverings

Carpeting is usually the choice for floor covering in the reception area and often in the physician's consultation room. Unsecured rugs should never be used in a medical facility. In the clinical areas, a smooth washable floor covering, such as vinyl or tile, is generally more satisfactory. If wax is used on the floor covering, specify that it be the nonskid variety.

Wallpaper can add a pleasant atmosphere in the reception area. In the administrative and clinical areas, a good quality wall paint in soft colors is attractive, easily cleaned, and long-lasting.

Traffic Control

The furnishings in the entrance and reception areas should be arranged to allow easy traffic without crowding in any one area. The reception desk must be placed so that anyone coming into the office can easily spot the desk, and so that the medical assistant at the desk can view the entire reception area (see Chapter 9). In the inner office, the doctor and the other members of the staff should be able to pass from one station to another without creating a roadblock.

Sound Control

Walls should be soundproof, if possible, to prevent voices and conversations from being heard from one room to another.

Privacy

Treatment rooms should be arranged so that the patient is out of view if it should be necessary to open the door to a hallway.

Efficiency

The physician and medical assistant must be able to move easily within each room and have access to equipment and supplies as needed.

Area Utilization and Care

The medical facility, whether large or small, is separated by utilization into these areas:

- Reception
- Administration
- Clinical activities
- Lavatories
- Storage and utility

The overall cleaning and maintenance of these areas is probably being done by an outside service under the direction of the medical assistant or office manager. However, additional individual attention is required by the staff. In some instances, particularly in rural areas, it may be the sole responsibility of the medical assistant.

Good housekeeping begins with having a place for everything and with keeping everything clean and ready for use. Good housekeeping saves time and energy, conserves property, and eliminates incorrect use of materials. Poor housekeeping holds potential dangers for patients, physicians, and assistants alike.

Reception Area

The importance of a neat, attractive reception room was discussed in Chapter 9, Patient Reception. Draperies, carpet, and upholstery should be cleaned at regular intervals in addition to the daily maintenance.

Administration Area

The administration area includes the reception desk, the records storage, telephone equipment, business machines such as typewriters, computer, calculators, photocopier, and so forth. This area should be separated from the reception room by a locked door. Records and business papers on the reception desk should be placed in desk trays where they will be safe and out of sight of visitors during

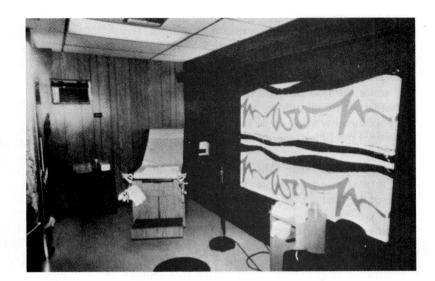

FIGURE 21-1. A clean, neat, and orderly patient examination room.

the day, and in locked files at night. Personal items should be put away in a drawer or locker.

Clinical Area

The clinical area includes the physician's consultation room, which is used for patient interviews and for the physician's private study; patient examination and treatment rooms; and a recovery room where patients may rest after therapy or minor surgery.

CONSULTATION ROOM. The physician's consultation room should always be kept neat and clean. Give this room a quick once-over after each patient visit and remove any evidence of the departing patient.

Follow the preferences of the physician with respect to straightening the desk or other furnishings.

EXAMINATION AND TREATMENT ROOMS. Examination/treatment rooms are designed for utility; only necessary equipment and supplies should be found here. Instruments, medications, and other supplies are in cabinets or drawers (Fig. 21-1). Supply cabinets should be checked daily before the first patient arrives (Fig. 21-2). The room must be straightened, and all counter tops and the sink should be wiped clean after each patient. Disposable gowns, towels, and tissues must be discarded, fresh linens provided, and the room left spotless. The temperature in these rooms is crucial to the comfort of the patients, who are often asked to disrobe and put on a gown.

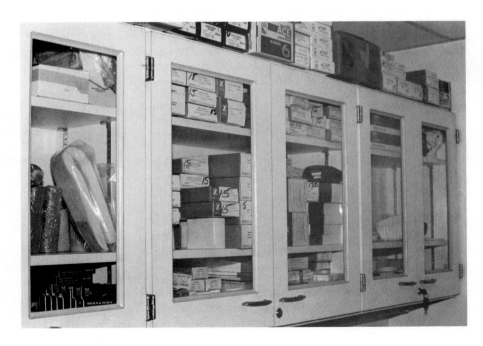

FIGURE 21-2. An example of a neat cabinet for orthopedic supplies.

LABORATORY. The laboratory may be anything from a small closet to a large room. It must be kept clean, with everything in its place, in order for accurate work to be accomplished.

Adequate ventilation in the laboratory is especially important. There are many odors from the laboratory to which the office staff becomes accustomed but which may be disagreeable to patients.

Contamination control must be exercised according to the current regulations of the Occupational Safety and Health Administration (OSHA), which are available from the U.S. Department of Labor in Washington, D.C. Some states have their own OSHA-approved occupational safety and health regulations, which may be even more stringent than the federal standard.

RECOVERY ROOM. The recovery room should be comfortable, clean, and quiet. Facilities should be provided so that patients can relax and keep warm. Interesting reading material will help the time pass more pleasantly. If the patient wishes to sleep, see that no one enters the room.

Lavatories

In the small solo practice office, the lavatory may be shared by staff and patients. In this situation, every member of the staff should be instructed to leave the room meticulously clean. Most medical facilities provide a separate lavatory for patients. This room must be checked by the medical assistant after each use to be certain it is left clean and that all supplies are replenished as needed.

Storage and Utility Rooms

There must be storage space for office and medical supplies, cleaning equipment and supplies, staff lockers or coat hooks, and so forth. The size of these spaces will vary, but whatever area is available must be kept organized and supplies and other items kept in order. Storage and utility rooms are generally closed to all except the staff.

MAINTENANCE

Responsibilities of Staff

One member of the staff, often the administrative medical assistant, is delegated the responsibility of overseeing the maintenance of the premises. The details should be outlined in the office policy and procedure manual (see Chapter 22).

Each member of the staff will probably wish to tidy and dust his or her own desk or work station, with the administrative medical assistant taking care of the physician's desk.

The clinical medical assistant is usually the one who periodically cleans the interior of cabinets and drawers in the examination/treatment rooms. This should be done only when there is time to complete the job. Do one shelf at a time, starting at the top.

1. Remove all items from the shelf and place them on a table in the same order as on the shelf.
2. Wash the shelf and rinse it well. Dry the shelf.
3. Clean and polish the instruments and check for faults. Examine hinges and blades.
4. Check all labels on containers for clarity. Reglue labels, if necessary. Examine supplies for expiration dates, quantity, and deterioration. Make a list of those items that should be reordered.
5. Replace the supplies in their original places on the shelf.

Clean the tops of cabinets and the undersides of towel and tape dispensers as necessary. These areas are frequently overlooked in the daily cleaning.

Maintenance services do not usually include as part of their service such tasks as cleaning mirrors, replacing light bulbs, cleaning the refrigerator, daily cleaning of sinks, straightening magazines, and watering plants. These and numerous other occasional as well as daily jobs are performed by the office staff.

Instructions to Maintenance Service

Every member of the staff must be alert to any problem of cleanliness or safety that might be overlooked by the maintenance service, and report the condition to the medical assistant in charge. The staff member who has the responsibility for instructing the maintenance service must be able to plan and be explicit in giving instructions:

- Prepare a written list of the services that you expect.
- Go over it with the service people.
- Be specific about any areas that are not to be entered or disturbed.
- Set up a regular schedule.
- Evaluate the service regularly.
- Communicate your pleasure or displeasure promptly to the person in charge of performing the service.

FURNITURE AND EQUIPMENT

The physician, individually or as a member of a group practice, has a large investment in the furnishings and equipment necessary to carry on a medical practice. The medical assistant has a responsibility to properly use and care for any piece of equipment in order to preserve its useful life.

Acquisition

When a new piece of equipment is acquired, read the instructions thoroughly and carefully. Do not attempt to assemble or use items that you have not first studied. Keep the purchase invoice on file. The date of purchase and the cost are required for insurance and for depreciation credit on income tax.

Warranty Requirements

If there is a warranty card with the item, copy the code number, fill in the blanks, and mail as instructed.

Service

Keep a service file for equipment that needs regular servicing. This file should contain:

- Warranty dates
- Frequency of service
- When and by whom the item was last serviced
- Cost of service

File all instructions in a special folder and save them for future reference or for your successors.

Inventory

It is good business to **inventory** all equipment and supplies once per year. If you have an office computer, keep the inventory on disk for easy access and updating.

First, list all **capital purchases,** such as furniture, medical and surgical instruments, sterilizers and autoclaves, laboratory equipment, business machines, and any major pieces of artwork or artifacts. These items are permanent and usually expensive. List the date of purchase for each item, along with the original price.

Next, list the smaller, less costly items that are considered **expendable,** such as small instruments, syringes, and thermometers.

Last, estimate the usable supplies and drugs on hand. Keep this inventory to check against the inventory for the coming year. An inventory is valuable in preparing income tax, and especially in case of office burglary or loss from other causes.

SUPPLIES

Selecting Supplies and Suppliers

Supplies are those items that are expendable and must be ordered more or less frequently. In the administrative functions of the practice, they include:

- Stationery and filing supplies
- Appointment books and cards
- Accounting supplies
- Small desk items, such as paper clips, staples, typewriter ribbons, pens, and pencils

In the clinical area, expendable supplies include:

- Examination/treatment items, such as disposable scopes, specula, lubricants, tongue blades, applicators, syringes and needles, dressings, and bandages
- Paper gowns, drapes, towels
- Autoclaving and sterilizing supplies

For general usage, you need to order:

- Soap and towels for lavatories
- Cleaning supplies
- Tissues
- Items for the staff lounge

In general, the person who will use the item is the best person to select what is to be ordered, but it is probably best for one person only to be in charge of ordering all supplies. The purchasing agent in the local hospital is a good source of information on supplies and their sources.

Since there is such a variety of supplies needed, you will have to use more than one supplier. Study the market and find the items that are best suited to the practice with respect to quality and packaging, and order from the suppliers who offer the best service and prices. You should make periodic price checks, but do not sacrifice convenience and service for the sake of saving a few pennies.

Ordering Supplies

There should be an established method for ordering supplies. Keep a list or running inventory from which you can note diminishing supplies and determine when to re-order (Figs. 21–3 and 21–4). Representatives of supply houses regularly call at physicians' offices and are often very helpful in suggesting new items and answering questions about what is available to meet your needs. Mail-order houses also send catalogs describing a great variety of equipment and supplies that can be ordered by mail.

It is advisable to establish good credit with several **reputable** supply companies, both local and mail-order, to provide a choice of vendors. However, do not shift your purchases from company to company without good reason. The loyal customer usually receives better service and may enjoy special privileges, such as being given the option of trying out a piece of equipment before actually agreeing to purchase it.

Attention to detail in ordering will speed delivery and assure greater accuracy. Use the actual title of the supply being ordered, including any special name, size, color, and so forth. The order should state whether payment is enclosed or whether the purchase is to be charged to the physician's account.

21

ORDER	(ITEM NAME)	3-ply Disposable Drape Sheets (white) 7459					**ON ORDER**				

ORDER QUANTITY ___300___   **REORDER POINT** ___100___

ORDER	QTY	REC'D	COST	PREPAID	ON ACCT	ORDER	QTY	REC'D	COST	PREPAID	ON ACCT
1/25	300	2/10	64.95	X							

INVENTORY COUNT

	JAN	FEB	MAR	APR	MAY	JUNE	JULY	AUG	SEPT	OCT	NOV	DEC
19 _94_	200											
19 ___												

ORDER SOURCE   **UNIT PRICE**

The Colwell Company   100 – $23.95

201 Kenyon Road   300 – $64.95

Champaign, IL 61820

FORM 2450 COLWELL CO., CHAMPAIGN, ILLINOIS

FIGURE 21-3. Preprinted form for maintaining a running inventory of medical supplies.

RED FLAG RE-ORDER TAG

when this inventory
point is reached,
its time to reorder

Product
Identification

The Colwell Company
Champaign, Illinois

FIGURE 21-4. A "flag" indicates when the supply of a particular item is low and replacement supplies must be ordered.

Prevention of Waste

In some cases, the unit cost of an item may be reduced by purchasing in larger quantities, but this is not always a saving. Make this decision only after considering the following questions:

- Will the supply be used in a reasonable length of time?
- Will it spoil or deteriorate?
- Is there sufficient space for storage?
- Will the practice continue to use the product?

Receiving and Storing

All orders should be placed in the storage area and opened only when you have time to check the contents. Compare the items in the package with your original purchase order and the invoice included with the shipment. Check for correct items, sizes, and styles as well as the number or amount received. Note any back orders and discrepancies. When you are satisfied that the order is correct and complete, make the necessary notations on the inventory and order cards and place the items in their designated storage areas.

If you have any questions regarding the order or if you have a complaint to make, gather the following information before contacting the supplier:

- Invoice number
- Date ordered
- Name of person who placed order

List on paper your questions and the information you desire. If a catalog was used in placing the order, open your copy to the correct page and secure any additional pertinent information. With all this information at hand, you can make a professional inquiry by letter or telephone.

Follow good housekeeping standards in storing supplies. Place supplies where they are most accessible yet protected from damage and exposure to moisture, heat, light, and air.

Most drugs and solutions should be stored in a cool, dark cupboard, because direct light and sunlight cause drug deterioration.

Poisons should be stored in a locked compartment and kept separate from products used routinely. Have a distinct label or cap for poisons. A bright red color for their labels or caps may be useful.

Narcotics must be stored in a secure place out of sight.

Acids and **caustics** should have special resistant lids; never use metal lids for these substances. Do not store strong acids next to alkalis.

Inflammable items must be stored away from heat.

If drugs and solutions are to be stored for some time, the stoppers should be dipped in paraffin to seal them from the air. Do not fill these bottles to the very top; leave a little room for expansion.

Caring for Labels

If a bottle is to be used for a long time, the label should be indestructible. The original label should

---

PROCEDURE 21-1 ESTABLISHING AND MAINTAINING A SUPPLY INVENTORY AND ORDERING SYSTEM

GOAL To establish an inventory of all expendable supplies in the physician's office and follow an efficient plan of order control using a card system.

EQUIPMENT AND SUPPLIES

File box
Inventory and order control cards
List of supplies on hand

Metal tabs
Re-order tags
Pen or pencil

PROCEDURAL STEPS

1. Write the name of each item on a separate card.
   Purpose: To establish a record of all items in inventory.

2. Write the amount of each item on hand in the space provided.
   Purpose: To establish beginning inventory.

3. Place a re-order tag at the point where the supply should be replenished.
   Purpose: The tag will serve as an alert that supply is low.

4. Place a metal tab over the *order* section of the card.
   Purpose: The metal tab will be a reminder to include this item in the next order.

5. When the order has been placed, note the date and quantity ordered and move the tab to the *on order* section of the card.

6. When the order is received, note the date and quantity in the appropriate column, remove the tab, and refile the card.
   Note: If the order is only partially filled, let the tab remain until the order is complete.

21

be treated for preservation when it is first received. When using the contents of the bottle, pour away from the label side to prevent any dripping on the label. Plastic screw caps protect the lip of the bottle and keep it clean.

When a label shows signs of wear or mutilation, or is difficult to read, replace the entire bottle and solution for safety purposes.

Drug Samples

Samples of drugs and medications that are suitable to the physician's practice should be organized **categorically** in a sample cupboard or drawer.

Place all similar drugs together, preferably in boxes of similar size and shape, with the tops open and plainly labeled on the outside. Clear plastic boxes are excellent for this type of storage. Color-coded labels are an additional help in identification.

Keep all the sedative samples in one box, all stimulant samples in another, and so forth. It is good practice to band together drug samples that have the same code number or expiration date. Rotate the drugs by placing the most recently received items in back of those that were previously on hand. At regular intervals, check all samples for expiration dates, and properly dispose of those that have expired.

THE DOCTOR'S BAG

Although the physician who makes housecalls has become a rarity, the practice is not entirely extinct and is even making a comeback in some areas. Any medical assistant who is given the responsibility of keeping the doctor's bag ready for use must regard it seriously and give it close and continual attention.

The items that are included in the bag depend on professional requirements, the kinds of emergencies that are responded to, and the personal preferences of the person using it. That person could be the physician, a physician's assistant, a nurse practitioner, or an emergency medical technician.

Following is a basic inventory of items commonly found in a physician's bag:

Blood pressure set	Sterile hemostatic forceps
Stethoscope	Sterile syringes and
Thermometers (oral and rectal)	needles (preferably disposable)
Flashlight or penlight	Sterile swabs
Sterile gloves and lubricant	Sterile dressings
Wooden applicators	Tongue depressors
Assorted bandages	Scissors
Adhesive tape (assorted widths)	Sterile dressing forceps
Safety pins	Aspiration equipment
Towel	Microscopic slides and fixative
Ballpoint pens	Containers for specimens
Prescription pads	Culture tubes for throat cultures

Sterile suture set	Medications:
Sterile scalpel	Adrenalin
Probe	Digitalis
Tourniquet	Antibiotics
Percussion hammer	Antihistamines
Illuminated diagnostic set (otoscope and ophthalmoscope)	Alcohol and/or skin disinfectant
Sterile tissue forceps	Sterilizing solution
	Spirits of ammonia

As a guide, keep an inventory of the bag's contents posted inside a cupboard above the place where you check and clean the bag. When checking the bag after a patient has been tended to, remove any specimens and see that they are properly labeled with the patient's full name, the date, and the type of test if the specimen is to be sent out for examination.

If any instruments or gloves have been used, remove them and replace with sterile ones. Even if this equipment has not been used, it should be sterilized weekly. Keep the containers of alcohol, germicides, and other substances filled, and check containers often for any leakage. Allow a small space for heat expansion in containers of fluid.

SAFETY AND SECURITY CONSIDERATIONS
Detection of Hazards

The physician and every member of the staff should continually monitor possible hazards to themselves and the patients.

The reception room and public areas of the facility are particularly vulnerable. Are the chairs in the reception room safe for children? . . . for an exceptionally heavy patient? . . . for a physically disadvantaged patient? Are there any exposed telephone or light cords that someone could trip on? . . . lamps that could tip?

In the examining rooms, be especially careful to put away any sharp instruments, hazardous liquids, or medications. Any spills on the floor should be wiped immediately to prevent a fall or slipping. Keep prescription pads out of sight.

Are the stairways and entrances to the facility well lighted and safe? Are there any known hazards in the parking area?

Drug Enforcement Administration (DEA) Regulations

A physician who has controlled substances (narcotics) stored on the premises must keep these drugs in a locked cabinet or safe. Any loss of controlled drugs by theft must be reported to the regional office of the DEA at the time the theft is discovered. The local police department and the State Bureau of Narcotic Enforcement should also be notified.

Smoke Alarms and Fire Extinguishers

Smoke alarms are required in all new buildings and should be installed in every existing medical facility. Their functioning must be checked regularly to ensure effectiveness if they should be needed. There should be a fire extinguisher readily accessible to any part of the facility.

Fire Exits

Fire exits should be clearly marked and the staff instructed on evacuation proceedings in case of fire.

Contact with Security Systems

If the doctor's office is located in a multiple unit building or medical complex, know whom to contact if a security emergency should occur. Have the telephone number handy for local fire and police departments (911 in many areas).

Routine Office Security

Within the office, all valuables should be kept out of sight. A frequent target of thieves is the medical assistant's handbag, which is often left under a desk or table, where it can be easily spotted by an intruder.

It is most important to secure all entrances — windows as well as doors. Have good double locks installed by a reliable locksmith. It may be well worth the cost to consult a professional security service and follow their advice. Making an office burglar-proof is impossible, but entry can be made difficult, and this in itself usually discourages the amateur.

Outside sensor lights with unbreakable shields are extremely helpful. Leaving a light burning and a radio playing inside the office are additional deterrents. Tell the local police or the building security force which lights will always be left on.

Alarms can be helpful if they are reliable and are not easily disconnected by an expert. Loud local alarms are usually sufficient to frighten off a prowler. It is possible, if greater security is needed, to install an alarm system that will ring in the local police station or at a special security office.

Police departments urge that all valuables be protected by etching them with personal identification, such as the owner's name or social security number. This is easily done with an electric engraving tool that cuts into the equipment, and the marking is practically impossible to eradicate. Even if an attempt is made to scratch it off, a sufficient impression will be left so that police, with the aid of a special chemical, can bring the engraved characters up again (Fig. 21–5).

The most effective step in protecting your premises against break-ins is to remember to check carefully at the end of every day to make certain that all doors and windows are doubly locked.

> # warning
> WE HAVE JOINED
> **OPERATION IDENTIFICATION**
> ALL ITEMS OF VALUE
> ON THESE PREMISES
> HAVE BEEN INDELIBLY MARKED
> FOR READY IDENTIFICATION
> BY LAW ENFORCEMENT AGENCIES

FIGURE 21–5. A sign for office window indicating that valuables have been marked for purposes of identification.

▶ **LEARNING ACHIEVEMENTS**

Are you able to:

1. Define the terms listed in the Vocabulary of this chapter?
2. List seven items to check in controlling the general environment of a medical facility?
3. Describe the ways in which the five main areas of a medical facility are used?
4. Establish and maintain a supply inventory and ordering system?
5. Discuss the importance of maintaining order and cleanliness in the medical facility?
6. Write a program of instructions for a maintenance service?
7. Explain what you would do with the instructions and warranties that are provided with new equipment purchases?
8. Cite the precautions to be observed in storing and disposing of poisons, narcotics, acids and caustics, and flammable items?
9. List at least six possible safety hazards in a medical facility?
10. Discuss ways of maintaining security of the premises?

REFERENCES AND READINGS

American Medical Association: *Physician's Office Laboratory Guidelines and Procedure Manual,* Chicago, American Medical Association, 1992.

American Medical Association: *Planning Guide for Physicians' Medical Facilities,* Chicago, American Medical Association, 1989.

American Medical Association: *OSHA Regulations: A Prescription for Compliance (12-minute video),* Chicago, American Medical Association, 1992.

Cody, J. P.: Materials Management: Developing an Inventory System, *The Professional Medical Assistant* 1991; January/February: 11–14.

Newsome, R.: OSHA Regulations for the Physician's Office, *The Professional Medical Assistant* 1991; January/February: 17–18.

21

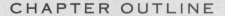

CHAPTER OUTLINE

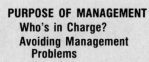

VOCABULARY

ancillary Subordinate; auxiliary.

appraisal Setting a value on or judging as to quality.

candid Frank; straightforward.

circumvention Going around or avoidance.

discrimination A distinction based on race, religion, sex, or some other factor, especially one resulting in unfair or injurious treatment of an individual belonging to a particular group.

disseminate To broadcast or spread over a considerable area.

insubordination Refusing to submit to authority.

meticulous Extremely careful of small details.

motivation Process of inciting a person to some action or behavior.

orientation The determination or adjustment of one's intellectual or emotional position with reference to circumstances.

philosophy The general laws that furnish the rational explanation of anything.

probationary Pertaining to a trial or a period of trial to ascertain fitness for a job.

recruitment The supplying of new members or help.

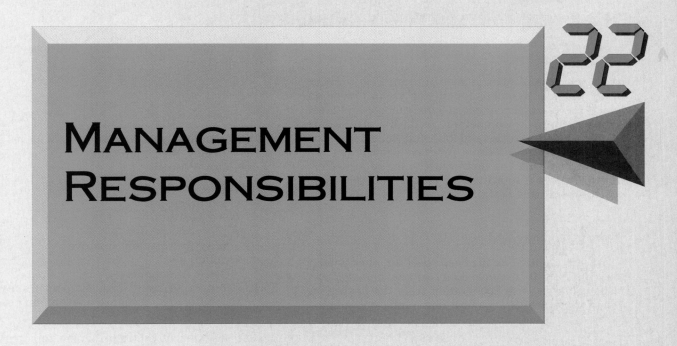

MANAGEMENT RESPONSIBILITIES

22

LEARNING OBJECTIVES

COGNITIVE

Upon successful completion of this chapter, you should be able to:

1. Define the terms listed in the Vocabulary.

2. State the purpose and goals of medical office management.

3. Discuss the desirable qualities of an office manager and their importance in the selection of a supervisor.

4. Identify the goals of an office policy manual and how they may be achieved.

5. Discuss the steps in the hiring and dismissal of employees.

6. List five kinds of staff meetings.

7. Explain how a procedure manual differs from a policy manual.

8. Discuss the concept of practice development and its importance.

9. List at least 10 features of a patient information folder.

10. State two advantages of patient instruction sheets.

11. Discuss the supervisor's role in financial management.

12. Identify the source of reference for information on employer taxes and deposit requirements.

PERFORMANCE

Upon successful completion of this chapter, you should be able to perform the following activities:

1. Interview an applicant for a position, utilizing the guidelines in this chapter.

2. Prepare an outline of contents for a basic office policy manual.

3. Write a procedure sheet for a specific task.

4. Outline a patient information folder.

5. Outline a financial policies folder.

6. Write a patient instruction sheet.

PURPOSE OF MANAGEMENT

The purpose of management in a medical practice is to provide a quiet, functional environment in which the physician or physicians can see and treat patients, provide competent medical care, safely store medical records, and bill and collect for services in order to continue practicing medicine. We have learned that the daily functioning of a medical office involves a multitude of details and that good management does not just happen.

Who's in Charge?

If there is only one medical assistant, that person must be able to assume many of the management responsibilities with cooperation from the physician. When there are two medical assistants, one administrative and one clinical, it is often the administrative medical assistant who is expected to take on the management duties. In the office with a larger staff, a line of authority must be established.

An office with three or more employees should have one person designated as supervisor or office manager. This individual should have management skills and the ability to deal with personnel matters. Other employees answer to the supervisor; the supervisor answers to the physician or physicians. This sets up an orderly way for:

- The office staff to consult with the doctor regarding administrative or technical problems, complaints, or grievances
- The doctor to check on the operation of the office, **disseminate** information on policy changes, and correct errors or grievances

Although the career of the medical assistant is more challenging than it has been in the past, it offers more opportunities for advancement today than ever before. The recently graduated medical assistant whose first position is as a receptionist may systematically be given more responsibilities and eventually become the office manager of a large staff. "The single most critical short supply in health manpower is executive level personnel, specifically individuals competent to develop and operate a health maintenance organization, or prepaid group practice." (Gettys and Zasa, 1977)

Avoiding Management Problems

Management problems can often be avoided by carefully defining the areas of authority and responsibility of each employee. Many physicians say that friction between workers is their most common personnel problem. A definite chain of command must be established, and the physician must not undermine the supervisor's authority by **circumvention.** When employees know what is expected of them, they can plan both their daily and long-term work more effectively.

QUALITIES OF A SUPERVISOR

What qualities should a supervisor have? Job experience may be important, but the supervisor should also possess:

- Leadership ability
- Good judgment
- Good health
- Ability to organize
- Ability to learn and improve
- Original ideas
- A sense of fairness
- Strength to stand firm on policy, but enough flexibility to recognize when an exception should be made

The selection of the right person to supervise the employees is critical. The supervisor may come from within the ranks or may be selected as a new member of the staff. Some employees do not wish to assume management responsibilities; others may not have the necessary qualifications.

Running the administrative side of a medical practice is a complex job that is getting more complex every day. The American Medical Association's Department of Practice Management offers workshops designed to help medical assistants hone their office skills. One workshop called "Team Building —A Better Way to Supervise" is especially designed to sharpen the supervisory skills needed by the medical office manager. Some practice management consultants conduct seminars for medical office personnel. These are often arranged through a chapter of the American Association of Medical Assistants or the local medical society.

MANAGEMENT DUTIES

Medical office administrative procedures fall into three broad categories: patient scheduling, medical recordkeeping, and practice management. We have dealt in detail with the first two categories in previous chapters. It is the third category—practice management processes—that concerns us here.

The practice manager's duties vary with the practice but may include any or all of the following:

Personnel management

- Preparing and updating policy and procedure manuals
- Recruiting
- Hiring
- Orientation and training
- Performance and salary review
- Dismissal

Business management

- Planning staff meetings
- Maintaining staff harmony
- Establishing work flow guidelines
- Improving office efficiency
- Supervising the purchase and care of equipment
- Patient education
- Eliminating time-wasting tasks for the physician
- Practice marketing

Financial management

- Supervising cash transactions
- Maintaining payroll records
- Taking care of employee benefits

Personnel Management

Office Policy Manual

An office policy manual may be a manager's best friend. It can serve as:

- An informational guide for the new employee
- A ready reference for a temporary employee
- A reminder of policies for the regular employee

A well-designed policy manual accomplishes several goals:

- It solidifies what may have been vague thoughts into definite statements of policy.
- It communicates these statements in exactly the same way to every employee.
- It provides a permanent record of these policies.

This does not mean that the policies can never be changed, but a well-formulated policy may be the difference between order and chaos. The manual must be:

- Designed for a specific office
- Comprehensive but flexible
- Easy to read
- In conformance with professional ethics
- Reviewed frequently and kept up-to-date as changes in policy occur

CONTENT OF POLICY MANUAL. A policy manual often has an opening statement of the **philosophy** of the practice, for example:

The patient is the most important person in this office, is the purpose of our being here, and shall receive our most courteous and attentive treatment at all times.

Follow the opening statement with a **personnel chart** that shows the line of authority and states who has authority to enforce the policies.

Include **professional information** regarding the physician's education and specialty board achieve-ments, hospital staff memberships, memberships in professional societies, state license number, and narcotic registry number.

Expectations regarding the personal appearance of employees should be established so that there is no misunderstanding. Guidelines regarding appropriate dress, use of makeup, nail polish, and perfume, cleanliness, grooming, and hygiene are difficult to discuss on a personal basis but can be matter-of-fact in an office manual.

Describe the work week, listing the daily office hours and any days off, the daily appointment schedule, and where the physician can be reached with messages or emergencies. Specify the time allowed each day for lunch and breaks and whether they must be taken at specific times.

What provisions exist for **sick leave**, emergency leave, and any other absences? Are medical services provided by the professional staff free to employees? Are they discounted? When is the employee eligible for benefits?

Describe the **vacation policy**, including how much vacation time the employee is allowed in terms of number of working days, who authorizes it, and whether there are any restrictions as to when vacation time may be taken. List the holidays observed.

Are there other **benefits** for employees, such as payment of professional dues, health insurance, uniform allowances, pension plan, profit sharing, and free parking?

Is time off given for education courses or for attending professional organization conventions or seminars? If so, is this time counted as paid time or as vacation time?

Does the office pay for courses, professional memberships, and expenses incurred at professional conventions?

When is payday? What is the policy on overtime? Are there annual bonuses? If so, on what are they based? What is the policy for performance reviews, salary reviews, and merit increases (Figure 22-1)?

How much notice is expected if an employee wants to quit? Can the employee who resigns receive severance pay? What are the grounds for immediate dismissal? How are complaints and grievances handled?

Recruitment

The office manager can be expected to initiate the **recruitment** and screening of prospective employees. Careful judgment and objectivity must be used in the search for an employee who is suitable for the practice.

Name _____ Soc. Sec. No. _____

Job Classification _____

Employment Date _____ Starting Salary _____

    Salary checks are issued every (week) (two weeks) (semi-monthly) (month)

on_____(day or date).

    Increase-in-pay review will be conducted six months after the completion
of three-month probationary period and each six months thereafter.

    Date of first pay review _____

    Current maximum salary for this job classification $_____

        Revised_____ $_____

        Revised_____ $_____

SALARY SCHEDULE

Date	Amount of Increase	Total Salary
_____	_____	_____
_____	_____	_____
_____	_____	_____
_____	_____	_____

FIGURE 22–1. Example of a page from an office policy manual.

PRELIMINARY STEPS. Before interviewing any applicant, one needs to know:

- What personal qualities and abilities the applicant must have
- What the duties of the position are
- Salary range
- How soon the position will be open

Add any other specifications for the position. Then, after reviewing the policy manual, prepare an outline to guide you in selecting prospective applicants. Here are a few suggestions:

- Do the applicant's appearance and personal grooming meet the standards set forth in the policy manual?
- Has the applicant been previously employed? What duties were performed?
- If previously employed, how long was the applicant in the last position? Why did the applicant leave?
- In what skills is the applicant proficient? Do these meet the requirements for the position as set forth in the office procedure manual? Does the applicant seem to accept and enjoy responsibility?
- What is the applicant's formal education? Certified Medical Assistant? If not certified, is the applicant interested in taking the certifying examination? Is the applicant a member of a professional organization? Does he or she attend meetings?

ARRANGING THE PERSONAL INTERVIEW. If the applicant sent a letter asking for an interview, note whether the letter was correctly typed, included the essential information, and provided a personal data sheet (see Chapter 7). Forget the applicant who sends a letter handwritten in pencil. By telephoning the applicant, you will have an opportunity to judge the telephone voice. If it is poor, you may not wish to consider the applicant further.

Set a time for the personal interview when you most likely will be able to give the applicant your undivided attention. However, an applicant who is being considered for employment should have an opportunity to see your office when there is a fairly normal amount of activity. The prospective employee who is interviewed in a peaceful, quiet office on the doctor's day out may not be prepared for the activity on a normal working day.

Before interviewing any applicant, make certain you are thoroughly familiar with the federal, state, and local fair-employment practice (FEP) laws affecting hiring practices. Both men and women are receiving protection from on-the-job **discrimination,** sexual harassment, mandatory lie detector tests, and unfair discharge.

Illegal questions are sometimes asked on employment applications or during interviews. Title VII of the Civil Rights Act of 1964, as amended by the Equal Employment Opportunity Act of 1972, prohibits inquiries into an applicant's race, color, sex, religion, and national origin. Inquiries regarding medical history, arrest records, or former drug use are also illegal. Most states have laws designed to protect the rights of job applicants, and these laws may impose additional restrictions.

Either send the applicant an application form to be completed and brought in at the time of the interview or allow ample time for its completion on the day of the interview. The application form can serve as a check of the applicant's penmanship and thoroughness as well as a permanent record for your files. If you wish it completed in the applicant's own handwriting, be sure to state this on the instructions. The applicant should be **meticulous** about following instructions and filling in all the blanks (Fig. 22–2).

THE INTERVIEW. First, make sure the applicant feels at ease. You might shake his or her hand and ask a few social questions before starting the interview. In general, follow good manners and see that the person to be interviewed is comfortable.

Begin with a few open-ended questions that cannot be answered with a simple "yes" or "no," such as "What did you do in your last employment?" When interviewing a recent graduate who does not have experience, you might ask, "What was your favorite class at _____ College?"

As you speak with the applicant, make a mental note of whether the applicant:

- Converses easily
- Is a good listener
- Is free of annoying mannerisms
- Has a ready smile
- Is interested enough to ask as well as to answer questions
- Appears interested in the office and in the doctor's specialty

Avoid questions that involve the applicant's privacy. Your questions should be related to the available position and the applicant's ability to do the job. An interview should be a two-way exchange of information between the applicant and the interviewer.

If the applicant appears to be one who will receive serious consideration, you have the responsibility of explaining what will be expected in the way of duties; office policies regarding appearance, working hours, overtime, time off, and vacations; what initial salary is offered and any fringe benefits; and the office policy on increases. If you fail to mention these items, the applicant may be hesitant to inquire.

Review the job description for the position being filled. This is essential if you are to be certain that the person being interviewed understands the required duties and responsibilities. Ask if the applicant has any questions, and close the interview on a positive note.

During the hiring proceedings, you may wish to invite the prospective employee to lunch with the staff or for coffee in the more relaxed atmosphere of the employee lounge. This permits an opportunity to discover whether the applicant's personality will mesh with the atmosphere of the office.

FOLLOW-UP ACTIVITIES. When the interview is over, take a few moments to immediately rate the applicant on your checklist. Jot down some notes to refresh your memory when you refer this applicant to the doctor for the final interview. Do not trust to memory, especially if several applicants will be interviewed. The following is a suggested checklist that may be modified to suit your own circumstances:

	Superior	Above Average	Average	Poor	Remarks
Name_____ Date_____ Time_____					
Appearance and grooming					
General health					
Voice and diction					
Mannerisms					
Poise					
Friendliness					
Interest in work					
Did applicant ask questions?					
Overall impression					

If your employer is a member of a credit bureau, it may be advisable to request the applicant's permission to check his or her credit rating, especially if handling office finances will be one of the responsibilities. It can be safely assumed that one who is unable to handle personal financial affairs will be a poor risk in handling office finances.

CHECKING REFERENCES. It is always advisable to carefully check all references and to follow through on any leads for information. It is best to use the telephone in checking references because people are sometimes less than **candid** in a letter; furthermore, letter writing is time-consuming, and you may not get a reply.

Prepare a checklist before you place the call. When you talk with the person called be sure to "listen between the lines." Note the tone of the replies to your questions. Here are some questions you might ask in your inquiry:

Applicant's name_____
Name of reference called_____
Telephone No._____
1. When did_____ work for you? How long?_____
2. What were the duties?
3. Why did the employee leave?
4. Would you rehire this person under the right circumstances?
5. Was there frequent absenteeism or tardiness?
6. Did the employee assume responsibility well?
7. Was there good rapport with other staff members?
8. Do you have any suggestions or advice about hiring this person?

EMPLOYMENT APPLICATION

Prospective employees will receive consideration without discrimination because of race, creed, color, sex, age, national origin or handicap.

PERSONAL INFORMATION

Last Name	First	Middle	Date
Street Address			Home Phone ( ) —
City, State, Zip			Business Phone ( ) —
Have you ever applied for employment with us? ☐ Yes ☐ No If Yes: Month and Year _____ Location _____			Social Security No.
Position Desired			At what salary do you expect to start?
Apart from absence for religious observance, are you available for full-time work? ☐ Yes ☐ No If not, what hours can you work?_____			
Are you legally eligible for employment in the United States?			When will you be available to begin work? _____
Other special training or skills (languages, machine operation, etc.)			Whom to notify in emergency:
How did you learn of our organization?			

EDUCATIONAL BACKGROUND

SCHOOL	NAME AND LOCATION OF SCHOOL		NO. OF YEARS COM-PLETED	DID YOU GRADUATE?	DEGREE
College				☐ Yes ☐ No	
High				☐ Yes ☐ No	
Elementary				☐ Yes ☐ No	
Other				☐ Yes ☐ No	

MEMBERSHIP IN PROFESSIONAL OR CIVIC ORGANIZATIONS

FIGURE 22-2. Example of application used in a medical facility. (Courtesy of Medical Consultants, Anaheim, CA.)

HIRING. When a decision has been reached to hire someone, notify the applicant of the decision and state when the applicant will be expected to report for work.

Remember to notify all others who have applied. They may have hesitated to accept other interviews in the hope of hearing from you. It is unfair to keep individuals who are seeking employment "on the string." Good etiquette requires that you drop them a note or call by telephone, and say that the position is filled. Thank the individual for applying, and say that you will keep his or her application on file.

PREVIOUS EMPLOYMENT

1

Company Name	Telephone ( ) –
Address	Employed (State Month and Year) From To
Name of Supervisor	Weekly Pay Start Last
State Job Title and Describe Your Work	Reason for Leaving

2

Company Name	Telephone ( ) –
Address	Employed (State Month and Year) From To
Name of Supervisor	Weekly Pay Start Last
State Job Title and Describe Your Work	Reason for Leaving

3

Company Name	Telephone ( ) –
Address	Employed (State Month and Year) From To
Name of Supervisor	Weekly Pay Start Last
State Job Title and Describe Your Work	Reason for Leaving

HOBBIES & OUTSIDE INTERESTS

_____

_____

Can you handle?

    1. Medicare and Medi-Cal billing forms?_____

    2. Compensation first reports and final billings?_____

    3. All other insurance billings?_____

    4. Disability Reports?_____

Typing speed:_____Bookkeeping abilities:_____

Computer experience_____Dictating equipment_____Transcription_____

Medical terminology_____Ability to complete neat, properly spaced,

and properly spelled letters_____

How long do you plan to work full time?_____

Date:_____   Signature_____

FIGURE 22-2 *Continued*

Orientation and Training

Recruitment does not end with the hiring. Some preliminary **orientation** and training will help new employees to understand what is expected and to develop their full potential. Introduce the new employee to:

- The rest of the staff
- The physical environment by a tour of the entire facility
- The nature of the practice and specialty by explaining what types of patients are dealt with and how the staff is expected to interact with them
- The office policies by having the employee read the policy manual and then discussing it
- Your long-range expectations, but not expecting that they will all be handled efficiently on the first day

Performance and Salary Review

A new employee should be granted a **probationary** period. Sixty to 90 days has been traditional, but many employers feel that 2 weeks is sufficient to determine whether the employee will be able to learn and adapt to the position.

A definite date for a performance review at the end of the probationary period should be set at the time of employment. This review should not be squeezed in between patient visits, or be given a token few minutes at the end of a day. There should be ample time to relax and talk. At this time, the new employee is told how well expectations have been met and whether there are any deficiencies. Then, give the employee an opportunity to ask questions. Sometimes an employee fails to perform because of never having been told what was expected.

The performance **appraisal** includes a judgment of both the quality and quantity of work, personal appearance, attitudes and team spirit, dependability, self-discipline, **motivation,** attendance, and any other qualities essential to satisfactory performance of the job in question.

Although the probationary period does not always allow time to fully train an individual for a specific position, it is fair to assume that the potential for being a satisfactory employee can be judged at this time. Now is the time to talk out any problems and make suggestions for improvement.

The supervisor is responsible for an ongoing performance appraisal of all employees, complimenting whenever possible and appropriate, and offering helpful criticism when necessary. A formal performance appraisal at the end of the probationary period and at regular 6-month intervals thereafter, with a report to the physician employer, is helpful in the employee's salary review.

Dismissal

The necessity of having to dismiss an employee is unpleasant at best, but if the ground rules are decided upon in advance, written into the policy manual, and explained to all employees, the problem is partially solved. The policies must be applied equally and impartially to all. The final decision for dismissal will probably be made by the physician but may be based on the recommendation of the office manager/supervisor. The person who does the hiring should do the firing.

PROBATIONARY EMPLOYEE. The probationary employee who does not prove satisfactory should be dismissed at the end of the probationary period with tact and a full explanation of the reasons for dismissal. In all fairness, an individual should be told why the employment is ended and not be given weak excuses or untruths that do not help to correct deficiencies. If you are not straightforward in telling an employee the reason for dismissal, you are not helping that person to grow.

LONG-TERM EMPLOYEE. An employee who has been in service for some time and is offering unsatisfactory performance should be warned and given an explanation of the specific improvements expected. If a second chance does not produce improvement in performance or attitude, then dismissal must follow. It should be done privately, with tact and consideration.

Most practice consultants believe that firing should come close to the end of the day, after all other employees have left, and that the break should be clean and immediate. If the office policy provides for 2 weeks' notice, give 2 weeks' pay. A fired employee should not be allowed to train or influence a replacement.

The exit meeting should be planned just as carefully as the employment interview. Be honest with the employee. Discuss the employee's assets as well as liabilities and give the reasons for the termination before you announce the dismissal. There is no need to dwell upon the employee's deficiencies. These should have been thoroughly discussed at the warning interview, and the employee need only be told that the necessary improvements have not been made. Do listen to the employee's feedback, however. This may reveal some important administrative problems that need correction.

After you dismiss an employee, do not leave that person in the office unattended. Request and get the office keys before giving a dismissed employee the final paycheck. And don't offer to give the employee a good reference unless you can do it sincerely.

Certain breaches of conduct, such as embezzlement and blatant **insubordination** or violation of patient confidentiality, are grounds for immediate dismissal without warning.

Dear_____:

    Since your decision to leave our employ a few weeks ago, I have been concerned about your reasons for doing so. There may have been more than one reason—and one of them may have been dissatisfaction with the working conditions.

    If there was in fact some reason for dissatisfaction that influenced your decision to leave our employ, I would appreciate your passing it along to me, so that I may avoid losing other valuable employees in the future.

    Please drop me a note, telephone, or come in if you wish. I assure you that any comments you care to make will be treated with respect and appreciation.

                     Cordially yours,

FIGURE 22-3. Example of a letter from physician to an employee who resigns suddenly.

Occasionally, an employee voluntarily terminates a job without giving a valid reason. The physician or office manager may wish to follow up with a letter to the former employee to seek out any problem that may have prompted the resignation (Fig. 22-3).

Office Management

Staff Meetings

There must be some formal mechanism for keeping the office manager and other key employees current on the daily business affairs of the practice. One of the most common complaints from office personnel is that of being unable to discuss problems with the doctor. The solution to this problem may be to hold regular staff meetings, which may be scheduled as frequently as weekly but should be no less often than quarterly. Some of the best ideas for improvement come from the office staff, and expressing ideas should be encouraged.

The simplest technique is to set aside a specific time for regular meetings at an hour when the most people can attend with the least disruption. The meetings need not be long or overly formal, but in order to be effective they must be planned and organized. There must be a leader, and a secretary should be appointed to take notes. The effectiveness of the leader, a person who can balance firmness with fairness, is an important aspect of the meeting. This is usually either the physician or the office manager/supervisor. All members of the staff should be encouraged to submit ideas for discussion.

Draw up a simple outline of the issues you want to discuss and prepare any supporting data needed for the meeting. There are many kinds of staff meetings. They may be purely informational, or problem solving, or brainstorming; they may be

work sessions for updating manuals; training seminars, or whatever is necessary to that practice. The staff should meet to discuss new ideas and any changes in office procedures and to resolve any problems. The staff meeting must not be allowed to deteriorate into a gripe session. Individual complaints should be handled privately.

The meeting must have a set agenda, with time for topics that need discussion on a regular basis, as well as time to handle any current problems. The agenda might be similar to that of any business meeting:

1. Reading of the last meeting's minutes
2. Discussion of any unfinished business
3. Discussion of any problems in the clinical area
4. Discussion of any problems in the administrative area
5. Discussion of any problems in common areas
6. Adjournment

Some physicians like to combine the staff meeting with a breakfast or lunch. The time or place is not important as long as it is "neutral" and suits the practice and the meetings are conducted regularly, democratically, and without interruption (Fig. 22-4).

There must be follow-up to the items discussed; otherwise, the only result will be frustration and a reluctance to discuss problems at future meetings.

Office Procedure Manual

The office procedure manual supplements the office policy manual. Sometimes the two are combined. The policy manual is informational; the procedure manual is a "how to" manual, containing a job description for each position in the practice and detailed steps for carrying out each task. Unfortunately, too few practices take the time to develop such a manual, and even those that do often neglect to use it and keep it up to date.

22

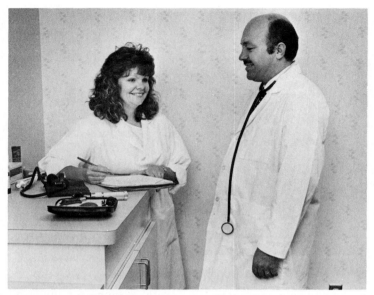

FIGURE 22-4. The office manager may discuss agenda items for a staff meeting with the physician.

JOB DESCRIPTIONS. A job description is a detailed account of the duties and the qualifications for a specific position (Fig. 22-5). In some cases, it should state both primary and secondary duties, emphasizing that the employee must be flexible. Job descriptions may change with personnel changes. No two people have the same capabilities and interests, and there is no need to try to mold a person to a job description when a simple shift in duties may accomplish a happier result. For instance, an administrative assistant might normally be expected to complete the computer sheets at the end of the day, but if a clinical assistant has a special aptitude for this and really enjoys the task, there is no reason

---

POSITION: Office Manager
RESPONSIBLE TO: Physician

The office manager is responsible for the coordination of all office activities, including recruitment and training of personnel, accounting and financial procedures.

SPECIFIC TASKS:

1. Preparing annual budget
2. Preparing monthly profit and loss statement
3. Approving of all expenditures
4. Reviewing and disposition of delinquent accounts
5. Approving of all write-offs
6. Maintaining liaison with accountant
7. Recruiting, hiring, and firing
8. Conducting performance appraisals and reporting to physician
9. Arranging personnel vacations and keeping records of leave days
10. Assisting in improving work flow and office efficiencies
11. Supervising purchase and repair of equipment
12. Purchasing and storage of supplies
13. Arranging for practice insurance
14. Supervising regular staff meetings
15. Keeping office policy manual current
16. Preparing patient education materials as needed

JOB QUALIFICATIONS: CMA or degree in business administration
                      Previous medical office experience
                      Supervisory experience helpful

FIGURE 22-5. Example of a job description.

this change in responsibility should not be made. Note it on the job description so that there is no confusion about who is responsible. Following the list of duties, there should be a procedure sheet for each task.

PROCEDURE SHEETS. A procedure sheet is a verbal flow chart that lists step-by-step the logical sequence of activities involved in a given task. An employee should be able to perform the task by following the written instructions (Fig. 22–6). Procedure writing is sometimes difficult because we tend to take for granted many of the simpler steps involved in performing a task once we become proficient. After a task has been learned, it is unnecessary to refer to the procedure sheet for instructions, but it is invaluable in training the new recruit and in assisting the temporary employee.

BENEFITS AND CONTENTS OF THE PROCEDURE MANUAL. Job descriptions and procedure sheets help the employee achieve expectations. Practice management specialists say that the most common remark from a discharged employee is "I didn't know I was supposed to. . . ." A written job description may also help avoid legal problems with an employee who is dismissed for not meeting performance standards.

A great deal of instruction can be incorporated into a procedure manual. Preferred performance procedures, both administrative and clinical, should be spelled out in detail, including the following information:

- A checklist of daily, weekly, monthly, quarterly, and yearly duties.

- How much time is allotted for new patients? Established patients? Postoperative patients?
- How are records prepared and filed? A description of the filing system may save the day if a temporary employee needs to find something in the file during the regular medical assistant's absence.
- How is the telephone to be answered? Which calls are put through to the doctor immediately, and which may the medical assistant handle? Include a list of the names and telephone numbers of persons you call often—for example, consulting physicians, hospitals, laboratories, and the physician's spouse.
- Billing and collection procedures. Is billing done weekly, twice monthly, monthly? Are the statements prepared in the office? By what method? Is a collection agency used? Which one?
- Completed samples of forms that need to be filled out and samples of correspondence (these provide excellent visual instruction).
- What kind of setup does the doctor prefer for office surgeries or treatments? Is there a card index showing these setups? If so, where is it kept?
- Where and how are supplies ordered and stored? Include the name, address, and telephone number of each supplier. Also include an inventory of major equipment with serial numbers, where and when the equipment was purchased, and a telephone number for servicing.
- Any special duties the doctor expects of the medical assistant, such as organizational activities or making travel arrangements.

PROCEDURE SHEET   PROCESS INCOMING MAIL

1. Assemble all necessary tools and supplies: letter opener, paper clips, stapler, mending tape, date stamp.

2. Open all mail except letters marked *personal.*

3. Check to be sure writer's address is on letter before destroying envelope. Staple envelope to letter if address is missing.

4. Paper clip enclosures to letter (or note their absence if they are not enclosed).

5. Date stamp the letter or piece of mail.

6. Set aside cash receipts for processing.

7. Route insurance claim forms and inquiries to insurance clerk.

8. Arrange mail with second and third class on bottom, then first class, with any personal mail on top.

9. Place entire stack in mail tray on right side of doctor's desk.

FIGURE 22–6. Example of a procedure sheet.

Management studies indicate that, in the multiple-employee office, it is good practice to have an understudy for each position who can substitute in an emergency. A well-documented procedure manual that is kept current ensures continuity when one employee must on occasion fill in for or assist another.

Development of a procedure manual is a good discussion item for staff meetings; the cooperation of the staff is essential if the project is to be successful. Keep it simple to update by using a three-ring binder. Include date of revision. Be sure to destroy old pages when revisions are made. One complete master copy should remain in the custody of the office manager and one with the physician. Each employee should have a copy of the portion that pertains to his or her particular job.

Practice Development

The office manager may play a large role in practice development, or "practice marketing" as it is often referred to. Practice development techniques are the outcome of a conscious need to improve the professional image, to increase exposure to the public, and to attract and keep patients.

As health costs continue to rise and patients become more demanding and selective in choosing their health care providers, practice survival may depend on good marketing techniques.

It may become necessary to make slight changes in office hours to accommodate the patient population, including, in some cases, providing for evening and weekend hours or even house calls.

The medical assistant with management responsibilities can encourage the physician to participate in community affairs, for example, by offering to give mass inoculations when needed, serving as a consultant in area health fairs, or speaking on health topics to civic and professional groups. Some physicians gain public exposure by writing articles or a question-and-answer column for an area newspaper. Local events may suggest other ways of promoting the practice.

Communication with the patient is essential. The practice with a computer or word processor can easily generate a newsletter several times a year containing information pertaining to the practice specialty or advances in health care in general. Letters to the patient and the patient's referring physician after a consultation are greatly appreciated by both and are easily and quickly accomplished with electronic equipment. Holiday and birthday remembrances are another easy way of keeping the patient aware of the practice and conveying your concern.

The first, last, and most important rule of marketing a medical practice, of course, is to treat the patients well, because the best source of patients consists of referrals from existing satisfied patients.

Patient Education

Patients have many common concerns about the doctor's policies, such as office hours, what is included in the doctor's specialty, directions for reaching the office, parking facilities, emergency services, answering service, cancellations, house calls, prescription renewals, payment of fees, and so forth. You can satisfy the patients' concerns and save your own time by putting these policies in writing and giving a copy to every new patient.

Many management experts recommend that two separate folders or pamphlets be prepared—one devoted to general office information and another to financial policies.

PATIENT INFORMATION FOLDER. Only an estimated 10% of practices have a booklet that explains the information basic to the operational and service aspects of the practice. Yet, a patient information folder can easily be compiled by the physician and staff cooperatively in a staff meeting. Experience has shown that if such a folder is given to every new patient, the number of incoming phone calls can be reduced by an average of 20 to 30%. It can also reduce misunderstanding and forgotten instructions. The folder must of necessity be tailored to the specific practice, but guidelines may be obtained free of charge from the American Medical Association's Department of Practice Management.

The patient information folder should be an introduction to the practice and, if possible, mailed to a new patient prior to the first visit. A supply may also be left with referring physicians' offices to be given to patients coming to your office. It should be designed to easily fit into a #10 business envelope.

The cover should show the name of the practice, its location, and the practice logo, if there is one. Consider using a photo of the medical building for easy identification by the new patient (Fig. 22–7A).

A statement of philosophy is frequently included in the introduction (Fig. 22–7B), followed by a description of the practice (Fig. 22–7C).

Describe the office policy regarding appointments and cancellations (Fig. 22–7D), telephone calls, and the function of the answering service. If a separate "business only" telephone line is available, be sure to include this information (Fig. 22–7E).

Describe any **ancillary** or laboratory services provided, how test results are reported, and your policy on prescription renewals (Fig. 22–7F).

Patients need to know the provisions for emergency procedures: What hospitals does the practice use regularly? What is the night and weekend coverage? Hospitalization procedures and postoperative care and follow-up may also be included (Fig. 22–7G).

List all physicians in the practice, their educational backgrounds, training, and board certifications, and define their specialties. List the names of

WELCOME TO OUR OFFICE

William C. McMaster, M.D.
Carl R. Weinert, Jr., M.D.
Samuel R. Rosenfeld, M.D.
Jeffrey L. Dobyns, M.D.

ORTHOPEDIC SURGERY

Providence Building
1310 West Stewart Drive
Suite 508
Orange, CA 92668

(714) 633-2111

A

What is orthopedics? Orthopedics involves the treatment of the skeletal system and its associated structures, mainly involving bones and joints, including muscles, tendons and ligaments. Orthopedic surgeons are medical doctors who have been specially trained in treatment of the skeletal system, both closed and surgical treatment. The doctors in this office can treat all types of orthopedic problems, including adult and children's orthopedics, fractures, congenital deformities or diseases, arthritis, hand and foot problems and other abnormalities involving the bones and joints. Methods of treatment can vary from simple evaluation and advice to casting, bracing and even surgery when necessary. Your initial evaluation will usually consist of a comprehensive history, physical examination, x-rays if necessary, and formation of an appropriate treatment plan. We have x-ray facilities in our office for your convenience. Treatment can then be started immediately following discussion of the long range plan, and will usually require follow-up visits to assess improvement. Treatment modalities used in orthopedic surgery may include alteration of activities, medication, heat or ice, stretching, exercises, formal physical therapy and if necessary, casting, bracing or surgery. Please be sure that all of your questions are answered prior to beginning the treatment plan as your full cooperation is essential. Your cooperation and understanding can have a strong, positive influence on the outcome of treatment.

Our practice is limited exclusively to the musculoskeletal system and its disorders. Therefore it is important for each patient to have a primary care physician such as a pediatrician, family physician or internist, to oversee the primary medical care for the entire patient. Our role is most effective as a consultant to your primary care physician.

C

WELCOME

The doctors and staff would like to welcome you to our office. We work as a team with the goal of providing prompt and thorough care of your orthopedic problems. We are always working to improve our care and service in any way possible.

B

FIGURE 22–7. *A*, Cover page on Patient Information Folder. *B*, Statement of philosophy. *C*, Description of practice.

Illustration continued on following page

APPOINTMENTS

We ask that you make an appointment if you need to see the doctor. We try to schedule our appointments so that each person can be seen as near to the appointed time as possible. In order to aid us in this, please allow 24 hours notice if cancelling an appointment. Cancelling without appropriate notice would cause other patients to be denied an appointment when they might otherwise be seen. We ask your cooperation and consideration in this matter. If you have an emergency situation, please call first as we do not see walk-in patients without an appointment. Patients who have an urgent or emergent problem will be scheduled to see the next available doctor. This may occasionally require you to see a doctor other than your own, however this is necessary to insure as prompt treatment as possible.

If you have seen any other physicians for your problem, please bring any available medical records, x-rays, other test results and the names of all medications you are currently taking. This will greatly aid in the accurate evaluation of your problem and may save unnecessary further testing or x-rays as well as any unnecessary delays in obtaining old records or x-rays.

OFFICE HOURS

Monday through Friday
9:00 a.m. to 5:00 p.m.

There are four doctors in this office and each individual doctor has a varying schedule. Please check with the receptionist regarding your particular doctor's schedule for the day in question.

D

TELEPHONE CALLS

This office has two receptionists available to answer phone calls during the regular office hours. The office is very busy and you will occasionally be asked to hold for a brief period. Please be patient with this. If you wish to speak to a doctor, your call will usually be returned during the next available break period or at the end of the office day. We receive many calls during the day and it is unfair to the patients who have scheduled appointments to continually interrupt the doctor for telephone calls. Therefore the receptionist will usually take a message and your call will be returned as soon as possible. Please inform the receptionist if your problem is urgent and she will let the doctor know this.

E

PRESCRIPTIONS

If you wish a new prescription you may call the office and leave a message with the receptionist. If you wish a refill of your prescription that you are already taking you should call the pharmacy and the pharmacist will call our office for an OK on the refill. For new prescriptions, please leave the phone number of your pharmacy with the receptionist. Prescriptions should be taken care of during regular office hours if possible. Prescription refills will only be handled during regular office hours.

F

EMERGENCIES

One of the doctors in the group is always on call for emergency situations. You may reach him by calling our office phone number, (714) 633-2111 and the answering service will put you in touch with the doctor on call at that time. Our doctors are on staff at St. Joseph Hospital of Orange, 633-9111 and for children, Childrens Hospital of Orange County, 997-3000. In case of an emergency, call 911.

SURGERY PATIENTS

If you are to have surgery you will be contacted by our Surgery Scheduling Coordinator, Linda, to schedule your surgery at a time convenient for both you and the doctor. This will usually be done at the end of your office visit. However, it can also be done by telephone if you need to make necessary arrangements or alterations in your schedule. Her telephone number is 633-1079. You will be asked to fill out forms regarding arrangements for surgery and also regarding insurance. Pre-operative lab testing is necessary and you will be given an appointment for this, usually 1-2 days prior to your scheduled surgical procedure. Some insurance companies require a second opinion for elective surgery. If you desire we will arrange this. Please inform our office as soon as possible if any last minute changes in your health occur prior to the surgery as these will occasionally require rescheduling of the surgery for your protection.

G

FIGURE 22-7 *Continued D*, Policy regarding appointments. *E*, Policy regarding telephone calls. *F*, Instructions to patient regarding prescriptions. *G*, Informs patient regarding emergency calls and hospitalization.

Our professional staff also includes: Pat, our registered nurse, and Jim, our x-ray technician. Martha and Elena are our receptionists.

Mary Ray is the office manager and if she can be of any help to you, she can be reached at (714) 541-0149.

For your convenience, we have two facilities in Orange County to serve your orthopedic needs. Our central Orange County facility is located in the city of Orange and is serviced by our entire staff of doctors.

The Irvine facility, staffed by Dr. Weinert and Dr. Dobyns, is located in the Centerstone Plaza, 4050 Barranca, Suite 200. The telephone number is (714) 633-2111.

We look forward to serving all your orthopedic needs.

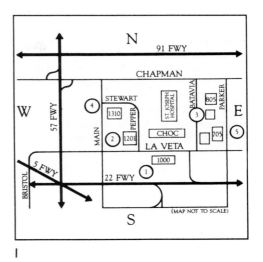

I

WILLIAM C. McMASTER, M.D.

Dr. McMaster graduated from Western Reserve University School of Medicine in 1966. He did his undergraduate studies at Yale University. He did his orthopedic residency at the University of California, Irvine. He is board certified with the American Board of Orthopedic Surgeons. He is a fellow of the American Academy of Orthopedic Surgeons and American College of Surgeons. He holds memberships with the American Academy of Orthopedic Surgeons, the American College of Surgeons, the Orange County Medical Assn., the California Medical Assn. and the Western Orthopedic Assn. Dr. McMaster is a clinical professor of orthopedic surgery at the University of California Irvine.

CARL R. WEINERT, JR., M.D.

Dr. Weinert completed college (1967), medical school (1971), and orthopedic residency (1976) at the University of Pittsburgh. He is board certified with the American Board of Orthopedic Surgeons and is a clinical associate professor of orthopedic surgery at the University of California, Irvine. He is a member of the Pediatric Orthopedic Society of North America, American Academy for Cerebral Palsy and Developmental Medicine, AMA, California Medical Association and Orange County Medical Assn. He has been chairman of orthopedic surgery at Childrens Hospital of Orange County since 1983 and chief of orthopedic surgery at Fairview State Hospital since 1979. His practice is limited to childrens orthopedics and orthopedic oncology.

H

FINANCIAL POLICY

We ask that our services be paid for at the time they are rendered. You will be provided with a Super Bill so that you may bill your insurance company and be reimbursed for services paid at the time of your visit. Simply attach the Super Bill to your insurance form and mail it to the insurance company. The appropriate diagnoses and charges will be on the Super Bill. There is usually a greater charge for the initial visit as this involves more time than follow up visits. If you are sent to an outside office for laboratory testing or special x-rays you will be billed separately from that office. We will be available to help if special circumstances arise involving difficulty with forms or receiving reimbursement. We will bill your insurance if you have a special situation such as surgery, pre-paid health plans, Medi-Cal, CCS or Senior Savers. We will complete disability papers as promptly as possible, however, you must obtain the necessary forms from your employer or the disability office.

J

22

FIGURE 22–7 *Continued* **H**, Information about office manager and the physicians' staff. **I**, Directions for reaching medical facility. **J**, Explanations of financial policy.

key clinical and administrative staff members, such as registered nurses and nurse practitioners, medical assistants, the office manager, the business manager, and so forth (Fig. 22–7*H*).

Provide the practice address, a map of how to get there, and information about the parking facilities (Fig. 22–7*I*). Include the financial policy of the practice (Fig. 22–7*J*), unless this information is placed in a separate folder.

Don't just stack these folders in the reception room for patients to pick up. Have the receptionist write the patient's name on the folder and hand it to the patient when he or she registers for the first appointment and suggest that the patient keep it for future reference.

FINANCIAL POLICIES FOLDER. A separate small folder of information covering the financial policies of the office can eliminate many questions and possible misunderstandings. Keep it small enough to fit into the billing envelope, and send it out with the first monthly statement.

Spell out policies regarding billing and collection procedures, and make it clear that patients are responsible for the uninsured portion of the fees. If you expect payment at the time of service, put this in the brochure. Include answers to the following questions:

- How can payment be made? For instance, are VISA and MasterCard accepted?
- Can time payments be arranged?
- Is there a charge for missed appointments?
- Is there a charge for completing insurance and disability forms? How much? Are there any exceptions?
- Note whether the doctor is a participating physician in Medicare, Medicaid, and other contract-service plans. Ask the patient to let you know if there are problems.
- Are there charges for other services such as telephone prescriptions, year-end statements, returned checks?

The financial policies folder should also clearly state that the ultimate responsibility for payment lies with the patient.

PATIENT INSTRUCTION SHEETS. In most medical offices there are patient procedures that occur over and over again. Instead of attempting to orally instruct a patient each time, why not develop clearly stated instruction sheets that you can review with the patient and then give the patient the written instructions to take home? The instruction sheets can include such procedures as:

- Preparation for x-ray or laboratory tests
- Preoperative and postoperative instructions
- Diet sheets
- Taking an enema
- Dressing a wound
- Taking medications

- Using a cane, crutches, walker, or wheelchair
- Care of casts
- Exercise therapy

In fact, anything for which patients are repeatedly given instructions can be written on these sheets.

Financial Management

The physician in a solo practice or small partnership may prefer to handle most financial aspects of the practice personally or may place that responsibility in the hands of a certified public accountant (CPA) or management consultant. In this situation, the medical assistant's involvement may be limited to the billing and bookkeeping activities discussed in previous chapters.

The medical assistant who is able to handle more responsibility will probably have the opportunity to do so. This could be the most challenging part of the position and may include any or all of the following activities:

- Supervising cash receipts:
  Banking
  Billing
  Collection
- Preparing periodic profit and loss statements
- Computing collection ratios
- Making provision for:
  Practice insurance
  Professional liability
  Workers' compensation
  Employee's health benefits
  Disability insurance
  Unemployment insurance
- Writing payroll checks
- Paying bills
- Preparing reports for governmental agencies
- Acting as a liaison with the accountant

Payroll Records

Handling payroll records, whether for one employee or dozens of employees, involves frequent reporting activities. If it were necessary only to write a check to each employee for the agreed upon salary for a given pay period, no discussion of payroll records would be necessary. But government regulations require the withholding of income taxes and payment of certain other taxes by both employee and employer.

In order to comply with government regulations, complete records must be kept for every employee. Such records include the following:

- Social Security number of the employee
- Number of exemptions claimed
- Amount of gross salary
- All deductions for Social Security taxes, federal, state, and city or other subdivision withholding taxes, state disability insurance, and state unemployment tax, where applicable

PRELIMINARY ACTIVITIES. Each employee and each employer must have a tax identification number. The Social Security number (000-00-0000) is the employee's tax identification number. Any person who does not have a Social Security number should apply for one using Form SS-5 available from any Internal Revenue Service or Social Security office and from most post offices.

The employer applies for a number for federal tax accounting purposes (00-0000000) from the Internal Revenue Service, using Form SS-4. In states that require employer reports, a state employer number must also be obtained.

Before the end of the first pay period, the employee should complete an Employee's Withholding Allowance Certificate (Form W-4) showing the number of exemptions claimed (Fig. 22–8). Otherwise, the employer must withhold on the basis of a single person with no exemptions.

The employee should complete a new form whenever changes occur in marital status or in the number of exemptions claimed. Each employee is entitled to one personal exemption and one for each qualified dependent. The employee may elect to take no exemptions, in which case the tax withheld will be greater and a refund may be due when the employee's annual tax report is filed.

A supply of all the necessary forms for filing federal returns, preprinted with the employer's name, will be furnished to an employer who has applied for an employer identification number. Extra forms may be obtained from the Internal Revenue office.

ACCOUNTING FOR PAYROLL. The simplest way to prepare the payroll checks and generate the necessary accounting records is by using a write-it-once combination check-writing system such as the one illustrated in Figure 22–9. This includes an employee compensation record (Fig. 22–10). The employee's compensation record is aligned with the first open line on the record of checks drawn, and a check with a carbonized strip is placed upon it. All information written on the check is automatically transferred to the compensation record, and the record of checks is drawn in one writing. The checks have a place for the address of the payee and can be mailed in a window envelope.

In practices with a number of employees, the summarization of the different categories for tax and reporting purposes is simplified, as the separate columns for different kinds of taxes on the record of checks drawn can simply be totaled at the end of the month (Fig. 22–11). If regular bank printed checks are used, the information for each employee must be posted to a separate record each time a payroll check is issued.

Income Tax Withholding

Employers are required by law to withhold certain amounts from employees' earnings and to report and forward these amounts to be applied toward payment of income tax. The amount to be withheld is based on the following:

Form **W-4** Department of the Treasury Internal Revenue Service

Employee's Withholding Allowance Certificate

▶ **For Privacy Act and Paperwork Reduction Act Notice, see reverse.**

OMB No. 1545-0010 **1992**

1 Type or print your first name and middle initial   Last name

2 Your social security number

Home address (number and street or rural route)

3 ☐ Single ☐ Married ☐ Married, but withhold at higher Single rate.
Note: *If married, but legally separated, or spouse is a nonresident alien, check the Single box.*

City or town, state, and ZIP code

4 If your last name differs from that on your social security card, check here and call 1-800-772-1213 for more information . ▶ ☐

5 Total number of allowances you are claiming (from line G above or from the Worksheets on back if they apply) **5**

6 Additional amount, if any, you want deducted from each paycheck . . . . **6** $

7 I claim exemption from withholding and I certify that I meet **ALL** of the following conditions for exemption:

- Last year I had a right to a refund of **ALL** Federal income tax withheld because I had **NO** tax liability; **AND**
- This year I expect a refund of **ALL** Federal income tax withheld because I expect to have **NO** tax liability; **AND**
- This year if my income exceeds $600 and includes nonwage income, another person cannot claim me as a dependent.

If you meet all of the above conditions, enter the year effective and "EXEMPT" here . . . ▶ **7** 19

8 Are you a full-time student? (**Note:** *Full-time students are not automatically exempt.*) . . . . **8** ☐ **Yes** ☐ **No**

Under penalties of perjury, I certify that I am entitled to the number of withholding allowances claimed on this certificate or entitled to claim exempt status.

Employee's signature ▶   **Date ▶** , 19

9 Employer's name and address (Employer: Complete 9 and 11 only if sending to the IRS)

10 Office code (optional)

11 Employer identification number

FIGURE 22–8. Employee's Withholding Allowance Certificate.

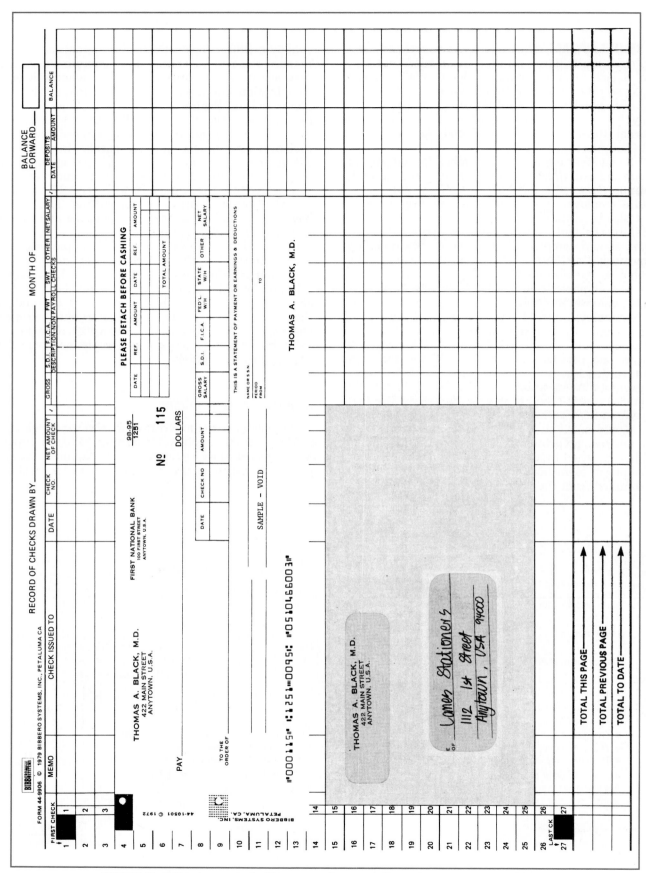

FIGURE 22-9. Write-it-once checkwriting system. (Courtesy of Bibbero Systems, Inc., Petaluma, CA.)

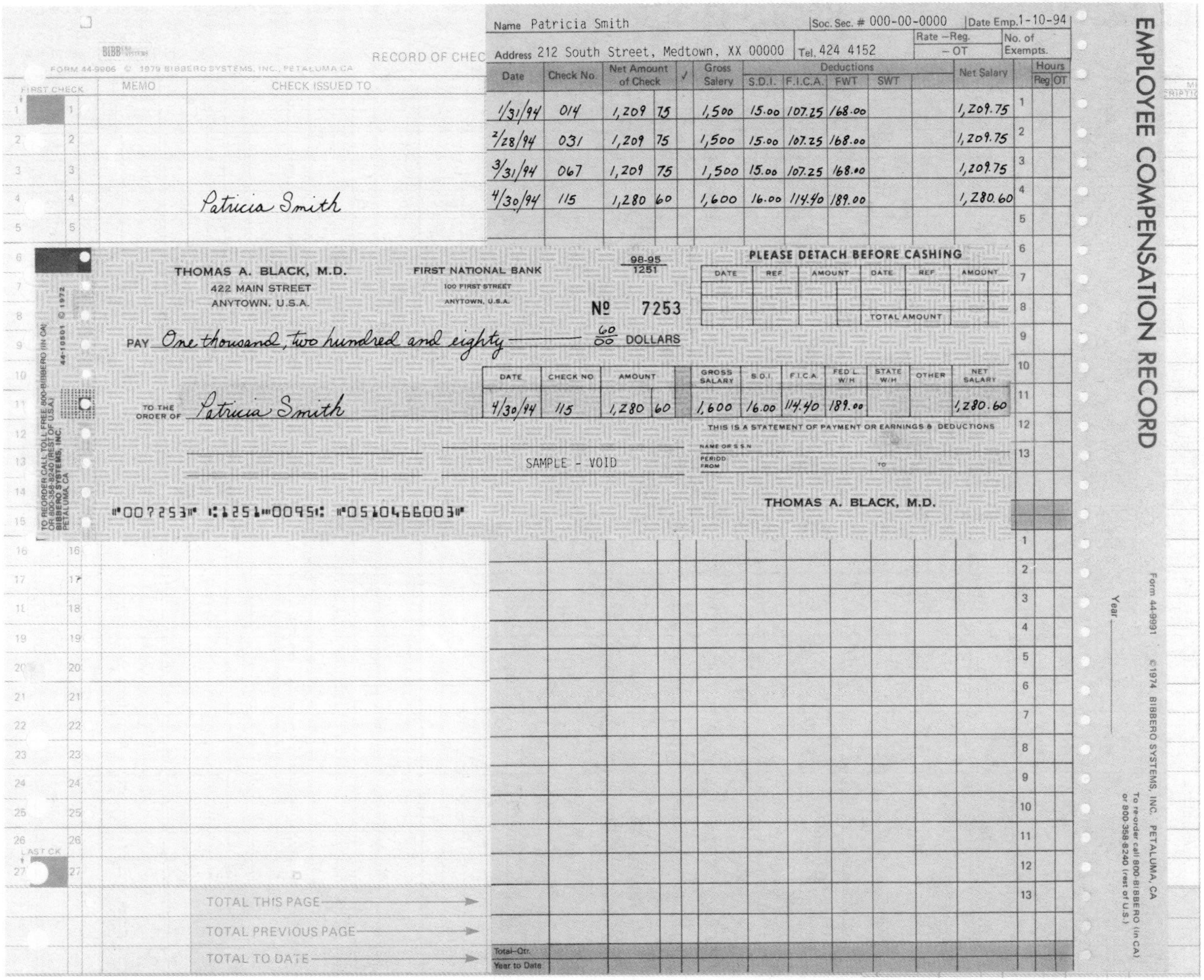

FIGURE 22–10. Employee compensation record for write-it-once checkwriting system. (Courtesy of Bibbero Systems, Inc., Petaluma, CA.)

EMPLOYEE COMPENSATION RECORD

Name	Patricia Smith									Soc. Sec. #	000-00-0000	Date Emp.	01-10-93		

Address 212 South Street, Medtown, XX 00000 | Tel. 424 4152 | Rate —Reg. / — OT | No. of Exempts.

Date	Check No.	Net Amount of Check		✓	Gross Salary	Deductions					Net Salary		Hours	
						S.D.I.	F.I.C.A.	FWT	SWT				Reg	OT
1/31/93	014	1,209	75		1,500	15.00	107.25	168.00			1,209.75	1		
2/28/93	031	1,209	75		1,500	15.00	107.25	168.00			1,209.75	2		
3/31/93	067	1,209	75		1,500	15.00	107.25	168.00			1,209.75	3		
4/30/93	115	1,280	60		1,600	16.00	114.40	189.00			1,280.60	4		
												5		
												6		
												7		
												8		
												9		
												10		
												11		
												12		
												13		
Total–Qtr.														
Year to Date														
												1		
												2		
												3		
												4		
												5		
												6		
												7		
												8		
												9		
												10		
												11		
												12		
												13		
Total–Qtr.														
Year to Date														

Year 1994

Form 44-9991 ©1974 BIBBERO SYSTEMS, INC. PETALUMA, CA

To re-order call 800-BIBBERO (in CA) or 800-358-8240 (rest of U.S.)

FIGURE 22-11. Payroll record for first quarter of year, one employee. (Courtesy of Bibbero Systems, Inc., Petaluma, CA.)

- Total earnings of the employee
- Number of exemptions claimed
- Marital status of the employee
- Length of the pay period involved

The Federal Employer's Tax Guide includes tables to be used in determining the amount to be withheld. Sample pages are shown in Figure 22–12. There is one table for single persons and unmarried heads of households, and one for married persons. The tables cover monthly, semimonthly, biweekly, weekly, and daily or miscellaneous periods.

EMPLOYER'S INCOME TAXES. The physician who is practicing as an individual is not subject to withholding tax but is expected to make an estimated tax payment four times a year. The accountant prepares four copies of Form 1040-ES, Declaration of Estimated Tax for Individuals, for the ensuing year when the annual income tax return is prepared. The first form and one-quarter of the estimated tax for the next year is filed at the same time as the tax return. The remaining three forms, with the estimated tax due, must be filed on June 15, September 15, and January 15. It may be the office manager's duty to see that these returns are filed when due.

SELF-EMPLOYMENT TAX. The employer also contributes to Social Security and Medicare in the form of a self-employment tax. The rate is slightly higher than that for an employee but less than the combined employee-employer contribution. This is computed and paid as a part of the income tax return.

In 1992, the self-employment tax was computed at 15.3%; 12.4% of this was for Social Security and applied only to the first $55,500 of income, and 2.9% was for Medicare applied to the first $130,200 of income.

SOCIAL SECURITY, MEDICARE, AND INCOME TAX WITHHOLDING. These taxes are imposed on both employers and employees under the Federal Insurance Contribution Act (FICA). The tax rate is reviewed frequently and is subject to change by Congress. In 1992, the FICA tax rate was 7.65%; 6.2% of this was for Social Security, and 1.45% was for Medicare. The Social Security portion applied only to the first $55,500 of income, but the Medicare portion was imposed on the first $130,200 of income.

DEPOSIT REQUIREMENTS. Generally, the employer must deposit income tax withheld, Social Security tax, and Medicare tax in an authorized financial institution or a Federal Reserve bank. The employer's deposit obligation is determined by the total amount of liability accumulated for the period. The rules are subject to change and are set forth in the Employer's Tax Guide previously referred to (Table 22–1).

TABLE 22–1. SUMMARY OF DEPOSIT RULES FOR SOCIAL SECURITY TAXES AND WITHHELD INCOME TAX

Deposit Rule	Deposit Due
1. If at the end of the quarter your total undeposited taxes for the quarter are less than $500:	No deposit is required. You may pay the taxes to IRS with Form 941 (or 941E), or you may deposit them by the due date of the return.
2. If at the end of any month your total undeposited taxes are less than $500:	No deposit is required. You may carry the taxes over to the following month.
3. If at the end of any month your total undeposited taxes are $500 or more but less than $3,000:	Within 15 days after the end of the month. (No deposit is required if you made a deposit for an eighth-monthly period during the month under rule 4. However, if this occurs in the last month of the quarter, deposit any balance due by the due date of the return).
4. If at the end of any eighth-monthly period (the 3rd, 7th, 11th, 15th, 19th, 22nd, 25th, and last day of each month) your total undeposited taxes are $3,000 or more:	Within 3 banking days after the end of the eighth-monthly period.

QUARTERLY RETURNS. Generally, all employers who are subject to income tax withholding or Social Security and Medicare taxes must file a quarterly return (Form 941) on or before the last day of the first month after the end of the quarter (Fig. 22–13). Due dates for this return and full payment of tax are April 30, July 31, October 31, and January 31. If deposits equaling full payment of taxes due have been made, the due date for the return is extended 10 days.

ANNUAL RETURNS. Form W-2 Wage and Tax Statement should be given to employees by January 31. Starting in 1991, the employer was required to report the amount of wages taxable under Social Security and under Medicare separately. In preparing the W-2 forms, these wages and taxes must also be reported separately. An example of a completed 1992 Form W-2 is shown in Figure 22–14.

The employer is required to furnish two copies of Form W-2 to each employee from whom income tax or Social Security tax has been withheld, or from whom income tax would have been withheld if the employee had claimed no more than one withholding exemption.

If employment ends before December 31, the employer may give the W-2 to the terminated employee any time after employment ends. If the employee asks for Form W-2, the employer should give the employee the completed copies within 30 days of the request or the final wage payment, whichever is later.

22

MARRIED Persons—MONTHLY Payroll Period

(For Wages Paid After December 1991)

And the wages are—		And the number of withholding allowances claimed is—										
At least	But less than	0	1	2	3	4	5	6	7	8	9	10
		The amount of income tax to be withheld shall be—										
$0	$320	$0	$0	$0	$0	$0	$0	$0	$0	$0	$0	$0
320	340	3	0	0	0	0	0	0	0	0	0	0
340	360	6	0	0	0	0	0	0	0	0	0	0
360	380	9	0	0	0	0	0	0	0	0	0	0
380	400	12	0	0	0	0	0	0	0	0	0	0
400	420	15	0	0	0	0	0	0	0	0	0	0
420	440	18	0	0	0	0	0	0	0	0	0	0
440	460	21	0	0	0	0	0	0	0	0	0	0
460	480	24	0	0	0	0	0	0	0	0	0	0
480	500	27	0	0	0	0	0	0	0	0	0	0
500	520	30	2	0	0	0	0	0	0	0	0	0
520	540	33	5	0	0	0	0	0	0	0	0	0
540	560	36	8	0	0	0	0	0	0	0	0	0
560	580	39	11	0	0	0	0	0	0	0	0	0
580	600	42	14	0	0	0	0	0	0	0	0	0
600	640	47	18	0	0	0	0	0	0	0	0	0
640	680	53	24	0	0	0	0	0	0	0	0	0
680	720	59	30	1	0	0	0	0	0	0	0	0
720	760	65	36	7	0	0	0	0	0	0	0	0
760	800	71	42	13	0	0	0	0	0	0	0	0
800	840	77	48	19	0	0	0	0	0	0	0	0
840	880	83	54	25	0	0	0	0	0	0	0	0
880	920	89	60	31	3	0	0	0	0	0	0	0
920	960	95	66	37	9	0	0	0	0	0	0	0
960	1,000	101	72	43	15	0	0	0	0	0	0	0
1,000	1,040	107	78	49	21	0	0	0	0	0	0	0
1,040	1,080	113	84	55	27	0	0	0	0	0	0	0
1,080	1,120	119	90	61	33	4	0	0	0	0	0	0
1,120	1,160	125	96	67	39	10	0	0	0	0	0	0
1,160	1,200	131	102	73	45	16	0	0	0	0	0	0
1,200	1,240	137	108	79	51	22	0	0	0	0	0	0
1,240	1,280	143	114	85	57	28	0	0	0	0	0	0
1,280	1,320	149	120	91	63	34	5	0	0	0	0	0
1,320	1,360	155	126	97	69	40	11	0	0	0	0	0
1,360	1,400	161	132	103	75	46	17	0	0	0	0	0
1,400	1,440	167	138	109	81	52	23	0	0	0	0	0
1,440	1,480	173	144	115	87	58	29	0	0	0	0	0
1,480	1,520	179	150	121	93	64	35	6	0	0	0	0
1,520	1,560	185	156	127	99	70	41	12	0	0	0	0
1,560	1,600	191	162	133	105	76	47	18	0	0	0	0
1,600	1,640	197	168	139	111	82	53	24	0	0	0	0
1,640	1,680	203	174	145	117	88	59	30	2	0	0	0
1,680	1,720	209	180	151	123	94	65	36	8	0	0	0
1,720	1,760	215	186	157	129	100	71	42	14	0	0	0
1,760	1,800	221	192	163	135	106	77	48	20	0	0	0
1,800	1,840	227	198	169	141	112	83	54	26	0	0	0
1,840	1,880	233	204	175	147	118	89	60	32	3	0	0
1,880	1,920	239	210	181	153	124	95	66	38	9	0	0
1,920	1,960	245	216	187	159	130	101	72	44	15	0	0
1,960	2,000	251	222	193	165	136	107	78	50	21	0	0
2,000	2,040	257	228	199	171	142	113	84	56	27	0	0
2,040	2,080	263	234	205	177	148	119	90	62	33	4	0
2,080	2,120	269	240	211	183	154	125	96	68	39	10	0
2,120	2,160	275	246	217	189	160	131	102	74	45	16	0
2,160	2,200	281	252	223	195	166	137	108	80	51	22	0
2,200	2,240	287	258	229	201	172	143	114	86	57	28	0
2,240	2,280	293	264	235	207	178	149	120	92	63	34	5
2,280	2,320	299	270	241	213	184	155	126	98	69	40	11
2,320	2,360	305	276	247	219	190	161	132	104	75	46	17
2,360	2,400	311	282	253	225	196	167	138	110	81	52	23
2,400	2,440	317	288	259	231	202	173	144	116	87	58	29
2,440	2,480	323	294	265	237	208	179	150	122	93	64	35
2,480	2,520	329	300	271	243	214	185	156	128	99	70	41
2,520	2,560	335	306	277	249	220	191	162	134	105	76	47
2,560	2,600	341	312	283	255	226	197	168	140	111	82	53
2,600	2,640	347	318	289	261	232	203	174	146	117	88	59
2,640	2,680	353	324	295	267	238	209	180	152	123	94	65
2,680	2,720	359	330	301	273	244	215	186	158	129	100	71
2,720	2,760	365	336	307	279	250	221	192	164	135	106	77
2,760	2,800	371	342	313	285	256	227	198	170	141	112	83

FIGURE 22–12. Pages from 1992 withholding tax table.

382

SINGLE Persons—MONTHLY Payroll Period

(For Wages Paid After December 1991)

And the wages are–		And the number of withholding allowances claimed is—										
At least	But less than	0	1	2	3	4	5	6	7	8	9	10
		The amount of income tax to be withheld shall be—										
$0	$110	$0	$0	$0	$0	$0	$0	$0	$0	$0	$0	$0
110	115	1	0	0	0	0	0	0	0	0	0	0
115	120	1	0	0	0	0	0	0	0	0	0	0
120	125	2	0	0	0	0	0	0	0	0	0	0
125	130	3	0	0	0	0	0	0	0	0	0	0
130	135	4	0	0	0	0	0	0	0	0	0	0
135	140	4	0	0	0	0	0	0	0	0	0	0
140	145	5	0	0	0	0	0	0	0	0	0	0
145	150	6	0	0	0	0	0	0	0	0	0	0
150	160	7	0	0	0	0	0	0	0	0	0	0
160	170	9	0	0	0	0	0	0	0	0	0	0
170	180	10	0	0	0	0	0	0	0	0	0	0
180	190	12	0	0	0	0	0	0	0	0	0	0
190	200	13	0	0	0	0	0	0	0	0	0	0
200	210	15	0	0	0	0	0	0	0	0	0	0
210	220	16	0	0	0	0	0	0	0	0	0	0
220	230	18	0	0	0	0	0	0	0	0	0	0
230	240	19	0	0	0	0	0	0	0	0	0	0
240	250	21	0	0	0	0	0	0	0	0	0	0
250	260	22	0	0	0	0	0	0	0	0	0	0
260	270	24	0	0	0	0	0	0	0	0	0	0
270	280	25	0	0	0	0	0	0	0	0	0	0
280	290	27	0	0	0	0	0	0	0	0	0	0
290	300	28	0	0	0	0	0	0	0	0	0	0
300	320	30	2	0	0	0	0	0	0	0	0	0
320	340	33	5	0	0	0	0	0	0	0	0	0
340	360	36	8	0	0	0	0	0	0	0	0	0
360	380	39	11	0	0	0	0	0	0	0	0	0
380	400	42	14	0	0	0	0	0	0	0	0	0
400	420	45	17	0	0	0	0	0	0	0	0	0
420	440	48	20	0	0	0	0	0	0	0	0	0
440	460	51	23	0	0	0	0	0	0	0	0	0
460	480	54	26	0	0	0	0	0	0	0	0	0
480	500	57	29	0	0	0	0	0	0	0	0	0
500	520	60	32	3	0	0	0	0	0	0	0	0
520	540	63	35	6	0	0	0	0	0	0	0	0
540	560	66	38	9	0	0	0	0	0	0	0	0
560	580	69	41	12	0	0	0	0	0	0	0	0
580	600	72	44	15	0	0	0	0	0	0	0	0
600	640	77	48	19	0	0	0	0	0	0	0	0
640	680	83	54	25	0	0	0	0	0	0	0	0
680	720	89	60	31	3	0	0	0	0	0	0	0
720	760	95	66	37	9	0	0	0	0	0	0	0
760	800	101	72	43	15	0	0	0	0	0	0	0
800	840	107	78	49	21	0	0	0	0	0	0	0
840	880	113	84	55	27	0	0	0	0	0	0	0
880	920	119	90	61	33	4	0	0	0	0	0	0
920	960	125	96	67	39	10	0	0	0	0	0	0
960	1,000	131	102	73	45	16	0	0	0	0	0	0
1,000	1,040	137	108	79	51	22	0	0	0	0	0	0
1,040	1,080	143	114	85	57	28	0	0	0	0	0	0
1,080	1,120	149	120	91	63	34	5	0	0	0	0	0
1,120	1,160	155	126	97	69	40	11	0	0	0	0	0
1,160	1,200	161	132	103	75	46	17	0	0	0	0	0
1,200	1,240	167	138	109	81	52	23	0	0	0	0	0
1,240	1,280	173	144	115	87	58	29	0	0	0	0	0
1,280	1,320	179	150	121	93	64	35	6	0	0	0	0
1,320	1,360	185	156	127	99	70	41	12	0	0	0	0
1,360	1,400	191	162	133	105	76	47	18	0	0	0	0
1,400	1,440	197	168	139	111	82	53	24	0	0	0	0
1,440	1,480	203	174	145	117	88	59	30	2	0	0	0
1,480	1,520	209	180	151	123	94	65	36	8	0	0	0
1,520	1,560	215	186	157	129	100	71	42	14	0	0	0
1,560	1,600	221	192	163	135	106	77	48	20	0	0	0
1,600	1,640	227	198	169	141	112	83	54	26	0	0	0
1,640	1,680	233	204	175	147	118	89	60	32	3	0	0
1,680	1,720	239	210	181	153	124	95	66	38	9	0	0
1,720	1,760	245	216	187	159	130	101	72	44	15	0	0
1,760	1,800	251	222	193	165	136	107	78	50	21	0	0

FIGURE 22–12 Continued

22

Form 941
(Rev. January 1992)
Department of the Treasury
Internal Revenue Service

4141

Employer's Quarterly Federal Tax Return
▶ See Circular E for more information concerning employment tax returns.
Please type or print.

OMB No. 1545-0029
Expires 5-31-93

Your name, address, employer identification number, and calendar quarter of return. (If not correct, please change.)
If address is different from prior return, check here ▶

Name (as distinguished from trade name)	Date quarter ended
Trade name, if any	Employer identification number
Address (number and street)	City, state, and ZIP code

T	
FF	
FD	
FP	
I	
T	

IRS Use

1 1 1   1 1 1 1 1 1   2   3 3 3 3 3 3   4 4 4

5 5 5   6   7   8 8 8 8 8   9 9 9   10 10 10 10 10 10 10 10

If you do not have to file returns in the future, check here . ▶ ☐   Date final wages paid . . . ▶ _____

If you are a seasonal employer, see **Seasonal employers** on page 2 and check here . . ▶ ☐

| 1 | Number of employees (except household) employed in the pay period that includes March 12th ▶ | 1 | |

2	Total wages and tips subject to withholding, plus other compensation . . . . . ▶	2	
3	Total income tax withheld from wages, tips, pensions, annuities, sick pay, gambling, etc. . ▶	3	
4	Adjustment of withheld income tax for preceding quarters of calendar year (see instructions) . ▶	4	
5	Adjusted total of income tax withheld (line 3 as adjusted by line 4—see instructions) . .	5	
6a	Taxable social security wages **(Complete line 7)** $_____ × 12.4% (.124) =	6a	
b	Taxable social security tips $_____ × 12.4% (.124) =	6b	
7	Taxable Medicare wages and tips . . . $_____ × 2.9% (.029) =	7	
8	Total social security and Medicare taxes (add lines 6a, 6b, and 7)	8	
9	Adjustment of social security and Medicare taxes (see instructions for required explanation) .	9	
10	Adjusted total of social security and Medicare taxes (line 8 as adjusted by line 9—see instructions) . ▶	10	
11	Backup withholding (see instructions)	11	
12	Adjustment of backup withholding tax for preceding quarters of calendar year	12	
13	Adjusted total of backup withholding (line 11 as adjusted by line 12)	13	
14	**Total taxes** (add lines 5, 10, and 13)	14	
15	Advance earned income credit (EIC) payments made to employees, if any . . . . . ▶	15	
16	Net taxes (subtract line 15 from line 14). **This should equal line IV below** (plus line IV of Schedule A (Form 941) if you have treated backup withholding as a separate liability) . . .	16	
17	**Total deposits for quarter,** including overpayment applied from a prior quarter, from your records . ▶	17	
18	**Balance due** (subtract line 17 from line 16). This should be less than $500. Pay to Internal Revenue Service . ▶	18	
19	**Overpayment,** if line 17 is more than line 16, enter excess here ▶ $_____ and check if to be:		

☐ Applied to next return **OR** ☐ Refunded.

Record of Federal Tax Liability (You must complete if line 16 is $500 or more and Schedule B is not attached.) See instructions before checking these boxes.
If you made deposits using the 95% rule, check here ▶ ☐   If you are a first time 3-banking-day depositor, check here . . ▶ ☐

Show tax liability here, **not deposits.** The IRS gets deposit data from FTD coupons.

Date wages paid		First month of quarter		Second month of quarter		Third month of quarter
1st through 3rd	A		I		Q	
4th through 7th	B		J		R	
8th through 11th	C		K		S	
12th through 15th	D		L		T	
16th through 19th	E		M		U	
20th through 22nd	F		N		V	
23rd through 25th	G		O		W	
26th through the last	H		P		X	
Total liability for month	I		II		III	

DO NOT Show Federal Tax Deposits Here

IV Total for quarter (add lines **I, II,** and **III**). **This should equal line 16 above** . . . . . . ▶

Sign Here
Under penalties of perjury, I declare that I have examined this return, including accompanying schedules and statements, and to the best of my knowledge and belief, it is true, correct, and complete.

Signature ▶ _____   Print Your Name and Title ▶ _____   Date ▶ _____

For Paperwork Reduction Act Notice, see page 2.   Cat. No. 17001Z

FIGURE 22–13. Employer's Quarterly Federal Tax Return.

1 Control number	22222	For Official Use Only ► OMB No. 1545-0008								

2 Employer's name, address, and ZIP code	6 Statutory employee ☐	Deceased ☐	Pension plan ☐	Legal rep. ☐	942 emp. ☐	Subtotal ☐	Deferred compensation ☐	Void ☐

Widget Company
11 Widget Lane
Anytown, US   54321

7 Allocated tips	8 Advance EIC payment
9 Federal income tax withheld **4576.00**	10 Wages, tips, other compensation **30000.00**

3 Employer's identification number **98-7654321**	4 Employer's state I.D. number	11 Social security tax withheld **1860.00**	12 Social security wages **30000.00**
5 Employee's social security number **123-45-6789**		13 Social security tips	14 Medicare wages and tips **30000.00**

19a Employee's name (first, middle initial, last) John E. Doe	15 Medicare tax withheld **435.00**	16 Nonqualified plans
12 South Street Southland, US 65432	17 See Instrs. for Form W-2	18 Other

19b Employee's address and ZIP code

20	21	22 Dependent care benefits	23 Benefits included in Box 10
24 State income tax	25 State wages, tips, etc.	26 Name of state	27 Local income tax	28 Local wages. tips, etc.	29 Name of locality

Copy A For Social Security Administration

Department of the Treasury—Internal Revenue Service

Form **W-2 Wage and Tax Statement 1992**

For Paperwork Reduction Act Notice and instructions for completing this form, see separate instructions.

FIGURE 22-14. Completed W-2 Wage and Tax Statement.

Employers must file Form W-3, Transmittal of Income and Tax Statement, annually, to transmit wage and income tax withheld statements (Forms W-2) to the Social Security Administration. These forms are processed by the Social Security Administration, which then furnishes the Internal Revenue Service with the income tax data that it needs from those forms. Form W-3 and its attachments must be filed separately from Form 941 on or before the last day of February following the calendar year for which the W-2 Forms are prepared.

Federal Unemployment Tax

Employers also contribute under the Federal Unemployment Tax Act (FUTA). Generally, credit can be taken against the FUTA tax for amounts paid into a State unemployment fund up to a certain percentage.

Employers are responsible for paying the FUTA tax; it must not be deducted from employees' wages. For 1992, the FUTA tax was 6.2% of the first $7,000 in wages paid to each employee during the calendar year.

FUTA DEPOSITS. For deposit purposes, the FUTA tax is figured quarterly, and any amount due must be paid by the last day of the first month after the quarter ends. The formula for determining the amount due is set forth in the Federal Employer's Tax Guide.

FUTA ANNUAL RETURN. An annual FUTA return must be filed on Form 940 on or before January 31 following the close of the calendar year for which the tax is due. Any tax still due is payable with the return. Form 940 may be filed on or before February 10 following the close of the year, if all required deposits were made on time and if full payment of the tax due is deposited on or before January 31 (Fig. 22-15).

State Unemployment Taxes

All of the states and the District of Columbia have unemployment compensation laws. In most states, the tax is imposed only on the employer, but a few states require employers to withhold a per-

Form **940**

Department of the Treasury
Internal Revenue Service

Employer's Annual Federal Unemployment (FUTA) Tax Return

▶ **For Paperwork Reduction Act Notice, see separate instructions.**

OMB No. 1545-0028

1991

T	
FF	
FD	
FP	
I	
T	

If incorrect, make any necessary change. ▲

┌ Name (as distinguished from trade name)

Calendar year ┐

Trade name, if any

Address and ZIP code

Employer identification number

A Did you pay all required contributions to state unemployment funds by the due date of Form 940? (If a 0% experience rate is granted, check "Yes" and see instructions.) . . . . ☐ **Yes** ☐ **No**

If you checked the "Yes" box, enter the amount of contributions paid to state unemployment funds ▶ $

B Are you required to pay contributions to only one state? . . . . ▲ . . . . . . ☐ **Yes** ☐ **No**

If you checked the "Yes" box: (1) Enter the name of the state where you have to pay contributions ▶

(2) Enter your state reporting number(s) as shown on state unemployment tax return. ▶

If you checked the "No" box, be sure to complete Part III and see the instructions.

C If any part of wages taxable for FUTA tax is exempt from state unemployment tax, check the box. (See the instructions.). . . . . ☐

If you will not have to file returns in the future, check here, complete, and sign the return . . . . . . ▲ ☐
if this is an Amended Return, check here . . . . ▲ ☐

Part I	**Computation of Taxable Wages** *(to be completed by all taxpayers)*

1 Total payments (including exempt payments) during the calendar year for services of employees. | **1** |

2 Exempt payments. (Explain each exemption shown, attach additional sheets if necessary.) ▶

Amount paid		
	2	

3 Payments of more than $7,000 for services. Enter only the amounts over the first $7,000 paid to each employee. Do not include payments from line 2. Do not use the state wage limitation . . .

| | **3** | |

4 Total exempt payments (add lines 2 and 3). . . . . ▲ | **4** |

5 **Total taxable wages** (subtract line 4 from line 1) . . . . ▲ | **5** |

6 Additional tax resulting from credit reduction for unpaid advances to the state of Michigan. Enter the wages included on line 5 above for that state and multiply by the rate shown. (See the instructions.) Enter the credit reduction amount here and in Part II, line 2, or Part III, line 5: Michigan wages _____ × .008 = _____ ▶ | **6** |

Cat. No. 11234O

Form **940** (1991)

Form 940 (1991)

Page **2**

Part II Tax Due or Refund (Complete if you checked the "Yes" boxes in both questions A and B and did not check the box in C.)

1	**FUTA tax.** Multiply the wages in Part I, line 5, by .008 and enter here.	1
2	Enter amount from Part I, line 6	2
3	**Total FUTA tax** (add lines 1 and 2) ▲	3
4	Total FUTA tax deposited for the year, including any overpayment applied from a prior year	4
5	**Balance due** (subtract line 4 from line 3). This should be $100 or less. Pay to the Internal Revenue Service. ▲	5
6	**Overpayment** (subtract line 3 from line 4). Check if it is to be: ☐ **Applied to next return,** or ☐ **Refunded** ▲	6

Part III Tax Due or Refund (Complete if you checked the "No" box in either question A or B or you checked the box in C.)

| 1 | Gross FUTA tax. Multiply the wages in Part I, line 5, by .062. | 1 |
| 2 | Maximum credit. Multiply the wages in Part I, line 5, by .054. | 2 |

3 Computation of tentative credit

(a) Name of state	(b) State reporting number(s) as shown on employer's state contribution returns	(c) Taxable payroll (as defined in state act)	(d) State experience rate period From To	(e) State experience rate	(f) Contributions if rate had been 5.4% (col. (c) x .054)	(g) Contributions payable at experience rate (col. (c) x col. (e))	(h) Additional credit (col. (f) minus col.(g)). If 0 or less, enter 0.	(i) Contributions actually paid to the state

| 3a | Totals ▲ | | | | | | | |

3b	Total tentative credit (add line 3a, columns (h) and (i) only—see instructions for limitations on late payments) ▲		
4	**Credit:** Enter the smaller of the amount in Part III, line 2, or line 3b	4
5	Enter the amount from Part I, line 6	5
6	**Credit allowable** (subtract line 5 from line 4). (If zero or less, enter 0.)	6
7	**Total FUTA tax** (subtract line 6 from line 1)	7
8	Total FUTA tax deposited for the year, including any overpayment applied from a prior year	8
9	**Balance due** (subtract line 8 from line 7). This should be $100 or less. Pay to the Internal Revenue Service. ▲	9
10	**Overpayment** (subtract line 7 from line 8). Check if it is to be: ☐ **Applied to next return,** or ☐ **Refunded** ▲	10

Part IV Record of Quarterly Federal Tax Liability for Unemployment Tax (Do not include state liability)

Quarter	First	Second	Third	Fourth	Total for year
Liability for quarter					

Under penalties of perjury, I declare that I have examined this return, including accompanying schedules and statements, and to the best of my knowledge and belief, it is true, correct, and complete, and that no part of any payment made to a state unemployment fund claimed as a credit was or is to be deducted from the payments to employees.

Signature ▲ _____ Title (Owner, etc.) ▲ _____ Date ▲ _____

FIGURE 22–15. Employer's Annual Federal Unemployment (FUTA) Tax Return.

22

centage of wages for unemployment compensation benefits.

An employer may be subject to federal unemployment tax and not subject to state unemployment tax. In some states, for instance, the employer with fewer than four employees is not subject to the state unemployment tax. The regulations for the individual state should be checked.

State Disability Insurance

Some states require that employees be covered by disability or sick-pay insurance. The employer may be required to withhold a certain amount from the employee's salary to pay for this insurance.

Special Duties

Before closing the chapter, we should mention certain events that do not occur with regularity but which may confront the office manager at some time.

Moving a Practice

The thought of moving into a shiny new spacious office can be exciting. Unless the move is planned in advance, however, moving day—and the weeks that follow—can be a nightmare.

PLANNING THE NEW QUARTERS. Do some careful measuring to see how the furniture and equipment you plan to move will fit into the new quarters. If possible, draw the rooms to scale and show where each item is to be placed by the mover. Include the location of available electrical outlets in your floor plan. If new furniture, carpets, or equipment are needed, try to have them in place before moving day. Don't expect to have the new carpet installed the day of your move.

ESTABLISHING A MOVING DATE. Decide what day you will move and whether you will close the office for one day or several. Select a mover and confirm the date. Patients must be notified of the move. As soon as the moving date is established, post a notice in the office and draw the patients' attention to it. You may want to send announcement cards to the active patients. Many doctors place a notice in the local newspapers.

NOTIFYING UTILITIES AND MAILERS. At least 60 days in advance of the move, start a change-of-address notification campaign. Notify publishers of journals and suppliers of catalogs. (Cards for changes of address are available from the post office.) Six weeks' notice is generally required on all subscriptions, and postage due on forwarded journals can be very expensive. Notify the telephone company and utility companies well in advance so that there will be no break in service. File a change of address card with the local post office. Order stationery and business cards with the new address.

PACKING. The moving company will supply packing cartons for you to use. Have each employee be responsible for packing and labeling the items from his or her own work area. Tag each carton with a number and keep a master list of what is in each numbered carton. This will help you find items that you need. Also, if a carton should be lost or mislaid, you will have a record of what was in it. If time allows, just before moving is a good time to cull material from the files and discard old journals, supply catalogs, and any obsolete supplies or equipment.

MOVING DAY STRATEGY. Prepare a written outline of the moving day strategy, indicating each person's responsibility, and give each member of the office staff a copy. It may be wise to work in shifts to avoid confusion, but have one person stationed at the new address to direct the movers when they arrive.

FOLLOW-UP. After the move, be sure to mention the new address when patients call for appointments. This is often neglected, especially after a few months have passed, and is very upsetting to the patient who tries to check in at the former address.

Closing a Practice

A medical practice may be closed because of retirement, death, a change in geographic location, or a change in profession. If the closing is unexpected, as in the case of sudden death of the physician, much of the burden falls on the staff. If the closing is voluntary and planned for, the physician may wish to consult an attorney or the local medical society for guidelines. The following information is useful in either event.

ADVANCE NOTICE TO PATIENTS. The physician who anticipates retirement can begin cutting back the practice months in advance. Patients can be notified as they come in that the practice will be closing on a specified date and asked to begin arrangements for care from another physician. The physician can also ask that patients pay at the time of service, to minimize accounts receivable at the time of retirement.

AVOIDING ABANDONMENT CHARGE. To avoid a charge of abandonment, the physician should notify active patients by letter that the practice is being discontinued. The letter should be sent out at least 3 months in advance, if possible. If a patient has been discharged or has not been in to see the doctor for at least 6 years, there is no obligation to send the notice.

PUBLIC ANNOUNCEMENT. About 1 month after the physician begins telling patients of the closing, an announcement should be placed in a local newspaper, giving the closing date of the office, explaining any arrangements made for continuing care, and thanking patients for their support in prior years.

OTHER NOTICES. Hospital affiliations should be informed early, particularly if the doctor will be leaving the community. If the office space is being rented, be sure to notify the landlord in observance of the rental contract if there is one. Insurance carriers must be advised of the change. The state medical licensure board should be contacted. If the practice is incorporated, an attorney should be consulted about disincorporation.

PATIENT TRANSFER AND PATIENT RECORDS. If another doctor is taking over the practice, tell the patient about the new doctor. However, be sure to explain that the patient's records will be transferred to any doctor the patient chooses and that the request for transfer of records must be in writing. For convenience, the doctor can have a form available that needs only the patient's signature.

Although the records belong to the physician, they can legally be transferred to another physician only with the consent of the patient. Any records not transferred should be stored, either in bulk or on microfilm, until the statutes of limitations for malpractice and abandonment have run out.

FINANCIAL CONCERNS. Income tax returns and supporting documents should be kept for at least 3 years after the tax return was filed. Appoint someone to take care of any remaining outstanding accounts receivable.

DISPOSITION OF CONTROLLED SUBSTANCES. Check with the Drug Enforcement Administration for current regulations on disposal of controlled substances and the physician's certificate of registration. Do not simply toss them out. The certificate will have to be sent to the DEA for cancellation and then it will be returned. It may be necessary to produce an inventory of all controlled substances on hand when the practice is terminated, along with duplicate copies of the official order forms that were used to obtain them. Return any unused forms to the DEA. Don't use leftover prescription blanks for note pads. Burn or shred them to avoid misuse.

PROFESSIONAL LIABILITY INSURANCE. The physician who is discontinuing active medical practice altogether can safely drop the professional liability insurance. However, do not destroy any of the previous policies. Most professional liability claims are covered by the policy that was in effect at the time the alleged act of negligence took place. The suit may be filed many years later and it is important that the old policy be available.

FURNISHINGS AND EQUIPMENT. Unfortunately, used office furniture and equipment do not bring much in the marketplace. If another physician is taking over the practice, the value of the furnishings and equipment can be negotiated. Many doctors donate their libraries to the local hospital and declare the gift as a deduction on their income tax. This is something to check with the accountant.

Some physicians reward loyal employees with severance pay. On the average, this equals at least 1 month's salary plus prorated compensation for any unused vacation time. A letter of reference is usually offered.

There are many details to take care of in closing a practice. Contact the local medical society for further guidance.

► **LEARNING ACHIEVEMENTS**

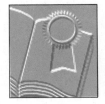

Are you able to:

1. Define the terms listed in the Vocabulary of this chapter?
2. State the goals of medical office management?
3. Describe the desirable qualities of an office manager?
4. Discuss the importance of having an office policy manual and how to develop the manual?
5. List and describe the steps in the hiring and dismissal of employees?
6. Briefly describe three kinds of staff meetings?
7. Explain how a policy manual differs from a procedure manual?
8. List at least 10 features of a patient information folder?
9. Discuss the office manager's role in financial management?
10. Identify the reference source for information on employer taxes and deposit requirements?
11. Prepare an outline of contents for a basic office policy manual?
12. Write a procedure sheet for a specific task?
13. Outline a financial policies folder?
14. Write a patient instruction sheet?

REFERENCES AND READINGS

American Medical Association: *The Business Side of Medical Practice,* Chicago, The Association, 1989.

Cotton, H.: *Medical Practice Management,* 2nd ed., Oradell, NJ, Medical Economics Books, 1977.

Department of the Treasury, Internal Revenue Service: Circular E, current edition.

For general information and Equal Employment Opportunity Commission publications, contact:

Office of Public Affairs
Equal Employment Opportunity Commission
2041 E Street N.W., Room 412
Washington, D.C 20507

SECTION 3

THE CLINICAL MEDICAL ASSISTANT

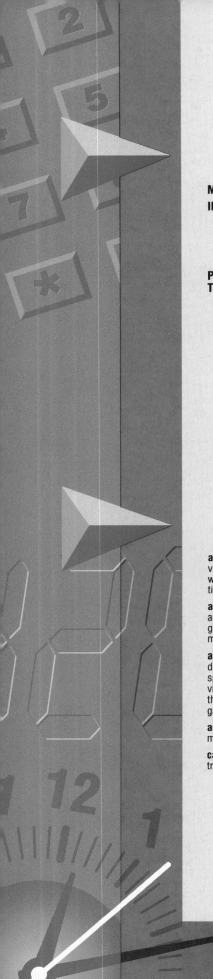

CHAPTER OUTLINE

MICROBIOLOGY

INFECTIOUS DISEASES

    Conditions That Favor Growth of Pathogenic Microorganisms

    The Chain of Infection

PREVENTION OF DISEASE TRANSMISSION

    The Inflammatory Response

    Nonspecific Defense Mechanisms

Specific Defense Mechanisms

    Antibody Formation

    Active Immunity

    Passive Immunity

CLASSIFICATION OF MICROORGANISMS

    Helminths

    Protozoa

    Fungi

    Bacteria

    Rickettsiae

    Viruses

MALFUNCTIONS OF THE IMMUNE SYSTEM

    Allergy

    Autoimmune Diseases

    Immune Deficiency Syndromes

ASEPSIS

    Medical Asepsis

    Procedure 23–1: Hand Washing for Assisting with Medical Aseptic Procedures

    Surgical Asepsis

LEGAL AND ETHICAL RESPONSIBILITIES

PATIENT EDUCATION

LEARNING ACHIEVEMENTS

VOCABULARY

acute Having a rapid onset and severe symptoms; usually subsiding within a relatively short period of time.

agar A substance extracted from algae and used in the laboratory to grow cultures of bacteria and other microorganisms.

antibody An immunoglobulin produced by lymphoid tissue in response to stimulus by bacterial, viral, or other antigens that protect the body from infection by that organism.

asepsis Absence of contaminated materials.

carrier Unaffected person who can transmit infection to another person.

chronic Persisting for a long period of time.

disease A definite pathologic process having a descriptive set of signs and symptoms.

infection Invasion and multiplication of microorganisms in body tissues causing injury and damage to the tissues.

latent Describing the seemingly inactive time between the exposure of tissue to an injurious agent and the time that response signs and symptoms begin to appear.

microorganisms Microscopic living parasites (also called *microbes*).

pathogens Disease-causing microorganisms.

spore A thick-walled reproductive cell formed within bacteria and capable of withstanding unfavorable environmental conditions.

toxin A poisonous material produced by pathogenic bacteria.

vaccines Weakened or dead microorganisms introduced into the body to produce immunity to specific disease.

virulent Describing any infectious agent that produces pathogenic effects.

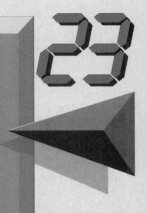

BASIC CONCEPTS OF ASEPSIS

LEARNING OBJECTIVES

COGNITIVE

Upon successful completion of this chapter, you should be able to:

1. Define and spell the terms in the Vocabulary.

2. List six conditions that favor the growth of microorganisms and give one preventive measure for each condition.

3. Define the five links in the "chain of infection."

4. Differentiate between direct and indirect transmission of disease and provide examples of each.

5. List the eight steps in the inflammatory process.

6. Distinguish between the nonspecific and specific defense mechanisms of the body.

7. Compare active and passive immunity.

8. List the six major classifications of microorganisms.

9. Name one disease for each subclassification of bacteria.

10. Differentiate between medical and surgical asepsis.

11. Discuss possible methods of patient education.

12. Explain legal and ethical implications of aseptic technique.

PERFORMANCE

Upon successful completion of this chapter, you should be able to:

1. Demonstrate the proper hand wash for assisting with medical aseptic procedures.

Medical microbiology and the principles of asepsis focus on the study of microorganisms that are disease-producing (pathogenic) and on the aseptic practices used for their control. In this chapter, you will study the concepts of disease transmission, the body's response to infection, and the natural defense mechanisms of the body, and you will be introduced to some of the more common pathogenic microorganisms that may invade the body. These concepts form the basis for understanding the importance of the first line of defense in preventing disease — the medical hand wash.

As you continue through the remainder of this textbook, you will always return to the fundamental concepts of this chapter. Every procedure begins with hand washing and is done with infection control in mind. The concepts in this chapter are basic to all clinical practice. Following them might save the life of a patient or a coworker and may even save your own life.

MICROBIOLOGY

Microbiology became a science in its own right with the work of such men as Louis Pasteur, Robert Koch, Joseph Lister, and many others. Pasteur was a French chemist. In about 1837, he was asked by wine makers to try to find out what was turning their wine sour. He discovered that it was a microorganism. This led him to work in other microbiologic areas. He perfected a treatment that prevented rabies in persons bitten by rabid animals. Later, he discovered the means for controlling anthrax, a disease of sheep.

Koch was a German physician who studied the causes and transmission of disease. He discovered the organism responsible for tuberculosis and developed techniques still used today for culturing (growing) and staining microorganisms for identification.

Lister, a Scottish surgeon, experimented with disinfection and sterilization techniques, especially for surgeons and operating room personnel. He proved that simple procedures, such as careful hand washing and the use of disinfectants, control the spread of disease-producing microorganisms. His principles for surgical asepsis have helped reduce surgical mortalities (deaths) from 50 per cent to less than 3 per cent and are still practiced.

After many years of research, medical microbiology now includes many classifications of disease-producing organisms. Viruses, which make up the last classification, are the smallest known microorganisms. They were not discovered until the powerful electron microscope, which uses a stream of electrons rather than light rays, was developed a few decades ago.

INFECTIOUS DISEASES

Disease may be defined as any sustained, harmful alteration of the normal structure, function, or metabolism (biochemistry) of an organism or cell. We recognize and categorize many different types of diseases: hereditary (genetic), drug-induced, structural, degenerative, and infectious, to name a few. Sometimes, a specific disease may fit two or more categories.

Infectious diseases are caused by **infection;** that is, the entrance of a living microbe into a cell or organism. Infection itself is not disease, for until the infected cell or organism shows a harmful alteration of its structure, physiology, or biochemistry, disease is either not detected or not considered present. In fact, a living microbe may be ingested, injected, or inhaled and never cause an infectious disease in that person. An unaffected person, however, could still transmit the infection to another person. In this case, we call the unaffected person a **carrier.**

Microbes that cause disease are called **pathogens.** The study of pathogens and their effects on the defense systems of the body is complex. Many factors determine the role of microbes in disease, the identification of microbes in the laboratory, and the ability of the body to maintain or recover health.

Microorganisms are almost everywhere. We carry them on our skin, in our bodies, and on our clothing. They are in ice, boiling water, the soil, and the air. The only places that are free of microorganisms are the insides of sterilized containers; inside fresh, unbruised fruits; and in certain internal body organs and tissues. Organs and tissues that do not connect with the outside by means of mucous-lined membranes are, in the normal state, free from all living microorganisms.

Conditions That Favor Growth of Pathogenic Microorganisms

Most pathogens prefer a fluid nutrient environment and an atmosphere full of oxygen. Pathogens that thrive in oxygen are called *aerobes*. Aerobes grow best when the following conditions are present:

- Oxygen
- Moisture (water)
- Nutrients from a living source, called a host (sometimes at the expense of the host), or from dead or decaying material
- Temperature of 98.6° Fahrenheit (F), or 37° centigrade (C)
- Darkness
- Neutral to slightly alkaline pH environment

Other pathogens prefer an environment without oxygen. These organisms are referred to as *anaerobes*. Anaerobes thrive in the dark, damp, warm, airless places inside the body. For example, the anaerobic bacterial pathogen *Clostridium tetani* causes *tetanus (lockjaw)*. Found in the soil or street dust, it is dormant and protected by a hard coating in what is called the **spore** stage. However, once inside human tissue, the protective spore becomes a living bacterium that releases **toxins.** The puncture wound that closes over and blocks out air (oxygen) is the perfect medium for growth. The bacterium rapidly multiplies and spreads through the bloodstream, causing the disease. In the same family of spore-forming bacteria is the *Clostridium perfringens* bacterium, which causes *gas gangrene.* The cycle is the same as for tetanus, except the infection is localized and often necessitates the amputation of a limb. Gas gangrene can result from contaminated surgical wounds. The third in this group of rod-shaped, spore-forming bacilli (bacteria) is the *Clostridium botulinum.* This organism grows in the oxygenless atmosphere of canned goods; when the can is opened, released toxins cause the disease known as *botulism.* Organisms that produce spores and release toxins are extremely dangerous, and these three diseases can be deadly.

The Chain of Infection

The life and growth of pathogens is a cycle, or chain. Break the chain, and you break the infectious process (Fig. 23–1).

The chain of infection starts at the *reservoir host.* A reservoir host may be an insect, animal, or human. Most pathogens must gain entrance into a host or else they will die. The reservoir host supplies nutrition to the organism, allowing it to multiply. The pathogen either causes infection in the host or exits from the host in great enough numbers to allow its transfer to another host.

The chain of infection continues with the *means of exit.* This is how the organism escapes. Exits include the mouth, nose, eyes, ears, intestines, urinary tract, reproductive tract, and open wounds.

After exiting the reservoir host, organisms spread by *means of transmission.* Transmission is either direct or indirect. *Direct transmission* occurs via contact with an infected person or with the discharges of an infected person, such as the feces or urine. *Indirect transmission* occurs from *droplets* in the air expelled from coughing, speaking, or sneezing; insects (called *vectors*) that harbor pathogens; contaminated food or drink; and contaminated objects (called *fomites*). Table 23–1 lists examples of direct and indirect means of transmission.

The next step is the *means of entry.* Now the transmitted organism will gain entry into a new host. The means of entry, like the means of exit, may be the mouth, nose, eyes, intestines, urinary tract, reproductive tract, or an open wound.

If the host is a *susceptible host,* that is, one that is capable of supporting the growth of the infecting organism, the organism will multiply. Factors affecting susceptibility include the location of entry, the dose of organisms, and the condition of the individual. If the conditions are right, the organisms reach infectious levels, the susceptible host becomes a *reservoir host,* and the cycle begins again.

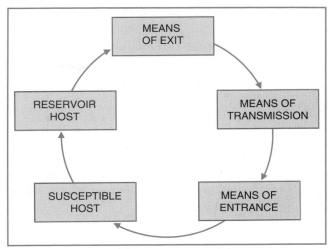

FIGURE 23–1. Chain of infection.

PREVENTION OF DISEASE TRANSMISSION

The best way to stop the growth and transmission of pathogens is to break the chain of infection. For example, with aerobes, remove the oxygen; or if pathogens thrive at 98.6°F, raise the temperature and most of them will die. If pathogens thrive in the dark, expose them to light. Many chemicals kill pathogens, provided the pathogens are exposed to the chemicals for a sufficient period of time. Spores are very resistant to chemicals, but some chemicals can even kill spores after 10 hours or more of exposure. Temperatures of 250°F (121°C) maintained for 20 minutes with at least 15 pounds of pressurized steam kill all life forms, including spores. This is the basis of the autoclave method of sterilization, which is discussed in Chapter 24. Good sanitization and housekeeping, sunshine and ventilation, universal blood and body-fluid precautions (see Chapter 25) and isolation techniques, and disinfection and sterilization are necessary to control and break the chain of infection in the medical office.

23

TABLE 23–1. DISEASE TRANSMISSION

Direct	Indirect
Contact with infected person	Contact with droplets (cough or sneeze) of infected person
Contact with infected person's discharges or excretions	Fomites (inanimate objects such as infected instruments, paper tissue, pens, forks, equipment, or clothes)
Sexual transmission	
Contact with infected blood through a break in the skin or with blood products	Vectors (e.g., bites from ticks, lice, and mosquitos)
	Contaminated food or drink

The Inflammatory Response

When pathogenic organisms invade through our protective mechanisms, our bodies respond in a predictable manner, called *inflammation* (Fig. 23–2). To defend itself, the body initiates the following eight specific reactions that destroy and remove pathogenic organisms and their byproducts or, if this is not possible, limit the extent of damage caused by pathogenic organisms and their byproducts:

- The blood vessels at the site of injury or invasion dilate, and the number of white blood cells in the area increases, causing redness.
- The white blood cells overpower and consume the pathogenic microorganisms in a process called *phagocytosis.*
- Fluids in the tissues increase, creating *edema,* which puts pressure on the nerves and causes pain.
- An increased blood supply to the area produces heat.

So far, this process characterizes the four classic symptoms of inflammation: redness (rubor), swelling (tumor), pain (dolor), and heat (calor). If the process is not reversed, it will continue through its course as follows:

- Destroyed pathogens, cells, and white blood cells collect in the area and form a thick, white substance called *suppuration* (pus).
- If the pathogenic invasion is too great for the white blood cells to control, the infection may collect in the body's lymph nodes, where more white blood cells are present to help fight the battle. This causes swollen glands.
- If the body is too weak or the number of pathogens is too great, the infection may spread to the bloodstream. This causes a systemic condition that could ultimately affect the entire body, called *septicemia* or blood poisoning.
- When the entire body is invaded, the condition is called general septicemia, or *pyemia.* Without appropriate medical intervention, death can occur. Antibiotics must be used to help the

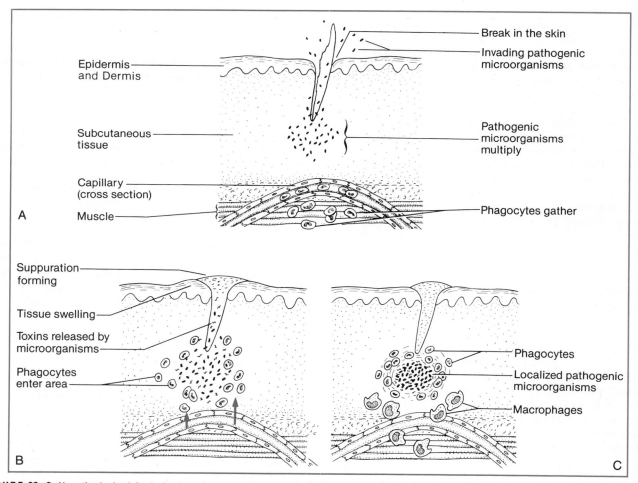

FIGURE 23–2. How the body defends itself against infection. *A,* Infection Stage. A break in the skin allows pathogenic microorganisms to enter and multiply within the tissues. As a defense, the body prepares to send phagocytes (white blood cells) to fight the invading pathogenic microorganisms. *B,* Inflammation Stage. As the pathogenic microorganisms multiply and die, toxins are released that destroy human tissue. Phagocytes have entered the infected area. Suppuration (liquified dead tissue, pathogenic microorganisms, and phagocytes, also called pus) causes swelling and pain. *C,* Phagocytosis. Phagocytes engulf and ingest the invading microorganisms, localizing the infection. Macrophages (specialized phagocytes) now enter the area to ingest and clean up all the dead tissue debris. When all the debris has been enveloped and digested, swelling and pain subside, and the wound closes and heals.

white blood cells bring the pathogenic invasion under control.

Nonspecific Defense Mechanisms

If microorganisms are everywhere, how do we avoid being ill most of the time? Fortunately, most microorganisms are not pathogenic. Most coexist with us and cause no harm. Some microorganisms are beneficial: microorganisms are responsible for fermenting wine and beer, the rising of bread, the manufacture of antibiotics, and the processing of waste in sewage treatment plants. Through the process of genetic engineering, bacteria are used to manufacture human insulin, human growth hormone, and other drugs in short supply much less expensively than the older, traditional processes.

While some pathogenic microorganisms dwell on people (since the human organism provides the perfect conditions for the growth and multiplication of pathogenic organisms), the human body has protective mechanisms to prevent the entry of microorganisms and disease.

The protection of the skin, mucous membranes, hair, and saliva; the washing effect of tears and stomach acid; and the lymphatic system all are parts of the *nonspecific defense system.* Transmission of disease depends on microorganisms finding entry through one of these barriers, and some pathogens cannot cause disease unless they gain entry by a specific route. As examples, the polio virus must enter through the gastrointestinal tract, and the gonococcus must enter through one of the mucous membranes to cause gonorrhea. The nonspecific defense system is our best defense against disease transmission; as long as it is working, pathogens are usually unable to make us ill.

Specific Defense Mechanisms

Immunity is the means of *specific defense.* It is called specific because a separate immune process takes place for each disease-producing organism that enters the body. However, the body is not able to build an immunity to every disease-producing organism, which is why it may be infected with some diseases again and again. The common cold is an example.

Immunity comes from antibody formation and can be *active* (the body produces the antibodies itself) or *passive* (the body borrows antibodies from others), and acquired either naturally or artificially.

Antibody Formation

Immunity means protection from disease and exists after the body forms substances called **antibodies.** Antibodies are formed in reaction to the presence of foreign substances, such as pathogens, in the blood. A foreign substance that stimulates the

formation of an antibody is called an *antigen.* When an antigen is introduced into the body, special white blood cells called *B lymphocytes* are programmed to produce antibodies. The antibodies then combine with the antigens and neutralize them, so that disease is arrested or, if early enough, prevented. In this process, a specific antibody always fights a specific antigen—they are paired.

Antigens can be living bacteria, viruses, or other microorganisms that gain entrance through a break in one of the body's protective barriers or mechanisms. Toxins, pollens, and drugs can also be considered antigens if the body reacts to them by forming antibodies. In addition, antigens include killed or *attenuated* (diluted) bacteria or viruses and attenuated toxins or pollens purposely introduced into the body through inoculations, commonly called immunizations.

Active Immunity

If long-term or permanent immunity is needed, the body must be stimulated to produce its own antibodies. This is called active immunity because the body is actively producing its own antibodies. The stimulus must come from the presence in the body of a disease-producing microorganism acting as a foreign substance. The stimulus can naturally occur from transmitted microorganisms gaining entrance into the body or from inoculation, which is the artificial means.

Inoculations contain microorganisms that have been killed or attenuated in a laboratory process. Their potency has been lessened so that they stimulate antibody formation but do not overpower the body and cause disease. Following immunization, a person frequently experiences inflammation at the site of the injection and generalized fever. This is because a less **virulent** disease process is going on in the body. Although the person may feel some of the effects of the disease, they are minimal. Some immunizations do not last a lifetime; in these cases, "boosters" are needed to restimulate ("boost") the B lymphocytes to produce antibodies again. Immunizations made from organisms are called **vaccines.** Immunizations made from the toxins of microorganisms are called *toxoids.*

Passive Immunity

Passive immunity results when antibodies that have been produced externally are introduced into the body, either across the placenta from mother to child (natural) or through inoculation (artificial). Passive immunity lasts only a short time: what we borrow, we cannot keep. Babies are born with immunity to many of the same diseases to which their mothers are immune. However, if these infants do not receive immunizations and actively produce their own antibodies, their passive immunity will gradually fade, and they will become susceptible to these diseases.

When people have been exposed to serious diseases and there is not enough time to wait for them to produce their own antibodies, preparations made from human or animal serum containing known antibodies can be administered for temporary protection. These products are called *antisera* or *immune serum globulins.* If the disease is caused by bacterial toxins rather than the bacteria itself, the products administered are called *antitoxins.*

One product, *immune human serum gamma globulin,* is most often administered to persons exposed to hepatitis. *Tetanus immune globulin (TIG),* or *tetanus antitoxin,* is administered to persons exposed to tetanus (lockjaw) organisms. TIG is made from human serum; tetanus antitoxin is manufactured from horse serum, which may cause serious reactions in people allergic to horses or horse hair. Antisera and antitoxins must be used with caution and are usually reserved for infectious diseases that could threaten life. Patients can be allergic to the derivatives in animal antisera and antitoxins, which is why human sera are preferred. *Antivenins* are also available for treating snake bites; the principle is the same.

CLASSIFICATIONS OF MICROORGANISMS

Microbes range in size from being visible to the naked eye, such as the tapeworm, to being visible only with the use of a microscope (e.g., bacteria and yeasts), to being so small that they are visible only with the use of the electron microscope (viruses). All microorganisms belong to one of the following six classifications. Some, such as bacteria, have subclassifications.

Helminths

Helminths are animal *parasites* called worms. A parasite is a plant or animal that lives upon or within another living organism and nourishes itself at the expense of the host organism. Helminths may live in animals or humans. They are usually transmitted through the soil or by infected clothing or fingernails, contact with infected persons, or contaminated food or water. Helminths go through the same life cycle as other worms. The adult worm lays eggs (ova). The ova develop into larvae. Larvae grow into adult worms, which lay eggs, and the cycle begins again. Diagnosis is usually based on microscopic examination of feces for ova and parasites and on patient signs and symptoms.

Prevention of Disease

The cycle of infection can be broken through cleanliness, proper preparation of foods, and the isolation of infected persons or animals.

Protozoa

Protozoa (singular—protozoon) are single-celled animals ranging in size from microscopic to *macroscopic* (visible to the naked eye). Protozoa are present in moist environments and in bodies of water such as lakes and ponds. Protozoa are transmitted through contaminated feces, food, or drink. Some pathogenic protozoa inhabit the bloodstream, whereas others inhabit the intestines and genital tract. Diagnosis is usually based on patient signs and symptoms and on microscopic examination of stool and blood (Table 23–2).

Prevention of Disease

The cycle of infection is broken by hand washing and by taking precautions when handling feces.

Fungi

Fungi (singular—fungus) are vegetable organisms and include *yeasts* and *molds.* Fungi are present in the soil, air, and water, but only a few species cause disease. Fungi thrive in warm, moist, dark places. They are transmitted by direct contact with infected persons, by prolonged exposure to a moist environment, or by inhalation of contaminated dust or soil. Diagnosis is usually based on the culturing or testing of skin scrapings, hair samples, or samples of sputum or mucous membranes (Table 23–3).

Prevention of Disease

The cycle of infection can be broken by isolating contaminated persons or animals and by avoiding places with contaminated dust and feces.

Bacteria

Bacteria (singular—bacterium), like plants, have cell walls, but unlike plants, they lack chlorophyll. Usually, pathogenic bacteria grow best at 98.6°F (37°C), in a moist, dark environment. Bacterial infections can be spread by any means of transmission. Bacteria live and reproduce in nutrients supplied by the body or in a laboratory culture medium, which is an **agar** preparation that simulates the body's condition. Since bacteria are the most commonly encountered pathogens, most of the laboratory procedures performed in the medical office deal with the isolation and identification of these microbes (see Chapter 31).

Humans host a variety of bacteria, both harmful and harmless, at all times. The skin, respiratory tract, and gastrointestinal tract are inhabited by a great variety of harmless bacteria, called *normal flora.* They are beneficial and protect the human host by aiding in metabolism and interfering with

TABLE 23–2. DISEASES CAUSED BY PROTOZOA AND OTHER PARASITES

Disease	Organism	Transmission	Symptoms	Tests/Specimens
Malaria	*Plasmodium* sp. (protozoa)	Bite of the *Anopheles* mosquito	Chills, fever (cyclic)	Blood: examination of stained film for parasites
Toxoplasmosis	*Toxoplasma gondii* (protozoa)	Fecal contamination (cat litter); congenitally	Febrile illness, rash; congenital: jaundice, enlarged liver and spleen, brain abnormalities	Skin test
Amebic dysentery	*Entamoeba histolytica* (protozoa)	Fecal contamination of food and water	Bloody diarrhea, cramping, fever	Stool for O & P
Giardiasis	*Giardia lamblia* (protozoa)	Common in intestinal tract opportunist; contaminated surface water	Asymptomatic to severe diarrhea and abdominal discomfort	Stool for O & P; intestinal biopsy; string test
Interstitial plasma cell pneumonia	*Pneumocystis carinii*	Widely prevalent in animals. Occurs in debilitated persons, immunosuppressed; common in AIDS	Pneumonia-like	Biopsy
Trichinosis	*Trichinella spiralis* (roundworm)	Ingestion of undercooked pork, bear meat	Nausea, fever, diarrhea, muscle pain and swelling, edema of face	Biopsy; blood tests
Tapeworm	*Taenia* sp.	Undercooked meats (beef and pork)	Abdominal discomfort, diarrhea, weight loss	Stool for O & P
	Diphyllobothrium latum	Undercooked fish; common among Norwegians, Japanese	As above; may become anemic	Stool for O & P
Pinworm	*Enterobius vermicularis* (roundworm)	Fecal-oral	Severe rectal itching, restlessness, insomnia	Scotch tape applied to perianal region for ova
Scabies	Itch mite: *Sarcoptes scabiei*	Direct contact; clothing, bedding	Nocturnal itching; skin burrows	Skin scrapings for parasites
Lice	*Pediculus humanus; Pthirus pubis* (crab)	Direct contact; clothing, bedding, furniture (can transmit other diseases via bite)	Intense itching; skin lesions	Finding adult lice or eggs (nits) on body or hair

Table courtesy of Kathleen Moody.
Abbreviations: sp: species; O & P: ova and parasites.

TABLE 23–3. SELECTED FUNGAL DISEASES

Disease	Organism	Predisposing Conditions and Transmission	Symptoms	Tests/Specimens
Thrush (oral yeast); *Candida* (vaginal yeast)	*Candida* species (yeast)	Oral: during birth; other: following antibiotic therapy, oral birth control, severe diabetes	White, cheesy growth	Swab for KOH prep, culture
Athlete's foot, jock itch, ringworm (tinea)	Several species of dermatophytes (skin fungi)	Opportunist; direct contact; clothing; prolonged exposure to moist environment	Hair loss, thickening of skin, nails; itching; red, scaly patches	Skin scraping for KOH prep; skin, hair for culture
Histoplasmosis	*Histoplasma capsulatum*	Inhalation of dust contaminated with bird or bat droppings	Mild, flu-like to systemic	Serologic
Cryptococcosis	*Cryptococcus neoformans*	Contact with poultry droppings	Cough, fever, malaise; can become systemic	Sputum culture
Sporotrichosis	*Sporothrix schenckii*	Farmers, florists, people exposed to soil	Skin lesions that spread along lymphatics; can become systemic	CSF culture, India ink direct examination, scrapings; serologic

Table courtesy of Kathleen Moody.
Abbreviations: CSF: cerebrospinal fluid; KOH: potassium hydroxide.

23

the harmful bacteria that may gain entrance. Occasionally, normal flora may become *opportunistic,* that is, cause infection. This occurs when one type of normal flora overgrows, usually as the result of an imbalance between it and the other normal flora, or when flora that is normal to one area invades another area, where it becomes pathogenic. One common example is *cystitis,* a urinary tract infection caused by contamination with *Escherichia coli,* a bacterium that is normal flora in the intestine.

One way of classifying bacteria is by *morphology* (size and shape). Spherical bacteria are called *cocci,* rod-shaped bacteria are called *bacilli,* and those shaped like threads are called *spirilla* or *spirochetes.* If any of these groups grow in pairs, the prefix *diplo* is used, as in *diplococci;* if in chains, the prefix *strepto* is used, as in *streptococci.* If they grow in clusters, like grapes, the prefix *staphylo* is used, as in *staphylococci* (Fig. 23–3).

Different kinds of bacteria tend to affect the various organs of the body in different ways, producing diseases, each with its own symptoms and effects (Tables 23–4 and 23–5).

Chlamydia and Mycoplasma

These are separately classified bacteria. Chlamydia are *obligate* parasites (unable to survive without a host) and the smallest of all bacteria. They are important because of their role in *sexually transmit-*

ted *disease (STD). Chlamydia trachomatis* is the most frequent cause of *pelvic inflammatory disease (PID)* and is considered the most prevalent STD today. Flies can also carry *Chlamydia trachomatis* and cause *trachoma,* the leading cause of infectious blindness (see Table 23–6).

Prevention for All Types of Bacterial Infections

Break the infection cycle through immunizations, proper sanitary conditions, isolation, and aseptic procedures.

Rickettsiae

Rickettsiae (singular — rickettsia) are microscopic parasites that are insect-borne and fever-producing. Rickettsiae are transmitted from rodents or other animals to humans by the bites of lice, fleas, ticks, and mites. These parasites attack the linings of small blood vessels. Usually, diagnosis is based on patient signs and symptoms and on blood testing (see Table 23–6).

Prevention of Disease

Break the infection cycle with control of rodent and insect populations and high sanitation standards.

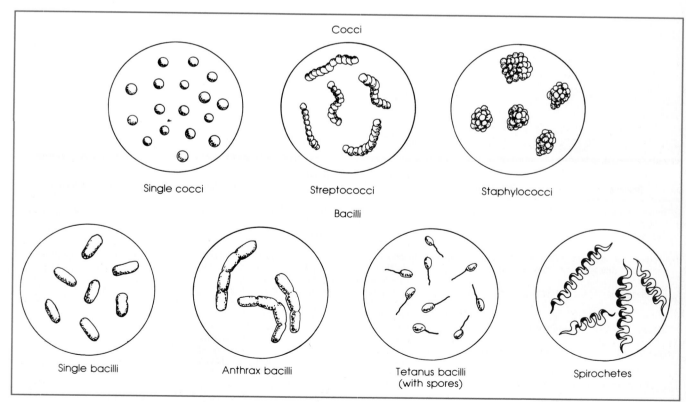

FIGURE 23–3. Drawings of various pathogenic microorganisms as they appear under the microscope.

TABLE 23–4. COMMON DISEASES CAUSED BY COCCI

Disease	Organism	Description	Transmission	Symptoms	Specimens	Tests
Pneumonia	*Streptococcus pneumoniae*	Gram-positive cocci in pairs	Direct contact, droplets	Productive cough, fever, chest pain	Sputum; bronchoscopy secretions	Culture, Gram's stain
Strep throat	*Streptococcus pyogenes* (group A strep)	Gram-positive cocci in chains	Direct contact, droplets, fomites	Severe sore throat, fever, malaise	Direct swab	Direct agglutination; culture, WBC and differential
Wound infection, abscesses, boils	*Staphylococcus aureus*	Gram-positive cocci in clusters	Direct contact, fomites, carriers; poor hand washing	Area red, warm, swollen; pus; pain; ulceration or sinus formation	Deep swab; aspirate of drainage	Culture and sensitivity (aerobic and anaerobic)
Staphylococcal food poisoning	*Staphylococcus aureus*	Gram-positive cocci in clusters	Poor hygiene and improper refrigeration of foods	Vomiting, abdominal cramps, diarrhea	Suspected food, stool	Culture
Toxic shock	*Staphylococcus aureus*	Gram-positive cocci in clusters	Use of absorbent packing materials (e.g., tampons, nasal packs)	Fever, headache, nausea, vomiting, delirium, low BP	Swab, blood	Culture and serology
Gonorrhea	*Neisseria gonorrhoeae*	Gram-negative cocci in pairs; intracellular in WBC	Sexually transmitted	*Females:* pelvic pain, discharge. May be asymptomatic. *Males:* urethral drip, pain on urination	Swab of cervix, urethra; rectal and pharyngeal swabs in homosexuals	Gram's stain; culture
Meningococcal meningitis	*Neisseria meningitidis*	Gram-negative diplococci	Respiratory tract secretions	High fever, headache, projectile vomiting, delirium, neck and back rigidity, convulsions, petechial skin rash	Nasopharyngeal swabs, CSF, blood	Gram's stain; culture; cell counts and chemistries

Table courtesy of Kathleen Moody.
Abbreviations: WBC: white blood cells; BP: blood pressure.

Viruses

Medical science has not yet conquered the control of viruses. Very few antiviral drugs have been introduced, and those that are used have limited effectiveness on specific viruses only. Invading viruses are difficult to treat chemically because the chemicals that effectively attack viruses also seriously damage human tissues.

Viruses can be treated easily in the external environment. Widely used chemicals such as chlorine (bleach), iodine, phenol, and formaldehyde easily and effectively destroy viruses on surfaces and objects coming into contact with the infected patient. These agents, however, are too toxic to be used internally.

Viruses can be seen only with the electron microscope. Each virus is an organism made up of a nucleic acid core covered with a coating of protein; but the nucleic acid core of the virus is unique in nature because it has either RNA (ribonucleic acid) or DNA (deoxyribonucleic acid), but never both. All other organisms have both RNA and DNA, which together form pairs of chromosomes that contain all the genetic codes necessary for protein synthesis and reproduction. Viruses, on the other hand, have a complete set of hereditary factors in half the number of chromosomes and, therefore, can reproduce only within living cells and only after a living host cell's enzymes dissolve the outer protein coating. A virus enters a host cell, and the host's enzymes wash away the virus's outer coating. Then the virus's nucleic acid is released into the cell's cytoplasm, where it mixes, and the virus is able to replicate itself. Once infected, the parasitized host cells die, while the multiplying viruses continue to "swarm" from the dying cells to invade and attack new cells and tissues.

Viruses cause many clinically significant diseases in humans. Unfortunately, most viral diseases can be treated only *symptomatically,* that is, for the symptom and not the infective cause. General antibiotics are ineffective in preventing or curtailing viral infections, and even the few drugs that are effective against some specific viruses have limitations because viruses often produce different types of infections in host cells (Table 23–7).

Prevention of Disease

Avoidance of the infection is the best approach. This includes staying away from public areas during the flu season and isolating patients known to be

TABLE 23-5. SELECTED DISEASES CAUSED BY BACILLI AND SPIRILLA

Disease	Organism	Description	Transmission	Symptoms	Tests/Specimens	Prevention and Immunization
Tuberculosis	*Mycobacterium tuberculosis*	Acid-fast beaded bacilli	Inhalation	Pulmonary: cough, hemoptysis, sweats, weight loss. May affect other systems	Sputum for culture; x-ray; skin tests	BCG vaccine
Urinary tract infections	*Escherichia coli, Proteus sp., Klebsiella sp., Pseudomonas aeruginosa*	Gram-negative bacilli	Ascends urethra; catheterization	Cystitis: frequency, burning bloody urine. Pyelonephritis: flank pain, fever	Clean-catch urine for culture and analysis	Good personal hygiene; always wipe from front to back
Syphilis	*Treponema pallidum*	Spirochete	Sexually; congenitally	*Primary:* painless sore. *Secondary:* generalized rash involving palms and soles of feet. *Congenital:* birth defects	Blood for serologic tests: VDRL, RPR, FTA-ABS	Avoidance of infected persons; use of condoms
Lyme disease	*Borrelia*	Spirochete	Tick bite	Fever, joint pain, red annular rash	Swab for culture	Eliminating animal vectors
Cholera	*Vibrio cholerae*	Gram-negative spirillum	Fecal contamination of food and water (warm climates)	Severe vomiting and diarrhea; dehydration	Stool for culture	Cholera vaccine; boiling water; cooking foods
Legionnaires' disease	*Legionella pneumophila*	Gram-negative bacillus (stains poorly with usual methods)	Grows freely in water (air conditioning systems)	Pneumonia-like symptoms	Sputum; blood	Isolation
Tetanus (lockjaw)	*Clostridium tetani*	Gram-positive spore-forming bacilli, anaerobic	Open wounds, fractures, punctures	Toxin affects motor nerves; muscle spasms, convulsions, rigidity	Blood	DPT in childhood; T or Td every 10 years
Gas gangrene	*Clostridium perfringens*	Gram-positive spore-forming bacilli, anaerobic	Wounds	Gas and watery exudate in infected wound	Swab, aspirate of wound for culture	Proper wound care
Botulism	*Clostridium botulinum*	Gram-positive spore-forming bacilli, anaerobic	Improperly cooked canned foods	Neurotoxin affects speech, swallowing, vision; paralysis of respiratory muscles, death	Contaminated food; blood	Botulinus antitoxin; boil canned goods 20 minutes before tasting or eating
Diphtheria	*Corynebacterium diphtheriae*	Gram-positive bacilli, club-shaped	Respiratory secretions	Sore throat, fever, headache, gray membrane in throat	Swabs; Gram's stain, culture; Schick test for immunity	DPT in childhood
Whooping cough	*Bordetella pertussis*	Gram-negative bacilli	Respiratory secretions	Upper respiratory tract symptoms; high-pitched, crowing whoop	Swabs for culture	DPT in childhood
Typhoid and paratyphoid fevers	*Salmonella sp.*	Gram-negative bacilli	Contaminated food, water, poor hygiene; carriers	Fever, headache, diarrhea, toxemia, rose spots on skin	Stool for culture	Typhoid/paratyphoid A and B vaccine
Plague	*Yersinia pestis*	Gram-negative bacilli	Via flea bite from infected rodents	Fever and chills, delirium, enlarged, painful lymph nodes	Sputum for culture; blood	Vaccine available; rodent control
Nonspecific vaginitis	*Gardnerella vaginalis*, with anaerobes	Gram-variable bacillus	Sexual	Vaginal irritation itching, fishy-smelling malodorous discharge	Swab; wet prep for "clue cells"	Avoidance of infected persons; good personal hygiene

Table courtesy of Kathleen Moody.

Abbreviations: BCG vaccine: Bacille Calmette-Guérin vaccine; VDRL: Veneral Disease Research Laboratory; RPR: rapid plasma reagin (test); FTA-ABS: fluorescent treponemal antibody absorption (test); DPT: diphtheria-pertussis-tetanus (vaccine); T: tetanus (toxoid); Td: tetanus and diphtheria (toxoids).

TABLE 23–6. DISEASES CAUSED BY *RICKETTSIA, CHLAMYDIA,* AND *MYCOPLASMA*

Disease	Organism	Transmission	Symptoms	Tests/Specimens
Rocky Mountain spotted fever	*Rickettsia rickettsii*	Tick bite	Headache, chills, fever, characteristic rash on extremities and trunk	Blood for serologic tests; skin biopsy for direct fluorescent microscopy
Typhus	*Rickettsia prowazekii*	Tick bite	Fever, rash, confusion	Blood for serology
Atypical pneumonia	*Mycoplasma pneumoniae*	Respiratory secretions	Fever, cough, chest pain	Blood, sputum
Nongonococcal urethritis and vaginitis	*Chlamydia trachomatis*	Sexual	May be asymptomatic	Swabs for culture and serologic testing
Inclusion conjunctivitis, pneumonia		Congenital	Severe conjunctivitis in newborns Afebrile pneumonia in newborns	

Table courtesy of Kathleen Moody.

TABLE 23–7. VIRAL DISEASES

Disease	Transmission	Symptoms	Tests	Prevention
Smallpox	Direct contact; fomites	Vesicles on entire body, including soles and palms		Eradicated (vaccine is still available)
Herpes I (cold sores, fever blisters)	Direct contact; fomites	Recurrent painful blisters on lips, mouth	Serologic	Avoid contact with active lesions
Herpes II (genital)	Sexual contact	Recurrent painful blisters on labia, penis, rectum	Serologic	Avoid sexual contact with persons having active lesions
Infectious mononucleosis	Direct and airborne	Sore throat, fever, malaise lymph gland involvement; hepatitis, enlarged spleen	Blood for Monospot	Avoid direct contact with known cases
Influenza	Droplet and fomites	Fever, body aches, cough		Immunization for old, young, debilitated
Warts	Direct and indirect contact	Circumscribed outgrowths on skin; most common on hands and feet		
Rabies	Contact with saliva of infected animal (dog, cat, skunk, fox, bat are usual)	Fever, uncontrollable excitement, spasms of throat, profuse salivation	Animal's brain tissue examined for Negri bodies	Vaccine available. Vaccinate pets
Mumps	Direct contact	Pain, swelling of salivary glands, fever	Acute and convalescent titers	MMR* vaccine
Measles	Direct contact; droplets	Fever, nasal discharge, red eyes; Koplik's spots, rash	Serologic	MMR vaccine
Rubella	Direct contact; droplets. Congenital	Rash, swollen lymph glands; causes severe birth defects	Serologic	MMR vaccine
Common cold	Direct; droplets; fomites	Headache, fever, runny nose, congestion		Good hygiene (hand washing)
Hepatitis A (infectious hepatitis)	Fecal-oral; contaminated food and water	Nausea, fever, weakness, loss of appetite, jaundice	Serologic	Good hygiene (hand washing)
Hepatitis B (serum hepatitis)	Blood and blood products; accidental needle sticks	Similar to hepatitis A, but more severe	Serologic	Vaccine is available. Avoid contact with blood from infected persons
AIDS	Sexual; drug abuse (needles); blood and body fluids	Poor immunity, resulting in disseminated viral, fungal, and protozoan infections; Kaposi's sarcoma	Serologic	Avoid casual sexual contact. Use extra caution when drawing and/or handling specimens
Polio	Direct contact; carriers. Enter via mouth	Fever, headache, stiff neck and back, paralysis of muscles		Trivalent oral polio vaccine (TOPV)

Table courtesy of Kathleen Moody.
*Measles, mumps, rubella.

23

infected with a virus. Patients must be vaccinated against polio (Sabin vaccine), German measles (rubella vaccine), measles (rubeola vaccine), and mumps (epidemic parotitis vaccine). High-risk patients can be vaccinated against some other viruses, such as flu and hepatitis. This is especially important for the elderly and the chronically ill (Table 23-7).

Acute Infection

In the **acute** viral infection, the host cell typically dies within a period of hours or days. Symptoms appear after the tissue damage begins to occur. Usually, the virus can be isolated only shortly before or after the first symptom appears. In most acute infections, such as the common cold, the body's defense mechanisms eliminate the virus within 2 to 3 weeks.

Chronic Infection

Persistent viral infections are those in which the virus is present for a long period of time; some may persist for life. The person may be asymptomatic and the virus undetectable; or, as in **chronic** viral *hepatitis B,* the patient is asymptomatic, but the virus may be detected and transmissible. Hepatitis B, or *serum hepatitis,* may be transmitted by blood or blood products and is a hazard to health care personnel. At one time hepatitis B was unpreventable, but blood tests now can determine the presence of certain antigens that identify a person as a carrier of hepatitis B, and a vaccine is available for protection against the disease.

Latent Infection

A **latent** infection is a persistent infection in which the symptoms and the virus come and go. *Cold sores (oral herpes simplex)* and *genital herpes* are latent viral infections. The virus first enters the body and causes the original lesion. It then lies dormant, away from the surface, in a nerve cell, until certain provocation (illness with fever, sunburn, or stress) causes the virus to leave the nerve cell and seek the surface again. Once the virus reaches the superficial tissues, it becomes detectable for a short time and causes another outbreak at that site. Another herpesvirus, *herpes zoster,* causes *chickenpox.* This virus then may lie dormant and later erupt as the painful disease *shingles.*

Slow Infection

Slow infections progress over very long periods of time. These conditions include the degenerative neurologic diseases, some with fatal outcomes. Generally, cures are not available; however, these diseases may enter remission for extended periods.

Viruses and Cancer

More and more, viruses are being implicated in cancer and other tumors. A virus enters a normal cell and incorporates itself into the cell's DNA, causing the uncontrolled growth that is characteristic of tumors. *Oncogenes (onco,* tumor), either inherited by the person or carried in the virus's genetic coding, may be responsible for the transformation of a normal cell into a tumor cell. Host cells infected with viruses may produce a substance called *interferon,* which protects nearby cells from invasion. The use of interferon in viral disease and cancer therapy has gained much attention lately as a possible treatment or preventive measure for viral diseases. Research continues to identify new cancer-related viruses and possible cures and vaccines.

MALFUNCTIONS OF THE IMMUNE SYSTEM

Allergy

Diseases of the immune system include allergy, autoimmune phenomena, and immune deficiencies. Allergy is the most common malfunction. In allergies, the usual antigen-antibody reaction is accompanied by harmful effects on the body, ranging from sneezing, coughing, and itching to anaphylactic shock and can occur for the first time at any age. The allergen can be inhaled, ingested, injected, or applied to the skin.

Anaphylactic Shock

Anaphylaxis is a life-threatening allergic reaction that can occur within minutes following the introduction of an allergen. Bee stings and medications are the usual causes. In the medical office, care must be taken to ascertain each patient's allergies and to keep the patient in the office 10 to 30 minutes after certain injections and inoculations. Anaphylactic reactions are possible in any patient following the administration of animal-derivative inoculations, certain injectable drugs such as penicillin, or allergy desensitization serum.

Symptoms include swelling, itching or burning of the throat and skin, choking, difficulty in breathing, hives, and a drop in blood pressure. If a reaction occurs, get the physician immediately and be prepared to administer basic life support (cardiopulmonary resuscitation). Anaphylactic shock is treated with intravenous epinephrine. Antihistamines or intramuscular corticosteroids may be administered in minor reactions (see Chapter 40).

Autoimmune Diseases

Autoimmune diseases occur when the body fails to recognize its own constituents *(autoantigens)* and produces antibodies to fight them. *Rheumatoid arthritis (RA)* and *systemic lupus erythematosus (SLE)* are two examples. In RA, the antibodies cause joint inflammation and bone and muscle deformity and may cause dysfunction of many organs, including the joints, heart, and kidneys. SLE is an autoimmune disease of connective tissue. A defect in the body's regulatory mechanisms is suspected. The body is not able to control a high level of autoantibodies, which attack the body's own cells. SLE is characterized by fever and injuries to the skin, mucous membranes, joints, kidneys, and the nervous system. It is found most often in women between 30 and 40 years of age.

Diagnosis of lupus and RA is based on laboratory identification of the antibody. The tests are performed on blood serum in a special laboratory. Some rheumatoid arthritis tests are simple and are performed in the medical office by the medical assistant.

Immune Deficiency Syndromes

Immune deficiency syndromes may be either inherited or acquired. The inherited deficiencies range from the inability to fight certain types of infections to the total inability to produce antibodies of any kind. Bone marrow transplants are helpful for some patients.

Acquired Immunodeficiency Syndrome (AIDS)

Acquired immunodeficiency syndrome is a major health threat. AIDS is caused by HIV (human immunodeficiency virus; formerly HTLV III), which is transmitted through blood and semen and may be present in other body fluids and tissues. AIDS was first recognized in 1979 among sexually active homosexual men living in the cities of New York, Los Angeles, and San Francisco. AIDS was originally confined to certain "H" groups: homosexuals, Haitians, hemophiliacs, and hypo abusers (drug addicts). However, it has now spread to the heterosexual population, throughout the United States and the world. Diagnosed cases have doubled every year since 1980, and health experts predict that over 40 million adults and children will have HIV by the turn of the century. Certain groups remain at high risk, including homosexual and bisexual males who have multiple sex partners, native Haitians who have recently emigrated from their country, individuals sharing drug injection needles, persons with hemophilia or others who are receiving large quantities of blood transfusions, and patients with renal disease being treated by machine dialysis (see Chapter 25).

ASEPSIS

Medical Asepsis

Asepsis means freedom from infection or infectious material. Medical asepsis is defined as the destruction of organisms *after they leave the body.* When we practice the principles of medical asepsis, we are directing our efforts at preventing reinfection of the patient or cross-infection of other patients or ourselves. The goal is to isolate microorganisms by following universal blood and body-fluid precautions (see Chapter 25), and disinfecting or sterilizing objects as soon as possible after they have been contaminated. This creates a nonsterile but clean environment.

As previously stated, the most effective barrier against infection is the unbroken skin. If the skin and mucous membranes are intact, medical asepsis can be practiced for most noninvasive (not penetrating through human tissues) procedures such as pelvic and proctologic examinations. Instruments and objects not breaking the skin must be sterilized before being used on another patient but then they may be stored and used under clean, nonsterile conditions. Clean hands and objects may touch the patient, although the routine use of nonsterile examination gloves is recommended (see Chapter 25). Gowns and masks may be used, but they are not presterilized; they are worn to protect the operator more than the patient. Hands are washed according to the principles of the medical aseptic hand wash.

Washing the Hands Is the First Line of Defense in the Practice of Medical Asepsis

Hands must be washed, using the correct technique, before and after each patient is examined or treated. It is not necessary to do an extended scrub each time, but the first scrub in the morning should be extensive. Subsequent hand washings may be brief unless your hands become excessively contaminated. A good surgical soap with chlorhexidine, such as Hibiclens, which has antiseptic residual action that will last several hours, should be used. Buy a good quality surgical soap that is gentle to the hands; purchasing inexpensive soap may be false economy. Each office sink should be equipped with a dispenser with surgical soap. Remember, dry, cracked skin can be a source of contamination.

Proper hand washing depends on two factors: running water and friction. Water should be tepid; water that is too hot or too cold will chap the skin. Friction means the firm rubbing of all surfaces of the hands and forearms. Remember that your fingers have four sides and fingernails. For the medical hand wash, all jewelry except a plain wedding band is removed. A wristwatch may be left on if it can be moved up on the forearm out of the wrist

23

area. Your hands are washed under running water, with the fingertips pointing downward. Soap and friction are applied only to the hands and wrists. Allow the water to wash away debris from your hands.

This procedure is used when you are performing medical procedures with patients. Your goal is to prevent cross-contamination of microorganisms from one patient to another. Use this procedure after you finish with one patient and before you go to attend another patient; after you finish handling one specimen and before you handle another specimen; before and after you use toilet facilities; whenever you touch something that causes your hands to become contaminated; and before you leave the office at the end of the day.

PROCEDURE 23-1   HAND WASHING FOR ASSISTING WITH MEDICAL ASEPTIC PROCEDURES

GOAL To wash your hands with soap, using friction and running water to sanitize your skin before and after assisting with nonsurgical procedures and whenever you have contaminated your hands.

EQUIPMENT AND SUPPLIES

A sink with running water
Soap in a dispenser (bar soap is not acceptable)
Paper towels in a dispenser

PROCEDURE

1. Remove all jewelry except your wristwatch and a plain gold ring.

2. Turn on the faucet and regulate the water temperature.

3. Allow your hands to become wet, apply soap, and lather with friction while holding your fingertips downward. Rub well between your fingers for 30 seconds (Fig. 23-4).
   Purpose: Friction removes soil and contaminants from your hands and wrists.

4. Rinse well, holding your hands so that the water flows from your wrists downward to your fingertips (Fig. 23-5).
   Purpose: Soil and contaminants will wash off you and down the drain.

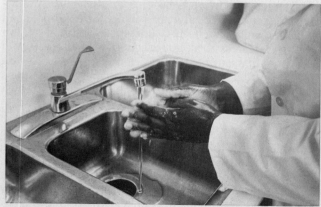

FIGURE 23-4.

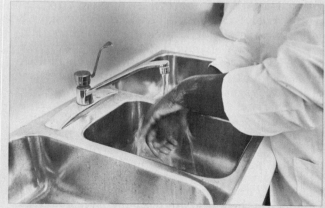

FIGURE 23-5.

Continued

5. Wet your hands again and repeat the scrubbing with soap for 15 seconds (Fig. 23–6).

6. Rinse your hands a second time and take time to inspect them (Fig. 23–7).
   Purpose: To ensure that the hands are really clean.

7. Dry your hands with a paper towel (Fig. 23–8).

8. Turn off the water faucet with the paper towel (Fig. 23–9).
   Purpose: The faucet is dirty and will contaminate your clean hands.

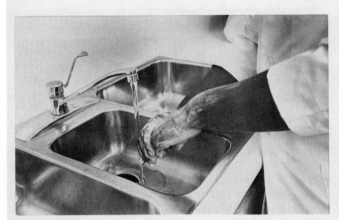

FIGURE 23-6.

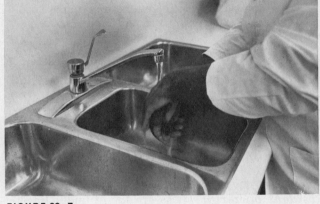

FIGURE 23-7.

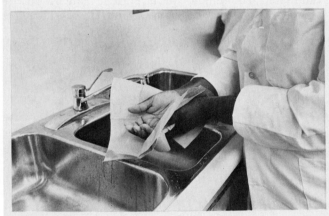

FIGURE 23-8.

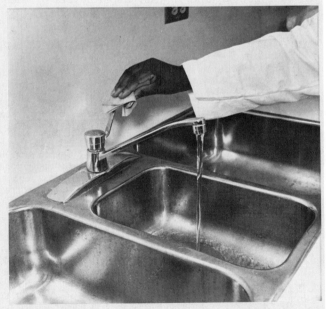

FIGURE 23-9.

9. Cover any hangnails or open wounds with Band-Aids. You should not perform any procedures that involve contact with a patient's blood or body fluids when you have open cuts on your hands.

23

Surgical Asepsis

Surgical asepsis is defined as the destruction of organisms *before they enter the body*. This technique is used for any procedure that invades the body's skin or tissues, such as surgery or injections. Any time the skin or mucous membrane is punctured, pierced, or incised (or will be during a procedure), surgical aseptic techniques are practiced. The surgical hand wash (scrub) must be used. Everything that comes into contact with the patient should be sterile, such as gowns, drapes, instruments, and the gloved hands of the surgical team. Minor surgery, urinary catheterizations, injections, and some specimen collections, such as blood and biopsies, are performed using surgical aseptic technique.

Because it is not possible to sterilize your hands, the goal of the hand scrub is to reduce skin bacteria by the use of mechanical friction, special surgical soaps, and running water. Normally, there are two types of bacteria on your skin:

Transient bacteria. These are surface bacteria that are introduced by fomites and remain with you a short time.

Resident bacteria. These are found under fingernails, in hair follicles, in the openings of the sebaceous glands, and in the deeper layers of the skin.

Resident bacteria in the deeper skin layers come to the surface with perspiration, which is why sterile gloves are used in addition to the surgical hand scrub. Some agencies recommend that you scrub for a specific number of minutes; others count the number of scrub strokes. Follow the guidelines of your employer and take periodic cultures from your scrubbed hands to determine whether or not your technique is effective (Table 23–8). This procedure will be explained in Chapter 35.

LEGAL AND ETHICAL RESPONSIBILITIES

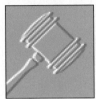

A number of legal and ethical concerns are related to medical asepsis in the medical office. Personal discipline is the primary concern in medical asepsis. Often, the assistant is alone when performing a medical aseptic procedure; if contamination occurs, no one may know except the medical assistant. It is the medical assistant's responsibility to begin the procedure again with clean supplies if it is believed that contamination has occurred. Allowing the physician to assume that the correct aseptic techniques have been employed in the preparation of equipment and allowing him or her to use contaminated equipment on a patient can result in claims of malpractice. Honesty on the part of the

---

TABLE 23–8. HOW TO DISTINGUISH BETWEEN MEDICAL AND SURGICAL ASEPSIS

	Medical Asepsis	Surgical Asepsis
Definition	Destruction of organisms *after* they leave the body	Destruction of organisms *before* they enter the body
Purpose	Prevent reinfection of the patient. Avoid cross-infection from one person to another	Care for open wounds; use in surgery
Technique	Universal blood and body-fluid precautions (Appendix C) Isolation techniques	Sterile technique
Procedure	Clean objects are kept from contamination Clean gloves and clean barriers used Objects disinfected as soon as possible after contact with the patient	Objects must be sterile Sterile gloves and articles used Objects must be sterilized before contact with the patient
When used	For examinations that do not involve open wounds or breaks in the skin or mucous membranes but do involve patient blood or body fluids; isolating infected persons from others	Surgery, biopsy, wound treatment, insertion of instruments into sterile body cavities
Hand wash technique	Hands and wrists washed for 1–2 min; soap, water, and plenty of friction used to remove oil and microorganisms from fingers Hands held downward, running water allowed to drain off fingertips, hands dried with paper towels	Hands and forearms scrubbed for 3–10 min; surgical soap, running water, friction, and sterile brush used; fingernails must be cleaned Hands held up, under running water, to drain off elbows. Hands dried with sterile towels

assistant builds self-respect and contributes to professional achievement.

▶ PATIENT EDUCATION

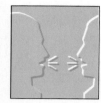

The competent medical assistant takes advantage of opportunities to help the patient learn about infection control, ways that bacteria and disease are transmitted, methods of prevention, and immunization procedures. There are many ways that the medical assistant can help the patient. Thinking up creative ideas for patient education might be a project for the office staff. Here are a few suggestions to educate and inform the patient about asepsis and infection control:

- Hang an information table in the waiting room with take-home pamphlets and literature.
- Mail a periodical newsletter to patients.
- Demonstrate and explain aseptic procedures to patients, inviting them to participate.

▶ LEARNING ACHIEVEMENTS

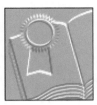

Upon successful completion of this chapter, can you:

1. Perform a 2-minute medical hand wash according to medical aseptic principles without missing a step or incorrectly performing a step?

REFERENCES AND READINGS

Compton, C.C.: *Pathologic Basis of Disease,* Philadelphia, W.B. Saunders Co., 1989.

Cooper, M.G., and Cooper, D.E.: *The Medical Assistant,* New York, McGraw-Hill Book Co., 1986.

Purtilo, R.B.: *Ethical Dimensions in the Health Professions,* Philadelphia, W.B. Saunders Co., 1993.

Shulman, S.T., Phair, J., and Sommers, H.M.: *The Biologic and Clinical Basis of Infectious Disease,* 4th ed., Philadelphia, W.B. Saunders Co., 1992.

Warden-Tamparo, C., and Lewis, M.A.: *Diseases of the Human Body,* Philadelphia, F.A. Davis Co., 1989.

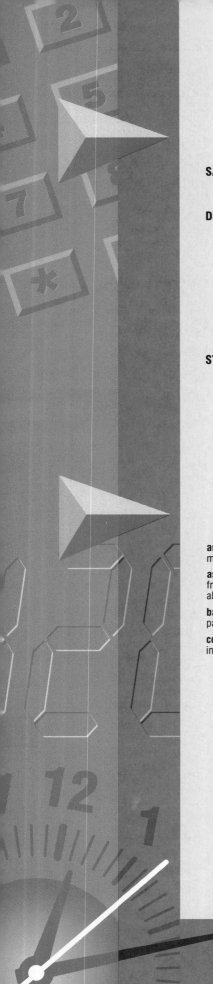

CHAPTER OUTLINE

VOCABULARY

antiseptic A substance that renders microorganisms harmless.

asepsis Condition of being free from infection or infectious materials.

bactericide Agent that destroys pathogenic organisms.

coagulable Capable of being formed into clots.

contamination Becoming soiled through contact with nonsterile material.

desiccation The act of drying.

disinfection Destruction of pathogenic organisms by chemical or physical means.

fumigation Using a gaseous agent to destroy organisms such as insects and vectors.

germicide See **bactericide.**

permeable Able to be passed or soaked through.

sanitization Reducing the number of microorganisms to a level that is relatively safe.

sterilization Complete destruction of all forms of microbial life.

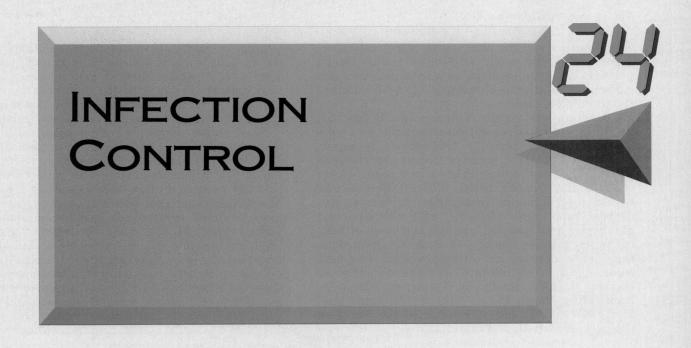

INFECTION CONTROL

24

LEARNING OBJECTIVES

COGNITIVE
Upon successful completion of this chapter, you should be able to:
1. Define and spell the terms in the Vocabulary.
2. List the criteria for choosing sanitization, disinfection, and sterilization.
3. Describe special precautions against cross-infection during sanitization.
4. Recall the physical methods for achieving sterilization.
5. Name five disinfectant agents.
6. List the advantages of moist heat sterilization.
7. Describe types of wrapping materials used for steam sterilization.
8. Name four places that indicators may be placed.

PERFORMANCE
Upon successful completion of this chapter, you should be able to:
1. Disinfect or sterilize instruments using a chemical disinfectant.
2. Wrap instruments and supplies for steam sterilization with an autoclave.
3. Sterilize instruments and supplies using an autoclave.

Sterilization and the attempts to reach and understand sterility are as old as recorded history. Many practices and theories have been tried and then discarded, but with each, something has been added to the total knowledge.

Cremation was known centuries ago. It has also been known that **desiccation** sometimes preserves body tissue and prevents the spread of sepsis. Moses, in about 1250 BC, gave the ancient Hebrews the first recorded sanitation laws. In a sense, Moses was our first "public health officer." The ancient Greeks used forms of **fumigation** to combat epidemics. Hippocrates (460–370 BC), who separated philosophy and medicine, realized the value of boiling water, washing hands, and using certain medications while dressing an infected wound. The next contribution of significance was the discovery of bacteria in 1683, chiefly by Anton van Leeuwenhoek. Then Joseph Lister (1827–1912), Louis Pasteur (1822–1895), and others started the world on the miraculous path of sterilization.

SANITIZATION

Detergents and Water

Instruments and other items used in office surgery, examination, or treatment must be carefully cleaned *before* proceeding with the steps of disinfection or sterilization. **Sanitization** is the careful scrubbing of materials, using brushes and specially formulated, blood-dissolving laboratory detergents that have a neutral pH and are low-etching and low-sudsing. Detergents that are very alkaline are corrosive to aluminum and also erode ground-glass surfaces. Strong alkaline detergents are also harmful to rubber. Most detergents are slightly alkaline and may be used for general purposes, but it is best to use the specially formulated laboratory detergents for cleaning glassware and rubber goods.

Detergents are mainly wetting agents that increase penetration and wetting power; they are sometimes called "soapless" soaps. Because of their ability to emulsify fats and oils, they aid in the mechanical removal of bacteria and tissue debris. Blood and debris must be removed so that later disinfection with chemicals or sterilization with steam, heat, or gases can penetrate to all the instrument's surfaces.

After washing, all items must be thoroughly rinsed in hot, running water, then in distilled water. Hot water is better for rinsing away detergent film; distilled water helps prevent mineral deposits from accumulating on instruments. Next, the items are placed on toweling or racks to dry, or they are hand-dried with a towel. Sanitization is a very important step, and it cannot be overlooked or done carelessly.

During a surgical procedure, a special receptacle is used to receive contaminated instruments. This is usually a basin of disinfectant solution placed within your reach. If a metal basin is used, you may want to line the bottom with gauze squares to prevent damage as you drop the instruments into the solution. After each procedure, immediately remove the basin to the cleaning and sterilization room.

Never allow blood or other **coagulable** substances to dry on an instrument. If immediate sanitization is not possible, leave the instruments soaking in the disinfecting solution or rinse them with cold tap water and place them to soak in a solution of detergent and cold water. You must know the manufacturers' recommendations for sanitizing the various types of instruments. For instance, stainless steel instruments should be sanitized immediately after use, or they may acquire a tarnish that is difficult to remove. Also, chrome-plated instruments may rust where there are minute breaks in the plating, if left to soak too long. If rust and stains develop, they may become a source of bacterial deposits and **contamination,** and the instruments must be discarded.

When you are ready to sanitize instruments, drain off the solution and rinse each instrument in cold, running water. Separate the sharp instruments from the others; other metal instruments may damage the cutting edges, or the sharp instruments may injure the other instruments or you. Clean all the sharp instruments at one time, when you can concentrate on avoiding the dangers of injury to yourself. Open all hinges, and scrub serrations and ratchets with a small scrub brush or toothbrush. Rinse the items, then check the instruments carefully for proper working order.

Rubber and plastic items may discolor some metals, so sanitize these items last. Some rubber and plastic items should not be soaked because they may discolor, become porous, or lose their glossy surfaces. These items must be sanitized immediately without soaking or cleaned by wiping dry with alcohol.

Because it is not possible to know whether or not every patient is free of hepatitis B or HIV (AIDS virus), extreme care must be taken when handling any item that has penetrated a patient's tissues. Whenever possible, you should minimize the need for sanitization and sterilization by using *disposable* instruments, needles, and syringes when working with human blood or giving injections. Many instruments are now available in the disposable form, but most are too expensive to throw away and must be sterilized for reuse. Reusable syringes and needles have become obsolete, and medical practice is discouraged from using them.

Ultrasonics

Sound waves can be used for sanitization of instruments by placing the instruments in a bath of ultrasonic cleaner and water and then passing ultrasonic waves through the bath. The sound vibrates and causes bubbling, which loosens the materials attached to the instruments. Ultrasonic cleaners do not damage even the most delicate instruments.

DISINFECTION

Disinfection is the freeing of an item from infectious materials. Disinfection is not always effective against spores, the tubercle bacilli, and certain viruses. In the medical office, the term usually refers to disinfecting instruments with chemicals or boiling water. Boiling water or very strong chemicals may kill microbes within a short time but are usually very hard on the instruments. Some chemicals are effective enough to kill all organisms, but the usual immersion time for these sterilants is 10 or more hours. When disinfecting with boiling water, time and temperature cannot be separated; strength is only a factor if chemicals are added to the boiling water. There are various methods of disinfection with varying degrees of effectiveness. It is important to know how to properly use each method, as well as its advantages, disadvantages, and the possible sources of error.

Chemical Disinfection

Chemical disinfectants and sterilants are convenient and often the agent of choice for materials that are damaged by heat (such as plastic or rubber products). A good chemical disinfectant is effective in a moderately low concentration and within a reasonable length of time. It should retain its potency in the presence of some dead organic matter, and it should not be too volatile (that is, rapidly evaporate).

Disinfectants are applied to inanimate objects, since they are too strong to be used on human tissues. Items that will *not* enter human tissue, the circulatory system, or a sterile body cavity may be disinfected. Items that come into contact with the skin or mucous membrane are immersed for longer periods of time in chemicals that are considered *sterilants,* but they must be rinsed with sterile water before use.

Disinfection is very difficult to verify, since there are no convenient indicators to ensure destruction of the organisms. Most commercial disinfectants kill staphylococci. Some claim to kill the tubercle bacilli, fungi, and even spores and viruses. Because you and the physician are not experts on chemical disinfectants, you should rely upon established manufacturers, who have rigid tests and standardization for their products and do not make false advertising claims.

Even when the manufacturer's directions for chemical strength and immersion times are followed, the following four common errors can cause chemicals to lose their effectiveness:

- Instruments are not thoroughly sanitized, and attached organic matter changes the action of the disinfectant. No chemical can kill unless it reaches the instrument's surfaces; therefore, complete sanitization is absolutely necessary.
- Sanitized instruments are not dried, and the wet instruments placed in the solution dilute it beyond the effective concentration.
- A solution is left in an open container, and evaporation changes its concentration.
- Solutions are not changed after the recommended period for use has expired.

Some of the more commonly used chemicals follow.

Soap

For many years, soap was considered the "all-purpose" disinfectant, but studies have shown that soap has very limited killing power. It is the scrubbing action and the running water that have real value, as in hand washing and sanitizing. The average household soap has limited effect, but since soap is not a single chemical, there are additives that do have lethal power. Although considerable controversy surrounds the effectiveness of germicidal or "surgical" soaps, there are some germicidal soaps that do kill organisms, mainly staphylococci, which are the greatest offenders on our skin. These germicidal soaps leave a film of disinfectant on the skin that lasts for several hours.

Alcohol

Alcohol is the most widely used antiseptic. Ethyl alcohol had been widely used in the past, but isopropyl alcohol has become more frequently used. It exhibits slightly greater germicidal action than does ethyl alcohol. It is an excellent fat solvent and, therefore, good for cleansing the skin, but continued use is hard on the hands. Iodine and other chemicals are sometimes added to alcohol to increase its lethal powers.

Acids

Acids in concentrated form are excellent **germicides** (also called **bactericides**) but are corrosive. The more they are diluted to decrease these hazards, the less valuable they are as disinfectants.

Phenol (carbolic acid) was first used as an **antiseptic** in 1865 by Joseph Lister. It is toxic to tissues in strong dilutions but is often added to other agents. Phenol is used as a standard for testing disinfectants.

24

Formaldehyde

Formaldehyde (formalin) has strong disinfectant properties and is used as a preservative of tissue (10% solution). A 5% solution is actively germicidal and sporicidal in the presence of organic matter. It is irritating to tissue, and any instrument disinfected with it must be thoroughly rinsed with sterile or distilled water before use. It should be used at room temperature, because cooling reduces its effectiveness.

Alkalies

A popular product that is used frequently today is plain household bleach. When mixed with water to form a 10% solution, it is an effective and noncaustic disinfectant. It is used to wipe laboratory table tops where human blood and other body-fluid samples are handled. It can be used for soaking reusable rubber goods before sanitizing. Bleach is used to disinfect dialysis equipment and is an effective disinfectant for surfaces that have come into contact with viruses, including the HIV (AIDS virus).

Ultraviolet Disinfection

Ultraviolet rays, found in sunlight and ultraviolet lamps, are used to prevent airborne bacteria from spreading in operating rooms, classrooms, bacteriologic laboratories, beauty salons, and barber shops. The destructiveness of the ray varies greatly with the distance from the source, the air it passes through, and the surface of the article it hits. This form of radiation is not considered a method of sterilization because of its limitations and lack of penetrating power.

Desiccation

Desiccation, or drying, is used to inhibit or preserve, especially bacterial cultures and foods. Spores are highly resistant to this method. Desiccation is extremely limited for sterilization and should be thought of as a disinfectant.

Disinfection by Boiling (Moist Heat)

Boiling (212°F, or 100°C) kills most vegetative forms of pathogenic bacteria, but bacterial spores and some viruses associated with infectious hepatitis are resistant to temperatures of 212°F and below. No matter how much heat is applied or how vigorous the boil, water will reach only 212°F at sea level. The higher the elevation, the lower the temperature required to obtain a boil (for example, in Denver, Colorado, water boils at 202°F). Because of these limitations, *boiling does not sterilize* and is used for disinfection only.

STERILIZATION

In the medical office, cleanliness takes the extreme form of sterilization. Sterilization reduces the perpetual threat of contamination to patients, to the physician, and to the medical assistant. To ensure proper sterilization as the end product of aseptic procedures, an area should be set aside in each office for just this purpose. The area should be divided into two sections. One section is used for receiving contaminated materials. This area should have a sink, as well as receiving basins, proper cleaning agents, brushes, sterilizer wrapping paper, envelopes and tape, sterilizer indicators, and disposable gloves. The other section should be reserved for receiving the sterile items after they are removed from the sterilizer. Clear, clean plastic bags in which to store sterile packs may be kept in the sterile area. Both areas should be spotlessly clean and well organized. Wear disposable gloves when handling contaminated items. If you have an open cut or wound on your hands, you should not clean or prepare instruments for sterilization.

Sterilization can be achieved by physical methods, such as radiation, dry heat, and steam heat, or by chemical methods, such as the gas sterilizer or the chemical glutaraldehyde.

Chemical Sterilization

True chemical sterilization is recommended for instruments that may be dulled by heat sterilization. Many chemicals are believed to be sterilants, but in reality very few are. The glutaraldehydes, such as Cidex (The 3M Company) or Glutarex (Surgikos), will sterilize non–heat-resistant equipment, provided the items are submerged for at least 10 hours. Instruments sterilized by this method must be rinsed with sterile water or sterile distilled water before use on human tissues. For sterile use, instruments sterilized in this manner must be used immediately after they are removed from the chemical solution.

Moist Heat Sterilization

Steam under pressure is the best and most accepted method of sterilization. It is the principal

PROCEDURE 24-1   STERILIZING OR DISINFECTING INSTRUMENTS WITH CHEMICALS

GOAL To clean or sterilize instruments by placing them in the appropriate chemical disinfectant or sterilant (sterilizing agent) in a covered tray for an appropriate length of time.

EQUIPMENT AND SUPPLIES

Blood and body-fluid precaution barriers (goggles, masks, and aprons or gowns), as necessary
A closed container (chemical sterilizer)

Nonsterile gloves
Assorted instruments
A chemical disinfectant or sterilant
Sterile water or sterile distilled water

PROCEDURAL STEPS

1. Put on gloves, and assemble the instruments and make sure they are clean and dry.
   Purpose: Water dilutes the chemical. Coagulants and oils inhibit the chemical action on the microorganisms.

2. Open hinged instruments and disassemble multiunit instruments (Fig. 24-1).
   Purpose: All surfaces must receive maximum exposure to the chemical.

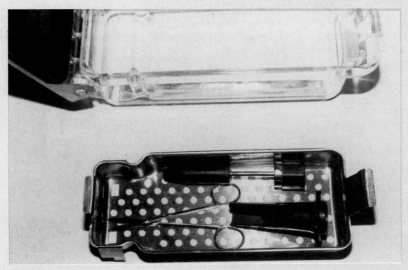

FIGURE 24-1.

3. Read the manufacturer's directions and prepare the chemical as directed.
   Purpose: Each product varies in preparation.

4. Place the instruments in the tray and cover them completely with the chemical (Fig. 24-2A).
   Purpose: All surfaces must receive maximum exposure to the chemical.

5. Close the lid (Fig. 24-2B).
   Purpose: Chemicals may have harmful or annoying fumes. These chemicals are harmful to the tissues of the body, and the lid helps to isolate the chemical by preventing spills and splashes.

Continued

PROCEDURE 24-1 *Continued*

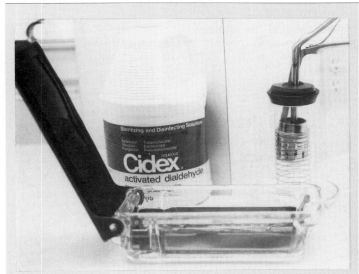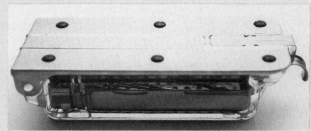

FIGURE 24-2.

6. Label the container with the name of the chemical.
   Purpose: To notify others of its contents.

7. Identify the instruments and the time of immersion on a clipboard.
   Purpose: Some disinfectants complete their action in 20 minutes; others, such as glutar-aldehydes, require 10 hours to sterilize.

8. At the end of the immersion period, transfer the items with transfer forceps to a sterile tray. Rinse the items thoroughly in sterile water or sterile distilled water, and use immediately (Fig. 24-3).
   Purpose: The chemicals are harmful to the skin and mucous membranes of both the medical assistant and the patient.

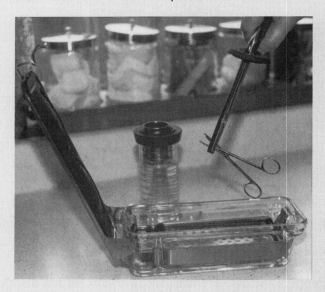

FIGURE 24-3.

9. Or rinse the items under hot running water, then dry with a towel or on a rack and store in a clean, covered area.

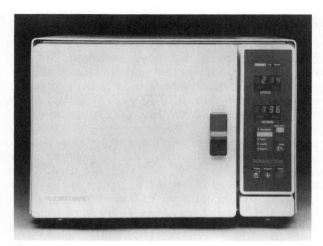

FIGURE 24-4. An automatic office autoclave. (Courtesy of Pelton and Crane, Charlotte, NC.)

moisture. Steam under pressure is capable of much faster penetration of fabrics and textiles than is dry heat, but it has definite limitations if the proper techniques are not followed.

Incorrect operation of an autoclave may result in *superheated* steam. If steam is brought to too high a temperature, it is literally dried out, and the advantage of a higher heat is diminished. *Wet* steam is another cause of incomplete sterilization. Wet steam results from failing to preheat the chamber, which results in excessive condensation in the interior of the chamber. Condensation is necessary, but too much prevents the sterilization process from coming to a proper completion. It can be compared to taking a hot shower in a cold bathroom, which results in heavily steamed mirrors, tile walls, and towels. If fabric packs become too saturated to dry during the drying cycle, the packs will pick up and absorb bacteria from the air or any surface they are placed on (Table 24–1). Cold instruments placed in a hot chamber also increase condensation. Other causes of wet steam include opening the door too wide during the drying cycle or allowing a rush of cold air into the chamber. Also, overfilling the water reservoir may produce this same effect.

The main cause of incomplete sterilization in the autoclave is the presence of residual air. Without the complete elimination of air, an adequately high temperature cannot be reached. Air and steam do not mix. Since air is heavier than steam, it will pool wherever possible. One tenth of 1% residual air trapped around an instrument will prevent complete sterilization. This is especially dangerous in older autoclaves that do not have a chamber thermometer separate from the pressure gauge. A certain chamber pressure does not guarantee a proper chamber tem-

operation of the *autoclave* (Fig. 24–4). Steam under pressure is fast, convenient, and dependable. The pressure allows a higher heat, and when combined with moisture, these two factors create a very effective mechanism for killing all microorganisms. When steam is admitted into the autoclave chamber, it simultaneously heats and wets the object, coagulating the proteins present in all living organisms. When the cycle is complete and the chamber cooled, the steam condenses and "explodes" the cells of microorganisms, thus destroying them. To be effective, all surfaces must be contacted by the

TABLE 24-1. STERILIZATION CHART

Article	Method	Temperature	Time
Gauze, small, loosely packed	Autoclave	250°F	30 min
Gauze, large, loosely packed	Autoclave	270°F	30 min
Gauze, small, tightly packed	Autoclave	250°F	40 min
Gauze, large, tightly packed	Autoclave	270°F	40 min
Gauze, tightly packed	Dry heat	320°F	3 h
Gauze, loosely packed	Dry heat	320°F	2 h
Glass syringes in tubes	Autoclave	250°F	30 min
Glass syringe in muslin	Dry heat	320°F	1 h
Instruments on tray, muslin under and over	Dry heat	320°F	1 h
Instruments on tray, muslin under and over	Autoclave	250°F	15 min
Solutions in flasks with gauze plug	Autoclave	250°F	30 min
Glassware unwrapped	Dry heat	320°F	1 h
Glassware wrapped	Autoclave	250°F	30 min
Petroleum jelly, 1-oz jar	Dry heat	340°F	1 h
Petroleum jelly, 1-oz jar	Dry heat	320°F	2 h
Petroleum gauze in instrument tray	Dry heat	320°F	150 min
Powder, 1-oz jar	Dry heat	320°F	2 h
Powder, small glove packs	Autoclave	250°F	15 min

Remember to always place an indicator in areas where there is doubt that the steam will penetrate.
Do not measure by chamber pounds. A thermometer and indicator are the reliable methods of judging a killing temperature.

24

perature. All release valves and discharge lines must be kept clean and free from dirt and lint.

Wrapping Materials

The maintenance of sterility is completely dependent upon the wrapper and its porosity as well as on the method of wrapping. The wrapping material must be **permeable** to steam but impervious to contaminants such as dust and insects. Muslin should be of 140-thread count, and a double thickness should be used. Canvas or duck fabric is not advisable because steam cannot penetrate it properly.

Acceptable wrapping materials for autoclaving are:

- A nonwoven disposable material such as Kim wrap
- Clear plastic with permeable paper facing envelope
- Permeable paper envelopes
- Rigid containers manufactured for autoclaving

The nonwoven disposable material is currently the best choice for the medical office. It is permeable to steam, resists contamination, and does not become brittle during storage. It can be used one time only. Transparent envelopes or clear plastic wrappers may be used, provided one side is made of a permeable paper that allows steam penetration (Fig. 24–5). They are convenient because they allow for the visibility of their contents. Regardless of which wrapping material is used, it should be folded in such a way that it may be opened easily without contaminating the contents. Chapter 36 contains instructions on how to open sterile packages.

Rigid containers, which were originally designed for hospital instrument sets, are becoming popular. They are expensive initially, but they pay for themselves by eliminating the need for costly wrapping materials.

Indicators

In 1881, Robert Koch tried using anthrax spores to see if the items had been sterilized, but this method was difficult to use and gave unreliable results. Also in the 19th century, a British physician used raw eggs in a load. If the eggs were hard at the end of exposure, he considered the load to be sterile. Even with these extremely poor and unreliable methods, it was realized that there was a need to determine sterility. To eliminate the constant doubt of complete sterilization, *indicators* are used. These indicators show, by melting or by changing color, that a certain temperature for a given period of time has been reached, irrespective of pressure. An indicator should be placed with each load in one of the following places:

- Buried deep in packs
- In constriction tubes
- In the bottoms of containers that cannot be turned on their sides
- In any other places that might be inaccessible to the flow of steam

Many feel that an indicator is not necessary if the chamber has a thermometer, but this tells you the temperature only where the tip of the thermometer is located and not in the aforementioned places. An indicator is also placed in the lower front near the air exhaust valve.

Read the accompanying instructions for the indicator you use. The dangers of incomplete sterilization are too great for you to be lax in your technique or in the care of the equipment.

A popular indicator that is easy to use is the OK Strip (Fig. 24–6). When the OK Strip has been exposed to 250°F for at least 15 minutes, the "OK" changes from tan to deep black. You must remember that this test is not a true indication of sterility. It merely means that the minimum tem-

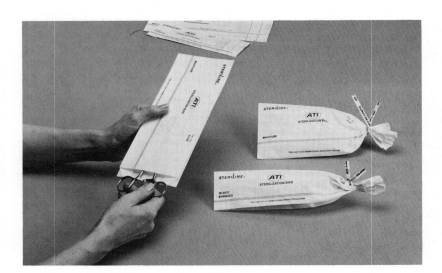

FIGURE 24–5. Instrument indicator bags have strips that change color when a minimum temperature is reached for a certain period of time. The translucency allows easy identification. (Courtesy of PyMaH Corporation, ATI Division, Somerville, NJ.)

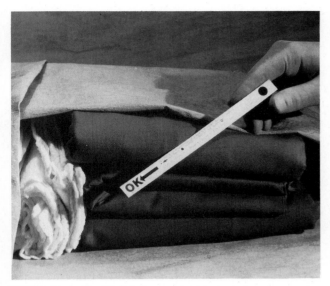

FIGURE 24-6. The OK Strip is used to detect whether pure pressure steam has penetrated the pack. It should be placed in the area judged most difficult for the steam to reach. In a complete exposure, the color change is to black and is as dark or darker than the standard reference color of the "O" in "OK." A color change that is incomplete (light tan to dark brown) is an indication of incomplete processing (exposure too short, temperature too low, and/or incomplete steam penetration). (Courtesy of Propper, Inc., New York, NY.)

perature has been maintained. There is no assurance of sterility of the load.

An example of an excellent system for testing the effectiveness of your office autoclave is the Attest system, manufactured by the 3M Company (Fig. 24-7A). It is a bioindicator that consists of a double-walled tube that, when broken, releases a microorganism into a culture medium. If the sterilization cycle is defective and the microorganism still lives, growth should occur within 24 hours. It can be cultured in an office water bath or a dry block incubator. Another method for determining the efficiency of sterilization processes is the indicator that contains dried bacterial spores of established, heat-resistant organisms (Fig. 24-7B). These bacterial spore strips are available commercially from reliable suppliers, but the indicators are not always practical for a physician's office because the strip, after autoclaving, must be sent to a bacteriology laboratory for sterility testing.

Autoclave or sterilizer tapes frequently have some form of indicator on them that changes after exposure to sterilization procedures. These tapes are excellent for securing packages and bags, but they are not to be used as sterilizer indicators. They never were intended for this purpose; they only indicate that the package has been processed, not that sterility has been reached.

Sterilization indicator bags are also very convenient. They are made of disposable paper or thermostable plastic, in which syringes, tubing, and many other items can be sterilized and stored. The paper or transparent material is permeable to steam

and provides a barrier against airborne bacteria during storage. Each bag has an indicator printed on it, similar to the sterilizer tape, which shows that the bag has been autoclaved but does not prove that its contents are sterile.

The Autoclave

The office autoclave is similar to the home pressure cooker. It operates on the principle of steam under pressure. Water in an outer chamber, or jacket, is heated to produce steam. The pressure in this outer jacket builds and forces steam into the inner chamber. As steam is forced in, air is forced out. Visualize the air flowing out of the chamber as water flowing down a sink drain. Read the manufacturer's instructions carefully. An autoclave usually has three gauges: (1) the jacket pressure gauge, which indicates the steam pressure in the outer chamber; (2) the chamber pressure gauge, which indicates the steam pressure in the inner chamber; and (3) the temperature gauge, which indicates the temperature in the inner chamber, where the items are sterilized. When the temperature gauge reaches 250°F (121°C) and the pressure gauge indicates 15 pounds of steam pressure, the load of articles to be sterilized can be timed for 20 to 30 minutes.

The autoclave chamber must be cleaned before each loading. If there has been boiling over of solutions, the water reservoir must be drained and thoroughly cleaned and rinsed. Check the manufacturer's instructions carefully and do not use a commercial cleaner unless advised by the manufacturer. A mild detergent may be used in the chamber, but make certain it is very thoroughly rinsed after any type of cleaner has been used.

The trays must also be kept clean and free of lint. Be sure to replace the bottom (chamber) tray after cleaning; it must be in place for proper steam circulation. The air exhaust valve is one of the most important parts of the autoclave and must be clean and free of lint, otherwise the air will not exhaust from the chamber. Unless proper care is taken of the autoclave, the dressings and instruments will have been *well heated but not sterilized.* Table 24-2 provides tips to improve autoclaving techniques.

LOADING THE AUTOCLAVE. Prepare all packs and arrange the load in such a manner to allow maximum circulation of steam and heat. Articles should be placed so that they rest on their edges, to permit proper permeation of the materials with moisture and heat. Under no conditions should you permit the crowding of packs into tight masses. Jars and containers should be placed on their sides. Instruments may be autoclaved unwrapped if they are to be used immediately or do not need to be sterile when used later. Perforated trays are used for sterilizing unwrapped instruments. Place a lint-free towel under and over the instruments to facilitate drying and to prevent contamination when removing them from the autoclave.

24

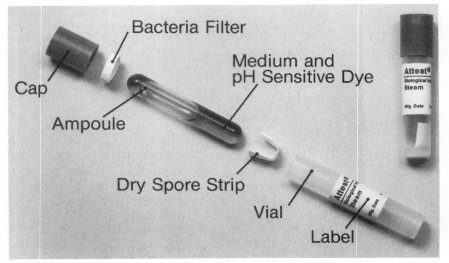

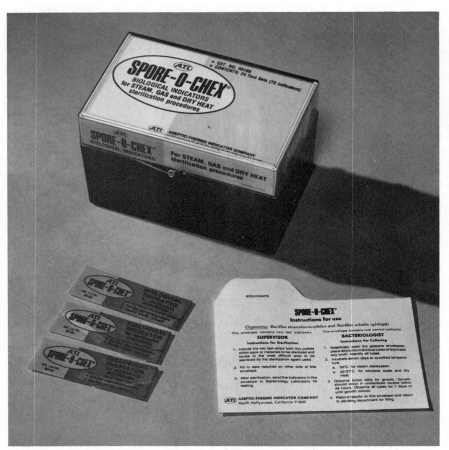

FIGURE 24–7. Biologic indicators that confirm sterility. *A,* The Attest system assures sterilization. The tube is cultured after the autoclaving cycle; if no organisms grow, sterility is assumed. (Courtesy of Medical Products Division: 3M, St. Paul, MN.) *B,* Spore-O-Chex, which contains bacillus spores. (Courtesy of Aseptic-Thermo Indicator Co., Simi Valley, CA.)

PROCEDURE 24-2 WRAPPING INSTRUMENTS AND SUPPLIES FOR STEAM STERILIZATION WITH THE AUTOCLAVE

GOAL To place dry, sanitized supplies and instruments inside appropriate wrapping materials for sterilization and storage without contamination.

EQUIPMENT AND SUPPLIES

Dry, sanitized items   Autoclave tape
Assorted wrapping materials   A waterproof pen

PROCEDURAL STEPS

1. Place the item(s) diagonally at the approximate center of the wrapping material. Make sure the size of the square is large enough for the items.
   Purpose: Each of the four corners must fold over and completely cover the item(s), with a few extra inches overlap for folding back a flap (Fig. 24-8).

2. With the squares that are cloth fabric, use two pieces if the cloth is single-layered, or one piece if the cloth is sewn together as a double layer.

3. If the square is paper or a synthetic product, follow the manufacturer's recommendation.

4. Open slightly any hinged instruments. If the instrument is sharp, its teeth or tip should be shielded with cotton or gauze.
   Purpose: To prevent puncture of the package or the operator.

5. Place a commercial sterilization indicator inside the package at the approximate center.
   Purpose: To ensure that the autoclave is reaching effective levels of heat and pressure.

6. Bring up the bottom corner of the wrap, and fold back a portion of it (Fig. 24-9).
   Purpose: You will use this flap as the "handle" to open the pack. This folded-back flap is the only part of each wrapper corner that can be touched when opening a sterile package.

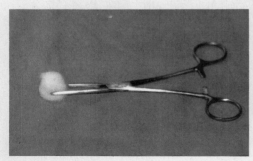

FIGURE 24-8.

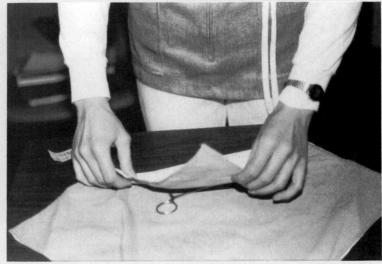

FIGURE 24-9.

24

Continued

PROCEDURE 24 – 2 *Continued*

7. Fold over the right corner, and turn back a portion of it (Fig. 24–10A).

8. Fold over the left corner, and turn back a portion of it (Fig. 24–10B).

9. Fold the covered area in half (Fig. 24–10C).

10. Bring down the top corner, and continue folding it around the pack as far as it will go.

11. Secure with autoclave tape (Fig. 24–10D).

12. Label the package with the date, contents, and your initials, or as instructed.
    Purpose: To know what is in the pack at a later date, whether or not the shelf life has expired (expiration date), and who performed the task. As a general rule, most office autoclaved packs are considered sterile (usable) for 30 days.

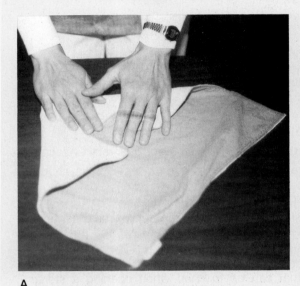

A

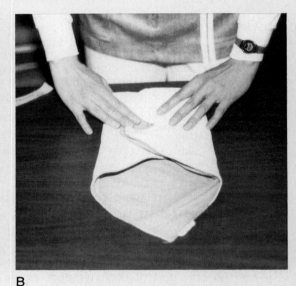

B

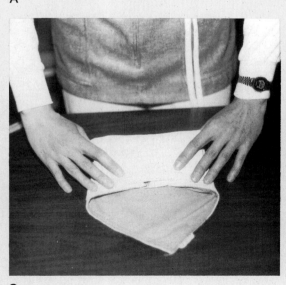

C

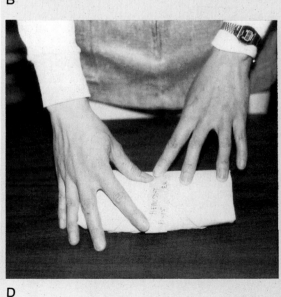

D

FIGURE 24–10.

TABLE 24-2. TIPS FOR IMPROVING AUTOCLAVING TECHNIQUES

Problem	Causes	How to Correct
Damp linens	Clogged chamber drain	Remove strainer, free openings of lint
	Goods removed from chamber too soon following cycle	Allow goods to remain in sterilizer an additional 15 min with door slightly open
	Improper loading	Place packs on edge, arrange for least possible resistance to flow of steam and air
Stained linens	Dirty chamber	Clean chamber with Calgonite solution; never use strong abrasives, such as steel wool; rinse thoroughly after cleaning
Corroded instruments	Poor cleaning; residual soil	Improve cleaning; do not allow soil to dry on instruments; sanitize first
	Exposure to hard chemicals (e.g., iodine, salt, and acids)	Do not expose instruments to these chemicals; if exposure occurs, rinse immediately
	Inferior instruments	Use only top-quality instruments
Spotted or stained instruments	Mineral deposits on instruments	Wash with soft soap and detergent with good wetting properties
	Residual detergents from cleaning	Rinse instruments thoroughly
	Mineral deposits from tap water	Rinse with distilled water
Instruments have soft hinges or joints	Corrosion or soil in joint	Clean with warm, weak acid solutions (10% nitric acid solution); rinse thoroughly
	Jaws and shanks out of alignment	Realignment by qualified instrument repair professional
Ebullition, or caps blow off solutions	Exhausing chamber too rapidly	Use slow exhaust, cool liquids, or turn autoclave off and let cool on its own—that is, let the pressure decrease at its own rate
Steam leakage	Worn gasket	Replace
	Door closes improperly	Reopen door and shut carefully; have serviced if unable to close door properly
Chamber door does not open	Vacuum in chamber (check chamber pressure gauge)	Turn on controls to starting steam pressure, wait until equalized, then vent and open door

UNLOADING THE AUTOCLAVE. When the sterilization cycle is complete, release the pressure with the control setting. Standing away from the door and with oven mits, slightly open the door about a quarter of an inch. Allow the load to dry for at least 5 minutes (this will vary according to the type of autoclave and the size of the load). *Capillary attraction* is the term describing the force that draws moisture through surfaces of materials. Materials act like a sponge. Any moisture outside the pack contains microorganisms, which, in turn, are drawn into the pack with the moisture. Touching a wet load will allow the microorganisms on your hands to penetrate the wrappings and to render the contents nonsterile. Dry, wrapped packs may be removed with clean, dry hands, but it is safer to wear oven mits to reduce the possibility of burns from the hot instruments inside the packs. Place the packs on a dry, dust-free surface for storage. Avoid cold surfaces, because the hot packs may cause condensation, and moisture will contaminate the contents.

Storage of Wrapped Supplies

Although experts do not agree upon the length of time that wrapped supplies remain sterile, the following shelf-life rules are fairly standard.

- Double-wrapped muslin and double-wrapped paper packs are considered sterile up to 28 days from the date of sterilization.
- Nonpermeable plastic-wrapped packs are considered sterile up to six months from the date of sterilization. (Most medical offices do not have the equipment to sterilize supplies in nonpermeable packages. Purchased nonpermeable packs will have expiration dates printed on the outside.)

All supplies should be stored on dry, dust-free, covered shelves or in drawers. Fabric wrappers must be relaundered. A damaged pack or a broken seal renders the package nonsterile. Spills of any fluid onto a package render the pack nonsterile. When a pack is no longer sterile because of a broken seal or an expiration date that has passed, the contents must be reprocessed starting with the sanitization process.

Gas Sterilization

Researchers report that gas sterilization could be the exclusive method of sterilization in the future, thereby eliminating the need for other methods. There is no doubt that gas sterilization has many advantages over all other methods in use today.

24

PROCEDURE 24-3   STERILIZING WITH THE STEAM AUTOCLAVE

GOAL   To sterilize supplies and instruments, using the autoclave.

EQUIPMENT AND SUPPLIES

An autoclave
Wrapped items, such as:
   a hemostat
   a thumb dressing forceps
   a glass syringe

cotton balls
applicators
gauze sponges
A jar containing gauze
A basin that can be autoclaved

PROCEDURAL STEPS

1. Check the water level in the reservoir and add distilled water as necessary.
   Purpose: Too much or too little water may alter the effectiveness of the equipment. Tap water will leave lime deposits in the chamber.

2. Adjust the control to "fill" to allow water to flow into the chamber. The water will flow until you turn the control to its next position. Do not let the water overflow.

3. Load the chamber with wrapped items, then space them for maximum circulation and penetration.

4. Close and seal the door. The door must be closed or the heated water in the chamber will evaporate.

5. Turn the control setting to "on" or "autoclave" to start the cycle.

6. Watch the gauges until the temperature gauge reaches at least 250°F (121°C) and the pressure gauge reaches 15 pounds of pressure.

7. Set the timer for the desired time, usually between 20 and 30 minutes.

8. At the end of the timed cycle, turn the control setting to "vent."
   Purpose: This releases the steam and pressure. The water at the bottom of the chamber will drain back into the reservoir.

9. Wait for the pressure gauge to reach zero.

10. Open the chamber door a quarter of an inch.
    Purpose: To allow steam to escape faster.

11. Leave the autoclave control at "vent" to continue producing heat.
    Purpose: To dry the items faster.

12. Allow complete drying of all articles.

13. Using heat-resistant gloves or pads, remove the items from the chamber.

14. Place the sterilized packages on dry, covered shelves.

15. Turn the control knob to "off," and keep the door slightly ajar.

There are considerable differences between the various gas sterilizers on the market, and each manufacturer has its own set of conditions necessary to achieve sterilization. The major disadvantages with the use of gas sterilization are time and the general hazards connected with using gas. The length of exposure time is usually 1 1/2 to 2 hours, although exposure times sometimes can be lessened by slightly increasing the temperature. Another disadvantage is the time required for aeration after sterilization. Sterilizers must be properly vented to reduce human exposure to the gas. In August 1984, standards were issued by the United States Occupational Safety and Health Administration (OSHA). If you work with ethylene oxide gas, you should have a copy of these standards on the premises. The human hazards of gas sterilization include the possibility of damage to the reproductive organs of the operator as well as the development of cancer from prolonged exposure to high concentrations of ethylene oxide.

Preparation and Wrapping

As for any type of sterilization, items are sanitized with care, and moisture is removed from all surfaces. Be sure that all surfaces of the items are exposed in the sterilizer; do not pack them too tightly. Almost all forms of wrapping materials are acceptable for gas sterilization, but the combination paper-plastic wrapper is preferred because the contents are visible and the package is easy to open under aseptic conditions. Always check and follow the manufacturer's directions and recommendations.

Indicators for Gas Sterilization

There are several excellent indicators on the market for gas sterilization, but the bacterial cultures are the superior method of checking that sterilization has taken place (Fig. 24–11).

STERILIZATION OF ITEMS USED IN THE MEDICAL OFFICE

Dressings

Dressings may be purchased in large bulk non-sterile packages and may be rewrapped in smaller packs for autoclaving. Presterilized individual packages can also be purchased. Most dressings and gauze sponges are made of cotton, silk, rayon, or cellulose (wood fibers). They are folded in various sizes and shapes, with all raw edges carefully placed inside the folds. Raveling from a raw edge could cling to a wound and act as a foreign body. Some dressings have a thin layer of synthetic material that will not adhere to a wound.

Dressings should be sterilized in the autoclave. Wrap them in small packets with sterilizer paper. Each packet should be firm enough to hold together during normal handling. Remember packages that are too tightly wrapped inhibit the flow of heat and steam. The packets are sealed with sterilizer tape, labeled, and dated.

An indicator should be placed in the thickest part of the pack. Since the sterilization time for dressings is different from that for instruments, it is best not to mix them with instruments when autoclaving.

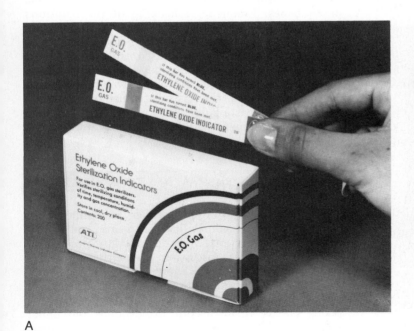

A

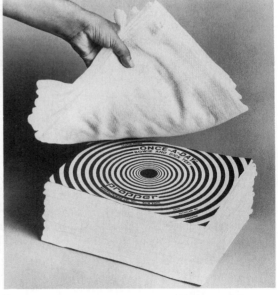

B

FIGURE 24–11. Indicators for gas sterilizers. *A*, Ethylene oxide indicators. (Courtesy of Aseptic-Thermo Indicator Co., Simi Valley, CA.) *B*, The Bowie and Dick Test. (Courtesy of Propper, Inc., New York, NY.)

Jars, Bottles, and Trays

Jars, bottles, and trays must be wrapped and placed on their sides if they are to be used to store sterile items. Covers on jars and containers should be put to one side or left ajar to allow steam to circulate. Extreme care must be taken not to contaminate the jars when replacing the lids after autoclaving is complete.

MECHANICAL AND PHYSICAL CAUSES OF INCOMPLETE STERILIZATION

- Inadequate sanitization. Steam cannot penetrate to the instrument surfaces in the presence of foreign substances such as soap film, blood, feces, or tissue debris.

- Improper wrapping.

- Using nonpermeable wrapping materials.

- Failure to preheat the chamber if the autoclave is cold.

- Incorrectly loading the autoclave chamber by:
  Overloading the chamber.
  Not placing jars on their edges.
  Blocking steam with small trays that do not have holes for circulation.
  Not placing thick packs vertically.
  Not using the autoclave bottom shelf.

- Starting the timer before correct temperature is reached.

- Too short an exposure time.

- Reading the gauges incorrectly or confusing one gauge for another.

- Too low a chamber pressure.

- Temperature too high (superheated steam) or not high enough (wet steam).

- Excessive condensation.

- Not allowing items to dry completely before removal from the chamber.

- Placing hot sterilized packages on a cold surface, causing condensation after sterilization and contamination of the packages.

- An unreliable autoclave.

- A dirty autoclave chamber or clogged exhaust lines.

- Resterilizing items in used wrappers.

Sterile Solutions

Some medical offices keep bottles of sterile distilled water or normal saline on hand for rinsing or irrigating purposes. Sterilization of these solutions may be done in an autoclave that has a slow-exhaust cycle only, otherwise the solution will boil over. Check the manufacturer's instruction guide regarding this procedure.

Rubber Materials

Rubber tubing and rubber goods are sterilized separately not only because they require a different sterilization time, but also because they discolor metals and may stick to them. Follow the manufacturer's recommendations.

THE MEDICAL ASSISTANT'S ROLE IN ASEPSIS

Medical **asepsis** is one of the very few procedures that directly affect the health of the patient, physician, and office staff. The spread of pathogens in the office can be controlled only through effective sterilization of all reusable equipment or with the use of disposable supplies and meticulous aseptic technique (see Mechanical and Physical Causes of Incomplete Sterilization).

The medical assistant must develop an inner sense for aseptic procedures. It is important that these techniques be done on such a routine basis that they become an unbreakable habit. Conscientious attention must be given to sterilizing *all* items at *all* times. Frequent rechecking of the solutions and techniques helps to ensure that the procedures employed are effective. The use of disposable items is highly recommended in the control of the infection process, and these items have become commonplace in many offices. However, when disposable equipment is used, the assistant must be conscious of pathogenic waste guidelines and provide the office and the environment with continuous protection.

LEGAL AND ETHICAL RESPONSIBILITIES

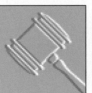 One of the medical assistant's main responsibilities is to carry out sterilization and disinfection procedures with precision and with total effectiveness. There is no room for compromise. Patients should have absolute assurance that they are being taken care of in an aseptic atmosphere and under aseptic conditions. This assurance is just as important for the protection of the physician and health staff as it is for the patient.

To have a good understanding of the subject, you must be aware of the different kinds of infectious agents that might be present in a doctor's office. You must become familiar with the various techniques of sterilization and disinfection. Ignorance or carelessness can be dangerous and is inexcusable before the law.

PATIENT EDUCATION

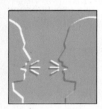

Many times, the patient is unfamiliar with the proper techniques of home sanitization and disinfection. They rely on the advertising that they see on television and read in magazines. The patient may feel too embarrassed to admit to the medical assistant that he or she does not understand or does not know how to minimize cross-contamination among family members or does not know what products will help keep every member in the family from infection when one member is ill. For these reasons, the medical assistant should take advantage of every opportunity to talk about family health and techniques that might be used to curb the spread of disease within the home. Sometimes in the course of a general conversation, the medical assistant can "pick up" hints of concerns that the patient has and can direct the conversation into a discussion of these concerns. A talented assistant is always listening to the patient and analyzing what the patient is saying. Always remember, the role of the medical assistant is to act as the patient's advocate and to help the physician to meet the physical and mental needs of the patient.

LEARNING ACHIEVEMENTS

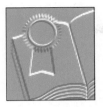

Upon completion of this chapter, can you in the time allowed by your evaluator:

1. Disinfect or sterilize a given group of instruments using safety precautions and correct immersion times (as determined by the manufacturer's directions) and by correctly completing every step of the procedure in the correct sequence?
2. Wrap and label a group of items for steam sterilization, completing each step of the procedure in the correct order?
3. Load, operate, and unload the steam autoclave (according to directions), completing each step of the procedure correctly and in the proper sequence?

REFERENCES AND READINGS

Bonewit, K.: *Clinical Procedures for the Medical Assistants,* 3rd ed., Philadelphia, W. B. Saunders Co., 1990.

Coates, H. W.: *Care and Handling of Surgical Instruments,* Chicago, V. Mueller Division, American Hospital Supply Corp., 1990.

Fuller, J. R.: *Surgical Technology Principles and Practices,* Philadelphia, W. B. Saunders Co., 1986.

Kirkis, E. J., and Grier, M.: *Nurse's Guide to Infectious Control,* Philadelphia, W. B. Saunders Co., 1988.

Walter, J. B.: *An Introduction to the Principles of Disease,* Philadelphia, W. B. Saunders Co., 1992.

24

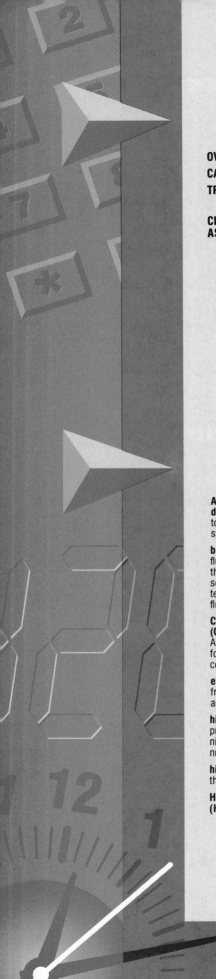

CHAPTER OUTLINE

VOCABULARY

Acquired Immunodeficiency Syndrome (AIDS) Disease involving the total collapse of the human immune system. Its cause is unknown.

body fluids External and internal fluids, secretions, and excretions of the human body, including blood, semen, vaginal secretions, saliva, tears, breast milk, cerebrospinal fluid, amniotic fluid, and urine.

Centers for Disease Control (CDC) National agency located in Atlanta, Georgia, that is responsible for the reporting of statistics for communicable diseases.

electrolyte imbalance A deviation from normal acid-alkaline base balance within the human body.

high-level disinfection A chemical procedure that kills vegetative organisms and viruses but not large numbers of bacterial spores.

histologic Pertaining to the study of the tissue cells of the body.

Human immunodeficiency virus (HIV) A virus that causes AIDS. It is transmitted through sexual contact and exposure to infected blood or blood components and from an infected mother to her fetus.

Kaposi's sarcoma A tumor of the walls of the blood vessels. It usually appears as pink or purple spots on the skin.

lymphoma A group of cancers that usually affect the lymph nodes; in HIV infections, they often affect other tissues.

meningitis An acute inflammation of the membranes of the spinal cord and the brain.

***Pneumocystis carinii* pneumonia (PCP)** A lung infection usually occurring in immunocompromised individuals. Caused by a protozoan that is present almost everywhere but is normally destroyed by healthy immune systems.

protozoal Pertaining to a pathogenic organism that can be ingested and transmitted through contact with contaminated feces. Hand washing and the observance of stool handling precautions are highly recommended.

T-cells (T-lymphocytes) Small circulating lymphocytes that are produced in the bone marrow. Their primary function is to indirectly aid cellular immune responses (i.e., the destruction of virus-infected cells and cancer cells).

thrush *(Candida albicans)* A yeast infection usually seen on the mucous membranes of the mouth and nose.

universal precautions A set of guidelines based on the assumption that every medical patient has a blood-borne infection that can be transmitted by blood, body fluids, or genital secretions.

wasting syndrome A decrease of total body mass seen in the HIV-infected patient, usually caused by lack of appetite and persistent watery stools.

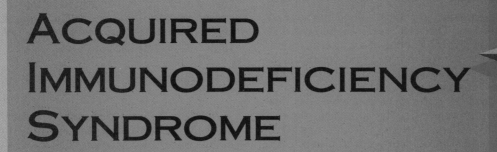

ACQUIRED IMMUNODEFICIENCY SYNDROME

TRANSMISSION AND PREVENTION

LEARNING OBJECTIVES

Upon successful completion of this chapter, you should be able to:

1. Define and spell the terms listed in the Vocabulary.

2. List the six recommendations included in the universal precautions for infection control.

3. Differentiate between HIV and AIDS.

4. List the possible portals of entry for HIV.

5. Discuss the specific diseases accompanying AIDS and HIV.

6. Describe the legal and ethical obligations involved in the treatment of the patient with HIV or AIDS.

7. Demonstrate routine barrier precautions used when contact with body fluids is anticipated.

Due to the serious nature of AIDS and HIV, this chapter has been written to assist you in understanding and coping with the problems they present. Before beginning, you should not forget that there are other diseases that are both blood-borne and sexually transmitted. Diseases such as hepatitis A and B, gonorrhea, syphilis, chlamydia, herpes simplex, herpes zoster, genital herpes, and tuberculosis are all potentially threatening to the health care provider. These diseases are a threat because of their etiology and symptomatology; each can be treated and possibly cured. On the contrary, there is no cure for AIDS. When someone is diagnosed with this dreaded disease, the only prognosis is death. In Chapters 28 and 29, blood and sexually transmitted diseases other than AIDS and HIV are discussed.

OVERVIEW

No other disease in the history of health care has had as large an impact worldwide as **Acquired Immunodeficiency Syndrome** (AIDS). It is one of the most frightening diseases currently known. The global AIDS epidemic is worsening faster than experts believed possible. Since it was first diagnosed in 1981, health concerns have steadily increased. The World Health Organization (WHO) predicted in 1988 that there would be a cumulative total of 15 million to 20 million adult AIDS infections by the year 2000. Now, they say that this total will be reached by 1995. Over 3 million new infections have occurred between 1989 and 1992. The WHO now feels that there will be over 40 million adults and children infected with the **human immunodeficiency virus** (HIV) by the turn of the century. Fear among some health care providers has been so great that they have chosen to leave their professions. This fear of AIDS is cited as being a major reason why enrollment in the caring professions has dropped. There is no doubt that AIDS is a primary issue in the medical profession and that it is causing revolutionary changes in every facet of the health care delivery system.

Figure 25–1 illustrates the dramatic increase over the last decade in the number of new AIDS cases reported each year and in the number of deaths due to AIDS in America. In 1992, the number of reported cases in the United States reached 365,656. Of this number, 62% have died. The medical assistant must join with other medical professionals and work to keep this disease from continuing to spread at its rapid pace. At present, the best tool we have for fighting AIDS is education.

It is predicted that AIDS will continue to have a serious impact on our lives for many years to come. This means that the members of the health care delivery system must become knowledgeable in the etiology and epidemiology of AIDS. If we are to provide safe and quality care to patients, we must arm ourselves with every available strategy.

In this chapter, the medical assistant is given the most current and accurate information on AIDS available at the time of publication. Since research on this dreaded virus is being conducted throughout the world, it is suggested that along with the presented material the medical assistant also contact the national or local AIDS hotline for additional information.

CAUSE

AIDS is a disease caused by a retrovirus that destroys a person's defenses against infections. These defenses are known as the *immune system.* The AIDS virus, known as HIV, can so weaken a person's immune system that he or she cannot fight off even mild infections. The patient eventually becomes vulnerable to life-threatening infections and cancers.

The exact origin of AIDS is unknown. The disease was first noted in the United States in the late 1970s and early 1980s. The tracing of AIDS began only when doctors had seen enough of it to recognize that they were faced with a serious and previously unknown disease. It was formally defined for the first time in 1982.

The AIDS virus attacks blood cells known as helper **T-cells,** or T-4 cells, that orchestrate the body's defenses against disease. The genetic information in the cells of most living things is made up of a chemical called *DNA.* However, the genes of the AIDS virus are made up of a substance called *RNA;* to take command of a T-cell, the virus must translate its genetic information into DNA by producing an enzyme called *reverse transcriptase.* A virus that can change genetic coding in this way is functioning on the level of creation and is capable of becoming a part of every body cell. Once the body accepts the virus' coding as part of a cell's DNA, the body's normal immune defense mechanisms can do nothing to stop it. The virus has destroyed the body's natural immune system—in other words, the patient has acquired an immune deficiency syndrome.

HIV is transmitted through contaminated **body fluids,** mainly blood and semen. An individual infected with HIV may first experience transient mononucleosis-like symptoms known as *acute HIV syndrome.* These symptoms include:

- fever
- pharyngitis
- myalgia
- arthralgia
- adenopathy

If these symptoms do occur, they usually subside, and the infected person normally has a long incubation period, sometimes lasting for years, during which he or she is asymptomatic. During this time, the carrier may not even realize that the HIV infection is present. The only evidence of HIV during this period is an antibody to HIV infection in the

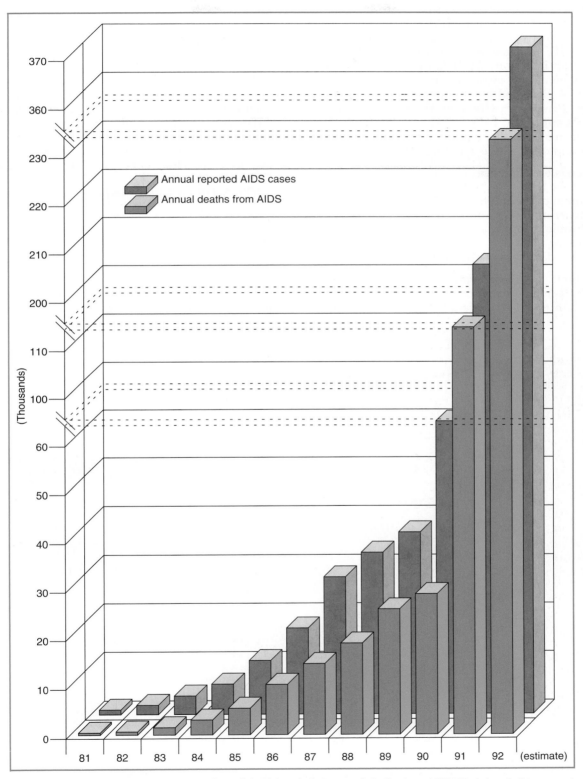

FIGURE 25-1. How AIDS is touching our lives. *Colored bars* indicate annual deaths from AIDS. *Black bars* indicate annual reported AIDS cases. (Data from Centers for Disease Control *Precaution Update*, 1991.)

25

blood. It is during this long incubation period that the HIV infection may be accidentally transmitted.

Current evidence indicates that 20 to 30% of the individuals infected with HIV will develop AIDS within a 5-year period. Some authorities predict that 80% of HIV carriers will develop AIDS within 10 years after infection. At this time, no one knows just how many will eventually develop the disease.

AIDS is identified by the presence of such disorders as ***Pneumocystis carinii* pneumonia** and **Kaposi's sarcoma;** before these conditions develop, HIV-infected persons may experience a group of lesser symptoms. These symptoms include:

- persistent diarrhea
- weight loss
- mononucleosis-like chronic fatigue
- recurring fevers and sweats
- chronic enlargement of the lymph nodes
- memory loss
- other disorders of the nervous system

In combination, these symptoms used to be known as *Aids Related Complex (ARC).* In 1987, the national **Centers for Disease Control** (CDC) ex-cluded the ARC classification in its revisions and now include most of the elements indicating progressive disease under the term *HIV wasting syndrome.*

In January 1991, the CDC adopted new guidelines for diagnosing the disease based on a patient's T-cell level. A healthy person has a T-cell (also called *CD4-cell*) level of 1000 per cubic millimeter of blood; an HIV-infected person with a count of 200 or fewer such cells (the others having been destroyed by the AIDS virus) is diagnosed as having AIDS. Washington, D.C. led the nation in the number of AIDS cases for the year ending June 1991, followed by Puerto Rico, New York, Florida, New Jersey, and California (Fig. 25–2).

The AIDS virus infection cycle has four stages:

1. Acute HIV infection
2. A period of asymptomatic incubation
3. ARC/AIDS wasting syndrome
4. The AIDS defining disorders

It is important to remember that all individuals infected may not experience every stage in the cycle.

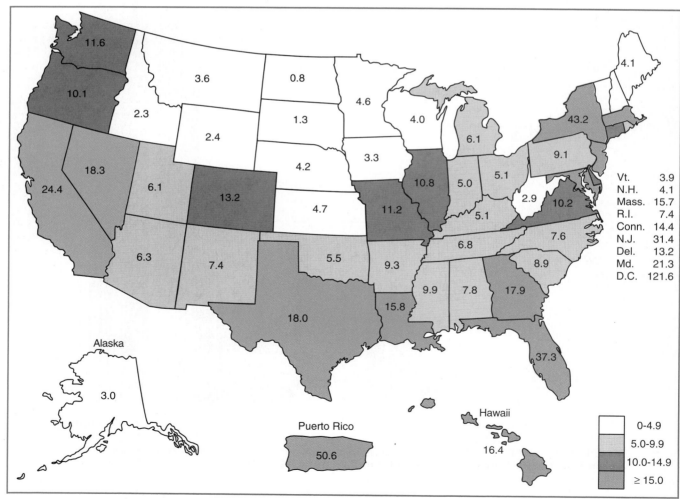

FIGURE 25–2. Number of AIDS cases per 100,000 persons in the United States from July 1990 to June 1991. (From Centers for Disease Control *Precaution Update,* 1991.)

TABLE 25-1. ESTIMATES OF RISK OF ACQUIRING HIV INFECTION BY PORTALS OF ENTRY*

Entry Site	Type Risk	Risk Gets to Site	Risk Virus Enters	Risk of Inoculation
Conjunctiva	Random	Moderate	Moderate	Very low
Oral mucosa	Random	Moderate	Moderate	Low
Nasal mucosa	Random	Low	Low	Very low
Respiratory	Random	Very low	Very low	Very low
Anus	Behavior	Very high	Very high	Very high
Skin (intact)	Accident	Very low	Very low	Very low
Skin (broken)	Accident	Low	High	High
Sexual				
Vagina	Behavior	Low	Low	Medium
Penis	Behavior	High	Low	Low
Ulcers (STD)	Behavior	High	High	Very high
Blood products	Behavior	High	High	High
Shared needles	Behavior	High	High	Very high
Accidental needle-stick	Accident	Low	High	Low
Traumatic wound	Accident	Modest	High	High
Perinatal	Accident	High	High	High

* Data from Centers for Disease Control *Precaution Update*, 1991.

TRANSMISSION OF AIDS

HIV cannot multiply outside of living cells. When infected cells leave the host and enter the environment, the virus is unable to survive for more than a few hours. Humans are the only known reservoir for HIV. Whether infected with HIV or suffering from full blown AIDS, the individual can transmit HIV. It is believed that the higher the concentration of the virus in the blood, the more contagious the fluids of the person become. The major portals of exit for HIV include:

- blood
- semen
- vaginal secretions with or without pus

Portals of Entry

The site where the HIV enters the body and gains access to the bloodstream is called the "portal of entry." The major portals of entry are breaks in the mucosa of the genitalia or anus and needle punctures in the skin (Table 25-1).

In the United States, AIDS has been reported most frequently among male homosexuals and intravenous drug users. The remaining cases of HIV infection are among recipients of contaminated blood transfusions, female sexual partners of other risk groups, and newborn babies of HIV-infected mothers.

CLINICAL MANIFESTATIONS ASSOCIATED WITH AIDS

Since the patient with AIDS is susceptible to multiple infections and cancers, it is important to familiarize yourself with the clinical manifestations of some of the most commonly occurring diseases.

Kaposi's sarcoma. The most common malignancy that is associated with AIDS is Kaposi's sarcoma, which occurs in approximately 11% of those with AIDS. Small, purplish-brown palpable lesions that are not usually painful can occur anywhere on the body, but they are most frequently seen on the skin; they can also develop in the lymph nodes, gastrointestinal tract, and lungs. Development in the lymph nodes frequently causes **lymphoma.** Kaposi's sarcoma is diagnosed by biopsy and **histologic** examination of one of the lesions.

Opportunistic infections. Infections from a variety of organisms account for the majority of clinical manifestations seen in AIDS. The infections can be **protozoal,** viral, fungal, or atypical bacterial. Often, a patient has more than one infection at the same time.

***Pneumocystis carinii* pneumonia.** *Pneumocystis carinii* pneumonia is a protozoal infection that occurs in about 60% of AIDS patients. The patient usually complains of tightness in the chest and shortness of breath that gradually worsen. A dry cough or a low grade fever, or both, may be present. As this worsens, there may be personality changes, mild confusion, and headaches. These symptoms then lead to encephalitis, seizures, and severe confusion. Any of these symptoms may also be indicative of other diseases, such as bacterial or viral pneumonia.

Cryptosporidium. *Cryptosporidium* is a parasite that causes gastroenteritis with diarrhea and abdominal discomfort. In AIDS, this illness ranges from mild diarrhea to watery stools, weight loss, and **electrolyte imbalance.** This is known as the **wasting syndrome.**

Candida albicans. This fungus causes a disorder commonly known as **thrush.** It is a yeast infection that appears on the mucous membranes of the mouth and nose. The patient usually complains of food "tasting funny." There may be mouth pain and difficulty in swallowing. The inside of the mouth appears to be covered with a cheese-like white exudate and is inflamed.

Bacterial infections. The most common bacterial pathogen is *Mycobacterium avium-intracellulare.* The usual structures involved are the lymph nodes, bone marrow, and, sometimes, the blood. This then manifests pathologic **meningitis,** pneumonia, and severe anemias. Other types of mycobacteria seen include those that cause tuberculosis.

Viral infections. Cytomegalovirus (CMV) infection is responsible for many symptoms seen in AIDS, including:

- fever
- fatigue
- weight loss
- enlargement of the lymph nodes
- visual impairment

CMV is also responsible for liquid stools, abdominal bloating, and weight loss. It can cause encephalitis, pneumonitis, adrenalitis, hepatitis, and colitis. Herpes simplex virus is usually present in the form of ulcer-like lesions in the perirectal area. However, the possibility always exists that these symptoms may be indicative of other sexually transmitted diseases, such as genital herpes or syphilis.

Some patients experience severe wasting syndrome for no definite reason. Weight loss is persistent and sometimes becomes extreme. The patient may become very thin and complain of dry itchy skin and rashes. He or she may develop eczema or psoriasis.

PRECAUTIONS AND CONTROL

The prevention of HIV infection in the medical setting depends on three major factors:

- appropriate precautions
- appropriate supplies being readily available
- proficiency in infection control

We should add that AIDS is not a casually-contacted disease. The general patient care procedures that are done in the medical setting are not the source of AIDS transmission. AIDS is not transmitted through coughing, sneezing, talking, touching, hugging, or using the same bathroom. Comparing all the sexually transmitted diseases that are now known, AIDS is the most difficult to contract.

Although the chances of contracting HIV are low, the serious nature of the infection and the probability of developing AIDS from the infection make it imperative that the medical assistant use precautionary procedures. Since many HIV carriers are asymptomatic and may not know that they even have the virus, procedures to minimize the risk of exposure to blood and body fluids should be taken with *all* patients at *all* times. These precautions are also recommended as a measure of protection against other blood-borne pathogens, such as hepatitis B. The CDC has issued a recommended set of universal precautions for all health care workers to follow and authorized the Occupational Safety and Health Administration (OSHA) to act as the enforcement agency.

Universal Precautions

The recommendations for preventing the transmission of HIV in health care settings emphasize that *universal blood and body-fluid precautions* be consistently used for *all* patients in *all* situations, including emergency care, when there is an increased risk of exposure to blood, and when the infectious status of the patient is unknown.

The **universal precaution** system differs from the traditional isolation precaution system. The traditional isolation precaution system is based on a specific isolation technique that is used for a specific diagnosis or in the known presence of a specific disease category. Some isolation techniques include the placing of signs on doors and warning labels on specimens.

The universal precaution system is a body-substance isolation system and is not dependent on knowing whether or not a patient is infected with AIDS or any other blood-borne pathogen, such as hepatitis B. Since we cannot reliably identify all patients infected with HIV or other blood-borne pathogens, these recommendations emphasize the need to treat the blood and body fluids of *all* patients as potentially infectious.

This very simple strategy is based on the consistent application of procedures for contact with body substances of *all* patients. Implementation of the universal precaution system eliminates the need for warnings. No additional precautions are necessary, even if the patient is known to be infectious. The only exception is for airborne infections. Diagnosed or suspected airborne infections still require the use of traditional isolation techniques with regard to the patient, including the segregation of the patient from other patients and the use of masks (although the effectiveness of masks in preventing the inhalation of airborne pathogens has not been proved).

Since medical history and examination cannot reliably identify all patients infected with HIV or other blood-borne pathogens, blood and body-fluid precautions should be consistently used for *all* patients. This approach, previously recommended by the CDC and referred to as "universal blood and body-fluid precautions" or "universal precautions," should be used in the care of all patients when the risk of contamination by body fluids exists. *Treat every patient as if he or she is infected with a blood-borne infection.*

The universal precaution system is designed to reduce the risk of cross-infection of *any* infective agent in *any* body substance in *any* patient. The result is greater protection for health care workers and patients.

Barrier Protection

Medical assistants should routinely use appropriate barrier precautions when contact with blood or other body fluids is anticipated.

If you have exudative lesions or weeping dermatitis, you should not perform any duties involving direct patient care or handle any equipment used in patient care until the condition resolves. Hands and skin surfaces should be washed:

- Immediately after gloves are removed
- Immediately and thoroughly after any accidental contact with blood or other body fluids
- Immediately after the completion of any specimen processing
- After completing daily clinical or laboratory activities

GLOVES. Gloves should be changed after contact with each patient and after the handling of each specimen. Gloves should be worn during the following activities and procedures:

- Touching a patient's blood and body fluids, mucous membranes, or skin that is not intact.
- Handling items and surfaces contaminated with blood and body fluids.
- Performing venipuncture and other vascular access procedures.
- Any invasive procedure. If a glove is torn or an injury occurs, the glove should be removed and replaced with a new glove as soon as safety permits. The instrument involved in the incident should be removed from the sterile field to a safe container.
- Dressing changes. Enclose small dressings inside the glove as you remove it, by grasping the dressing as you pull the glove off inside out.
- Handling and processing all specimens of blood and body fluids.
- Cleaning and decontaminating spills of blood or other body fluids.
- Disposing bulk blood, suctioned fluids, excretions, and secretions down a drain connected to a sanitary sewer.

GOWNS AND APRONS. Cover gowns or disposable plastic aprons should be worn:

- If it is probable that your clothing will be soiled with body substances.
- When procedures are likely to generate splashes of blood or other body fluids.
- When cleaning and decontaminating spills of blood or other body fluids.

Masks and Eye Protection

Use masks and protective eyewear (eyeglasses are considered an effective barrier) when:

- Procedures are likely to generate droplets of blood or body fluids.
- Mucous-membrane contact with blood or body fluids is anticipated during the handling of blood or body-fluid specimens.
- High-speed suctioning or evacuation equipment is likely to generate aerosol contamination.
- Laboratory procedures have a high potential for generating droplets (for example, blending, ultrasonic procedures, centrifugation, and vigorous mixing).

Needles and Sharp Instruments

Special care must be taken to prevent injuries caused by needles and sharp instruments during procedures, when cleaning used instruments, and during the disposal of instruments. These precautions should be followed:

- Do not recap used needles and scalpel blades.
- Do not bend or break needles and scalpel blades.
- Do not remove used needles from syringes.
- Do not otherwise manipulate used needles by hand.
- Do not remove used scalpel blades from handles by hand. Use a hemostat to remove the blade.
- Immediately after use, dispose of syringes and needles, scalpel blades, and other sharp items in puncture-resistant containers. The containers must be located as close as possible to the area where the instruments are used.
- Immediately after use, place reusable sharp materials in a puncture-resistant container for transport to the reprocessing room.
- If a needle cap must be replaced during work with specimens, recap with only one hand. Place the cap on a clean surface, and insert the needle into it using the scoop method (Fig. 25–3). This technique is done with *extreme* caution.

Laboratory Specimens

All blood and other body fluids from every patient should be considered infective. The following precautions should be taken when handling specimens:

- Place all specimens in well-constructed containers with secure lids. Place this in a second container, such as an impervious bag, for transport. Check the bag for cracks or leaks.
- Avoid contaminating the outside of the container or the label with the specimen substance. If the outside is contaminated, the

25

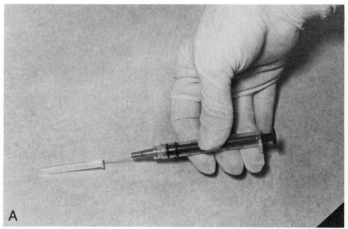

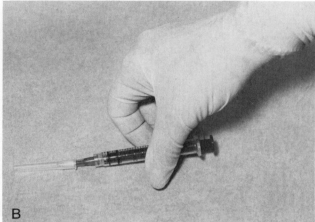

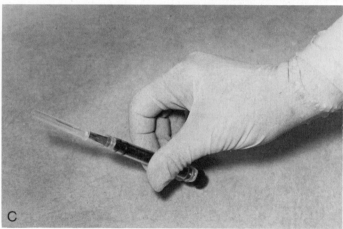

FIGURE 25–3. Scoop method of recapping a used needle.

container should be disinfected, for example with 1:10 dilution of 5.25% sodium hypochlorite (household chlorine bleach and water), and placed in an impervious bag for transport.

- Biologic safety cabinets should be used if procedures that generate droplets or spattering are performed.
- Mouth pipetting must not be done.
- Laboratory work surfaces must be immediately decontaminated with a disinfectant (such as sodium hypochlorite) after accidental spills of blood or body fluids and at the end of each procedure.
- Contaminated test materials should be decontaminated before reprocessing or should be placed in impervious bags and disposed of according to policy.
- Equipment that has been contaminated with blood or body fluid should be decontaminated before being repaired in the office or transported to the manufacturer.

ENVIRONMENTAL CONSIDERATIONS

There is no documentation of the transmission of HIV through the environment mode. However, certain precautions should be consistently practiced with *all* patients.

Sterilization and Disinfection

Current standards for sterilization and disinfection techniques are considered satisfactory for sterilizing and disinfecting items contaminated with blood and body fluids from patients infected with blood-borne pathogens, including HIV.

- Instruments that invade the tissues or the vascular system should be sterilized before reuse.
- Instruments and equipment that come into contact with the mucous membranes should be sterilized or receive high-level disinfection.

- HIV is rapidly inactivated after being exposed to common household bleach (sodium hypochlorite), prepared daily, in dilutions ranging from 1:100 to 1:10, depending on the amount of blood or body fluid present on the surface to be cleaned and disinfected. This method is inexpensive and effective.
- Many commercial germicides are effective and may be more compatible with certain medical devices and equipment that might be corroded by exposure to household bleach. Read the manufacturers' recommendations.

Housekeeping

Walls, floors, and other surfaces that are not in direct contact with treatment routines are not considered a source of infection. The strategies for cleaning and disinfecting these areas do not need to be changed. Below are standard guidelines:

- Cleaning and removing soil should be routine.
- Horizontal surfaces in the patient treatment areas should be cleaned on a regular basis, after spills, and after each patient.
- Scrubbing is as important as the disinfectant or detergent used.

Blood or Other Body-Fluid Spills

Follow the steps below to clean up all spills involving blood or body fluids:

1. Use proper barrier protections (gloves, apron, goggles, and mask).
2. First, remove the visible material with disposable towels.
3. Place the spilled material and the towels immediately into an impervious bag, at the spill site.
4. Decontaminate the area with chemical germicides that are approved for use as "hospital disinfectants." The label should state that the disinfectant is tuberculocidal when used at room temperature. Household bleach (1:10 dilution of 5.25% sodium hypochlorite with water) may be used.
5. If the spill is large, the contaminated area should be flooded with a liquid germicide and then cleaned and decontaminated with fresh germicidal chemical.
6. Dispose of all materials, including your gloves, apron, and mask, in a second impervious bag.
7. Clean your goggles, and wash your hands thoroughly.

Laundry

The risk of HIV transmission from soiled linen is negligible. Good hygienic procedures are adequate.

Wear gloves and other protective clothing, as necessary.

- Handle soiled linen as little as possible.
- Handle linens with minimum agitation to prevent airborne transmission of microorganisms.
- Bag linens where they are used. Do not sort them.
- Linens soiled with blood or body fluids should be bagged and transported in bags that will not leak.

Infective Waste

Every office should develop written policies for the removal of infective materials from the facility.

- Contaminated materials should be decontaminated before being placed in bags and disposed of.
- Infective waste should be autoclaved before disposal in a sanitary landfill or by incineration.
- Bulk blood and body fluids may be carefully poured down a drain connected to a sanitary sewer.
- Biohazardous waste must be collected in impermeable *red* polyethylene or polypropylene bags and sealed.
- Disposal methods include treatment by heat, incineration, steam sterilization, chemical treatment, or other equivalent methods that render the waste inactive.

Special Ophthalmic Considerations

- Contact lenses used for trial fittings should be disinfected with a hydrogen peroxide contact lens disinfecting system or heat (172.4 to 176.0°F, 78 to 80°C) for 10 minutes.
- Gloves should be worn during eye examinations, and procedures involving contact with tears, or hands should be washed immediately after such examinations and procedures.

Miscellaneous Considerations

- Pregnant health care workers should be extremely familiar with and should strictly adhere to the precautions associated with HIV transmission because the infant is at risk of infection during a pregnancy.
- Although saliva has not been implicated in HIV transmission, mouthpieces, resuscitation bags, and other ventilation devices should be available for use in cardiopulmonary resuscitation (CPR).

25

OSHA Blood-borne Pathogen Standards

In July 1992, OSHA began enforcing work practice controls regarding blood-borne pathogens. These controls include mandatory employee education on blood-borne disease transmission and training in universal precautions. In addition, employers must formally record all occupational injuries and be responsible for the labeling of all hazardous material located in the workplace.

OSHA has determined that employees face a significant health risk as the result of occupational exposure to blood and other potentially infectious materials because these materials may contain blood-borne pathogens, including hepatitis B virus (HBV) and HIV. OSHA concluded that this exposure can be minimized or eliminated by a combination of engineering and work practice controls, the use of personal protective clothing and equipment, training, medical surveillance, HBV vaccination, and the use of warning signs and labels.

Owing to the prevalence of HIV infection among health care workers who are exposed to blood and other potentially infectious materials in the workplace, it is not possible to estimate an "observed" infection rate. Hence, it is not possible to qualify the risk of exposure. It is known that the virus is present only in blood and certain blody fluids and that exposure to these fluids from an HIV-infected person places one at risk for HIV infection.

The best way to reduce occupational risk of infection is to follow the universal precautions. Health care workers must take adequate nondiscriminatory precautions to protect themselves. Universal precautions should apply to the handling of blood, synovial fluid, pleural fluid, peritoneal fluid, and amniotic fluid. To ensure compliance with these rules, a state-designated agency is required to inspect all biohazardous wastes and all waste generators as often as needed. *A violation of OSHA's blood-borne pathogen standards may result in fines or penalties to the employer of up to $7000 per violation multiplied by the number of employees. (For interactive training support, call 1-(800)-547-0308.)*

CARING FOR THE HIV-INFECTED PATIENT

The patient who becomes chronically ill must cope with the emotional, physical, and psychologic aspects of his or her illness. When an individual is diagnosed with an HIV infection, the emotional reactions from family, friends, and health care workers are even more prevalent. These patients are often rejected and feared and are aware of such feelings among health care professionals. As a result, the HIV-infected patient often does not seek medical help. Medical assistants need to be aware of their own feelings before they can focus on the patient's needs.

All interactions with the HIV-infected patient should be based on honesty and fairness. The patient's needs and concerns should be the focal point. When a patient is coping with a life-threatening disease, making him or her feel socially isolated places an unwarranted psychologic burden.

Many HIV-infected patients may be either homosexual or bisexual, and prejudice toward them based on their lifestyle can have a negative impact on the manner in which they are treated. The medical assistant should not view the HIV-infected patient in a negative fashion. You may feel that this patient deserves the illness and deserves to die, but these feelings must remain personal and not be reflected in the quality of the care given.

As health care workers, we must remember that the HIV-infected person has a legal right to total health care. Every patient needs to be given comfort and compassion when afflicted with chronic and possibly terminal illnesses. The medical assistant can be the patient's advocate and an aid to the physician by showing genuine concern for the welfare of the HIV-infected patient and by gaining the trust and the cooperation of the patient.

For more than a century, it has been a recognized fact that infections and infectious body specimens pose an occupational hazard to the health care worker, but never has any disease posed a more serious threat than AIDS. Fear and hysteria are commonplace, and many competent health care workers have left the profession as a result.

Every paper, magazine, and professional journal that you read has at least one article on HIV or AIDS. Many of these articles contradict each other, leaving the reader to wonder what the truth is and who can be believed.

The medical assistant *must* learn to follow the universal precautions and not attempt a "short cut" in order to complete a task more quickly. Integrity and honesty must be the prime virtues in coping with this disease and with the patients who have it. It is only through education that this disease can be brought under control, and only when it is under control can the health care worker claim victory.

AIDS is a very sensitive subject for all of us, but it may not disappear for a long time to come. In the very near future, every medical practice will include an HIV-positive patient. If you have a problem working with AIDS and HIV-infected patients, it may be wise for you to reconsider your vocational goal of working in the medical field.

LEGAL AND ETHICAL RESPONSIBILITIES

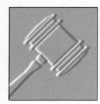

The laws and regulations regarding HIV and AIDS are constantly changing and vary from state to state. The safest approach for the medical assistant regarding information on the status of a patient is *never to disclose* his or her name or any other confidential information. Upon written order from the physician, public agencies may be given the names of HIV-positive patients. Refer all inquiries to the physician at all times.

The medical assistant's responsibility to all patients is to preserve their rights to privacy and informed consent. To perform these tasks, the assistant needs to have current knowledge of local regulations and of state and federal laws and guidelines. Every medical office should have a clear and concise policy on informed consent, and this policy should be carefully followed.

As with all sensitive patient information, there is an ethical and legal obligation to weigh the patient's right to privacy against the rights of caregivers and other third parties that require information for legitimate purposes.

▶ PATIENT EDUCATION

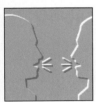

HIV patients need to understand how this disease may progress, the testing available to them, possible treatment, names and numbers of support groups, and methods of protecting themselves from new viruses and infections. These patients should be given all the latest information about their infection so that they remain well informed and can feel involved in their treatment.

The names and numbers of some groups that can provide you with information on AIDS and HIV are listed here for your use. Additional local numbers can be found in your local telephone directory.

National STD Hotline/American Social Health Association 1-(800)-227-8922
Public Health Service AIDS Hotline: 1-(800)-342-2437
AIDS Drug Assistance Program: 1-(800)-542-AIDS

National AIDS Network
Suite 300
129 8th Street, SE
Washington, D.C. 20003

With the cooperation of the physician and other medical staff, the HIV-positive patient should be taught to:

- See the doctor on a regular basis.
- Seek psychologic counseling.
- Never donate blood or other body tissues.
- Refuse to share intravenous drugs.
- Use a condom with spermicide during sexual activity.
- Refrain from oral-genital sex.
- Refrain from sharing toothbrushes, razors, or anything that may be blood-contaminated.
- Postpone pregnancy, and discuss this with a physician.
- Inform physicians, dentists, and other health care workers associated with their care of their condition.
- Inform sexual contacts of their HIV infection before becoming intimate.
- If abusing drugs, enter a drug treatment program.
- If using needles and syringes to inject insulin or other substances, soak these items in a 1:10 bleach solution and then discard in a tamper-proof container to avoid recovery and reuse by others.

REFERENCES AND READINGS

Baker, L. S.: *You and HIV . . . ,* Philadelphia, W. B. Saunders Co., 1991.
Bonewit, K.: *Clinical Procedures for Medical Assistants,* 3rd ed., Philadelphia, W. B. Saunders Co., 1990.
Hopp, J., and Rogers, E.: *AIDS and the Allied Health Professions,* Philadelphia, F. A. Davis Co., 1989.
Centers for Disease Control: Recommendations for prevention of HIV transmission in health care settings, *MMWR* 1987; 36:3S.
Centers for Disease Control: Universal precautions for prevention of transmission of HIV, hepatitis B virus, and other blood-borne pathogens in health-care settings. *MMWR* 1988; 37:377.
Lane, K.: *Aids Concepts for Medical Assistants,* Chicago, American Association of Medical Assistants, 1990.
Nash, G., and Said, J. W.: *Pathology of AIDS and HIV Infection,* Philadelphia, W. B. Saunders Co., 1992.
Shulman, S. T., Phair, J., and Sommers, H. M.: *The Biologic and Clinical Basis of Infectious Diseases,* 4th ed., Philadelphia, W. B. Saunders Co., 1992.

25

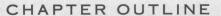

CHAPTER OUTLINE

VOCABULARY

apnea The absence or cessation of breathing.

arrhythmia Irregular pulse rhythm.

bounding pulse One characterized by increased tension.

bradycardia A slow heart beat; a pulse below 60 beats per minute.

bradypnea Respirations that are regular in rhythm but slower than normal in rate.

dyspnea Difficult or painful breathing.

elastic pulse One with regular alterations of weak and strong beats without changes in cycle.

essential hypertension Hypertension that develops for no apparent reason. Its cause is unknown. Sometimes called *primary hypertension.*

hyperpnea Increased rate of respiration.

hypertension High blood pressure (systolic pressure consistently above 160 mm Hg, and diastolic pressure above 90 mm Hg).

hyperventilation Abnormally prolonged and deep breathing usually associated with acute anxiety or emotional tension.

hypotension Blood pressure that is below normal (systolic pressure below 90 mm Hg, and diastolic pressure below 50 mm Hg).

intermittent pulse A pulse in which occasional beats are skipped.

irregular pulse A pulse that varies in force and frequency.

meniscus The concave or convex surface of a column of liquid in a tubular or cylindrical container.

orthopnea Breathing in an upright position.

orthostatic blood pressure Blood pressure measurement taken with the patient in a standing and erect position.

pulse deficit Difference between the apical pulse and the radial pulse.

pulse pressure Difference between the systolic and the diastolic blood pressures. Fewer than 30 points or more than 50 points is considered normal.

rales Abnormal or crackling chest sounds during breathing.

remittent fever Fever in which temperature fluctuates greatly but never falls to the normal level (see Fig. 25–1C).

rhonchi Rattling noises in the throat that may resemble snoring.

stertorous Describing a deep snoring sound that occurs with each inspiration.

secondary hypertension Elevated blood pressure due to another condition. *Prenatal hypertension:* Elevation of a mother's blood pressure during pregnancy; when the pregnancy terminates, blood pressure returns to normal.

tachypnea Respirations that are regular in rhythm but faster than normal in rate.

thready pulse A pulse that is scarcely perceptible.

unequal pulses Difference felt between right and left radial and/or femoral pulse counts.

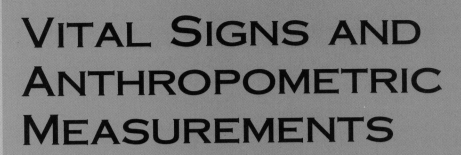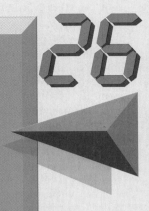

Vital Signs and Anthropometric Measurements

LEARNING OBJECTIVES

COGNITIVE

Upon completion of this chapter, you should be able to:

1. Define and spell the words in the Vocabulary.

2. Cite the normal values of body temperatures, pulse rates, respiratory rates, and blood pressure.

3. List five factors that cause body temperature to increase or decrease.

4. Locate seven pulse sites.

5. Describe pulse volume and rhythm.

6. List four factors that cause the pulse rate to increase or decrease.

7. List five factors affecting blood pressure.

8. Differentiate between essential and secondary hypertension.

9. Describe the different Korotkoff phases.

10. Cite two reasons for obtaining fat-fold measurements.

11. Discuss patient education possibilities.

12. Describe ethical and legal obligations to yourself, the physician/employer, and the patient.

PERFORMANCE

Upon successful completion of this chapter, you should be able to perform the following activities:

1. Measure the oral, axillary, and tympanic body temperatures of adults and children.

2. Determine pulse rates in adults and children.

3. Determine respiration rates in adults and children.

4. Determine a patient's blood pressure.

5. Measure a patient's height and weight.

6. Measure a patient's deltoid fat-fold.

The measurement of vital signs is an important aspect of almost every visit a patient makes to the medical office. These signs are the human body's indicators of wellness and disease and represent the general state of health of the patient. Since the medical assistant is chiefly responsible for obtaining these measurements, it is imperative for you to have confidence in both their theoretical and practical applications. When the principles of and the reasons for these measurements are understood, you will become a valuable asset to any medical office.

The vital signs are the patient's temperature, pulse, respiration, and blood pressure. These four signs are abbreviated *TPR* and *BP* and may be referred to as *cardinal signs*. It is essential to understand the significance of the vital signs in health and disease and to be able to accurately measure and record them. Anthropometric measurements are not considered vital signs but are usually obtained at the same time as the vital signs. Therefore, the procedure for measuring height, weight, and other body measurements is included in this chapter.

Asepsis (cleanliness techniques used to prevent the transmission of disease-causing microorganisms) is discussed in Chapter 23, Basic Concepts of Asepsis. This basic concept is of extreme importance and is the foundation on which all medical procedures begin.

The medical assistant must make a habit of washing his or her hands prior to seeing each patient and after each potentially infectious situation. Since you move from one patient to another, assist with examinations and treatments, and handle instruments, supplies, and body fluid specimens, the potential for cross-contamination is significant.

The aseptic technique of hand washing precedes the measurement of vital signs, the preparation of a patient for an examination or treatment, the gowning of a patient, and the actual placement of hands on a patient.

The vital signs are influenced by many factors, both physical and emotional. A patient may have rushed to arrive at the office on time or may have consumed a hot or cold beverage just before the examination. A patient may be angry or afraid of what the doctor may find. Most patients, for one reason or another, are apprehensive during an office visit. These emotions may alter the vital signs, and it is necessary for the medical assistant to help the patient relax before taking any readings. It sometimes is necessary to obtain some measurements a second time, after the patient is calmer or more comfortable. To obtain a better picture of the patient's vital signs, you may be asked to record the vital signs three times: at the beginning of the visit, during the visit, and just before the patient leaves the office.

Accuracy is essential. A change in one or more of the patient's vital signs may indicate a change in general health. Variations may indicate the presence or disappearance of a disease process and, therefore, a change in the treatment plan. Although you will obtain vital signs routinely, it is not a routine task. These findings are crucial to a correct diagnosis, and you should never perform them with indifference or casualness. In addition to accurate measurement, you must use extreme care when charting your findings on the patient's medical record.

TEMPERATURE

Physiology

Body temperature is defined as the balance between the heat lost and the heat produced by the body. It is measured in degrees. The process of chemical and physical change within our bodies that produces heat is called *metabolism*. Body temperature is a result of this process. Examples of the factors that may elevate body temperature include respiration, muscle activity, emotional changes, and sexual and reproductive activities. Temperature elevation may also be caused by external factors, such as the temperature of the environment. A healthy person's temperature varies slightly during the day, depending on both internal and external stimuli.

In illness, the individual's metabolic activity is increased; this causes internal heat production to increase. This in turn increases body temperature. The increase in body temperature is thought to be the body's defensive reaction, as heat is believed to inhibit the growth of some bacteria and viruses.

When a fever is present, superficial blood vessels near the surface of the skin constrict. The small papillary muscles at the bases of hair follicles also constrict and cause "goosebumps." Chills and shivering follow, causing internal heat to be produced. As this process repeats itself, more heat is produced, and body temperature becomes elevated or increases above normal levels. When more heat is lost than is produced, the opposite effect occurs, and body temperature drops below normal levels.

A variation from the patient's normal range of body temperature may be the first warning of an illness or change in the patient's present condition.

The Fahrenheit (F) scale has been used most frequently in the United States to measure body temperature, but many doctors and hospitals are now using the centigrade (or Celsius) scale (Table 26–1).

Normal body temperature varies from person to person and is at different levels at different times in each person. The daily average oral temperature of a healthy person may vary from 97.6° to 99°F (36.4° to 37.3°C). The lowest body temperature occurs in the early morning (from 2 AM to 6 AM). The highest body temperature occurs in the evening (from 5 PM to 8 PM). Body temperature may vary to a greater degree, and is generally higher in an infant or young child than in an adult (see Table 26–2).

TABLE 26–1. TEMPERATURE CONVERSION SCALE: FAHRENHEIT TO CELSIUS*

F	C	F	C	F	C
95.0	35.0	100.2	37.9	105.4	40.8
95.2	35.1	100.4	38.0	105.6	40.9
95.4	35.2	100.6	38.1	105.8	41.0
95.6	35.3	100.8	38.2	106.0	41.1
95.8	35.4	101.0	38.3	106.2	41.2
96.0	35.5	101.2	38.4	106.4	41.3
96.2	35.6	101.4	38.5	106.6	41.4
96.4	35.7	101.6	38.6	106.8	41.5
96.6	35.9	101.8	38.7	107.0	41.6
96.8	36.0	102.0	38.8	107.2	41.8
97.0	36.1	102.2	39.0	107.4	41.9
97.2	36.2	102.4	39.2	107.6	42.0
97.4	36.3	102.6	39.3	107.8	42.1
97.6	36.4	102.8	39.4	108.0	42.2
97.8	36.5	103.0	39.5	108.2	42.3
98.0	36.6	103.2	39.6	108.4	42.4
98.2	36.8	103.4	39.7	108.6	42.5
98.4	36.9	103.6	39.8	108.8	42.6
98.6	37.0	103.8	39.9	109.0	42.7
98.8	37.1	104.0	40.0	109.2	42.9
99.0	37.2	104.2	40.1	109.4	43.0
99.2	37.3	104.4	40.2	109.6	43.1
99.4	37.4	104.6	40.3	109.8	43.2
99.6	37.5	104.8	40.4	110.0	43.3
99.8	37.6	105.0	40.5		
100.0	37.7	105.2	40.6		

* To convert degrees F to degrees C, subtract 32, then multiply by 5/9. To convert degrees C to degrees F, multiply by 9/5, then add 32.

Fever usually accompanies infection and many other disease processes (Fig. 26–1). Fever is present when the oral temperature is 100°F (38.8°C) or higher. Temperatures of 104°F (40°C) or higher are common in serious illnesses.

Normal Temperature Readings

A clinical thermometer is used to measure body temperature and is calibrated in either the Fahrenheit or Celsius scale. The thermometer is placed under the tongue, in the rectum, or in the axilla, because large blood vessels are near the surface at these points. The normal temperature values for these three sites, based on statistical average, are:

- Oral: 98.6°F, or 37°C
- Rectal: 99.6°F, or 37.6°C
- Axillary: 97.6°F, or 36.4°C

Rectal temperatures, when taken accurately, are approximately 1°F or 0.6°C higher than oral readings. Axillary temperatures are approximately 1°F or 0.6°C lower than accurate oral readings. Rectal temperature measurement is considered the most accurate because the mucous membrane lining of the rectum with which the thermometer comes in contact is not exposed to the air and because the

rectal environment does not vary as does that of the mouth or the axilla.

When obtaining temperatures orally using the oral method of measurement, you do not have to indicate this when recording the reading. You do record an "R" for rectal and an "A" for axillary readings. In pediatrics, it is assumed that the temperature reading is obtained by the rectal method, and the "R" is omitted. An "O" is used for an oral reading.

Types of Thermometers

Glass/Mercury

An oral thermometer has a long slender mercury bulb that allows the greatest surface contact with tissues when it is placed in the mouth under the tongue or in the axilla. A short, blunt bulb is used to obtain the rectal temperature because this shape is less traumatic during rectal insertion and is se-

TABLE 26–2. CAUSES OF CHANGES IN BODY TEMPERATURE*

Increase in Body Temperature

Condition	Cause
Illness	Bacterial infection, producing fever
Activity	Increased muscular activity leading to increased body temperature
Food intake	Increased metabolism, resulting in increased body temperature
Emotions	Stress and strong emotional reactions, causing increased body temperature
Exposure to heat	Increase in heat, producing increased body temperature
Pregnancy	Increased metabolism, leading to increased body temperature
Drugs	Some drugs increase body temperature by increasing metabolism or muscular activity
Age	Infants have body temperatures that are 1–2°F higher than those of adults.

Decrease in Body Temperature

Condition	Cause
Illness	Viral infection, resulting in subnormal body temperature
Activity	Decreased muscular activity, causing decreased body temperature
Fasting	Decreased metabolism, producing decreased body temperature
Emotions	Depression and shock, leading to decreased body temperature
Exposure to cold	Decrease in heat, resulting in decreased body temperature
Drugs	Some drugs decrease body temperature by decreasing metabolism or muscular activity
Age	Elderly have decreased metabolism

* Average temperature = 98.6°F (37°C). Normal variations from 97° to 99.6°F (36.1° to 37.5°C).

26

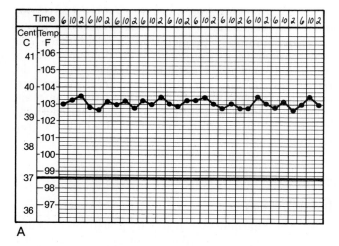

A

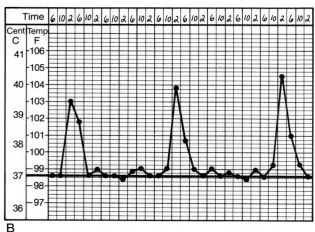

B

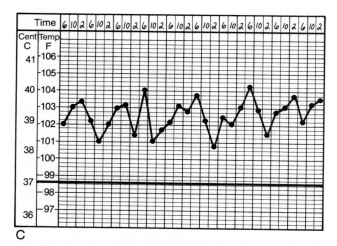

C

FIGURE 26-1. Temperature charts illustrating specific fevers. *A,* Continuous fever. *B,* Intermittent fever. *C,* Remittent fever.

curely held by the rectal mucosa (Fig. 26-2). The upper tips of both types are usually colored for clear identification (red is used for rectal measurement, and blue is used for oral measurement).

The mercury in the bulb of the glass thermometer rises upon contact with warm body tissue. After a

designated period of time, the mercury registers its highest reading and no longer rises. This is usually in about 3 to 5 minutes. The reading is obtained by viewing the calibration scale on the thermometer and noting the highest point reached by the mercury.

The longest lines on all thermometers represent 1° of temperature. On the Fahrenheit scale, the shorter lines represent 0.2° increments, and on the Celsius scale, the lines represent 0.1° increments (Fig. 26-3).

STORING GLASS THERMOMETERS. Glass thermometers should be stored in separate, clean containers, either dry or soaking in 70% isopropyl alcohol or other suitable disinfectant solution. The choice of a solution should be based on its disinfecting effectiveness and safety for use on human tissues. After use, a thermometer should not be returned to its container until it has been sanitized, then separately disinfected. At least once each week, the containers should be thoroughly cleaned and the solutions, if any, changed. Label the container as to the thermometer type, that is, oral or rectal. Patients are very alert to and apprehensive about the type of thermometer being used, where it was used last, and its cleanliness. Even though your thermometers are disinfected, you can add more protection by using a disposable sheath that slips over the entire length of the thermometer. Patients feel more at ease knowing that the thermometers do not come into contact with their bodies.

PREPARING THE GLASS/MERCURY THERMOMETER. Hold your fingers under running water to check that the water temperature is cool. Warm water will cause the mercury to rise, and you will need to shake down the mercury before using the thermometer. Hot water will break the thermometer. Rinse the thermometer clean before use. Lower the mercury column to below 95°F (35°C) by shaking with a snap of the wrist. Be sure to hold the thermometer tightly between your thumb and forefinger at the end opposite the bulb. Be careful not to strike the thermometer against a hard object, as the glass will break and the mercury will spill. Such spills require special handling, as mercury is a poisonous substance.

Electronic

Electronic thermometers are becoming increasingly popular and are available in both Fahrenheit and Celsius scales. They come equipped with disposable covers and are used to obtain both oral and rectal readings. Readings are recorded in approximately 10 seconds, and since the instrument that comes in contact with the patient is sheathed, the risk of cross-infection is greatly reduced (Fig. 26-4).

FIGURE 26-2. *A*, The cross section of the clinical thermometer is triangular-shaped. The lens must be held at eye level to see and read the level of mercury. *B*, Illustration of the construction of the bulbs. The rectal thermometer is stubby. The security thermometer is often used for the measurement of axillary temperatures. The oral thermometer has a longer, more slender bulb.

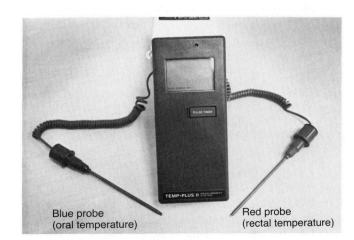

Tympanic/Surface

The tympanic membrane of the ear can also be used for the quick, accurate, and safe assessment of a patient's temperature. It shares the blood supply that reaches the hypothalamus, which is the brain's thermoregulatory control. Since the ear canal is lined with skin rather than mucous membrane, the risk of spreading communicable diseases during temperature measurement is greatly reduced.

Because clinical body temperatures are not identical at different measurement sites, the tympanic/surface measurement system allows you to optionally program a "temperature equivalence" that is applied to the actual measurements obtained in the tympanic membrane mode. For example, if you have been using the electronic or glass/mercury oral method, by selecting the oral equivalence, the tympanic membrane readings will approximate to readings to which the staff is accustomed.

The tympanic/surface measurement system consists of a processor unit, a probe module, a charger base, and a disposable speculum. When the probe gently seals the external opening of the ear canal, the infrared energy emitted by the tympanic membrane is gathered. This signal is then digitalized by the processor unit and shown on the display screen (Fig. 26-5).

Disposable

Disposable thermometers (those that are used only once) are also available for obtaining body temperatures. They are frequently used in the home on small children. The reading is obtained by a heat-

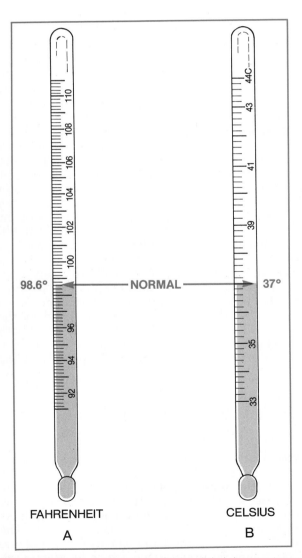

FIGURE 26-3. The Fahrenheit and Celsius clinical thermometers compared to show the difference in scales and normal body temperature, which is about 98.6°F or 37°C when measured orally.

FIGURE 26-4. IVAC digital thermometer.

Blue probe (oral temperature)

Red probe (rectal temperature)

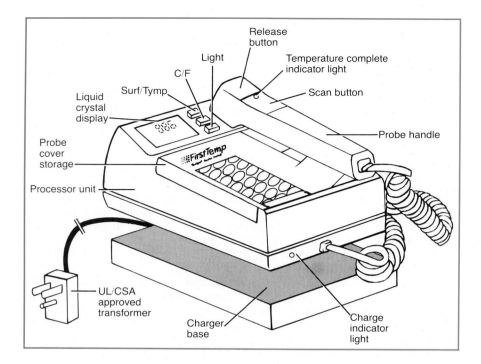

FIGURE 26-5. FirstTemp tympanic/surface thermometry system. (Courtesy of I.M.S., Carlsbad, CA.)

sensitive material that changes color according to the elevation of body temperature.

Disposable sheaths are available for use over all glass thermometers. Sheaths are used only once, thus limiting the necessity for continuous cleaning. They are uncomfortable to the patient while under the tongue and require careful lubrication when used rectally.

OBTAINING TEMPERATURE READINGS

TIPS FOR OBTAINING TEMPERATURES

- Do not take an oral temperature within 30 minutes after the patient has eaten, drunk, or smoked.

- Label containers to differentiate thermometers that are contaminated or soaking from those that are clean.

- Label rectal thermometers carefully. If you are not using the different bulb types for identification, mark the stem ends of the rectal thermometers with red nail polish.

- Keep rectal thermometers in solutions separate from the oral and axillary thermometers.

- Use separate security-tipped bulbs for obtaining axillary temperatures.

Obtaining Temperatures Rectally

The rectal method is usually required for the very young patient, patients with breathing difficulties, or patients who are uncooperative or unconscious. The procedure is the same as for the oral method, except the bulb must be lubricated with a water soluble jelly. The patient's temperature will register on the thermometer within 2 minutes. Stay with the patient or have the parent stay with the patient. Adults should be kept in the prone or Sims position until the thermometer is removed. Place an infant in the supine position. Hold the legs straight up with one hand, and hold the thermometer in place with the other. Alternatively, restrain the small child in the prone position with one hand at the buttocks, and hold the thermometer in place with the other. You must never leave a thermometer in an infant or child without you or the parent holding onto it.

Obtaining Temperatures by the Axillary Method

Recent studies reveal that the axillary temperature may be as accurate as the other methods. For example, the presence of feces in the bowel may cause a falsely elevated rectal temperature, and the rectal method is not the best choice for patients with hemorrhagic diseases such as leukemia. The axillary method is gaining in popularity in geriatrics. Axillary temperatures take more time to register the correct body temperature, but the method is safe, simple, and easily accessible.

PROCEDURE 26-1   DETERMINING ORAL TEMPERATURE USING A GLASS/MERCURY THERMOMETER

GOAL   To determine and record a patient's temperature as part of the patient assessment.

EQUIPMENT AND SUPPLIES

An oral Fahrenheit thermometer
A supply of tissues

PROCEDURAL STEPS

1. Read the directions before you begin.

2. Gather the necessary equipment and supplies.

3. Wash your hands and follow the universal blood and body-fluid precautions.

4. Introduce yourself and correctly identify your patient (Fig. 26-6).
    Purpose: To make sure that you have the correct patient.

5. Rinse the chosen thermometer under cool running water, letting the water run from the bulb to the tip (Fig. 26-7).
    Purpose: To remove antiseptic solution, which may produce a bitter taste.

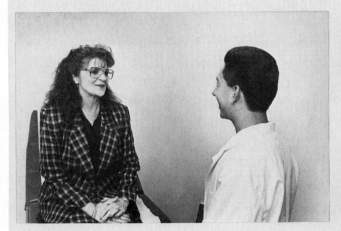

FIGURE 26-6.

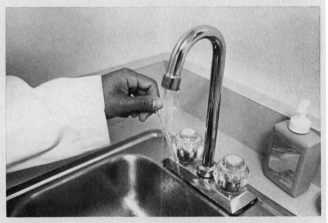

FIGURE 26-7.

6. Shake down the thermometer, allowing yourself enough room so that you do not strike it against an object and break it (Fig. 26-8).
    Purpose: To allow the column of mercury to fall to 95°F or lower.

7. Place the thermometer under the patient's tongue, and ask the patient to keep his or her lips firmly closed and to breathe through the nose (Fig. 26-9).
    Purpose: Air seeping into the mouth interferes with an accurate body temperature reading.

26

Continued

PROCEDURE 26-1 *Continued*

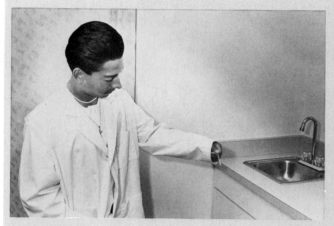

FIGURE 26-8.

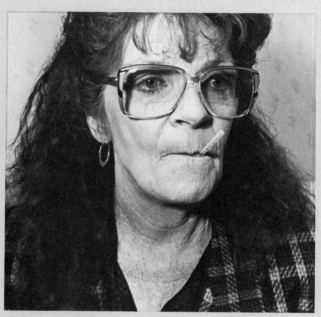

FIGURE 26-9.

8. Advise the patient that the thermometer needs to be held in place for at least 5 minutes (Fig. 26-10).
   Purpose: This is the required time to obtain an accurate oral reading.

9. Remove the thermometer and wipe it dry from stem to bulb with a tissue.
   Purpose: Wiping with a tissue cleans the surface for visibility and reduces the risk of cross-contamination.

10. Read the thermometer, making certain that you hold it at eye level. Look for the silver column of mercury, and follow it until it ends. Align the end of the column to the scale marked in degrees (Fig. 26-11).
    Purpose: Holding the thermometer at eye level facilitates an easier and more accurate reading.

11. Shake down the mercury column to 95°F.

12. Rinse the thermometer and then sterilize it by soaking it in a chemical sterilant for an amount of time prescribed by the manufacturer. After complete sterilization, dried thermometers may be stored in a dry container or in containers filled with antiseptic solution (Fig. 26-12).
    Purpose: Thermometers must be thoroughly sterilized and dried before being returned to their containers for use with another patient.

13. Record the temperature reading on the patient's medical record. Record the temperature first, followed by pulse and then respiration measurements.

Continued

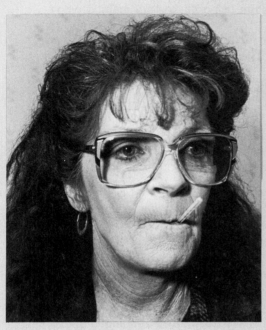

FIGURE 26-10.

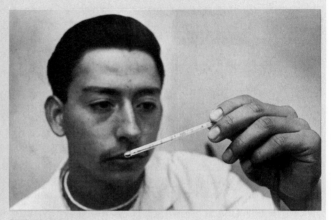

FIGURE 26-11.

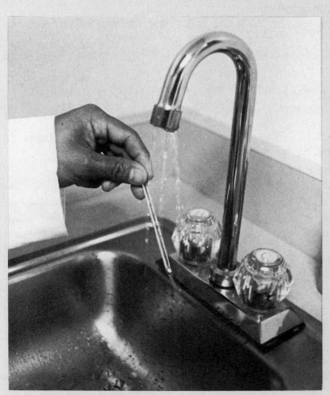

FIGURE 26-12.

PROCEDURE 26-2   DETERMINING AN AXILLARY TEMPERATURE

GOAL   To determine a patient's axillary temperature using the axillary method when requested by the physician.

EQUIPMENT AND SUPPLIES

A security-tipped clinical Fahrenheit thermometer
A supply of tissues
A towel to dry the axilla
Alcohol sponge

PROCEDURAL STEPS

1. Gather the necessary equipment and supplies.

2. Wash your hands. Follow universal blood and body-fluid precautions.

3. Introduce yourself and correctly identify your patient.
   Purpose: To make sure that you have the right patient.

4. Rinse a short-bulbed clinical thermometer under cool running water, letting the water run from the stem to the bulb.
   Purpose: To remove antiseptic solution, which may be irritating to the patient's skin.

5. Check the reading on the thermometer, and shake down if the reading is above 95°F.
   Purpose: Mercury must be at 95°F or below for an accurate reading.

6. Place the thermometer in a safe place while you prepare the patient. Use a tissue to protect the bulb.

7. Pat the patient's axilla area dry with a towel.
   Purpose: To ensure an accurate reading. Do not rub area, as this may cause an elevated reading.

8. Place the bulb of the thermometer into the center of the armpit, pointing the stem to the upper chest.

9. Instruct the patient to hold the arm snugly against the ribs with the other hand.

10. Inform the patient that the thermometer needs to be held in place for at least 10 minutes.
    Purpose: The axilla is an area where air may enter, so the time needed to obtain an accurate reading must be extended.

11. Remove the thermometer and wipe it dry from stem to bulb with a tissue.
    Purpose: Wiping with a tissue cleans the surface for visibility and prevents cross-contamination.

12. Read the thermometer, making sure that you hold it at eye level. Look for the silver column of mercury and follow it until it ends. Align the end of the column to the scale marked in degrees.
    Purpose: Holding the thermometer at eye level facilitates an easier and more accurate reading.

13. Read and record the axillary temperature on the patient's medical record; for example, "99.6°(A)," or "37.5°(A)."

14. Shake down the mercury column to 95°F (35°C).

15. Rinse the thermometer with cool running water, then soak it in a separate soap solution. Later, you can sanitize and rinse the thermometer and then sterilize it by soaking it in a chemical solution for the amount of time prescribed by the manufacturer. After complete sterilization, dried thermometers may be stored in a dry container or in a container of antiseptic solution.

Using the Electronic Thermometer

Electronic thermometers record rapidly, usually within 5 seconds, and claim an accuracy of ±0.2°F (Fig. 26–13). They have color-coded disposable tips for both oral and rectal use. The temperature reading on the dial remains displayed until it is released, which allows ample time to read and record the findings. Electronic thermometers require adjustment, and care must be taken to have the dial at eye level while adjusting it. Many models are available, and some require additional fine adjustments. Be certain to follow the manufacturer's instructions to ensure accuracy.

PULSE RATE

Determining the pulse rate is such a routine part of the physical examination that it is often taken in a mechanical way, and some of the finer aspects are neglected. The pulse rate is a method of counting the heartbeat by feeling the pulsing of an artery. What is felt is the expansion and relaxation of the artery in response to the pressure changes of each heart beat. When the heart contracts, pressure throughout the arteries increases, and the arteries expand. When the heart relaxes, arterial pressure decreases, and the arteries relax. Each constriction and relaxation of the heart muscle is a heartbeat, and each resulting expansion and relaxation of the arteries is the pulse rate. Normally, heartbeat (rate) and pulse rate are the same. The pulse rate varies from person to person. It is affected by the individual's activities and illnesses.

Since the body must balance heat loss by increasing circulation (a faster heart rate), the pulse rate is proportionate to the size of the body. The smaller the body, the greater the heat loss and the faster the heart must pump to compensate. Therefore, infants and children normally have a faster pulse than do adults.

When you are taking a pulse, there are four important characteristics to note:

- rate
- rhythm
- volume of the pulse
- condition of the arterial wall

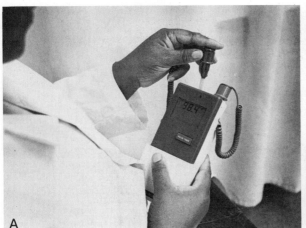
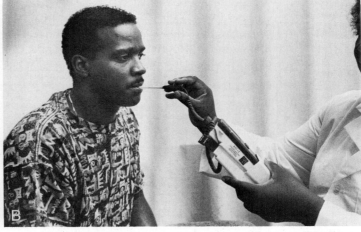
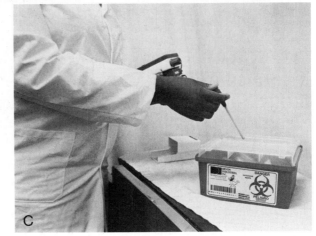

FIGURE 26–13. *A,* The electronic thermometer registers a patient's temperature within 5 seconds. *B,* Special care is taken so that the probe is inserted under the tongue. *C,* Probe cover is ejected into a biologic waste container. The medical assistant's hands never touch the probe cover.

26

PROCEDURE 26-3   DETERMINING A PATIENT'S TEMPERATURE USING THE TYMPANIC/SURFACE SYSTEM

GOAL To determine and record a patient's temperature using the tympanic membrane.

EQUIPMENT AND SUPPLIES

A tympanic/surface system thermometer
Disposable probe covers

PROCEDURAL STEPS

1. Read the directions before you begin.

2. Gather the necessary equipment and supplies.

3. Wash your hands following universal blood and body-fluid procedures as necessary.

4. Introduce yourself and correctly identify your patient.
   Purpose: To make sure that you have the right patient.

5. Explain the procedure that you will be doing.
   Purpose: To lower the anxiety level of the patient and enhance cooperation during the procedure.

6. Select "TYMPANIC" mode on instrument panel (Fig. 26–14).
   Purpose: The mode changes the general operation from tympanic (clinical temperature measurement) to surface (surface or soft tissue measurement).

7. Remove probe from the charger and wait for "READY" to appear on the display.

8. Grasp the probe at finger grips and lift it from the cradle (Fig. 26–15).

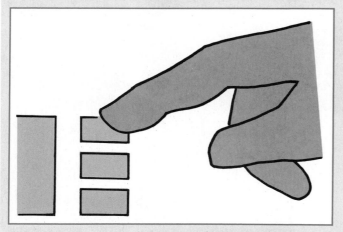

FIGURE 26-14.

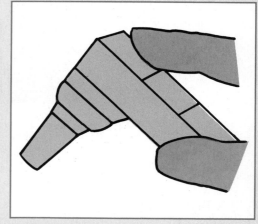

FIGURE 26-15.

9. Place disposable probe cover on probe, avoiding sharp edges (Fig. 26–16).
   Purpose: To ensure a clean surface and prevent cross-contamination.

Continued

10. Place the probe into the ear canal far enough to "seal" the opening. Do not apply pressure (Fig. 26–17).
    Purpose: Air seeping around the probe interferes with an accurate body temperature reading.

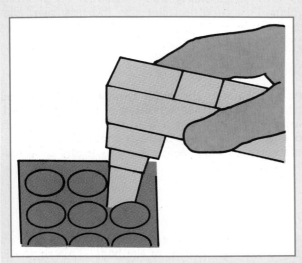

FIGURE 26–16.

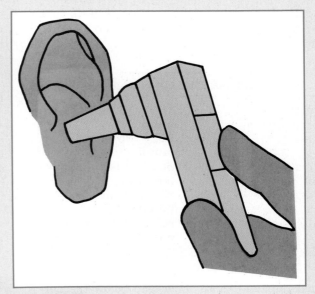

FIGURE 26–17.

11. Press the "SCAN" button on the probe.
    Purpose: To activate the system.
12. Wait for the intermittent beep to sound and the red light on the probe to illuminate (1–2 sec).
13. Read temperature on the display screen (Fig. 26–18).

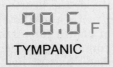

FIGURE 26–18.

14. Press the blue "RELEASE" button to discard the probe cover.
15. Replace the probe in the cradle.
16. Replace the unit on the charger base. The charge light must be on.
17. Wash your hands.
18. Record temperature results on the patient's medical record.

26

These characteristics depend on the size and elasticity of the artery, the strength of the contraction of the heart, and the tissues surrounding the artery. A patient's pulse may reveal valuable information regarding abnormalities of the circulation of the heart.

Rate

The rate of the pulse is the number of beats (pulsations) that occur in 1 minute (See chart of Average Pulse Rates).

AVERAGE PULSE RATES	
At birth	130–160 beats per minute
Infants	110–130 beats per minute
Children ages 1–7 years	80–120 beats per minute
Children over 7 years	80–90 beats per minute
Adults	60–80 beats per minute

Abnormal rates are those above and below the normal range.

Pulse rates normally vary as a result of a person's age, body size, sex, and health status. The rate is usually faster in women (70–80 beats per minute) than in men (60–70 beats per minute). Children tend to have more rapid pulse rates than do adults. When sitting, the rate is more rapid than when lying down, and it increases when standing and walking or running. During sleep or rest, the pulse rate may drop as low as 45 to 50 beats per minute. Athletes also tend to have very low resting pulse rates.

Rhythm

The rhythm is the time between each pulse beat. In a normal rhythm pattern, the time intervals between the beats are of equal duration. Abnormal rhythm is described according to the rhythm pattern you detect with your hand, and the terminology for the possible patterns is listed in this chapter section. Skipping an occasional beat (**intermittent pulse**) occurs in all normal individuals and may be more noticeable during exercise or after drinking a beverage containing caffeine. If there are frequent skipped beats or if the beats are markedly irregular, the physician should be advised, as this may indicate heart disease. It is sometimes helpful to count the radial pulse for 1 minute and then count the apical pulse for 1 minute. Record both readings. The

difference between the two is called the **pulse deficit.**

Volume

The volume of the pulse refers to the strength of the beat and is described as full, strong, feeble, **thready,** weak, hard, or soft. The force of the heartbeat and the condition of the arterial walls influence the volume. It is possible for the pulse to vary only in intensity and otherwise be perfectly regular. This condition can also indicate heart disease.

Condition of the Arterial Wall

As you palpate the pulse through the skin, you must also evaluate the condition of the arterial wall. Normally, the wall would be described as being soft and elastic. Abnormal findings include hard, ropelike, knotty, or wiry-feeling vessels, or any combination of these.

Pulse Sites

A pulse rate may be counted anyplace where an artery is near the surface of the body. This rhythmic throbbing may be felt at the following arteries: radial, brachial, carotid, temporal, femoral, popliteal, and dorsalis pedis (Fig. 26–19).

The radial artery is the most frequently used site for counting the pulse rate. It is best found on the thumb side of the wrist, 1 inch above the base of the thumb.

The brachial pulse is felt at the inner (antecubital) aspect of the elbow. It is the artery heard and felt when taking a blood pressure. It is also felt in the groove between the biceps and triceps muscles on the inner surface of the arm, just above the elbow.

The apical heart rate, or the heartbeat at the apex of the heart, is heard with a stethoscope. It is frequently the method of choice for infants and young children. An apical count may be requested if the patient is taking cardiac drugs or has **bradycardia** (slow heartbeat) or a rapid, irregular pulse at one of the other pulse sites. The physician may listen to the apical beat while you count the pulse at another site. This is to determine equal pulse between the heartbeat and the artery. The stethoscope is placed just below the left breast. Count for 1 minute, and note the method by placing an "AP" beside the recorded count.

The apex of the heart is located in the left fifth intercostal space on the midclavicular line, that is, between the fifth and sixth ribs on a line with the midpoint of the left clavicle, usually just below the nipple.

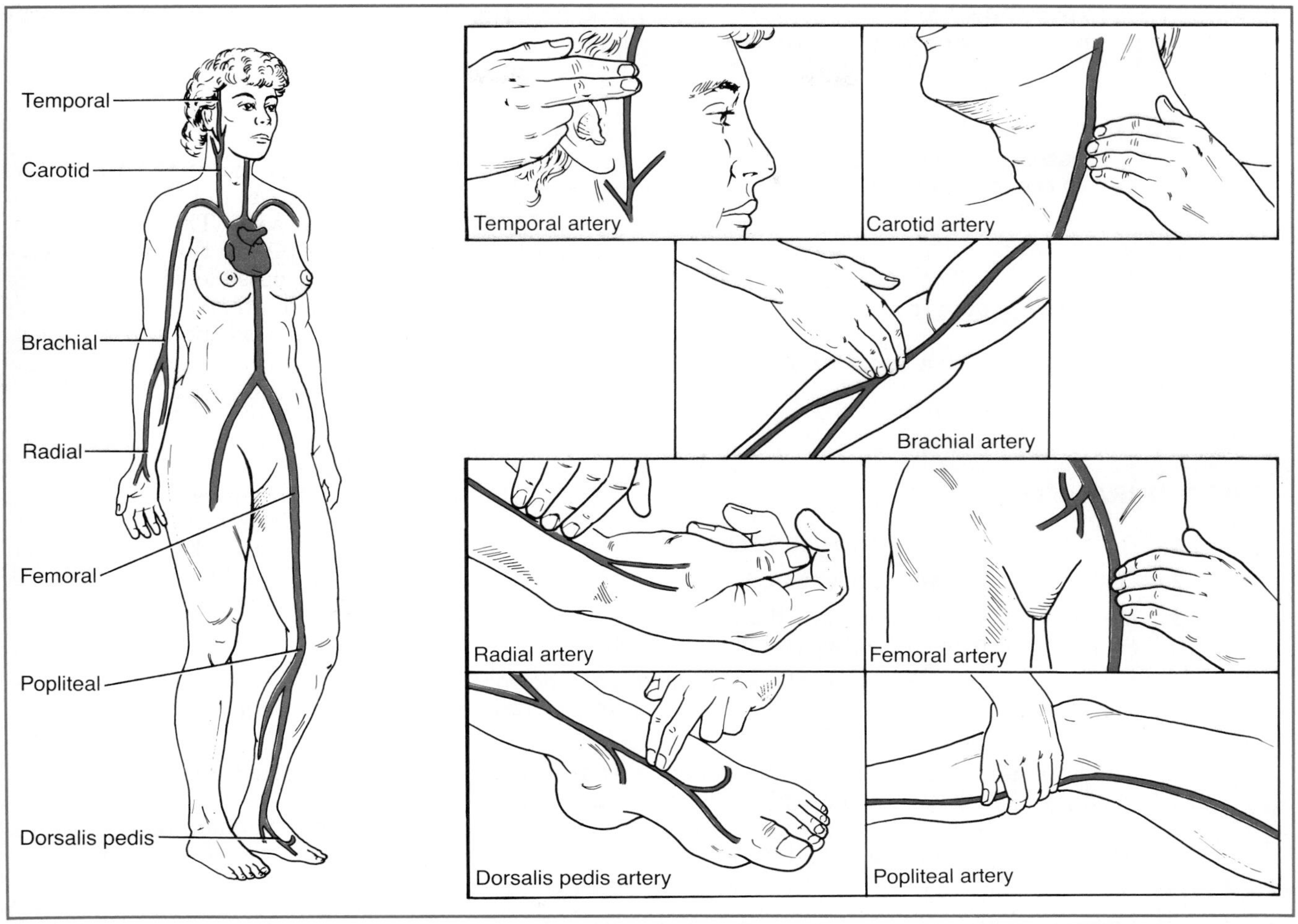

FIGURE 26-19. The pulse sites. Although the radial artery is the most frequently used, it is important for the medical assistant to be able to obtain a pulse rate from any of the alternative sites.

The carotid artery is located between the larynx and the sternocleidomastoid muscle in the front and to the side of the neck. It is most frequently used in emergencies and during cardiopulmonary resuscitation (CPR). It can be felt by pushing the muscle to the side and pressing against the larynx.

The femoral pulse is located at the site where the femoral artery passes through the groin. One must press deeply below the inguinal ligament. The popliteal pulse is found at the back of the knee. The patient must be in a recumbent position, with the knee slightly flexed. The popliteal artery is deep and difficult to feel. This artery is palpated and listened to with the stethoscope when a leg blood pressure reading is necessary. The dorsalis pedis artery is felt on the top of the foot, just slightly lateral to the midline, beside the extensor tendon of the great toe. This pulse may be congenitally absent in some patients. A good pulse rate at this site is an indicator of normal lower limb circulation and arterial sufficiency.

Determining Pulse Rate

The patient should be in a comfortable position, with the artery to be used at the same level as or lower than the heart. The limb should be well supported and relaxed. The patient may be lying down or sitting. As with all pulse readings, the pads of your first three fingers are placed over the artery with slight pressure. The pulse is counted for 1 minute, and any irregularities or variations from the normal quality, such as **arrhythmias** or pulses that are **thready, elastic, intermittent, irregular, bounding,** or **unequal** are noted and recorded. Some pulses are more difficult to feel than are others, and the correct pressures to be used for each patient and site require practice and experience. Both you and your patient should be in relaxed positions. The sensitivity in your counting fingers is greatly reduced if you are in an awkward position. Too much pressure obliterates the patient's pulse and too little pressure prevents detection of irregu-

26

PROCEDURE 26-4   DETERMINING PULSE RATE

GOAL To determine and record a patient's pulse rate as part of the general physical assessment procedure. (Note: When TPR measurements are ordered, it is advisable to count the patient's pulse while the thermometer is in his or her mouth.)

EQUIPMENT AND SUPPLIES

A watch with a second hand

PROCEDURAL STEPS

1. Read the directions before you begin.
2. Gather the necessary equipment.
3. Introduce yourself and identify the patient.
   Purpose: To make sure that you have the right patient.
4. Place the patient's arm in a relaxed position, palm downward.
   Purpose: The patient's radial artery is more easily palpated when the patient is relaxed and in this position.
5. Gently grasp the palm side of the patient's wrist with your first three fingertips approximately 1 inch above the base of the thumb (Fig. 26-20).
   Purpose: This position puts your fingertips directly over the artery. If you press too hard, you will occlude the artery and feel nothing.

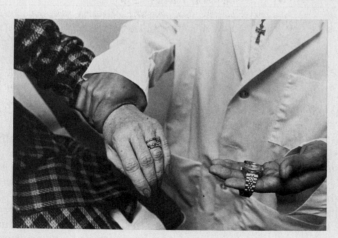

FIGURE 26-20.

6. Count the beats for 1 minute, using a watch with a second hand.
   Purpose: Counting for the full minute allows you to obtain an accurate count, including any irregularities in rhythm and volume.
7. Record the count and any irregularities on the patient's medical record. Pulse is usually recorded immediately after the temperature.

THE HUMAN BODY

Highlights of Structure and Function
Plate 1 ■ SKELETAL SYSTEM

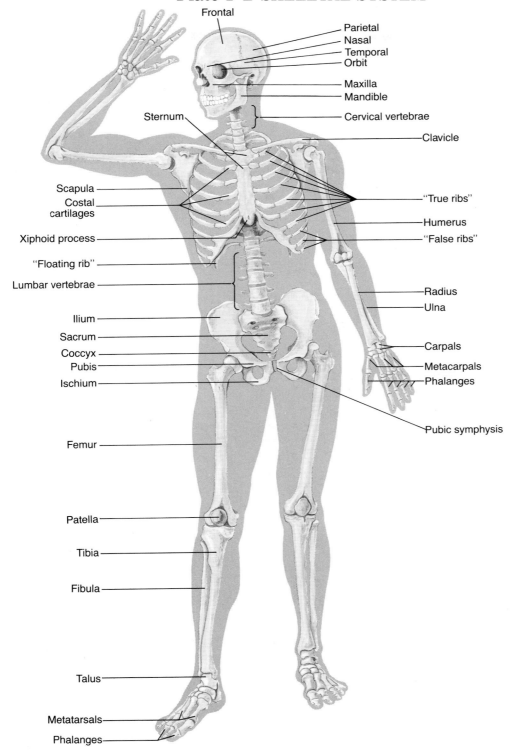

Frontal
Parietal
Nasal
Temporal
Orbit
Maxilla
Mandible
Cervical vertebrae
Clavicle
Sternum
Scapula
Costal cartilages
"True ribs"
Humerus
"False ribs"
Xiphoid process
"Floating rib"
Lumbar vertebrae
Radius
Ulna
Ilium
Sacrum
Coccyx
Carpals
Pubis
Metacarpals
Ischium
Phalanges
Pubic symphysis
Femur
Patella
Tibia
Fibula
Talus
Metatarsals
Phalanges

Plate 2 ■ SKELETAL SYSTEM Continued

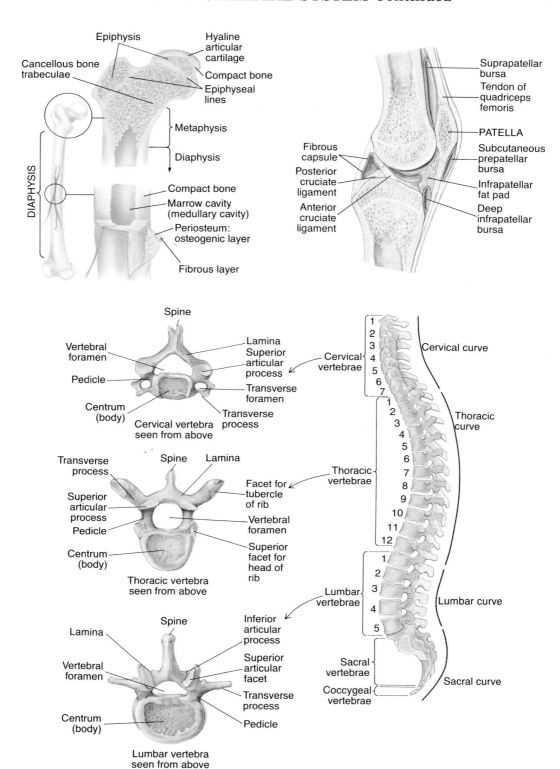

Epiphysis

Hyaline articular cartilage

Cancellous bone trabeculae

Compact bone

Epiphyseal lines

Metaphysis

Diaphysis

DIAPHYSIS

Compact bone

Marrow cavity (medullary cavity)

Periosteum: osteogenic layer

Fibrous layer

Suprapatellar bursa

Tendon of quadriceps femoris

PATELLA

Fibrous capsule

Subcutaneous prepatellar bursa

Posterior cruciate ligament

Infrapatellar fat pad

Anterior cruciate ligament

Deep infrapatellar bursa

Spine

Vertebral foramen

Lamina

Superior articular process

Pedicle

Transverse foramen

Centrum (body)

Transverse process

Cervical vertebra seen from above

Transverse process

Spine

Lamina

Superior articular process

Facet for tubercle of rib

Pedicle

Vertebral foramen

Centrum (body)

Superior facet for head of rib

Thoracic vertebra seen from above

Lamina

Spine

Inferior articular process

Vertebral foramen

Superior articular facet

Transverse process

Centrum (body)

Pedicle

Lumbar vertebra seen from above

Cervical vertebrae
1 2 3 4 5 6 7

Cervical curve

Thoracic vertebrae
1 2 3 4 5 6 7 8 9 10 11 12

Thoracic curve

Lumbar vertebrae
1 2 3 4 5

Lumbar curve

Sacral vertebrae

Coccygeal vertebrae

Sacral curve

Plate 3 ■ ANTERIOR SUPERFICIAL MUSCLES

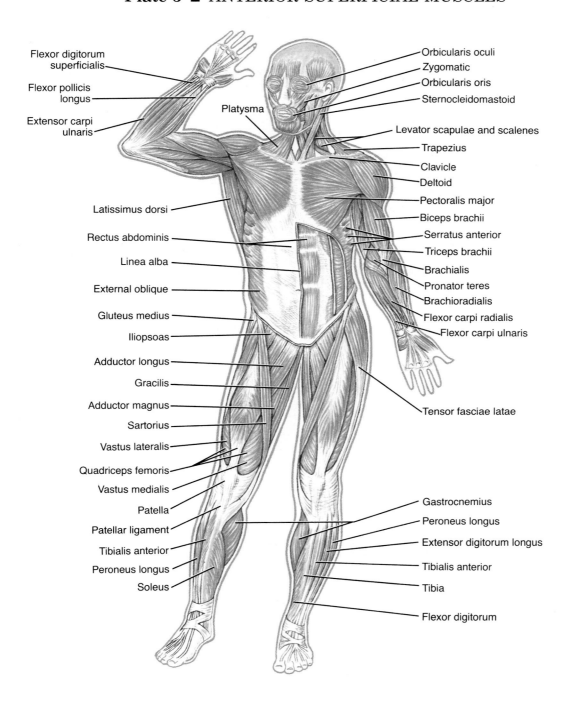

Flexor digitorum superficialis

Flexor pollicis longus

Extensor carpi ulnaris

Platysma

Latissimus dorsi

Rectus abdominis

Linea alba

External oblique

Gluteus medius

Iliopsoas

Adductor longus

Gracilis

Adductor magnus

Sartorius

Vastus lateralis

Quadriceps femoris

Vastus medialis

Patella

Patellar ligament

Tibialis anterior

Peroneus longus

Soleus

Orbicularis oculi

Zygomatic

Orbicularis oris

Sternocleidomastoid

Levator scapulae and scalenes

Trapezius

Clavicle

Deltoid

Pectoralis major

Biceps brachii

Serratus anterior

Triceps brachii

Brachialis

Pronator teres

Brachioradialis

Flexor carpi radialis

Flexor carpi ulnaris

Tensor fasciae latae

Gastrocnemius

Peroneus longus

Extensor digitorum longus

Tibialis anterior

Tibia

Flexor digitorum

Plate 4 ■ ANTERIOR DEEP MUSCLES

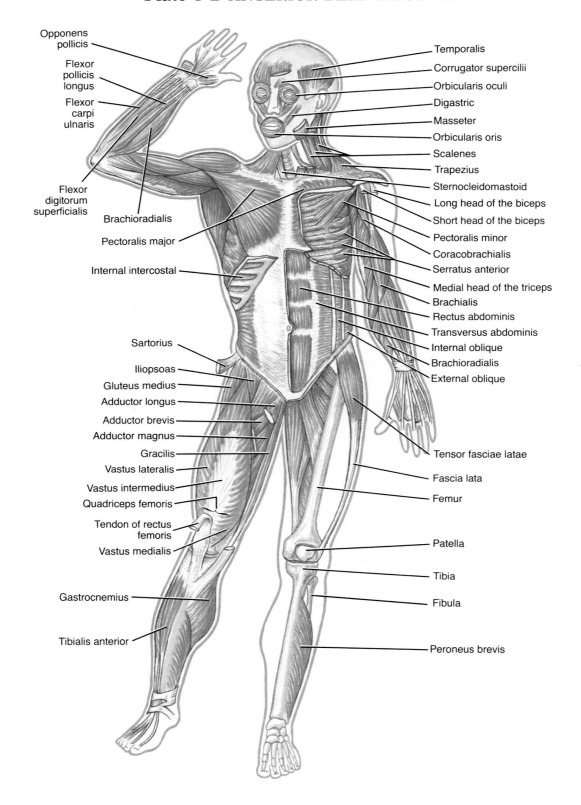

Opponens pollicis

Flexor pollicis longus

Flexor carpi ulnaris

Flexor digitorum superficialis

Brachioradialis

Pectoralis major

Internal intercostal

Sartorius

Iliopsoas

Gluteus medius

Adductor longus

Adductor brevis

Adductor magnus

Gracilis

Vastus lateralis

Vastus intermedius

Quadriceps femoris

Tendon of rectus femoris

Vastus medialis

Gastrocnemius

Tibialis anterior

Temporalis

Corrugator supercilii

Orbicularis oculi

Digastric

Masseter

Orbicularis oris

Scalenes

Trapezius

Sternocleidomastoid

Long head of the biceps

Short head of the biceps

Pectoralis minor

Coracobrachialis

Serratus anterior

Medial head of the triceps

Brachialis

Rectus abdominis

Transversus abdominis

Internal oblique

Brachioradialis

External oblique

Tensor fasciae latae

Fascia lata

Femur

Patella

Tibia

Fibula

Peroneus brevis

Plate 5 ■ POSTERIOR SUPERFICIAL MUSCLES

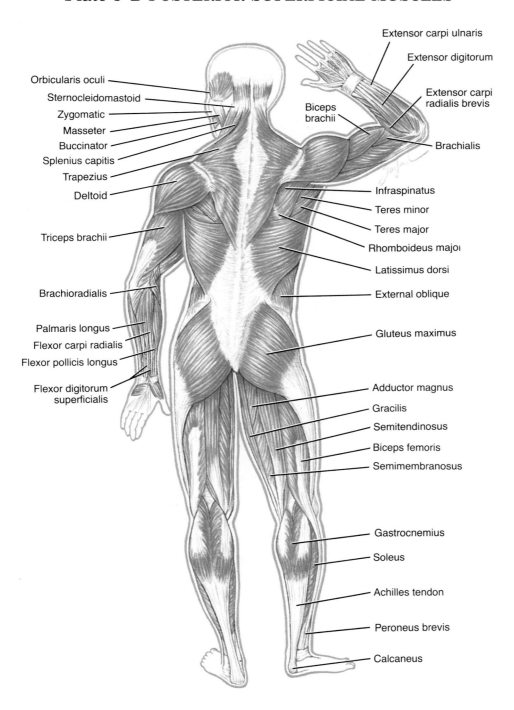

Orbicularis oculi

Sternocleidomastoid

Zygomatic

Masseter

Buccinator

Splenius capitis

Trapezius

Deltoid

Triceps brachii

Brachioradialis

Palmaris longus

Flexor carpi radialis

Flexor pollicis longus

Flexor digitorum
superficialis

Extensor carpi ulnaris

Extensor digitorum

Extensor carpi
radialis brevis

Biceps
brachii

Brachialis

Infraspinatus

Teres minor

Teres major

Rhomboideus major

Latissimus dorsi

External oblique

Gluteus maximus

Adductor magnus

Gracilis

Semitendinosus

Biceps femoris

Semimembranosus

Gastrocnemius

Soleus

Achilles tendon

Peroneus brevis

Calcaneus

Plate 6 ■ POSTERIOR DEEP MUSCLES

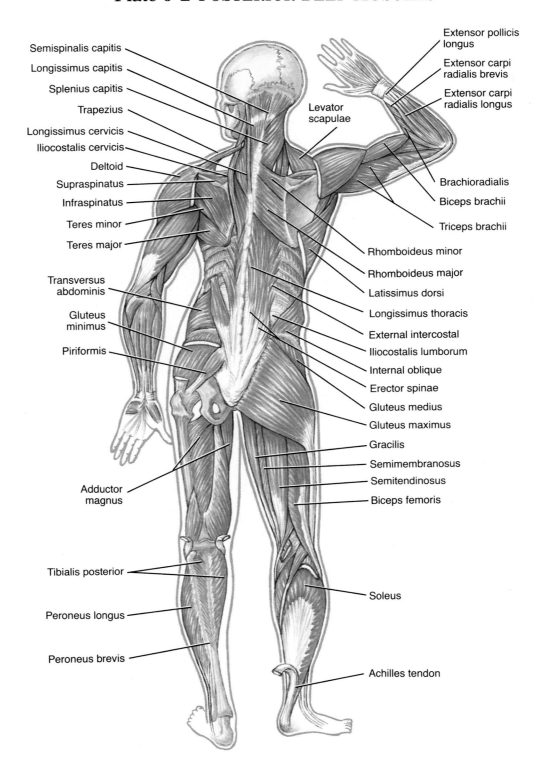

Semispinalis capitis

Longissimus capitis

Splenius capitis

Trapezius

Longissimus cervicis

Iliocostalis cervicis

Deltoid

Supraspinatus

Infraspinatus

Teres minor

Teres major

Transversus abdominis

Gluteus minimus

Piriformis

Adductor magnus

Tibialis posterior

Peroneus longus

Peroneus brevis

Levator scapulae

Extensor pollicis longus

Extensor carpi radialis brevis

Extensor carpi radialis longus

Brachioradialis

Biceps brachii

Triceps brachii

Rhomboideus minor

Rhomboideus major

Latissimus dorsi

Longissimus thoracis

External intercostal

Iliocostalis lumborum

Internal oblique

Erector spinae

Gluteus medius

Gluteus maximus

Gracilis

Semimembranosus

Semitendinosus

Biceps femoris

Soleus

Achilles tendon

Plate 7 ■ HEART AND RESPIRATORY SYSTEM

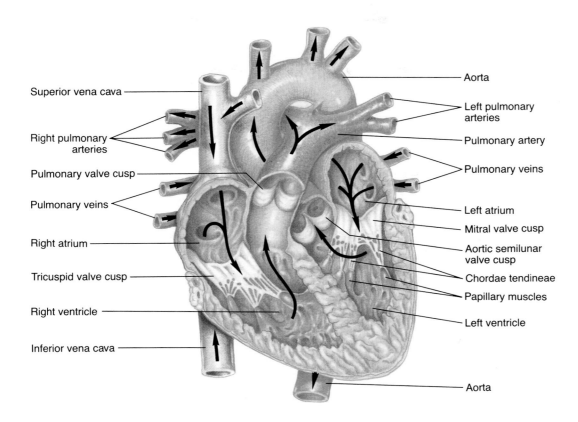

Superior vena cava

Right pulmonary arteries

Pulmonary valve cusp

Pulmonary veins

Right atrium

Tricuspid valve cusp

Right ventricle

Inferior vena cava

Aorta

Left pulmonary arteries

Pulmonary artery

Pulmonary veins

Left atrium

Mitral valve cusp

Aortic semilunar valve cusp

Chordae tendineae

Papillary muscles

Left ventricle

Aorta

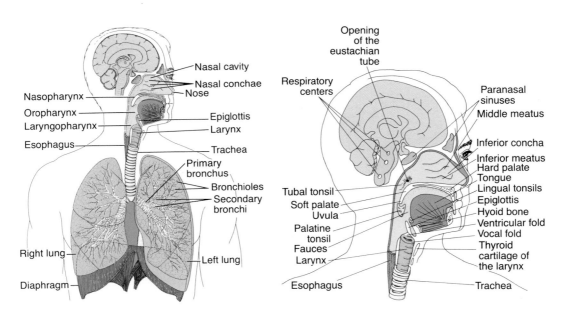

Nasal cavity

Nasal conchae

Nose

Nasopharynx

Oropharynx

Laryngopharynx

Esophagus

Epiglottis

Larynx

Trachea

Primary bronchus

Bronchioles

Secondary bronchi

Right lung

Left lung

Diaphragm

Opening of the eustachian tube

Respiratory centers

Paranasal sinuses

Middle meatus

Inferior concha

Inferior meatus

Hard palate

Tongue

Lingual tonsils

Epiglottis

Hyoid bone

Ventricular fold

Vocal fold

Thyroid cartilage of the larynx

Trachea

Tubal tonsil

Soft palate

Uvula

Palatine tonsil

Fauces

Larynx

Esophagus

Plate 8 ■ CIRCULATORY SYSTEM—BLOOD

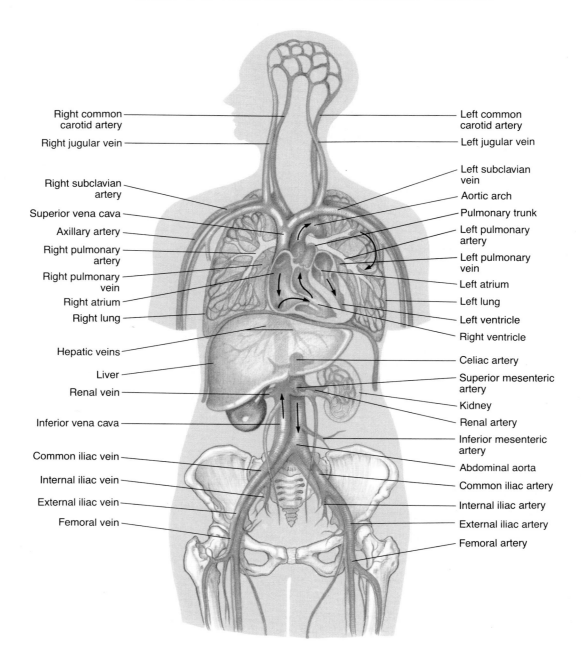

Right common carotid artery

Right jugular vein

Right subclavian artery

Superior vena cava

Axillary artery

Right pulmonary artery

Right pulmonary vein

Right atrium

Right lung

Hepatic veins

Liver

Renal vein

Inferior vena cava

Common iliac vein

Internal iliac vein

External iliac vein

Femoral vein

Left common carotid artery

Left jugular vein

Left subclavian vein

Aortic arch

Pulmonary trunk

Left pulmonary artery

Left pulmonary vein

Left atrium

Left lung

Left ventricle

Right ventricle

Celiac artery

Superior mesenteric artery

Kidney

Renal artery

Inferior mesenteric artery

Abdominal aorta

Common iliac artery

Internal iliac artery

External iliac artery

Femoral artery

Plate 9 ■ CIRCULATORY SYSTEM—LYMPH

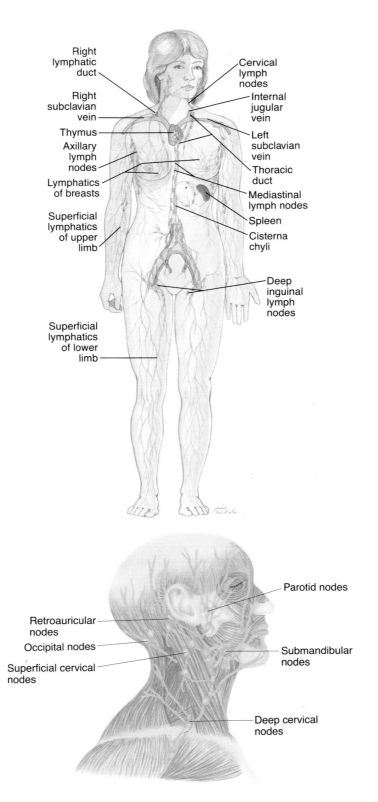

Right
lymphatic
duct

Right
subclavian
vein

Thymus

Axillary
lymph
nodes

Lymphatics
of breasts

Superficial
lymphatics
of upper
limb

Superficial
lymphatics
of lower
limb

Cervical
lymph
nodes

Internal
jugular
vein

Left
subclavian
vein

Thoracic
duct

Mediastinal
lymph nodes

Spleen

Cisterna
chyli

Deep
inguinal
lymph
nodes

Retroauricular
nodes

Occipital nodes

Superficial cervical
nodes

Parotid nodes

Submandibular
nodes

Deep cervical
nodes

Plate 10 ■ DIGESTIVE SYSTEM

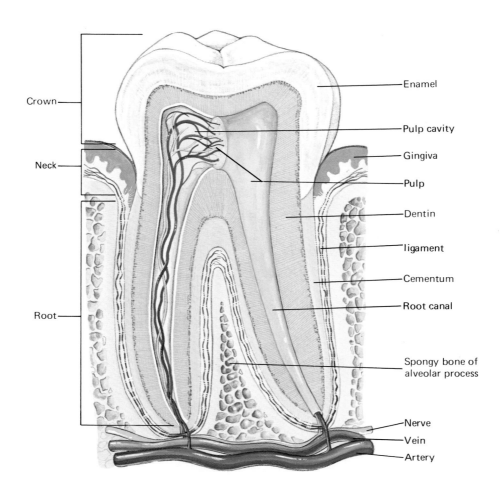

Crown

Neck

Root

Enamel

Pulp cavity

Gingiva

Pulp

Dentin

ligament

Cementum

Root canal

Spongy bone of
alveolar process

Nerve

Vein

Artery

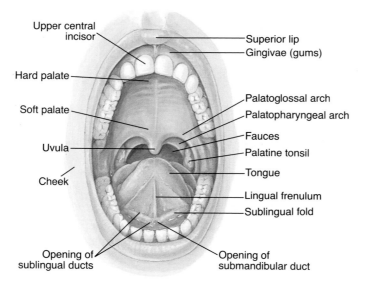

Upper central
incisor

Hard palate

Soft palate

Uvula

Cheek

Opening of
sublingual ducts

Superior lip

Gingivae (gums)

Palatoglossal arch

Palatopharyngeal arch

Fauces

Palatine tonsil

Tongue

Lingual frenulum

Sublingual fold

Opening of
submandibular duct

Plate 11 ■ DIGESTIVE SYSTEM Continued

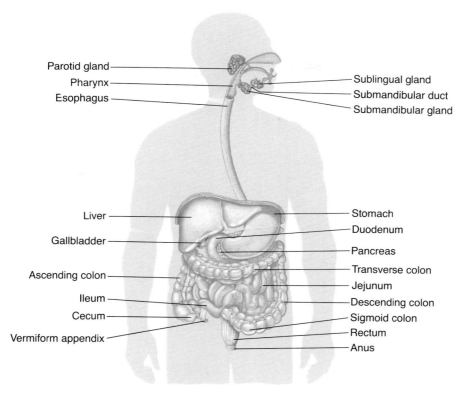

Parotid gland
Pharynx
Esophagus

Sublingual gland
Submandibular duct
Submandibular gland

Liver
Gallbladder
Ascending colon
Ileum
Cecum
Vermiform appendix

Stomach
Duodenum
Pancreas
Transverse colon
Jejunum
Descending colon
Sigmoid colon
Rectum
Anus

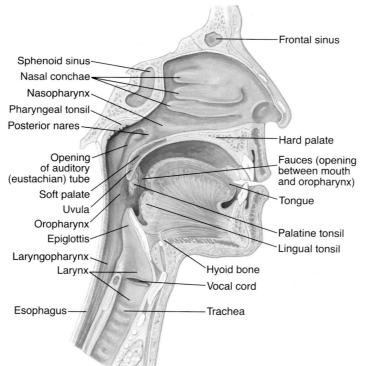

Frontal sinus

Sphenoid sinus
Nasal conchae
Nasopharynx
Pharyngeal tonsil
Posterior nares

Opening
of auditory
(eustachian) tube
Soft palate
Uvula
Oropharynx
Epiglottis
Laryngopharynx
Larynx

Esophagus

Hard palate
Fauces (opening
between mouth
and oropharynx)
Tongue

Palatine tonsil
Lingual tonsil

Hyoid bone
Vocal cord

Trachea

Plate 12 ■ GENITOURINARY SYSTEM

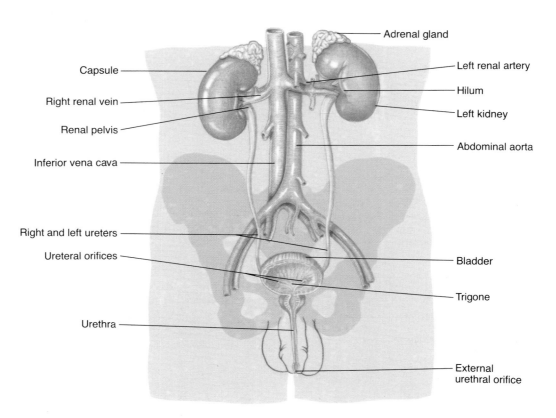

Adrenal gland

Capsule

Left renal artery

Right renal vein

Hilum

Renal pelvis

Left kidney

Inferior vena cava

Abdominal aorta

Right and left ureters

Ureteral orifices

Bladder

Trigone

Urethra

External
urethral orifice

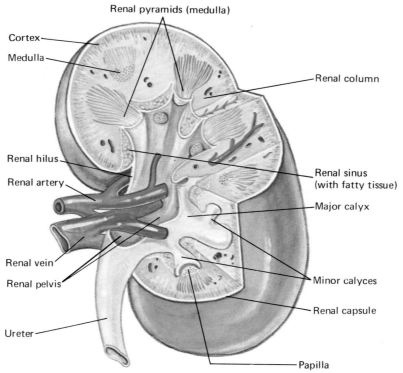

Renal pyramids (medulla)

Cortex

Medulla

Renal column

Renal hilus

Renal sinus
(with fatty tissue)

Renal artery

Major calyx

Renal vein

Renal pelvis

Minor calyces

Ureter

Renal capsule

Papilla

Plate 13 ■ GENITOURINARY SYSTEM Continued

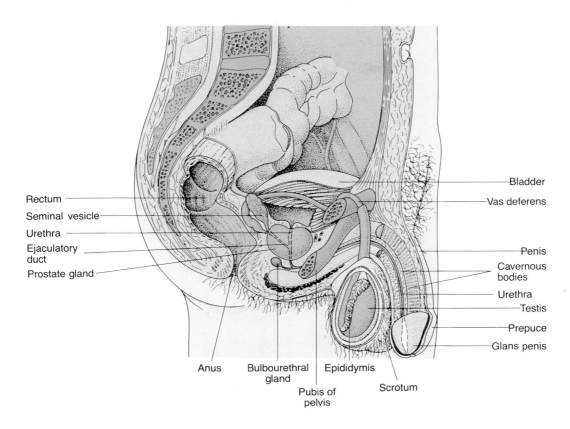

Rectum

Seminal vesicle

Urethra

Ejaculatory
duct

Prostate gland

Bladder

Vas deferens

Penis

Cavernous
bodies

Urethra

Testis

Prepuce

Glans penis

Anus   Bulbourethral   Epididymis
                  gland

Pubis of
pelvis

Scrotum

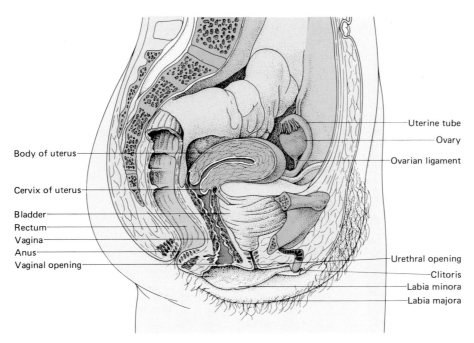

Body of uterus

Cervix of uterus

Bladder

Rectum

Vagina

Anus

Vaginal opening

Uterine tube

Ovary

Ovarian ligament

Urethral opening

Clitoris

Labia minora

Labia majora

Plate 14 ■ NERVOUS SYSTEM

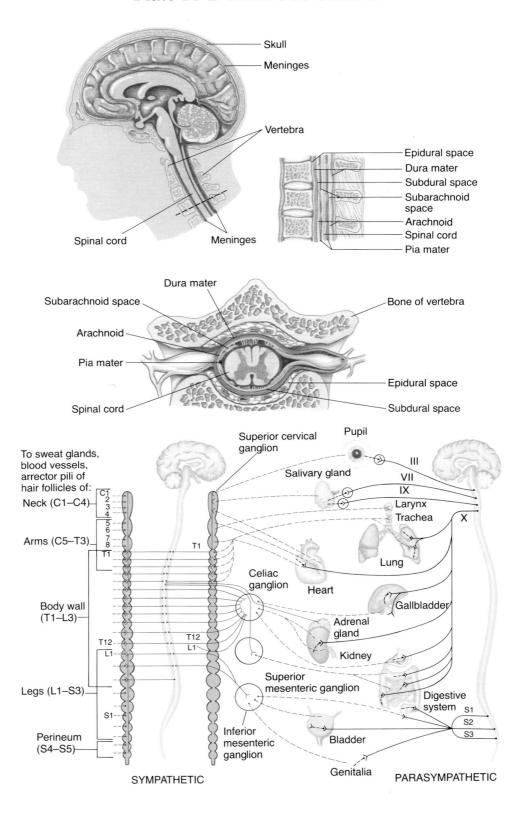

Skull

Meninges

Vertebra

Epidural space

Dura mater

Subdural space

Subarachnoid space

Arachnoid

Spinal cord

Pia mater

Spinal cord

Meninges

Dura mater

Subarachnoid space

Bone of vertebra

Arachnoid

Pia mater

Epidural space

Spinal cord

Subdural space

To sweat glands, blood vessels, arrector pili of hair follicles of:

Superior cervical ganglion

Pupil

Salivary gland

III

VII

IX

Larynx

Trachea

X

Neck (C1–C4)

C1
2
3
4

Arms (C5–T3)

5
6
7
8
T1

T1

Body wall (T1–L3)

Celiac ganglion

Heart

Lung

Gallbladder

Adrenal gland

Kidney

T12

L1

T12
L1

Legs (L1–S3)

Superior mesenteric ganglion

Digestive system

S1

S1
S2
S3

Perineum (S4–S5)

Inferior mesenteric ganglion

Bladder

Genitalia

SYMPATHETIC

PARASYMPATHETIC

Plate 15 ■ NERVOUS SYSTEM Continued

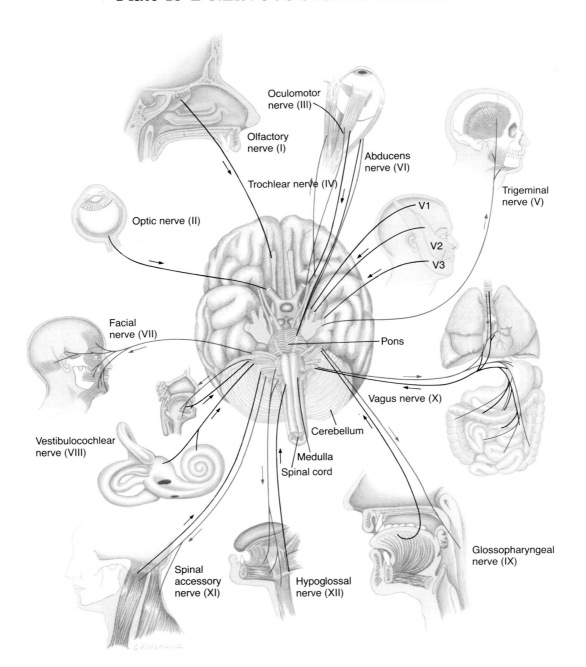

Oculomotor
nerve (III)

Olfactory
nerve (I)

Abducens
nerve (VI)

Trochlear nerve (IV)

Trigeminal
nerve (V)

V1

V2

V3

Optic nerve (II)

Facial
nerve (VII)

Pons

Vagus nerve (X)

Cerebellum

Vestibulocochlear
nerve (VIII)

Medulla

Spinal cord

Spinal
accessory
nerve (XI)

Hypoglossal
nerve (XII)

Glossopharyngeal
nerve (IX)

Plate 16 ■ NERVOUS SYSTEM Continued

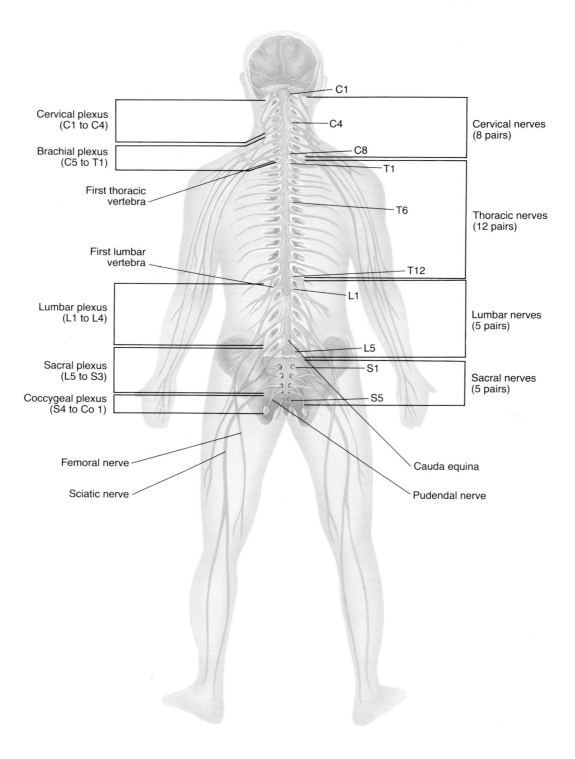

Cervical plexus
(C1 to C4)

Brachial plexus
(C5 to T1)

First thoracic
vertebra

First lumbar
vertebra

Lumbar plexus
(L1 to L4)

Sacral plexus
(L5 to S3)

Coccygeal plexus
(S4 to Co 1)

Femoral nerve

Sciatic nerve

C1

C4

C8

T1

T6

T12

L1

L5

S1

S5

Cauda equina

Pudendal nerve

Cervical nerves
(8 pairs)

Thoracic nerves
(12 pairs)

Lumbar nerves
(5 pairs)

Sacral nerves
(5 pairs)

Plate 17 ■ ORGANS OF SPECIAL SENSE

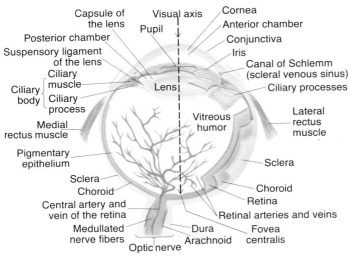

Capsule of the lens
Visual axis
Cornea
Pupil
Anterior chamber
Posterior chamber
Conjunctiva
Suspensory ligament of the lens
Iris
Ciliary muscle
Canal of Schlemm (scleral venous sinus)
Ciliary body
Lens
Ciliary process
Ciliary processes
Medial rectus muscle
Vitreous humor
Lateral rectus muscle
Pigmentary epithelium
Sclera
Sclera
Choroid
Central artery and vein of the retina
Retina
Choroid
Retinal arteries and veins
Medullated nerve fibers
Dura
Fovea centralis
Optic nerve
Arachnoid

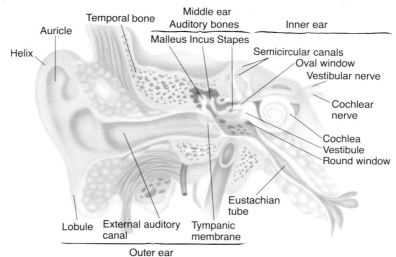

Temporal bone
Middle ear
Auditory bones
Inner ear
Auricle
Malleus Incus Stapes
Helix
Semicircular canals
Oval window
Vestibular nerve
Cochlear nerve
Cochlea
Vestibule
Round window
Eustachian tube
Lobule
External auditory canal
Tympanic membrane
Outer ear

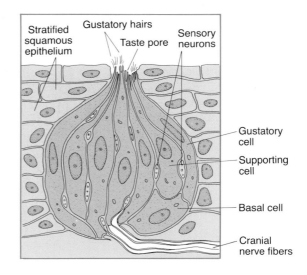

Stratified squamous epithelium
Gustatory hairs
Taste pore
Sensory neurons
Gustatory cell
Supporting cell
Basal cell
Cranial nerve fibers

Plate 18 ■ SALIVARY AND ENDOCRINE GLANDS AND SKIN

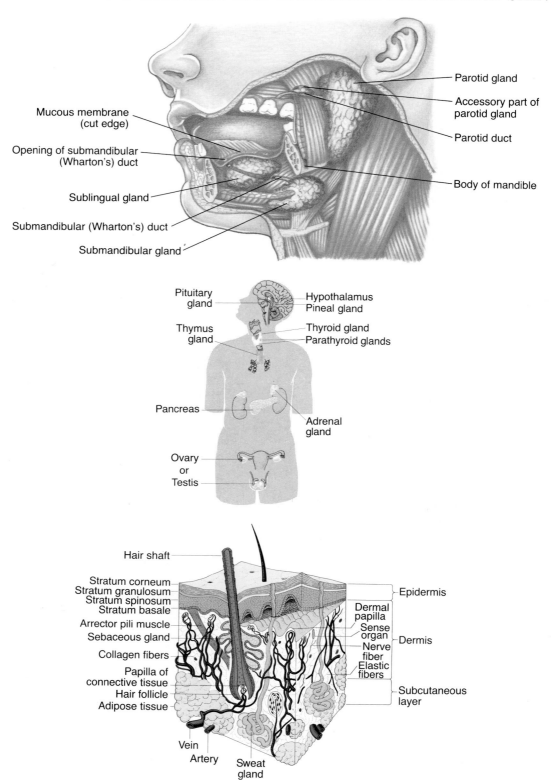

Parotid gland

Accessory part of parotid gland

Parotid duct

Mucous membrane (cut edge)

Opening of submandibular (Wharton's) duct

Body of mandible

Sublingual gland

Submandibular (Wharton's) duct

Submandibular gland

Pituitary gland

Hypothalamus

Pineal gland

Thymus gland

Thyroid gland

Parathyroid glands

Pancreas

Adrenal gland

Ovary
or
Testis

Hair shaft

Stratum corneum

Stratum granulosum

Stratum spinosum

Stratum basale

Arrector pili muscle

Sebaceous gland

Collagen fibers

Papilla of connective tissue

Hair follicle

Adipose tissue

Epidermis

Dermal papilla

Sense organ

Nerve fiber

Elastic fibers

Dermis

Subcutaneous layer

Vein

Artery

Sweat gland

larities or all of the beats. Record the number of beats counted in 1 minute. If the pulse rate is counted at any site other than the radius, the site should be recorded.

RESPIRATION

The purpose of respiration is to provide for the exchange of oxygen and carbon dioxide between the atmosphere and the blood. Oxygen is taken into the body to be used for life-sustaining body processes, and carbon dioxide is released as a waste product.

One complete inspiration and expiration is called a *respiration*. During the inspiration phase, the diaphragm contracts, causing the lungs to expand and fill with air. Then, during the expiration phase, the diaphragm returns to its normal position, causing the lungs to expel the waste air back into the atmosphere.

Respiration is both internal and external. *External respiration* refers to the exchange of oxygen and carbon dioxide in the lungs. *Internal respiration* occurs at the cell level, when the oxygen in the bloodstream is utilized and the cells release carbon dioxide as a waste product to be transported back to the lungs for exhalation.

When there is build-up of carbon dioxide in the blood, a message is sent to the medulla oblongata, which is located in the brain between the top of the spine and the brain stem. This control center sends a message to trigger respiration.

Respiration is controlled by the involuntary nervous system; this means we breathe automatically. Since a person can control respiration to a certain extent, it is also a voluntary body function. Breathing is ultimately under the control of the medulla oblongata, which is why we can hold our breaths only for a given length of time. Once the blood carbon dioxide level increases to the point at which cells become oxygen-starved, a stimulus is sent, and breathing begins involuntarily.

When determining the respiratory rate of a patient, three important characteristics must be noted:

- rate
- rhythm
- depth

Rate

The rate of respiration refers to the number of respirations per minute. It is described as *normal, rapid,* or *slow.* The adult norm is 12 to 20 cycles per minute; the clinical average for infants is 30 to 60 cycles per minute, and that for children 1 to 7 years of age is 18 to 30 cycles per minute.

Rhythm

The rhythm refers to the breathing pattern. A *regular* breathing pattern is normal in adults; however, the breathing pattern for infants is *irregular.* Automatic interruptions, such as sighing, are also considered normal.

Depth

The depth of respiration refers to the amount of air being inhaled and exhaled. When a patient is at rest, normal respirations have a consistent depth, which can be noted as you watch the rise and fall of the chest. Rapid, shallow breathing at rest occurs in some disease states.

Normally, no noticeable breath sounds occur during the breathing process; the one exception is snoring. Noticeable breath sounds are a symptom of certain diseases. When referring to breath sounds, the descriptive characteristics are represented by the use of specific terminology, such as **rales, rhonchi,** and **sterterous.** The term matching the description should be noted on the chart.

When an individual cannot inspire enough oxygen to supply all of the body's cells with oxygenated blood, the normal skin coloring—particularly around the mouth and the nail beds—turns a bluish, dusky color. This color represents the increased level of carbon dioxide that is present in the blood and is termed *cyanosis.*

Respiration Rate

The normal adult respiration rate is 16 to 20 respirations per minute. The respiration rate is usually in proportion to the pulse rate, at the ratio 1:4. It is somewhat slower in older persons and faster in infants and children. The respiration rate generally increases as the body temperature rises. Examples of the respiration, pulse, and temperature ratios follow.

Respiration	Pulse	Temperature
16	64	98.6°F
20	80	99.0°F
24	96	101.0°F
28	112	104.0°F

Variations occur in the respiratory rate (fast or slow), volume (deep or shallow), and rhythm (regular or irregular) (Fig. 26–21). There are specific medical terms to describe the character of a person's breathing. **Dyspnea,** meaning difficult breathing, occurs in patients with pneumonia or asthma. It also occurs after physical exertion or at very high altitudes. Other alterations in breathing are **bradypnea** (abnormally slow respiration), **apnea** (temporary cessation of respiration), **tachypnea** (excessively rapid breathing), and **hyperpnea** (increased depth of breathing). Hyperpnea is usually accompanied by **hyperventilation** and is frequently found

26

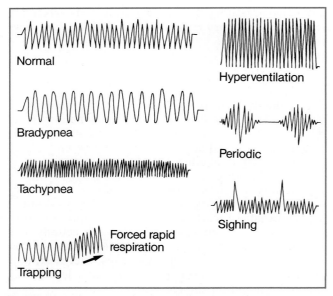

FIGURE 26-21. Various breathing patterns called spirograms, which are recorded using a spirometer.

in emotional conditions. **Orthopnea** is difficulty in breathing while lying down, as found in patients with congestive heart failure.

Counting Respirations

Because the respiration rate is easily controlled and patients self-consciously alter their breathing rates when they are being watched, it is best to count the respirations while appearing to count the pulse. Keep your eyes alternately on the patient's chest and your watch while you are counting the pulse rate, and then, without removing your fingers from the pulse site, determine the respiration rate. It may be easier to count the respirations first, as that number is not as hard to remember. If the patient is lying down, the arm may be crossed over the chest so the respirations can be felt with the rise and fall of the chest. Count the respirations for 1 minute, noting any variation or irregularity in the rate. Record both the pulse and respiration counts on the medical record at the same time.

PROCEDURE 26-5   DETERMINING RESPIRATIONS

GOAL To determine and record a patient's respirations as part of the physical assessment procedure. (Note: If you are taking TPR on a patient, the respiration count is done before or after the pulse count. Remember that the respiration count may be altered if the patient is aware that you are counting his or her breaths.)

EQUIPMENT AND SUPPLIES

A watch with a second hand

PROCEDURAL STEPS

1. Place the patient's arm in the same position as it was when you were counting the pulse.
   Purpose: This position allows you to feel the rise and fall of the chest wall.

2. Count the respirations for 1 minute, using a watch with a second hand.
   Purpose: Counting for one full minute allows you to obtain an accurate count and determine any irregularities in rhythm or depth or unusual breathing patterns, such as apnea or dyspnea.

3. Release the patient's wrist and record the respirations on the patient's medical record immediately after the pulse recording.

The pulse and respiration rates are usually counted while an oral temperature is being obtained. Doing the three procedures together is very efficient, and the patient cannot distract you with conversation. After recording the pulse and respiration counts, remove the thermometer and record that reading.

BLOOD PRESSURE

Blood pressure is the pressure of the blood against the walls of the arteries. Each time the ventricles contract, blood is pushed out of the heart and into the aorta and pulmonary artery, exerting pressure on the walls of the arteries. There are actually two blood pressure readings; the *systolic* pressure is the highest pressure level that occurs when the heart is contracting and the pulse beat is felt. The *diastolic* pressure is the lowest pressure level when the heart is relaxed and no pulse beat is felt. *Systole* (heart contraction) and *diastole* (heart relaxation) together make up the *cardiac cycle*.

Blood pressure is read in millimeters of mercury, abbreviated mm Hg. However, the abbreviations are not necessary when recording the reading on the patient's medical record. Blood pressure is recorded as a fraction, with the systolic reading the numerator (top) and the diastolic reading the denominator (bottom), for example, 130/80. The average normal blood pressures follow.

Newborn	50–52/25–30
6 years of age	95/62
10 years of age	100/65
16 years of age	118/75
Adult	120/80
Older adult	138/86

The normal adult range is: $\dfrac{100-140}{60-90}$

Factors Affecting Blood Pressure

The physiologic factors that determine the blood pressure include volume, peripheral resistance of blood vessels, vessel elasticity, and the condition of the heart muscle.

Volume is the amount of blood in the arteries. An increased blood volume increases the blood pressure, and a decreased blood volume decreases blood pressure. If a hemorrhage occurs, the blood volume drops, and so does the pressure.

Peripheral resistance of blood vessels refers to the relationship of the lumen of the vessel and the amount of blood flowing through it. The smaller the lumen, the greater the resistance to the bloodflow.

Blood pressure is high with a small lumen and low with a large lumen. Vessels affected by fatty cholesterol deposits result in increased blood pressure due to the narrowing of their diameters or *lumina* (plural of lumen).

Vessel elasticity refers to a vessel's capability to expand and contract in order to supply the body with a steady flow of blood. With age, vessel elasticity lessens, and the arterial walls become resistant; as a result, blood pressure increases.

Heart muscle condition is of primary importance to the volume of blood flowing through the body. A strong, forceful pump works efficiently and tends to keep blood pressure within normal limits. If the muscle becomes weak, blood pressure begins to increase.

Pulse pressure is the difference between the systolic and diastolic pressures and is an important measurement in diseases and trauma of the nervous system, especially of the spinal cord and brain. The average pulse pressure is 40 mm Hg. If the blood pressure is 120/80, then the pulse pressure is 40 (resulting in a 3:2:1 ratio). Conditions such as brain tumors and cerebral vascular accident (stroke) greatly increase pulse pressure.

When tracking a patient's blood pressure, frequent readings should be taken about the same time of day and by the same person. A person is said to have **hypertension** (elevated blood pressure) if the pressure is persistently above normal. Hypertension may have no known cause **(essential hypertension),** or it may be associated with some other disease **(secondary hypertension).** Essential hypertension is common among Americans. Secondary hypertension often accompanies renal diseases, pregnancy, endocrine imbalances, obesity, arteriosclerosis, atherosclerosis, and brain injuries. Temporary hypertension may occur with stress, pain, and exercise.

Hypertension has been called the silent disease because it has no symptoms, and persons may go for long periods of time without knowing that they have a problem. Often, hypertension is discovered by accident during the medical or dental treatment of another problem. Long-term, untreated hypertension is suspected to be a major cause of strokes.

Hypotension is abnormally low blood pressure and may be caused by shock, both emotional and traumatic; hemorrhage; central nervous system disorders; and chronic wasting diseases. Persistent readings of 90/60 mm Hg or below are usually considered hypotensive. *Orthostatic,* or *postural,* hypotension is the temporary fall in blood pressure that occurs when a person rapidly changes from a recumbent position to a standing position or when a person stands motionless in a fixed position, such as standing at attention. Some medications can cause orthostatic hypotension. The patient may feel suddenly dizzy and have blurred vision or may actually faint.

26

Measuring Blood Pressure

The instrument used to measure blood pressure is called the *sphygmomanometer*. The term *manometer* refers to an instrument used to measure the pressure of a liquid or a gas. *Sphygmo* means pulse. Thus, sphygmomanometer means an instrument used for measuring blood pressure in the arteries. The instrument consists of an inflatable cuff, an inflatable bulb with a control valve, and a pressure gauge. There are two common types of pressure gauges: the mercury column (Fig. 26–22A) and the aneroid dial (Fig. 26–22B). Sphygmomanometers are delicately calibrated instruments and must be handled carefully. They should be recalibrated regularly, either by you or a medical supply dealer. Check your sphygmomanometers for accuracy. The recording needle on the aneroid dial sphygmomanometer should rest within the small square at the bottom of the dial. The **meniscus** of mercury on the mercury column sphygmomanometer should rest at zero (0). Inexpensive models are available in drug stores and retail stores for patients to use to measure their own blood pressure at home. More sophisticated electronic and computerized sphygmomanometers are also available for home use.

The sphygmomanometer must be used with a stethoscope. The objective of the procedure is to use the inflatable cuff to obliterate (cause to disappear) circulation through an artery, similar to when using a tourniquet. The stethoscope is placed over the artery just under the cuff, and then the cuff is slowly deflated to allow the blood to flow again. As blood flow is resumed, the cardiac cycle sounds may be heard again through the stethoscope, and gauge readings are taken when the first and last sounds are heard.

Heart Sounds

There are two basic heart sounds produced by the functioning of the heart during the cardiac cycle. The first sound produced at systole (contraction) is dull, firm, and prolonged and is heard as a "lubb" sound. The second sound, produced at diastole (relaxation) when the heart valves close, is shorter and sharper and is heard as a "dupp" sound. The "lubb–dupp" is the sound of one heartbeat.

Korotkoff Sounds

The Korotkoff sounds are the sounds heard during the measurement of blood pressure. These sounds are thought to be produced by the vibrations of the arterial wall as the wall suddenly distends

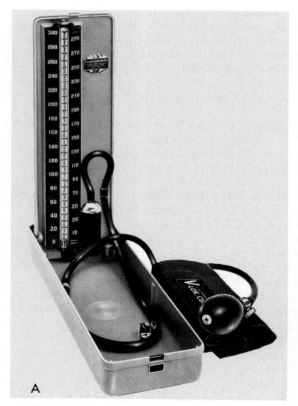
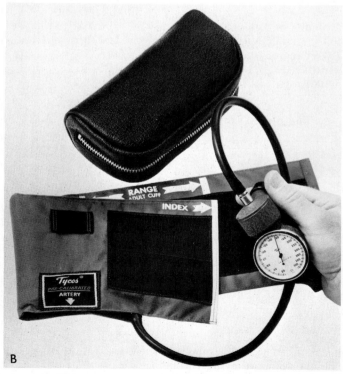

FIGURE 26–22. *A*, Baum mercury manometer. (Courtesy of Baum Co., Copiaque, NY.) *B*, Tycos aneroid manometer. (Courtesy of Tycos Co., Asheville, NC.)

PROCEDURE 26-6 DETERMINING A PATIENT'S BLOOD PRESSURE

GOAL To perform a blood pressure measurement that is correct in technique and accurate and comfortable to the patient.

EQUIPMENT AND SUPPLIES

Sphygmomanometer
Stethoscope
Antiseptic wipes

PROCEDURAL STEPS

1. Read the directions before you begin.

2. Assemble the equipment and supplies needed.

3. Wash your hands.

4. Introduce yourself and correctly identify the patient.
   Purpose: To make sure that you have the correct patient.

5. Explain the procedure to the patient.
   Purpose: Knowing what you are going to do will help the patient relax and lessens the chance for an incorrect measurement.

6. Have the patient sit or lie down for 5 minutes with legs uncrossed.
   Purpose: To promote relaxation and aid you in obtaining a true reading.

7. Determine the correct cuff size.
   Purpose: An incorrect cuff size prevents accurate measurement of blood pressure.

8. Palpate the brachial artery in both arms. If one arm has a stronger pulse, use that arm; if the pulses are equal, select the right arm.
   Purpose: A stronger pulse is easier to measure; the right arm is the universal arm of choice.

9. Roll up the sleeve to about 5 inches above the elbow, or have the patient remove the arm from his or her sleeve.
   Purpose: Tight clothing interferes with an accurate reading.

10. Support the patient's arm at heart level or slightly lower.

11. Center the cuff bladder over the brachial artery, with the connecting tube away from the patient's body and the tube to the bulb close to the body.

12. Place the lower edge of the cuff about 1 inch above the natural crease of the inner elbow and wrap it snugly and smoothly.

13. Position the gauge of the sphygmomanometer so that it is at eye level.
    Purpose: The dial is calibrated to be read in this position.

14. Check the patient's pulse rate for 1 minute, using the radial pulse, and mentally add 40 mm to the reading.
    Purpose: This is to determine the maximum inflation level needed to find phase I of the Korotkoff sounds.

15. Insert the ear pieces of the stethoscope turned down and forward into your ears.

26

Continued

PROCEDURE 26-6 *Continued*

16. Palpate the brachial artery and place the stethoscope diaphragm over the artery firmly enough to obtain a seal but not so tightly that you constrict the artery (Fig. 26–23).

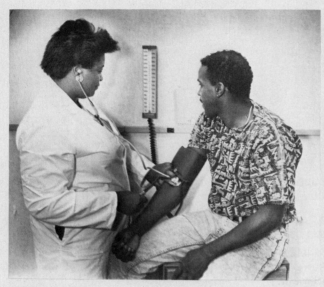

FIGURE 26–23.

17. Close the valve, and squeeze the bulb to inflate the cuff at a rapid but smooth rate to the maximum inflation level that was previously determined.

18. Open the valve slightly and deflate the cuff at the constant rate of 2 mm Hg per second. **Purpose:** Careful, slow release allows you to listen to all of the sounds.

19. Listen throughout the entire deflation until the sounds have stopped for at least 10 mm Hg.

20. Remove the stethoscope from your ears, and record the systolic and diastolic readings as "BP systolic/diastolic" (e.g., BP 120/80).

21. If you are uncertain of your reading, release the air from the cuff, wait 1 to 2 minutes, then repeat the process. It is advisable to have the patient gently wiggle his or her fingers during the waiting period. **Purpose:** This waiting time allows circulatory congestion to dissipate.

22. Remove the cuff from the patient's arm and return it to its proper storage area. Clean the ear pieces of stethoscope with alcohol and return to storage.

---

when compressed by the blood pressure cuff. However, it has not been determined whether the sounds come from within the wall itself or from the blood passing through the vessel. The sounds were first discovered and classified into five distinct phases by Nicolai Sergeevich Korotkoff, a Russian neurologist.

PHASE I. This is the first sound heard as the cuff deflates. The blood is resurging into the patient's artery and can be heard quite clearly as a sharp, tapping sound. Note the gauge reading when this first sound is heard. Record this as the *systolic pressure.*

PHASE II. As the cuff deflates, even more blood flows through the artery. The movement of the blood makes a swishing sound. If proper procedure is not followed in inflating the cuff, these sounds may not be heard because of their soft quality. Occasionally, blood pressure sounds completely disappear during this phase. The loss of the sounds and their reappearance later is called the *auscultatory gap*. The silence may continue as the needle or the column of mercury falls another 30 mm Hg. Auscultatory gaps occur particularly in hypertension and certain heart diseases. So, if you notice such a gap, be certain to report it to the physician.

PHASE III. A great deal of blood is now pushing down into the artery. The distinct, sharp tapping sounds return and continue rhythmically. If you do not inflate the cuff enough, you will miss the first two phases completely, and you will incorrectly interpret the beginning of phase III as the systolic blood pressure (phase I).

PHASE IV. At this point, the blood is flowing easily. The sound changes to a soft tapping, which becomes muffled and begins to grow fainter. Occasionally, these sounds continue to zero (0). This may occur in children, after exercise, with a fever, or in pregnancy if anemia is present. The American Heart Association recommends that the beginning of phase IV be recorded as the diastolic reading for a child. Some physicians call the change at phase IV

the "fading sound" and want it recorded between the systolic and the diastolic recordings (for example, 120/84/70, with the "84" representing the gauge reading when the sounds of phase III have ended and those of phase IV are beginning. Other physicians consider phase IV the true diastolic pressure.

PHASE V. All sounds disappear in this phase. Note the gauge reading when the last sound is heard. Record this as the *diastolic pressure.*

Palpatory Method

The systolic pressure may be checked by feeling the radial pulse rather than hearing (auscultatory method) it with the stethoscope. Place the cuff in the usual position and palpate the radial pulse, noting the rate and rhythm. Now inflate the cuff until the pulse disappears, and then add 30 mm more of inflation to get above the systolic pressure. Do not remove your fingers from the pulse or change the pressure of your fingers. Now, slowly release the pressure in the cuff, and wait for the pulse to be felt again. Note the reading on the gauge, and record the first pulse felt as the systolic pressure. The diastolic and the Korotkoff phases cannot be determined by this method, and its use, other than in combination with the auscultatory method, is not recommended.

ANTHROPOMETRIC MEASUREMENT

Anthropometry is the science that deals with the measurement of the size, weight, and proportions of the human body. These measurements are not routinely included in the initial measurement of the vital signs unless requested by the physician. Since they are indicators of the state of health and well-being of the patient, these measurements are discussed as part of the vital signs.

Measuring Height and Weight

The patient's height and weight are often helpful in diagnosis, and the medical assistant must determine these readings with accuracy and empathy. Some patients are sensitive or secretive about their body weight. Your manner and approach are very important in keeping many patients from feeling embarrassed or shy.

Although weight measurement is not routinely done in all medical settings, there are certain medical specialties and specific medical problems that require continuous monitoring of weight. Hormone disorders (e.g., diabetes), growth patterns (seen in children), and eating disorders (e.g., obesity and bulimia) necessitate accurate weight checks as part of every medical visit. In addition, maternity patients and patients with fluid retention difficulties also need weight monitoring.

COMMON CAUSES OF ERRORS IN BLOOD PRESSURE READINGS

The limb being used is not at the same level as the heart. (It is not necessary for the manometer to be at the same level as the heart.)

The rubber bladder in the cuff has not been completely deflated before starting or retaking a reading.

The mercury column is allowed to drop too rapidly, resulting in an inaccurate reading.

The patient is nervous, uncomfortable, or too anxious, which may cause a reading higher than the patient's actual blood pressure.

The cuff is improperly applied:
The cuff is too large or too small.
The cuff is not placed around the arm smoothly.
The cuff is too loose or too tight.
The bladder is not centered over the artery.
The rubber bladder bulges out from the cover.

Failing to wait 1 to 2 minutes between measurements.

Defective instruments:
Air leaks in the valve.
Air leaks in the bladder.
Dirty mercury column.
Mercury column or aneroid needle that is not calibrated to zero.

Some scales are calibrated in kilograms, while others are in pounds. When it is necessary to convert a weight, use the following formulas:

TO CONVERT KILOGRAMS TO POUNDS:

1 kilogram = 2.2 pounds
Multiply the number of kilograms by 2.2
Example: If a patient weighs 68 kilograms, multiply 68 by 2.2 (68 × 2.2 = 149.6 pounds)

TO CONVERT POUNDS TO KILOGRAMS:

1 pound = 0.45 kilogram
Multiply the number of pounds by 0.45
Example: If a patient weighs 120 pounds, multiply 120 by 0.45 (120 × 0.45 = 55.00 kilograms)

The location of the scale should be considered. Whether your patients are obese, petite persons who do not want their weight known to others, or handicapped with appliances that must be removed, make certain that your office scale is placed in an area of privacy.

It is not necessary to remove shoes and clothing if patients are consistently weighed and measured with them on. Although the exact weight and height may not be determined, changes in the patient's weight and height can be detected and analyzed (Table 26–3).

Do not comment on a patient's progress in a weight program; this is the physician's or counselor's responsibility. When the physician prescribes weight measurement at home, make certain that the patient understands the importance of weighing himself or herself each day at the same time in clothing of similar weight. Body weight may vary considerably from early morning to late afternoon. Teach the patient how to record the weight on a graphic record and how to make any other important notations.

TABLE 26–3. MEAN HEIGHTS AND WEIGHTS AND RECOMMENDED ENERGY INTAKE*

Category	Age (years)	Weight (kg)	Weight (lb)	Height (cm)	Height (in)	Energy Needs (with range) (kcal)	Energy Needs (with range) (MJ)
Infants	0.0–0.5	6	13	60	24	kg × 115 (95–145)	kg × .48
	0.5–1.0	9	20	71	28	kg × 105 (80–135)	kg × .44
Children	1–3	13	29	90	35	1300 (900–1800)	5.5
	4–6	20	44	112	44	1700 (1300–2300)	7.1
	7–10	28	62	132	52	2400 (1650–3300)	10.1
Males	11–14	45	99	157	62	2700 (2000–3700)	11.3
	15–18	66	145	176	69	2800 (2100–3900)	11.8
	19–22	70	154	177	70	2900 (2500–3300)	12.2
	23–50	70	154	178	70	2700 (2300–3100)	11.3
	51–75	70	154	178	70	2400 (2000–2800)	10.1
	76+	70	154	178	70	2050 (1650–2450)	8.6
Females	11–14	46	101	157	62	2200 (1500–3000)	9.2
	15–18	55	120	163	64	2100 (1200–3000)	8.8
	19–22	55	120	163	64	2100 (1700–2500)	8.8
	23–50	55	120	163	64	2000 (1600–2400)	8.4
	51–75	55	120	163	64	1800 (1400–2200)	7.6
	76+	55	120	163	64	1600 (1200–2000)	6.7
Pregnant						+300	
Lactating						+500	

Reprinted with permission from Recommended Dietary Allowances, 10th Edition, c. 1989 by the National Academy of Sciences. Published by National Academy Press, Washington, D.C.

* The data in this table have been assembled from observed median heights and weights of children, together with desirable weights for adults for the mean heights of men (70 inches) and women (64 inches) between the ages of 18 and 34 years as surveyed in the U.S. population (HEW/NCHS data).

The energy allowances for the young adults are for men and women doing light work. The allowances for the two older groups represent mean energy needs over these age spans, allowing for a 2% decrease in basal (resting) metabolic rate per decade and reduction in activity of 200 kcal/day for men and women between 51 and 75 years, 500 kcal for men over 75 years, and 400 kcal for women over 75. The customary range of daily energy output is shown in parentheses for adults, and is based on a variation in energy needs of ±400 kcal at any one age, emphasizing the wide range of energy intakes appropriate for any group of people.

Energy allowances for children through age 18 are based on median energy intakes of children of these ages followed in longitudinal growth studies. The values in parentheses are 10th and 90th percentiles of energy intake, to indicate the range of energy consumption among children of these ages.

PROCEDURE 26-7 MEASURING A PATIENT'S HEIGHT AND WEIGHT

GOAL To accurately weigh and measure a patient as part of the physical assessment procedure.

EQUIPMENT AND SUPPLIES

A balance scale with a measuring bar

PROCEDURAL STEPS

1. Introduce yourself and correctly identify the patient.

2. Explain what you are going to do to the patient.

3. If the patient is to remove his or her shoes for weighing, place a paper towel on the scale platform.

4. Check to see that the balance bar pointer floats in the middle of the balance frame when all weights are at zero (Fig. 26-24).
Purpose: A floating pointer indicates that the scale is properly adjusted and in balance.

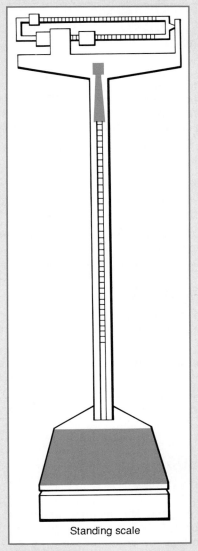

Standing scale

FIGURE 26-24.

Continued

PROCEDURE 26-7 *Continued*

WEIGHT

5. Help the patient onto the scale. Be sure that the female patient is not holding a purse and that the male patient has removed any heavy objects from his pants pockets.

6. Move the large weight into the groove closest to the estimated weight of the patient. The grooves are calibrated in 50-lb increments. If you chose a groove that is more than the patient's weight, the pointer will immediately tilt to the bottom of the balance frame. You then must move it back one groove (Fig. 26–25).

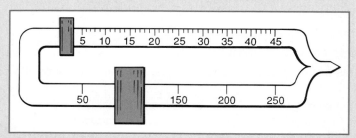

FIGURE 26–25.

7. While the patient is standing still, slide the small upper weight to the right along the 1/4-pound markers until the pointer balances in the middle of the balance frame.
   Purpose: The pointer will float between the bottom and the top of the frame when both lower and upper weights together balance the scale with the patient's weight.
   Leave the weights in place.

HEIGHT

8. Ask the patient to stand up straight and to look straight ahead.

9. Adjust the height bar so that it just touches the top of the patient's head.
   Leave the bar set.

10. Assist the patient off the scale. Be sure all items removed for weighing are given back to the patient.

11. Read the weight scale. Add the numbers at the markers of the large and the small weights and record the total to the nearest 1/4 pound on the patient's medical record (e.g., Wt: 122 1/2).

12. Record the height. Read the marker at the movable point of the ruler, and record the measurement to the nearest quarter inch on the patient's medical record (e.g., Ht: 64 1/2).

13. Return the weights and the measuring bar to zero.

MEASURING OF BODY FAT

At the physician's request, the medical assistant may be asked to perform body fat measurements on a patient. The percentage of body fat may be an indicator of cardiovascular disease and overall health, vitality, and appearance.

In general, a range of 15 to 19% fat for men and 22 to 25% fat for women is considered a normal body level. The bodies of some sedentary men are as much as 40% fat. Muscular athletes typically weigh more than sedentary men and women of the same height, but their percentage of body fat is considerably lower.

Measuring body fat is more complicated than stepping on a scale. Scientists have developed so-

PROCEDURE 26-8   DETERMINING FAT-FOLD MEASUREMENTS

GOAL   To determine and record a measurement of body fat.

EQUIPMENT AND SUPPLIES

Fat-fold body calipers

PROCEDURAL STEPS

1. Read the directions before you begin.
2. Gather the equipment and supplies needed to complete the procedure.
3. Identify the patient.
    Purpose: To make sure that you have the right patient.
4. Explain the procedure to the patient.
    Purpose: To provide assurance to the patient.
5. Using the deltoid process of the lower part of the upper arm, grasp the skinfold with thumb and index finger. Make sure that the fold is in a parallel angle by keeping the thumb and index finger in line with one another. Be sure you do not grasp muscle tissue or pinch too tightly (Fig. 26–27).
    Purpose: Other sites may be used, but this one is convenient and affords a quality measurement.

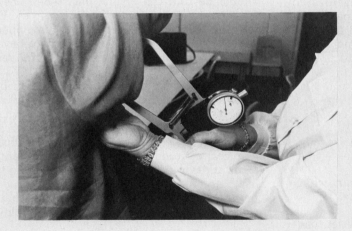

FIGURE 26-27. Fat-fold measure.

6. Place calipers over the fold and measure.
7. Record the results.
    Purpose: The physician can compare patient's readings with established normal measurements. Physician may discuss the results of the test with the patient.
8. Return equipment to its proper place.
9. Wash your hands.

26

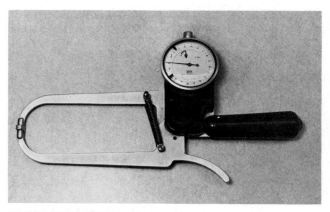

FIGURE 26–26. Skinfold calipers.

phisticated methods that use an electric current or radioactive isotopes to scan the body. These methods are generally not available in the medical office, so physicians rely on measurements using skin calipers (Fig. 26–26). The skin calipers pinch skinfolds at the arms, waist, and back. The measurement appears on the dial of the calipers.

The location of body fat is also very important. Studies conducted in the United States and in Sweden indicate that the body has two different fat stores: one at the hips and the other in the abdomen. Fat at the hips, which is more common in women and more difficult to lose, is primarily stored for special purposes, such as to provide extra energy during pregnancy and nursing. Abdominal fat, which is easier to lose, seems to be more dangerous to overall health. Measure the waist and hips of the patient and correlate the waist-to-hip ratio (the bigger the belly, the higher the ratio). Normal ratios are less than 0.75 in women and are 0.9 to 0.95 in men.

GLOSSARY OF ADDITIONAL TERMS

acrotism The absence of a pulse.
aerophagia The swallowing or gulping of air, which results in rapid and/or irregular breathing.
afebrile Without fever.
benign hypertension Hypertension of slow onset, usually without symptoms.
bigeminal pulse Two regular pulse beats followed by a pause.
continuous fever Body temperature is elevated and remains at an elevated level with little or no fluctuation within a 24-hour period.
crisis A sudden drop of a high body temperature to a normal or subnormal level generally within a 24-hour period.
eupnea Normal breathing.
febrile Referring to a fever; *Fever:* elevation of body temperature above normal. It is sometimes classified as follows: low—99° to 100°F (37.2° to 38.3°

C); moderate—101° to 103°F (38.3° to 39.5° C); high—103° to 105°F (39.5° to 40.6° C).
hypoxia Reduction in the amount of oxygen transported to body tissue.
intermittent fever Fever in which body temperature is elevated at certain times within a 24-hour period but which falls to normal or even subnormal levels during the same period of time (see Fig. 26–1*B*).
malignant hypertension Hypertension that develops rapidly and may be fatal if not treated immediately.
onset Beginning.
slow pulse Between 40 and 60 beats per minute. May be noted in athletes and the aged during rest.
tachycardia A rapid heart rate; a pulse greater than 100 beats per minute.

LEGAL AND ETHICAL RESPONSIBILITIES

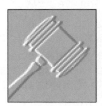

The medical assistant must always remember that as the physician's agent, he or she plays an important role in preventing legal claims against the physician and the medical office. The medical assistant must always function within the legal boundaries of the profession. When obtaining vital signs, you must carefully select your response to a patient who asks about the results. Patients should be told the results *only* when the physician has given the assistant consent to do so. Even when the physician has given consent, remember that you are *never* to diagnose, that is, you are never to evaluate or give an opinion of what the results may mean.

Always be very accurate in the transcribing of the results onto the patient's chart. If the results are incorrectly entered, there is a chance that the patient will be incorrectly diagnosed or treated. This can result in legal action that may implicate you. A careless attitude toward the assessment of vital signs and toward documentation can lead to possible legal entanglement. Cultivate a sensitivity toward proper conduct and performance so that you can protect yourself and your physician/employer.

▶ PATIENT EDUCATION

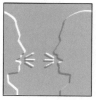

All patients should know how to use a thermometer safely and how to read a thermometer accurately. Since many types of temperature reading equipment are sold, ask the patient what type of equipment he or she uses at home to obtain temperature readings. By talking with the patient, you will be able to determine whether the patient understands how to use a thermometer.

When instructing a patient in methods of pulse assessment, it is important to remember not only to count the beats but also to determine the rate, rhythm, and regularity of the beat.

If a patient is to keep track of his or her own respirations, he or she will need assistance in counting; however, the patient can be taught self-assessment of impending complications as well as preventive breathing exercises.

Monitoring blood pressure at home has become very common in the past several years. Have the patient bring his or her equipment to the office and practice with it. In this way, you can be sure that the patient can correctly hear the diastolic and systolic beats using his or her own stethoscope and sphygmomanometer and record the results accurately in a record book.

Weight management can be a trying and emotional experience for a patient. Understanding how weight is affected by the time of day, by a particular activity, or by the type of scale used can help the patient to maintain a positive attitude.

► LEARNING ACHIEVEMENTS

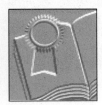

Upon completion of this chapter, can you in the time allowed by your evaluator:

1. Obtain and record a patient's oral temperature within ±0.2°F (or ±0.1°C) of your evaluator's reading?
2. Obtain and record a patient's axillary temperature, adhering to acceptable principles of medical asepsis, patient safety, and good communication, within ±0.2°F (or ±0.1°C) of your evaluator's reading?
3. Obtain and record a tympanic membrane temperature correctly within ±0.2°F (or ±0.1°C) of your evaluator's reading without missing a step?
4. Determine and record a patient's pulse rate within ±2 beats of your evaluator's count?
5. Count and record the respiration rate of a patient, following accepted procedures while observing the principles of patient safety and good communication?
6. Determine a patient's blood pressure within ±4 mm Hg of your evaluator's reading and record the reading on the patient's medical record with 100% accuracy?
7. Obtain a patient's height and weight within 1/4 inch and 1/4 pound of your evaluator's measurement?
8. Determine a patient's percentage of body fat within ±5% of your evaluator's measurements?

REFERENCES AND READINGS

Bonewit, K.: *Clinical Procedures for Medical Assistants*, 3rd ed., Philadelphia, W.B. Saunders Co., 1990.

DeWit, S.: *Keane's Essentials of Medical-Surgical Nursing*, 3rd ed., Philadelphia, W.B. Saunders Co., 1992.

Kirkendall, W. M.: *Recommendations for Human Blood Pressure Determination by Sphygmomanometers, Report of a Subcommittee of the Postgraduate Education Committee of AHA*, Dallas, American Heart Association, 1980.

Lane, K.: *Saunders' Manual For Medical Assisting*, Philadelphia, W.B. Saunders Co., 1992.

Miller, B. F., and Keane, C. B.: *Encyclopedia and Dictionary of Medicine, Nursing, and Allied Health*, 5th ed., Philadelphia, W.B. Saunders Co., 1992.

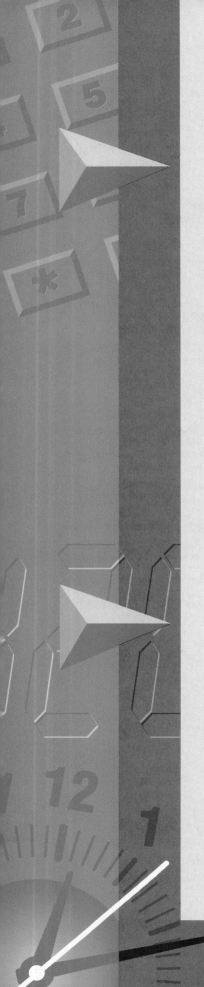

CHAPTER OUTLINE

VOCABULARY

acidosis Chemical imbalance caused by a decrease in the alkaline content of body fluids.

atrophy Wasting away; a decrease in size from normal.

bilirubin The orange-yellow pigment that is formed from the breakdown of hemoglobin in old red blood cells.

bruit An abnormal sound or murmur heard on auscultation of an organ, vessel, or gland.

cyanosis A bluish coloration of the skin and mucous membranes caused by a decreased level of oxygen to the cell.

emphysema A pathologic accumulation of air in the tissues or organs in which the bronchioles become plugged with mucus and lose elasticity.

endogenous Produced or caused by factors within the body.

exogenous Produced or caused by factors outside the body.

exophthalmos An abnormal protrusion of the eyes.

jaundice Yellow color of the skin, sclera, and secretions resulting from increased levels of bilirubin.

myxedema A condition resulting from advanced hypothyroidism.

nevi Round moles or birthmarks varying in color from yellow-brown to black.

pallor The absence of color to the skin and mucous membranes.

passive manipulation Moving or exercising a body part by an externally applied force.

resonance Sound or echo produced by percussion of a body part or cavity.

symmetry Relative correspondence of opposite sides of the body and its parts to each other with respect to size, form, and arrangement.

tinnitus Ringing in the ears.

uremia A toxic renal condition characterized by an excess of urea, creatinine, and other nitrogenous end products in the blood.

vertigo The sensation of moving around in space; dizziness.

vitiligo White patches to the skin caused by loss of melanin.

Assisting with Routine Examinations

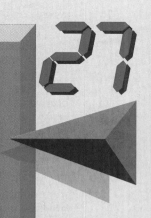

27

LEARNING OBJECTIVES

COGNITIVE
Upon successful completion of this chapter, you should be able to:

1. Define and spell the words in the Vocabulary.

2. List seven parts of the medical history.

3. Differentiate between signs and symptoms.

4. Describe each of the four parts of the Problem-Oriented Medical Record.

5. Describe the six methods of examination and give an example for each.

6. Describe the basic principles of properly draping a patient for examination.

7. List eight positions used in the physical examination.

8. List the sequence of a routine physical examination.

9. Plan a possible patient teaching session.

10. Discuss the legal and ethical implications of the physical examination.

PERFORMANCE
Upon successful completion of this chapter, you should be able to perform the following activities:

1. Obtain patient information and record it in the medical history.

2. Prepare the examination room for the routine physical examination.

3. Assist in the positioning and draping of the patient.

4. Assist with a routine physical examination.

Clinical responsibilities vary widely, depending on the physician's specialty and the extent of reliance upon the medical assistant. Some physicians are reluctant to delegate clinical duties; however, the physician who does utilize the assistant appreciates how time is saved and how professional skills can be enhanced. The medical assistant can ease the roles of both the physician and the patient in many clinical procedures.

To be effective, you must develop the ability to

- Communicate with the patient and the physician easily and professionally.
- Evaluate patient needs and respond to these needs.
- Follow the physician's instructions quickly, accurately, and confidentially.

The purpose of the physical examination is to determine the overall state of well-being of the patient. All major organs and all body systems are checked during a physical examination. As the physician examines the entire body, the findings are interpreted, and by the time the examination is completed, the physician has formed an initial diagnosis regarding the patient's condition. Frequently, laboratory and other diagnostic tests are ordered to supplement the physician's initial diagnosis. The results of these tests are often used to aid the physician in planning a treatment for the patient, in maintaining drug therapy, or in evaluating the patient's progress.

There is much the medical assistant can do to facilitate the quality of patient care and the physician's schedule. The successful medical assistant orchestrates a routine that is organized yet flexible enough to adjust to the individual problems that may arise.

PREPARING FOR THE PHYSICAL EXAMINATION

Patient care does not start with the physical examination; it begins when the patient makes first contact with the office. Even before the examination, you have the opportunity to interact with and react to the patient to ensure that he or she feels comfortable during the process and that all the necessary information is obtained.

Attitude Toward the Patient

More than ever, medicine emphasizes the importance of communicating with the patient and providing a warm and caring environment. Positive reactions and interactions with the patient are essential to providing good patient care. As the patient progresses through the various stages of health care, all members of the medical team must exercise a variety of special skills to enhance the process. These skills are not all technical and medical in nature; many involve the art of caring for the patient as a human being. Because medical care is of an extremely personal nature, the medical assistant must always remember that each patient is an individual with certain anxieties. These anxieties often cause people to act and react in different ways, and effective verbal and nonverbal communication with each patient is essential.

You can do much to put a patient at ease through the tone of your voice and the ease and confidence of your movements and by showing a sincere interest. Give the patient your undivided attention, and let each patient know you *want* to give him or her your attention. The patient is not concerned with the problems of the office staff, nor are you there to impress the patient with your medical knowledge. You are there for one purpose — to give each patient the best possible care.

The Medical Record

When a new patient calls or comes in for an appointment, some medical offices ask him or her to complete a special self-history form (Fig. 27–1). Besides being useful for diagnosing and treating the patient, the self-history allows the patient more participation in the process. The form may be mailed to the patient's home a week before the appointment or may be completed in the office during the first visit.

If you are responsible for taking a portion of the medical history, do it in an area free from outside interference and beyond the hearing range of other patients. Patients will not talk freely where they may be overheard or interrupted. The room should be physically comfortable and conducive to confidential communications.

Listen to the patient. Do not express surprise or displeasure at any of the patient's statements. Remember, you are there not to pass judgment but to gather medical data. Your responses should show interest and concern and should not be judgmental. Report the information gained to the physician in an organized manner, exactly as given by the patient, without opinion or interpretation.

In some medical offices, the physician takes the medical history, during the patient's initial interview. The physician will correlate the physical findings with the information in the history. Questioning the patient is the usual method of obtaining this vital information. The complete medical history and the physical examination cannot be separated and are the first basic skills of the medical profession.

FIGURE 27–1. Example of a patient self-history, which may be mailed to the patient the week before the initial visit. The self-history includes a family history as well as the patient's own medical history. ▶

U.S. MEDICAL CLINIC
University Blvd., S.E.
Yourtown, USA 90000
(123) 456-7899

Date _____

☐ Single
☐ Divorced
☐ Married
NAME _____ ☐ Widowed

S. S. No. _____ Date of Birth _____

OCCUPATION _____ YEARS OF HIGH SCHOOL_____ COLLEGE ____
POSTGRADUATE ____

DATE OF LAST PHYSICAL _____

ARMED SERVICES? _____ WHEN & WHERE _____

WEIGHT TODAY _____ 1 YEAR AGO _____ MAXIMUM WEIGHT _____ MINIMUM ADULT WEIGHT _____

Please answer the following questions. Where boxes are provided to check, place a check mark in front of the disease or condition which you have had. If you do not understand the question fully, the nurse will assist you. **This form must be completed and returned to the clinic at least 1 week prior to your appointment.**

FAMILY HISTORY:

Relative	Living? (Give Present Age)	If Deceased At What Age?	Cause of Death
Father			
Mother			
Brothers: 1			
2			
3			
4			
5			
or more			
Sisters: 1			
2			
3			
4			
5			
or more			

HAS ANY RELATIVE EVER HAD? (Check boxes)

WHICH RELATIVE?

☐ Cancer _____
☐ Tumor _____
☐ Leukemia _____
☐ Bleeding problems _____
☐ Anemia _____
☐ Diabetes _____
☐ Gout _____
☐ Rheumatism or arthritis _____
☐ High blood pressure _____
☐ Heart disease _____
☐ Strokes _____
☐ Epilepsy _____

WHICH RELATIVE?

☐ Ulcers _____
☐ Kidney disease _____
☐ Kidney stones _____
☐ Gall stones _____
☐ Lung disease _____
☐ Mental disorders _____
☐ Sucide _____
☐ Typhoid disease _____
☐ Migraine _____
☐ Tuberculosis _____
☐ Asthma _____
☐ Allergies _____

HAVE YOU HAD A FAMILY HISTORY OF: (Check the ones that apply)
☐ Hay fever   ☐ Asthma   ☐ Emphysema   ☐ Bronchiectasis

27

FIGURE 27–1. *See legend on opposite page.*

Illustration continued on following page

PERSONAL HISTORY:

PAST ILLNESSES: (Check the ones you have had)

- ☐ Measles
- ☐ Chicken pox
- ☐ Whooping cough

- ☐ Scarlet fever
- ☐ Rheumatic fever
- ☐ Diphtheria

- ☐ Thyroid fever
- ☐ Asthma
- ☐ Nephritix (Bright's Disease)
- ☐ Poliomyelitis

MEDICAL ILLNESSES OR HOSPITALIZATIONS: (Please describe briefly)

_____ What Year _____
_____ _____
_____ _____
_____ _____

SURGICAL OPERATIONS: _____ What Year _____
_____ _____
_____ _____

BROKEN BONES OR ACCIDENTS: _____ What Year _____
_____

HAVE YOU EVER HAD: ☐ Sweats   ☐ Fevers   ☐ Bleeding

HAVE YOU EVER HAD ANY ALLERGIES AND/OR DRUG REACTIONS?   ☐ Yes   ☐ No

If yes, to what agent or drug? _____

DRUGS: (CHeck the ones you have taken or are taking)
- ☐ Laxatives
- ☐ Sedatives
- ☐ Tranquilizers

- ☐ Digitalis
- ☐ Thyroid
- ☐ Stimulants

- ☐ Sleeping Pills
- ☐ Aspirin
- ☐ Cortisone

- ☐ Insulin
- ☐ Hormones
- ☐ Birth control pills

IMMUNIZATIONS: (Shots - check the ones you have had)
- ☐ Smallpox vaccination in the last 6 years.
- ☐ Tetanus (not antitoxin) in the last 2 years.
- ☐ Polio in last 2 years.

EXAMINATIONS: (Check the ones you have had)
- ☐ Chest x-ray last year
- ☐ ECG (Heart Tracing)   When _____
- ☐ UGI (X-ray stomach)   When _____
- ☐ Proctoscopic   When _____
- ☐ Barium enema   When _____
- ☐ IVP (Kidney X-ray)   When _____
- ☐ BMR   When _____
- ☐ Thyroid studies   When _____

HABITS: (Check the ones you have)
- ☐ Tobacco   ☐ Alcoholic beverages   ☐ Coffee   ☐ Tea   Other _____

GENERAL: Do you have or have you had? (Check those that apply).
- ☐ Frequent sweats, fevers or chills
- ☐ Night sweats
- ☐ Recent weight loss

- ☐ Nervousness
- ☐ Recent weight gain
- ☐ Intolerance to heat or cold

- ☐ Allergies
- ☐ Drug reactions

HAVE YOU HAD EXPOSURE TO: (Check the ones that apply).
- ☐ Dust
- ☐ Mold

- ☐ Hay
- ☐ Silage

- ☐ Stonecutting
- ☐ Sandblasting

- ☐ Foundry work
- ☐ Metal polishing

- ☐ Fumes

REVIEW OF SYSTEMS: (Head, eyes, ears, nose and throat) (Check any that apply to you.)
- ☐ Headache
- ☐ Loss of hair
- ☐ Excessive tearing
- ☐ Dryness of the eyes
- ☐ Pain behind the eyes
- ☐ Pain in the eyes
- ☐ See flashing lights
- ☐ See black spots

- ☐ Bothered by bright lights
- ☐ Blurring of vision
- ☐ Loss of vision
- ☐ Have you worn glasses?
- ☐ Painful red eyes
- ☐ Ringing in the ears
- ☐ Loss of hearing
- ☐ Drainage from ears

- ☐ Itching ear canals
- ☐ Fullness or popping in the ears
- ☐ Nasal stuffiness
- ☐ Loss of smell or taste
- ☐ Nosebleeds
- ☐ Sneezing
- ☐ Postnasal drip
- ☐ Sinus infections

- ☐ Hoarseness
- ☐ Change of voice
- ☐ Difficulty swallowing
- ☐ Bleeding gums
- ☐ Pyorrhea
- ☐ Trench mouth
- ☐ Sores in mouth

FIGURE 27–1 *Continued*

LUNGS: (Check the items that apply)
☐ Morning cough ☐ Cough during the day ☐ Pleurisy ☐ Wheezing
☐ Evening cough ☐ Sputum with cough ☐ Cough up blood ☐ Frequent colds
☐ Blood clot to lungs (embolus)

HEART: (Check the items that apply)
☐ Fatigue, (tired feeling) with work ☐ Pain in chest when working
☐ Shortness of breath with walking ☐ Rapid beating of the heart
☐ Shortness of breath with work ☐ Irregular beating of the heart
☐ Shortness of breath lying down ☐ Nightmares
☐ Awake at night with cough ☐ Pain or numbness in legs when walking
☐ Cough on lying down ☐ Pain, or whiteness, of hands in cool weather (or in cool water)
☐ Awake at night short of breath ☐ Awake at night with tightness in chest
☐ Awake at night with pain in chest ☐ Swelling of hands
☐ Pain in chest on walking ☐ Swelling of feet or legs
☐ Pain in chest on running ☐ Sleep on more than one pillow
☐ Pain in chest after meals

BLOOD, BLOOD VESSELS AND SKIN: (Check the items that apply)
☐ Bruise easily ☐ Anemia, history of ☐ History of lymphoma ☐ Psoriasis
☐ Red spots on hands - feet ☐ Bleed easily ☐ History of pernicious anemia ☐ Hives
☐ Swollen glands ☐ History of leukemia ☐ Skin rash ☐ Fungus infection

STOMACH, INTESTINES AND COLON: (Check the items that apply)
☐ Appetite poor ☐ "Heartburn" or "Indigestion" ☐ Intolerance to fried, fatty, greasy foods or milk ☐ Jaundice ☐ Gaseousness
☐ Nausea, upset stomach ☐ Bloating ☐ Pain in abdomen ☐ Passage of gas
☐ Vomiting ☐ Belching ☐ Hunger pains ☐ Colic ☐ Fissure
☐ Fever, recurrent ☐ Diarrhea ☐ Mucus in bowel movements ☐ Grease in bowel movements ☐ Hemorrhoids
☐ Chills, recurrent ☐ Constipation ☐ Blood in bowel movements ☐ Fistula
☐ Change in bowel habits or stools ☐ Black bowel movements ☐ Pain with bowel movements
☐ Vomit blood

BLADDER AND SEX ORGANS: (Fill in the blanks & check the items that apply)
Number of times of urination daily _____ Number of times of urination nightly _____
☐ Blood in urine ☐ Colic, kidney ☐ Loss of urine with cough, laughing, straining, etc. ☐ Satisfied with sex
☐ Burning on urination ☐ Pain in flank ☐ Completely emptying bladder after urination
☐ Discharge ☐ Pain in side ☐ Soiling undergarments
☐ Kidney stone ☐ Desire to urinate, but unable to pass urine ☐ Venereal disease

FOR MEN ONLY: (Check the items that apply)
☐ Decreased force of stream ☐ Straining ☐ Difficulty with erection ☐ Difficulty with production of sperm
☐ Small stream ☐ Stream starts and stops ☐ Dribbling

FOR WOMEN ONLY: (Check the items that apply & fill in the blanks)
Menses, onset, age _____ ☐ Bleeding after or pain with intercourse
Menses, stopped, age _____ No. of pregnancies _____
Last period began _____ No. of live births _____
Period prior to this one began _____ No. of miscarriages _____
No. of pads or Tampons per period _____ No. of dead births _____
Light ____ Heavy ____ Soaked ____ ☐ Toxemia with pregnancy
No. of days flow _____ ☐ Family history of cancer of the breast
No. of days between periods _____ ☐ Mass in the breast
☐ Any discharge between periods ☐ Discharge from the nipple
☐ Pain with menses
☐ Bleeding between periods

BONES, MUSCLES AND JOINTS: (Check the items that apply)
☐ Aching muscles ☐ Trick knee ☐ Infection in the bones ☐ Sciatica
☐ Aching joints ☐ Had gout ☐ Popping in the joints ☐ Lumbago
☐ Swollen joints ☐ Had rheumatoid arthritis ☐ Pain in hips, knees, ankles, and with walking ☐ Rheumatism
☐ Red and swollen joints ☐ Had lupus erythematosus ☐ Had other _____
☐ Joint stiffness in the A.M. ☐ Infection in the joints

BRAIN AND NERVES: (Check the items that apply)
☐ Fits or convulsions ☐ Weakness of arms or legs ☐ Memory loss ☐ Tremors or shaking
☐ Coma or unconsciousness ☐ Pins and needles sensation ☐ Poor coordination ☐ Muscular twitching
☐ Fainting spells ☐ Inability to feel pain ☐ Difficulty concentrating ☐ Head injury
☐ Dizziness ☐ Inability to feel cold ☐ Difficulty buttoning shirts ☐ Encephalitis (sleeping sickness)
☐ Loss of balance ☐ Inability to feel heat ☐ Difficulty tying shoelaces ☐ Meningitis
☐ Paralysis (can't move arm or leg) ☐ Personality change

FIGURE 27-1 *Continued*

27

CHARTING

Charting may vary from office to office depending on the physician's preference. The SOAP method is the most utilized charting method (see Fig. 14–4). Regardless of the method used in the office, certain procedures have been standardized to meet the necessary legalities of maintaining medical records in an accurate and concise manner.

- Check the name on the record and be certain that the information you are charting is recorded on the correct form on the correct patient's chart.
- All charting is done in black ink—*do not use pencil.*
- Write in a clear, legible manner.
- When you enter information on a patient's chart, you must sign or initial the entry. The month, day, and year must precede the entry.
- Carefully enter all diagnostic procedures, treatments, medications, and results (including unexpected reactions).
- All unusual complaints, symptoms, or reactions are noted in detail. If patient comments are entered in the patient's own words, then enclose them in quotation marks (" ").
- Learn to be observant and to note anything that seems to be pertinent.
- Spelling, abbreviations, symbols, and terminology used *must* always be correct and accurate.
- Never scribble, erase, or white-out an error. Correct the error by drawing one line through it; write "err," the date, and your initials above the lined-out error.

Medical terminology differs from our ordinary language. Whenever an unfamiliar word is used, you must learn its meaning, how to spell it correctly, its pronunciation, and its proper usage. Learning medical terminology is an ongoing process of vocabulary building. Consistent use of a good medical dictionary is essential. To aid you in learning, a terminology glossary has been provided in the back of this textbook. It is your responsibility to make each new term a working part of your overall medical knowledge.

Charting Terminology

Chief complaint (CC): Usually the reason for the patient's seeking medical care. Often, it is recorded in the patient's own words. It is a list of the patient's current symptoms.

Diagnosis: *Initial:* The physician's temporary impression (i.e., he or she has not reached a definite conclusion); sometimes called a *working diagnosis. Final:* The conclusion the doctor reaches after evaluating all findings, including laboratory and other testing results.

Family history (FH): Details regarding the patient's mother and father, their health, and, if deceased, the cause and age of death. Hereditary tendencies are recorded here and may include information about siblings and offspring.

Past history (PH) or past medical history (PMH): Covers the dates and questions regarding the patient's *usual childhood diseases (UCD or UCHD),* major illnesses and operations, allergies, accidents, and immunizations.

Present illness (PI): An amplification of the chief complaint. It is usually written in chronologic sequence with dates of onset.

Problem-Oriented Medical Record (POMR). This method of medical record keeping introduced a logical sequence to recording the information obtained from the patient. It is based on the scientific method and was designed to "solve a problem." The medical history and the physical examination fit into a special format designed to clarify each patient problem. The format includes supporting data that aid in solving the patient's problem. Because the POMR is universally organized, it is clear to anyone who reads the record. It lends to better audit of the medical record. The POMR is said to be the tool that revolutionized communication among the members of the health team caring for the patient. The system is designed for and easily adapted to computerized medical records systems.

Dr. Lawrence L. Weed is credited with bringing this logical system of patient record keeping to the medical profession. The POMR system includes four basic parts:

- *Database.* The record of the patient's history, physical examination, and initial laboratory findings. As new information is added, it becomes a part of this database.
- *Problem List.* A list of the identified patient problems kept in the front of the patient's chart. It is the "Table of Contents" or the "Index" of the chart. Each problem entered here is numerically listed and dated and is supported by the database. If the problem is resolved, the date of problem resolution is entered next to the problem.
- *Initial Plan.* A written plan for each problem identified on the problem list, outlining further studies, treatments, and patient education.
- *Progress Notes.* Structured notes that correspond to each problem on the problem list, including (1) subjective data, (2) objective data, (3) assessment of the problem, and (4) plans (diagnostic studies, treatments, and patient education). The first letters of each part of the progress note add up to SOAP; therefore, this portion of the POMR system is called "soap notes."

Further information on the POMR system may be found in Chapter 14, Medical Records Management.

Signs and Symptoms. Many times, you will hear that certain findings and conclusions in a medical history are either objective or subjective. Sometimes, these two terms are confused, as are the terms *signs and symptoms,* which may be used interchangeably with objective and subjective, respectively.

Subjective findings, or symptoms, are perceptible only to the patient; they are what the patient feels. An ache, pain, or dizziness is felt only by the patient, and only the patient can tell you it exists. The patient tells the physician about these symptoms, and the physician records them as subjective findings or symptoms. Symptoms of the greatest significance in identifying a disease are called *cardinal symptoms.*

Objective findings, or signs, are perceptible to a person other than the patient, specifically the physician. They are the signs that a physician detects when examining a patient. The physician feels, sees, or hears the signs that are often associated with a certain disease or abnormal condition. Objective findings are dependent upon another person's senses. A mass that a physician feels in the patient's abdomen is an objective finding. It is a sign of an abnormal condition.

Other terms that require understanding are the words functional and physical (organic). When a condition or disease is functional, it means that the disease is without discoverable, or organic, cause, that is, the organ appears normal but its function is not normal. A functional disease is any disease that alters the body functions but is not associated with any apparent organic, or physical, reason. A physical, or organic, disease or condition is one in which the abnormality can be seen or felt.

Social history (SH): Social history includes the patient's eating, drinking, smoking, and sleeping habits; hobbies; interests; and methods of exercise. The physician may wish to inquire about the patient's *occupational history (OH).*

Systems review (SR) or review of systems (ROS): A guide to general health; tends to detect conditions other than those covered in the present illness. It is obtained by a logical sequence of questions, beginning with the head and proceeding downward.

PROCEDURE 27-1 OBTAINING A MEDICAL HISTORY

GOAL To obtain an acceptable written background from the patient to help the physician determine the etiology and effects of the present illness. This includes the chief complaint, present illness, past history, family history, and social history.

SUPPLIES AND EQUIPMENT

A history form
Two pens, red and black ink

A quiet, private area

PROCEDURAL STEPS

1. Greet and identify the patient in a pleasant manner. Introduce yourself and explain your role.
   Purpose: To make the patient feel at ease.

2. Find a quiet, private area for the interview, and explain to the patient the need for the requested information.
   Purpose: An informed patient is more cooperative and, thus, more likely to contribute useful information.

3. Complete the history form by asking appropriate questions. A self-history may have been mailed to the patient prior to the visit. If so, review the self-history for completeness.
   Purpose: The self-history is designed to save time and to involve the patient in the process.

Continued

PROCEDURE 27-1 *Continued*

4. Speak in a pleasant, distinct manner, remembering to keep eye contact with your patient.
   Purpose: Positive nonverbal behavior creates a friendly atmosphere.

5. Record the following statistical information on the patient information form:
   - Patient's full name, including middle initial.
   - Address, including apartment number and ZIP code.
   - Marital status.
   - Sex (gender).
   - Age and date of birth (DOB).
   - Telephone number.
   - Employer's name, address, telephone number.

6. Record the following medical history on the patient history form:
   - Chief complaint.
   - Present illness.
   - Past history.
   - Family history.
   - Social history.
   Purpose: This is information that the physician needs to know to make an accurate assessment and diagnosis. The physician usually completes the review of systems during the pre-examination interview.

7. Ask about allergies to drugs and any other substances, and record them in red ink on every page of the history form.
   Purpose: The presence of an allergy may alter medication and treatment procedures.

8. Record all information legibly and neatly, and spell words correctly. Print rather than write in longhand. Do not erase; if you make an error, draw a single line through the error and initial the correction.
   Purpose: To maintain a medical record that is understandable and defensible in a court of law.

9. Check for accuracy by repeating back to the patient the spelling of the name and the address, ZIP code, and phone number.

10. Thank the patient for cooperating, and direct him or her back to the reception area.

11. Review the record for errors before you hand it to the physician.

12. Use the information on the record to complete the patient's chart as directed by the physician. Keep the information confidential.
    Purpose: All facts and information concerning the patient must remain in the office. This information may be legally and ethically discussed with only the physician.

ASSISTING WITH THE PHYSICAL EXAMINATION

Methods of Examination

Examinations are performed as both a routine confirmation of the absence of illness and a means of diagnosing disease. There are six methods of examining the human body. All six methods are part of every complete physical examination.

Inspection

This is the art of observation: the ability to detect significant physical features (Fig. 27-2A). The focus of this method of examination ranges from the patient's general appearance—the general state of health, including posture, mannerisms, and grooming—to the more detailed observations that may include body contour, **symmetry,** visible injuries and deformities, tremors, rashes, and color changes.

Palpation

This method uses the sense of touch (Fig. 27–2B). A part of the body is felt with the hand for the purpose of determining its condition or that of an underlying organ. It may include touching the skin or the more firm feeling of the abdomen for underlying masses. This technique involves a wide range of perceptions: temperature, vibrations, consistency, form, size, rigidity, elasticity, moisture, texture, position, and contour. Palpation is performed with one hand, both hands (bimanual), one finger (digital), the fingertips, or the palmar aspects of the hand. A pelvic examination is done bimanually, whereas an anal examination is performed digitally. Do not confuse palpation with *palpitation,* which is a throbbing pulsation.

Percussion

This tapping or striking of the body, usually with the fingers or a small hammer to elicit sounds or vibratory sensations, aids in the determination of

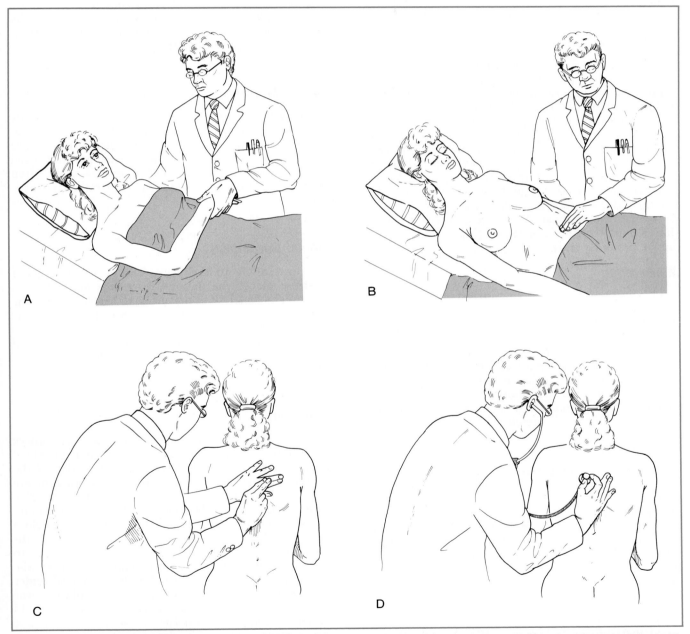

FIGURE 27–2. Four standard methods of physical examination. *A,* Inspection: The art of observation. The physician is inspecting the patient's hand with his eyes for any visible signs of abnormality. *B,* Palpation. The physician may use the sense of touch to determine the size of a part or the presence of abnormal growths. Palpation may be performed with two hands (bimanually) or the fingers (digitally). *C,* Percussion. A part of the body is tapped with the hands or a percussion hammer. *D,* Auscultation. The sense of hearing is used to listen to a body sound. The stethoscope amplifies what can be heard.

the position, size, and density of an underlying organ or cavity. The effect of percussion is both heard and felt by the examiner. It is helpful in determining the amount of air or solid matter in an underlying organ or cavity. The two basic methods of percussion are *direct* and *indirect*. Direct (immediate) percussion is performed by striking the body with a finger. Indirect (mediate) palpation is used more frequently and is done by the examiner placing his own finger on the area and then striking the placed finger with a finger of the other hand (Fig. 27–2C). Both a sound and a sense of vibration are evident here. The examiner will speak of sounds in terms of pitch, quality, duration, and **resonance.**

Auscultation

This is the process of listening to sounds arising from the body—not the sound produced by the examiner as in percussion, but sounds that originate within the patient's body. This is a difficult method of examination because the examiner must distinguish between a normal and an abnormal sound. A stethoscope is usually used to amplify sounds (Fig. 27–2D). Auscultation is particularly useful in appraising sounds arising from the lungs, heart, and abdomen and in distinguishing **bruits,** murmurs, rhythms, durations, and quality. Indirect listening is done with the stethoscope, whereas direct auscultation is done by the examiner placing the ear directly on the patient's body.

Mensuration

This is the process of measuring. Measurements are taken of the length and diameter of an extremity, the extent of flexion or extension of an extremity, or the pressure of a grip. The expansion of the chest or the circumference of the head can be measured. The patient's height and weight are measurements. Hearing and vision are measured, and measuring is done for pregnancy. Measurements are taken using tape measures or small rulers and are usually reported in centimeters.

Manipulation

This is the forceful, **passive** movement of a joint to determine the range of extension or flexion of a part of the body. Manipulation may or may not be grouped with palpation. It is usually considered separate from the four standard methods of examination (inspection, palpation, percussion, and auscultation) and is grouped with mensuration, especially by the orthopedist and the neurologist. Insurance and industrial reports often request this information in detail.

Positioning and Draping for Physical Examinations

There are various positions in which a patient may be placed to facilitate a physical examination.

The medical assistant instructs the patient about, and assists the patient into, these positions with as much ease and modesty as possible. The medical assistant helps the patient to maintain a position during the examination with as little discomfort as possible.

Draping with an examination sheet protects the patient from embarrassment and keeps the patient warm, but the sheet must be positioned so that it allows complete visibility for the examiner and does not interfere with the examination. During the general examination, each part of the body is exposed one portion at a time. For gynecologic and rectal examinations, the sheet may be positioned on the diagonal across the patient. The following positions are used for medical examinations.

Horizontal Recumbent (Supine)

Recumbent means lying down; supine means lying down with the face upward. Either term is used to describe the patient who is lying flat with the face upward (Fig. 27–3A). These terms are not used when instructing the patient; they are most often used when transcribing surgical and radiological reports.

Dorsal Recumbent

Dorsal refers to the back. The dorsal recumbent position places the patient lying face upward, with the weight distributed primarily to the surface of the back (Fig. 27–3B). This is accomplished by flexing the knees so that the feet are flat on the table. This position relieves muscle tension in the abdomen and is used for examination of the abdomen and for resting.

Lithotomy

The patient is placed on the back, with the knees sharply flexed, the arms placed at the sides or folded over the chest, and the buttocks to the edge of the table. The feet are supported in table stirrups or are hung in hammocklike knee supports (Fig. 27–3C). The stirrups should be placed wide apart and somewhat away from the table. If the heels are too close to the buttocks, the possibility of leg cramps is increased, and it is more difficult for the patient to relax the abdominal muscles. Make sure that the stirrups are locked in place. A towel is placed under the patient's buttocks, and a drape is placed over the patient's abdomen and knees. The drape should be large enough to cover the breasts if the patient is not wearing a gown. The drape must be long enough to cover the knees and touch the ankles, and wide enough to prevent the sides of the thighs from being exposed. The physician will push the drape away from the pubic area when the examination begins.

Trendelenburg

The patient is supine on a table that has been raised at the lower end about 45 degrees (Fig. 27–3*D*). This places the patient's head lower than the legs. The patient's legs are then flexed over the end. This position is sometimes used in cases of shock or low blood pressure. Recent studies in emergency care question the value of lowering the patient's head, and experts are suggesting that this position is no longer necessary for shock victims. It is also a position for abdominal surgery because the abdominal viscera gravitate upward and out of the way of the surgical procedure. A sheet is placed over the patient, covering from the underarms to below the knees.

Fowler

The patient is sitting on the examination table with the head elevated. The head usually is raised to a level of about 90 degrees. This position is useful for examinations and treatments of the head, neck, and chest. The drape will vary according to the exposure of the patient, but the female breasts should be covered and the drape should extend to the feet (Fig. 27–3*E*).

Jackknife

The patient is placed on the back with the shoulders slightly elevated and the legs flexed sharply up over the abdomen (Fig. 27–3*F*). This places the thighs at right angles to the abdomen, and the lower leg at right angles to the thighs. This position, also called the *reclining* position, is used for the passing of a urethral sound. Placement of the drape is similar to that for the lithotomy position. (The proctologic position is often incorrectly referred to as the jackknife position.)

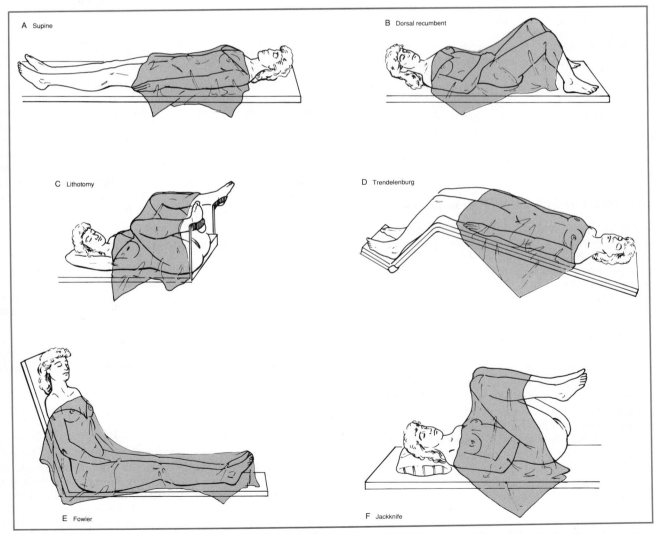

FIGURE 27–3. The basic positions and draping. *A*, The horizontal (supine) position. *B*, The dorsal recumbent position. *C*, The lithotomy position is preferred for the gynecologic examination. *D*, The Trendelenburg position is usually used for hospital surgery. *E*, Fowler position. *F*, The jackknife position has long been confused with the proctologic position. It is used in urologic procedures.

27

Prone

The patient is lying face down on the table, on the ventral surface of the body (Fig. 27–4A). This is the opposite of the supine position and is another one of the recumbent positions. The patient is covered with a drape large enough to cover from the midback to below the knees. The drape on the female patient should extend high enough to cover the breasts if she is to be turned over to the dorsal recumbent position during the examination.

Sims

This position is sometimes called the *lateral* position. The patient is placed on the left side, with a towel or small pillow under the left cheek. The left arm and shoulder are drawn back behind the body so that the body's weight is predominantly on the chest. The right arm is flexed upward for support. The left leg is slightly flexed, and the buttocks are pulled to the edge of the table. The right leg is sharply flexed upward (Fig. 27–4B). A towel is placed on the upper left thigh, just below the perineal area. A sheet is placed over the patient, extending from under the arms to below the knees. The physician will raise a small portion of the sheet from the back of the patient to sufficiently expose the rectum. The remaining portion of the sheet will cover the patient's chest area and thighs. This position is used for rectal examinations, since the rectal ampulla is dropped down into the abdominal cavity; this facilitates entrance to and examination of the rectum. It is also used for perineal and some pelvic examinations.

Proctologic Position on a Proctologic Table

This position requires an examining table that can be elevated and tilted in the center and lowered at the head and legs. The patient's head and legs are at an angle lower than the buttocks. It must be stressed that the patient's body is flexed at the hip joint and not at the waist (Fig. 27–4C). If this flexion is not correct, the patient will experience considerable discomfort, and the bowel will not be displaced forward. A fenestrated drape is best, but a single sheet may be draped in a "U" around the anal area. Do not bind the patient's legs together with the drape because it may be necessary to separate the legs during the examination. This position is the superior choice for a sigmoidoscopic examination because it straightens the rectosigmoid area and displaces the lower bowel. It is a convenient position for examining the perineal area, the anus, and hemorrhoids.

Knee-chest

As the term implies, the patient rests on the knees and the chest (Fig. 27–4D). The head is turned to one side, with one arm flexed under the abdomen and the other hanging over the side of the table, or both arms extended along the sides of the body. The thighs are perpendicular to the table and are slightly separated. The patient's back should not be rounded, but curved inward somewhat to an anterior convexity. The patient will need assistance in order to obtain this position correctly, and it is a difficult position for most patients to maintain. If the correct knee-chest position cannot be obtained, the patient may have to be placed in a knee-elbow position. This position puts less strain on the patient and is easier to maintain. The knee-chest position is also known as the *genupectoral;* the knee-elbow is also called the *genucubital.* These positions are used for the same types of examinations as the proctologic positions. An aperture (opening) drape is used, or a single sheet may be draped in a "U" and pinned over the patient's back at the sacral area. Two smaller sheets may be used, with one sheet over the patient's back and the other from the curve of the buttocks down over the thighs. It will be necessary to join the two sheets together on each side of the examination area with towel clamps.

Basics of the Routine Physical Examination

Examinations vary greatly, depending on the physician's specialty and the reason for the examination. There may also be a variance in the sequence of an examination as individual patient needs are addressed. This chapter reviews an average routine that an examiner might follow. It gives an overview of the process, with some of the terminology and descriptive pathology that are commonly used or seen. Since each physician has individual preferences, only basic instruments are described.

Presenting Appearance (General Appearance)

The physical examination really starts as soon as the patient appears before the examiner. Either of the terms *presenting appearance* and *general appearance* may be used on the medical record. These terms note whether or not the patient appears well and in good health. The patient may appear disoriented or in distress. The patient's responses to the opening remarks or questions may show an alertness or dullness.

Gait

The patient's gait, that is, the manner or style of walking, will often give some information. The patient may limp, walk with the feet wide apart, or have difficulty in maintaining his or her balance. The analysis of gait is usually done with the patient walking a straight line or may be done without the patient knowing that he or she is being observed. Some of the terms used are *ataxic* (which describes an unsteady, uncoordinated walk over a wide base), *slapping* or *steppage* (in which the advancing leg is

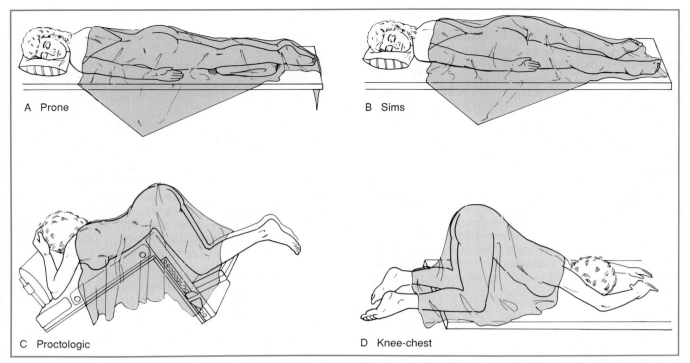

FIGURE 27–4. The basic positions with the patient lying face down. *A,* The prone position. *B,* The Sims (or lateral) position. *C,* The proctologic position. *D,* The knee-chest position.

lifted high enough for the toes to clear the ground), *drag-to* (in which the feet are dragged rather than lifted), and *spastic* (in which the legs are held together and move in a stiff manner, the toes seeming to drag and catch).

Stature

The patient's height is measured. The physician notes the body build and proportions. Any gross (immediately obvious; taking no account of details, or *minutiae*) deformities are recorded. Sometimes, abnormalities in height or body proportion may be due to hormonal imbalances.

Posture

A patient's posture may indicate an area of pain. A rigid posture may indicate a fixed spine, and an altered posture may result from an extremity with limited motion. The patient may say that he cannot sleep unless in a sitting position (frequently seen in heart and lung diseases). *Torticollis (wryneck)* may be present as a result of a spasm or the shortening of the neck and chest muscles. Examination of the spine may show abnormal curvatures such as *kyphosis* (humpback), *scoliosis* (curvature of the spine), or *lordosis* (abnormal or exaggerated curvature of the lumbosacral area, which causes the buttocks to protrude excessively).

Body Movements

These may be classed as voluntary or involuntary. The voluntary movements are the patient's normal habits and have limited clinical value, unless they are the result of an abnormal condition. Involuntary movements are frequently *tics,* which may be habit spasms (usually found around the eyes, neck, or face) or the result of various conditions. Tics are involuntary, rhythmic movements by a group of muscles that goes into spasm at irregular intervals. A *tremor* is an involuntary trembling or quivering. A tremor may be the beating of the thumb against a flexing finger or a rhythmic oscillation of the head, as may occur in old age.

Speech

In addition to social history, speech may reveal an abnormal condition. Some basic speech defects are *aphonia,* the inability to speak because of a loss of the voice, commonly seen with severe laryngitis or overuse of the voice; *aphasia,* the loss of the power of expression through speech, writing, or sign due to injury or disease of the brain centers; and *dysphasia,* a lack of coordination and failure to arrange words in proper order, usually due to a brain lesion. Other comments concerning speech may include *incoherent, jumbled,* or *slurred.*

27

Breath Odors

These may or may not be diagnostic, although they often are associated with poor oral hygiene or dental care. **Acidosis** will give the strong odor of acetone, which is sweet and fruity. Acidosis may result from diabetes mellitus, starvation, or renal disease. A musty odor is usually associated with liver disease, and the odor of ammonia may be found in cases of **uremia.**

Nutrition

Charts are published containing what is considered normal weight for the age and height of females and males. A patient is generally thought of as being overweight or underweight in comparison with these accepted averages. Obesity may be due to one of two origins: **exogenous,** involving excessive caloric intake in relation to the expenditure of calories, or **endogenous,** involving certain endocrine imbalances.

Edema is the accumulation of fluid in the intercellular tissue spaces of the body. Edema must be differentiated from fat by the simple test of pressing a finger on the skin over a bony area, such as the ankle, and observing whether or not a pit or depression remains. Edema will leave a whitened pit for a few moments and is recorded as *pitting edema.* Fat does not pit but returns to skin level immediately after the finger is removed.

Skin

Comments on the skin are included as a part of the general appearance, unless the chief complaint involves a condition related to the skin. If so, then the skin is listed as a separate category. In the physical examination, the skin is considered a separate organ of the body. Concerns include abnormal coloring such as redness, **cyanosis, pallor,** or excessive brown patches. **Jaundice** may indicate an increase in the level of **bilirubin** in the blood. Decreased pigmentation is found in **vitiligo,** which is the acquired loss of melanin and is characterized by white patches. Lesions, ulcers, and bruises may be the result of pathologic conditions. Skin texture refers to smoothness, roughness, and scaling. Loss of elasticity is when the skin does not return immediately to normal when it has been pulled or stretched. This can occur as an inherited condition or from prolonged injury, such as excessive exposure to the sun.

Fingernails and toenails often give some indication of a person's health. Brittle, grooved, or lined nails may indicate either local infection or systemic disease. *Clubbing* of the fingertips is associated with some congenital heart diseases. *Spooning* of the nail is seen in some severe iron deficiency anemias. *Beau's lines* appear after an acute illness but will grow out and disappear.

Hair Distribution

The distribution or the lack of hair and hair texture is important. Excessive hair, especially facial hair in the female, indicates some bodily change. Heavy abdominal or thigh hair may be an indication of a pathologic condition.

Instruments and Equipment Needed for Physical Examination

The instruments most commonly used for the basic examination are described below and shown in Fig. 27–5. These instruments help the physician to inspect, see, feel, and test parts of the body. It is the medical assistant's responsibility to inspect each piece of equipment before placing it on the examination tray for the physician's use.

Nasal speculum: Instrument used to inspect the lining of the nose, nasal membranes, and internal septum. Nasal specula are wide and short may be reusable or disposable.

Ophthalmoscope: Instrument used to inspect the inner structures of the eye.

Otoscope: Instrument used to examine the ear canal and tympanic membrane. A light is focused through a magnifying lens and ear speculum. Specula are long, narrow, and numbered according to size of the lumen. Some offices prefer to use disposable specula.

The previously described three instruments may all work off of a common base unit, and only the examination end is changed for each part of the examination.

Tongue depressor: Flat, wooden blade used to hold down the tongue when examining the throat.

Stethoscope: Listening device used when auscultating certain areas of the body, particularly the heart and lungs.

Gloves: Disposable gloves are used to protect the physician and the patient from possible microorganisms while the oral, rectal, and vaginal (female only) cavities are examined.

Reflex hammer: Medical instrument with a rubber, triangularly shaped head used to test neurologic reflexes of the knee and elbow.

Tuning fork: Used to check a patient's auditory acuity. Produces a humming sound perceived by the ear drum.

Lubricant: A water-soluble form is used on the glove when the rectum or vaginal cavity is examined.

Tape measure: Used to assess developmental progress or determine the size of an abnormality found during an examination.

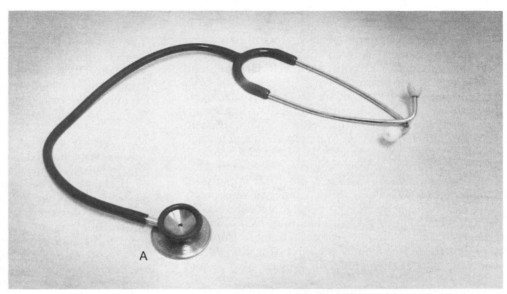

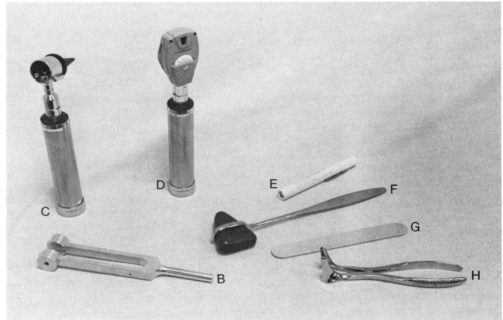

FIGURE 27-5. Instruments used in physical examination. *A*, Stethoscope. *B*, Tuning fork. *C*, Otoscope. *D*, Ophthalmoscope. *E*, Pen-light. *F*, Percussion hammer. *G*, Tongue depressor. *H*, Nasal speculum.

Headlight or flashlight: Used only if additional light is needed to visualize.

Vaginal speculum: Instrument used to expand the vaginal orifice and allow the physician to examine the vagina and cervix or to obtain a cytologic specimen for the Pap test.

Cervix scraper: Wooden instrument designed to remove cervical secretions from the cervical os and from the cervical cuff. Used to obtain secretions for the Pap test.

Fixative: An agent used in preserving a histologic or pathologic specimen to maintain its normal structure.

Certain supplies, such as gauze flats, glass slides, cervix scraper, fixative, and cotton-tipped applicators, should be on the tray or easily accessible for use during the examination.

Sequence of the Routine Physical Examination

There is a routine, or sequence, to the physical examination of the patient. The following descriptions of the process will have variations depending on the examiner.

27

Preparing the Patient

After the physician interviews the patient, you prepare the patient for the physical examination. Usually, you take the patient's height, weight, and vital signs at this time. Give your patient a brief explanation of the type of examination to be done. Patients are more cooperative and less anxious if they understand what is expected of them. Remain with the female patient throughout the examination unless the physician excuses you from the room. A female assistant in the room during the examination of the female patient can avert potential lawsuits. If a patient objects to disrobing, then you must tactfully explain the necessity of adequate exposure in order to facilitate a careful examination. Failure to properly prepare the patient often leads to unnecessary delays and difficulties for the physician. Do not ask the patient to disrobe in an area that is not private.

Rapport is accomplished by conversation, but as soon as the physician begins the examination, keep your conversation to a minimum and remain inconspicuous. When the patient is properly positioned and draped, notify the physician that you are ready.

The examination usually starts with the patient seated on the examining table. If the physician uses reflected light, then the light source should be behind the patient's right shoulder. If illuminated instruments are used, then the standard overhead lights are sufficient. Be careful not to shine a light directly into the patient's eyes. Turn on lights while they are directed away from the patient, and then carefully move the light toward the area to be examined.

Head

The patient's head and face are usually the starting place for the examination. The face reflects the patient's state and tells the examiner a great deal. It may appear puffy, especially the eyelids, giving the appearance that the patient has just awakened. The puffiness may be due to **myxedema** or a medication such as cortisone. With scleroderma, the facial skin is characteristically tight and **atrophied.** *Lipid* or fatty patches that collect in the eyelids, usually near the center, are called *xanthelasma*. These appear as yellowish white, slightly elevated small patches and may or may not be associated with disease.

Neck

The neck is examined for *range of motion* (ROM) by having the patient move the head in various directions. One limitation that may appear is torticollis. *Bounding* is an involuntary slight nodding of the head synchronized with the pulsation of the heart. The thyroid gland is given special attention for symmetry, size, and texture. The examiner manually palpates the thyroid area, and the patient is asked to swallow several times. The medical assist-

ant may help by giving the patient a small amount of water in a paper cup. The examiner palpates the thyroid gland both anteriorly and posteriorly. The carotid artery is palpated and auscultated for possible bruit. The lymph nodes are palpated. Swollen lymph nodes usually are present when there is infection in the face, head, or neck.

Eyes

Eyes are checked for reaction to light into the pupils; this is known as *light and accommodation* (L & A). The color of the sclera may be abnormally red or yellow. The movements of the eyes are tested by having the patient follow the examiner's finger. **Exophthalmos** is an important observation that is seen in some cases of hyperthyroidism or of a tumor or fat pad behind the eyeballs. Intraocular pressure is checked using the tonometer in most individuals past the age of 35. Pressure within the eyeball could indicate the presence of glaucoma, which results in pathologic changes in the optic disc, visual defects, and eventual blindness.

Ears

The ears are examined using the otoscope. Symptoms of the ear include deafness, pain, discharge, **vertigo,** and **tinnitus.** The external ear is first checked for redness of the ear canal or the presence of ear wax (cerumen). The tympanic membrane (eardrum) may be seen in most patients and appears pearly gray. Scars appearing on the eardrum are frequently the result of earlier, chronic ear infections or perforations. The color of the eardrum is important to the diagnosis because it may indicate fluids such as blood or pus behind the drum in the middle ear. The patient may be asked to swallow several times in order to observe movement of the tympanic membrane, which occurs on pressure changes in the eustachian tube. The eustachian tube equalizes air pressure between the middle ear and the throat.

Mouth and Throat

The mouth, or oral cavity, is usually thought of in terms of oral hygiene and dental care. A history of sore throats, bleeding gums, tooth extractions, or voice changes requires careful examination. The status of dental hygiene includes the condition of the teeth, how the patient cares for the teeth and gums, and whether or not the teeth of the upper and lower jaws meet properly (occlude) for chewing. Normal gums are pale pink, glossy, and smooth and do not bleed when pressure from a tongue depressor is applied. *Pyorrhea*, the discharge of pus from the dental periosteum, is a progressive condition. It is also called *periodontitis*. The palatine tonsils are usually visible. Tonsils may be enlarged and pitted. The pharyngeal tonsils (adenoids) are not easily accessible but may be visualized using the mouth mirror. The examiner will use a tongue depressor and a piece of gauze to grasp the tongue for careful examination of it. The floor of the mouth is examined by both inspection and palpation for enlarged lymph nodes, salivary gland function, and ulcerations. The insides of the cheeks are also examined for any abnormal marks or color.

Nose

The nasal cavity and the nasopharynx may reveal the presence of a discharge from the sinuses known as a *postnasal drip* (PND), a common occurrence. Other abnormalities may be obstructions, a deviated septum, polyps, or ulcerations. The nasal cavity basically requires an examination of the color and texture of the mucosa. When a patient has a nosebleed, it is correctly called *epistaxis*. The sinus meatus cannot be seen, but the frontal and maxillary sinuses may be examined by the application of pressure over the area and transillumination.

Chest

While the patient is still in the sitting position, the chest, heart, lungs, and breasts are examined. The chest is examined for symmetric expansion. A tape measure may be used, especially if there is a variation between the upper and lower chest expansion. A patient with a history of **emphysema** may display a chest that is barrellike.

With the stethoscope to the patient's back, the examiner listens to the lung sounds. The patient is asked to take deep and regular breaths during this examination. This may produce a slight dizziness, which is not abnormal; the patient may be assured that it is only the result of the deep respirations and will rapidly pass. The types of respiration are noted. Some common variations in respiration can be found in Chapter 26, Vital Signs. Chest sounds heard by the physician may be described as various types or as *rales* (abnormal sounds that vary from coarse musical sounds to the whistling or squeaking sounds frequently heard in asthma or bronchitis). The term *stridor* describes a wheezing sound or a shrill, harsh, or crowing sound. Next, the examiner will tap (percuss) the patient's back at various points to determine the resonance of the chest and diagnose possible tuberculosis. The patient may be asked to take more deep breaths at this time.

Syncope (fainting) and chest pains warrant careful examination. Much of the examination of the cardiovascular system also depends on data gained from the vital signs (Chapter 26). Because it takes considerable concentration to interpret the heart sounds, it is necessary to have complete silence when the examiner is listening to the patient's heart. The heart is examined using a stethoscope from both the anterior and posterior approaches to the patient. Further examination may include auscultation on the left, lateral side. In cases of heart disease, the examiner may spend an extended period of time listening to the heart sounds.

Reflexes

The patient's reflexes are checked with the patient in the sitting and supine positions. While the patient is sitting, the biceps are checked with the patient's arm flexed and supported by the examiner. The knee-jerk (patellar reflex) and the ankle-jerk (Achilles reflex) are checked using tapotement with either the fingers or the reflex hammer. The plantar reflexes (Babinski and Chaddock reflexes) are tested with the patient in either the sitting or the lying position.

Breasts

A careful breast examination is part of the examination of every female, whether or not the patient is symptomatic. The patient is usually examined in the sitting position, but may be examined later in the supine position. Breast cancer is the most common malignancy occurring in women, and early detection is the key to successful treatment (see Chapter 28 for more detailed examination procedures).

Abdomen

The patient is lowered to the dorsal recumbent position, and the drape is lowered to the pubic hair line. The gown is raised to just under the breasts. A towel should be placed over the female breasts if a gown is not worn. Whether right- or left-handed, the examiner stands to the patient's right side. The patient's arms may be placed at the side, or the hands may be crossed over the chest. If the table is narrow and the patient cannot relax completely, it may help to have the patient tuck the thumbs under the buttocks in order to relax the shoulders. Relaxation of the abdominal muscles is absolutely essential for the abdominal examination. It sometimes helps to place a small pillow under the patient's head or the knees. If the patient exhibits ticklishness, it is best to disregard it and try to continue the examination by changing the routine.

It is important to know the topography of the abdomen and the underlying organs. Mentally divide the abdomen into quadrants (Fig. 27–6A). The vertical line extends from the xiphoid process of the sternum to the symphysis pubis; the horizontal line crosses the abdomen at the level of the umbilicus (navel). Another method of dividing the abdomen is by regions, or sections (Fig. 27–6B). Note that the right and left hypochondriac regions are composed almost entirely of the costal margins. This is because the abdomen extends up under the rib cage to the dome of the diaphragm. The liver and spleen are located in these two regions.

Abdominal symptoms that a patient may give during the history include *dyspepsia* (indigestion),

27

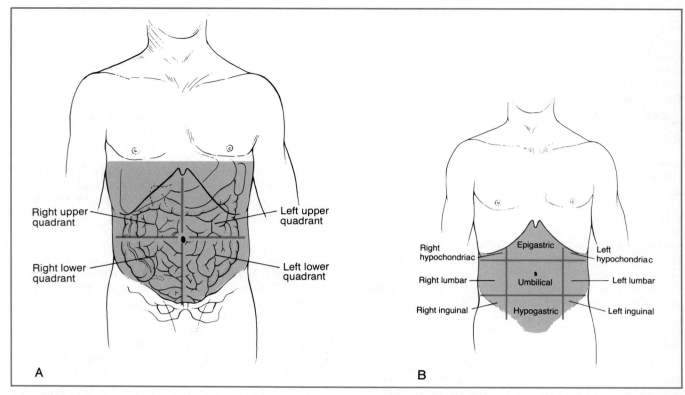

FIGURE 27–6. *A*, Quadrants of the abdomen. *B*, Regions of the abdomen. (From Swartz, M. H.: Textbook of Physical Diagnosis: History and Examination. Philadelphia, W. B. Saunders Co., 1989, p. 320)

dysphagia (difficulty in swallowing), a change in bowel habits, excessive *flatulence* (gas), nausea, and vomiting. General abdominal discomfort is common, since abdominal pain is frequently referred pain, that is, pain that is felt in the abdomen but is actually being generated from an organ elsewhere.

The inspection of the abdomen begins with noting any change in skin color such as jaundice. *Striae* (silver stretch marks), *petechiae* (small purple hemorrhagic spots), cutaneous *angiomas* (spider **nevi**), scars, and visible masses may be observed. The contour of the abdomen may be flat, rounded, or bulg-

PROCEDURE 27–2   ASSISTING WITH A ROUTINE PHYSICAL EXAMINATION

GOAL   To help the physician examine patients by preparing the necessary equipment and ensuring patient safety and comfort during the examination.

EQUIPMENT AND SUPPLIES

Stethoscope
Sphygmomanometer
Ophthalmoscope
Otoscope
Scale
Tape measure
Tongue depressors
Gauze sponges
Cotton balls
Head mirror

Examination light
Pen-light
Percussion hammer
Nasal speculum
Lubricating gel
Examination gloves
Vaginal speculum
Blood and body-fluid protection barriers (goggles, masks, and aprons or gowns) as necessary.

Continued

PROCEDURAL STEPS

1. Prepare the examining room according to acceptable medical aseptic rules.
   Purpose: Room must be aseptically clean.

2. Wash your hands. Follow universal blood and body-fluid precautions.

3. Locate the instruments for the procedure. Set them out in the sequence that the examiner will follow.

4. Identify the patient, and determine whether the patient understands the procedure. If the patient does not understand, explain what you and the physician will be doing.
   Purpose: To increase patient cooperation during the examination.

5. Measure and record the patient's vital signs, height, and weight. Report any unusual findings to the physician as soon as possible.
   Purpose: To gather data needed before the examination begins.

6. If a specimen is needed, instruct the patient on how to collect the specimen, and hand the patient the proper specimen container.
   Purpose: To obtain a specimen that can be tested.

7. Direct the patient to the lavatory, and have the patient empty his or her bladder. Label the collected specimen.
   Purpose: To have the patient's bladder empty for the examination.

8. Hand the patient a gown and sheet. Instruct the patient on how to put the gown on and to use the sheet. Tell the patient to have a seat on the examination table after putting on the gown. Help patient with undressing as needed; however, most patients prefer to undress in privacy, if possible.

9. Assist during the examination by handing the physician each instrument as it is needed.

10. If the physician requires a specific position, explain to the patient what you want him or her to do, and assist the patient into that position.

11. If the examination includes a pelvic examination, help the patient into the lithotomy position, and have a warmed speculum ready for the physician.

12. Listen to the patient and help diminish his or her fears. Apply a hand to his or her shoulder, or hold hands if needed.

13. If specimens are taken, label them immediately.

14. When the physician has completed the examination, allow the patient to rest for a moment, then help the patient from the table. Assist with dressing, if necessary.

15. Remove all soiled equipment to the proper area.

16. Change the paper goods or linens with minimal movements to prevent stirring the dust and air.

17. Clean table-top surfaces with disinfectant or bactericide.

18. Prepare specimens for transport or examination.

19. Dispose of blood and body-fluid protection barriers, and wash your hands.

20. Record the necessary notes on the patient's chart and forward it to the physician for further notations.

21. Return to the patient and ask him or her if there are any questions. Give the patient any final instructions, and schedule the next appointment if that is appropriate.
    Purpose: To clarify directions, eliminate any misunderstandings, and allow the patient to discuss any concerns. If there are misunderstandings or concerns beyond your scope of experience or skill, you must arrange for the physician to speak with the patient again.

27

ing in localized areas. A bulging in the right and left lumbar regions (the flanks) may be the result of the presence of free abdominal fluid *(ascites)*. Abdominal hernias are examined with the patient in the supine and standing positions. To complete the abdominal examination, the patient may be placed in the knee-elbow position to better determine the presence of free abdominal fluid. The Sims position may also be used for this purpose.

The examination of the male and female reproductive systems is covered in Chapter 28, Specialty Examination.

Rectum

The rectal examination usually follows the abdominal examination or may be part of the examination of the male and female genitalia. The patient's comfort and dignity are vital. The examination is limited to an area of within 6 to 8 cm (2.5 to 3.5 in). The examiner needs one to two finger cots or an examining glove and lubricating jelly. A good light must be directed at the perineal area.

The routine physical examination is the backbone of medical practice. It is this examination that establishes a beginning diagnosis and treatment plan for the patient. For that reason, at no time should this examination be considered "routine." Every examination is unique, just as is every patient's personality; each patient's needs differ from those of others. The medical assistant must learn to foresee the patient's needs and be prepared to assist whenever needed. Now that you have learned the theory of the physical examination, it is time to practice the procedures learned. Once you feel confident, demonstrate your skills and knowledge to your instructor by accurately preparing for and assisting with the routine physical examination.

LEGAL AND ETHICAL RESPONSIBILITIES

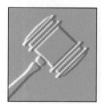

The medical assistant must recognize that a legal and ethical contract exists between the patient and the physician. In Chapters 4 and 5, you learned how a contract is formed and why it is necessary for everyone in the office to be aware of the role that he or she plays in medical law and ethics. It is imperative that the assistant remember that information gained during the physical examination is confidential and must remain that way. The assistant has a responsibility to the patient, to the physician, to himself or herself, and to society to uphold the ethical responsibilities as written in the AAMA Code of Ethics: to render service, respect confidential information, and uphold the honor and high principles of the profession.

▶ PATIENT EDUCATION

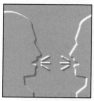

In order to improve the overall health status of individuals and to enlist the patient as an ally in the examination process, the medical assistant must educate the patient in many different ways. Patient education is an important function of the profession, the procedure process, and the concepts of holistic health.

The physical examination process is an excellent time for the medical assistant to assess the need for patient education. This assessment should be performed to identify the best way to meet the needs of the patient. When identifying these needs, consider the following:

- the information that the patient needs to know
- how to convey the information so that the patient will understand
- how the patient will use the information once he or she has it

Develop a plan to teach the patient. Think about the different modalities available, such as pamphlets, pictures, films, demonstrations, and community resources. The more interesting you make your information, the more fun you will have presenting it to the patient, and the more enjoyment the patient will get out of learning. Always share your teaching strategy plans with your physician/employer so you will proceed with full consent. Remember that your physician may have some additional ideas that will make this teaching plan even more exciting.

When planning patient education, it is helpful to follow an outline. An outline will help you remember everything you want to tell the patient, and it will assist you to present material in an orderly manner so that the patient is able to understand and learn. An outline might contain the following subdivisions:

A. Goal (what do you want to accomplish?)
B. Intervention (how do you plan to accomplish this?)
C. Evaluation (how will you know that the teaching was successful?)

After you have completed the teaching session with the patient, you need to evaluate your effectiveness.

- Did you cover all the items on your plan?
- Did the patient learn?
- How do you feel about your performance?
- Are you willing to try it again?
- How did the patient receive the information?

Developing patient teaching materials can be time-consuming. However, sharing meaningful and helpful information with the patient is a gift that can have positive repercussions throughout the patient's life.

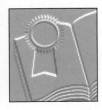

▶ LEARNING ACHIEVEMENTS

Upon completion of this chapter, can you in the time allowed by your evaluator:

1. Interview and obtain an accurate and useful patient medical record that is complete in scope and depth, legible, and without spelling errors?

2. Position and drape a patient in six different examining positions with ease while mindful of patient modesty?

3. Prepare the examination room and instruments, and assist in the physical examination of a patient, correctly completing each step of the procedure in the proper sequence?

READINGS AND REFERENCES

Carlson, J. H., Craft, C. A., McGuire, A. D., and Popkess-Vawter, S.: *Nursing Diagnosis: A Case Study Approach,* Philadelphia, W. B. Saunders Co., 1991.

Frew, M. A., and Frew, D. R.: *Comprehensive Medical Assisting,* 2nd ed., Philadelphia, F. A. Davis Co., 1990.

Ignatavicius, D. D., and Bayne, M. V.: *Medical and Surgical Nursing,* Philadelphia, W. B. Saunders Co., 1992.

Miller, B. F., and Keane, C. B.: *Encyclopedia and Dictionary of Medicine, Nursing, and Allied Health,* 5th ed., Philadelphia, W. B. Saunders Co., 1992.

Purtilo, R.: *Health Professional and Patient Interaction,* 4th ed., Philadelphia, W. B. Saunders Co., 1990.

VOCABULARY

cervix The narrow lower end of the uterus. Sometimes called the *neck of the uterus*.

chancre The primary lesion of syphilis occurring at the site of entry of the infection.

congenital Present at and existing from birth.

ejaculation Ejection of the seminal fluid from the male urethra.

epididymis Oblong coiled body on top of the testis that stores the sperm cells.

fallopian tubes Tubes that capture the expelled ova and transport them to the uterus. Usual location of fertilization. Also called the *oviducts*.

foreskin Loose skin covering the end of the penis.

glans penis The cone shaped glans at the end of the penis; covered by the foreskin in the uncircumcised male.

hydrocephaly An elargement of the crainum caused by abnormal accumulation of cerebrospinal fluid within the cerebral system.

labia majora Two folds of adipose tissue that extend from the mons pubis to the perineum in the female.

labia minora The two thin folds of epithelial tissue between the labia majara and the opening of the vagina.

mammary glands The breasts.

menarche The onset of the menstrual cycle.

menopause The biologic end of the reproductive cycle of the female. Also called *climacteric*.

menstruation The cyclic shedding of the lining (endometrium) of the uterus.

microcephaly A small size of the head in relationship to the rest of the body.

mons pubis The fat pad that covers the symphysis pubis.

multiparous Describing women who have had two or more pregnancies.

ovaries A pair of almond-shaped organs located at the distal end of the fallopian tubes that are responsible for the production and release of ova and a large percentage of female hormones.

penis The male organ of copulation.

prostate A fluid-secreting gland that surrounds the neck of the urethra.

scrotum The double pouch that contains the testicles and epididymides.

semen Thick whitish secretion containing spermatozoa.

seminal vesicles A pair of structures located at the base of the bladder that produce the fluid portion of semen.

spermatozoa The mature male sex cells or germ cells.

testicle The male gonad.

urethra The canal through which urine is discharged.

uterus A pear-shaped organ located in the pelvic cavity between the bladder and the rectum and attached to the cervix. Holds the fetus during pregnancy.

vagina A collapsible tube extending from the vaginal opening to the cervix.

vas deferens The testicular duct that carries sperm from the epididymis to the ejaculatory duct. Also called *ductus deferens*.

vasectomy Sterilization procedure for the male.

void To urinate.

vulva The external female genitalia. It begins at the mons pubis and terminates at the anus.

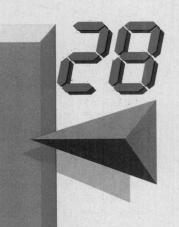

SPECIALTY EXAMINATION

PART 1: OBSTETRICS, GYNECOLOGY, UROLOGY, AND PEDIATRICS

LEARNING OBJECTIVES

COGNITIVE

Upon successful completion of this chapter, you should be able to:

1. Define and spell the words listed in the Vocabulary.

2. Outline the procedure for female and male reproductive system examinations.

3. List 10 disorders of the female reproductive system and 5 of the male reproductive system.

4. Describe the signs and symptoms of sexually transmitted diseases in males and females.

5. List the female and male diagnostic tests performed in the office.

6. Compare the three trimesters of pregnancy.

7. Outline the sterilizing procedures in obstetrics, gynecology, pediatrics, and urology.

8. Discuss methods of family planning.

9. Describe changes in the examination procedure when the patient is a child.

10. Define the medical assistant's legal and ethical obligations.

PERFORMANCE

Upon successful completion of this chapter, you should be able to:

1. Assist with the examination of the female reproductive system.

2. Assist with the examination of the male reproductive system.

3. Assist with the physical examination of a child.

4. Instruct a patient in self-examination procedures for breast or testicular abnormalities.

5. Perform a Denver Developmental Screening Test on a preschool-age child.

In this chapter, the disciplines of obstetrics, gynecology, urology, and pediatrics are discussed. The sexual and reproductive health of the parent and the health maintenance of the child are the primary topics.

Sexual health includes the maintenance of one's freedom from physical and psychologic impairment. The medical assistant can assist the physician in a variety of situations to promote sexual health and to prevent sexual dysfunctions that are related to illness and injury throughout the life of the patient.

The assessment of the male and female reproductive systems is an important part of health care. Often, patients are hesitant and uncomfortable with talking about sexual matters and wait until symptoms are intolerable or disease is advanced before seeking medical care. It is important that the medical assistant be aware of the patient's emotional state and give support as needed.

In pediatrics, the child is usually joined by one or both parents during visits to the physician. The health of the child is the concern of both parents, and the medical assistant is usually confronted with the parents' questions and comments concerning their child. Parents need to have reinforcement, praise, and understanding in dealing with the health and welfare of their child, and they expect to receive such support from the pediatrician and the office staff.

OBSTETRICS AND GYNECOLOGY

The branch of medicine that deals with pregnancy, labor, and the puerperium is known as *obstetrics,* and the branch of medicine that deals with diseases of the genital tract in women is called *gynecology.* Frequently, a physician practices both specialties and is known as an "OB/GYN" physician.

An annual pelvic examination is recommended for women after the age of 20 years (before this age if they are sexually active) and if birth control medications are prescribed.

Examination of the female reproductive system is done to assure normality of the reproductive organs or to diagnose and treat abnormalities of these organs. A gynecologic history includes age at **menarche;** regularity of the menstrual cycle; amount and duration of the menstrual flow; menstrual disturbances such as dysmenorrhea; intermenstrual or postmenstrual bleeding; and the presence of vaginal discharges. The first prenatal visit is rather extensive, with a complete history and physical examination and a pelvic examination that includes pelvic measurements, serologic tests, and routine laboratory tests. Follow-up prenatal visits include urinalysis, weight, and blood pressure measurement, and advice on diet and health habits. Any concerns of the patient are alleviated at this time.

The examining room must be adequately equipped, and the surroundings pleasant. A dressing area with an adjacent toilet should be provided. The dressing area should assure privacy and should be equipped with tissues and sanitary protection items. Disposable examination gowns are also placed in this room. Supplies should be checked frequently throughout the day.

EXAMINATION OF THE FEMALE REPRODUCTIVE SYSTEM

The patient should be instructed to empty her bladder and rectum, completely disrobe, and put on an examination gown. Unless contraindicated, the patient should have been advised at the time the appointment was made not to douche or have sexual intercourse for 24 hours prior to the examination in order to properly evaluate vaginal discharges and to ensure accurate results of cytologic studies.

Breast Examination

The examination of the reproductive system usually begins with the **mammary glands.** The patient is advised to sit at the end of the examination table in Fowler's position. The drape should be arranged so that only the breast tissue is exposed. The physician then examines the breasts by inspection and palpation. Afterward, the assistant is instructed to assist the patient into a supine position so that the remainder of the breast examination may be performed. When the examination is completed, the gown is readjusted to cover the breast tissue.

Abdominal Examination

Following the examination of the breasts, the physician palpates the abdomen to confirm normal symmetry and the presence of possible masses. In the case of pregnancy, the uterine enlargement is also evaluated. For this examination, the patient's arms should be placed at her sides to achieve better relaxation of the abdominal muscles.

The Pelvic Examination

The medical assistant should remain in the examining room to provide reassurance to the patient as well as offer legal protection to the physician while the **vagina** and perineal areas are being examined. Furthermore, the patient should be given assistance in getting on and off the table. The lithotomy position is very awkward to get into unassisted and is embarrassing to the patient.

First, the physician inspects the external genitalia and palpates the perineal body, Bartholin's and Skene's glands, and the urethral meatus. The patient may be asked to "bear down" in order to show any muscular weaknesses that may be the result of lacerations of the perineal body during childbirth. A third-degree laceration may have involved the rectal sphincter and may cause rectal incontinence.

Next, the vaginal speculum is inserted for examination of the **cervix** and the vaginal canal (Fig. 28–1). The normal cervix points posteriorly and is smooth, pink-colored squamous epithelium. The abnormalities most frequently seen are ulcerations (erosions), nabothian cysts, and cervical polyps. Since erosions cannot be palpated, inspection is the only method of knowing their presence. Healed lacerations resulting from childbirth are common in the multiparous patient. Pregnancy increases the size of the cervix, and hormone deficiency causes it to atrophy. The vaginal wall is reddish pink and has a corrugated appearance. Vaginal infections change the appearance of the vaginal mucosa.

After the vaginal speculum has been removed, the physician does a bimanual examination; that is, the minor hand is lubricated and inserted into the vaginal canal and the major hand palpates the abdomen over the pelvic organs and the **mons pubis** (Fig. 28–2). The **uterus** is examined for shape, size, and consistency. The position of the uterus is noted. The normal uterus is freely movable with limited discomfort (Fig. 28–3). A laterally displaced uterus is usually the result of pelvic adhesions or displacement caused by a pelvic tumor. The uterine adnexa (**fallopian tubes** and **ovaries**) are evaluated. The normal tubes and ovaries are difficult to palpate. The physician may now complete the examination by rectovaginal abdominal examination. This is done when the middle finger of the minor hand is inserted into the rectum and the index finger is in the vaginal canal. The rectum is checked by the index finger inserted into the rectum.

Disorders of the Female Reproductive System

Spontaneous Abortion

Spontaneous abortion (miscarriage) is the loss of a pregnancy before the 20th week of fetal development. Common causes are defective development of the embryo, abnormalities of the placenta, endocrine disorders, malnutrition, infection, drug reaction, blood group incompatibilities, severe trauma, and shock. Symptoms include vaginal bleeding of varying degrees of severity and lower abdominal cramping progressing to cervical dilatation with rupture of membranes and complete expulsion of the products of conception. An incomplete abortion results from the partial retention of these products, necessitating a D & C (dilatation and curettage.)

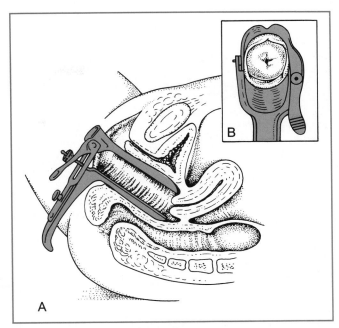

FIGURE 28–1. *A,* Proper position of inserted speculum for examination of the cervix uteri. *B,* Normal parous cervix as seen through a speculum.

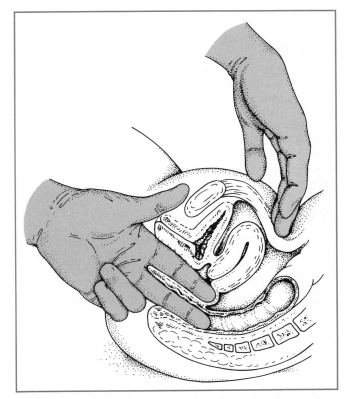

FIGURE 28–2. Bimanual pelvic examination. The hand on the abdomen brings more of the pelvic contents into contact with the inserted fingers. This technique provides a more adequate palpation of the pelvic viscera than can be accomplished by vaginal examination alone.

28

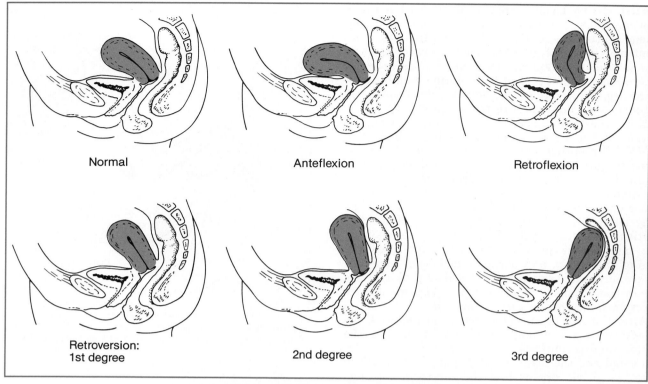

Normal | Anteflexion | Retroflexion

Retroversion: 1st degree | 2nd degree | 3rd degree

FIGURE 28-3. Positions of the uterus in sagittal section.

Cervicitis

Cervicitis is an inflammation of the cervix caused by an invading organism. The main symptom is a thick, purulent, whitish discharge with an acrid odor. Dysuria may also be present. Cervicitis is common after vaginal delivery, resulting from infection of cervical lacerations. Treatment consists primarily of antibiotics, although cauterization, or electrocoagulation, may be indicated when cervical erosion exists.

Cervical Polyps

Polyps are the second most common lesion of the cervix. They are most prevalent during the reproductive years. The most common symptom is genital bleeding following intercourse, douching, or tampon insertion. Treatment consists of surgical removal of the polyps in the office.

Cystocele

A cystocele is a protrusion of the bladder into the vagina. A diagnosis can be made by requesting the patient to bear down as the vaginal opening is examined. Cystoceles may result from injury during childbirth, obesity, heavy lifting, chronic coughing, and poor musculature due to aging.

Dysmenorrhea

Dysmenorrhea consists of lower abdominal and pelvic pain associated with **menstruation.** It is one of the most common gynecologic disorders among young females, although it tends to decrease with maturity. The pain is spasmodic. It usually begins 12 to 14 hours prior to the onset of menses and lasts 24 to 48 hours. Dysmenorrhea may be associated with headaches, dizziness, nausea, vomiting, fatigue, low back pain, and diarrhea. The cause of dysmenorrhea is unknown. However, dysmenorrhea may be a symptom of an organic disease, and in this case, must be corrected. Treatment includes analgesics, heat, drugs to decrease uterine contractions, and hormones to suppress ovulation.

Endometriosis

Endometriosis is characterized by the presence of endometrial tissue outside the uterus. It is commonly found in the pelvic area attached to the **vulva,** urinary bladder, uterus, fallopian tubes, ovaries, intestines, and peritoneum. The cause is unknown, but it is believed to be the result of recent surgery on the uterus, retrograde tubal flow of menstrual fragments, poor nutrition, intercourse during menstruation, or hormonal influences. Use of tampons has also been suggested as a possible cause. Dysmenorrhea and contact pain in the lower abdomen, pelvis, vagina, and back beginning 7 days before menses and lasting 3 days after onset characterize this condition. Other symptoms can include profuse menses, hematuria, rectal bleeding, nausea, vomiting, and abdominal cramps. Treatment includes analgesics, hormonal therapy, and surgery.

Fibrocystic Breast Disease

Fibrocystic breast disease is the presence of multiple, palpable lumps in the breast, usually associated with pain and tenderness that fluctuate with the menstrual cycle. The lumps may be fibrous tumors that have degenerated or sacs filled with fluid. Women with the disease are believed to be at greater risk of developing breast cancer, but this has not been proved.

Fibroid Tumors

Uterine fibroids are benign tumors composed mainly of smooth muscle and some fibrous connective tissue. Fibroids are the common pelvic tumor in women. Their cause is unknown. Menorrhagia (excessive menstruation) is the primary symptom, although the patient may experience bladder or rectal pressure, pelvic pressure, pain, abdominal distortion, and infertility. Treatment consists of surgical removal of small masses, but a hysterectomy (removal of uterus) is indicated when there is greater involvement.

Ovarian Cysts

Ovarian cysts are sacs of fluid or semisolid material located on the ovary. Most cysts are nonmalignant, small, and asymptomatic. They can occur in the follicle or the corpus luteum at any time between puberty and **menopause.** Large or multiple cysts may cause discomfort, low back pain, nausea, vomiting, and abnormal uterine bleeding. Surgery may be indicated if rupture of the cyst occurs.

Pelvic Inflammatory Disease (PID)

PID is any acute or chronic infection of the reproductive system ascending from the vagina (vaginitis), cervix (cervicitis), uterus (endometritis), fallopian tubes (salpingitis), and ovaries (oophoritis). The most common cause of PID is gonorrhea. Uterine infection can also develop following the insertion of an intrauterine device (IUD). Other causative factors include pelvic surgery, tubal examinations, and abortion. Symptoms include a purulent vaginal discharge, fever, malaise, dysuria, lower abdominal pain, bleeding, and nausea and vomiting. PID can be treated with antibiotics, analgesics, and bed rest.

Premenstrual Syndrome (PMS)

PMS is a number of symptoms that appear 1 to 2 weeks before menstruation and that usually subside close to the onset of menses. Symptoms include irritability, nervousness, fatigue, depression, headache, dizziness, numbness of extremities, fainting, asthma, rhinitis, constipation, diarrhea, breast tenderness and enlargement, water retention, backache, palpitations, temporary weight gain, change in appetite, and abdominal bloating. PMS is believed to be a result of salt retention. Treatment consists of diuretics and salt restriction.

Rectocele

A rectocele is a protrusion of the rectum into the vagina. Diagnosis can be made by requesting the patient to bear down as the vaginal opening is examined. Rectoceles are most common in postmenopausal women. Rectoceles may result from pregnancies, instrument deliveries, prolonged labors, obesity, chronic coughing, and lifting heavy objects.

Malignancy of the Reproductive System

The majority of the problems encountered with the female reproductive organs are related to abnormal cell growth. Early screening and preventive intervention are essential. Most malignant tumors require surgical removal. Radiation, chemotherapy, and hormone therapy may be alternative treatment choices. Uterine cancer is the most common reproductive organ cancer, usually affecting women between the ages of 50 and 60 years. The first signs of uterine cancer include uterine enlargement and unusual bleeding. The only reliable diagnostic procedure is a biopsy. Cervical cancer is asymptomatic until the malignancy has penetrated through the membranes and spread. The earliest symptoms include abnormal vaginal bleeding, persistent discharge, and bleeding and pain during intercourse. Cervical cancer can be detected early by a Papanicolaou (PAP) smear. The American Cancer Society recommends that all women under the age of 40 years of age have a smear performed every 3 years and that women over 40 years of age have annual smears. Other cancers of the female reproductive organs include endometrial, ovarian, vulvar, and vaginal cancers, and carcinoma of the fallopian tube.

Malignancy of the Breast

Breast cancer is the most common malignancy among females and the leading cause of death among women between 35 and 55 years of age. Although the cause is unknown, other predisposing factors include family history of breast cancer, early menarche and late menopause, first pregnancy after the age of 35 years or no pregnancy, high socioeconomic status, obesity, stress, high-fat diet, extensive use of oral contraceptives, and other cancers. The incidence of this cancer is highest among white patients.

Breast cancer appears most commonly in the upper outer quadrant of the left breast. It spreads through the lymphatic and circulatory systems to other parts of the body. Specific signs include

- A lump in the breast
- Changes in breast shape and size
- Change in the appearance of the skin
- Change in skin temperature
- Drainage or discharge
- Change in the nipple

Diagnosis is made through routine monthly breast self-examinations, mammography, ultrasonography, needle aspiration, and surgical biopsy. Treatment consists of

- A lumpectomy (removal of tumor only)
- Simple mastectomy (removal of breast only)
- Modified radical mastectomy (removal of breast and axillary nodes)
- Radical mastectomy (removal of breast, axillary nodes, and muscle of chest wall)

Invasive mammary carcinoma has been classified into four clinical stages:

Stage I: Breast tumors less than 2 cm in diameter.

Stage II: Breast tumors 2 to 5 cm in diameter, or cancers with small mobile axillary lymph node metastases.

Stage III: Breast tumors over 5 cm in diameter with lymph node metastases or skin involvement.

Stage IV: Distant metastases.

Noninvasive mammary carcinomas are classified as Stage TIS (tumor in situ).

Sexually Transmitted Infections

Herpes Simplex Virus (HSV)

HSV is a virus that is spread by direct skin-to-skin contact with another lesion. There are two strains of the virus, HSV-1 (Type 1) and HSV-2 (Type 2). HSV-1 causes the typical cold sore on the lip or edge of the nose, whereas HSV-2 is the more frequent cause of genital infection. Painful genital fluid-filled vesicles appear on the cervix, **labia,** vulva, vagina, perineum, or buttocks 3 to 7 days after contact with infected secretions. After the lesions heal, the virus becomes dormant, but additional attacks may recur throughout life. There is some evidence that HSV-2 may cause spontaneous abortion and premature delivery. Newborns can be infected with herpes through active lesions in the birth canal during vaginal deliveries. Brain damage, blindness, or death of the newborn may occur. Most

physicians choose to perform a cesarean section when a woman has active lesions at the time of birth.

Diagnosis is made by observation of the characteristic vesicles, from patient history, and from virologic tests. Treatment consists of a combination of antiviral medications such as acyclovir, sulfa-based creams to ease discomfort, and antibacterial agents to combat secondary infections. These herpes lesions are highly contagious, and the medical assistant must avoid contact with all secretions.

Gonorrhea

Gonorrhea is among the most common sexually transmitted diseases. It is widespread throughout the world. It occurs most frequently among lower socioeconomic groups. The causative organism of gonorrhea is the bacterium *Neisseria gonorrhoeae.* The organism is quite fragile and can survive only in a moist, dark, warm area of the body. The most common sites are the vagina, **penis,** rectum, mouth, and throat. The disease is spread only through direct sexual contact. Infants can become infected during birth if the mother has the disease. Women are usually asymptomatic, but they may develop a greenish-yellow discharge from the cervix. Preliminary diagnosis may be made by microscopic examination using Gram's stain and viewing intracellular or extracellular Gram-negative diplococci. To confirm the diagnosis, the gonococci from the discharge are cultured. Large doses of penicillin or tetracycline are the recommended treatment.

Syphilis

Syphilis is of unique importance among the sexually transmitted infections because its early lesions heal without treatment and become a major risk to the patient. Since the patient has no symptoms, he or she thinks the infection has disappeared. Syphilis is caused by a delicate bacterium called a *spirochete,* which inhabits the warm moist areas of the genitals and rectum. Syphilis is spread by direct sexual contact or by prenatal transmission to the fetus via the placenta, resulting in an infant with **congenital** syphilis.

The disease progresses through four stages. Symptoms vary according to the stage of involvement. The primary stage (first stage) begins with the organism entering the mucous membranes or the genitals as a result of sexual contact with an infected person. Three or four weeks later, a lesion called a **chancre** appears at the site of organism entrance. Secondary syphilis (second stage) develops 6 to 8 weeks after the chancre. Skin, mucous membranes, and lymph nodes are involved. This stage is characterized by a generalized, painless, nonitching rash. Systemic manifestations include appetite, hair, and weight loss; fever; sore throat; headache; nausea; constipation; and bone, muscle, and joint pain. Without treatment, the disease becomes asymptomatic in 2 to 6 weeks. Early latent syphilis (third stage) is asymptomatic and may last for years. The organism is invading the blood vessels, brain, spinal cord, and the bones. After 1 year, the disease is no longer infectious. Late latent syphilis (fourth stage) is characterized according to the type of involvement, such as internal organs, heart and major blood vessels, and brain and spinal cord.

Syphilis must be diagnosed by darkfield examination of the spirochete or by a blood test called VDRL (Venereal Disease Research Laboratory). Diagnosis is confirmed with the FTA-ABS (fluorescent treponemal antibody with absorbed serum) blood test or the TPHA (treponemal pallidum hemagglutination) test. Penicillin is the treatment for syphilis.

Trichomoniasis

Trichomonas vaginalis is the parasitic organism responsible for the infection. The infection can be passed back and forth between sexual partners; therefore, both persons must be treated. The prime and discriminating symptom is a foul, profuse, yellowish, frothy discharge that may be identified by visual examination or during routine urinalysis or microscopic examination. Diagnosis is made by placing a drop of the secretion on a slide and microscopically identifying the organism. Metronidazole is the drug of choice.

Candidiasis

Candida albicans is the yeastlike fungus responsible for this infection. Candida organisms are commonly part of the normal flora of the mouth, skin, intestinal tract, and vagina. Overgrowth of the organism can be caused by long-term antibiotic use, high estrogen levels, diabetes mellitus, and the wearing of tight clothing. Symptoms include itching; dry, bright-red vagina; and vaginal discharge thick with curds that are identified during the microscopic examination of the routine urinalysis. Diagnosis is made by microscopic examination of the discharge mixed with 10% potassium hydroxide on a slide. Miconazole cream is the drug treatment of choice.

Chlamydia

Chlamydia trachomatis produces a wide variety of illnesses, including infertility, urethritis, proctitis, endometritis, pneumonitis, and epididymitis. The infections are primarily sexually transmitted. *Chlamydia trachomatis* was the most commonly transmitted bacterium in the United States in 1988.

Transmission of the bacterium to the newborn can occur during vaginal delivery, resulting in neonatal eye infections and pneumonia. An estimated 155,000 infants are infected yearly. About 75% of women with the infection may have no symptoms. Some experience a vaginal discharge, dysuria, urinary frequency, and soreness in the affected area. In men, the symptoms are the same except that the discharge is usually present only in the morning after waking.

Diagnostic Testing

Diagnostic testing seen in the medical office includes the following procedures.

Breast Self-Examination

Routine monthly breast self-examinations are the best and most reliable means of detecting breast cancer. Over 90% of all initial findings of breast cancer are made by the patient. The American Cancer Society provides excellent pamphlets and films demonstrating the procedure (Fig. 28–4).

Ultrasonogram

Ultrasound is a technique that uses high-frequency sound waves to produce images of solid organs of the body and of accumulations of fluid. Ultrasound can distinguish between cysts and tumors. It is used during pregnancy to determine the number of fetuses, age and sex of the fetus, fetal abnormalities, and position of the placenta.

Mammogram

This is an x-ray film of the breast performed almost exclusively for the detection of breast cancer. The American Cancer Society recommends a single baseline mammogram for all women between 35 and 40 years of age, to be followed by annual mammograms after the age of 50 years.

Papanicolaou (PAP) Test

A PAP smear is the single most important test performed in the OB/GYN office. A PAP smear is the removal of cells from the cervix and upper vagina to detect the presence of cancer. These cells are scraped from the cervix with a cervical spatula, are spread on a slide, and are sprayed with a commercial fixative of 50% alcohol and 50% ether. The slide is then labeled and sent to the cytology laboratory (Figs. 28–5 and 28–6).

The descriptive terminology currently preferred by physicians and Papanicolaou's classification of cytologic findings are as follows:

28

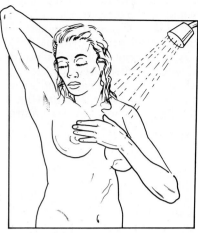

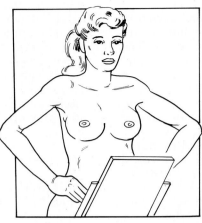

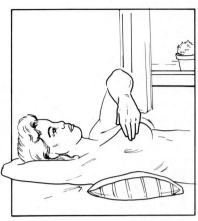

In the shower.
Raise one arm. With fingers flat, touch every part of each breast, gently feeling for a lump or thickening. Use your right hand to examine your left breast, your left hand for your right breast.

Before a mirror.
With arms at your sides, then with arms raised above your head, look carefully for changes in the size, shape, and contour of each breast. Look for puckering, dimpling, or changes in skin texture.

Gently squeeze both nipples and look for discharge.

Lying down.
Place a towel or pillow under your right shoulder and your right shoulder and your right hand behind your head. Examine your right breast with your left hand.

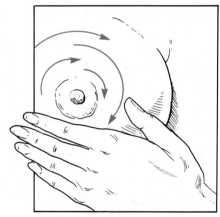

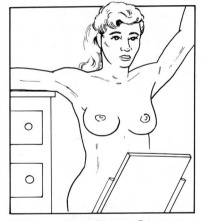

Fingers flat, press gently in small circles, starting at the outermost top edge of your breast and spiraling in toward the nipple. Examine every part of the breast. Repeat with left breast.

With your arm resting on a firm surface, use the same circular motion to examine the underarm area. This is breast tissue, too.

This self-exam is not a substitute for periodic examinations by a qualified physician.

FIGURE 28-4. Performing a monthly breast self-examination. (Redrawn with permission of Albert Einstein Healthcare Foundation, Philadelphia, PA.)

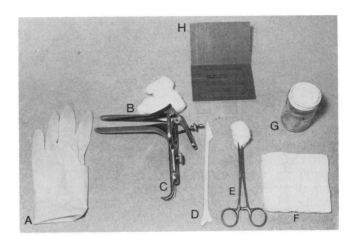

FIGURE 28-5. Typical set-up for a Papanicolaou smear. *A*, Nonsterile glove. *B*, Rayon balls. *C*, Vaginal speculum. *D*, Cervix scraper. *E*, Uterine sponge forceps. *F*, 4″ × 4″ Gauze flats. *G*, Fixative. *H*, Slides and laboratory request.

Current Descriptive Terminology

- Normal
- Metaplasia
- Inflammation
- Minimal atypia koilocytosis
- Mild dysplasia
- Severe dysplasia, carcinoma in situ
- Invasive carcinoma

Papanicolaou's classification

Class 1: Absence of atypical or abnormal cells

Class 2: Atypical cytologic results but no evidence of malignancy

Class 3: Cytologic results suggestive of, but not conclusive for, malignancy

Class 4: Cytologic results strongly suggestive of malignancy

Class 5: Cytologic results conclusive for malignancy

If a woman's smear has demonstrated atypical cells, she should be encouraged to have follow-up testing.

Pregnancy Testing

Most pregnancy tests are designed to detect the hormone *human chorionic gonadotropin (HCG),* normally found in the serum and urine of pregnant women about 1 week after the first missed menses. Urine testing and blood testing are commonly performed. The urine test should be conducted on the first urine specimen voided in the morning, because the hormone is most concentrated at this time. (Pregnancy testing is covered in Chapter 33.)

Pregnancy

The medical assistant should also be knowledgeable about the pregnant female, since many of the OB/GYN patients are pregnant. Pregnancy is de-

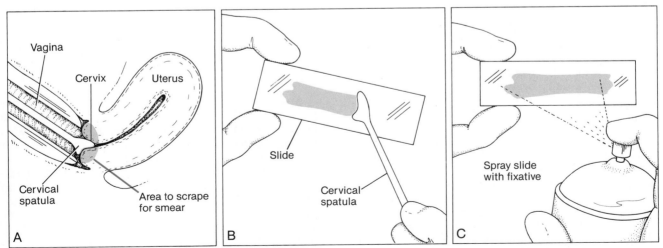

FIGURE 28-6. Collecting a Papanicolaou smear. *A*, Scrape a small portion of the musosa from the cervical os using a wooden cervical spatula. *B*, Transfer the specimen onto a slide by moving the spatula over the surface. *C*, Fix the slide with an aerosol "fixative" or hair spray.

fined as the condition of carrying a developing embryo in the uterus. The duration of pregnancy is approximately 280 days and is divided into first, second, and third trimesters.

First Trimester

The *first trimester* is the period from the beginning of the last menstrual period through the 14th week. It is a period of multiple physical and psychologic changes for the female. For the fetus, it is a crucial period of organ development. It is during this time that the obstetrician obtains a complete health history of the patient, including family, medical, menstrual, and obstetric histories. The patient also undergoes a complete medical and obstetric examination. Diagnostic testing at this time includes:

- Complete blood count
- Blood type and Rh factor
- Serologic test for syphilis
- Rubella titer
- Sickle cell trait or disease (for black patients)
- Blood glucose (for high-risk patients)
- PAP smear
- Smears for infections (when indicated)
- Urinalysis
- Pregnancy test

Second Trimester

The *second trimester* is the period from the 15th through the 28th week after the last menstrual period. The uterus has enlarged to above the umbilicus, and the first fetal movements are felt by the patient. In addition to the basic health history and physical examination, assessment by abdominal palpation and fetal heart monitoring are conducted. Diagnostic testing during this period may include amniocentesis, ultrasonography, and x-ray films.

Third Trimester

The *third trimester* is the period from the end of the 28th week until the time of delivery. This is a period marked by rapid fetal growth. The patient continues to be closely monitored. Childbirth preparation classes usually begin during this time.

Labor

Labor is the physiologic process by which the uterus expels the fetus and the placenta. Labor is divided into three stages:

Stage I: Period from onset of labor through complete dilatation of the cervix.
Stage II: Period from complete dilatation of the cervix through the birth of the fetus.
Stage III: Period from the birth of the fetus through the expulsion of the placenta and the membranes.

Family Planning

Family planning refers to the process of deciding whether to have children, how many to have, and when to have them. Choices of whether or not to use a contraceptive method, which to use, and how to use it may be influenced by many external factors and internal feelings.

Permanent methods of contraception include the surgical procedures of **vasectomy** for the male and tubal ligation for the female. Tubal ligation is a surgical procedure in which the fallopian tubes are occluded to prevent the passage of future ova. It can be performed using several different surgical techniques, each of which produces the same result. A woman needs to be fully informed about sterilization before she gives consent for the procedure. The U.S. Department of Health and Human Services has set up the following guidelines for federally funded sterilizations to make sure that a woman fully understands the procedure:

- The risks, benefits, and alternatives of the procedure must be explained.
- A statement that describes sterilization as a permanent and irreversible method of birth control is given to the patient.
- A 30-day waiting period is required between the time of consent and the surgery.
- The consent forms must be in the woman's native language, or provisions for an interpreter must be provided.

Sterilization does not stop the normal menstrual cycle nor does it cause any changes in physiologic or sexual responses.

There are many effective methods of contraception available to the couple that wants to plan a family. Table 28–1 provides information on the most commonly used methods of temporary contraception used in family planning.

STERILIZATION PROCEDURES

Any instrument that comes in contact with a patient should be sterilized in an autoclave for 15 to 20 minutes at 15 pounds of pressure and at 250°F, or with a germicide chemical before it is used for another patient. If the instrument does not penetrate tissue, it may be stored under clean or medically aseptic conditions. Some physicians prefer to use disposable specula for routine pelvic examinations. Instruments that penetrate the tissue *must be sterilized and stored under sterile conditions*. Such instruments include the uterine biopsy punch, uterine tenaculum, cervical dilators and sounds, and any item used for the insertion of an intrauterine device.

TABLE 28–1. COMMONLY USED METHODS OF CONTRACEPTION

Method	Description	Possible Side Effects	Advantages
Norplant implants	Implanted by the doctor once every 5 y.	Menstrual	Convenient; long-term effectiveness; safe for women who should not take estrogen.
The pill	Prescribed by doctor; taken daily.	Weight gain, nausea, headache; increased risk of stroke, cardiovascular disease for women over 35 y of age who smoke.	Easy to use; protects against endometrial and ovarian cancers, pelvic inflammatory disease; alleviates common menstrual disorders.
Mini pill	Prescribed by doctor; taken daily.	Menstrual irregularities; increased risk of ectopic pregnancy.	Safe for women who should not take estrogen.
Intrauterine device (IUD)	Inserted by doctor every 1–6 y.	Increased menstrual bleeding, often with pain; increased risk of infection, infertility, ectopic pregnancy, and pelvic inflammatory disease.	Convenient; long-term effectiveness.
Diaphragm cervical cap (with spermicide)	Fitted by doctor; inserted by woman prior to intercourse.	May increase risk of bladder infections; spermicide may cause vaginal irritation.	No apparent health risks; some protection against sexually transmitted diseases.
Condom	Applied prior to intercourse.	None.	Helps protect against some sexually transmitted diseases.
Spermicide	Applied prior to intercourse.	Vaginal irritation.	No apparent health risks.
Rhythm method	Abstinence for 1/3 to 1/2 of menstrual cycle.	None.	No apparent health risks.
Sterilization	One-time surgical procedure.	None.	Permanent; no long-term health risks.

MEDICAL ASSISTANT'S ROLE IN THE FEMALE REPRODUCTIVE SYSTEM EXAMINATION

The female medical assistant should be in attendance while the patient is exposed, including during the examination. The male medical assistant is usually not in the room during the examination except when it is necessary to assist with a procedure. The physician makes the decision regarding the male assistant's role in the female reproductive system examination. When in attendance, it is your responsibility to support the patient and to assist the physician during the procedure. The procedure should be fully explained to the patient to avoid unnecessary embarrassment and discomfort. During the explanation, the assistant has the opportunity to do some patient teaching.

Begin the examination by placing the patient into a sitting position and by adjusting the gown so that the breast tissue can be easily exposed. The physician will instruct the patient to place her arms above her head, and the assistant should be present to assist the patient if she has difficulty in following these instructions. When the patient is instructed to assume a supine position, the assistant helps the patient and adjusts the gown and drape as needed for the physician and for the patient's comfort. A small pillow may be placed under the patient's head for comfort, and a second may be placed under the breast that is being examined to distribute the tissue more evenly.

When the physician is ready to perform the pelvic examination, the assistant places the patient into the lithotomy position and adjusts the drape so that only the perineum is exposed. The speculum should be at body temperature for the patient's comfort. The assistant should be ready to hand the physician the equipment and supplies needed as the examination is performed. Always watch the patient for signs of anxiety or pain; if you note such signs, report this to the physician immediately. After the PAP specimen is obtained, the medical assistant may be responsible for applying the fixative agent to the glass slide and preparing the specimen for transport to the cytology laboratory. Be sure to follow the laboratory instructions in the preparation to avoid possibly repeating the examination to obtain another specimen.

Once the examination is concluded, the medical assistant instructs the patient to take several deep, even breaths slowly through the mouth to help her to relax. The assistant then helps her back into a sitting position and into the dressing room if needed.

Remove all of the examination equipment and supplies while the patient is dressing so that when the physician returns to talk to the patient, the room is aesthetically neat. Once the patient has left, the room should be cleaned and restocked as necessary and made ready for the next patient.

28

PROCEDURE 28-1   ASSISTING WITH A PELVIC EXAMINATION

GOAL   To assist the physician in a routine pelvic examination.

EQUIPMENT AND SUPPLIES

Patient gown
Drape sheet
Vaginal speculum
Lubricant
Examination light
Uterine sponge forceps
4" × 4" Gauze flats

Vaginal spatula (cervix scraper)
Disposable gloves
Laboratory slips
Microscopic slides
Fixative for Pap smear
Blood and body-fluid protection barriers, as necessary

PROCEDURAL STEPS

1. Wash your hands. Follow universal blood and body-fluid precautions. Glove yourself with nonsterile gloves.

2. Assemble the materials needed, and prepare the room.

3. Identify the patient, and briefly explain the procedure.
   Purpose: Explanations help gain patient cooperation and alleviate apprehension.

4. Instruct the patient to empty the bladder and collect a urine specimen if needed.
   Purpose: Organ palpations are performed on an empty bladder.

5. Instruct the patient to disrobe completely and to put on a gown. Explain proper gown opening (front or back).

6. Assist the patient into the lithotomy position, and apply a drape.
   Purpose: To avoid exposing the patient unnecessarily.

7. Direct the light source into the vaginal speculum.

8. Assist the physician with gloving.

9. Assist the physician with preparation of the smear, its labeling, and its transportation to the laboratory.

10. Pass the proper instruments to the physician in proper sequence.

11. Apply the lubricant to the physician's fingers.

12. Place the soiled instruments in a basin.

13. Instruct the patient to breathe deeply through the mouth with hands crossed over the chest.
    Purpose: Helps relax muscles.

14. Assist the patient off the table.

15. Instruct the patient to dress.

16. Clean up the room immediately.

17. Wash your hands.

PEDIATRICS

Pediatrics deals with the development and care of children and with the treatment of childhood diseases. The age range of the pediatric patient is from birth to puberty. Some practices continue to see the child until he or she is 14 to 16 years of age. A large percentage of the patients in the pediatric office are "well-baby" or "well-child" care patients. The role of the physician and the medical office staff is to supervise and help maintain the health of these patients. An increasing number of auxiliary health care personnel are being involved in the health services provided to young patients. Parents of these young patients must be involved with their care and development. The medical assistant can help a great deal in the communications between the patient, the parents, and the medical staff. The confidence a child develops in the care and the consideration received in the physician's office is the basis of good medical care.

Pediatric care actually starts before the child is born, with the promotion of the mother's good general health before conception and during pregnancy. The confidence and enthusiasm of the parents also affect the infant's physical and emotional wellbeing.

The newborn's first physical assessment comes at the time of delivery, when the pediatrician assesses the newborn's ability to thrive outside the uterus. The Apgar score is a system of scoring the infant's physical condition at 1 and 5 minutes after birth (Table 28-2). The heart rate, respiration, muscle tone, response to stimuli, and color of the infant are each rated 0, 1, or 2. The maximum total score is 10. Those infants with low scores must be given immediate attention.

The frequency of the well-child visits varies with the physician and the community. It may follow this pattern: 2 weeks, 7 weeks, 4 months, 1 year, 2 years, 5 years, 10 years, and 15 years. Immunizations and illnesses significantly increase the frequency of these visits.

As with any other physical examination, the medical history is an essential guide to the pediatric examination. With the infant, the physician is dependent on the parent for the history, but as the child gets older some history may be obtained from the child and clarified or amplified by the parent. Generally, the child is extremely honest regarding the facts of the illness. Close observation also gives the physician considerable information. A wince may indicate tenderness, and the facial expression associated with nausea should alert the physician and the staff.

Explaining what is to be done and showing the child the instruments to be used often contribute to his or her cooperation. The instruments and the examiner's hands should be warm.

The duties of the medical assistant are to weigh and measure the infant, to record this information on the patient's chart and on the parent's records, and to check whether immunizations are due (Table 28-3).

The sequence of the examination varies and is frequently adapted to the cooperation of the child. Leave until last the areas to which the patient may object the most and in which the patient may be the least cooperative. Sometimes, a tongue depressor in each little hand keeps an infant from grabbing the stethoscope.

The physician is concerned with the patient's growth and development. The child's alertness and responses tell the physician a considerable amount. In infancy (birth to 2 y) and in the young child of preschool age (2-6 y), the parent is closely questioned about the child's eating, sleeping, and elimination habits. The school-age child (6-12 y or to puberty) is usually a little more cooperative during an examination and can answer most questions

TABLE 28-2. THE APGAR SCORING SYSTEM*

Clinical Sign	Assigned Score		
	0	*1*	*2*
Heart rate	Absent	Under 100	Over 100
Respiratory effort	Absent	Slow and irregular	Good and crying
Muscle tone	Limp	Some flexion of the arms and legs	Active movement
Reflex irritability	No response	Grimace	Coughing and sneezing
Color	Blue and pale	Body pink, and extremities blue	Pink all over

* The readings are taken by the pediatrician at 1-minute and 5-minute intervals after birth. At *1 minute*, if the score is 7 or less, some nervous system problems are suspected. If the score is below 4, resuscitation is usually necessary. At *5 minutes*, if the score is at least 8, the pediatrician can conduct a complete examination. The child is probably reacting normally.

28

PROCEDURE 28-2   MEASURING THE CIRCUMFERENCE OF AN INFANT'S HEAD

GOAL   To obtain an accurate measurement of the circumference of an infant's head.

EQUIPMENT AND SUPPLIES

Flexible tape measure   Patient's chart
Growth chart   Pen or pencil

PROCEDURAL STEPS

1. Wash your hands.
2. Identify the patient.
3. Gain infant cooperation through conversation.
4. Place the infant in the supine position on the examination table; alternatively, the infant may be held by the parent.
5. Hold the tape measure with the zero mark against the infant's forehead, above the eyebrows.
6. Bring the tape measure around the head, just above the ears, to meet at the mid-forehead (Fig. 28-7).

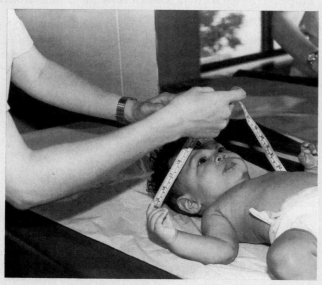

FIGURE 28-7.

7. Read to the nearest 0.01 cm.
8. Record the measurement on the growth chart and the patient's chart.
9. Clean the work area.
10. Wash your hands.

without parental assistance. The adolescent (onset of puberty to the cessation of growth, or roughly 12–19 y of age) is in a difficult period of life. These patients are usually sensitive, are easily embarrassed, and are concerned about their health and appearance. More physicians are now specializing in adolescent medicine.

Well-Baby Examination

Examination of the child during routine well-baby care includes the measurement of the circumference of the infant's head. The head of the infant is measured to determine normal growth and development. If the circumference of the head deviates greatly from normal measurements, **hydrocephaly** or **microcephaly** may be suspected. It is important to discover these conditions as early as possible so that appropriate treatment measures can be initiated. Measurement of head circumference should be performed during routine office visits until the child is 36 months old. The medical assistant measures the head at the time that the weight and height measurements are determined.

Ross Laboratories has made growth charts available to physicians for many years (Figs. 28–8 and 28–9). These charts use the *National Center For Health Statistics* (NCHS) system for evaluating and comparing young children's growth rates with those of similar children of similar ages. Slowed growth patterns and nutritional variances are easily detected. Because boys and girls differ in normal growth rates, separate charts are used. There are charts for two age groups: birth to 36 months, and ages 2 to 18 years. Frequently, medical assistants are asked to plot a growth pattern (Table 28–4).

Many medical offices evaluate young children's rates of growth and development with the *Denver Developmental Screening Test*. This test helps detect delays in development and documents normal development in the preschool child. It is a simple screening test and is easy to use. The directions for screening and the scoring system are published with the test. It does not test intelligence but rather focuses on four basic categories: gross motor, fine motor-adaptive, language, and personal-social development. If unusual or unexplained delays are detected, the child can be referred for more detailed diagnosis by a specialist (Fig. 28–10).

Restraints for Children

For routine examinations, begin by taking time to explain the procedure to the child and by gaining his or her confidence. If you maintain a positive and reassuring attitude, restraints are usually not needed. A small child may be held on an adult's lap, with the child's right arm tucked under the adult's left arm. The child's left arm may be held in place by the adult's right hand. The adult's left hand is then free to support the child's head.

TABLE 28–3. SCHEDULE FOR ACTIVE IMMUNIZATION OF NORMAL INFANTS AND CHILDREN IN THE UNITED STATES

DPT Vaccine
Diphtheria—produces toxin that damages the heart, kidneys, and nerves. One of every 10 children with diphtheria dies.
Tetanus—causes painful muscle contractions. Two to 6 of every 10 children with tetanus die.
Pertussis (whooping cough)—may cause pneumonia and seizures. May result in death.

MMR Vaccine
Measles—may cause pneumonia or ear infections. One of every 1000 children with measles develops deafness, seizures, or brain disorders.
Mumps—may cause permanent deafness and temporary brain disorder.
Rubella—may cause miscarriage, stillbirth, and birth defects such as deafness and heart disease.

Oral Polio Vaccine
Polio—causes paralysis of the arms and legs; interferes with breathing. One of every 10 children with paralysis dies.

HIB Vaccine
Hemophilus influenza bacteria—a bacteria that is the most common cause of blood, bone, and joint disease and the most common cause of meningitis in infants and young children.

Hepatitis B Vaccine
Hepatitis B—10 to 15% of hepatitis B cases occur in children.

Recommended Immunization Schedule

Age	Vaccine
2 mo	DPT, Oral Polio, HIB (Hep. B)
4 mo	DPT, Oral Polio, HIB (Hep. B)
6 mo	DPT, HIB (Hep. B)
12 mo	Measles, Mumps, and Rubella
15 mo	DPT, Oral Polio, HIB
18 mo	Any vaccine not previously given
4–6 y	DPT, Oral Polio

From the Centers for Disease Control, Atlanta, GA.

For examination and treatment of the ears, eyes, nose, or throat, place the child on the examination table. Immobilize the head as gently as possible. Try to gain the child's cooperation. Ask the parent to assist. The parent can frequently help restrain the child. A familiar face and voice can help to calm children's anxieties and fears.

When restraining a crying child, check your own position and that of the child. Sometimes a child cries from the pain of too tight a hold rather than from the pain of the examination. For example, when holding an infant's legs to expose the buttocks, place your index finger between the ankles to reduce pressure.

When more extensive examinations are necessary, place the child on a large sheet that has been folded lengthwise, keeping the top of the sheet even with the shoulders and the bottom just below the feet. Leave a greater portion of the sheet on the left side of the child. Now bring this longer side back over the left arm and under the body and right arm. Next, bring the sheet back over the right arm and under the body again. The two arms will be com-

28

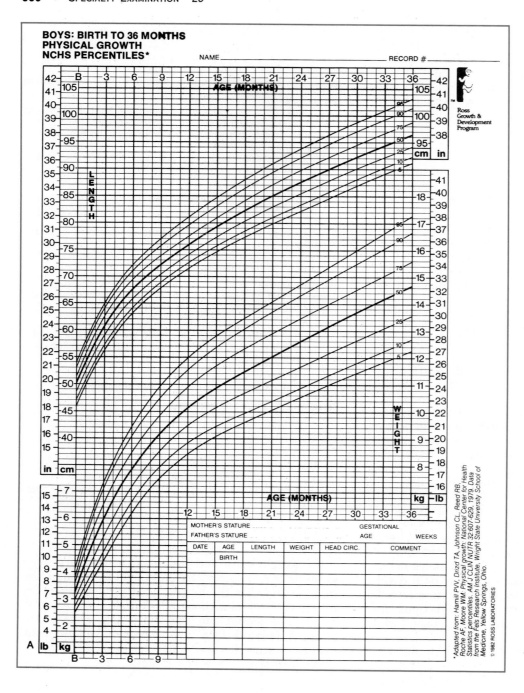

BOYS: BIRTH TO 36 MONTHS PHYSICAL GROWTH NCHS PERCENTILES*

NAME _____ RECORD # _____

Adapted from: Hamill PVV, Drizd TA, Johnson CL, Reed RB, Roche AF, Moore WM. Physical growth: National Center for Health Statistics percentiles. AM J CLIN NUTR 32:607-629, 1979. Data from the Fels Research Institute, Wright State University School of Medicine, Yellow Springs, Ohio.

© 1982 ROSS LABORATORIES

FIGURE 28–8. National Center for Health Statistics (NCHS) Physical Growth Percentile Chart for boys. (Courtesy of Ross Laboratories, Columbus, OH.)

pletely restrained, leaving the abdomen exposed. When restraining the entire body, bring the right portion of the sheet over the abdomen, and tuck it securely under the entire back and out again on the right side.

Another method of restraint is the mummy style (Fig. 28–11). Fold the sheet into a triangle, and place it on the examining table. The distance from the fold to the lower corner of the sheet should be twice the length of the child. Place the child on the

sheet, with the fold slightly above the shoulders. Loosen tight clothing and straighten the child's arms and legs. Bring the lower corner of the sheet up over the child's body. The left corner is brought over the body and tucked under the body snugly, leaving the arm exposed. Bring the opposite corner over the exposed arm and under the child's body.

This restraint can be quickly and easily made and can be used to leave either arm exposed while securing the opposite arm and also the legs and body.

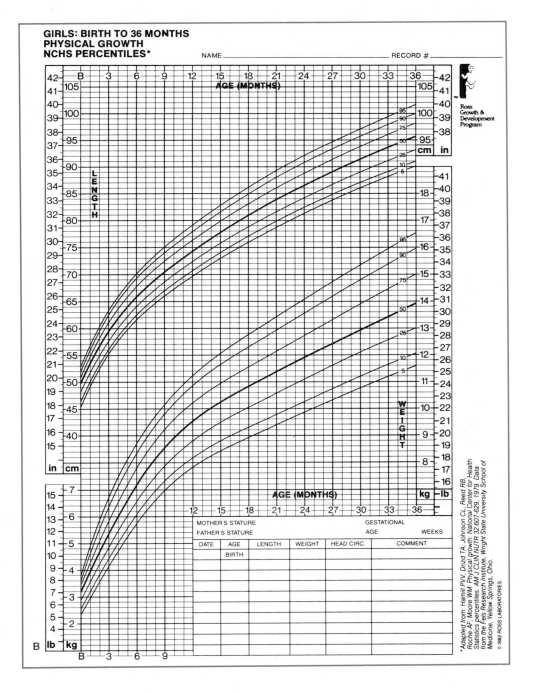

FIGURE 28-9. NCHS Physical Growth Percentile Chart for girls. (Courtesy of Ross Laboratories, Columbus, OH.)

It may be pinned if necessary. Elbow restraints may be made by using a blood pressure cuff or a towel wrapped around the elbow several times.

To prevent a small child or infant from rolling the head from side to side, stand at the head of the table and support the child's head between the hands, making certain not to press on the ears or on the anterior or posterior fontanel. The reverse of this may be restraining a child with your body by taking the place of the physician, and the physi-

cian's working from above the child's head. This may be used for an examination of the child's eyes. A small infant may be placed crosswise on the table that has both the head and base raised slightly, forming a large V in the table. This prevents the infant from rolling, as might happen on a flat surface.

It is not necessary to drape an infant, but the older child's modesty should be respected. Sincere respect and friendly conversation at the child's level

28

TABLE 28-4. HOW TO USE THE NCHS GROWTH CHARTS

1. Look at the vertical column to find *stature, length,* or *weight.*
2. In the horizontal column find your patient's age.
3. Mark an "X" at the spot on the graph where the items in number 1 meet.
4. Next, find the percentile in which your patient places as compared with children of the same age.
   a. Trace the percentile line up to the value listed on the right side of the chart.
   b. Remember to alter the percentile if it is not located exactly on the line.
5. Report the result to your physician immediately if it is above or below the normal range.

accomplish a great deal. Always be patient with children. Be certain that they understand what is expected. Always involve the parents as much as possible.

Medical Assistant's Role in the Pediatric Examination

The examination of the pediatric patient follows the same pattern as that for the adult, with the exception that the examination is altered to focus on normal growth and development. Since the child is continuously growing and changing, his or her physiologic and psychologic growth patterns must be carefully noted and recorded. Depending on the age of the child, the physician may make changes in the routine examination procedure. The medical assistant must be flexible and ready to adapt to changes in order to assist the physician and the patient. It is important that the assistant be knowledgeable of the major problems that affect children in different age groups and develop the skills needed to identify possible areas of concern.

If the pediatrician has pamphlets available for parents that offer advice and assistance in caring for their child, the medical assistant should discuss them with the parents. You should answer questions whenever possible or alert the physician so that questions can be answered during the office visit. It is important that you make the most of every opportunity to teach parents about sound health care.

Sterilization in Pediatrics

It has been known for many years that the main source of cross-infection in pediatrics has been the thermometer. Because it is used so frequently, some carelessness in sanitizing the thermometer before chemical sterilization can occur. The chemical sterilant may not be changed or the container sterilized as frequently as it should be. Sometimes, alcohol

alone is used, and this solution is not a sporocide or virucide, especially for the hepatitis virus. Thermometers used by patients with hepatitis should be discarded and should not be used again. The use of disposable thermometers prevents cross-infection. Single-use thermometer sheaths are available in both oral and rectal types and are easy to use.

Carelessness may also be involved in removing small foreign objects from the skin (e.g., splinters). Sterile procedures and sterile instruments must always be used when entering the skin, regardless of how uncooperative the patient may be.

UROLOGY

The urologist treats diseases of the urinary tract in the female and diseases of both the urinary tract and the reproductive system in the male. Urologists use a wide variety of medical treatments, including surgery, if necessary.

Urinary Tract Diagnosis

Much of the diagnosis of urinary dysfunction is dependent on the patient's history, which may include frequency or urgency of urination, dysuria, or incontinence. Cystitis and renal calculi are frequency disorders of the urinary tract.

A major part of the urologic examination is the urinalysis. The medical assistant must be able to instruct the patient in how to obtain a clean-catch urine specimen (see Chapter 32). It is best to have the patient **void** in the physician's office so that the specimen can be examined immediately. Most urologists prefer to examine a catheterized specimen, which is collected using a sterile technique. A small catheter is introduced into the bladder, and the urine is collected in a sterile container. This procedure is usually done by the physician, but in some states, the medical assistant can perform catheterization procedures if specially trained to do so. This procedure should never be performed by the medical assistant who does not have the necessary training in the sterile technique and knowledge of the responsibilities of catheterization.

Major complaints presented to the urologist involve changes in the frequency of urination. This is the symptom of several conditions, including *cystitis, diabetes mellitus,* and *diabetes insipidus.* This symptom may or may not be accompanied by painful or difficult urination (dysuria). Urgency is another very annoying symptom, since it is the inability to control the release of urine after the desire to urinate occurs. Similar to this is incontinence, the involuntary loss of urine. Stress incontinence is the loss of urine during physical stress, such as during coughing, sneezing, or laughing. This is commonly seen in

DATE:
NAME:
BIRTHDATE:
HOSPITAL NO.

DIRECTIONS

1. Try to get child to smile by smiling, talking, or waving to him or her. Do not touch the child.
2. When child is playing with a toy, pull it away. Pass if he or she resists.
3. Child does not have to be able to tie shoes or button in the back.
4. Move yarn slowly in an arc from one side to the other, about 6 inches above the child's face. Pass if eyes follow 90 degrees to midline (Past midline; 180 degrees.)
5. Pass if child grasps rattle when it is touched to the backs or tips of fingers.
6. Pass if child continues to look where yarn disappeared or tries to see where it went. Yarn should be dropped quickly from sight from tester's hand without arm movement.
7. Pass if child picks up raisin with any part of thumb and a finger.
8. Pass if child picks up raisin with the ends of thumb and index finger using an over-hand approach.

9. Pass any enclosed form. Fail continuous round motions.

10. Which line is longer (not bigger)? Turn paper upside-down and repeat. (3/3 or 5/6)

11. Pass any crossing lines.

12. Have child copy first. If failed, demonstrate.

When giving items 9, 11, and 12, do not name the forms. Do not demonstrate 9 and 11.

13. When scoring, each pair (2 arms, 2 legs, etc.) counts as one part.
14. Point to picture and have child name it. (No credit is given for sounds only.)

15. Tell child to: Give block to Mommie; put block on table; put block on floor. Pass 2 of 3. (Do not help child by pointing or moving head or eyes.)
16. Ask child: What do you do when you are cold?...hungry?...tired? Pass 2 of 3.
17. Tell child to: Put block on table; under table; in front of chair, behind chair. Pass 3 of 4. (Do not help child by pointing or moving eyes.)
18. Ask child: If fire is hot, ice is ?; Mother is a woman, Dad is a ?; A horse is big, a mouse is ? Pass 2 of 3.
19. Ask child: What is a ball?...lake?...desk?...house?...banana?...curtain?...ceiling?...hedge?...pavement? Pass if defined in terms of use, shape, what it is made of or general category (such as banana is fruit, not just yellow). Pass 6 of 9.
20. Ask child: What is a spoon made of?...a shoe made of?...a door made of? (No other objects may be substituted.) Pass 3 of 3.
21. When placed on stomach, child lifts chest off table with support of forearms and/or hands.
22. When child is on back, grasp his hands and pull him to sitting. Pass if head does not hang back.
23. Child may use wall or rail only, not person. May not crawl.
24. Child must throw ball overhand 3 feet to within arm's reach of tester.
25. Child must perform stranding broad jump over width of test sheet. (8-1/2 inches)
26. Tell child to walk forward, heel within one inch of toe. Tester may demonstrate. Child must walk 4 consecutive steps, 2 out of 3 trials.
27. Bounce ball to child who should stand 3 feet away from tester. Child must catch ball with hands not arms, 2 out of 3 trials.
28. Tell child to walk backward, toe within 1 inch of heel. Tester may demonstrate. Child must walk 4 consecutive steps, 2 out of 3 trials.

DATE AND BEHAVIORAL OBSERVATIONS (how child feels at time of test, relation to tester, attention span, verbal behavior, self-confidence, etc.):

FIGURE 28-10. The Denver Developmental Screening Test, which is used in most medical offices. (Reprinted with permission, ©1969, William K. Frankenburg, M.D., and Josiah B. Dodds, Ph.D., University of Colorado Medical Center.)

Illustration continued on following page

28

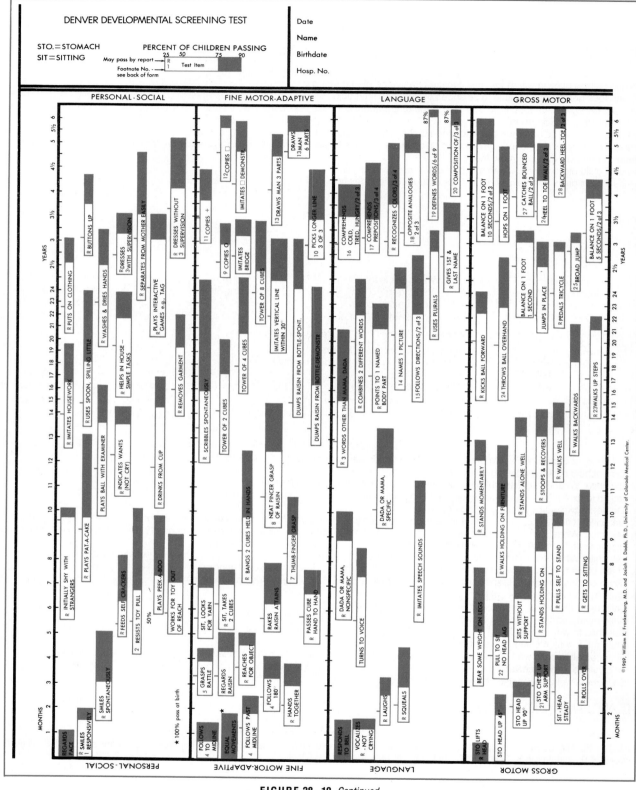

FIGURE 28-10. *Continued*

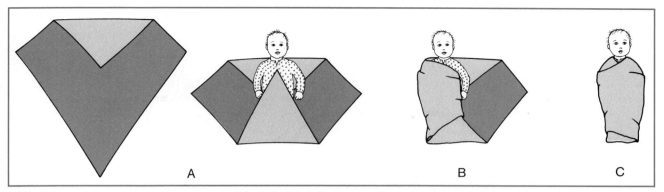

FIGURE 28–11. A very safe method of restraining an infant. The baby's blanket can serve as the restraining device. *A, B,* and *C* show how to wrap the blanket around the child.

the **multiparous** woman with a *cystocele* or *urethrocele.*

Many diagnostic aids are used in urology, and a complete urinalysis is probably the most common. Renal function tests include determination of serum creatinine and blood urea nitrogen levels. An excretory test is the phenosulfonphthalein test. Frequently employed radiographic studies are the *intravenous pyelogram* and the *retrograde pyelogram.* For the detection of calculi, an x-ray film of the abdomen may show the kidneys, ureters, and bladder. Radioisotopic studies as well as sonography are useful.

Cystoscopy is the examination of the bladder by means of a cystoscope passed through the **urethra** and into the bladder. The cystoscope illuminates the bladder interior. By means of special lenses and mirrors, the bladder mucosa is examined for inflammation, tumors, and calculi. A catheter can be passed through the cystoscope and on into the ureters and kidneys to obtain samples of urine or to introduce an opaque substance for x-ray films.

No special instrument setup is required for a routine urologic examination unless a special procedure, such as obtaining a catheterized urine specimen, is done. Most offices use prepackaged disposable units for catheterization and for bladder irrigation.

Both male and female patients are disrobed and given a gown. The female is placed in the lithotomy position. The male patient is seated on the examining table, and the physician instructs the patient to do what is needed.

THE MALE REPRODUCTIVE SYSTEM

The male reproductive system consists of the **testicles, vas deferens, seminal vesicles, prostate gland,** urethra, and the penis (Fig. 28–12). The act of sexual intercourse is made possible through vas-

cular engorgement of the penile vessels, which causes the penis to become erect. Through the stimulation of the nervous system, the male then experiences lubrication followed by emission and **ejaculation.**

As with all systems in the human body, the male reproductive system undergoes physiologic changes with aging. Most male reproductive problems are one of the following: changes in urination, urethral discharge, impotence, infertility, or the presence of masses. Prostatic enlargement is common and often produces symptomatic changes when urinating. The patient may have problems in urinating or in maintaining a stream while urinating. In the geriatric patient, urine samples may contain elevated post-ejaculation sperm levels.

Examination of the Male Reproductive System

The patient is usually asked to empty his bladder before the examination. He is asked to disrobe, and a drape sheet is placed over his chest and abdomen. The medical assistant (if male) assists the physician with the drape to facilitate the examination. A female medical assistant assists *only* if it is requested by the physician. The physician inspects the **foreskin** (if patient is not circumcised) and the **glans penis.** He then palpates the penis and the **scrotum** for possible masses and tenderness. If the physician uses a transilluminator, the assistant may be asked to darken the room. The assistant then assists the patient into a standing position for the examination of the prostate gland. This is done by digital insertion into the rectum, with the patient standing using the table for support. At this time, the physician may also check the patient for possible inguinal hernias.

When the examination has been completed, the assistant aids the patient as needed.

28

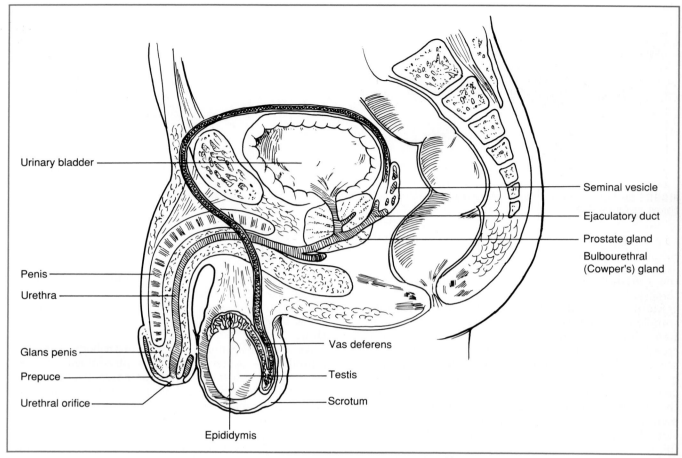

FIGURE 28-12. Sagittal view of the male reproductive system.

Disorders of the Male Reproductive System

Epididymitis

Inflammation of the **epididymis** is usually caused by some form of bacterial infection. It may be the result of an infection in the prostate or of long-term catheter use. The patient usually complains of pain along the inguinal canal and the vas deferens. Swelling is usually seen in the groin and the scrotum, and a slight fever is present. The treatment consists of antibiotics and bed rest. The patient may place a pillow under the scrotum to relieve pain and swelling. If untreated, the patient may experience a marked decrease in **spermatozoa.** If an abscess develops, and an orchiectomy may be necessary.

Prostatitis

Prostatitis is an inflammation of the prostate gland that can be viral or infectious. It most commonly occurs after a viral illness. Infectious organisms are believed to reach the gland via the urethra or bloodstream. Prostatitis is treated with antibiotics and bed rest. Prostatitis can become a chronic problem, and the medical assistant should instruct the patient as to how to recognize the early signs of urinary tract infections.

Testicular Cancer

Testicular cancer is rare and represents only about 2% of all cancers in men. Testicular cancer strikes men between the ages of 20 and 40 years. Treatment starts with early detection and chemotherapy intervention. Testicular cancer has now become one of the most curable cancers (Fig. 28-13).

Prostate Cancer

Prostate cancer is the most common type of cancer among American men and the third leading cause of cancer deaths. Black men seem to develop prostate cancer twice as frequently as and at a younger age than do white men. Its cause is still being researched, but it is believed that heredity and diet are important factors. The most common form is *adenoma,* but other forms, including *sarcomas,* are found. Surgical treatment is the treatment of choice, followed by chemotherapy and hormone therapy.

A simple 3 minute self-examination, once a month, can detect one of the cancers most common among men aged 15-34. If detected early, testicular cancer is one of the most easily cured.

The best time to check yourself is in the shower or after a warm bath. Fingers glide over soapy skin making it easier to concentrate on the texture underneath. The heat causes the skin to relax, making the exam easier.

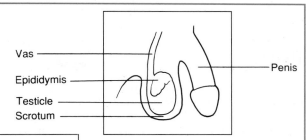

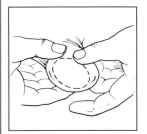 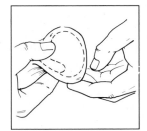 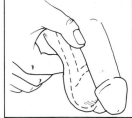

1. Start by examining your testicles. Slowly roll the testicle between the thumb and fingers, applying slight pressure. Try to find hard, painless lumps.

2. Now examine your epididymis. This comma-shaped cord is behind each testicle. It may be tender to the touch. It's also the location of the most noncancerous problems.

3. Continue by examining the vas (the sperm-carrying tube that runs up from your epididymis). The vas normally feels like a firm, movable smooth tube.

Now repeat the exam on the other side.

What are the symptoms?

In early stages testicular cancer may be symptomless. When symptoms do occur they include:

- Lump on the testicle
- Slight enlargement of one of the testes
- Heavy sensation in the testicles or groin
- Dull ache in lower abdomen or groin

If you find any hard lumps or nodules, see your doctor promptly. Only your doctor can make a diagnosis.

FIGURE 28-13. Performing a testicular self-examination. (Redrawn with permission of St. Agnes Medical Center, Fresno, CA.)

The new surgical procedures enable the surgeon to remove the growth without injuring the nerves that enervate an erection; thus, the patient is usually not impotent after the surgical procedure is performed.

Impotence

Impotence is the inability to achieve or maintain an erection, or both. The cause is believed to be physical in about 50% of patients. Nonsurgical management of the dysfunction includes psychosocial therapy and medication. In cases of penile nerve damage, an implant can be surgically placed to enable the penis to become erect when the prosthesis is pumped just behind the glans.

Sexually Transmitted Diseases

AIDS, chlamydia, genital warts, gonorrhea, syphilis, and viral herpes are common sexually transmitted diseases seen in both the male and the female.

Their symptoms and treatments were discussed earlier in this chapter.

Medical Assistant's Role in the Male Examination

The primary function of the medical assistant in the male reproductive system examination is to understand the male reproductive system and to be supportive. It is impossible to guess what meaning a particular dysfunction may have on an individual. Being a good listener and offering support whenever possible are the assistant's primary goals.

If the assistant is male, he may be needed to assist the physician with the examination and aid the patient with draping and positioning. The assistant should watch the patient for signs of discomfort and anxiety; if these signs are noted, he should notify the physician immediately. Answering the patient's questions and reenforcing understand-

28

ing of the physician's orders are among the assistant's responsibilities.

DIAGNOSTIC TESTS

A tissue biopsy may be ordered if a mass is detected by the physician when the reproductive organs are palpated. Obtaining the biopsy specimen is usually done at the hospital on an outpatient basis. Instructions should be given to the patient both verbally and in writing. If the physician orders a **semen** specimen for fertility testing, the assistant gives the patient a specimen container along with instructions on how to collect the specimen at home. The assistant also provides the patient with the laboratory forms to take along with the specimen to the testing center. Other procedures may include drawing blood, making microscopic smears on glass slides, or sending the patient to a laboratory with request forms for specific tests to be performed.

STERILIZATION IN THE UROLOGY OFFICE

Items used for urethral insertion and for bladder instillation *must* be sterile. To ensure sterility, disposable syringes, catheters, and solution bowls are used. Medical supply companies offer sterile prepackaged procedure kits for the urology office. Irrigating solutions and instilled medications are commercially prepared and ready to use. Only syringes used for chemotherapy are reusable, since chemotherapeutic drugs are so caustic that they dissolve plastic syringes. When glass syringes are used, it is your responsibility to clean and sterilize them according to procedural guidelines and the manufacturer's recommendations.

If cystoscopic examinations are done in the office, extreme care must be taken to maintain sterility. A majority of cystoscopic procedures are now done in the hospital. Office vasectomies must be performed with sterile operating room technique to prevent contamination.

LEGAL AND ETHICAL RESPONSIBILITIES

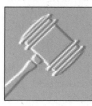

The medical assistant's legal and ethical responsibilities in the specialty practice involve many of the basic principles that apply in the general practice. You must maintain confidentiality as well as act as the patient's advocate and the physician's agent.

When working in a specialty office, the medical assistant must be very careful to ensure that patients have given informed consent for the procedures to be performed. When the patient refuses a procedure, the assistant needs to have the patient sign the appropriate informed refusal forms; these forms are then included in the medical record. All patient education should be done after the doctor has completed the explanation and has given the assistant instructions to do so. Never diagnose, prescribe, or offer comment about a patient's condition. Remember that as the physician's agent, your comments can be considered as those of the physician.

The medical assistant must provide a safe environment for children. Children should never be left alone in the examination room; they are always inquisitive and often touch or taste whatever they see. Be sure to include the parent in all explanations to the child, and remember to provide for the child's privacy and comfort in the same manner as you would for the adult patient.

Medical assistants who overstep their professional boundaries may place the doctor and themselves in legal jeopardy. Remember that the informed patient who is legally informed and satisfied with the care received is less likely to find the need to take legal action against the physician and the assistant.

When assisting in the specialty areas of male, female, and child health care, the medical assistant must develop diverse skills if he or she is to benefit both the physician and the patient. These skills help the assistant anticipate the needs of the physician and ascertain the needs of the patient. There is a strong need for patient education in the specialty areas, and the medical assistant should see this need as an opportunity to become a greater asset to the physician/employer, the patient, and the profession. The greater the interest taken in the needs and desires of the patients, the greater the personal reward.

▶ LEARNING ACHIEVEMENTS

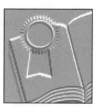

Upon completion of this chapter, can you in the time allowed by your evaluator:

1. Assist in a simulated pelvic examination, completing each step correctly and in the proper order?
2. Measure and record the head circumference of an infant to within 1/8 inch of the actual reading?
3. Assist in a simulated examination of the male reproductive system?
4. Assist with the physical examination of a child?
5. Instruct a female patient in self-examination of the breasts?
6. Instruct a male patient in testicular self-examination?
7. Perform a Denver Developmental Screening Test on a preschool-age child?
8. Answer questions regarding methods of contraception?

REFERENCES AND READINGS

Bonewit, K.: *Clinical Procedures for Medical Assistants*, 3rd ed., Philadelphia, W.B. Saunders Co., 1990.

Frew, M., and Frew, D.: *Comprehensive Medical Assisting*, 2nd ed., Philadelphia, F. A. Davis Co., 1988.

Ignatavicius, D., and Bayne, M.V.: *Medical Surgical Nursing*, Philadelphia, W.B. Saunders Co., 1991.

Kinn, M.: *Medical Terminology*, New York, Delmar Publishers, 1990.

Lane, K.: *Saunders Manual For Medical Assisting*, Jarrettville, MD, Education Management Resources, 1992.

28

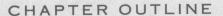

CHAPTER OUTLINE

VOCABULARY

amenorrhea Absence of menstrual period.

ankylosis Immobility of a joint owing to disease or injury.

anoscope Instrument used to examine the anus.

arrhythmia Variation from the normal heart rhythm.

asthma Spasmodic constriction of the bronchi.

bariatrics Field of medicine dealing with obesity.

benign Noncancerous (as when describing a mass or tumor).

cancer Any cellular tumor or neoplastic disease in which there is a transformation of normal body cells into malignant cells.

colitis Inflammation of the colon.

contraindication A condition that renders a treatment improper or undesirable.

diplopia Double vision.

eczema A common allergic reaction in children; atopic dermatitis.

erythema Redness or inflammation of the skin.

eustachian tube A narrow tube leading from the middle ear to the pharynx.

flatus Gas expelled through the anus.

hemoccult Hidden blood; a test for occult blood in the stool.

incontinence Inability to control excretory functions.

induration An abnormally hard spot or place.

jaundice Yellow discoloration of the skin and mucous membrane.

leukoderma White patches on the skin.

myringotomy Incision of the tympanic membrane.

neoplasia New growth of cells (used interchangeably with the term *cancer*).

otitis Inflammation of the ear canal.

presbyopia Diminution of accommodation of the lens of the eye occurring normally with aging; results in farsightedness.

pruritus Itching.

ptosis Drooping of the upper eyelid.

rhinitis Inflammation of the nasal membranes.

sigmoidoscope Instrument used to examine the sigmoid colon; may be rigid or flexible.

tinnitus Ringing in the ears. It is a symptom of labyrinthitis, eighth cranial nerve damage, or cerebral arteriosclerosis.

vertigo The sensation of dizziness.

vesiculation Formation of blister-like sacs on the skin.

vitiligo A loss of pigment in areas of the skin.

wheal A localized area of edema on the skin that is usually accompanied by itching.

SPECIALTY EXAMINATION

PART 2: ALLERGOLOGY, DERMATOLOGY, ENDOCRINOLOGY, SURGERY, INTERNAL MEDICINE, NEUROLOGY, ONCOLOGY, OPHTHALMOLOGY, ORTHOPEDICS, OTORHINOLARYNGOLOGY, AND PROCTOLOGY

LEARNING OBJECTIVES

COGNITIVE
Upon successful completion of this chapter, you should be able to:

1. Define the words in the Vocabulary.

2. Discuss the signs and symptoms of allergy.

3. List and explain the types of allergy testing.

4. Elaborate on the medical assistant's responsibilities in the dermatology and endocrinology specialty offices.

5. List the four specialties within the field of internal medicine.

6. Compare and contrast the specialties of neurology and oncology.

7. List four eye tests that may be performed in the ophthalmology office.

8. Describe the common disorders of the ear.

9. List three diseases and disorders seen in the proctology office.

10. Discuss legal and ethical issues that are pertinent to the specialty office.

PERFORMANCE
Upon successful completion of this chapter, you should be able to:

1. Administer a tuberculin tine test.

2. Test distance acuity using a Snellen distance visual acuity chart.

3. Locate and identify an ear drum using an otoscope.

4. Irrigate an ear using an ear syringe.

5. Position a patient for a sigmoidoscopy examination.

6. Test color acuity using the Ishihara test.

7. Irrigate a patient's eyes.

8. Instill medication into a patient's eyes.

Protocols exist for the various physical examinations performed in the medical office; however, particular methods of examination and treatment vary among physicians, based on individual needs and habits.

In the specialist's office, emphasis is given to a specific area of the body or a particular complaint. Medical assistants perform many specialty procedures and must assist in the specialty examination.

This chapter discusses, in alphabetical order, each specialty and its most commonly used procedures. Specific diseases and diagnostic aids such as x-rays and laboratory tests are also mentioned as they apply to the specialty.

ALLERGOLOGY

The specialty of allergology concerns the diagnosis and treatment of allergic conditions. It is difficult to separate allergology and immunology; to understand one, it is necessary to have a degree of understanding of the other. In a normal immune reaction, an antigen promotes the production of lymph cells or other white blood cells (called *antibodies*) and results in the elimination of the harmful antigen. An allergic reaction is the same, but the interaction of the antigen and the antibody is accompanied by a harmful effect on the body tissue and by excessive release of a substance called *histamine*. This abnormal immune response is referred to as "hypersensitive reaction," and the diseases arising from it are called "diseases of hypersensitivity." Among such diseases are allergy, hay fever, serum sickness, and transfusion reactions.

Symptoms of an allergy can occur for the first time at any age. The substances that produce an allergic response can be eaten, inhaled, injected, or applied topically to the skin. The response to these antigens, or *allergens,* as the allergists prefer to call them, bears no relationship to the type of material involved. For example, foods may cause **eczema, rhinitis,** or **asthma.** Pollens may also cause any of these conditions. When rhinitis is caused by a pollen, it is given a special name, *hay fever,* although "hay" is not necessarily the causative agent.

An allergic reaction does not usually occur on the first contact with the allergen, because the antibodies have not yet been produced by the body. It may occur on the second contact, when the antibodies have been released and are in reserve in the body tissues. The reaction may not occur until later in life, when contact with the allergen suddenly develops into a sensitivity. An allergy is said to be a reaction to a substance that ordinarily is harmless to most people. There are almost as many allergens, such as pollens, foods, plants, animal fur, insect bites, and chemicals, as there are substances. Reactions range from mild sneezing to severe serum sickness, or *anaphylactic shock,* which can be fatal unless immediate emergency measures are taken.

The diagnosis of an allergy is made by taking a very careful history from the patient, performing a careful and complete physical examination, and following this up with selected laboratory tests, which may include x-ray studies, blood and urine examinations, and skin tests. This history and physical examination are always made by the physician, but the skin tests and laboratory tests may be the responsibilities of a medical assistant or laboratory technician. Since skin tests are potentially very hazardous to perform, they should always be conducted under supervision of a physician. It should be emphasized that skin tests by themselves are not strictly diagnostic of an allergy, but when combined with a careful history and other factors, they are helpful in establishing the diagnosis. Skin tests are ordinarily performed by one or more of several methods: scratch, intradermal, ophthalmic, or patch.

Scratch Test

The least satisfactory test is the scratch and puncture test. It is most popular because it is rapid and simple to perform. The tests may be performed on any smooth surface of the skin, but the arm and back are most popular. The arm is safer (either the outer surface of the upper arm or the palmar surface of the lower arm), since a serious reaction may be limited by the application of a tourniquet above the site. However, the back is favored in infants and in young children because of the large area of skin available. It is also easier to immobilize the child in this position.

A reaction usually occurs within 10 to 30 minutes. If the reaction is positive, a **wheal** (hive) will be formed at the site of the scratch. The interpretation of the test should always be based on a comparison of this reaction with that of the control, which is a scratch with a plain base fluid free of any allergy-producing extract.

The interpretation, or reading, of the skin tests is performed by the physician. However, a few doctors delegate this step to the trained skin tester. Reactions are commonly graded from 2 to 4. No precise definition of a reaction can be given, and indeed the intensity may vary among individuals. However, as a general rule, a 2 reaction implies a wheal that is definitely larger than that of the control. A larger wheal is interpreted as a 3, whereas the presence of pseudopods (finger-like extensions around the periphery of the wheal) may be read as a 4. Carefully wipe off the extract to stop the reaction when a strong reaction is occurring. **Erythema,** or reddening, around the wheal is usually disregarded in the interpretations. Frequently, the large or significant reactions are accompanied by local itching. The degree of sensitivity is measured on a numeric scale (shown in color on the inside cover of this book).

Intradermal (Intracutaneous) Test

This test is more sensitive than the scratch test. Extracts are injected into the skin, with the usual sterile technique, in a dose of 0.01 to 0.02 ml. This method is used for the tuberculin (purified protein derivative, or PPD) test and the Valley Fever coccidiomycosis test. The reaction time is identical to that of the scratch test; however, the antigen is more dilute. Remember that the extract cannot be wiped off as in the scratch method. This method is always done on the anterior aspect of the patient's forearm. This is a safety measure. In a severe reaction, apply a tourniquet immediately above the reaction area in order to retard absorption of the extract. Immediately prepare epinephrine to be administered on the physician's orders.

Tine Test

The tine tuberculin test is administered with a sterile, simple, multiple-puncture, disposable intradermal device for the detection of tuberculosis infection. Each test unit consists of a stainless steel disc attached to a plastic handle. Projecting from the disc are four triangular-shaped prongs (tines) that are 2 mm long and approximately 4 mm apart. The tines have been dipped in a sterile solution containing substances extracted from tuberculosis

cultures. The substance on the tines is called *old tuberculin* (OT).

The preferred site for the tine test is the upper third of the anterior forearm. Avoid areas with excessive hair, scarring, or any other abnormality of the skin surface. Alcohol, acetone, or ether may be used to cleanse the skin. The area must be thoroughly dry before application of the tines.

The results should be read at 42 to 78 hours after the test is given. **Vesiculation** or the extent of **induration** is the determining factor in reading the results: redness without induration is of no significance. The reading should be made in good light, with the forearm slightly flexed. The size of the induration is determined in millimeters by inspection, measuring, and palpation. The tests come with cards for measuring and reading. Interpretation of readings is as follows: vesiculation—positive reaction; induration of 2 mm or more—doubtful reaction, further testing needed; induration less than 2 mm—negative. There are no known **contraindications** for this test; however, testing should be done with caution in patients with tuberculosis. Adverse reactions include pain, itching, and discomfort at the test site. Rarely, bleeding may occur at the puncture site, but it is of no significance.

PROCEDURE 29-1   ADMINISTERING A TUBERCULIN TINE TEST

GOAL   To administer a tuberculin tine test following correct procedural guidelines.

EQUIPMENT AND SUPPLIES

Alcohol preps
Nonsterile gloves

Tine test disc
Patient instruction leaflet

PROCEDURAL STEPS

1. Read the directions for administering the test, and gather the needed supplies and equipment.

2. Wash your hands.

3. Identify your patient and explain the procedure.

4. Check the patient's arm and select an appropriate site to administer the tine test. The anterior surface of the forearm halfway between the antecubital space and the wrist is recommended. Hairy or traumatized areas are to be avoided.
   Purpose: The use of skin areas that are hairy or traumatized makes it difficult to read the results.

5. Prepare the site by cleansing the area with alcohol or other appropriate cleansing agent (Fig. 29-1).
   Purpose: The skin surface should be made as free from organisms as possible.

Continued

29

PROCEDURE 29-1 *Continued*

6. Put on gloves. Remove the protective cap from the disc, exposing the four tines. Use a twisting, pulling motion to remove the cap (Fig. 29-2).
   Purpose: Gloves provide the correct barrier protection.

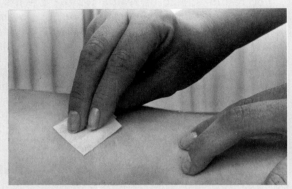

FIGURE 29-1. (From Bonewit, K.: *Clinical Procedures for Medical Assistants*, 3rd ed., Philadelphia, W.B. Saunders Co., 1990, p 262.)

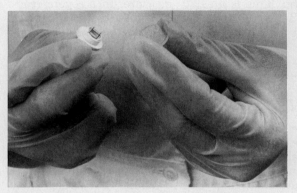

FIGURE 29-2. (From Bonewit, K.: *Clinical Procedures for Medical Assistants*, 3rd ed., Philadelphia, W.B. Saunders Co., 1990, p 262.)

7. Grasp the forearm immediately beneath the site where the test is to be given and stretch the skin tightly to create a smooth site for the tines to slightly puncture the skin (Fig. 29-3).
   Purpose: Stretching the skin allows for easier insertion of the tines.

8. While holding the skin tightly, gently but firmly place the tines' tips on the patient's skin and hold in place for 2 seconds to allow for puncture (Fig. 29-4).
   Purpose: The tines must puncture the patient's skin so that the tuberculin on the tines is introduced into the skin.

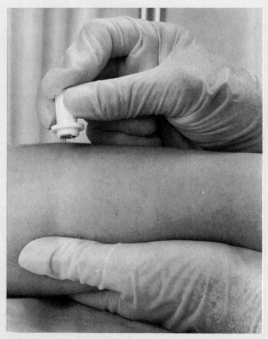

FIGURE 29-3. (From Bonewit, K.: *Clinical Procedures for Medical Assistants*, 3rd ed., Philadelphia, W.B. Saunders Co., 1990, p 263.)

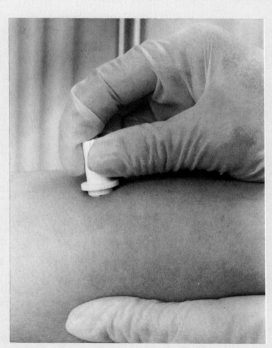

FIGURE 29-4. (From Bonewit, K.: *Clinical Procedures for Medical Assistants*, 3rd ed., Philadelphia, W.B. Saunders Co., 1990, p 263.)

Continued

9. Relax the tension from your grasp and remove the testing unit. Do not rub the testing site after application.
    Purpose: Rubbing the site causes the tuberculin to be absorbed into the tissue.

10. Place the used tine disc into a pathogenic waste container, remove your gloves, and wash your hands.

11. Advise the patient to return to have the test read in 48 to 72 hours, or instruct the patient in assessing the test at home and calling in the results.
    Purpose: Optimal results occur within the 48 to 72 hours. The test *must* be read during that time span for clinically acceptable results to be obtained.

12. Record the type of test given and the administration site on the patient's medical record. Include the date and time if not previously recorded. Initial or sign the entry.
    Purpose: It is your legal and ethical responsibility to record procedure data on the patient's medical record.

Patch Test

This method of testing is of some value in diagnosing dermatitis. In the patch test, the suspected material is placed on the skin (near the original lesion, if possible), covered with a small square of cellophane, and held down with strips of adhesive or transparent tape or even collodion. The reaction is read within 1 to 4 days (Fig. 29–5).

RAST (Radioallergosorbent Test)

This laboratory procedure measures minute quantities of specific antibodies against foods with the

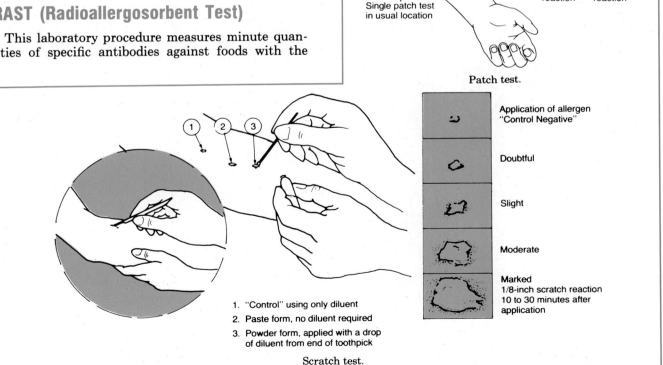

FIGURE 29-5. Technique for the patch test for skin allergies. (From Miller, B.F., and Keane, C.B.: *Encyclopedia and Dictionary of Medicine, Nursing, and Allied Health,* 5th ed., Philadelphia, W.B. Saunders Co., 1992, p 1376.)

use of radioisotopes. A venipuncture is performed, and a blood specimen is collected, which is then sent to a specialized laboratory. The RAST generally provides no more information than direct skin testing, which is less expensive and provides immediate results.

Environmental Control

Patients with allergies are encouraged to make their surroundings as free as possible from the offending allergens and are instructed in the various methods of doing so. One way is the elimination of animals, feathers, and dust-collecting items within the house. The garden is checked for offending grasses and pollens. Foods that cause problems are best eliminated. Contact allergens such as soaps and cosmetics are avoided.

DERMATOLOGY

This specialty deals with the diagnosis and treatment of skin diseases. The human skin, also called the *integument* or *integumentary system,* is the largest organ of the body. It has many different func-

tions: it aids in controlling body temperature, is a barrier to most bacteria, furnishes a sensory system, and is an insulator against outside elements. Both the term "dermis" (Greek) and the term "cutis" (Latin) are used when referring to the skin. Dermatitis and cutitis are synonymous for inflammations of the skin, but dermatitis is by far the preferred term.

The skin has an outer layer, the *epidermis,* and an inner layer, the *dermis,* or *corium.* Blood vessels and nerves, as well as sweat glands, hair roots, and the nail bed, are located in the dermis (Fig. 29–6). Normality of the skin depends on the person's age, sex, and physical and emotional health. The skin reflects both internal and external contact reactions. Examination of the skin is basically inspection followed with detailed examination by palpation, diascopy, and special tests. The *diascope* is a glass plate held against the skin to permit observation of changes produced in the underlying areas by the pressure. The impairments that most frequently bring a patient to the dermatologist's office are the cosmetic disfigurements caused by a skin disease, pain and **pruritus,** and interference with sensations or movements. The possibility that a skin lesion is the result of a systemic condition is sometimes a major concern.

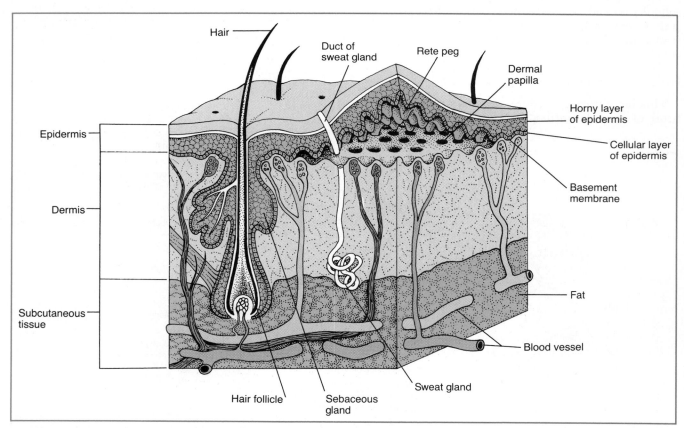

FIGURE 29–6. The histologic anatomy of the skin and its appendages. (From Ignatavicius, D.D., and Bayne, M.V.: *Medical–Surgical Nursing: A Nursing Process Approach,* Philadelphia, W.B. Saunders Co., 1991, p 1134.)

Inspection of the skin may reveal color changes such as **erythema, leukoderma, jaundice,** or **vitiligo.** Localized red or purple changes may be the result of vascular neoplasms, birthmarks, or subcutaneous hemorrhages (petechiae and ecchymoses). Palpation is used to confirm and amplify findings seen by inspection. Inspection and palpation are interrelated in confirming diagnoses. Palpatory findings may be texture, elasticity, or edema.

One disorder of the skin is *seborrheic dermatitis,* a chronic inflammation of the scalp, commonly called *dandruff.* It may spread to the face, neck, and body. *Acne vulgaris* is also a disorder of the sebaceous glands and presents as pustules, blackheads (comedones), and cysts. *Furuncles* (boils) and *carbuncles* (clusters of furuncles) are often seen.

Disorders of the skin may be divided into primary and secondary lesions. *Primary lesions* are those that appear immediately. Macules, papules, plaques, nodules, comedones, cysts, wheals, and pustules are all primary lesions. *Secondary lesions* never appear originally but are the result of alterations in a primary lesion. Examples of secondary lesions are scales, crusts, fissures, erosions, ulcerations, and scars. A burn gives a blister. The blister is the primary lesion; the blister breaks and an ulceration forms; then healing ends in a scar. The ulceration and the scar are secondary lesions (Fig. 29–7).

Draping a patient for a skin examination depends on the area to be examined. Remember to expose the area adequately but protect the patient's privacy. Try to make the patient as comfortable as possible, and offer support when it is needed.

One dermatology test performed in the dermatologist's office is the *Wood's light examination.* This is a visual examination of the skin made in a darkened room with the ultraviolet lamp. Differences in the ultraviolet light absorption and fluorescence bring out characteristics of some mycologic skin diseases, such as *tinea capitis (ringworm).*

ENDOCRINOLOGY

Endocrinology is the study of the function and dysfunction of the glands of internal secretion. Changes due to an endocrine disease may cause alterations in body contour, size, fat distribution, skin texture and pigmentation, and circulation and may have considerable effect on the nervous system. The endocrinologist must be able to distinguish between endocrine dysfunction and the patient's hereditary pattern. This dysfunction in hormone production falls into two categories: deficiency (hypoproduction) and excess (hyperproduction).

Inspection and palpation are the most common methods employed in examining the patient, with inspection being the more prevalent. Of the six endocrine glands in the body, the thyroid and the testes are the most accessible to palpation. The ovaries are palpable to a degree.

Eponyms are used more frequently in endocrinology than in other specialties, but they are slowly being replaced with true anatomic or pathologic terms. Many endocrine disorders are also seen and treated in other specialties. The gynecologist sees the patient with the ovarian changes of **amenorrhea** and menopause. The internist may examine an enlarged thyroid gland that has resulted from an iodine deficiency, or *myxedema* from severe *hypothyroidism.* The ophthalmologist may examine the patient with *exophthalmic goiter,* which gives the appearance of bulging eyes.

Besides the complete physical examination, the physician is aided in diagnosis by a great variety of tests. Some of these tests are x-rays, radioisotopes, and blood chemistry tests.

The medical assistant in an endocrinologist's office will be called upon to participate in the routine physical examination and the collection of blood and urine specimens for diagnostic testing of these glandular disorders. Some of these tests are discussed in Chapter 31.

GENERAL SURGERY

A surgeon's practice is what may be called a "referral specialty." That is, patients are usually referred to the surgeon from other specialties or by the family physician. The procedure to be followed in the evaluation of the patient and the comprehensive preoperative examination requires teamwork between the surgeon and the referring physician. An effective working arrangement between these two physicians sometimes depends on the cooperation of the medical assistant. The referring physician frequently takes care of the initial physical examination and basic preoperative laboratory tests, and then the referring physician's knowledge of the patient's past medical and family history is shared with the surgeon. The surgeon will then have a clear understanding of the objectives of surgery and the patient's preoperative status. The surgeon may offer the patient a simple and understandable description of the operation, its rationale, and possible complications. (This is the basis of "informed consent.")

The psychologic preparation of the patient is also shared by the referring physician and the surgeon. Anxieties of the patient are normal and inevitable and can be somewhat lessened by the attitude of a good medical assistant. The medical assistant in the surgeon's office can identify the patient with special needs and, with the surgeon's consent, can reduce some of these anxieties with simple explanations and reports.

Assisting the surgeon may include assisting with preoperative examinations and postoperative office visits. Physical examinations would follow the outline given in Chapter 27. The office postoperative care may include dressing changes and suture removal. These are described in Chapter 35.

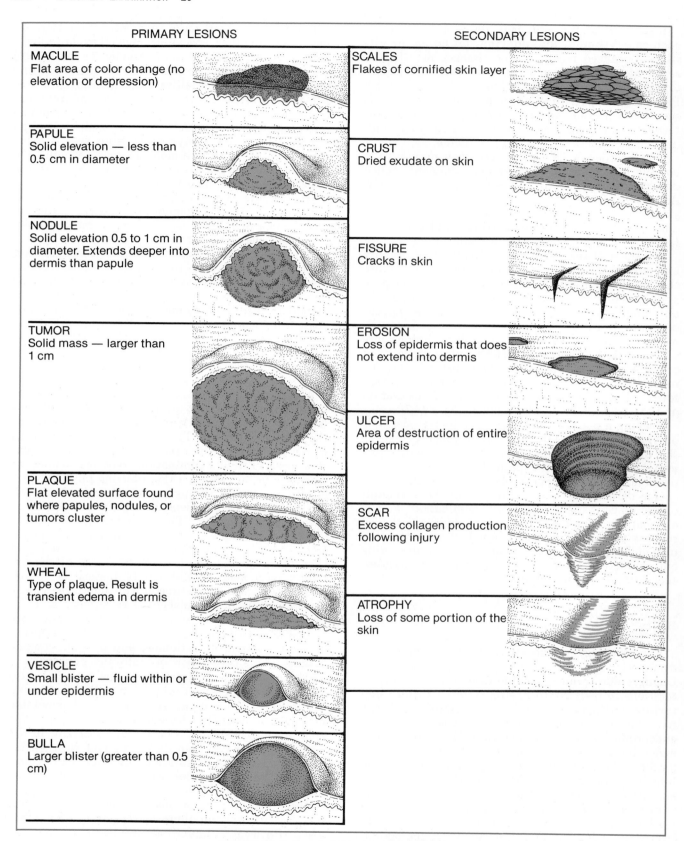

PRIMARY LESIONS	SECONDARY LESIONS

MACULE
Flat area of color change (no elevation or depression)

PAPULE
Solid elevation — less than 0.5 cm in diameter

NODULE
Solid elevation 0.5 to 1 cm in diameter. Extends deeper into dermis than papule

TUMOR
Solid mass — larger than 1 cm

PLAQUE
Flat elevated surface found where papules, nodules, or tumors cluster

WHEAL
Type of plaque. Result is transient edema in dermis

VESICLE
Small blister — fluid within or under epidermis

BULLA
Larger blister (greater than 0.5 cm)

SCALES
Flakes of cornified skin layer

CRUST
Dried exudate on skin

FISSURE
Cracks in skin

EROSION
Loss of epidermis that does not extend into dermis

ULCER
Area of destruction of entire epidermis

SCAR
Excess collagen production following injury

ATROPHY
Loss of some portion of the skin

FIGURE 29-7. Characteristics of common skin lesions.

INTERNAL MEDICINE

Internal medicine is a nonsurgical specialty with several subspecialties, such as gastroenterology, rheumatology, cardiology, pulmonary diseases, and **bariatrics.** Internists are often known as the "diagnosticians of medicine" as well as frequently being considered the "family physicians." The physical examination frequently follows the outline given in Chapter 27.

Gastroenterology

This specialty covers an extremely wide area that includes the stomach, the small intestine, and the bowel down to the rectum. Proctology is concerned with disorders of the rectum and anus.

A patient with a gastrointestinal (GI) problem may complain of such things as nausea, anorexia, or abdominal pain as well as numerous other symptoms. It may be difficult for the medical assistant to organize a patient's complaints when a patient first contacts the office by telephone for an appointment. The patient may say he has a "belly ache" when the discomfort is really in the stomach area; the "belly" is the central portion of the entire abdominal cavity. Or the patient may say he has a stomach ache when the discomfort is in the hypogastric area and not in the epigastric area. Careful questioning will guide the patient to a more precise description of the symptoms.

Emotional factors play an important part in many GI problems, often making the separation of functional disorders and organic disorders difficult. Abdominal pain may be classified as chronic or acute. The "chronic abdomen," or chronic pain, may or may not be abdominal in origin. It may originate in the thoracic cavity or musculoskeletal system. The "acute abdomen" may demand immediate attention, as in acute appendicitis or acute gastritis with possible hemorrhage. Both may demand surgical therapy.

In order to isolate an abdominal problem, it is frequently necessary for the physician to do a sigmoidoscopic examination as well as a pelvic examination on the female patient. The accessory organs of the digestive system also play an important role. These are the liver, the gallbladder, and the pancreas. Jaundice is a sign of liver disease, or obstructive jaundice due to *choledocholithiasis* (a calculus in the common bile duct). *Acute pancreatitis* produces diffuse pain and tenderness in the epigastrium.

Many of the diagnostic tests for GI symptoms are noninvasive in nature. The patient may be asked to have various roentgenograms (x-ray films) taken of the digestive system. These include barium swallow, upper GI series, and barium enema. The gallbladder is viewed by cholecystography. Liver function is checked by various laboratory procedures. The SGOT (serum glutamic-oxaloacetic transaminase),

SGPT (serum glutamic-pyruvic transaminase), and chemistry profiles are commonly performed blood tests. The urine is tested for bilirubin and urinary amylase. The stool is tested for occult blood, intestinal parasites and organisms, fat excretion, and color.

Pulmonary Medicine

Patients with respiratory problems may present with chronic or acute symptoms. A common complaint seen in this specialty, the upper respiratory infection (URI), may be, like the others, either chronic or acute. Other infections involving the so-called lower respiratory system, the lungs, also present as chronic or acute problems. Many of the infections of the lungs are in the wide group of pneumonias. It is estimated that there are over 50 different causes of pneumonia, ranging from bacteria, viruses, and fungi to chemical irritants. The term *pneumonitis* is synonymous with pneumonia. The diagnosis of lobar pneumonia refers to an infection involving a segment or lobe of the lung.

Diagnostic aids vary with the possible diagnosis. The most frequently used are x-ray film of the chest, blood count, TB skin tests, and analysis of sputum. Arterial blood tests, pulmonary function tests (discussed in Chapter 39), and lung scans are also done.

If a patient in the waiting room is coughing very much or if the cough is productive, it would be advisable to have this patient wait for the physician in an examining room. Provide this patient with ample tissues and show him or her where the waste receptacle is located.

Aseptic Procedures in Pulmonary Medicine

The most common source of contamination in pulmonary medicine is the pulmonary function test equipment. These machines are difficult to sterilize, and asepsis is frequently ignored in their use. The interior of the apparatus is not accessible and cannot be sterilized except by gas sterilization. The parts that are nearest to the patient should be autoclaved or carefully sterilized in a chemical sterilant. Disposable parts such as mouthpieces and tubes are commonly used to protect the patient and ensure asepsis.

Cardiology

Heart disease is the major cause of death in the United States, as well as the cause of many chronic illnesses. People are concerned and apprehensive about their hearts. No physician would consider examining a patient without checking the patient's heart. Patients seem to derive some therapeutic value from just having a physician "listen to their heart." Auscultation is the primary method of examining the heart.

Examination starts by observing the general appearance of the patient. The physician may notice a degree of cyanosis, facial edema, clubbing of the fingertips, a cough, or shortness of breath. Cardiac disease has many symptoms and many etiologies; hypertension, arteriosclerosis of the coronary arteries, and rheumatic fever are the leading causes. *Congestive heart failure* is the inability of the heart to maintain sufficient circulation to meet the body's needs. **Arrhythmia** may or may not be associated with congestive heart failure. *Angina pectoris* is acute chest pain resulting from a decrease in the blood supply to the heart muscles; it is not a disease but a symptom. The topographic landmarks of the chest (Fig. 29–8) are helpful in describing the heart's location and borders during the examination.

Other diagnostic procedures that aid the physician in the study of the heart include x-ray films; the resting electrocardiogram; exercise ECGs (stress tests) such as the Master's two-step, treadmill, or bicycle ergometer test (an apparatus for measuring the amount of work done by the patient); and blood tests such as the cardiac risk panels and triglyceride studies. The cardiologist also uses such tests as cardiac catheterization and angiocardiogram (see Chapter 30). Cardiac catheterization is accomplished by introducing a small flexible catheter into a vein of the arm, usually the left antecubital, under fluoroscopic guidance, and gently passing it into the right atrium, right ventricle, and on to the pulmonary artery. The pressure of the blood is measured in these vessels and heart chambers. Samples of the blood are also withdrawn from these areas to determine their oxygen content. The angiocardiogram is a special x-ray procedure that uses an opaque dye to show the heart and its major blood vessels.

To assist in attaining complete relaxation during the cardiac examination, the medical assistant should instruct the patient to void prior to the examination. The room must be warm, since the patient will be disrobed. Silence is a must while the physician is listening to the heart. The assistant should have any available laboratory and x-ray results on hand prior to the examination.

NEUROLOGY

As in other physical examinations, a careful history provides valuable clues in diagnosing neurologic malfunctions. These may be seizures, syncope, **diplopia, incontinence,** and subjective sensations. The patient's general health often complicates a neurologic diagnosis. The purposes of a neurologic examination are to determine whether a nervous system malfunction is present, discover its location, and identify its type and extent. During the history-taking, the physician may determine the patient's emotional status, intellectual performance, and general behavior, which may be evident in the patient's grooming and mannerisms. The patient's ability to communicate is also observed at this time.

Each cranial nerve is checked. For example, the first cranial nerve, the *olfactory nerve,* is examined by determining the patient's ability to identify familiar odors, such as coffee, tobacco, or cloves. The fifth cranial nerve, the *trigeminal nerve,* is checked by the patient's differentiating between warm and cold objects held on his or her right and left cheeks.

The motor system is examined by observing the patient's muscular strength and movements. The diameters of the upper arms and the calves of the legs are measured for muscular atrophy. The sensory system is examined by noting the patient's ability to perceive superficial sensations, such as a wisp of cotton brushed on the skin, a light pinprick, or hot and cold touching certain areas. Several reflexes, such as the patellar and Achilles reflexes, are examined. A stroke with a dull instrument on the lateral aspect of the sole of the foot may produce the Babinski reflex, in which the great toe dorsiflexes, whereas the smaller toes fan out.

Some other tests include skull x-ray films, angiograms, myelograms, and brain scans. An electroencephalogram (EEG) also is performed. The medical assistant may wish to remind patients to wear some sort of head covering after the EEG, because there may be some contact paste left on the scalp. Conditions such as stroke (cerebral vascular accident, or CVA), cerebral aneurysm, a brain tumor or abscess, Parkinson's disease, or multiple sclerosis (MS) and

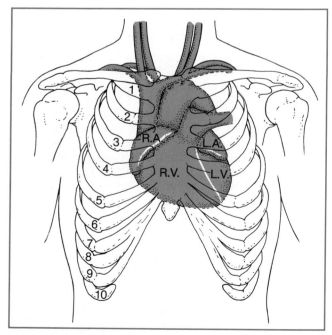

FIGURE 29–8. Topography of the chest. (*R.A.:* right atrium; *R.V.:* right ventricle; *L.A.:* left atrium; *L.V.:* left ventricle.)

Alzheimer's disease are often seen by the neurologist.

ONCOLOGY

Oncology is the medical specialty that concerns the diagnosis and treatment of tumors and masses. Most of the patients who are seen by oncologists have some form of **cancer**, or **neoplasia**, and exhibit changes in body function that are directly or indirectly related to changes in cell development.

Cancer can occur at any age, but it is most common among the elderly. It strikes approximately three of every four families in the United States. In 1990, more than 1 million people were diagnosed as having cancer (ACS, 1990).

The major responsibility of the medical assistant in the oncology practice is to monitor the patient's responses to body changes. Although these changes cannot always be seen clinically, the primary focus should be understanding the process and how these changes affect the patient and the family.

The number of people with cancer who are now considered "cured" is steadily increasing. New ways of treating and curing cancer are being found every day. At one time, cancer diagnosis was considered a death sentence, but this is no longer true. Major advances in the prevention, detection, diagnosis, and treatment of cancer have improved the survival rates and the quality of life of patients with the disease. The medical assistant should be aware of the treatments and procedures used in cancer management, as this awareness will aid in supporting the patient during treatment. Listening and counseling skills are also important. The American Cancer Society offers classes and pamphlets for cancer patients and their families to help in understanding the disease. You can also benefit from these classes.

OPHTHALMOLOGY

A complete examination of the eye is technical and requires expensive equipment, but the practitioner of general medicine does become involved with some examinations and treatments of the eye with the use of basic office equipment. The use of the ophthalmoscope to examine the retina of the eye is an essential part of every complete physical examination. The eye often reflects an individual's general health or may be involved in a systemic disease or injury. The eye may react to a systemic medication the patient is taking.

The most routine eye test, other than the use of the ophthalmoscope, is the distance acuity test, usually given with the *Snellen chart* (Fig. 29–9). This test may be administered by the medical assistant, who may also check the patient's near vision with the *Near-Vision Acuity chart* (Fig. 29–10). This is

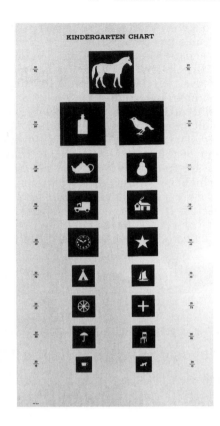

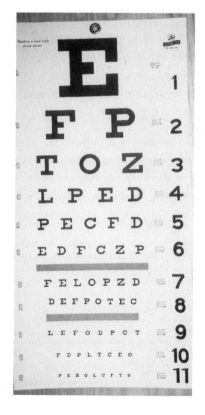

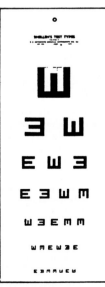

FIGURE 29–9. *A,* Special chart for children who are too young to read. *B,* The Snellen eye chart. *C,* The "E" chart, which can be used for children or for persons unable to read English.

29

especially done on the patient older than 40 years of age for possible **presbyopia.**

Testing a patient's color vision is important, especially if the patient is in certain occupations. By the age of five, all children should be checked with color vision charts (Fig. 29–11).

The eyelids are examined for edema, which may be the result of nephrosis, heart failure, allergy, or thyroid deficiency. **Ptosis** of the eyelid may be an involvement of the third cranial nerve. Infections of the eyelids are frequently a sty (an infected eyelash follicle), which is painful, or a chalazion (a beady nodule in the eyelid), which is usually not painful unless infected. If the lacrimal ducts are obstructed, the patient has constant tearing, known as *epiphora.* The *conjunctiva* of the eye is the delicate membrane covering the eyeball and lining the eyelids. Inflammation of the conjunctiva may be bacterial or viral, and there is a highly contagious conjunctivitis commonly called *pinkeye.*

The corneal reflex or corneal sensitivity is tested by touching the cornea of the eye quickly with a wisp of cotton. The patient will blink. The pupils of the eyes are normally round and equal in size. Normal pupils constrict rapidly in response to light and during accommodation. This is seen by shining a bright pinpoint light into one eye from the side of the patient's head. The pupil of the illuminated eye constricts, and the pupil of the other eye constricts equally. This test is called *light and accommodation (L & A).* An older patient's eyes do not accommodate as well as a younger person's. Each eye is

---

60

Nothing can take the place of "the only pair of eyes you will ever have." That is why you are exercising such good judgment in taking care of them as you are now doing.

50

For this reason, you will welcome the suggestion about lenses which are designed and made to give you "greater comfort and better appearance." In man's earliest days he had little use for glasses. He used his eyes chiefly for long distance.

40

He worked by daylight and at tasks with little detail. But now, you use your eyes for much close work—reading, writing, sewing and many other uses which the eyes of primitive man did not know. Now your eyes meet all sorts of lighting conditions, artificial and natural.

30

Many of these conditions produce "overbrightness" or glare. Sometimes it is the direct or reflected glare of sunlight; often it is direct or reflected from artificial light. And very often this glare is uncomfortable—impairs your efficiency. But special lenses, developed by America's leading optical scientists, combat this glare.

25

These lenses give you more comfortable vision and blend harmoniously with your complexion. These lenses are less conspicuous. We are glad to rec- ommend them because they will give you greater comfort and better appearance. Thousands of satisfied wearers testify to their real benefits.

20

You are wise in taking good care of "the only pair of eyes you will ever have." You know how valuable they are, that you can never have another pair. For this reason, you will welcome the suggestion about lenses which are designed and made to give you "greater comfort and better appear- ance." In man's earliest days he had little use for glasses.

The above letters subtend the visual angle of 5' at the designated distance in inches.

B-858 **BAUSCH & LOMB** ▼ Printed in U.S.A.
Mark of Leadership

FIGURE 29–10. The Near-Vision Acuity Chart for persons older than 40 years of age who have difficulty with accommodation (adjusting to changes in distance) because the eye muscles no longer respond quickly.

checked this way. Then, the patient is asked to look at the physician's finger as it is moved directly toward the patient's nose.

The ophthalmoscope is used for examining the interior of the eye. It projects a bright narrow beam of light that permits the physician to examine the interior parts of the eye and retina through the lens of the eye. It is helpful in detecting disorders of the eyes as well as disorders of other organs, the conditions of which are reflected in the condition of the eyes.

Intraocular pressure has been checked by ophthalmologists for many years, but today many general-practice physicians also check their patients for intraocular pressure. Elevated intraocular pressure, known as *glaucoma,* causes pressure on the nerve fibers and thus may possibly result in blindness. The tonometer is used to measure this intraocular pressure. The patient is placed in a reclining position or sits with the head resting back on a support. A topical anesthetic is instilled in each eye. After 1 minute, the patient is instructed to fix his or her vision on a spot on the ceiling. The physician then touches the sterile footplate of the tonometer to the cornea of the eye. The tonometer is an extremely delicate instrument requiring particular care and storage. After each use, it must be sterilized and returned to its stand. Read the manufacturer's instructions and follow them carefully.

Strabismus, or crossed eyes, is seen predominantly in a small percentage of young children because it is diagnosed early in life and is treated as early as possible. There are several problems that cause eyes to turn, but most commonly the condition is due to weakness of an extraocular muscle. Evaluation of patients with strabismus includes a cover test, measurement of visual acuity, and a careful ophthalmoscopic examination.

Special techniques employed in the ophthalmologist's office include the use of a *slit-lamp biomicroscope.* This is used to view the fine details in the anterior segments of the eye. It is also used to view a corneal foreign body because it gives a well-illuminated and highly magnified view of the area. The patient with exophthalmia (abnormal protrusion of the eye due possibly to an overactive thyroid or to a tumor behind the eyeball) is checked with the *exophthalmometer.* This instrument is designed to measure the pressure of the central retinal artery. It is helpful in patients with circulatory disease because it measures the blood pressure in the retinal artery.

Distance Visual Acuity

Distance visual acuity is frequently part of a complete physical examination. It is widely used in schools and industry. To date, it is the best single test available for visual screening. Many cases of myopia, astigmatism, or hyperopia have been de-

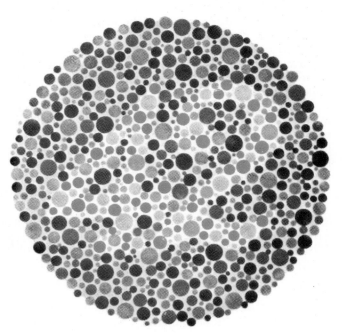

FIGURE 29–11. Ishihara color graph testing.

tected by this routine test. The most common chart used is the *Snellen Alphabetical* chart (see Fig. 29–9B). This chart has various letters of the alphabet and is for general use. Patients with limited knowledge of the English alphabet can be tested with the *"E" chart* (see Fig. 29–9C). In addition, there is a chart available that uses pictures as symbols (see Fig. 29–9A). This chart is also used for preschool patients, slow learners, or mentally retarded children who have not yet learned the English alphabet. The symbol on the top line of the chart can be read by persons of normal vision at 200 feet. In each of the succeeding rows, from the top down, the size of the symbols is reduced so that a person with normal vision can see them at distances of 100, 70, 50, 40, 30, and 20 feet.

The patient must not be allowed to study the chart before the test. The room or hall should be long enough so that the 20-foot distance can be marked off accurately. The chart should be hung at eye level and illuminated with maximum light, without glare on the chart. The patient may be standing or sitting with the chart at eye level.

Most adults do not need the chart explained, but the assistant must have the patient's cooperation. With the "E" chart, for example, an explanation must be given as to how the E's are to be read. The patient may point up or down, or right or left. The patient may prefer to hold three fingers in the same direction that the letter is facing. Use the same routine each time the patient is tested, by starting with the right eye. If the patient is wearing glasses, the physician may want the eyes tested first with the glasses on and then without them. Indicate on the patient's record "with" or "without." Test one eye at a time. Both eyes are to be kept open during the test, but the eye not being tested is to be covered with a paper cup or a piece of cardboard. The paper cup is best because it does not touch the eye. Under no circumstances should the patient use fingers to hold the eye closed.

Allow a moment between changing eyes. The medical assistant should stand beside the chart and point to the line to be read. Start with the line having the larger symbols, then proceed to the lower lines. Record the smallest line that the patient can read without a mistake, and also record any behavioral observations such as squinting, straining, tearing, or turning of the head. Record the responses of each eye separately. The response is recorded as a fraction. The numerator (top number) is the distance of the patient from the chart, the denominator (bottom number) is the lowest line read satisfactorily by the patient. For example, if the patient reads the 20 line at 20 feet, the fraction 20/20 is recorded for that eye. Make certain the record reads "right eye" (O.D.) and "left eye" (O.S.).

PROCEDURE 29-2   MEASURING DISTANCE VISUAL ACUITY USING THE SNELLEN CHART

GOAL To determine the patient's degree of visual clarity at a measured distance, using the Snellen chart.

EQUIPMENT AND SUPPLIES

Snellen eye chart   Pen or pencil and paper
Eye cover

PROCEDURAL STEPS

1. Wash your hands.
2. Prepare the examination room. Make sure that (1) the room is well lighted, (2) a distance marker is 20 feet from the chart, and (3) the chart is placed at eye level.
3. Assemble the materials needed.
4. Identify the patient, and explain the procedure.
   Purpose: Explanations help gain patient cooperation and alleviate apprehension.
5. Position the patient in a standing or sitting position at the 20-foot marker.
   Purpose: Twenty feet is the standard testing distance.
6. Position the Snellen chart at eye level to the patient.
7. Instruct the patient to cover the left eye.
   Purpose: The right eye is traditionally tested first.
8. Stand beside the chart, and point to each row as the patient orally reads down the chart, starting with the 20/200 row.
   Purpose: Starting with larger letters allows the patient to gain confidence.
9. Record any patient reactions in reading the chart.
   Purpose: Reactions such as squinting, leaning, tearing, or blinking may indicate that the patient is experiencing difficulty with the test.
10. Record the smallest line that the patient can read without making a mistake.
11. Repeat the procedure on the other eye.

PROCEDURE 29-3   ASSESSMENT OF COLOR ACUITY

GOAL   To correctly assess a patient's color acuity and record the results.

EQUIPMENT AND SUPPLIES

Appropiate room area with natural light   Pen, pencil, and paper
Ishihara Color Plate Book

PROCEDURAL STEPS

1. Assemble the necessary equipment and prepare the room for testing. The room should be quiet and illuminated with natural light.
   Purpose: For testing colors to be seen correctly, natural light is needed.

2. Identify the patient and explain the procedure. Use a practice card during the explanation and be sure that the patient understands that he or she has 3 seconds to identify each plate.
   Purpose: An informed patient is a cooperative patient. The first plate is a practice plate and is designed to be read correctly.

3. Hold up the first plate at a right angle to the patient's line of vision and 30 inches from the patient. Be sure both eyes are kept open during the test (Fig. 29-12).

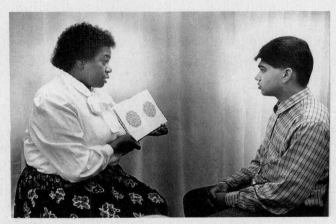

FIGURE 29-12.

4. Ask the patient to tell you what number is on the plate, and record the patient's answer.

5. Continue this sequence until all of the plates have been read. If the patient cannot identify the number on the plate, place an "X" in the record for that plate number. Your record should look like this:
   Plate 1 = 12   Plate: 2 = 8   Plate: 3 = x   Plate 4 = 70

6. Include any unusual symptoms in your record, such as eye rubbing, squinting, or excessive blinking. Initial your results.

7. Return the book to its storage space. The Ishihara book needs to be stored in a closed position away from external light to protect the colors.

Eye Irrigation

The purpose of eye irrigation is to relieve inflammation, promote drainage, dilute chemicals, or wash away foreign bodies. Sterile technique and equipment must be used to avoid contamination.

When an eye irrigation is ordered by the physician, the assistant may perform the procedure, provided that he or she has completed proper training and is competent in the application of the technique. The solution should be warmed to between 95° and 105°F. Follow the procedure as prescribed, making sure that the patient is comfortable. Always record the treatment on the patient's record immediately after completing it.

PROCEDURE 29-4   IRRIGATING A PATIENT'S EYES

GOAL To cleanse the eye(s), as ordered by the physician.

EQUIPMENT AND SUPPLIES

Prescribed sterile irrigation solution
Irrigating bulb syringe
Basin for solution
Basin for drainage
Sterile cotton balls
Disposable drape

Towel
Nonsterile gloves
Blood and body-fluid protection barriers (goggles, masks, and aprons or gowns), as necessary

PROCEDURAL STEPS

1. Wash your hands. Follow universal blood and body-fluid precautions. Glove yourself with nonsterile gloves.

2. Check the physician's orders to determine which eye(s) require irrigation.
    Purpose: To check the abbreviations: O.D. (right eye), O.S. (left eye), O.U. (both eyes).

3. Assemble the materials needed.

4. Read the label of the solution three times.
    Purpose: To follow the rules for administering medications.

5. Identify the patient, and explain the procedure.
    Purpose: Explanations help gain patient cooperation and alleviate apprehension.

6. Assist the patient into a sitting or supine position, making certain that the head is turned toward the affected eye. Place the disposable drape over the patient's neck and shoulder.
    Purpose: This causes the solution to flow away from the unaffected eye so as to reduce the chances for cross-contamination of the healthy eye.

7. Place or have the patient hold a drainage basin next to the affected eye to receive the solution from the eye. Position a towel under the basin to avoid getting the solution on the patient (Fig. 29-13).

8. Moisten a cotton ball with solution, and cleanse the eyelid and lashes. Start at the inner canthus (near nose) to the outer canthus (farthest from nose) and dispose of the cotton ball.
    Purpose: Debris on the lids or lashes must be cleansed away before exposing the conjunctiva.

9. Pour the required volume of irrigating solution into the basin, and withdraw solution into the bulb syringe.

10. Separate eyelids with the index finger and thumb of one hand, and hold.

11. With the other hand, place the syringe on the bridge of the nose parallel to the eye.
    Purpose: To support and steady the syringe.

Continued

12. Squeeze the bulb, directing the solution toward the inner contour of the eye and allowing the solution to flow steadily and slowly. Do not allow the syringe to touch the eye or eyelids (Fig. 29–14).
Purpose: Prevents possible injury to the eye.

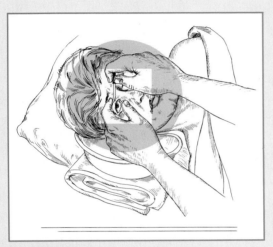

FIGURE 29–13.

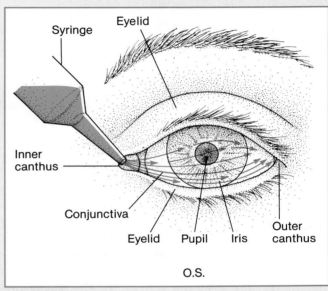

FIGURE 29–14.

13. Dry the eyelid with a cotton ball.

14. Record the procedure on the patient's chart.

15. Clean up the work area.

16. Wash your hands.

Eye Instillation

The purpose of eye instillation is to apply medication. Instillation may also be performed to dilate the pupils prior to examination.

Aseptic Procedures in Ophthalmology

The major concern is in the careless use of eyedrops and careless handling of the medicine dropper.

The use of stock solutions has been discouraged because of the dangers of the solution becoming a culture for pathogenic bacteria. Eye ointments present a similar problem. Sterile solutions must be used if there is a laceration or ulceration of the eye. Instruments used for the removal of a foreign body should be sterile. It is advisable to reserve a medication for the patient for whom it is prescribed and not to use it on other patients.

29

PROCEDURE 29-5   INSTILLING MEDICATION INTO A PATIENT'S EYES

GOAL   To apply medication to the eye(s), as ordered by the physician.

EQUIPMENT AND SUPPLIES

Sterile medication with dropper
Disposable drape
Gauze squares

Nonsterile gloves
Blood and body-fluid protection barriers

PROCEDURAL STEPS

1. Wash your hands. Follow universal blood and body-fluid precautions. Gather supplies. Glove yourself with nonsterile gloves.

2. Check the physician's order to determine which eye(s) require medication.
   Purpose: To check the abbreviations.

3. Assemble the materials needed.

4. Read the label of the medication three times.
   Purpose: To follow the rules for administering medications.

5. Identify the patient, and explain the procedure.
   Purpose: Explanations help gain patient cooperation and alleviate apprehension.

6. Assist the patient into a sitting or supine position with the head tilted backward and "looking up."

7. Pull the lower conjunctival sac downward with a gauze square (Fig. 29-15).
   Purpose: Gauze prevents your fingers from slipping.

8. Insert the prescribed number of drops into the eye, directly over the center of the lower conjunctival sac while holding the dropper parallel to the eye and 1/2 inch away.
   Purpose: Never point the dropper toward the eye or touch the eye with the dropper (Fig. 29-16).

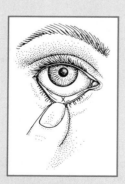

FIGURE 29-15.

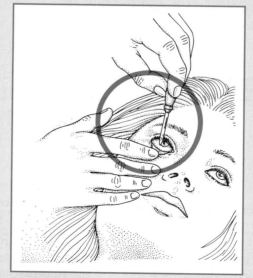

FIGURE 29-16.

Continued

9. Instruct the patient to close the eye immediately and to rotate the eyeball.
   Purpose: Rotating the eyeball distributes the medication.

10. Dry any excess drainage.

11. Record the procedure on the patient's chart.

12. Clean up the work area.

13. Wash your hands.

ORTHOPEDICS

An orthopedist is concerned with the body's mobility and with diagnosing and treating diseases and abnormalities of the musculoskeletal system. A considerable part of this practice may be caring for fractures, dislocations, strains, sprains, and ruptures.

A common complaint heard in the orthopedist's office is "low back pain." Other diseases seen are rheumatoid arthritis, osteoarthritis, gout, and bursitis.

Besides a careful history, the examination covers basically the back and the extremities. The physical examination of the musculoskeletal system is performed largely by inspection, but palpation and mensuration are also done. The orthopedic physician wants to determine the condition of the muscles, joints, and bones. A large part of the examination is done to determine the direction and the range of active and passive motion in the joints.

The first step is usually inspection of the patient's posture in the standing, sitting, and supine positions. A lateral view of the patient in a standing position shows the position of the head in relation to the trunk of the body. Normal or rigid curves of the cervical, thoracic, and lumbar spine may be seen. Abnormalities such as kyphosis and lordosis are seen in this lateral inspection. Scoliosis is seen from the posterior view. To determine the patient's

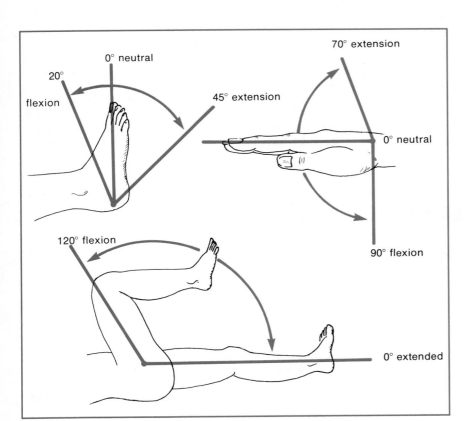

FIGURE 29–17. Flexion and extension measured in degrees.

29

gait, the physician asks the patient to walk. The physician may observe a limp, possibly due to **ankylosis,** or a scissor gait, as seen in spastic paraplegia.

Each major joint of the body is inspected for range of motion. A goniometer is used for precise measurement of a joint's flexion and extension. Muscles are examined for hypertrophy or atrophy. The measurement of the circumference of an extremity at a given point, such as the calf of the leg or the biceps of the arm, is compared with that of the opposite side. The tendon reflexes are checked.

The spine, or vertebral column, is referred to in divisions. The first 7 vertebrae are the cervical spine, the next 12 are the thoracic spine, and the next 5 are the lumbar spine. These are the 24 movable vertebrae. Below the lumbar vertebrae are the sacrum and coccyx. When referring to the movable spine, the physician may say C-5, meaning the fifth cervical vertebra, or L-3, meaning the third lumbar vertebra.

Physicians specializing in industrial medicine and worker's compensation cases have special terminology and methods for recording and measuring the musculoskeletal system. The American Academy of Orthopedic Surgeons has published a guide called *Joint Motion: Method of Measuring and Recording.*

The medical assistant must be familiar with such terms as *extension,* which is a movement that increases the angle between the ends of a jointed part, such as the straightening of a limb. The opposite of this is *flexion,* which is the act of bending or decreasing such an angle. The amount of bending is recorded in degrees (Fig. 29–17). Other terms used are *abduction,* meaning lateral movement away from the middle plane. *Adduction* is movement toward the middle plane.

Radiographs are the most common diagnostic aid used in the orthopedic office. Urinalysis and blood tests are ordered when there is joint involvement or severe pain and swelling. Physical therapy and rehabilitation are also a major part of the therapy.

OTORHINOLARYNGOLOGY

This is the medical specialty that deals with the ear, nose, and throat. It is frequently referred to as otolaryngology or even as a single specialty of otology or laryngology. Usually, the specialty otorhinolaryngology is referred to simply as ear, nose, and throat (ENT). The anatomic point at which the ENT examination begins varies with the physician. Most of the involved area is visible to the physician, with the exception of the nasal accessory sinuses and the middle and inner ear. A large part of this examination consists of the inspection of the mucosa.

If the ears are examined first, the external auditory canal is viewed with an otoscope or a light and ear speculum. The normal external canal contains a small amount of cerumen (wax). Cerumen is a protective secretion produced to ward off microorganisms. Patients who attempt to remove the wax by using cotton-tip applicators often push the wax farther into the canal, which causes the wax to lodge and harden. This impacted wax is uncomfortable and eventually impairs hearing. Patients can have the impacted wax removed to avoid further discomfort or possible ear damage. A softening solution may be instilled into the impacted ear and then followed by irrigation to remove the excess ear wax.

Aseptic Procedures in Otorhinolaryngology

Routine examination instruments are sterilized after use and stored in a clean area. Surgical asepsis must be practiced when changing dressings, placing packs, and performing minor surgery. Dressing forceps must be sterilized after their use with each patient. Medicines, such as ear and nose drops, must be handled carefully to avoid contamination.

PROCEDURE 29–6   IRRIGATING A PATIENT'S EARS

GOAL   To remove excessive or impacted cerumen from a patient's ear(s).

EQUIPMENT AND SUPPLIES

Irrigating solution
Basin for irrigating solution
Bulb syringe
Gauze squares

Otoscope
Drainage basin
Disposable drape
Cotton-tip applicators

Continued

Ear Irrigation

Ear irrigation is performed to remove excessive or impacted cerumen. When an ear irrigation is ordered by the physician, the assistant may perform the procedure provided that proper training has been completed and that the assistant is competent in the technique. The solution should be warmed to between 95° and 105°F. Follow the procedure as prescribed, making sure that the patient is comfortable. Always chart the treatment immediately after completing it.

PROCEDURAL STEPS

1. Wash your hands.
2. Assemble the materials needed.
3. Check the physician's orders.
4. Check the label of the solution three times.
5. Prepare the solution as ordered. The solution temperature should be between 95° and 105°F.
   Purpose: Warm solutions are most comfortable to the patient.
6. Identify the patient, and explain the procedure.
7. View the affected ear with an otoscope to locate impaction or a foreign object.
8. Drape the patient.
   Purpose: Draping protects the patient's clothing.
9. Position the patient with the head slightly tilted toward the affected side.
   Purpose: This position allows gravity to help the solution flow from the ear to the basin.
10. Place the drainage basin next to the affected ear.
    Purpose: To prevent the solution from running down the patient's neck.
11. Wipe any particles from the outside of the ear with gauze squares.
    Purpose: Prevents the introduction of foreign materials into the ear canal.
12. Fill the syringe.
13. Pull up the auricle of the ear gently with one hand.
14. With the other hand, place the tip of the syringe into the meatus of the ear (Fig. 29–18).

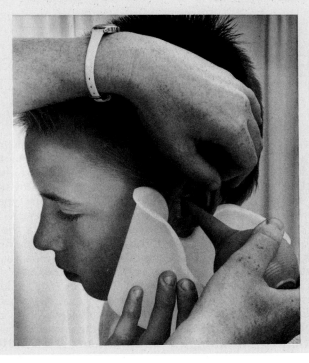

FIGURE 29–18.

Continued

PROCEDURE 29-6   *Continued*

15. Direct the flow of the solution gently upward (Fig. 29-19).

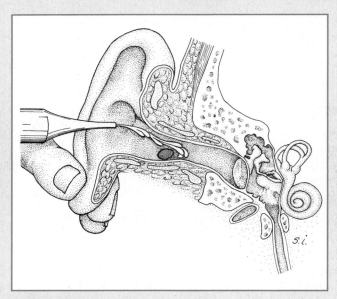

FIGURE 29-19.

16. Dry the patient's external ear with gauze squares.

17. Dry the ear canal gently with cotton-tip applicators.

18. Inspect the ear with an otoscope to determine the results.

19. Record the procedure on the patient's chart.

20. Clean up the work area.

21. Wash your hands.

Disorders of the Ear

The patient may be given a hearing test with an *audiometer* (Fig. 29-20) to disclose any hearing loss. There are three types of hearing loss: conductive, sensorineural, and central. *Conductive* hearing loss (external or middle ear disorders) occurs when sound cannot reach the cochlea because of blockage of the ear canal or disorders of the eardrum or ossicles. Factors causing this type of hearing loss include foreign body or cerumen impaction, perforated tympanic membrane, exudate in the middle ear, otosclerosis, and adhesions of the ossicles. *Sensorineural* hearing loss (perceptive hearing loss) occurs when there is damage to the cochlea or eighth cranial nerve, which conducts sound from the inner ear to the brain. The deafness may be caused by heredi-

tary factors, German measles, trauma, noise, drugs, tumors, aging, and infection. *Central* hearing loss (brain stem and cerebral hemispheres) is uncommon and usually is characterized by loss of speech rather than of pure tone perception. This type of hearing loss is usually due to lesions or tumors.

The anatomic differences between the adult's and the child's **eustachian tube** make children far more susceptible to middle ear infections (**otitis** media). Occasionally, it may be necessary to do a **myringotomy** to drain the exudate from the middle ear.

The inner ear can be invaded by bacteria, especially as a complication of acute otitis media. **Vertigo** (the sensation of dizziness) may be a symptom of some diseases of the inner ear. **Tinnitus** (ringing in the ears) is also a subjective symptom. It may be

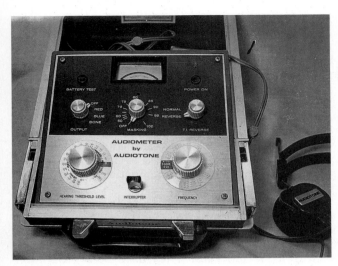

FIGURE 29-20. The audiometer is used to screen patients who have possible hearing loss.

present in labyrinthitis, damage to the eighth cranial nerve, or cerebral arteriosclerosis.

Other disorders of the ear follow.

Otitis externa (swimmer's ear). Otitis externa is a bacterial or fungal infection caused by swimming in contaminated water or heavily chlorinated swimming pools.

External canal blockage. External canal blockage is caused by a collection of cerumen or by a foreign body. This may result in reduced hearing, direct tissue damage, or perforation of the eardrum.

Perforation of the eardrum. Perforation of the eardrum can result from chronic infection, burns, direct blows to the side of the head, insertion of bobby pins and toothpicks, blast injury, and careless use of cotton swabs.

Meniere's syndrome. Meniere's syndrome is a dysfunction of the ear labyrinth resulting in swelling and loss of equilibrium. This condition may be caused by infection, allergies, tumors, arteriosclerosis and atherosclerosis, stress, genetic disorders, and poisoning.

Otosclerosis. Otosclerosis consists of ossification of the stapes against the oval window, resulting in a diminished transmission of sound to the inner ear. The cause is unknown. This condition occurs primarily in females.

Motion sickness. Motion sickness is caused by a disturbance within the inner ear. This condition results from any type of motion via transportation (train, car, bus, boat, or plane).

Examination of the Nose and Throat

Examination of the nasal cavity is mainly inspection of the mucous membrane. The common cold and allergies are the main causes of changes in the mucosa. Because the physician cannot see the nasal sinuses, they are examined by palpation and transillumination. If the mucosa is swollen, it may be necessary to spray the area with a vasoconstrictor.

The throat is the area that includes the larynx and pharynx and is viewed with the aid of a mirror and a tongue depressor or piece of gauze to grasp the tongue. In the nasopharynx, the physician looks for enlarged adenoids (pharyngeal tonsils) and for the orifice of the eustachian tube. It may be necessary to grasp the tongue with the aid of a piece of gauze in order to view the laryngopharynx. Spraying the throat with a topical anesthetic helps with the gagging patient.

In the oral cavity, the patient's teeth and gums are carefully examined. The palatine (faucial) tonsils (if present) are checked for size and the presence of crypts. The lingual tonsils are also checked. The salivary glands are palpated.

PROCTOLOGY

Proctology is the branch of medicine concerned with the disorders of the rectum and anus. Proctoscopy is an examination of the lower rectum and anal canal through a 3-inch-long proctoscope or **anoscope.** The proctoscope permits detection of hemorrhoids, polyps, fissures, fistulae, and abscesses (Fig. 29-21). The patient may need an enema for this procedure. Sigmoidoscopy is an examination used to view the lower portion of the sigmoid and rectum

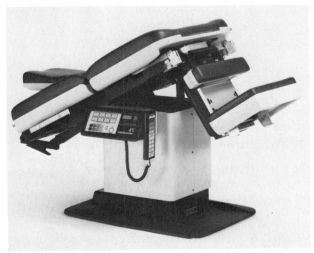

FIGURE 29-21. A special examination table for proctologic examinations. (Courtesy of Ritter, Liebel-Flarsheim, a division of Sybron Corp., Cincinnati, OH.)

29

through a 10- to 12-inch-long **sigmoidoscope.** The patient is examined in a knee-chest position or on a special jackknife table. The sigmoidoscope aids in the diagnosis of infection, inflammation, and ulcerative conditions and permits actual viewing of tumors and polyps. The patient must follow a precise preparation procedure 24 to 48 hours prior to the examination.

Other diagnostic aids used in the diagnosis of colon and rectum disorders include gastrointestinal series (x-ray films), stool cultures, and tests for **hemoccult,** or occult blood, in feces.

Disorders and Diseases

Rectocolonic cancer comprises 15% of all cancer and accounts for 20% of cancer deaths. It usually occurs after the age of 55 years. In younger patients, it is often associated with ulcerative **colitis.** Rectal cancer is more common in men, whereas colon cancer is more common in women. Its incidence appears to be associated with low-fiber diets, high-carbohydrate diets, high-fat diets, and genetic factors. At least 70% of rectocolonic cancers are anatomically within reach of the sigmoidoscope (10 in), and approximately 13% are found within digital reach (3.2 in). The American Cancer Society guidelines for early detection of colorectal disorders include a routine annual digital rectal examination beginning at 40 years; an annual stool guaiac rectal test beginning at age 50 years; and after age 50 years, a sigmoidoscopy every 3 to 5 years after two negative sigmoidoscopy examinations have been performed 1 year apart.

Both the lower portion of the rectum and the anal canal contain vertical folds of mucous membrane called rectal and anal columns. The veins in the mucosa of these folds frequently become dilated, resulting in *hemorrhoids*. They have been associated with standing for long periods, diarrhea, pregnancy, constipation, vomiting, coughing, loss of muscle tone, anorectal infections, hepatitis, and alcoholism.

PROCEDURE 29-7   ASSISTING WITH PROCTOSIGMOIDOSCOPY

GOAL To assist the physician with the examination of the rectum and colon, to collect specimens as requested, and to promote patient comfort and safety.

EQUIPMENT AND SUPPLIES

Examination table
Sigmoidoscope
Anoscope
Light source
Suction pump
Insufflator
Rectal dressing forceps
Finger cots
Gloves
Lubricating jelly

Basin of water
Biopsy forceps
Drape sheet
Patient gown
Towel
Cotton balls
Gauze squares
Tissues
Specimen bottle with preservative

PROCEDURAL STEPS

1. Wash your hands. Follow universal blood and body-fluid precautions. Glove yourself with nonsterile gloves.
2. Assemble the materials in the proper order.
    Purpose: To position the instruments according to the physician's preferred order.
3. Test the equipment for proper functioning.
    Purpose: To make certain that the suction device is functioning properly.

Continued

Polyps are growths protruding from the mucous membrane of the GI tract. There are several varieties, of which most are **benign.** Most types develop in adults over 45 years of age. Predisposing factors include age, heredity, diet, and infection. Polyps are difficult to diagnose because they are usually asymptomatic and are discovered during sigmoidoscopy or on lower GI x-ray films. The most common symptom is rectal bleeding.

Pruritus ani is itching around the anus that is associated with irritation and burning. Contributing factors include excessive rubbing with soap and cloth, poor hygiene, excessive perspiration, the consumption of spicy foods, diabetes, the use of perfumed toilet paper or colored paper, coffee, alcohol, food preservatives, fungal and parasitic infections, anorectal disease, and certain skin diseases.

Colorectal Examination

Many patients are apprehensive about colorectal examinations. The patient's feelings and concerns must be considered. Most patients suffer from a great deal of anxiety from the moment they enter the examining room. It is important that the assistant create an atmosphere of confidence and calm.

In an attempt to alleviate apprehension, the patient needs to know exactly what to do before the examination begins and may need to be reminded as the examination continues. Let the patient know that the examination is not usually painful, but some discomfort such as cramping can be experienced. Furthermore, the sensations of expelling **flatus** or of an impending bowel movement may be present. Explain that these sensations are caused by the instruments.

4. Identify the patient, and explain the procedure.

5. Instruct the patient to empty his or her bladder.

6. Give the patient a gown, and instruct him or her to remove all clothing from the waist down and to put the gown on with the opening in the back.

7. Assist the patient into the desired position.
   Purpose: Proper positioning is very important for the comfort of the patient and for the accessibility of the rectum and sigmoid colon. The best position can be attained with an adjustable table constructed for this purpose. Special proctologic tables allow the contents of the abdomen to drop forward. The "S" curve of the sigmoid colon is thus allowed to straighten out somewhat, which better accommodates the insertion of the sigmoidoscope.

8. Cover the patient with a drape immediately.
   Purpose: To avoid exposing the patient unnecessarily.

9. Assist the physician as needed. Hand the physician the various instruments and equipment.
   - Lubricate the physician's gloved finger and instruments.
   - Attach the inflation bulb to the scope.
   - Attach the light source to the scope.
   - Adjust the light source.
   - Turn on the suction machine.
   - Hand the biopsy forceps to the physician.
   - Label the specimen bottle.

10. Observe the patient during the procedure for any undue reactions such as fatigue or fainting, and be ready to offer assistance.

11. Wipe the anal area with tissue at the completion of the examination.

12. Assist the patient into a supine position.

13. Instruct the patient to get dressed.

14. Send the specimen to the laboratory, if collected.

15. Clean the work area.

16. Wash your hands.

29

THE MEDICAL ASSISTANT'S RESPONSIBILITIES IN THE SPECIALTY OFFICE

In all medical offices, you need to be prepared to assist the physician in all procedures performed. It is also your responsibility to meet the needs of the patient.

Patients are seen in the specialty office for specific disorders and problems. As health problems become more severe, so do anxieties and fears. You must be ready to address the patient's needs with empathy and compassion. You will need to develop a concerned attitude but also remain firm in your professional commitment.

The needs of the physician vary considerably from specialty to specialty. Some specialties require you to complete additional training in testing and performing procedures. As you learn new skills and take on greater responsibilities, you become a valued member of the health care team and an asset to your coworkers and employer.

GLOSSARY OF OTHER SPECIALTY PRACTICE TERMS

dysplasia Abnormal development of cells and tissues.

hyperplasia Increase in the number of cells.

malignant Having properties of metastasis; resulting in death.

melanosis Unusual deposits of black pigment on the skin.

primary tumor Tumor at the site of origin.

rales Abnormal respiratory sounds heard on inspiration.

rhonchus Abnormal sound heard when the airway is obstructed; also known as a *wheeze*.

staging A means to describe the extent of cancer spread in the body.

stridor High-pitched harsh sound heard when the larynx is obstructed.

xeroderma Dry skin.

LEGAL AND ETHICAL RESPONSIBILITIES

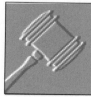

Working in a busy medical specialty practice is at times more demanding than working in the quiet general or family practice office. Specialists are expected to provide a higher degree of care quality than are family practice or general practice physicians. Your legal obligations to the physician, yourself, and your profession are the same regardless of the nature of the specialty practice where you are em-

ployed. Adhering to the code of ethics is difficult but necessary. Although the work of the medical assistant does not usually involve making life-or-death decisions, it does involve interpersonal interaction with patients and their families before and after decisions are made. You also need to support and aid the physician who must make these difficult decisions. It is important for the medical assistant to know how he or she can contribute to the physician's difficult decision-making process.

PATIENT EDUCATION

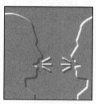

The most important contribution you can make to the welfare of the patient is to reinforce the care and treatment prescribed by the physician and to teach preventive health measures. You should help the patient recognize the signs and symptoms of his or her disorder, stress the importance of regular examinations to detect changes, and advise the patient and his or her family of any support groups that might be of service.

Medical advances have helped significantly to extend life expectancy. As a result, the number of chronically ill patients has also increased. Because many of these patients live independently and assume responsibility for their own care, they need to become willing partners in its planning. Your responsibility is to teach patients self-care in a way that encourages collaboration with health care professionals as well as effective problem solving. For example, in teaching a diabetic patient about proper nutrition and exercise, you must recognize the patient's dietary and physical activity preferences.

Patient education in all medical facilities—particularly in specialty practices—is a team effort. Plans should be made as to how information is to be presented and what is to be emphasized. Always remember that the patient must be a participant in this planning and that the physician must give the final approval.

LEARNING ACHIEVEMENTS

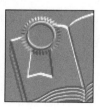

Upon completion of this chapter, can you in the time allowed by your evaluator:

1. Perform a tine tuberculin test on a patient, completing each step correctly and in the proper sequence?
2. Test and record your findings for the Ishihara test for color blindness, completing each step correctly and using accepted recording symbols?
3. Record distance visual acuity for both eyes,

using the Snellen chart and completing each step in proper sequence?

4. Irrigate a patient's eye(s), completing each step correctly and in proper sequence?

5. Instill appropriate medication into a patient's eye(s), using the proper technique?

6. Irrigate a patient's ear(s), completing each step in proper sequence while providing for the patient's comfort and safety?

7. Assist in a simulated proctosigmoidoscopic examination, completing each step carefully, completely, and in proper sequence while remembering the needs of the patient?

REFERENCES AND READINGS

Bonewit, K.: *Clinical Procedures for Medical Assistants,* 3rd ed., Philadelphia, W.B. Saunders Co., 1990.

Frew, M., and Frew, D.: *Comprehensive Medical Assisting,* 2nd ed., Philadelphia, F.A. Davis Co., 1988.

Ignatavicius, D., and Bayne, M.V.: *Medical–Surgical Nursing:* A Nursing Process Approach, Philadelphia, W.B. Saunders Co., 1991.

Kinn, M.: *Medical Terminology,* New York, Delmar Publishers, 1990.

Lane, K.: *Saunders Manual of Medical Assisting Practice,* Philadelphia, W.B. Saunders Co., 1992.

29

CHAPTER OUTLINE

THE HEART'S NATURAL PACEMAKER

THE CARDIAC CYCLE AND ELECTROCARDIOGRAPHY

THE ELECTROCARDIOGRAM
Electrocardiograph Paper
Electrodes and Electrolytes
Leads
Standard, or Bipolar, Leads
Augmented Leads
Chest, or Precordial, Leads
Standardization
Artifacts
Wandering Baseline
Somatic Tremor
Alternating Current
Baseline Interruption

OBTAINING THE ELECTROCARDIOGRAM

Preparing the Room and the Patient
Applying the Electrodes and Lead Wires
Recording the Electrocardiogram
Limb Leads
Chest Leads

MULTIPLE-CHANNEL ELECTROCARDIOGRAPH

AUTOMATIC LEAD CONTROL SWITCH

TELEPHONE TRANSMISSION

INTERPRETIVE ELECTROCARDIOGRAPHS

POST-TEST PROCEDURES
Equipment Maintenance
Mounting an Electrocardiogram

OBTAINING A 12-LEAD ELECTROCARDIOGRAM
Procedure 30–1: Obtaining a 12-Lead ECG
Interpretation of the Electrocardiogram
Heart Rate
Heart Rhythm

CARDIAC STRESS TESTING

VECTORCARDIOGRAPHY

ECHOCARDIOGRAPHY

HOLTER MONITOR CARDIOGRAPHY

ADDITIONAL VOCABULARY USED IN ELECTROCARDIOGRAPHY

LEGAL AND ETHICAL RESPONSIBILITIES

LEARNING ACHIEVEMENTS

VOCABULARY

arrhythmia An abnormality or irregularity in heart rhythm.

atrioventricular node (AV node) Part of the conductive system located between the atria and the ventricles near the septum. It receives the impulses from the SA node and sends them down the bundles of His and the bundle branches.

atrium One of the upper chambers of the heart.

bundle of His Atrioventricular bundle of impulse-conducting fibers in the myocardium.

cardiac arrest Total cessation of a functional heartbeat.

defibrillator An apparatus used to produce a brief electroshock to the heart through electrodes placed on the chest wall.

dyspnea Difficult or painful breathing.

erythema Redness of the skin caused by congestion of the capillaries in the skin layers.

sinoatrial node (SA node) Pacemaker of the heart located in the right atrium.

ventricle One of the lower chambers of the heart.

vertigo Sensation of rotation or movement; dizziness.

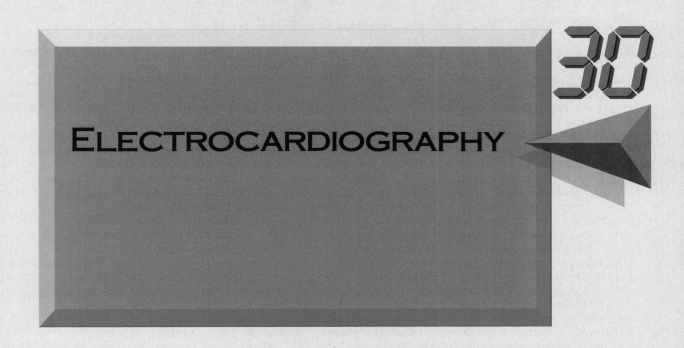

ELECTROCARDIOGRAPHY

30

LEARNING OBJECTIVES

COGNITIVE

Upon successful completion of this chapter you should be able to:

1. Define and spell the terms in the Vocabulary.

2. Trace the electric conduction system through the heart.

3. Match the contractions of the heart with the deflections on the ECG tracing.

4. State the meaning of the horizontal and vertical lines on the ECG paper.

5. List four types of artifacts commonly seen and explain the probable cause for each.

6. List the 12 leads recorded on an ECG; state the electrical activity of each; and identify the coding used for each.

7. State the purpose for using an electrolyte.

8. Discuss the process of standardizing the ECG.

9. Recognize the differences between patient preparation of the basic ECG and the stress test.

10. Describe placement of electrodes for the Holter monitor.

PERFORMANCE

Upon successful completion of this chapter, you should be able to:

1. Prepare the patient for the ECG.

2. Apply ECG electrodes and lead wires.

3. Record a 12-lead ECG tracing.

4. Clean up after the ECG procedure.

5. Mount the ECG tracing.

6. Apply a Holter monitor.

Electrocardiography is frequently used in the diagnosis of heart disease. It is a painless and safe procedure. To perform electrocardiography, cables with electrodes are attached to the patient. The machine, called an *electrocardiograph,* magnifies many times the natural electric currents generated by the action of the heart. A pattern of the heart waves is traced on heat-sensitive graph paper with a balanced tracing pen, or stylus. This tracing, called an *electrocardiogram* (ECG; or, commonly, EKG), is an exact graphic representation of the heart's rhythm and other heart muscle actions. The tracing is then mounted in a predesigned folder for the physician to examine and as a permanent record. In many offices, the medical assistant is responsible for both obtaining and mounting the electrocardiogram.

In order for the recording to depict the true cardiac activity, the medical assistant must have an understanding of normal cardiac function and its relationship to the ECG markings. It is the medical assistant's responsibility to ensure that the patient has been prepared mentally and physically and that the equipment is set up properly. When performing the test, the medical assistant must be able to recognize electric interference and to make needed corrections or adjustments. The validity of the test depends on the accuracy and skill of the technician.

THE HEART'S NATURAL PACEMAKER

The heart is a hollow, muscular organ situated in the chest between the lungs. It weighs approximately 9 ounces and is only a little larger than a fist. Its function is to circulate the blood throughout the body.

The heart is really a double pump. On the right side, one pump receives blood that has just come from the body after delivering nutrients and oxygen to the tissues. The right side pumps deoxygenated blood to the lungs, where the carbon dioxide is exchanged for a fresh supply of oxygen. The pump on the left side of the heart receives this fresh oxygenated blood from the lungs and pumps it out through the aorta, to be distributed to all parts of the body.

The heart is divided into four chambers by partitions. The two upper chambers, called the right **atrium** and left atrium are the receiving chambers. The two lower chambers, called the right **ventricle** and left ventricle, are the pumping chambers. Valves located between each upper and lower chamber open and close to permit the flow of blood in one direction. The tricuspid valve is located between the right atrium and ventricle. The bicuspid, or mitral, valve is located between the left atrium and ventricle. The wall of the heart possesses three layers: the outer epicardium, the middle **myocardium,** and the inner endocardium (Figs. 30–1 and 30–2; Table 30–1).

A sophisticated electric conduction system, controlled by the autonomic nervous system and located in the myocardium, stimulates the heart muscle contractions, which makes blood move through the chambers of the heart and the rest of the body. Each electric impulse moves through the heart muscle in a twisting, spiral motion. These rhythmic waves cause the heart to "beat."

The cardiac impulse originates in specialized muscle tissue called the **sinoatrial (SA) node.** The SA node is located in the right atrium, just at the junction of the superior vena cava and the atrium. This wave spreads in concentric circles over the atrial wall, and the atria contract.

The wave then passes through a second area of specialized muscle tissue between the atrium and the ventricle, called the **atrioventricular (AV) node.** In the AV node, the cardiac impulse moves through a band of cardiac muscle that connects the atria with the ventricles. This band, or collection, of tissue is called the **bundle of His.**

From the bundle of His, the transmission of the cardiac wave continues through a mass of cardiac muscle fibers known as the *Purkinje fibers.* The Purkinje fibers end in the muscles of the ventricles, where the cardiac wave causes the ventricles to contract.

This conduction system is so highly organized that transmission is slightly delayed at the AV node, thus allowing time for the atria to first contract and then empty their contents into the ventricles before the ventricles begin to contract.

The transmission of the cardiac impulse from the SA node to the muscles in the ventricles is called *depolarization.* A period of electric *recovery,* called *repolarization,* then occurs. The heart returns to resting *(polarization),* and the entire cycle begins again. The normal cardiac cycle consists of atrial contraction, ventricular contraction, and then recovery and heart rest. This cycle maintains the normal 70 to 90 beats per minute (BPM) and a normal heart rhythm.

THE CARDIAC CYCLE AND ELECTROCARDIOGRAPHY

The term *cardiac cycle* refers to one complete heartbeat, which consists of depolarization (contraction), repolarization (recovery), and polarization (relaxation). The cardiac impulse can be transferred to a machine that records this natural electric activity. This is the physiologic basis of electrocardiography. The electrocardiogram measures the normal conductive mechanism of the heart muscle and detects any disturbances or disruptions of heart rhythm.

The ECG records a series of waves, or deflections, above or below a baseline. Each deflection corresponds to a particular part of the cardiac cycle (Table 30–1). The normal ECG cycle consists of wave forms that have been arbitrarily labeled the *P* wave, the *Q* wave, the *R* wave, the *S* wave, and the *T* wave. The Q, R, and S waves are frequently iden-

The Cardiac Cycle

On the electrocardiogram, one complete heartbeat is recorded as PQRSTU.

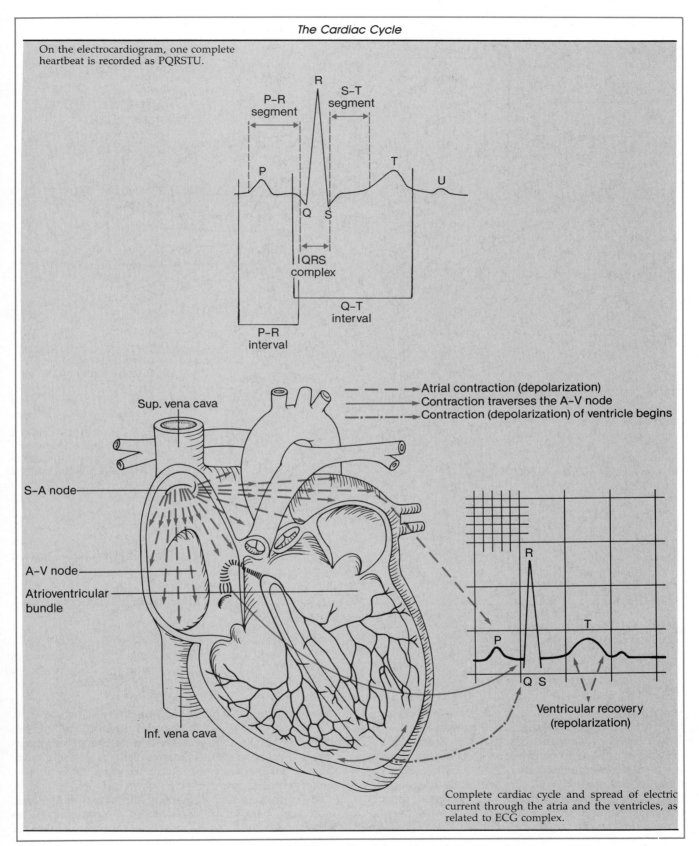

Complete cardiac cycle and spread of electric current through the atria and the ventricles, as related to ECG complex.

FIGURE 30-1. The cardiac cycle.

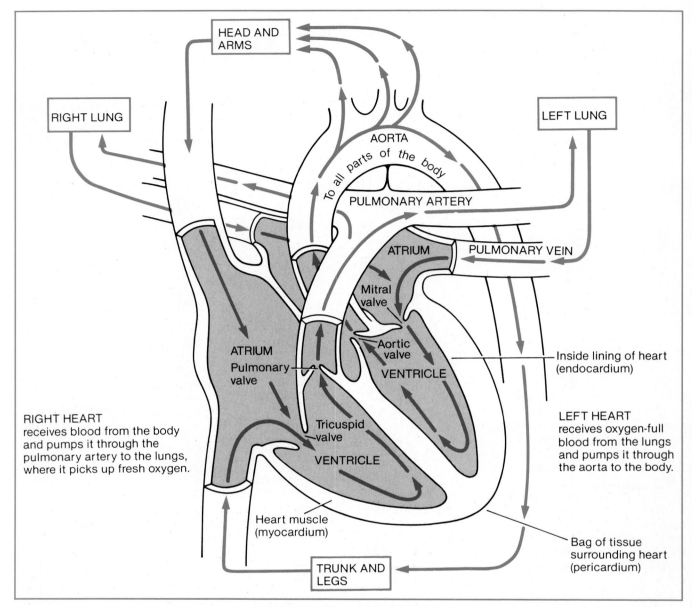

FIGURE 30–2. The heart and its function.

tified as the *QRS complex*. The *P wave* reflects contraction of the atria (beginning depolarization). The *P-R interval* reflects the time it takes from the beginning of the atrial contraction to the beginning of the ventricular contraction. The *QRS complex* reflects the contraction of the ventricles (depolarization of both ventricles). The *S-T segment* reflects the time interval from the end of the ventricular contraction to the beginning of ventricular recovery. The *T wave* reflects ventricular recovery (repolarization of the ventricles). After the T wave, there is a period of heart rest (polarization), and the tracing shows a straight line, indicating the resting state of the heart. This flat horizontal line is called the *baseline*. Occasionally, after the T wave, another small *U wave* is seen. It may appear in patients who have a low serum potassium level and other metabolic disturbances.

By observing and measuring the actual configuration and location of each wave in relation to the other waves and to the baseline, as well as the intervals and segments, the physician is able to detect rhythmic disturbances of the heart and to distinguish different types of cardiac disorders.

TABLE 30-1. THE CARDIAC CYCLE

Stage	Heart Activity	Electric Current
P wave*	Atrial contraction	Atrial depolarization
P-R segment†	Contraction traversing the A-V node	Depolarization traversing the A-V node
QRS complex‡	Ventricular contraction	Ventricular depolarization
S-T segment	Time interval between ventricular contraction and the beginning of ventricular recovery	Time interval between ventricular depolarization and ventricular repolarization
T-wave	Ventricular contraction subsides	Ventricular repolarization (electric recovery)
U wave (not always present)	Associated with further ventricular relaxation	Associated with further ventricular repolarization
Baseline§	The heart at rest	Polarization
P-R interval‖	Time interval between atrial contraction and ventricular contraction	Time interval between atrial depolarization and ventricular depolarization
Q-T interval	Time interval between the beginning of ventricular contraction and the subsiding of ventricular contraction	Time interval between the beginning of ventricular depolarization and ventricular repolarization (electric recovery)

* Wave—a uniformly advancing deflection (upward or downward) from a baseline on a recording.
† Segment—a portion of an ECG recording between two consecutive waves. Represents the time needed for an electric current to move on.
‡ Complex—the portion of the ECG tracing that represents the sum of three waves (contraction of the ventricles).
§ Interval—the lapse of time between two different ECG events.
‖ Baseline—a neutral line against which waves are valued as they deflect upward (positive) or downward (negative) from the line.

THE ELECTROCARDIOGRAM

Electrocardiograph Paper

Electrocardiograph paper is heat-sensitive and pressure-sensitive. The recording or writing device of the electrocardiograph is called a *stylus*. When the machine is on, the heated stylus moves along a horizontal line and burns the paper. Since the paper is also pressure-sensitive, it must be handled carefully to avoid any markings that would blemish the tracing.

Electrocardiograph paper is graph paper with internationally accepted increments for measuring the cardiac cycle (Table 30-2). These universal measurements allow physicians anywhere, anytime to interpret the significance of each person's ECG in the same manner. The medical assistant needs to know the size and the meaning of each square to understand its significance.

Each small square measures 1 mm by 1 mm. Every fifth line (both vertical and horizontal) is darker than the other lines and defines a square measuring 5 mm by 5 mm. As the electrocardiograph paper advances, the stylus moves along one horizontal line and intersects with a vertical line every 0.04 second. Therefore, every fifth line intersected represents 0.2 second (0.04 second per line × 5 lines = 0.2 second) in time. Routinely, the electrocardiograph paper advances at a speed of 25 mm per second (5 lines per 0.2 second = 25 lines per second). In 1 minute, the paper advances 300 5-mm increments (Fig. 30-3).

Electrodes and Electrolytes

Metal *electrodes* are placed on the patient's limbs and chest to pick up the electric activity of the heart. The cardiac impulses are transmitted to the electrocardiograph by metal tips and wires that are attached to the electrodes (Fig. 30-4). The standard 12-lead electrocardiograph has five electrodes. Two electrodes are attached to the fleshy part of the arms and two to the fleshy part of the legs. The fifth electrode is moved to six different positions on the chest (Fig. 30-5).

The cardiac impulses travel from the metal electrodes and wires to an amplifier, where they are magnified (Fig. 30-6). The magnified impulses are then converted into mechanical action by a *galvanometer* and are recorded on the electrocardiograph paper by the stylus.

The skin is a poor conductor of electricity. To aid in the conduction of this electric current, an *electro-*

TABLE 30-2. THE STANDARD MARKING CODES

	Electrodes Connected	Marking Code
Standard or Bipolar Limb Leads		
Lead 1	LA and RA	·
Lead 2	LL and RA	· ·
Lead 3	LL and LA	· · ·
Augmented Unipolar Limb Leads		
AVR	RA and (LA-LL)	—
AVL	LA and (RA-LL)	— —
AVF	LL and (RA-LA)	— — —
Chest or Precordial Leads		
V	C and (LA-RA-LL)	V1 — ·
		V2 — · ·
		V3 — · · ·
		V4 — · · · ·
		V5 — · · · · ·
		V6 — · · · · · ·

(Courtesy of Burdick, Inc., Schaumberg, IL.)

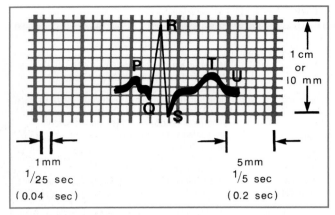

FIGURE 30-3. Measurements of squares on the ECG paper.

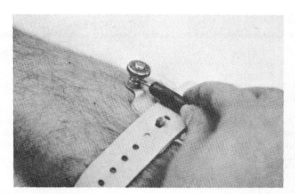

FIGURE 30-4. Electrode hook-up on a patient's leg. (From *Electrocardiography: A Better Way*, Burdick, Inc., Schaumberg, IL.)

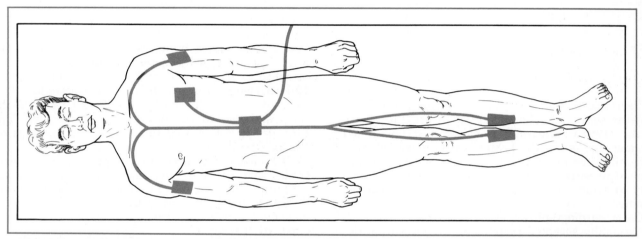

FIGURE 30-5. Standard placing of the limb leads and chest leads for the running of the limb lead tracings and augmented voltage lead tracings.

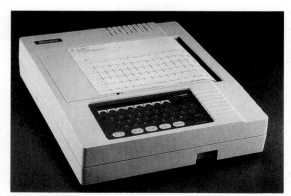

FIGURE 30-6. Electrocardiograph. (Courtesy of Burdick, Inc., Schaumberg, IL.)

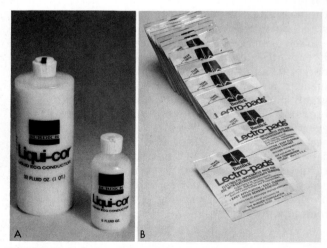

FIGURE 30-7. Forms of electrolytes. *A*, Electrolyte paste. *B*, Presaturated electrolyte pads. These pads are often preferred because they are not as messy and because they ensure that identical amounts of electrolyte are at each electrode while eliminating the need for prepping swabs. (Courtesy of Burdick, Inc., Schaumberg, IL.)

lyte is applied to each electrode. Electrolyte products are available in the form of pastes, gels, or pads saturated with electrolyte solution (Fig. 30–7).

Leads

The standard ECG consists of 12 separate *leads,* or recordings, of the electric activity of the heart, from different angles. Each lead must be marked, or coded, for the physician to know the angle recorded. Machines automatically mark the 12 leads as the *lead selector switch* is turned. However, there may be times when the assistant will be required to mark or code each lead manually. A certain coding system is used to identify each lead recorded. Codes consist of a series of dots and dashes. One standard marking code is illustrated in Table 30–2.

Standard, or Bipolar, Leads

The first three leads recorded are called the standard, or *bipolar,* leads. They are referred to as bipolar because they each use two limb electrodes to record the electric activity. Roman numerals are used to designate these leads (Fig. 30–8).

- Lead I records the electric activity between the right arm and the left arm.
- Lead II records the electric activity between the right arm and the left leg.
- Lead III records the electric activity between the left arm and the left leg.

TRACING AN ERROR IN PLACEMENT OF THE BIPOLAR LIMB LEADS

- If there is interference in limb leads I and II, check the electrode connection on the patient's right arm.
- If there is interference in limb leads I and III, check the electrode connection on the patient's left arm.
- If there is interference in limb leads II and III, check the electrode connection on the patient's left leg.

Augmented Leads

The next three leads recorded are the augmented leads. They are AVR, AVL, and AVF. The AV

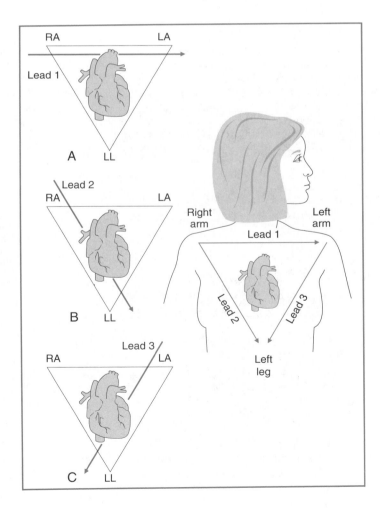

FIGURE 30–8. The standard limb leads record the electric activity of the heart from three angles. *A,* Limb lead I. The angle recording the heart's voltage between the right arm and the left arm. *B,* Limb lead II. The angle recording the heart's voltage between the right arm and the left leg. *C,* Limb lead III. The angle recording the heart's voltage between the left arm and the left leg.

stands for augmented voltage, the R for right arm, the L for left arm, and the F for foot. These leads are unipolar.

- *Lead AVR* records the electric activity from the midpoint between the left arm and the left leg to the right arm (Fig. 30–9*A*).
- *Lead AVL* records the electric activity from the midpoint between the right arm and the left leg to the left arm (Fig. 30–9*B*).
- *Lead AVF* records the electric activity from the midpoint between the right arm and the left arm to the left leg (Fig. 30–9*C*).

Chest, or Precordial, Leads

The last six leads are the chest, or *precordial,* leads. These leads are unipolar and are designated as V1, V2, V3, V4, V5, and V6. Each number signifies the position of the electrode on the chest (Fig. 30–10). Leads V1 through V6 record the electric activity between six points on the chest wall and a point within the heart.

Standardization

Standardization has been determined by an international agreement to ensure that an ECG can be interpreted anywhere in the world. It assumes that the electrocardiograph used has been calibrated according to universal measurements. Before recording a patient's tracing, you must make certain that the machine is correctly standardized.

When a machine is "in standard" (1 STD), 1 millivolt (mV) of electricity causes the stylus to move vertically 10 mm. Thus, it is possible to calculate electric voltages by the vertical movement of the stylus on the paper. The stylus should deflect exactly 10 mm when the *standardization button* is depressed with a quick pecking motion. The standardization should be 2 mm wide and rectangular in shape. Each manufacturer's manual explains the method of adjustment to obtain a perfect standardization.

Most machines have three standard (STD) positions that may be used. They are 1/2 STD, 1 STD,

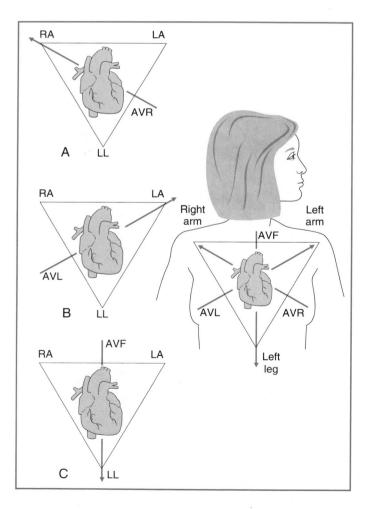

FIGURE 30–9. The augmented leads. When two leads are joined together, the machine "thinks" it is recording halfway between the electrodes, thus giving a picture of the heart. *A, AVR* is the recording made from the midpoint between *LA* and *LL* to *RA. B, AVL* is the recording made from the midpoint between *RA* and *LL* to *LA. C, AVF* is the recording made from the midpoint between *RA* and *LA* to *LL.*

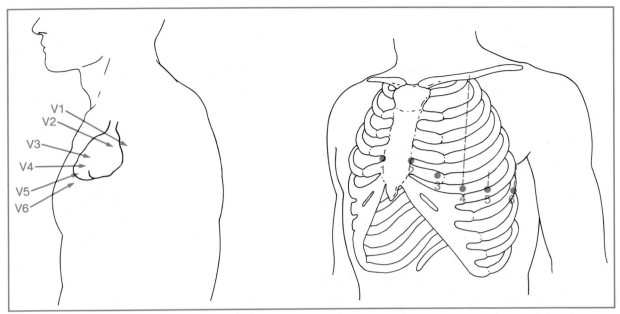

FIGURE 30-10. *A,* Chest leads. The chest leads record an additional six views of the heart. From the total of 12 recordings that make up an ECG series—three standard, three augmented, and six chest leads—the physician is able to determine much about the status of the heart. *B,* The anatomic placement for each individual chest electrode: *V1,* fourth intercostal space at right margin of sternum; *V2,* fourth intercostal space at left margin of sternum; *V3,* midway between position *2* and position *4; V4,* fifth intercostal space at junction of left midclavicular line; *V5,* at horizontal level of position *4* at left anterior axillary line; *V6,* at horizontal level of position *4* at left midaxillary line.

and 2 STD. When recording 1/2 STD, 1 mV causes the stylus to deflect 5 mm. If the amplitude (height) of the QRS complex is too high and is causing the stylus to move off the paper, the machine should be put on 1/2 STD. If the amplitude of the QRS complex is too small, the machine should be put on 2 STD, causing the stylus to deflect 20 mm. Figure 30-11 shows the three standard positions. Make note of any variation from the normal 1 STD. Standardization is usually performed at the beginning of the first lead recording, although some physicians require a standardization within each of the 12 lead recordings.

As mentioned, the universal standard for recording an electrocardiogram is at a speed of 25 mm per second. If the patient's heart rate is very rapid or if certain parts of the complex are too close together, it may be necessary to adjust the paper run to 50 mm per second. This will double the speed of the paper run and extend the recording to twice its normal length (Fig. 30-12). Again, make certain that this is noted on the tracing.

FIGURE 30-11. Sensitivity control. *A,* Correct standardization of 1 cm (10 mm). *B,* One half is at half sensitivity of 0.5 cm (5 mm). *C,* Two is double the sensitivity of 2 cm (20 mm). (From Bonewit, K.: *Clinical Procedures for Medical Assistants,* 3rd ed., Philadelphia, W. B. Saunders Co., 1990, p 446.)

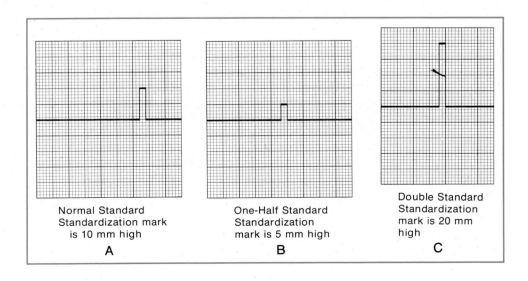

Normal Standard
Standardization mark
is 10 mm high

A

One-Half Standard
Standardization
mark is 5 mm high

B

Double Standard
Standardization
mark is 20 mm
high

C

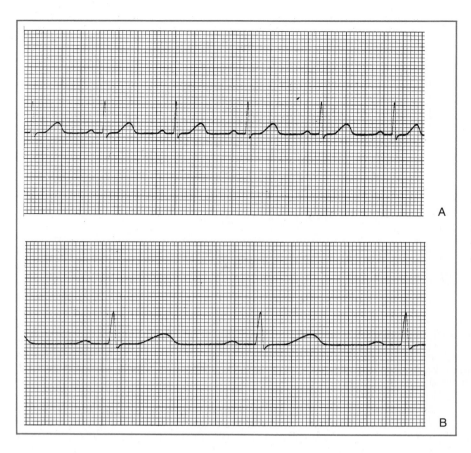

FIGURE 30–12. Paper run. *A*, Run 25 is normal speed for recording, 25 mm per second. *B*, Run 50 mm per second. It is used when the heart rate is very rapid and the complexes are too close together. This extends the complexes twice as far apart.

Artifacts

An artifact is unwanted movement of the stylus on the paper produced by outside electric interference. The electrocardiograph is extremely sensitive to any kind of electric activity. Artifacts on the tracing make the interpretation of the recording difficult. The medical assistant should have a thorough understanding of the causes of, and remedies for, these artifacts. The types of artifacts include wandering baseline, somatic tremor, alternating current, and baseline interruption.

Wandering Baseline

This artifact is a gradual shifting of the stylus away from the center of the paper, usually resulting from unnoticed movement of the patient (Fig. 30–13). If this occurs, remind the patient to remain still. Other causes include electrodes that are corroded or dirty or have been applied too loosely or too tightly; tension on the electrode from a dangling cable; poor-quality electrolyte paste, or too little applied to the electrode; and improper preparation of the patient's skin prior to applying the electrolyte.

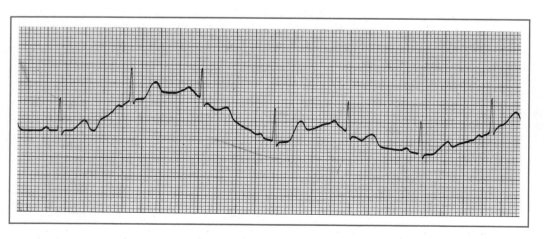

FIGURE 30–13. Wandering baseline. (Courtesy of Burdick, Inc., Schaumberg, IL.)

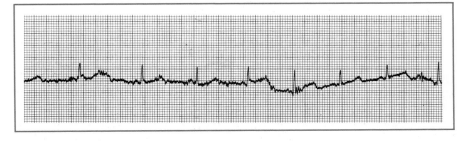

FIGURE 30-14. Somatic tremor. (Courtesy of Burdick, Inc., Schaumberg, IL.)

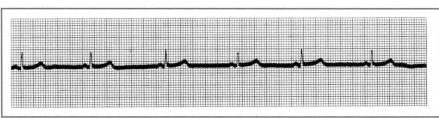

FIGURE 30-15. AC interference. (Courtesy of Burdick, Inc., Schaumberg, IL.)

Somatic Tremor

Somatic tremor means "muscle movement." Natural electric voltage from muscle movement causes additional stylus movement across the paper. This results in a recording with jagged peaks of irregular height and spacing, and a shifting baseline (Fig. 30-14). Usually, this is because the patient is uncomfortable, apprehensive, moving or talking, or suffering from a disorder that causes body tremors. Explaining the procedure beforehand alleviates apprehension and relaxes the patient. Reposition the patient comfortably, or offer the patient a pillow. Sometimes it helps to place the patient's hands under the buttocks or to ask the patient to take slow, deep breaths. Chills cause somatic tremor; check the room temperature. The physician may prescribe a sedative for the patient who is having great difficulty in relaxing.

Alternating Current

Commonly known as alternating current (AC) interference, this artifact appears as a series of uniform, small spiked lines on the paper (Fig. 30-15). Alternating current present in nearby equipment or wires can radiate small amounts of energy into the room where the ECG is being performed. Some of this energy can be detected by the sensitive electro-cardiograph. Unplug other electric appliances in the room. Move the patient table to another area of the room, or turn the table around. Move the table away from the wall, since the interference may be in the electric wiring in the wall or in an adjoining room. Make certain that your patient is not touching anything off the patient table. If necessary, turn off the overhead fluorescent lights.

If none of these procedures eliminates the AC interference, check the machine for proper grounding. You may need to use an external ground wire provided with the machine. Be certain to follow the manufacturer's directions. Check to see that the lead wires are not crossed. Also check that the electrodes are clean.

Baseline Interruption

Baseline interruption occurs when the electric connection has been interrupted. The stylus moves onto the margin of the paper (Fig. 30-16). The stylus moves violently up and down, or it may record a straight line across the top or the bottom of the paper. Most baseline interruption is caused by noticeable patient movement jarring the electrodes. Other causes can be a broken wire in the patient cable or cable tips that are attached too loosely to the electrodes.

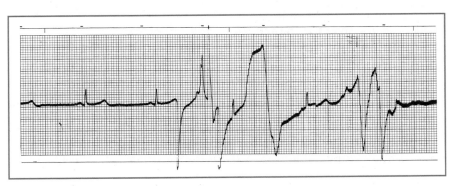

FIGURE 30-16. Baseline interruption. (Courtesy of Burdick, Inc., Schaumberg, IL.)

OBTAINING THE ELECTROCARDIOGRAM

Preparing the Room and the Patient

The room should be free from interruptions, and the machine should be as far away from other electric equipment as possible. This includes x-ray machines, diathermy equipment, centrifuges, electric fans, refrigerators, and air conditioners. The room should be quiet and warm.

The treatment table should be comfortable and wide enough to avoid muscle movement. The table should be wood or have some form of insulation between metal legs or surfaces. It is best to position the table so that you are working from the patient's left side.

Small pillows are helpful in relaxing the patient. One pillow may be used under the patient's head, but it should not be pressing down on or elevating the patient's shoulders. A small pillow placed under the patient's knees may also help relax the muscles of the abdomen and the lower extremities.

The patient should be supine, with arms at the sides, and the legs not touching one another. If this is not possible, the patient may be placed in a semi-Fowler position or may be seated on a wooden chair. In the sitting position, the patient's feet should be on the floor on a rubber mat or on a wooden footstool or a stack of books. The legs must not hang free, nor should there be any pressure on the back of the lower thighs. If the patient is in a sitting or semi-Fowler position, note this on the patient's recording.

The patient should disrobe to the waist, and the lower legs should be exposed. A patient gown should be put on, with the opening in the front. Shoes and nylons must be removed. Loosen all tight clothing.

It is advisable to have the patient rest for at least 10 minutes prior to the recording. Check to determine whether the patient was able to follow the instructions given (Fig. 30–17). Note on the patient's record any medications taken.

Explain to the patient the nature and purpose of the electrocardiogram. Chat with the patient while preparing for the procedure. Stress the importance of not moving during the entire procedure, and assure the patient that no electric shock will be felt. (When you tell patients to lie still, make sure that their breathing remains normal. Frequently, when you tell patients to lie still they tend to hold their breath.) Allow time for the patient to ask questions or to express any concerns before you begin the tracing.

Applying the Electrodes and Lead Wires

Before beginning, turn the power switch on to allow the machine to warm up. Expose the patient's arms and legs. Attach an electrode strap to each electrode, then place a small amount of electrolyte or an electrolyte pad on each electrode. Make certain that you have the same amount on each electrode. With the electrode, rub the electrolyte into the skin on the fleshy part of the arms and legs. Rub the skin's surface until a slight **erythema** appears. Wipe off any excess electrolyte. Do not allow your hands to carry the electrolyte from the patient to the equipment. Unequal amounts of electrolyte or the spreading of it to the wires and equipment may cause artifacts.

Position the electrodes with the lead connectors pointing toward the hands and the feet. Place the electrodes on the prepared skin areas. Place each strap around the limb until the hole just meets the hook. Then move the strap one hole tighter, and fasten it. This should provide the correct tension. An accurate tracing cannot be made if the straps are too loose or too tight.

Place the disc-shaped chest electrode in the first chest lead position (V1). It will be moved to the other chest points, one lead at a time, during the procedure. A *Welch electrode* is bulb-shaped and may be used for the chest leads. Many multichanneled ECGs use Welch electrodes, which are all connected at the same time. Locate each of the chest lead sites. Squeeze a dab of electrolyte on each electrode site and pinch the bulb slightly. Take care that the bulbs do not touch each other.

Insert the tips of the lead cords into the lead connector holes of the leg and arm electrodes. Check to make certain that you have connected the correct lead terminal into the corresponding electrode. Say out loud what you are doing, for example, "right arm electrode into right arm terminal." The lead cords are color-coded, but it is still easy to confuse the patient's right and left sides. Make sure all wires lie on the patient's body because this will reduce interference and prevent drag on the cable, which can cause an improper electrode connection. Check that each lead cord terminal is tight. Plug the patient cable into the patient cable jack on the machine, making certain that it is pushed in all the way.

Recording the Electrocardiogram

You are now ready to record the patient's electrocardiogram.

Limb Leads

Check the manufacturer's instructions for the specific amount of warm-up time needed. Set the *lead selector control* to STD. Turn the *recorder control* to ON and then to RUN. Using the *position control knob*, center the *stylus* on the baseline. Check the standardization by pressing the *standardization button* to a height of 10 mm.

INSTRUCTIONS FOR PATIENT BEFORE TAKING AN ELECTROCARDIOGRAM

Name: _____

Your cardiogram appointment is _____, _____ at _____ AM / PM
                                  Day   Date   Time

These instructions are simple, but it is important that you follow them. Please call us if you are unable to follow these instructions or keep your appointment so we may make another appointment.

1. There is no discomfort or sensation in taking an electrocardiogram. No electricity is put into the patient in any way. Small metal plates are placed on the calf of each leg and on each arm and at different places on the chest. The minute impulse generated by your heart is simply picked up by these plates and recorded by the machine.

2. You will be asked to lie down on a comfortable table while the test is being performed by the technician.

3. For your convenience, it is best to wear loose clothing. You will be asked to disrobe to your waist to expose the chest. It will also be necessary to expose your lower legs from the knees down and the upper arms just below the shoulders.

4. The actual test only takes about 5 minutes, but you will be asked to rest for about one-half hour before the test. It is best you do not have a heavy meal for about 2 hours before the test. You should not consume any cold drinks or ice cream or smoke just before the test. It is also advisable to refrain from excessive exercise just prior to the test. Do not take any medications without the physician's usual instructions and knowledge.

5. During the test, you will be asked to lie absolutely still and relax, as the slightest movement interferes with an accurate tracing. Do not talk.

6. The skin on the legs, arms, and chest must be free from skin ointments, oils, and medications.

7. The technician taking the test is specially trained to perform the test but is unable to tell you the results of the test, as he or she is neither trained nor authorized to make any interpretations of the cardiogram. This is the task of the physician.

FIGURE 30-17. Example of an instruction sheet that is given to the patient at the time the appointment is made for an ECG.

After obtaining a proper standardization, turn the *lead selector control* to *lead I*. Code the lead immediately unless the machine does so automatically. Run 8 to 12 inches of the tracing. Switch to *lead II* and *lead III,* and repeat the same steps. Run 4 to 6 inches of *AVR, AVL,* and *AVF.* Turn the machine to OFF while preparing to record the chest leads (see Fig. 30–5).

Chest Leads

Locate and apply the electrolyte over the six chest locations on the patient. The run begins with the chest electrode over the chest lead V1. Turn the *lead selector control* to either *V* or *V1,* depending on the machine, and the *recorder switch* to RUN. Run 4 to 6 inches of recording. Standardize and code the lead. Turn the *recorder switch* to OFF; this prevents excessive movement of the stylus. Move the chest electrode to V2, V3, V4, V5, and V6, repeating the steps. Having completed all chest leads, slowly turn the *lead selector control* back to *STD,* one lead at a

time, to avoid possible stripping of the gears in the dial. Run a straight baseline, and turn the *recorder switch* to OFF. Unplug the machine.

MULTIPLE-CHANNEL ELECTROCARDIOGRAPH

An electrocardiograph with a three-channel or six-channel capability can simultaneously record three or six different leads. For these machines, there are six chest electrodes and all are placed into position before the test is run. Once started, some machines run through all 12 leads automatically and mark each lead with its identifying letters instead of the dot-dash coding seen on the single-channel tracing. These tracings are shorter when they are produced and need no special mounting when placed into the patient's chart. Figure 30–18 shows an example of a three-channel ECG recording.

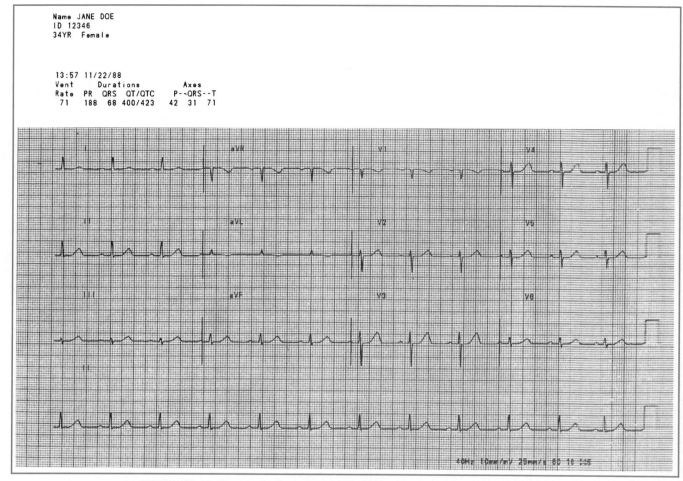

Name JANE DOE
ID 12346
34YR Female

13:57 11/22/88
Vent   Durations   Axes
Rate PR QRS QT/QTC   P--QRS--T
71   188 68 400/423   42 31 71

FIGURE 30-18. Example of a three-channel ECG. (Courtesy of Burdick, Inc., Schaumberg, IL.)

AUTOMATIC LEAD CONTROL SWITCH

Both single-channel and multiple-channel electrocardiographs may be equipped with automatic sequencing ability. This connects the correct electrode combinations without having to advance a control. In the single-channel machine, the 12 leads automatically record one at a time until all 12 are recorded; in the multichannel machines, three or six leads record one at a time until all leads have been recorded. A standardization mark is also automatically recorded on the tracing. Most of these machines also have a manual recording capability that can be used when longer tracings are required for interpretations. If the machine has a "copy" capability, it can produce an accurate copy of the last ECG recorded.

TELEPHONE TRANSMISSION

An electrocardiograph with telephone transmission capabilities can transmit a recording over the telephone line to an ECG data interpretation center.

The machine is equipped with a connector well in which a telephone headset is placed. The recording is interpreted by a computer at the data center, and a printout with the computer-assisted interpretations is mailed back to the sender by return mail. Patient information that may be important to the interpretation, such as age, sex, height, weight, blood pressure, and medications, may also be relayed either verbally or by computer to the center.

INTERPRETIVE ELECTROCARDIOGRAPHS

Interpretive electrocardiographs are equipped with a built-in computer, which analyzes the recording as it is being run. With this capability, immediate information on the heart's activity is available and can help in earlier diagnosis and treatment. It is necessary to enter patient baseline data into the computer *before* the tracing is taken. The computer analysis of the ECG and the reason for each interpretation is printed out on the top of the recording.

POST-TEST PROCEDURES

Equipment Maintenance

Tear off the tracing from the machine. Immediately label the tracing with the patient's name, the date, and your initials. Roll the tracing loosely with the recording on the inside, and secure with a small rubber band. Do not roll tightly, and do not attach the paper clip over any part of the tracing. Tracings scratch easily and should be carefully handled. Set the tracing aside.

Remove the tips of the lead wires from the electrodes, unfasten the rubber straps, and remove the electrodes from the patient. Clean the electrode sites with a warm, wet paper towel, and dry. Assist the patient to a sitting position, but let the patient remain on the table for a few moments. After the patient rests, assist the patient off the table and with dressing, if needed. Change the table paper, and discard any used disposable materials.

Clean the rubber straps with a mild detergent, and dry them. The electrodes must be cleaned with a mild detergent first, then polished with a fine grade of scouring powder. Do not use steel wool or any metal-base polish because it will interfere with the tracing and cause artifacts. Always rinse the electrodes well and let them dry before storing them. Use an applicator to clean the connecting holes and the inside of the suction-type chest electrode.

Mounting an Electrocardiogram

Today, there are many different types of mounts. An office should select the mount that is best adapted to its needs. It is advisable to select a mount that can be easily read in its entirety on one surface. Because tracings are usually a series of records over a period of years, a mount that will last with the passing of time should be selected.

The slotted-type folder best protects the tracings. It can be mounted on one surface and has a longer limb lead, but it is more expensive and takes more filing space. The slotted-folder also takes longer to mount than some of the other styles.

Paper clips and staples should not be used, because they will scratch a tracing. Clear tape can be used, but some tape becomes sticky or yellow with time. Copy machines can be used to make a single-sheet copy of the tracing without damaging the original record. Photocopies take up less filing space.

Regardless of the style of mount used, each ECG should be neatly and carefully mounted, with complete information recorded on each one. The following information must appear on the mount:

- Patient's full name
- Sex
- Age
- Date of ECG
- Medications
- Variation from normal STD and variation from a machine speed of 25 mm per second

A notation should be made of any variation from the routine, such as a very nervous patient, a different position of the patient, lack of rest before the test, or smoking immediately before the test. If the lead placements were different from the routine, this also should be noted.

Extreme care should be taken when mounting. Do not allow your desk to become cluttered with tracing trimmings. Discard the trimmings into a waste container as you trim them off. Most tracings are easily scratched, so be careful not to damage the tracing with finger rings or sleeve buttons. Do not stack other items on top of the open-faced type of mount.

Do not cut off the lead coding until you are ready to mount that particular lead. Double-check each lead code with the mount placement. Some mounts place the precordial leads horizontally, whereas others place them vertically. Take great care not to mount a lead upside down. If you have been requested to show the STD in a lead, be careful not to cut it off. Do not cover the tips of the QRS complexes with the sides of the slotted-type mount. Place the mounted ECG tracing on the physician's desk for evaluation with the patient's medical record and any previous ECG tracings.

OBTAINING A 12-LEAD ELECTROCARDIOGRAM

The procedure for running a 12-lead ECG is based on the conventional single-channel electrocardiograph that uses one chest electrode. The type of equipment may vary from office to office, but the basic techniques of patient preparation, placement of the limb and chest leads, attachment of the lead wires, and elimination of the artifacts remain the same. The medical assistant should be able to operate different types of ECG equipment with the knowledge of the basic unit.

Interpretation of the Electrocardiogram

Two important heart functions that can be determined by the physician when interpreting the electrocardiogram are heart rate and heart rhythm.

Heart Rate

On the ECG tracing, all heartbeats consist of P waves, QRS complexes, and T waves. It is possible to calculate heart rate by counting the number of 5-mm boxes between two R waves. Divide this number into 300. Your answer will be the BPM.

PROCEDURE 30-1   OBTAINING A 12-LEAD ELECTROCARDIOGRAM

GOAL   To prepare the patient, correctly obtain the tracing, and properly mount the results.

EQUIPMENT AND SUPPLIES

Electrocardiograph with paper inserted   Drape sheet
Electrodes   Patient cable
Electrolyte   Chest lead strap
Patient gown

PROCEDURAL STEPS

1. Wash hands.

2. Explain procedure to the patient.
    Purpose: To gain patient cooperation and alleviate apprehension.

3. Ask patient to disrobe from the waist up and to remove shoes and stockings.

4. Position patient on ECG table and drape properly.
    Purpose: To ensure the safety, modesty, and comfort of the patient.

5. Turn on the machine to warm stylus.

6. Work on the patient's left side with power cord running away from the patient.
    Purpose: These precautions help reduce AC interference.

7. Attach the rubber straps to the electrodes and prepare the skin with an electrolyte using equal amounts at each site (Figs. 30–19 and 30–20).
    Purpose: Unequal amounts of electrolyte can cause a wandering baseline.

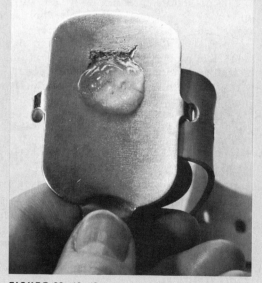

FIGURE 30–19. (Courtesy of Burdick, Inc., Schaumberg, IL.)

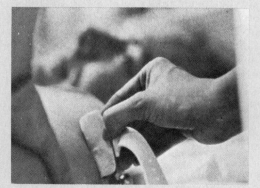

FIGURE 30–20. (From Bonewit, K.: *Clinical Procedures for Medical Assistants*, 3rd ed., Philadelphia, W.B. Saunders Co., 1990, p 459.)

Continued

8. Place the electrode on the fleshiest portion of the upper arms and lower legs. Keep lead connections pointing toward the fingers and toes (Figs. 30–21 and 30–22).
   Purpose: Placing the electrodes on the fleshiest parts of the upper arms and lower legs minimizes chances for somatic tremors.

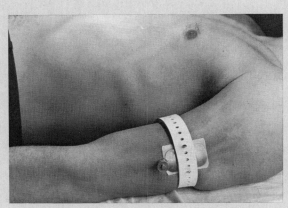

FIGURE 30–21. (Courtesy of Burdick, Inc., Schaumberg, IL.)

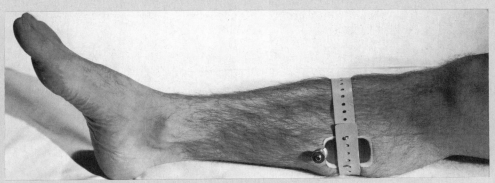

FIGURE 30–22. (Courtesy of Burdick, Inc., Schaumberg, IL.)

9. Wrap a rubber strap around each limb until the hole in the strap just meets the hook. Then, stretch the strap one hole tighter, and fasten it (Fig. 30–23).
   Purpose: Electrodes that are too tight or too loose could result in artifacts.

10. Apply the electrolyte to the chest electrode and place it in the first chest lead position (Fig. 30–24).

11. Adjust the chest strap (if a flat chest electrode is used) so the strap weight rests near the right anterior axillary line. Place its plastic anchor plate under the patient's chest at the level of V4, V5, and V6. The free end of the strap should be placed across the patient's chest while holding the electrode in proper position (Fig. 30–25).

12. Attach the lead wires of the patient cable to the electrodes.

13. Double-check all electrodes and cables for proper placement and connection. Make sure that the lead cable loosely follows the contour of the patient's body (Fig. 30–26).
    Purpose: Large cable loops or cable drag causes AC artifacts or a wandering baseline.

Continued

PROCEDURE 30-1 *Continued*

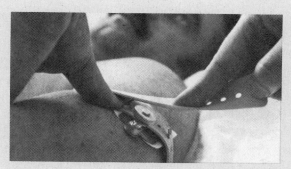

FIGURE 30-23. (From Bonewit, K.: *Clinical Procedures for Medical Assistants,* 3rd ed., Philadelphia, W. B. Saunders Co., 1990, p 459.)

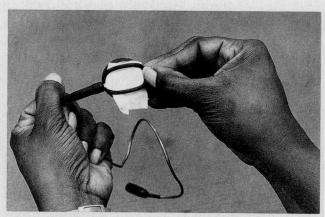

FIGURE 30-24.

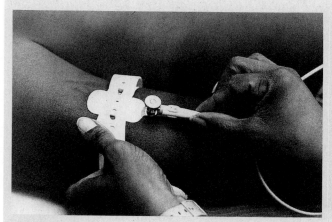

FIGURE 30-25.

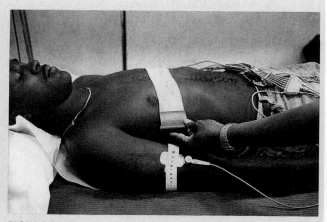

FIGURE 30-26.

14. Set the lead selector to STD and the recorder switch to ON.

15. Turn the recorder switch to RUN 25 and center the baseline.

16. Depress the standard button and note if standardization deflection is 10 mm.
    Purpose: The universal standard of ECG measurement is ensured.

17. Run leads I, II, III, AVR, AVL, and AVF. Run a 5- to 10-inch strip of each lead. Correct any artifacts. If the machine does not have automatic coding, code the beginning of each lead with the dot-dash coding system.

18. Turn machine to OFF.

19. Check the position of the chest lead for V1 running.
    Purpose: Turning off machine while placing electrode in proper position for chest lead tracings prevents stylus from thrashing about.

20. Turn selector switch to RUN 25 and record tracing. Turn machine to OFF.

21. Move the chest electrode to the next position and repeat the previous step.

Continued

22. Turn the selector switch to STD and run out until only a baseline appears. Turn the machine to OFF.

23. Remove all sensors and clean skin with a soft cloth.
    Purpose: To prevent skin irritation.

24. Assist patient from the table and to the dressing area.

25. Clean and dry electrodes and straps.

26. Return equipment and room to its original condition.

27. Mount ECG tracing using the mounting supplies that are made for the equipment you are using.

28. Enter "test taken" notation on the patient's medical record and initial the entry.

Heart Rhythm

Heart rhythm is determined to be either regular or irregular. The horizontal distance between the P waves is measured first. If the distance is the same, atrial rhythm is regular, and if not, it is irregular. Next, measure the horizontal distance between the R waves. If the distance is the same, ventricular rhythm is regular, and if not, it is irregular.

CARDIAC STRESS TESTING

Cardiac stress testing is conducted to observe and record the patient's cardiovascular response to measured exercise challenges. Stress testing is performed to diagnose cardiac disease that cannot be detected by the standard resting ECG, to determine an individual's energy performance capacity, or to prescribe a specially designed exercise plan. The stress test is done while the patient is exercising on either a bicycle or a treadmill and under careful supervision.

After you have carefully recorded a patient's history, inform the patient of the details of the procedure. The purpose of the test is to increase physical exertion until a *target heart rate* is reached or signs of deficiency of blood supply to the heart appear. The patient must read and sign a consent form. Some offices publish information booklets for their patients (Fig. 30–27).

The chest electrodes are placed on the patient and are connected to the cable wires. One team member demonstrates how to walk on the treadmill. The patient's blood pressure and heart rate are recorded before the test begins. The treadmill is turned on, and a continuous ECG is run during the exercise (Fig. 30–28). The patient's blood pressure and heart rate are also monitored. Immediately after the ter-

mination of the test, the blood pressure and heart rate are again recorded. A post-resting ECG is then run on the monitor for 5 minutes before the patient is discharged.

Stress testing can cause **cardiac arrest.** The medical assistant must be able to recognize symptoms of **dyspnea, vertigo,** extreme fatigue, severe **arrhythmia,** and other abnormal ECG readings that may develop during the stress test or during the rest period immediately following the exercise.

All members of a cardiac stress testing team must be trained in cardiopulmonary resuscitation and must be prepared to terminate testing immediately if the patient is unable to continue or when abnormalities appear on the monitor. It is imperative that the physician be present during this procedure. Besides the monitoring equipment, oxygen, a **defibrillator,** and emergency cardiac medications must be available in case of cardiac crisis.

The medical assistant must receive additional schooling before preforming the following tests. Be sure to check with your state scope of practice regarding requirements in your area.

VECTORCARDIOGRAPHY

The vectorcardiograph portrays graphically, by elliptical curves called *vector loops,* the direction and strength of the electric forces during the heartbeat. The machine projects these loops onto an oscilloscope screen, and photographs are taken of the projections for the patient's permanent record.

ECHOCARDIOGRAPHY

Echocardiography makes use of ultrasound to measure the structure and movement of the various

Cardiac Stress Test

Cardiac stress testing (also known as an exercise tolerance test or treadmill test) is a means of observing, evaluating, and recording your heart's response during a measured exercise test. This test determines your capacity to adapt to physical stress.

There are various reasons that your physician may suggest this test for you:

1. To aid in determining the presence of suspected coronary heart disease.
2. To aid in the selection of therapy.
   a. For angina pectoris (tightness or pain in the chest).
   b. Following a myocardial infarction (heart attack).
   c. Following coronary bypass surgery (open heart surgery).
3. To determine your physical work capacity.
4. To authorize participation in a physical exercise program.

Preparation for the Test

1. Avoid eating a heavy meal within 2 hours of your appointment.
2. Take your medications as you usually do, unless your doctor advises you not to take them.
3. Wear a shirt or blouse that buttons down the front with slacks, a skirt, jogging pants, or shorts.
4. Do not wear one-piece undergarments, jumpsuits, or dresses.
5. Tennis shoes are ideal if you have them. Otherwise, wear comfortable flat or low-heeled shoes. Do not wear clogs, sling-backs, crepe soles, boots, or high heels, as they make walking on the treadmill more difficult.

The Procedure

When you arrive in the Cardiology Department, areas of your chest may be shaved (men only) to allow the electrodes to adhere tightly to your chest. A blood pressure cuff will be wrapped around your arm, and an electrocardiogram (ECG) is taken while you are at rest. The technician will then demonstrate how to walk on the treadmill and will answer any questions you may have.

You will then perform a graded exercise test on a motor-driven treadmill. You will begin walking very gradually at a rate you can easily accomplish. Progressively throughout the test, the speed and grade of the treadmill will be increased, and you will be walking at a faster pace up a slight incline. At no time will you be asked to jog or run, nor will you be asked to exercise beyond your capabilities.

At all times during the test, trained personnel are in the room with you, monitoring your heart rate and blood pressure and observing you for signs of fatigue or discomfort. We do not wish to exercise you to a level that is medically unsafe or physically distressing.

An ECG is taken again when you finish walking. Your cardiologist will immediately interpret the results of the test and explain his or her findings to you. If necessary, medications or treatment will be discussed. A letter with the results of the stress test will be sent to your referring physician.

The entire procedure will take 1 to 1 1/2 hours. If you have any questions regarding the cardiac stress test or any problems with your appointment, please contact us.

FIGURE 30–27. Information booklet that may be given to the patient prior to testing.

parts of the heart. It can be done in two or three dimensions. The patient is placed in a supine position, and the transducer is held against the chest wall. The sound waves are sent out and echoed back through the transducer into the machine where they are converted into a picture that shows the exact size and movement of the parts of the heart that are being measured. The use of the echogram is convenient; it has the advantage of providing an immediate visualization of what is happening inside the heart without the complication of an invasive heart catheterization procedure.

HOLTER MONITOR CARDIOGRAPHY

A Holter monitor is a portable monitoring system for recording cardiac activity of a patient over a 24-hour period (Fig. 30–29A). This machine is lightweight so the patient can wear it while doing usual daily activities. The Holter monitor can be programmed to take a continuous recording for the 24-hour period, or only at certain points of the time span. It can also be set to record when activated by the patient when symptoms occur or during periods of stress.

It is very important that the patient keep a written diary of all activities during the day that cause stress, such as driving in rush hour traffic, bowel movements, intercourse, stair climbing, and other symptoms associated with possible heart problems. This diary should be explained completely to the patient so that proper entries can be made during the monitoring period, along with the time of each entry. Some machines are capable of recording the patient's voice while he or she describes the activi-

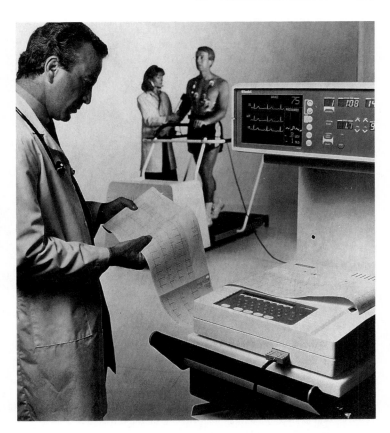

FIGURE 30-28. Stress test. The medical team in this picture is conducting a stress test. The patient uses the treadmill as directed by the physician, and the patient's heart reaction is displayed on the monitor and recorded. (Courtesy of Burdick, Inc., Schaumberg, IL.)

ties and symptoms experienced during the 24-hour monitoring. Although the majority of the monitoring periods last 24 hours, there are instances when the patient needs to wear the monitor for a longer period, for example, when only certain symptoms are being monitored by a patient activating the machine.

Many physicians have Holter monitors in their offices, so the medical assistant is responsible for preparing the patient, applying and removing the equipment, and instructing the patient in the guidelines of the procedure. The number of electrodes and leads varies with the number of channels on the machine. The electrode positions may not be any of the standard locations. The usual placement of the leads is shown in Figure 30-29*B*, but the assistant should always check with the physician regarding placement before attaching the electrodes. Because electrodes must be firmly placed, it may be necessary to shave the sites for secure placement. The lead wires are run from the electrodes to the monitor, which is usually attached to a belt that is worn diagonally over the shoulder or around the waist. The patient is taught how to use the monitor. If the monitor is equipped with an event marker, the patient is shown how to use this in case a significant symptom is experienced. This marker alerts the

technician when the tape is being interpreted. If the marker is used, the patient must also make note of the significant symptom in the diary. The patient can only sponge bathe during the test period because the equipment must not get wet.

At the end of the monitoring time, the patient returns to the office, and the machine is disconnected and removed. The tape and diary covering the testing period are placed into a Holter scanner or computer by a trained technician who analyzes the results. Any portion of the tape can be printed out for further study.

ADDITIONAL VOCABULARY USED IN ELECTROCARDIOGRAPHY

bradycardia Slow heart beat.
infarction An area of tissue that has died because of lack of blood supply.
ischemia Temporary deficiency of blood supply to a tissue or organ.
myocardium The middle layer of the walls of the heart muscle.
pericardium The sac that surrounds the heart.
tachycardia Fast heartbeat.

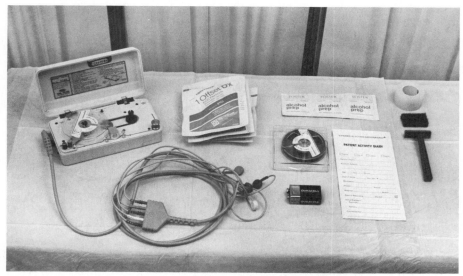

A

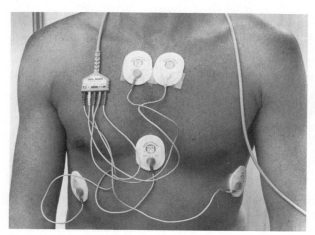

B

FIGURE 30-29. *A*, Holter monitor, including the supplies required for its application. (From Bonewit, K.: *Clinical Procedures for Medical Assistants,* 3rd ed., Philadelphia, W. B. Saunders Co., 1990, p 463.) *B*, Usual placement of electrodes. (From Bonewit, K.: *Clinical Procedures for Medical Assistants,* 3rd ed., Philadelphia, W. B. Saunders Co., 1990, p 467.)

LEGAL AND ETHICAL RESPONSIBILITIES

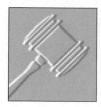

In order for the doctor to be able to interpret the ECG tracing and establish its value in diagnosing the patient's problem, the medical assistant has the ethical obligation to complete the task as it is assigned and required. This diagnostic procedure can have a marked effect on the patient's treatment. There is no room for error or improper technique. To ensure the integrity of the physician and the assistant, accuracy, neatness, and proper handling of the patient and equipment are of the utmost importance.

Electrocardiography is a valuable diagnostic tool. It is one of the primary procedures used in the treatment of the patient with a possible heart problem. The cardiologist compares and measures the patient's heart activity with known values by using the ECG tracing. He or she can also note changes in the patient's heart condition by comparing previous ECGs with current tracings. Using this valuable tool requires precise skill and knowledge. The medical assistant who is competent in performing this procedure will be a valuable asset to the physician and the medical practice served.

▶ LEARNING ACHIEVEMENTS

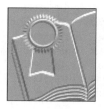

Upon successful completion of this chapter, can you in the time allowed by your evaluator:

1. Properly prepare the room and the patient for a 12-lead ECG by correctly completing each step of the procedure in the proper order?

2. Obtain an ECG tracing by completing each step of the procedure in the correct sequence?
3. Clean and return the ECG machine to its original state using the correct cleaning procedures and following the manufacturer's recommendations?
4. Properly mount the tracing on the correct mounting board with all waves correctly identified and in the correct position?

REFERENCES AND READINGS

Bonewit, K.: *Clinical Procedures for Medical Assistants,* 3rd ed., Philadelphia, W. B. Saunders Co., 1990.

Marcus, M., Schelbert, H., Skorton, D., Wolf, G.: *Cardiac Imaging,* Philadelphia, W. B. Saunders Co., 1991.

Wellens, H. J.: *The ECG in Emergency Decision Making,* Philadelphia, W. B. Saunders Co., 1992.

Wiederhold, R.: *Electrocardiography: The Monitoring Lead,* Philadelphia, W. B. Saunders Co., 1989.

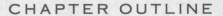

CHAPTER OUTLINE

VOCABULARY

agglutination The clumping together of particles (antigens and antibodies) resulting from their interaction with specific antibodies (or antigens); used in laboratory tests for blood typing and many other pathologic tests.

aliquot A portion of a well-mixed sample that is removed for testing.

antibody An immunoglobulin produced by lymphoid tissue in response to substances interpreted as foreign invaders gaining entry into the body.

anticoagulant A substance added to a blood sample that prevents coagulation.

cerebrospinal fluid Fluid within the subarachnoid space, the central canal of the spinal cord, and the four ventricles of the brain.

colony The visible growth on a culture plate, usually resulting from a single bacterium.

endotoxin A poisonous substance found in certain bacteria that is released after the death of the bacteria, causing fever, chills, and other symptoms.

fast(ing) To go without solid food for a specified period of time.

hematoma A localized collection of clotted blood caused by a broken blood vessel.

hemolysis The destruction of red blood cells.

hemolyzed A blood sample in which the red cells have been ruptured.

inoculate To place a specimen in a culture medium to allow it to grow so that it can be identified.

mordant A chemical (Gram's iodine) used to make the primary stain adhere to the cells it stains.

occult Hidden; not visible with the eye alone.

photometer An instrument that measures the intensity of a beam of light passing through it. The intensity of a beam is directly related to the concentration of the substance the beam passes through.

preservative A substance added to a specimen to prevent deterioration of cells or chemicals in the specimen.

quality assurance A law-enforced program that guarantees quality patient care.

quality control The operational procedures used to implement the quality assurance program.

reference laboratory A large laboratory that accepts specimens from smaller laboratories to perform tests not done by smaller laboratories.

reference values The listings of accepted ranges for normal values for routine hematology tests.

requisition A formal written request from the physician, authorizing a laboratory to perform procedure.

screening test A laboratory test done on large numbers of people to detect occult diseases.

specimen A sample of body fluid, waste product, or tissue that is collected for analysis.

stat Do immediately (from the Latin word *statin,* meaning "at once").

toxin A poisonous protein substance produced by some plants, animals, and pathogenic bacteria that builds up in the body as the microorganisms multiply.

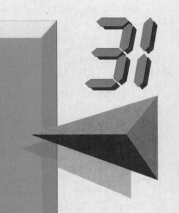

MICROBIOLOGY IN THE PHYSICIAN'S OFFICE

LEARNING OBJECTIVES

COGNITIVE

Upon successful completion of this chapter, you should be able to:

1. Define and spell the terms in the Vocabulary.

2. Discuss your role in coordinating laboratory tests and results.

3. List the 12 departments found in most laboratories.

4. State the safety rules for the laboratory.

5. Define the objective of quality assurance and equipment maintenance.

6. Identify the parts of a microscope.

7. Give five reasons that physicians order laboratory tests.

8. Cite the morphologic differences of bacteria.

9. Describe the difference between selective and nonselective media.

10. Discuss legal and ethical issues in laboratory testing.

PERFORMANCE

Upon completion of this chapter, you should be able to perform the following:

1. Focus a microscope under low power, high power, and oil immersion.

2. Collect a throat culture for either immediate testing or transportation to a laboratory.

3. Perform an occult blood test on a stool specimen.

4. Inoculate media for cultures.

5. Prepare direct smears and indirect smears from culture.

6. Examine stained smears for the presence of microorganisms.

7. Perform slide agglutination testing for infectious mononucleosis.

THE ROLE OF THE MEDICAL ASSISTANT

Laboratory tests are an essential part of a medical diagnosis, an aid to treatment, and, frequently, a control of medication. Only a physician may request laboratory testing for a patient. The medical assistant is responsible for a number of these laboratory testing procedures. The assistant must know the normal range of these tests, proper patient preparation, and the procedure for each. The assistant must carefully follow all laboratory instructions in obtaining and labeling the specimens and sending them to the laboratory. There must be good communication among the patient, the office staff, and the laboratory personnel. The assistant should make patients feel more at ease with these procedures and, thus, elicit more cooperation.

It is the medical assistant's responsibility to alert the physician to any abnormal results or findings. This may be accomplished by either circling or underlining the abnormality in red. Laboratory results are not filed until they are reviewed by the physician. Usually, the assistant contacts the patient concerning reports, follow-up procedures, and office visits.

THE LABORATORY

The laboratory is the place where specimens are tested, analyzed, and evaluated. Precise measurements are made, and the results are then calculated and interpreted. Tests are performed manually (by hand) or through automation (by using specialized instruments). These tests are performed by professionally trained medical technologists, medical laboratory technicians, and other allied health personnel. The *medical technologist (MT)* has a bachelor's degree and 1 year of clinical training. The *medical laboratory technician (MLT)* has 1 year of college and 1 year of clinical training. Both become certified by the successful completion of a national certifying examination. In addition to certification, many states monitor laboratory personnel by requiring state licensure.

Medical laboratories are located in either hospitals or nonhospital facilities. Nonhospital facilities include physician's offices, clinics, public health departments, health maintenance organizations (HMOs), and private **reference laboratories.** The head of a laboratory is the *pathologist,* a physician specially trained in the nature and cause of disease. The laboratory is divided into various departments, which may include hematology, chemistry, microbiology, specimen collection and processing, blood bank, coagulation, serology, histology, cytology, toxicology, urinalysis, and special chemistry. The laboratory in the physician's office usually performs procedures in hematology, chemistry, microbiology, and urinalysis.

Hematology. Whole blood is the specimen used for the majority of the tests performed. The numbers of *leukocytes* (white blood cells), *erythrocytes* (red blood cells), and *thrombocytes* (platelets) are actually counted. Observation is also made of the size, shape, and maturity level of these blood components. The results of these tests are used to diagnose anemias, leukemias, and clotting disorders.

Chemistry. Tests are usually performed on *serum,* the liquid part of blood left after a clot has formed. Urine and other body fluids may also be tested. The most common procedures performed measure levels of glucose (to determine blood sugar levels), enzymes (to determine heart damage), and electrolytes (to determine sodium, chloride, potassium, and bicarbonate levels).

Microbiology. Organisms are grown and identified from blood, urine, sputum, and wound specimens. Susceptibility testing is then performed on these organisms to determine proper antibiotic therapy. Microbiology deals with the study of bacteria, fungi, yeasts, parasites, and viruses.

Urinalysis. Urinalysis includes the physical, chemical, and microscopic examination of urine. In the physical examination, the color, transparency, and specific gravity are noted. Chemical analysis is performed to measure levels of glucose, protein, ketones, blood, bilirubin, urobilinogen, nitrites, and pH. Microscopically, the urine is examined for the presence of red, white, and epithelial cells; mucus; casts; crystals; yeasts; parasites; and bacteria.

Laboratory Safety

Basic safety rules must be observed at all times in the laboratory to avoid personal injury and to prevent equipment damage. Any accident must be reported to the physician or supervisor. Hazards in the laboratory can be classified as either physical, chemical, or biologic.

Physical Hazards. Physical hazards include fires resulting from electrical malfunction or alcohol lamps. Open flames are no longer used in modern laboratories. All personnel must be familiar with the location of fire extinguishers and fire escape routes. Keep all electric equipment in proper repair, and always follow manufacturers' instructions.

Chemical Hazards. Chemical hazards include contact with corrosives and toxic or carcinogenic substances. Caution should be taken in handling all chemicals and specimens to avoid spills and splashes. Skin or eyes that come into contact with any chemicals must be immediately washed with water for at least 5 minutes. Pipetting should be performed only with safety bulbs or filters.

Biologic Hazards. Biologic hazards can result from the use of specimens and reagents capable of transmitting disease. The laboratory work area must be disinfected before and after each use when dealing with biologicals. Eating, drinking, smoking, or mouth pipetting is not allowed. Gloves should be worn. Laboratory aprons or coats should be worn. Specimens and any contaminated materials must be disposed of through sterilization or incineration. Hands must be washed before and after every procedure. Extreme caution and common sense are essential at all times in the laboratory. Regulations and precautions must be followed consistently (see Laboratory Rules).

LABORATORY RULES

- No eating, drinking, or smoking.
- Keep pens, pencils, and fingers away from mouth and eyes.
- Pull long hair back and up.
- No mouth pipetting.
- Report all accidents to physician or supervisor.
- Wear laboratory coat or apron.
- Wipe spills and splashes immediately.
- Wash hands before and after every procedure.
- Follow manufacturer's instructions for equipment operation.
- Know the location of all safety equipment and supplies and fire escape routes.
- Wear protective gloves and safety glasses.
- Avoid wearing chains, rings, bracelets, and other loose hanging jewelry.
- Clean work area before and after every procedure.
- Disinfect or sterilize specimens and materials contaminated with blood or microorganisms.
- No storage of food and beverages in laboratory refrigerator.
- Repair malfunctioning equipment immediately.
- Be familiar with appropriate first-aid procedures.
- Properly ground all electric equipment.
- Clearly label all reagents and solutions.
- Be a professional at all times.

Quality Assurance

Quality assurance (QA) is a comprehensive set of policies and procedures developed to ensure the quality of laboratory testing. It includes quality control, personnel orientation, laboratory documentation, knowledge of laboratory instrumentation, and enrollment in a proficiency testing program. QA focuses on establishing a series of operating procedures to produce reliable laboratory results for the benefit of the patient, the physician, and the medical assistant who does the laboratory testing.

These policies benefit the physician by reducing the liability for inaccurate reporting of test results. In order for a physician to use a laboratory test in diagnosing, the results must be compared with **reference values.** The QA system enables the laboratory to assess, verify, and document the quality of the test results.

Quality Control

The objective of **quality control** in the laboratory is to ensure the *accuracy* of test results while detecting and eliminating error. Quality control is a major part of the routine in most medical laboratories. Mandated by law, quality control programs monitor all aspects of laboratory activity, from specimen collection through the processing, testing, and reporting steps. Programs check supplies, reagents, machinery, personnel, and actual test performance. Equipment performance and maintenance are also monitored. Specially prepared quality control samples are tested along with patient samples. The results of testing performed on the quality control samples must be within a pre-established range before the patient results can be reported. The quality control samples, called *controls,* are usually supplied with prepackaged kits intended for use in the small laboratory. The controls should be analyzed at specified intervals. For example, positive and negative controls supplied with pregnancy test kits should be performed with each patient specimen. Urinalysis dipsticks (used for chemical examination of urine) should be checked daily and each time a new container is opened. Controls for automated chemistry analyses should be performed at specified intervals during the day. Consistent results of controls ensure constant conditions throughout the testing sequence.

Equipment Maintenance

Continuous care of your laboratory instruments is important to ensure proper operation and accurate test results. Preventive maintenance prolongs the life of your equipment and reduces breakdowns; it includes daily cleaning and adjusting and replacing parts when necessary. Each instrument should have a log or worksheet to record all changes, including daily maintenance. The following guidelines are provided for a preventive maintenance program:

- Follow the manufacturer's instructions for calibration of instruments.
- Read and understand instructions for routine instrument care.
- Perform all preventive maintenance provided by manufacturer's instructions.
- Keep all spare parts available for immediate use.
- Record the name, address, and phone number of a contact person for maintenance or repair.
- Create a maintenance form or use the one provided.

THE MICROSCOPE

Every medical laboratory is equipped with a microscope. This indispensable instrument is used to view objects too small to be seen with the naked eye (Fig. 31–1). The microscope is helpful in identifying microorganisms in urine sediment and other body fluids. The microscope is employed to evaluate stained blood smears, urine sediment, and microbacterial throat smears, and to determine blood cell counts. Since the microscope is an expensive and technical instrument, special care must be taken in its operation, care, and storage.

Microscopes are either *monocular* or *binocular*. A monocular microscope has one eyepiece for viewing, and a binocular has two. The *eyepiece*, or *ocular*, is located at the top of the microscope and contains a lens to magnify what is being seen. The usual magnification is 10 times (×10). The ocular is attached to a barrel or tube that is connected to the microscope *arm*. Under the arm is the *revolving nosepiece*, to which are attached the *objectives*. Most microscopes have three objectives; each has a different magnifying power. The shortest objective has the lowest power (×10). Low power is used to scan the field of interest and then focus on a particular object. Greater detail is observed with the next longest objective, which is high power (×40). The longest objective, oil immersion (×100), allows for the finest focusing of the object.

The arm of the microscope connects the objectives and oculars to the *base,* which supports the microscope and contains its light source. Together,

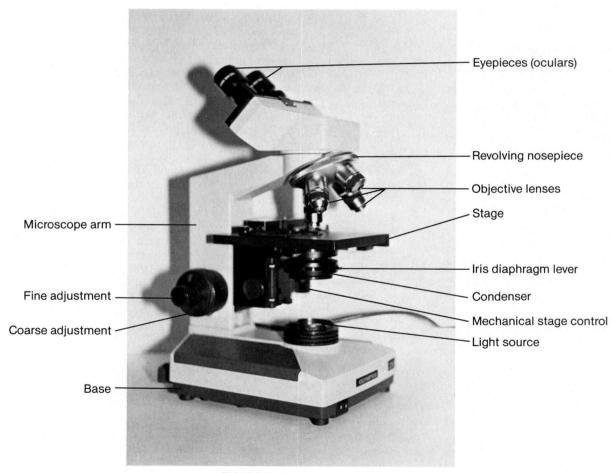

FIGURE 31–1. Parts of a microscope.

Eyepieces (oculars)

Revolving nosepiece

Objective lenses

Stage

Iris diaphragm lever

Condenser

Mechanical stage control

Light source

Microscope arm

Fine adjustment

Coarse adjustment

Base

PROCEDURE 31-1   USING THE MICROSCOPE

GOAL To focus the microscope properly, using a prepared slide, under low power, high power, and oil immersion.

EQUIPMENT AND SUPPLIES

Microscope   Lens cleaner
Lens tissue   Slide containing specimen

PROCEDURAL STEPS

1. Wash your hands.
2. Gather the materials needed.
3. Clean the lenses with lens tissue and lens cleaner.
4. Adjust seating to a comfortable height.
5. Plug the microscope into an electric outlet, and turn on the light switch.
6. Place the slide specimen on the stage and secure it.
7. Turn the revolving nosepiece to low power.
8. Carefully raise the stage while observing with the naked eye from the side.
9. Focus the specimen, using the coarse-adjustment knob.
10. Switch to fine adjustment, and focus the specimen in detail.
11. Adjust the amount of light by closing the iris diaphragm and lowering the condenser.
12. Turn the revolving nosepiece between the high power objective and oil immersion.
13. Place a small drop of oil on the slide.
14. Carefully swing the oil immersion objective into place.
15. Adjust the focus with the fine-adjustment knob.
16. Increase the light by opening the iris diaphragm and raising the condenser.
17. Identify the specimen.
18. Return to low power.
19. Lower the stage.
20. Center the stage.
21. Remove the slide.
22. Switch off the light and unplug the microscope.
23. Clean the lenses with lens tissue, and remove oil with lens cleaner.
24. Wipe the microscope with a cloth.
25. Cover the microscope.
26. Clean the work area.
27. Wash your hands.

the *condenser* and the *iris diaphragm* direct and regulate the light up through the objective. Just above the base are the focusing knobs. The *coarse adjustment* is used only with low power, and the *fine adjustment* is used with high power and oil immersion. The *stage* of the microscope holds the slide to be viewed.

Microscopes are very precise and expensive instruments that require careful handling. The amount of routine maintenance depends on the amount of daily use. Dirt is the enemy of the microscope, which must be kept scrupulously clean at all times. The microscope should always be stored in a plastic dust cover when not in use. Lenses should be cleaned before and after each use with lens paper and lens cleaner. Any other type of tissue scratches the lenses or leaves lint residue behind. The use of solvent cleaners, such as xylene, is not recommended on a routine basis because they may loosen lenses. Xylene can be used to remove oil that has dried on the lenses. Oil, makeup, dust, and eye secretions all can obstruct vision through the lens and cause the possible transmission of infection. Finally, the body of the microscope should be dusted with a soft cloth.

Microscopes should be placed in a permanent location in the laboratory, on a sturdy table in an area where they cannot be bumped. If a microscope must be moved, it should be carried securely, with one hand supporting the base and the other holding the arm. When storing the microscope, it should be left with the low power objective in the lowest position. The stage should be centered.

SPECIMEN COLLECTION

The medical assistant is responsible for the collection of many different types of **specimens.** It is important to recognize that all clinical laboratory results are only as good as the specimen received. The most common specimens are blood, urine, and swabs for culture. Less often, feces, gastric contents, **cerebrospinal fluid (CSF),** tissue samples, semen, and aspirates, such as synovial fluid or amniotic fluid, are submitted for testing. These specimens are analyzed for levels of many chemicals and drugs, types and numbers of cells present, and the presence of microorganisms.

Results of Testing

The results of these tests, along with other diagnostic testing, patient history, and physical examination, lead the physician to diagnose or rule out a particular disease. Management of the patient's condition may require repeated testing, such as routine glucose level determinations in the diabetic patient. If a patient is receiving medication, the physi-

cian may request therapeutic drug monitoring to be certain that the patient is actually taking the medication and to detect possible toxic levels. Patients being given diuretics for the treatment of high blood pressure may need to have their potassium levels checked on a routine basis. Occasionally, the physician may request a test to determine the patient's baseline level, for comparison with the results of future tests.

Screening tests, such as routine urinalysis, are performed to detect hidden disease in otherwise apparently healthy individuals. A urinalysis may reveal the presence of diabetes, liver disease, or pathology of the urinary tract. Some screening tests are required by law in certain states. Persons applying for a marriage license may be required to have a Venereal Disease Research Laboratory (VDRL) test to detect syphilis, and a rapid plasma reagin (RPR) to determine the rubella titer may also be requested. Some states require screening of newborns for hereditary metabolic defects such as phenylketonuria (PKU) and hypothyroidism. Tests may reveal the extent of disease or degree of damage done to an organ or body system. For example, the measurement of the rise of certain enzymes after a heart attack can indicate the amount of heart damage, whereas the measurement of the level of the HIV **antibody** is an accurate assessment of the risk of AIDS transmission. Repeated testing can allow the physician to follow the course of a disease and assess the effectiveness of the treatment. A person diagnosed as having leukemia will have daily white blood cell counts performed before receiving chemotherapy.

Achieving Accurate Results

The importance of specimen collection cannot be overemphasized. If not performed correctly, it can easily lead to inaccurate results. If the tests are to be accurate indicators of the patient's state of health, it is imperative that the concepts of specimen collection be understood and followed exactly.

Using Proper Equipment

The correct specimen must be collected in the correct container; for example, blood may be collected using a vacuum tube system (Fig. 31–2). These tubes are available in a variety of sizes with and without **preservatives** and **anticoagulants.** The tubes are color-coded so that the color of the stopper denotes which, if any, additive is present (Table 31–1).

The medical assistant should always check the laboratory's specimen requirements manual for any unfamiliar tests. The manual lists all specimen collection information. Any unanswered questions should be resolved by calling the laboratory before collection of the specimen.

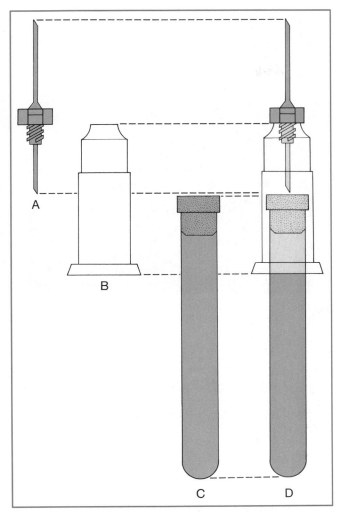

FIGURE 31-2. Vacuum tube blood-collecting system. *A*, Needle; *B*, holder; *C*, vacuum tube; *D*, assembled unit.

Avoiding Contamination

Care must be taken to avoid contamination of the specimen or the assistant. The correct collection and handling of the specimens used in various microbiology procedures are absolutely essential if the results are to be of any value in the diagnosis of the disease and the treatment of the patient. Expiration dates on swabs, tubes, transport media, and other collection containers should be checked before these items are used.

An improperly handled specimen may become contaminated or may contaminate the surrounding environment. Follow the universal blood and body-fluid precautions. All blood and other body fluids from *all* patients should be considered infective. See Chapter 25.

Providing Sufficient and True Representative Samples

Sufficient samples should be collected for the tests requested by the physician. Amounts may vary based on the methods used. If a report is returned from the laboratory with the term *"insufficient sample"* (QNS), it indicates a request for an additional specimen. Be certain to clarify any questions concerning the previous specimen by calling the laboratory before collecting a new one.

The specimen collected must be a true representative sample. A swab for a wound culture collected from the surface of the wound generally does not yield the same results as one taken from the depths of the wound. A **hemolyzed** blood specimen, or one taken from an atypical area, such as a **hematoma** or the area above an intravenous (IV) hookup, shows marked differences in many tests. If a large volume of specimen is collected, such as a 24-hour urine or fecal fat specimen, the total volume or weight must be carefully measured and recorded. The specimen must be well mixed before an **aliquot** is removed and submitted for testing.

Providing Proper Instructions to Patients

Many testing procedures require that patients be given a specific set of instructions to follow. For example, patients may be required to **fast** 8 to 12 hours prior to the collection of blood and urine. They may need to follow a high-carbohydrate diet for several days prior to a *glucose tolerance test*. The consumption of some foods and medication must be discontinued. The physician will discuss medication alternatives with the patient. Sometimes, it might not be medically advisable to discontinue the medication; this must be noted on the laboratory **requisition**. The laboratory will then be alerted to the possible drug interferences, and it may be able to use an alternative test method.

TABLE 31-1. VACUUM TUBE BLOOD-COLLECTING SYSTEM

Stopper Color	Anticoagulant in Tube	Use of Tube
Red	None	For clotting blood; obtaining serum, chemistry studies
Purple	EDTA	For whole blood hematology studies
Blue	Sodium citrate	For plasma coagulation studies
Green	Heparin	For special plasma chemistry tests

Proper Handling, Processing, and Storage

The specimen must be handled, processed, and stored according to the instructions, to avoid causing any alterations that would affect test results. Check whether the specimen needs to be kept warm or cool. Specimens such as urine require chilling if the testing is not going to be done immediately. Some cultures or specimens need to be kept at body temperature after collection. *Neisseria* gonococcal (CC) cultures and semen analysis are two such examples, since cooling kills the gonococci and sperm. When required, serum must be separated from the cells as soon as possible after the specimen has clotted, to prevent alterations caused by the metabolism of the cells. Specimens for bilirubin testing must be protected from light. Some specimens need to be frozen to prevent chemical constituents from changing. Consult the laboratory specimen requirements to be certain that each specimen is handled and processed properly.

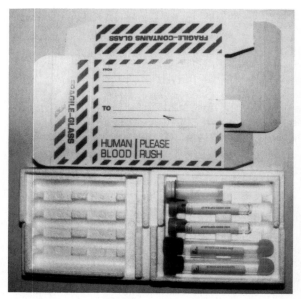

FIGURE 31–3. Example of good mailing package for specimen. It is made of plastic foam for protection of the contents.

Requisition for Laboratory Testing

A completed requisition must accompany each specimen sent to the laboratory. The information must be carefully printed in ink. All copies must be legible. Be sure to complete all necessary items on the requisition. The following information is usually required when specimens are sent to the laboratory:

1. Physician's name, account number, address, and phone number.
2. Patient's full name, surname first.
3. Patient's address.
4. Patient's insurance information.
5. Patient's age, date of birth, and sex.
6. Source of specimen.
7. Date and time of collection.
8. Specific test requested.
9. Medications the patient is taking.
10. Possible diagnosis.
11. Indication of whether test is **stat** (needed immediately).

If the specimen is to be mailed, it must be carefully packaged to prevent breakage, damage, or contamination by all persons handling it. Containers of liquid specimens may be wrapped in absorbent material and inserted in unbreakable tubes with safe-top lids. The lids are taped shut so that no leakage occurs if the specimen container breaks. Place all specimens in a second container, such as an impervious bag, for transport. The completed requisition goes inside the outermost wrap. Usually, Styrofoam mailers (Fig. 31–3) are used because they cushion the sample and also provide insulation. Styrofoam inserts can be shaped to fit around the specimen containers. A warning label specifying the etiologic agent or biologic specimen is affixed to the outside of the container. The specimen should be given to the laboratory courier or mailed at a post office immediately so that it is not exposed to temperature extremes.

Collection of Microbiology Specimens

Medical assistants are often called upon to collect specimens for the identification of possible microorganisms. A microbiology specimen must contain as few contaminants as possible and must be composed of material from the actual site of the infection. Microbiology specimens are most often contaminated by normal flora (bacteria) from the site of collection, such as normal skin flora from a wound site. Wound swabs should be taken from the depths of the wound; surface organisms may not be the true cause of the infection.

Optimal Collection Times

Knowledge of the optimal collection times is necessary for the best chance of recovery of the causative organisms or collection of positive serologic specimens. Urinary tract infections are best diagnosed from the first specimen voided in the morning, since the specimen has been incubating in the bladder overnight. In addition, this specimen is most likely to have a high number of microorganisms. Blood for serologic testing is usually collected during the acute stage of the disease and again during the convalescent stage. The results of the two are compared; a rise in antibody titer is usually diagnostic.

Sufficient Sample

A sufficient sample must be obtained to perform all tests requested. For example, in cases of suspected mycobacterial infection, which causes tuberculosis (TB), the physician may order a sputum specimen to be collected for a Gram stain, acid-fast stain, and acid-fast culture for aerobes and anaerobes. The patient must be instructed to collect at least 10 ml of a first morning sputum specimen.

Proper Equipment and Procedures

The proper collection containers, media, and procedures must be used. These include sterile, non-breakable containers with tight-fitting lids; polyester (not cotton) swabs (Fig. 31–4); appropriate transport media for aerobic and anaerobic cultures; and the immediate inoculation of swabs for gonococcus cultures onto prewarmed modified Thayer-Martin agar. If possible, obtain specimens for culture before antibiotics are given. This is particularly important for throat and gonococcus cultures. If an antibiotic has been given, note it on the requisition, and send the specimen to the laboratory immediately for inoculation onto the media. Even small amounts of the antibiotic interfere with the culture.

Types of Specimens Collected in the Physician's Office

Throat and urine specimens are frequently collected in the physician's office to assist in the diagnosis of "strep throat" and urinary tract infections.

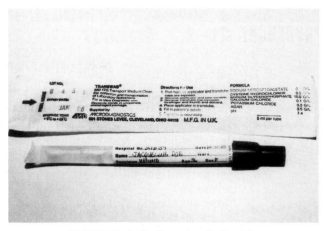

FIGURE 31–4. Sterile swab collection tube.

Strep throat is caused by an organism called *Streptococcus* and, if left untreated, can cause serious complications such as rheumatic fever, rheumatic endocarditis, and glomerulonephritis. The organism most commonly isolated in the urine is *Escherichia coli*. The medical assistant collects the throat culture specimen and instructs the patient to collect a clean-catch urine specimen.

Throat cultures are collected by gently swabbing the back of the throat and the surfaces of the tonsils with a sterile swab. The mouth and tongue should not be touched. This prevents contamination of the swab with the normal flora of the mouth. This procedure can be accomplished best by depressing the tongue and instructing the patient to say "ah."

PROCEDURE 31–2 COLLECTING A SPECIMEN BY SWAB FOR THROAT CULTURE AND FOR DIRECT SLIDE TESTING

GOAL To collect a throat culture, using sterile technique, for either immediate testing or transportation to the laboratory.

EQUIPMENT AND SUPPLIES

For on-site testing:
Sterile swab
Sterile tongue depressor

For transport:
Sterile swab
Sterile tongue depressor
Transport medium

PROCEDURAL STEPS

1. Wash and dry your hands. Follow universal blood and body-fluid precautions. Glove yourself with nonsterile or sterile gloves.
   Purpose: To reduce the spread of infection.

Continued

PROCEDURE 31-2   *Continued*

2. Gather the materials needed.

3. Position the patient so that the light shines into the mouth.
   Purpose: Visualization of the area to be swabbed.

4. Remove the sterile swab from the sterile wrap with your dominant hand, and grasp the sterile tongue depressor with your nondominant hand.
   Purpose: Better control of the swabbing process.

5. Instruct the patient to open the mouth and to say "ah." Depress the tongue with the depressor.
   Purpose: Saying "ah" helps elevate the uvula and reduces the tendency to gag. The tongue is depressed so that you can see the back of the throat.

6. Swab the back of the throat between the tonsillar pillars and especially the reddened, patchy areas of the throat and the tonsils (Fig. 31–5).
   Purpose: Pathogenic organisms are found in the back of the throat and on the tonsils.

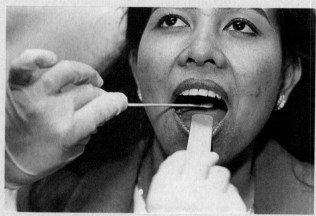

FIGURE 31–5.

7. Place the swab into the transport medium, label it, and send it to the laboratory. If testing is performed in the office, inoculate a blood agar plate and label it. If direct slide testing is requested, return the labeled swab to the laboratory.
   Purpose: Transport media prevent the swab from drying. Labeling immediately after collection prevents mixing up specimens.

8. Dispose of contaminated supplies.
   Purpose: Prevents the spread of infection.

9. Disinfect the work area.

10. Wash your hands.

Occult Blood

Screening tests for **occult** blood in the stool are routinely performed to detect bleeding in the intestinal tract, which may indicate cancer, polyps, or other lesions of the colon or rectum. The test can be performed in the office during a rectal examination, or the patient may be instructed to collect a sample at home. Most test procedures use a paper impregnated with a gum resin called *guaiac,* which turns blue when a developer is added and blood is present. Home tests are also available. The test paper impregnated with the reagents is dropped into the toilet bowl after a bowel movement. The patient then watches for the color change, as explained in the instructions.

The guaiac tests are subject to interferences. Vitamin C in large doses causes false negatives. Iron, red meats, and certain raw, leafy vegetables can cause false positives. Contamination with menstrual blood or collection of the specimen when hemorrhoids are present results in a positive test result. If patients are collecting specimens at home, they must be given supplies and instructions. *Hemoccult* slides (Smithkline Diagnostics, Sunnyvale, CA) come in packets of three for collection on three consecutive bowel movements. The patient should be free of vitamin C and be on a nonmeat diet for 2 days prior to the beginning of collection. The stool should be passed into a clean container, and then a small sample should be smeared on the paper in the appropriate windows of the slide with the wooden applicator provided. Oxidizing cleaning agents present in the toilet bowl can cause false positives if the sample is retrieved from the bowl. It is convenient to place the labeled slides, applicators, and instructions in an envelope addressed to the office. After the specimens have been collected, the slides may be mailed back to the office. The testing of specimens collected in the office is often done using rolls of guaiac paper. A sample from the glove following a rectal examination is also sufficient for testing.

Collection of Semen

Semen analysis is usually performed for fertility studies, especially after vasectomies to establish the effectiveness of the *vasectomy.* The patient is ad-

---

PROCEDURE 31-3   PERFORMING AN OCCULT BLOOD TEST

GOAL   Collection of a stool specimen and performance of an occult blood test on the specimen obtained.

EQUIPMENT AND SUPPLIES

Collection slides
Applicator sticks

Developer
Written instructions

PROCEDURAL STEPS

1. Supply the patient with an addressed envelope containing slides, applicator sticks, and written instructions including diet restrictions. Tell the patient to return the slides to the office (Fig. 31–6).
    Purpose: Most screening for occult blood is done on samples collected at home.

2. Wash and dry your hands. Follow universal blood and body-fluid precautions. Glove yourself with nonsterile or sterile gloves.

3. Open test window on the back of the slide, and add two drops of developer to each test area. Look for the development of a blue color, which indicates a positive test for hidden blood.

4. Add developer to the on-slide performance monitor at the bottom of the slide window. Look for correct reactions in the positive and negative control circles. If the on-slide monitor does not perform as expected, the results of the patient test are invalid. Do not report them. If the on-slide monitor shows the developer is reacting as expected, the patient results may be reported (Fig. 31–7).
    Purpose: The monitors are a form of quality control of the procedure to ensure that the guaiac paper and developer react as expected.

Continued

PROCEDURE 31-3   *Continued*

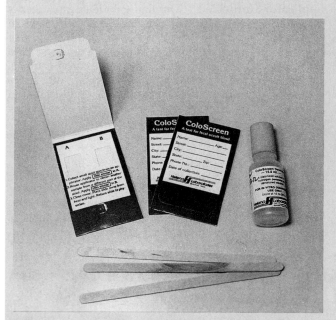

FIGURE 31-6. (Courtesy of Wampole Laboratories, a division of Carter-Wallace, Inc., Cranbury, NJ.)

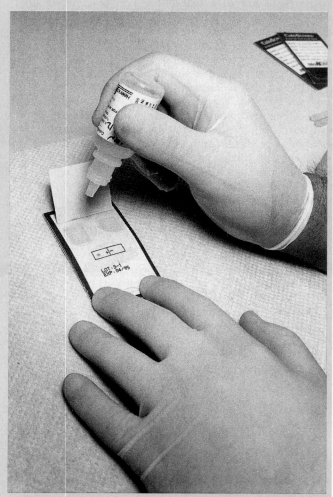

FIGURE 31-7.

5. Record the results of the patient and the on-slide monitor.

vised to refrain from intercourse for 2 to 4 days before the sample is collected. Instruct the patient to collect the total specimen in an opaque glass container. Masturbation or coitus interruptus may be employed as methods of obtaining the specimen, but if the latter is used, great care must be taken to collect the entire ejaculate. Condoms should never be employed, because the latex has definite spermicidal qualities. The cap of the container must be tightly closed, with the patient's name, the date, and the time of ejaculation written on the label. The specimen must be kept at body temperature and must be delivered to the laboratory within 3 hours after collection.

BLOOD CHEMISTRY TESTS

Blood Glucose

The most common blood chemistry test performed in the laboratory of the physician's office is the blood glucose level. It is used in the diagnosis of diabetes and as an aid in the control of the diabetic patient. It may also be requested in screening for hypoglycemia (low blood sugar). If the laboratory does not perform other chemistry tests, the enzymatic glucose stick methods produced by Bio-Dynamics (Chemstrip bG) and Ames (Glucostix and Visidex) will probably be the method used because the sticks can be read with the naked eye and require no additional instruments for testing. However, if the physician chooses, a portable meter can be purchased to mechanically determine the reading. The meter gives a more accurate reading than can be obtained by visual comparison of the colors. This **photometer** measures the amount of light reflected off the reacted reagent pad and converts the measurement into a digital readout of the blood glucose level. The photometers are designed for use with one particular reagent manufacturer's strips and are not interchangeable.

Other blood chemistry tests commonly ordered by the physician include tests for serum calcium, uric acid, blood urea nitrogen, and cholesterol.

Serum Calcium. Calcium is essential in the formation of bone tissue, in muscular activity, and in blood coagulation. When there is a deficiency of calcium, tetany occurs. This condition is characterized by a twitching of muscle fibers and tetanic convulsions. An increase of serum calcium is found in hyperparathyroidism, multiple myeloma, and some respiratory diseases.

Uric Acid. This test is used basically to aid in the diagnosis of gout, a metabolic disease marked by acute arthritis and inflammation of the joints. An increase in uric acid levels is also seen in severe kidney damage, toxemias of pregnancy, and electrolyte imbalance.

TABLE 31–2. PANELS AND PROFILES

Panel/Profile	Tests Included	Requirement	Expected Range Male (16–65)	Units
Chemistry panel	Glucose	2 ml serum: 1 serum-separation tube	75–125	mg/dl
	BUN (blood urea nitrogen)		6–25	mg/dl
	Creatinine		0.6–1.5	mg/dl
	Uric acid		4.0–8.5	mg/dl
	SGOT (ASG) (aspartate aminotransferase)		0–50	mU/ml*
	Cholesterol		135–300	mg/dl
	Triglycerides		30–175	mg/dl
	LDH (LD) (lactate dehydrogenase)		100–225	mU/ml*
	Total bilirubin		0.1–1.1	mg/dl
	Albumin		3.2–5.2	g/dl
	GGT (gamma glutamyltransferase)		0–60	mU/ml*
	Alkaline phosphate		15–100	mU/ml*
	Calcium		8.2–10.5	mg/dl
	Phosphorus		2.1–5.0	mg/dl
	Iron		30–180	μg/dl
	Sodium (Na^+) ⎫		136–145	mmol/L
	Potassium (K^+) ⎬ Electrolytes		3.2–5.5	mmol/L
	Chloride (Cl^-)		98–108	mmol/L
	Bicarbonate (HCO_3^-) ⎭		22–32	mmol/L
Electrolyte panel	Sodium (Na^+)	1 ml serum: 1 serum-separation tube, no hemolysis	136–145	mmol/L
	Potassium (K^+)		3.2–5.5	mmol/L
	Chloride (Cl^-)		98–108	mmol/L
	Bicarbonate (HCO_3^-)		22–32	mmol/L
Lipid profile	Triglycerides	3 ml serum: 1 serum-separation tube. Cannot be done on lipemic serum because of triglyceride interference with HDL. Fasting specimen required.	30–175	mg/dl
	Cholesterol		130–300	mg/dl
	HDL (high-density lipoprotein) Cholesterol		30–70	mg/dl (M)
			40–90	mg/dl (F)
	LDL (low-density lipoprotein) Cholesterol		60–180	mg/dl
Thyroid panel	Triiodothyronine (T_3) uptake	1 ml serum: 1 serum-separation tube	35–49% (M)	
			33–46% (F)	
	Thyroxine (T_4) radioimmunoassay (RIA)		4.0–11.0	μg/dl
	T_7 (calculated)		1.4–5.4 (M)	
			1.3–5.1 (F)	
OB profile	ABO	2 red top tubes: spin unopened and send intact. Positive RPR results in additional tests and cost.		
	Rh factor			
	Antibody screen		Negative	
	Rubella			
	RPR (rapid plasma reagent)		Negative	

Blood Urea Nitrogen (BUN). This is a kidney function test. Normally, the kidneys excrete urea. This major product of the kidneys is the end product of protein metabolism. In some kidney diseases, the kidneys do not excrete urea sufficiently, so the urea nitrogen in the blood increases.

Cholesterol. Cholesterol is normally found in the blood, but in some disease states, the cholesterol concentration is increased or decreased. An elevated reading may aid in the diagnosis of liver malfunction, hypothyroidism, and a possibility of atherosclerosis. A decrease is found in hyperthyroidism, anemias, cachexia, and acute infections.

Many times, the physician may order a *panel* or *profile* on a patient. This is a group of tests relating to a particular organ or system. Cardiac, liver, and thyroid profiles are common. Panels may include 20 or more tests relating to a number of different body systems. Panels are performed on sophisticated automated machinery and provide maximum information with minimum sample and cost (Table 31–2).

INTRODUCTION TO MICROBIOLOGY

Microbiology is the study of microorganisms, including bacteria, fungi, viruses, rickettsiae, mycobacteria, and parasites. The main objective of microbiologic procedures is to identify the organisms responsible for illness so that the physician can properly treat the patient. These procedures are performed either in the physician's office or in the microbiology department of a medical laboratory.

Bacteria

The study of bacteria is called *bacteriology.* Bacteria are one-celled plant microorganisms. There are numerous ways of identifying bacteria, including their morphology (form and structure), their ability to retain certain dyes, their growth in different physical environments, and the results of certain biochemical reactions.

Bacteria exist in three main forms: round-shaped *cocci,* rod-shaped *bacilli,* and spiral-shaped *spirilla.* They can occur singly, in pairs, in clusters, or in long chains and are widely distributed in the air, soil, water, living animals and plants, and dead organic matter. The *Gram stain* is a method of staining that differentiates bacteria according to the chemical composition of their cell walls. *Gram-positive* bacteria stain purple, and *Gram-negative* bacteria stain red. Microanaerobic bacteria grow best in an atmosphere of reduced oxygen tension. Aerobic bacteria grow under conditions of either normal or reduced oxygen. The most important

classification of bacteria pertains to the toxic effects they have on the body. *Pathogenic* (disease-causing) bacteria attack the body by secreting **toxins** while they are growing, or they release **endotoxins** when they die. After an incubation period, these poisons cause the symptoms of the disease.

The skin, respiratory tract, and gastrointestinal tract are inhabited by a variety of harmless, normal flora. An infection occurs when bacteria occurring naturally in one part of the body invade another part of the body and become harmful. A common example is the bacterium *Escherichia coli* (normal flora of the intestinal tract) causing a urinary tract infection. Pathogenic bacteria can be transmitted from person to person by many mechanisms, including direct contact (by means of airborne infections, contact with animals, or transmission by insects) and indirect contact (through drinking water or food products or on inanimate objects). Another example is the bacterium *Staphylococcus epidermidis,* normally found on the surface of the skin. When bacteria of this type invade the body, as with a cut, they usually produce an infection.

Fungi

Mycology is the study of fungi and the diseases they cause. Fungi are larger than bacteria and have rigid cell walls. Fungal infections are resistant to antibiotics used in the treatment of bacterial infections and must be treated with drugs active against the unusual cell walls of this organism. Fungi are present in the soil, air, and water, but only a few produce disease. These infections may be quite superficial, affecting only the skin, hair, or nails. However, some fungi can penetrate the tissues of the internal body structures and produce serious diseases of the mucous membranes, heart, lungs, and other organs. Among the fungal diseases are *ringworm, athlete's foot* (tinea pedis), *thrush* (oral candidiasis), *histoplasmosis, coccidioidomycosis,* and *blastomycosis.*

Mycobacteria

Mycobacteria have been important agents of disease throughout the world since before the time of recorded history. There are 54 species of mycobacterium, and 14 of these cause diseases in humans. *Mycobacterium tuberculosis* is the cause of tuberculosis.

World Health Organization reports indicate that tuberculosis kills 3 million people annually in underdeveloped countries. Since the mid-1980s, there has been an increase in new active cases in the United States. Part of the increase is related to the acquired immunodeficiency syndrome (AIDS) epidemic, and part of it is due to the introduction of new, more resistant strains by immigrants from underdeveloped countries.

Physicians are dependent on the assistance clinical microbiology laboratories supply in the diagnostic testing, treatment, and monitoring of mycobacterial disease.

Viruses

Viruses, the smallest infectious microorganisms, can be seen only with the aid of an electron microscope. Study of viruses and their diseases is known as *virology.* Viruses cannot be grown on artificial culture media and cannot be destroyed by antibiotic drugs. Viral diseases are transmitted by direct contact, insects, blood transfusion, contamination of food or water, and inhalation of droplets expelled by coughing or sneezing. Some of the more than 50 known viral diseases include the *common cold, smallpox, chickenpox, influenza, poliomyelitis, measles, mumps, German measles, cold sores, shingles, viral hepatitis, rabies, infectious mononucleosis, croup, viral encephalitis, yellow fever,* and *AIDS.*

Rickettsiae

Rickettsiae are microorganisms found in the tissue cells of lice, fleas, ticks, and mites and are transmitted to humans by the bite of these insects. Rickettsial diseases include *Rocky Mountain spotted fever, typhus, Q fever,* and *trench fever.* These diseases are not common in communities with good sanitary conditions. They can be prevented by insecticides, vaccines, and antibiotics.

Parasites

In contrast to the previously mentioned microorganisms, the protozoa are animals, not plants. Depending on the protozoon, transmission can occur through insect bites, blood transfusion, sexual contact, and fecal contamination. Pathogenic protozoa include *Plasmodium* (malaria), *Trichomonas* (vaginitis), *Entamoeba histolytica* (dysentery), and *Toxoplasma gondii* (encephalitis).

MICROBIOLOGY PROCEDURES COMMONLY PERFORMED IN THE PHYSICIAN'S OFFICE

Some physicians prefer to perform some of the simple screening procedures in their offices and refer the more complex tests to special laboratories. Others collect specimens in the office and send all of them to larger laboratories for analysis. The basic microbiology procedures most frequently encountered in the small physician laboratory include preparation of direct smears; staining; microscopic examination of smears, wet preps, and potassium hydroxide (KOH) preps; **screening tests** for strep throat and infectious mononucleosis; and screening for urinary tract infections. Many types of tests are available in kit form. The kits supply all needed reagents and most equipment. Directions for the entire test procedure are contained in the kits and must be followed carefully. Known controls are also included to ensure accurate testing. To perform microbiologic procedures in the office, the following equipment is needed: a microscope, an incubator, a staining rack and materials, slides, culture media, inoculation loops, a Bunsen burner, and sterile supplies for specimen collection.

Preparation of Smears

A smear is made on a glass slide that is stained and examined under the microscope. A direct smear is made from a swab of the infected area; a culture smear is taken from a single cluster of organisms **(colony)** growing on a plate of solid media or in a tube of liquid broth, using a loop. The material must be applied thinly or the resulting smear is too thick to study under the microscope. Slides should be labeled before the infectious material is applied. This prevents possible incorrect labeling and contamination of hands with infectious organisms. Smears are dried, heat-fixed, and stained.

Staining

Most bacteria are so small and possess so little color that they are difficult to observe. Staining allows the microorganisms to be clearly seen under the microscope. The Gram stain is used most often. This staining procedure consists of applying a sequence of dye, **mordant,** decolorizer, and counterstain to the bacteria. The dyes are taken up differently according to the chemical composition of the cell walls. This serves to classify organisms according to their reactions to the stain and separates them into Gram-positive, which stain purple, and Gram-negative, which stain red.

Types of Media

A variety of growth media is available to promote the optimum growth of microorganisms. A growth medium may be liquid, semisolid, or solid. Liquid broth can be solidified by adding *agar,* a seaweed extract. The agar broth may come in tubes or plates, also called *Petri dishes.* Media can be *selective* or *nonselective.* Selective media allow the growth of specific bacteria while inhibiting the growth of others. *Eosin–methylene blue (EMB), MacConkey,* and *Thayer-Martin* are examples of selective media. Nonselective media support the growth of most bacteria. Generally, this medium is blood agar. This contains *sheep blood* and *tryptic soy broth (TSB).* These media have undergone extensive quality control testing for both sterility and appropriate reactions with certain organisms. An expiration date appears on each tube or plate. The used containers are autoclaved and then disposed.

Blood agar is used for performing throat cultures. The organism that causes strep throat *(Streptococcus)* is able to use the red blood cells in the agar for growth. This growth results in a detectable change in the medium called **hemolysis.** For urine cultures, two types of media are used: EMB or MacConkey and blood agar. The organism *Escherichia coli* is commonly isolated from urine.

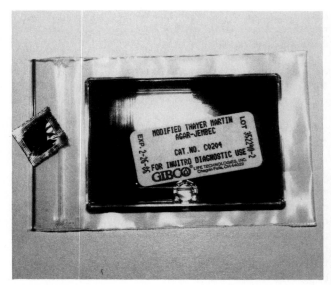

FIGURE 31–8. Transport plate of modified Thayer-Martin agar for growth of the organism that causes gonorrhea. The plate is inoculated with a swab and labeled, and the CO$_2$-generating tablet contained in the foil packet is placed in a well in the plate. The plate is sealed in the plastic pouch and kept in the incubator until picked up by the courier. (Courtesy of Life Technologies, Chagrin Falls, OH.)

Cultures

A culture is **inoculated** by passing a swab or loop lightly over the surface of an agar medium in a zigzag pattern. Broths are inoculated by swirling the swab or loop in them. The inoculated tubes or plates are incubated at 37°C for 24 hours and are then examined for growth.

Some organisms require a high concentration of carbon dioxide (CO$_2$) for growth. Transport plates of chocolate agar or Thayer-Martin agar have a CO$_2$-generating tablet that is placed in a well in the plate immediately after inoculation (Fig. 31–8). Without this special atmosphere, organisms such as the *Neisseria gonorrhoeae,* which causes gonorrhea, would die. Alternatively, the plate is placed in a sealed jar with a lighted candle. The burning of the candle generates CO$_2$.

Antimicrobial Sensitivity Testing

Isolating the infectious agent from a patient is only the first step in successful treatment. Most bacteria exhibit resistance to antimicrobial agents. These patterns of resistance are continuously changing; therefore, they cannot be predicted.

Shifting patterns of resistance require testing of individual bacteria against the appropriate antimicrobial agent.

The appropriate antimicrobial agent is the one:

- With the most activity against the infectious agent.
- That has the least toxicity to the patient.

- That has the least impact on the normal flora of the body.
- That has the desired pharmacologic characteristics.
- That is the most economical.

The clinical microbiology laboratory can only recommend antimicrobial agents based on their in vitro activity. The final therapeutic outcome is the decision of the physician. The physician bases this decision on numerous factors, including the test results, physical examination, and the knowledge of the patient. The expertise of a pharmacologist can be very helpful in choosing the most effective antimicrobial agent for the patient.

Procedures for Inoculating Specimens and Preparing and Examining Smears

Aseptic techniques must be strictly observed in the following procedures to ensure safety and good results.

PROCEDURE 31-4   INOCULATING A BLOOD AGAR PLATE FOR CULTURE OF STREP THROAT

GOAL   To inoculate a blood agar plate for culture of strep throat.

EQUIPMENT AND SUPPLIES

Blood agar plate
Bacitracin disk or strep A disk
Bunsen burner

Inoculating loop
Permanent marker
Swab from patient's throat
Forceps

PROCEDURAL STEPS

1. Wash and dry your hands. Follow the universal blood and body-fluid precautions. Glove yourself with nonsterile gloves.

2. Remove the swab from the container. Grasp the plate by the bottom (media side), and lift the cover, or lift the cover while the plate is on the table.
   Purpose: To make handling the plate easier and to prevent contamination of the plate.

3. Roll the swab down the middle of the top half of the plate, then use the swab to streak the same half of the plate. Dispose of the swab properly (Fig. 31-9, left).
   Purpose: Rolling the swab ensures contact with the surface of the agar.

4. Sterilize the loop in the Bacti-cinerator, and allow it to cool.
   Purpose: Loops must be sterilized before and after use, to prevent cross-contamination of specimens.

5. Streak for isolation of colonies in the third and fourth quadrants, using the loop. Use the loop to make three slices in the agar in the area of heavy inoculum. Sterilize the loop (Fig. 31-9).
   Purpose: Isolated colonies are needed for observation of colony morphology. The agar is sliced where the disk is to be placed, to allow for detection of subsurface hemolysis.

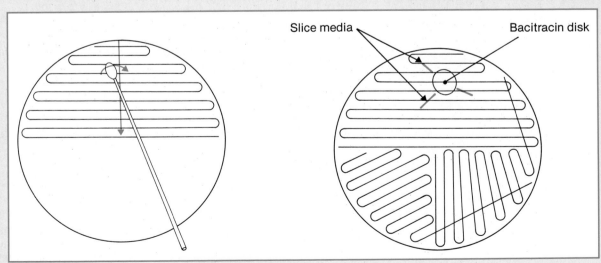

FIGURE 31-9.

Continued

PROCEDURE 31 – 4   *Continued*

6. Sterilize the forceps and remove one disk from the vial. Place the disk on the agar between the cuts. Sterilize the forceps.
   Purpose: Group A beta-hemolytic streptococci are presumptively identified by their sensitivity to the disk.

7. Label with permanent marker the agar side of the plate with the patient's name and identification number and the date.
   Purpose: Labeling the agar side of dish prevents mixing up specimens.

8. Place the plate in the incubator, with the agar side of the plate on the top.
   Purpose: Placing the plate with the agar side up prevents accumulation of moisture on the surface of the agar.

9. Record all information in the laboratory log and on the patient's chart.
   Purpose: Laboratories must keep records of all tests performed, and these tests are assigned an identifying accession number.

10. Incubate for 24 hours and then examine. Incubate negative cultures for an additional 24 hours.
    Purpose: Some hemolysis patterns are not well-defined after 24 hours of growth.

11. Clean the work area.

12. Wash your hands.

PROCEDURE 31 – 5   STREAKING PLATES FOR QUANTITATIVE CULTURES

GOAL To inoculate two plates with urine, using quantitative streaking methods.

EQUIPMENT AND SUPPLIES

Urine specimen
Bacti-cinerator
Calibrated inoculating loop

Blood agar plate or biplates, which are plates having both blood agar and either EMB or MacKintex in a single plate

PROCEDURAL STEPS

1. Wash and dry your hands. Follow the universal blood and body-fluid precautions. Glove yourself with nonsterile gloves.

2. Mix the urine specimen thoroughly by swirling.
   Purpose: Microorganisms settle to the bottom of the specimen when the specimen is allowed to stand.

3. Sterilize the calibrated loop, cool, and dip the tip into the specimen.
   Purpose: The loop must be allowed to cool, or the heat will destroy the microorganisms as the loop comes into contact with the urine specimen, resulting in falsely low colony counts on the culture. Urine on the shaft of the loop will run down the shaft and increase the size of the specimen deposited on the plate, resulting in a falsely elevated colony count on the culture.

Continued

4. Deposit the specimen on the plate, as indicated in Figure 31–10. Use the loop to streak as shown in Figure 31–10.
   Purpose: Careful streaking of the plates is necessary for an accurate estimate of the organisms present.

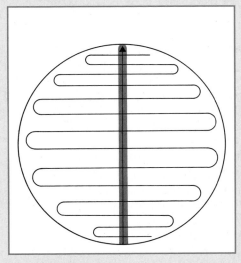

FIGURE 31–10.

5. Inoculate the second plate in the same manner.
6. Label the bottom of the plates with the patient's name and identification number, and the date.
   Purpose: Labeling the bottom of the plates prevents mixing up of the specimens.
7. Record all information in the laboratory log and on the patient's chart.
8. Place the plates in the incubator, with the agar sides of the plates facing up.
9. Incubate for 24 hours, then identify organisms.
10. Clean the work area.
11. Wash your hands.

PROCEDURE 31-6   PREPARING A DIRECT SMEAR OR CULTURE SMEAR FOR STAINING

GOAL   To prepare a smear for staining from a clinical specimen or from a culture medium.

EQUIPMENT AND SUPPLIES

Clean glass slides
Diamond-tip pen or permanent marker

Bacti-cinerator
Saline solution
Specimen

Continued

PROCEDURE 31 – 6   *Continued*

PROCEDURAL STEPS
DIRECT SMEAR

1. Wash and dry your hands. Follow the universal blood and body-fluid precautions. Glove yourself with nonsterile gloves.

2. Label the slide with a diamond-tip pen.
   Purpose: Other labels are destroyed in the staining process.

3. Prepare a thin smear by rolling the swab on the slide. Make certain that all areas of the swab touch the slide (Fig. 31 – 11).
   Purpose: Rolling the swab ensures that all parts of the swab come in contact with the slide so that the organisms collected are deposited on the slide. Thin smears are needed for evaluation.

4. Allow the smear to air-dry. Do not wave it or heat-dry it.
   Purpose: Waving the slide spreads pathogens. Overheating organisms distorts them.

5. Hold the slide with the smear up. Heat-fix the slide using a Bacti-cinerator. Check the heating process by touching the slide to the back of the hand (Fig. 31 – 12). The slide should feel warm, not hot. Check it often by touching the back of the slide to the back of the hand. Cool the slide.
   Purpose: Heat-fixing causes materials to adhere to the slide.

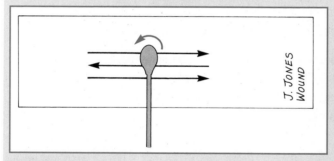

FIGURE 31 – 11.

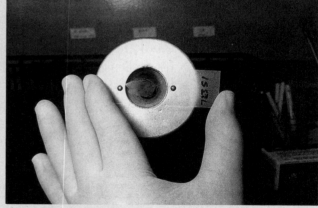

FIGURE 31 – 12.

CULTURE SMEAR

1. Wash and dry your hands. Follow the universal blood and body-fluid precautions. Glove yourself with nonsterile gloves.

2. Identify the colonies to be stained by circling them on the back of the plate and numbering them with a permanent marker. Label the slide accordingly (Fig. 31 – 13, left).
   Purpose: This allows accurate identification of colonies.

3. Apply a small drop of saline solution to the slide, using a loop.
   Purpose: Liquid is needed to emulsify the colony. Large drops require a longer drying time.

Continued

4. Touch, with a sterile loop, only the top of the colony chosen. Transfer the material picked up to the appropriate area of the slide, and spread it in a circular motion to the size of a dime. Repeat for each colony chosen (Fig. 31–13, right).
Purpose: Only a small amount of colony is needed for staining.

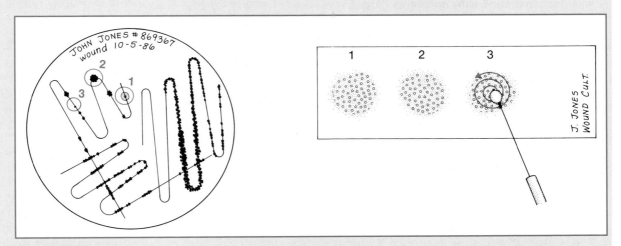

FIGURE 31–13.

5. Allow the smear to air-dry.
6. Heat-fix the smear.
7. Clean the work area.
8. Wash your hands.

PROCEDURE 31–7   STAINING A SMEAR WITH GRAM STAIN

GOAL To stain a slide, using Gram stain, so that the organisms present are colored appropriately (neither overcolorized nor too strongly decolorized).

EQUIPMENT AND SUPPLIES

Gram stain reagents
Staining rack
Forceps

Wash bottle of water
Prepared smear for staining
Absorbent paper

Continued

PROCEDURE 31-7 *Continued*

PROCEDURAL STEPS

1. Wash and dry your hands. Follow the universal blood and body-fluid precautions. Glove yourself with nonsterile gloves.

2. Place the slide face up on a level staining rack.
    Purpose: If the slide is face down, the organisms will not be stained. If the rack is uneven, the stain will run off the slide surface.

3. Flood the slide with *crystal violet.* Time for 30 seconds. Figure 31-14 shows the entire staining process.
    Purpose: Crystal violet is the primary stain and colors everything purple.

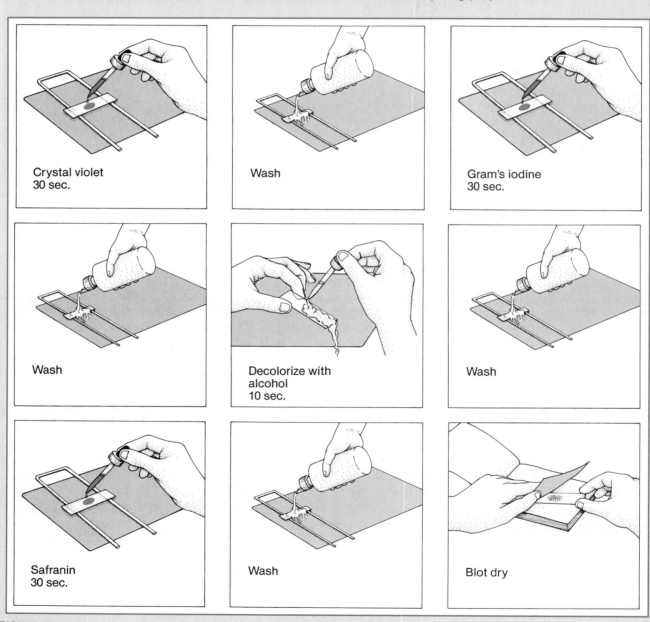

Crystal violet
30 sec.

Wash

Gram's iodine
30 sec.

Wash

Decolorize with
alcohol
10 sec.

Wash

Safranin
30 sec.

Wash

Blot dry

FIGURE 31-14.

Continued

4. Flood the stain off with a sharp stream of water from the wash bottle. With forceps, tip the slide to remove the water.
   Purpose: Using forceps keeps your fingers clean.

5. Flood the slide with *Gram's iodine* (mordant). Time for 30 seconds.
   Purpose: Gram's iodine causes the stain to set in the organisms that are Gram-positive.

6. Flood the iodine off with water. Grasp the slide with forceps, and hold it nearly vertical.

7. Decolorize by running the *decolorizer* (alcohol) down the slide until the smear stops giving off purple stain in all but the thickest portions (about 10 seconds).
   Purpose: This is the critical step. The decolorizer removes stain from the organisms that are Gram-negative.

8. Rinse the slide with water, and return it to the staining rack.

9. Flood the slide with *safranin,* and time for 30 seconds.
   Purpose: Safranin is the counterstain and stains red everything that decolorized.

10. Rinse the slide well with water.

11. Wipe off the back of the slide with an alcohol tissue.
    Purpose: The back of the slide is cleaned to remove traces of stain, which make examination of the smear difficult.

12. Blot the slide dry between sheets of absorbent paper.

13. Clean the work area.

14. Wash your hands.

Slide Agglutination Test

The procedure for performing the *Mono-Test* (Wampole Laboratories, Cranbury, NJ) for infectious mononucleosis is included here because it is performed routinely in many small laboratories. The kit contains all the supplies and reagents needed (Fig. 31–15).

The test is an example of **agglutination** reactions found in many testing procedures. In agglutination tests, antigen-coated red cells (or latex particles) and **antibodies** are combined in a test tube or on slides. The test suspension is rocked for a specified amount of time and is observed for the presence of clumping. The visible clumps indicate a positive test. Known positive and negative controls are run at the same time as the patient's sample.

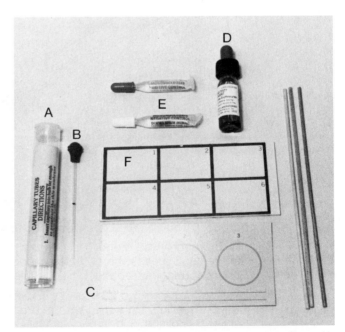

FIGURE 31–15. Materials contained in a Mono-Test kit. *A,* Disposable capillary pipettes; *B,* reusable bulb; *C,* reusable glass slide; *D,* Mono-Test reagent; *E,* positive and negative controls; *F,* disposable cardboard slide. (Trademark of Wampole Laboratories, a division of Carter-Wallace, Inc., Cranbury, NJ.)

PROCEDURE 31-8   MONO-TEST FOR INFECTIOUS MONONUCLEOSIS

GOAL To perform and interpret a slide test for infectious mononucleosis.

EQUIPMENT AND SUPPLIES

Mono-test kit
Blood specimen (serum or plasma)

PROCEDURAL STEPS

1. Wash and dry your hands. Follow the universal blood and body-fluid precautions. Glove yourself with nonsterile gloves.

2. Remove the test kit from the refrigerator, and allow the reagents to warm to room temperature. Check the expiration date of the kit.
   Purpose: Outdated or cold reagents do not react as expected.

3. Fill a disposable capillary tube to the calibration mark with serum or plasma (see Chapter 33 for collection of blood). Using the rubber bulb included in the kit, deposit the specimen in the middle circle of the clean glass slide also provided in the kit (Fig. 31–16).
   Purpose: The capillary tube measures the exact amount of sample for accurate testing.

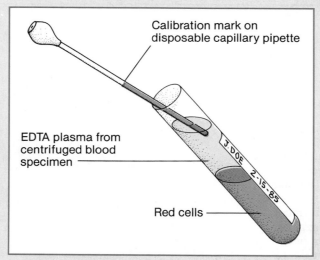

Calibration mark on disposable capillary pipette

EDTA plasma from centrifuged blood specimen

Red cells

FIGURE 31-16.

4. Place one drop of negative control in the right circle and one drop of positive control in the left circle.
   Purpose: Known controls ensure that reagents are functioning properly.

5. Mix thoroughly the Mono-Test reagent by rolling the bottle gently between the palms of the hands. Squeeze the enclosed dropper to mix all the contents of the bottle.
   Purpose: Reagent red blood cells settle on standing and must be mixed before use.

6. Hold the dropper in a vertical position, and add one drop of Mono-Test reagent to each area of the slide. Do not touch the dropper to the slide.
   Purpose: Holding a dropper vertically ensures delivery of the same size drop. If the dropper touches other materials, it becomes contaminated, and results will be inaccurate.

Continued

7. Using separate stirrers, quickly and thoroughly mix each area, spreading each area out to 1 inch in diameter (Fig. 31–17).
   Purpose: Failure to use a clean stirrer for each area would invalidate the test because of cross-contamination.

8. Rock the slide gently for exactly 2 minutes; observe immediately for agglutination. A dark background is best for viewing.
   Purpose: Timing is always important.

9. Interpret the test results, and record them. Agglutination is positive, and no agglutination is negative (Fig. 31–18).

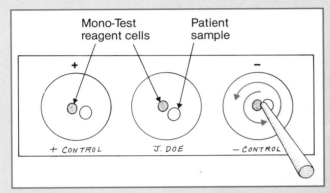

FIGURE 31–17.

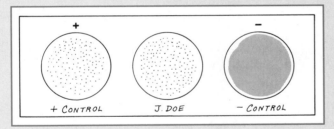

FIGURE 31–18.

10. Clean the work area.

11. Wash your hands.

Rapid Culture Methods

Several companies manufacture rapid culture methods designed for use in small laboratories. The tests selected depend upon the number of tests performed per month and the amount of refrigerator space available for storage. Dry media such as *Microstix-3* for urine culture plus nitrite testing, and *Biocult GC,* for gonorrhea (both produced by Ames Company), and *Bacturcult,* for urine (Wampole Laboratories, Cranbury, NJ), have a long shelf life,

do not require refrigeration, and occupy little incubator space (Fig. 31–19A and B). *Respirastick,* for strep screening, and *Uricult,* for urine culture (both produced by Medical Technology Corporation), are small, screw-top vials containing media on paddles (Fig. 31–19C). The vials are self-standing for growth in any conventional incubator and do not require refrigeration before use. *Isocult* systems (SmithKline Diagnostics, Sunnyvale, CA) offer tests for strep screening; urine culture; and yeast, gonococcus, and *Trichomonas* culturing. The long plastic

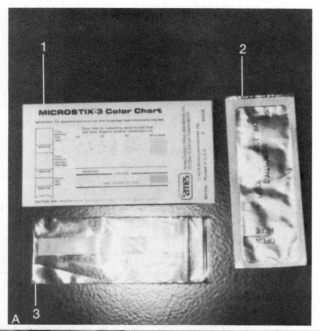

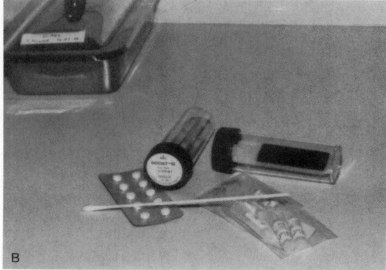

FIGURE 31–19. *A,* Microstix-3 urine culture kit. *1,* Color chart for the interpretation of the nitrite test and bacterial colony count; *2,* Microstix-3 foil packet; *3,* Microstix-3 in incubation pouch. *B,* Biocult GC for the detection of gonorrhea.

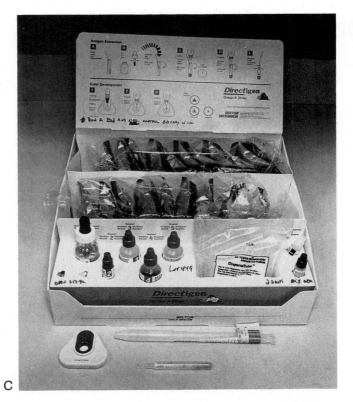

C

FIGURE 31–19. *Continued C,* Directigen Group A Strep System used as rapid method for identifying streptococci. (Courtesy of Becton Dickenson Microbiology Systems, Cockeysville, MD.).

containers can be used in their own incubator or in a conventional incubator. They must be refrigerated before use. The rapid culture methods offer only presumptive identification of most organisms. Further specialization and sensitivity testing require additional materials and procedures.

Interpretation of Throat Culture

Group A beta-hemolytic streptococci (Streptococcus pyogenes) cause septic sore throat and are capable of producing severe complications if not diagnosed and treated. Complications include scarlet fever, rheumatic fever, and glomerulonephritis. Group A beta-hemolytic streptococci may be identified by placing an antibiotic disk, bacitracin, on a streaked plate and observing inhibition of any bacterial growth after 24 hours of incubation (Fig. 31–20). Complete clearing of the agar around the colonies indicates beta-hemolysis.

Several slide and tube tests have been developed for the detection of group A streptococci directly from throat cultures. The tests can be performed while the patient waits. The patient's throat is swabbed, the swab is placed in a tube, reagents are added at timed intervals, and a liquid extract is expressed from the swab onto a slide. Reagents are added and mixed. The slide is gently rocked and then examined for agglutination after a specified time. Agglutination indicates the presence of group A streptococci. The entire procedure can be performed in less than 15 minutes.

A color-change tube test (Ventrescreen, Ventrex Laboratories, Hybritech Incorporated, San Diego, CA) for group A streptococci identification directly from a throat swab is also available. The swab is placed in a coated test tube, and extraction reagents are added at timed intervals. The tube is incubated, washed five times with water, and a color reagent is added. Any blue color developing within 2 minutes is a positive test.

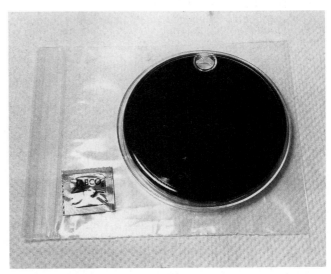

FIGURE 31–20. Bacterial growth after 24 h of incubation. Note clearing indicating beta-hemolysis.

These tests are available in kits that contain all the needed supplies. Performance should be checked routinely using known controls.

LEGAL AND ETHICAL RESPONSIBILITIES

Maintaining a laboratory in the office increases the physician's liability. By testing patients' specimens in the office, the physician assumes responsibility for the interpretation and accuracy of the results. As the person in the office who runs the tests and notes the results on the patient's chart, it is your responsibility to maintain optimal accuracy in the testing results. A *quality assurance* (QA) program for *physicians' office laboratories* (POL) may reduce the risks involved and still allow the patient to benefit from the convenience of office testing.

QA is being mandated by the government, and pressures are increasing to control POLs. Upon implementation of the Clinical Laboratory Improvement Amendment of 1988 (CLIA 88), all laboratories are required to participate in a recognized proficiency testing program for laboratory tests performed. POLs that have established QA programs, with written policies and procedures that govern their laboratory testing and ensure that these policies are implemented, are in compliance. If the office where you are employed does not have laboratory guidelines, suggest developing testing guidelines. The following programs are available for information and assistance:

- American Association of Bioanalysts (AAB): AAB Proficiency Testing Service
- American Academy of Family Physicians (AAFP): AAFP-PT
- American Society of Internal Medicine (ASIM): Medical Laboratory Evaluation (MLE)
- College of American Pathologists (CAP): External Comparative Evaluation for Laboratories (EXCEL)

▶ PATIENT EDUCATION

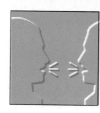

Microorganisms such as bacteria, viruses, fungi, and parasites are responsible for most human diseases. Patient education plays an important role in helping the patient and the patient's family to control the spread of infection.

The following is a list of teaching topics that will help you in educating the patient in infection control:

- An explanation of the patient's type of infection—bacterial, viral, fungal, or parasitic
- How infection spreads
- Normal barriers to infection
- Risk factors for infection
- Preparation for cultures and serologic, hematologic, and imaging tests, as necessary
- The patient's role in specimen collection
- Self-care measures, such as applying dry dressings and using mouthwashes and gargles
- Hand washing, proper storage and cleaning of personal items, and disposal of contaminated supplies

Explain to the patient that infection does not always occur at the entry site; for example, measles can be transmitted through the respiratory tract or through the conjunctivae by touching an affected patient and then rubbing the eye.

Reinforce the need for strict adherence to the prescribed antimicrobial therapy by pointing out the possible complications of noncompliance, such as relapse or systemic involvement. Explain to the patient that inadequate drug therapy (not taking the medication as prescribed) may cause the infection to worsen and spread.

Above all, always listen to the patient; be sure that the questions asked are answered. Don't try to answer questions that you are unsure of. Notify the physician of the patient's concerns so that the doctor can include the answers and explanations in the patient's consultation.

▶ LEARNING ACHIEVEMENTS

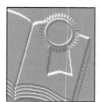

Upon completion of this chapter, can you in the time allowed by your evaluator:

1. Focus a microscope under low power, high power, and oil immersion?
2. Collect a throat culture and prepare it for immediate examination?
3. Collect a throat culture and prepare it for transportation to a laboratory?
4. Perform an occult blood test on a stool specimen?
5. Inoculate media for cultures?
6. Prepare a direct smear from a culture?
7. Prepare an indirect smear from a culture?
8. Examine a stained smear for microorganisms?
9. Perform a slide agglutination test for infectious mononucleosis?

REFERENCES AND READINGS

Ames Company: *Modern Urinary Chemistry, A Guide to the Diagnosis of Urinary Tract Diseases and Metabolic Disorders.* Revised Reprint. Elhart Indiana, 1992.

Bonewit, K.: *Clinical Procedures for Medical Assistants,* 3rd ed., Philadelphia, W.B. Saunders Co., 1990.

Calbreath, D.F.: *Clinical Chemistry,* Philadelphia, W.B. Saunders Co., 1992.

Feingold, S.M., and Baron, E.J.: *Bailey and Scott's Diagnostic Microbiology,* St. Louis, C.V. Mosby Co., 1986.

Henry, J.B.: *Clinical Diagnosis and Management by Laboratory Methods,* 18th ed., Philadelphia, W.B. Saunders Co., 1991.

Wedding, M.E., and Toenjes, S.A.: *Medical Laboratory Procedures,* Philadelphia, F.A. Davis Co., 1992.

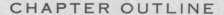

CHAPTER OUTLINE

VOCABULARY

anuria Complete suppression of urine formation by the kidney.

catheterization The insertion of a tube through the urethra and into the urinary bladder to withdraw urine from the bladder.

casts Fibrous or protein materials that are thrown off into the urine in kidney disease.

enzymatic reaction A chemical reaction controlled by an enzyme.

glycosuria The presence of glucose in the urine.

hematuria The presence of blood in the urine.

human chorionic gonadotropin (HCG) a hormone secreted in large amounts by the placenta during gestation to stimulate the formation of interstitial cells.

ischemia Decreased bloodflow to a body part or organ, caused by constriction or plugging of the supplying artery.

myoglobinuria Abnormal presence of a hemoglobin-like chemical of muscle tissue in urine, which results in muscle deterioration.

nosocomial Pertaining to or originating in a hospital.

phenylalanine An essential amino acid found in milk, eggs, and other foods.

proteinuria An excess of serum protein in the urine.

residual Urine left in the bladder after urination.

void Same as urinate.

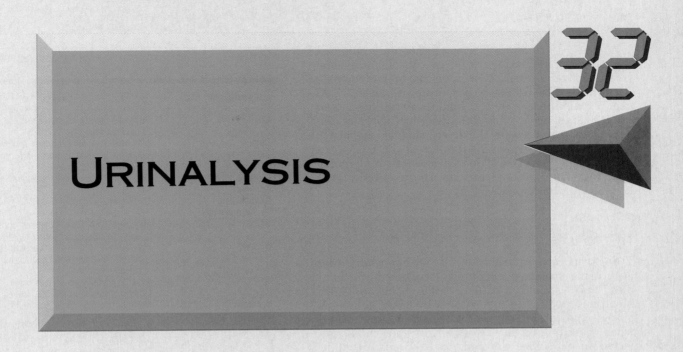

URINALYSIS

LEARNING OBJECTIVES

COGNITIVE

Upon completion of this chapter, you should be able to:

1. Define and spell the words in the Vocabulary.
2. State seven types of urine specimens used.
3. Discuss reasons for catheterization.
4. Describe the physiology of urine formation.
5. Describe the tests in the physical examination of urine.
6. Describe the tests in the chemical examination of urine.
7. List five materials found in urine sediment microscopically.
8. Define urinary quality control.

PERFORMANCE

Upon successful completion of this chapter, you should be able to perform the following activities:

1. Instruct a patient in the collection of a timed urine specimen.
2. Instruct a patient in the collection of a clean-catch midstream urine specimen.
3. Perform a complete urinalysis.
4. Perform a macroscopic quality control on urine.
5. Demonstrate glucose testing using the Clinitest method.
6. Demonstrate the use of precipitation testing for protein in urine.
7. Describe the proper usage and care of testing equipment.
8. Demonstrate the methods of pregnancy testing.

A routine *urinalysis* is one of the more common laboratory examinations used in the diagnosis and treatment of disease. It can be easily and quickly performed. The results of a routine urinalysis (UA) can reveal diseases of the bladder or kidneys, systemic metabolic or endocrine disorders such as diabetes, and diseases of the liver, such as hepatitis, cirrhosis, or obstruction of the bile ducts. Urinalysis is routinely performed on all patients undergoing physical examinations and on those entering the hospital for treatment.

COLLECTING URINE SPECIMENS

For accurate information, it is important that each urine specimen be properly collected and handled. You should routinely follow the universal blood and body-fluid precautions by using nonsterile gloves and other appropriate barrier precautions when handling urine. Most urine specimens collected in the office are *random specimens,* that is, collected at different times during the day. Since the makeup of urine changes constantly, depending on a person's activity, random specimens are used only for routine screening and initial evaluation.

First morning specimens are preferred as they are usually the most concentrated. They are best for pregnancy testing, culturing, and microscopic examination. *Timed specimens* are submitted when more specific information is needed for proper diagnosis. *Two-hour postprandial urine specimens,* collected 2 hours after a meal, are used in diabetic screening and for home diabetic-testing programs. *Twenty-four-hour urine specimens* are collected over a period of 24 hours to give quantitative chemical analyses, such as hormone levels and creatinine clearance rates (a procedure for evaluating the glomerular filtration rate of the kidneys).

Proper handling of specimens is essential. The chemical and cellular components of urine change if they are allowed to stand at room temperature (Table 32–1). These changes can be avoided by refrigerating the specimen if the analysis cannot be performed within 30 minutes after collection. Occasionally, preservatives must be added.

Routine (random) specimens are collected in nonsterile disposable containers. The container is always labeled with the patient's name before it is given to the patient to use.

A clean-catch midstream specimen may be ordered when the urine is to be cultured or examined for microorganisms. The purposes of the clean-catch are to remove microorganisms from the urinary meatus by thoroughly cleansing the area around the meatus and to flush out the distal portion of the urethra. Since the specimen is collected in the medical office by the patient, the medical assistant needs to give complete, understandable instructions to the patient on the method of collection. Failure to do so may mean that the patient will have to

TABLE 32–1. CHANGES IN URINE AT ROOM TEMPERATURE

Constituent	Change
Clarity	Becomes cloudy as crystals precipitate and bacteria multiply
Color	May change if pH becomes alkaline
pH	Becomes alkaline as bacteria form ammonia from urea
Glucose	Decreases as bacteria metabolize it
Ketones	Decrease
Bilirubin and urobilinogen	Undergo degradation in light
Blood	May hemolyze. False-positives possible due to bacterial peroxidase
Nitrite	May become positive as bacteria convert nitrate. Can become negative as bacteria metabolize nitrite.
Casts	Lyse or dissolve in alkaline urine
Cells	Lyse or dissolve in alkaline urine
Bacteria	Multiply twofold every 20 minutes
Yeast	Multiply
Crystals	Precipitate as urine cools. May dissolve if pH changes

return to the office to allow the collection of another specimen. Once the specimen has been collected, it should be tested immediately. If this cannot be done, the specimen should be refrigerated, or a preservative should be added to the specimen. For culturing, urine should be collected by catheterization or the clean-catch method into a sterile container.

Catheterization

Catheterization is the introduction of a catheter through the urethra into the bladder for the purpose of withdrawing urine. A *catheter* is a tube used to inject or remove body fluids. The following are common reasons for performing a urinary catheterization:

- To relieve urinary retention
- To obtain a sterile urine specimen from a woman
- To measure the amount of **residual** urine in the bladder: The patient is first asked to **void** and is then catheterized to determine how much urine stays in the bladder after normal voiding. An amount over 50 ml is considered abnormal.
- To obtain a urine specimen when it cannot be secured satisfactorily by other means
- To empty the bladder before and during surgery and before certain diagnostic examinations

In recent years, the value of catheterization has become increasingly suspect in view of the hazards involved. It is now considered the most prominent cause of **nosocomial** infections. Therefore, whenever possible, it is recommended that catheterization be avoided. When deemed necessary, it should be performed with careful technique by a fully trained and competent technician. In some states, the medical assistant cannot perform catheterization. Be sure to check your state guidelines regarding the training and the legality of performance.

Pediatric specimens are more difficult to collect. A sterile pouch is taped to the cleansed perineum or around the penis (Fig. 32–1). The infant may be coaxed into urinating by placing its feet in cool water.

Instructing Patients to Collect a Urine Specimen

Most patients understand the procedure for collecting a routine (random) urine specimen. However, they do need special instructions for collecting a timed specimen and a midstream clean-catch specimen. The following set of instructions is to help you teach patients how to collect urine specimens.

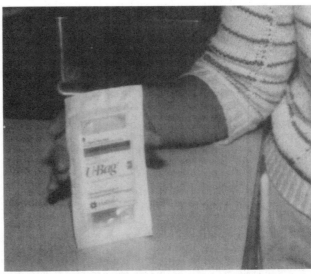

FIGURE 32–1. Sterile pouch for the collection of pediatric specimens. The pouch is taped to the cleansed genital area. Urination is stimulated by placing the infant's feet in cool water. The specimen is emptied into a container by removing a tape plug and allowing the urine to drain. This prevents contamination of the specimen by organisms that may be adhering to the taped opening of the pouch.

PATIENT INSTRUCTIONS FOR OBTAINING A URINE SPECIMEN

1. Upon arising in the morning, urinate into the toilet. Empty your bladder completely. Do not save this urine. Note exact time, and write it down on the container.

2. Collect all urine voided after this time for exactly 24 hours. Remember that all urine passed at night or during the day in this time period must be saved.

3. Remember to keep the urine cool.

4. At exactly the same time the following morning, urinate completely again. Save this sample. Add it to the collection container. This completes your 24-hour collection.

5. Take all specimens from the 24-hour collection to the medical office, or to the place designated, as soon as possible, maintaining the cool temperature in transit by placing the specimen in a portable cooler or insulated bag.

PATIENT INSTRUCTIONS FOR OBTAINING A CLEAN-CATCH MIDSTREAM SPECIMEN

FEMALE PATIENT

1. Wash hands and remove underclothing.

2. Expose the urinary meatus by spreading apart the labia with one hand.

---

3. Cleanse each side of the urinary meatus with a front-to-back motion, from the pubis to the anus. Use a fresh cotton ball on each side. (If the midstream specimen kit is used, an antiseptic wipe is provided to cleanse each side of the meatus.)

4. Cleanse directly across the meatus, front-to-back, using a third cotton ball or antiseptic wipe.

5. Rinse with water to remove traces of the soap used to prevent its entrance into the specimen.

6. Dry the area with a clean cotton ball using front-to-back motion. If a midstream kit has been used, the rinsing and drying procedure can be omitted.

7. Hold the labia apart throughout this procedure.

8. Void a small amount of urine into the toilet.

9. Move the specimen container into position and void the next portion of urine into it. Remember this is a sterile container. Do not put your fingers on the inside of the container.

10. Remove the cup and void the last amount of urine into the toilet. (This means that the first part and the last part of the urinary flow have been excluded from the specimen. Only the middle portion of the flow is included.)

11. Wipe in your usual manner, redress as needed, and return the sterile specimen to the place designated by the medical facility.

MALE PATIENT

1. Wash hands and remove underclothing.

2. Retract the foreskin of the penis (if not circumcised).

3. Cleanse the area around the glans penis (meatus) and the urethral opening by washing each side of the glans with a separate cotton ball. If a midstream kit is used, antiseptic wipes are provided.

4. Cleanse directly across the urethral opening using a third cotton ball or antiseptic wipe.

5. If soap and cotton balls are used, rinse with water to remove all traces of soap.

6. Dry the area using a front-to-back motion.

7. Void a small amount of urine into the toilet or urinal.

8. Collect the next portion of the urine in the *sterile* container without touching the inside of the container with hands or penis.

9. Void the last amount of urine into the toilet or urinal.

10. Wipe and redress as usual.

11. Return the specimen to the designated area provided.

GUIDELINES FOR CARING FOR A URINE SPECIMEN

- Do not add anything but your urine into the bottle.

- Do not pour out any liquid or powdered preservative from the container.

- If you accidentally spill some of the preservative on you, immediately wash with water and call the testing center or designated laboratory.

- Always keep the collection bottle refrigerated or cool. Refrigerate or keep in an ice-filled cooler or pail.

- Keep the cap on the container.

- You may find it more convenient to urinate into the smaller container provided, and then pour the urine into the larger collection bottle.

PHYSIOLOGY OF URINE FORMATION

To understand the meaning of urinalysis results, it is necessary to have a general understanding of the physiology of urine formation and the normal components of urine. Normal body functions and good health depend on homeostasis. Various organ systems supply the body cells with substances, such as oxygen and nutrients needed for metabolism, and help eliminate the waste products of metabolism, such as carbon dioxide. To function normally, body cells need more than a supply of nutrients and the elimination of waste products. Cells need to exist in a stable internal environment, where the composition of the extracellular fluids is constant. The urinary system functions to maintain this composition and, thus, the physiochemical properties of the internal environment.

The urinary tract is composed of paired kidneys located behind the peritoneum, on either side of the lumbar spine. Each drains through a ureter into the bladder. Urine is stored in the bladder until *micturition,* or voiding, when it passes out of the body through the urethra.

Inside each kidney are millions of nephrons, the functional unit of urine formation. In the nephron, blood from the body passes through the afferent arteriole and enters the glomerulus, where the first step of urine formation, called filtration, occurs. Water and dissolved chemicals in plasma filter through the glomerulus into Bowman's capsule. Normally, platelets, cells, and larger molecules, such as protein and certain drugs, do not pass across the glomerular membrane and are not found in the filtrate.

As the filtrate passes through the proximal convoluted tubule, loop of Henle, and distal convoluted tubule, reabsorption of needed chemical substances such as glucose, secretion of excess chemicals, and concentration of the filtrate occur to form urine.

Normally, water constitutes about 95% of urine. The other 5% includes dissolved chemicals such as urea, uric acid, creatinine, sodium chloride, calcium, sulfates, phosphates, hydrogen ions, and urochrome. The proportion of water and chemicals varies greatly, depending on the time of day, diet, metabolism, hormones, fluid intake, and nonurine fluid loss. Disease states alter urine volume and change physical, chemical, and microscopic constituents.

A urinalysis consists of a physical, chemical, and microscopic examination. Deviation from normal in any of these three areas assists the physician in the diagnosis and assessment of the patient's condition and treatment regimen.

PHYSICAL EXAMINATION OF URINE

The first part of a complete urinalysis is the assessment of the physical properties and the measurement of selected chemical constituents of diagnostic importance (Table 32–2).

Color and Turbidity

Normal urine color is a shade of yellow ranging from pale straw to yellow to amber. Color depends on the concentration of the pigment *urochrome* and the amount of water in the specimen. A dilute specimen should be pale, and a more concentrated specimen should be a darker yellow. Variations in color may be caused by diet, medication, and disease. Abnormal colors may be pathologic or nonpathologic (Table 32–3).

Both normal and abnormal urine specimens may range in appearance from clear to very cloudy. Cloudiness may be caused by cells, bacteria, yeast, vaginal contaminants, or crystals. Often, a urine specimen that was clear when voided will become cloudy as it cools when crystals form and precipitate.

Volume

The amount of urine is rarely measured on a random specimen. With a timed specimen, volume is

TABLE 32–3. URINE COLORS

Color	Pathologic Cause	Nonpathologic Cause
Straw	Diabetes	Diuretics; high fluid intake (coffee, beer)
Amber	Dehydration	Excessive sweating; low fluid intake
Bright yellow		Carotene, vitamins
Red	Blood, porphyrins	Beets, drugs, dyes
Orange-yellow	Bile, hepatitis	Pyridium (phenazopyridine hydrochloride), dyes, drugs
Greenish yellow	Bile, hepatitis	Senna, cascara, rhubarb
Reddish brown	Old blood, methemoglobin	
Brownish black	Methemoglobin, melanin	Levodopa
Salmon pink		Amorphous urates
White (milky)	Fats, pus	Amorphous phosphates
Blue-green	Biliverdin, infection with *Pseudomonas*	Vitamin B, drugs, dyes

measured by pouring the entire collection into a large graduated cylinder. Generally, it is not accurate enough to use the markings on the side of the collection container. Once the volume is measured and recorded, a portion of well-mixed specimen, called an *aliquot,* is removed for testing. The remainder is discarded or stored, depending on the preference of the laboratory.

The normal volume of urine produced every 24 hours varies according to the age of the individual. Infants and children produce smaller volumes than adults. The normal adult volume is 750 to 2000 ml in 24 hours, with an average of about 1500 ml. Excessive production of urine is called *polyuria.* It is common in diabetes and certain kidney disorders. *Oliguria* is insufficient production of urine and can be caused by dehydration, decreased fluid intake, shock, or renal disease. The absence of urine production, **anuria,** occurs in renal obstruction and renal failure.

Foam

Normally, the presence of foam is not recorded, but careful observation of this property can be a significant clue to an abnormality. White foam can indicate increased protein. Yellow foam can mean bilirubinuria. Foam is the presence of small bubbles that persist for a long time after the specimen has been shaken; they must not be confused with bubbles that rapidly disperse.

TABLE 32–2. COMPONENTS OF THE MACROSCOPIC URINALYSIS

Physical Property	Chemical Property Measured by Dipsticks
Color	Protein
Clarity	Glucose
Specific gravity	Ketones
Amount*	Bilirubin
Odor*	Blood: intact RBCs, hemoglobin, myoglobin
Foam*	Nitrite
	Urobilinogen
	Leukocyte esterase
	Specific gravity†
	pH†

* Not always assessed.
† Physical properties measured on dipsticks.

PROCEDURE 32-1   ASSESSING URINE FOR COLOR AND TURBIDITY

GOAL   To assess and record the color and clarity of a urine specimen.

EQUIPMENT AND SUPPLIES

Blood and body-fluid protection barriers   Urine specimen
Nonsterile gloves   Centrifuge tube

PROCEDURAL STEPS

1. Wash and dry your hands. Follow the universal blood and body-fluid precautions. Glove yourself with nonsterile gloves.

2. Mix the urine by swirling.
   Purpose: Suspended substances settle when urine stands. If urine is not mixed prior to assessing appearance, the finding will be incorrect.

3. Label a centrifuge tube if a complete urinalysis is being done.
   Purpose: If a complete urinalysis is being done, a portion of the specimen will be centrifuged for microscopic examination. The centrifuged specimen must be labeled to avoid specimen confusion.

4. Pour the specimen into a standard-size centrifuge tube.
   Purpose: Standard-size containers are a better quality control for assessing color and clarity results.

5. Assess and record the color (see Table 32–3):
   Pale straw
   Yellow
   Dark yellow
   Amber

6. Assess and record clarity:
   Clear—No cloudiness
   Slightly cloudy—Can see light print through tube
   Moderately cloudy—Can see only dark print through tube
   Very cloudy—Cannot see through tube

7. Clean the work area.

8. Wash your hands.

Odor

Like foam, odor is not normally recorded but can be an important clue. Normal urine odor is said to be aromatic. Changes in the odor of urine may be due to disease, the presence of bacteria, or diet. The odor of the urine of a patient with uncontrolled diabetes is described as fruity because of the presence of ketones, which are the products of fat metabolism. An ammonia smell in the urine can be due to an infection. The bacteria break down the urea in the urine to form ammonia. Infection usually imparts a putrid odor. Foods such as asparagus and garlic can also produce an abnormal odor in the urine.

Specific Gravity

Specific gravity (SG, or sp gr) is the weight of a substance compared with the weight of an equal volume of distilled water. In urinalysis, it is the rough measurement of the concentration, or amount, of substances dissolved in urine. The spe-

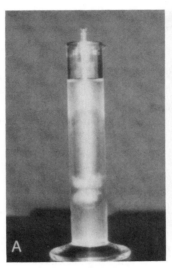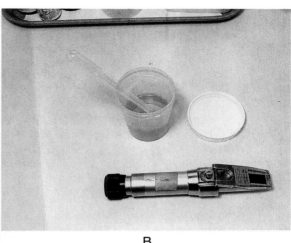

FIGURE 32-2. *A*, A urinometer floating in a clear glass cylinder. The specific gravity reading is taken on the stem of the urinometer as it slowly turns in the specimen. *B*, A refractometer is filled with a drop of the urine, the hinged lid is closed, and the specific gravity is read by reading the scale inside of eye piece.

cific gravity of distilled water is 1.000. Normal specific gravity of urine ranges from 1.005 to 1.030, depending on the fluid intake of the patient. Most samples fall between 1.010 and 1.025. Urine specific gravity indicates whether or not the kidneys are able to concentrate the urine and is one of the first indications of kidney disease. The presence of glucose, protein, or x-ray contrast media used in diagnostic studies may also increase the specific gravity of urine. To measure the specific gravity of urine, laboratories use dipstick, urinometer, or refractometer methods.

The *urinometer* is a sealed glass float with a calibrated paper scale in its stem (Fig. 32-2A). With a slight spinning motion, it is placed into a cylinder containing a urine sample, and the value is read at the meniscus of the urine. It requires a quantity of

urine sufficient to freely suspend the float, usually around 20 to 25 ml. If the sample is insufficient to float the urinometer, use a refractometer (see following) or record as QNS (quantity not sufficient).

The urinometer is fragile, and jarring can cause the paper scale in the stem to shift, resulting in erroneous readings. Occasionally, a damaged urinometer loses its calibration. Thus, the calibration of the urinometer should be checked daily with distilled water. The specific gravity of the distilled water should calibrate at 1.000 at 20°C (room temperature). (For example, if the urinometer reads 1.002 in distilled water, 0.002 must be subtracted from the urine readings. However, it is better to replace the instrument.) For each 3°C that the water temperature measures above 20°C, 0.001 must be added to the reading. For each 3°C that the

---

PROCEDURE 32-2   MEASURING SPECIFIC GRAVITY USING A URINOMETER

GOAL   To calibrate the urinometer to perform a quality control check and to obtain duplicate specific gravity readings.

EQUIPMENT AND SUPPLIES

   Blood and body-fluid protection barriers   Distilled water
Nonsterile gloves   Urinometer and cylinder
Urine specimen

PROCEDURAL STEPS

CALIBRATION

1. Wash and dry your hands. Follow the universal blood and body-fluid precautions. Glove yourself with nonsterile gloves.

Continued

PROCEDURE 32-2   *Continued*

2. Fill the glass cylinder two-thirds full with distilled water at 20°C (room temperature).
    Purpose: A quantity of 20 to 25 ml is needed to allow the urinometer to float.

3. Read the specific gravity of the distilled water.
    Purpose: If the urinometer does not read 1.000, a correction factor or a new urinometer is necessary.

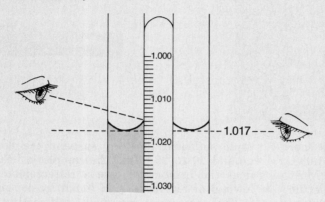

FOR CLOUDY URINE:
1. Read at top of meniscus
2. Add 0.002 to reading
   1.015
 + .002
   1.017

FOR CLEAR URINE:
Read at bottom of
meniscus at eye level

FIGURE 32-3.

SPECIMEN

1. Wash and dry your hands. Follow universal blood and body-fluid precautions. Glove yourself with nonsterile gloves.

2. Allow the specimen to come to room temperature if it was refrigerated.
    Purpose: Specific gravity measured by the urinometer is temperature dependent.

3. Mix the specimen well by swirling.

4. Pour the specimen into the clean glass cylinder to two-thirds to three-quarters full.
    Purpose: A sufficient sample must be present to allow the urinometer to float freely.

5. If the sample is insufficient to float the urinometer, record as QNS (quantity not sufficient).

6. With the cylinder on a level surface, gently float the urinometer in the specimen with a spinning motion.

7. While the urinometer is slowly rotating in the specimen, read the lower curve of the meniscus, at eye level.
    Purpose: For accurate results, the urinometer must be read at eye level. Adjust your line of vision to the urinometer: do not hold the cylinder in your hand.

8. Obtain duplicate readings. (Repeat steps 5 and 6.)
    Purpose: Duplication of test results is a means of quality control of the procedure.

9. Record the results on the laboratory form or on the patient's chart.

10. Clean and dry the equipment, and return it to proper storage.
    Purpose: Urine salts dried on the equipment cause erroneous readings in later tests.

11. Clean the work area.

12. Wash your hands.

water temperature measures below 20°C, 0.001 must be subtracted from the reading. Use a laboratory thermometer to determine the water temperature.

The *refractometer* measures the refraction of light through solids in a liquid. The result is called the *refractive index,* which, for our purposes, is the same as specific gravity (Fig. 32–2*B*). The refractometer is both faster and easier to use than the urinometer and requires only a drop of urine. One drop of well-mixed urine is placed under the hinged cover of the instrument, and the value is read directly from a scale viewed through an ocular. The refractometer must be calibrated daily with distilled water.

CHEMICAL EXAMINATION OF URINE

Tests can be performed on urine to detect the presence of certain chemicals that can provide valuable information to the physician. In certain situations, these chemical test results can be critical to the diagnosis.

Reagent strips (dipsticks) are the most widely used technique of detecting chemicals in the urine and are available in a variety of types (Table 32–4). Reagent strips are plastic strips to which one or more pads containing chemicals are attached. Tests are available for pH, specific gravity, vitamin C, leukocytes, protein, ketones, glucose, blood, bilirubin, nitrite, urobilinogen, phenylketones, and others. The presence or absence of these chemicals in the urine provides information on the status of carbohydrate metabolism, liver and kidney function, and the acid-base balance of the patient.

These reagent strips are designed to be used once and then discarded. The directions for each strip are located in the package, and these instructions must be followed exactly to obtain accurate results. A color-comparison chart is located on the label of the container. In addition to reagent strips, various tablet tests are available. Quality controls are also available to ensure reliable test results.

All strips and tablets must be kept in tightly closed containers and should only be removed im-

TABLE 32–4. URINALYSIS REAGENTS

	pH	Protein	Glucose	Ketones	Blood	Bilirubin	Urobilinogen	Nitrite	Leukocytes	Specific Gravity	Phenylketones	Dipstick	Tablet
Multistix 10 SG*	•	•	•	•	•	•	•	•	•	•		•	
Multistix 9*	•	•	•	•	•	•	•	•	•			•	
Chemstrip 9†	•	•	•	•	•	•	•	•	•			•	
Multistix 9 SG*	•	•	•	•	•	•		•	•	•		•	
Chemstrip 8†	•	•	•	•	•	•	•	•				•	
Chemstrip 7	•	•	•	•	•	•	•					•	
Multistix 8*	•	•	•	•	•	•		•	•			•	
Multistix 8 SG*	•	•	•	•	•			•	•	•		•	
Chemstrip 6†	•	•	•	•	•		•					•	
Multistix 7*	•	•	•	•	•			•	•			•	
Chemstrip 5*	•	•	•	•	•							•	
Uristix 4*		•	•					•	•			•	
Chemstrip GP†		•	•									•	
Multistix 2*								•	•			•	
Chemstrip LN†								•	•			•	
Clinitest*			•										•
Acetest*				•									•
Ictotest*						•							•
Phenistix*											•	•	

* Product of Ames Co.
† Product of BMC.

mediately prior to testing. Reagents should be stored in a cool, dry area. Ames and Bio-Dynamics manufacture the majority of the urinalysis materials used in testing today.

pH

The pH is a measurement of the degree of acidity or alkalinity of the urine. A urine specimen with a pH of 7 is neutral. Less than 7 is acid, and greater than 7 is alkaline. Normal, freshly voided urine may have a pH range of 5.5 to 8.0. Urinary pH varies with an individual's metabolic status, diet, drug therapy, and disease. Colors on the pH reagent pad usually range from yellow-orange for an acid pH to green-blue when the pH is alkaline.

Protein

Protein in the urine in detectable amounts is called **proteinuria** and is one of the first signs of renal disease. We normally excrete a small amount of protein every day, but our testing procedures are designed to detect only pathologic levels in the urine. Proteinuria may be light to heavy, constant, or sporadic. It may be postural (affected by posture) in nature. In orthostatic proteinuria, protein is excreted only when the patient is in an upright position. Generally, first morning specimens from these patients are negative, but protein is found in urine passed throughout the day. Proteinuria is a common finding in pregnancy. It is almost always present after heavy exercise. Colors on the protein reagent pad usually range from yellow for negative to yellow-green or green for positive.

Glucose

Glucose is filtered at the glomerulus, but under normal conditions, most of it is reabsorbed by the tubules. The minute quantities normally present are not detected by strips and tablets. Detectable **glycosuria** occurs whenever the renal tubules cannot reabsorb the filtered glucose load. A positive glucose finding is common in urine from diabetic patients and may be the first indication of the disease.

The reagent-strip glucose testing method is **enzymatic.** It detects only glucose; in other words, it is *specific* for glucose. None of the other sugars that can occur in urine are detected by the reagent strips, but *Clinitest* tablets (Ames Company, Elkhart, IN) do detect glucose and many other sugars. Clinitest is a *nonspecific* glucose test. Colors on the reagent strip range from green (low concentration of glucose) to brown (high concentration of glucose).

Ketones

Ketone bodies are the end product of fat metabolism in the body. Acetoacetic acid, acetone, and beta-hydroxybutyric acid are collectively referred to as ketone bodies, or ketones. *Ketonuria* is common in starvation, low-carbohydrate diets, excessive vomiting, and diabetes mellitus. Since ketones evaporate at room temperature, urine should be tested immediately, or it should be tightly covered and refrigerated if not tested promptly. Color reactions on the strip range from pink to maroon when ketones are present. *Acetest* tablets (Ames Company) provide an alternative to strip testing.

Blood

The presence of blood in the urine may indicate infection or trauma to the urinary tract, or bleeding in the kidneys. The blood test pad on the reagent strip reacts with three different blood constituents: intact red blood cells, hemoglobin from red blood cells, and myoglobin, a hemoglobin-like molecule that transports oxygen in muscle tissue.

Hematuria is the presence of intact red blood cells in urine. The color reaction on the reagent strip ranges from orange through green to dark blue when hematuria is present. Hematuria can be due to irritation of the ureters, bladder, or urethra. It is also a common finding in cystitis and in persons passing kidney stones.

Hemoglobinuria is the presence of hemolyzed red blood cells. True hemoglobinuria is rare. It occurs as the result of intravascular red blood cell destruction and can be caused by transfusion reactions, malaria, drug reactions, snake bites, and severe burns. **Myoglobinuria** occurs when muscle tissue is damaged or injured, such as in crushing injuries, myocardial infarctions, and contact sports. Muscular dystrophy patients often exhibit myoglobinuria. Hemoglobinuria cannot be distinguished from myoglobinuria by strip testing.

Bilirubin and Urobilinogen

Bilirubin is a product of the breakdown of hemoglobin (Fig. 32–4). Hemoglobin is released from old red blood cells destroyed in the reticuloendothelial system. It is gradually converted to bilirubin in the liver and then further to urobilinogen in the intestines. Bilirubin is a bile pigment not normally found in urine. Its presence in urine is one of the first signs of liver disease or other disease in which the liver may be involved, such as infectious mononucleosis.

Bilirubinuria can occur even before jaundice or other symptoms of liver disease are evident. It is the

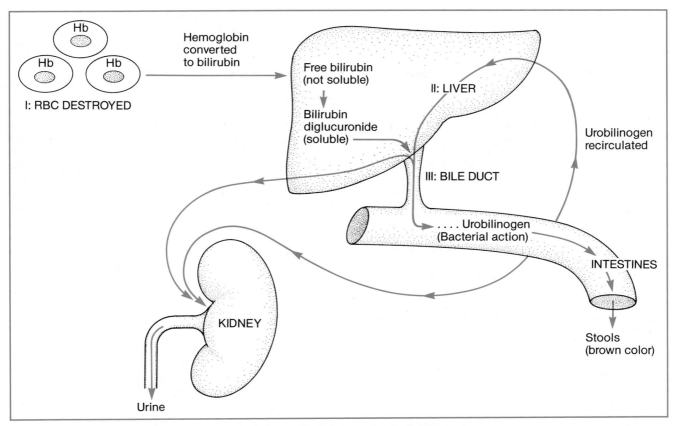

FIGURE 32–4. Detection of bilirubin and urobilinogen in urine.

result of liver cell damage or obstruction of the common bile duct by stones or neoplasms (tumors). Excessive bilirubin colors the urine yellow-brown to greenish-orange. Since direct light causes decomposition of bilirubin, urine samples must be protected from light until testing is complete. *Ictotest* tablets (Ames Company) are more sensitive to bilirubin than are the strips and are often easier to interpret when the urine is highly colored.

Urobilinogen is normally present in urine in small amounts. Increases are seen when there is increased red blood cell destruction and in liver disease. When there is total obstruction of the bile duct, no urobilinogen is formed in the intestines, none is reabsorbed into the circulation, and, hence, none is present in the urine. Strip methods cannot detect a decrease in urobilinogen. The reagent strip for positive testing results in color changes from orange through green to dark blue.

Nitrite

Nitrite occurs in urine when bacteria break down nitrate. A positive nitrite test indicates a urinary tract infection. However, not all bacteria are able to reduce nitrate to nitrite. Negative nitrite tests can also occur when there are insufficient bacteria present, or when the urine has not incubated in the bladder long enough for the reaction to occur. *Escherichia coli,* the organism that causes the majority of urinary tract infections, is nitrite positive. False positives can occur if a specimen is allowed to sit at room temperature and contaminating bacteria multiply. False negatives occur if the bacteria further metabolize the nitrite they have produced.

Leukocytes

Leukocytes occur in urine in infections of the urinary tract. They can also be contaminants from the vagina. The *leukocyte esterase test* on reagent strips detects intact and lysed polymorphonuclear white blood cells. However, it does not detect mononuclear white blood cells, which are occasionally present during infections. The test does not react with the small numbers of white blood cells found in normal urine.

Specific Gravity

Reagent strips are available that report specific gravity by the use of colored pads. The individual test pads on the strip give readings every 0.005 on the specific gravity scale from 1.005 to 1.030.

Phenylketones

Phenistix (Ames Company) are reagent strips used to detect the presence of phenylketones in the urine. This condition is called *phenylketonuria* (PKU). In this genetically inherited disorder, the body is unable to properly metabolize the nutrient **phenylalanine.**

As high levels of the phenylketones accumulate in the bloodstream, mental retardation occurs. Phenyl-ketonuria is easily treated by limiting dietary intake of phenylalanine in childhood. Since individuals who are properly treated for the disease do not suffer mental retardation, early detection is very important.

Ascorbic Acid (Vitamin C)

Ascorbic acid normally is not found in urine in quantities large enough to interfere with chemical urine tests. However, in persons who habitually consume large quantities of vitamin C, the urine levels of ascorbic acid may affect results of nitrite, glucose, bilirubin, and occult blood tests. STIX reagent strips (Ames Company) or any of the combination strips available detect interfering levels of the drug. If an elevated level is found, the patient should be instructed to discontinue vitamin C intake for 24 hours, and then another urine specimen should be collected for testing.

PROCEDURE 32-3   TESTING URINE WITH CHEMICAL REAGENT STRIPS

GOAL To perform chemical testing on a urine sample.

EQUIPMENT AND SUPPLIES

    Blood and body-fluid protection barriers   Reagent strips
Urine specimen   Timer

PROCEDURAL STEPS

1. Wash and dry your hands. Follow the universal blood and body-fluid precautions. Glove yourself with nonsterile gloves.

2. Check the time of collection, the container, and the mode of preservation.
   Purpose: Proper specimen identification and screening of specimens for appropriate collection containers and collection procedures prevents testing of inappropriate specimens.

3. If the specimen has been refrigerated, allow it to warm to room temperature.
   Purpose: Certain tests are temperature-dependent. Testing of cold specimens may cause false-negative results.

4. Check the reagent strip container for expiration date.
   Purpose: Do not use expired reagents.

5. Remove the reagent strip from the container. Hold it in your hand, or place it on a clean paper towel. Recap the container tightly.
   Purpose: Test strips are sensitive to moisture and must be stored in tightly sealed containers. Contamination from chemical residues on counter tops can affect results.

Continued

6. Compare nonreactive test pads with the negative color blocks on the color chart on the container.
   Purpose: Discolored pads have not been properly stored and must not be used for testing.

7. Thoroughly mix the specimen by swirling or inverting.
   Purpose: If settling occurs, certain elements may not be detected.

8. Following manufacturer's directions, note the time, and simultaneously dip the strip into the urine and remove.
   Purpose: Tests are time-dependent. Positive tests result in darkening with time.

9. Draw the strip across the lip of the container to remove excess specimen.
   Purpose: Excess urine on the strip, or prolonged dipping time, affects test results.

10. Hold the strip horizontally. At the exact time, compare the strip with the appropriate color chart on the reagent container.
    Purpose: Holding the strip horizontally prevents runover from one test pad to another and prevents interference from the mixing of chemicals in the test pads.

11. Read the concentration, and record it on the laboratory report form (Fig. 32–5*A*). Reagent strip with automated reaction readings are available as an alternative to manual reading. Automation gives more consistent results, since it eliminates timing and color perception as variables (Fig. 32–5*B*).
    Purpose: Timing is critical.

12. Clean the work area.

13. Wash your hands.

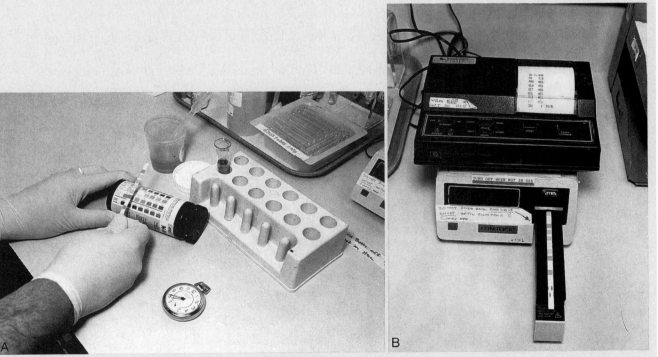

FIGURE 32–5.

Confirmatory Testing

Positive reagent strip testing should be confirmed by further testing whenever possible. Verification with a different procedure is preferred over repeating the same procedure to rule out any false reactions that may have been caused by interfering substances on the dipstick.

Positive protein tests should be confirmed by an *acid precipitation test.* Glucose-positive results should be confirmed with Clinitest tablets. Bilirubin-positive results should be confirmed with Ictotest tablets, especially since the dipstick test pad used for bilirubin is often difficult to interpret in highly colored urines. Acetest tablets are used to confirm positive ketone tests.

New tests are constantly being developed and marketed, and existing tests are constantly undergoing improvement. It is important to read the product insert to be aware of changes made in the testing procedure and of product performance.

PROCEDURE 32-4   TESTING URINE FOR GLUCOSE USING CLINITEST TABLETS

GOAL   To perform confirmatory testing for glucose in the urine using the Clinitest procedure for reducing substances.

EQUIPMENT AND SUPPLIES

Blood and body-fluid protection barriers
Nonsterile gloves
Urine specimen
Clinitest tablet
Clinitest tube

Distilled water
Test tube rack
Color chart
Timer

PROCEDURAL STEPS

1. Wash and dry your hands. Follow the universal blood and body-fluid precautions. Glove yourself with nonsterile gloves.

2. Holding a Clinitest dropper vertically, add 10 drops of distilled water and then 5 drops of urine to a Clinitest tube.
   Purpose: Holding the dropper vertically prevents altering the size of the drops.

3. With dry hands, remove a Clinitest tablet from the bottle by pouring the tablet into the bottle cap (Fig. 32–6).
   Purpose: Clinitest tablets react with moisture and become caustic. Handling tablets with moist hands could result in hydroxide burns.

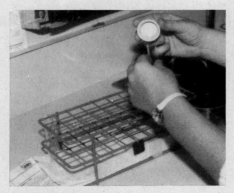

FIGURE 32-6.

Continued

4. Compare the color of the tablet with an unreacted tablet on the color chart.
   Purpose: If the tablet is discolored, it has degenerated and must not be used for testing.

5. Tap the tablet into the test tube, and recap the container.

6. Hold the test tube at the top.
   Purpose: The tube becomes hot as the reaction progresses.

7. Observe the entire reaction to detect the "rapid pass through" phenomenon. (See step no. 10).
   Purpose: If "pass through" occurs but is not detected, the reading will be falsely low.

8. When boiling ceases, time exactly 15 seconds; then gently shake the tube to mix the entire contents.

9. Immediately compare the color of the specimen with the "five-drop" color chart, and record your findings (Fig. 32–7).
   Purpose: Color darkens with time. For accurate results, time carefully.

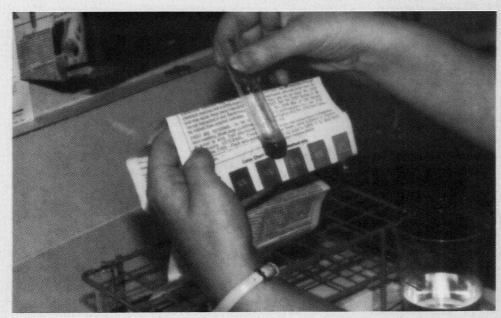

FIGURE 32–7.

10. If an orange color briefly develops during the reaction, "rapid pass through" has occurred, and the test must be repeated using the "two-drop" color chart.

11. Repeat the test, using ten drops of water and two drops of urine.

12. Compare the specimen color to the "two-drop" color chart.
    Purpose: The five-drop and the two-drop color charts are not interchangeable.

13. Clean the work area.

14. Record the results:
    Negative—Clear
    Trace—Slightly cloudy
    1+—Can see light print through tube
    2+—Can see dark print through tube
    3+—Cannot see through tube
    4+—Large, fluffy precipitate forms and settles, on standing

15. Wash your hands.

PROCEDURE 32–5 TESTING URINE FOR PROTEIN USING THE SULFOSALICYLIC ACID (SSA) PRECIPITATION TEST

GOAL To perform the sulfosalicylic acid (SSA) precipitation test for the presence of protein in the urine.

EQUIPMENT AND SUPPLIES

Blood and body-fluid protection barriers
Urine specimen
3% sulfosalicylic acid

Centrifuge tube and centrifuge
Test tube and rack
Dropper

PROCEDURAL STEPS

1. Wash and dry your hands. Follow the universal blood and body-fluid precautions. Glove yourself with nonsterile gloves.

2. If the urine is cloudy, filter the specimen or use a centrifuged specimen.
   Purpose: If the urine is already turbid (cloudy), the test will be difficult to interpret.

3. In a clear test tube, mix equal volumes of urine and 3% SSA.

4. Observe for cloudiness and record:
   Negative—Clear
   Trace—Slightly cloudy
   1+—Can see light print through tube
   2+—Can see dark print through tube
   3+—Cannot see through tube
   4+—Large, fluffy precipitate forms and settles on standing
   Purpose: This result gives a rough estimation of the protein concentration of the urine.

5. Clean the work area.

6. Wash your hands.

MICROSCOPIC EXAMINATION OF URINE SEDIMENT

The microscopic examination of urine consists of categorizing and counting cells, casts, crystals, and miscellaneous constituents of the sediment obtained when a measured portion of urine is centrifuged. The clear upper portion of the specimen is called the supernatant. It is poured off, and a drop of the well-mixed sediment is examined under a microscope. This part of the urinalysis gives the physician information about the course and progress of renal disease and detects the presence of infection.

Casts

Casts are formed when protein accumulates and precipitates in the kidney tubules and is washed into the urine. The protein takes on the size and shape of the tubules, hence the term *casts*. Casts are cylindric, with flat or rounded ends, and are classified according to the substances observed in them. Certain types of casts are associated with renal pathologic conditions; others are physiologic and are generally caused by strenuous exercise.

Casts are counted and reported under low-power magnification, but occasionally high-power magnification is needed to identify the type. Since casts tend to migrate to the edges of the coverslip, this area should be examined closely. Casts dissolve in alkaline urine on standing; therefore, examination of a fresh urine specimen is very important (Fig. 32–8).

Hyaline casts are pale, transparent cylindric structures that have rounded ends and parallel sides. Hyaline casts will be missed entirely if subdued light is not used. They are formed when urine flow

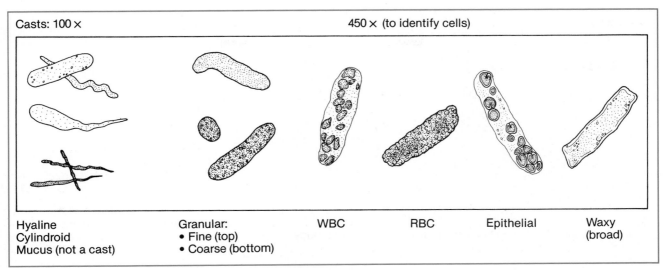

Casts: 100 ×		450 × (to identify cells)			
Hyaline Cylindroid Mucus (not a cast)	Granular: • Fine (top) • Coarse (bottom)	WBC	RBC	Epithelial	Waxy (broad)

FIGURE 32–8. Urine casts.

through individual nephrons is diminished. They can be found in kidney disease but can also be found in urine specimens of normal subjects who have exercised heavily. Occasionally, hyaline casts have granular or cellular inclusions. Cylindroids are hyaline casts with long, thin tails.

Finely and coarsely granular casts may be due to exercise but, when present in increased numbers, may indicate renal disease. On close examination, granular casts show a hyaline matrix with coarse or fine granular inclusions. The granules are thought to be due to protein aggregation or degeneration of cellular inclusions.

Red blood cell casts are always pathologic and highly diagnostic. Red blood cell casts occur in glomerulonephritis. They are hyaline casts with embedded red cells, and their presence indicates damage to the glomerular membrane. They may appear brown as a result of the color of the red blood cells present.

White blood cell casts are hyaline casts that contain leukocytes. White blood cells usually have a multilobed nucleus, which differentiates them from renal tubular epithelial cells, which have single, round nuclei. White blood cell casts are seen in pyelonephritis.

Renal tubular epithelial cell casts contain embedded renal tubular epithelial cells. These casts are easily confused with white blood cell casts, particularly if the cells have started to degenerate. Renal tubular epithelial cell casts are found when there is excessive damage. Causes are shock, renal *ischemia,* heavy-metal poisoning, certain allergic reactions, and nephrotoxic drugs.

Waxy casts are rarely seen. They appear as glassy, brittle, smooth, homogeneous structures. They are usually yellowish, have cracks or fissures, and have squared or broken ends. They are considered to be degenerated cellular casts and are found in severe renal disease.

Broad casts are from two to six times as wide as other casts. They are formed in the collecting tubules and indicate decreased urine output in several adjacent nephrons.

Occasionally, more than one type of cell will be found in a single cast. Mixed cellular casts have been reported. Absolute identification of the cell types present may be difficult. Be as specific as possible.

Cells

Cells that are found in urine include epithelial cells, which are derived from the lining of the genitourinary tract. Other cells in urine include red blood cells (RBCs) and white blood cells (WBCs) from the bloodstream. Cells are classified and counted under high-power magnification (Fig. 32–9).

Red blood cells may enter the urinary tract at any point where there is inflammation or injury. They may be found in normal urine in small numbers, usually less than 1 to 2 high-power field (HPF). Persistent hematuria should be investigated. Red blood cells are pale, round, nongranular, and flat or biconcave. They are smaller than white blood cells and have no nucleus. In hypotonic, or dilute, urine, they swell and burst. In hypertonic, or concentrated, urine, they may crenate and wrinkle. When they crenate, they can be mistaken for white blood cells, since the wrinkled surface makes them appear granular. They are often confused with yeast, oil droplets, and droplets of lens cleaner.

White blood cells may occasionally be found in normal urine, but increased numbers, usually greater than 5/HPF, are associated with inflammation or contamination of the specimen during collection. White blood cells are larger than red blood cells, have a granular appearance, and usually contain a

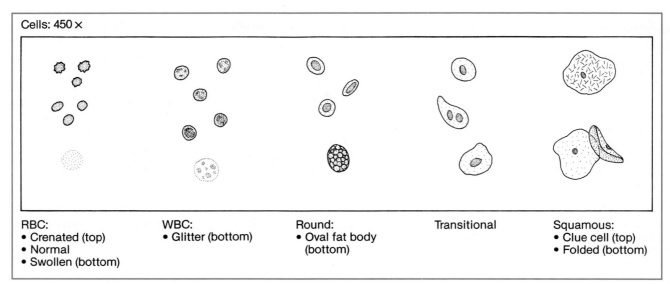

Cells: 450 ×

RBC:
• Crenated (top)
• Normal
• Swollen (bottom)

WBC:
• Glitter (bottom)

Round:
• Oval fat body
  (bottom)

Transitional

Squamous:
• Clue cell (top)
• Folded (bottom)

FIGURE 32-9. Red and white blood cells in urine.

multilobed nucleus, although nuclear detail may not be evident.

Renal tubular or round epithelial cells are somewhat larger than white blood cells, are round to oval, and have a single, large, oval, and sometimes eccentric nucleus. A few may be found in normal urine specimens, but their presence in increased numbers indicates tubular damage.

Transitional epithelial cells line the urinary tract from the renal pelvis to the upper portion of the urethra. They vary in size from slightly larger than a round epithelial cell to smaller than a squamous epithelial cell. They are round to oval and may have a tail. Occasionally, two nuclei are seen. When transitional cells are present in large numbers, a pathologic condition may exist.

Squamous epithelial cells line the lower portion of the genitourinary tract. When present in large numbers in females, they usually indicate vaginal contamination. Squamous epithelial cells are large, flat, irregular cells and are easily recognized under low-power magnification. They have a single, small, round, centrally located nucleus and often occur in sheets or clumps. Because of their flat nature, the edges of the cells are often rolled or folded.

In identifying epithelial cells, it is helpful to remember the appearance of eggs; round epithelial cells resemble hard-boiled eggs that have been cut in half. Transitional forms resemble poached eggs, and squamous cells resemble fried eggs with large, runny whites.

Crystals

Crystals are common in urine specimens, particularly if they have been allowed to cool. Cooling causes the solid crystals to precipitate out of the urine. The presence of most crystals is not clinically significant unless they are found in large numbers in patients with kidney stones. Occasionally, pathologic crystals are found. Identification of crystals begins with the determination of the pH of the urine. From there, one looks at color, shape, and refractility. Often, a history of drug intake is helpful. Consult Table 32-5 for nonpathologic and pathologic urine crystals. It is not always possible to identify crystals without additional chemical testing.

Miscellaneous Findings

Oval fat bodies (see Fig. 32-9) are formed when renal tubular epithelial cells or macrophages absorb fats. The fat droplets contained in the cells vary in size and are quite refractile. Oval fat bodies are characteristic of the nephrotic syndrome.

Yeast in urine may indicate vaginal contamination or infection of the urine with yeast. It is common in the urine of diabetic patients. Yeasts are easily confused with red blood cells, are usually oval, may show budding, and are more refractile. To differentiate yeast from red blood cells, a drop of sediment is placed on the blood test pad of a reagent strip. Yeast does not react, but red blood cells do. Red blood cells dissolve when a drop of dilute acetic acid (regular white vinegar) is added to the sediment. The yeast remains intact (Fig. 32-10).

A few *bacteria* may be found in normal urine specimens. Heavy bacterial concentrations in the absence of white blood cells may indicate that the specimen was allowed to sit at room temperature and the bacteria multiplied. Urine specimens with a

TABLE 32–5. CRYSTALS OF URINE

Nonpathologic Acid pH	Crystal	Description and Occurrence
	Calcium oxalate	Clear, colorless, bipyramidal or envelope-shaped. Occasionally, shaped like dumbbell or safety pin. Very common.
	Uric acid*	Pleomorphic, clear to yellow-brown, flattened, often four-sided, football-shaped, often in rosettes. Quite common.
	Hippuric acid	Elongated, six-sided, colorless to yellow-brown, often in clusters.
	Amorphous urates	Seen as salmon-pink precipitate in the centrifuge tube. Microscopically: shapeless, sand-like; brownish in color if heavy. Can be dispersed by warming tube prior to centrifugation. Very common.
	Sodium urate	Colorless to yellow, long, thin, blunt-ended needles, often in rosettes or clumps.
Alkaline pH		
	Triple phosphate	Colorless "coffin lid" six-sided prisms, often very large. Common in alkaline urines.
	Amorphous phosphate	Seen in centrifuge tube as a white precipitate. Microscopically, shapeless, whitish, granular "sand." Can be dispersed by adding acetic acid to the sediment. Fairly common.
	Calcium phosphate	Flat plates; long, thin needles or prisms; stars, crosses, or rosettes. Not very common.
	Ammonium biurate	Brown "thorn apples" or greasy brown spherules; rare.
Pathologic **All Found at an Acid pH**		
	Tyrosine needles	Colorless to yellow, fine, silky needles in sheaves, rosettes. Found in severe liver damage, often with leucine.
	Leucine spheres	Yellow, radially or concentrically striated spheres. Seen in liver disease.
	Bilirubin	Brownish cubes, rhombic plates, or needles in pompom ball arrangement. Free bilirubin stains sediment brown.
	Cholesterol plates	Colorless, flat plates with parallel sides and a characteristic notched corner. Seen in some renal diseases.
	Cystine	Clear, colorless, hexagonal plates. Seen in the congenital disorder cystinosis.
Other		
	Radiocontrast dyes	Colorless, long, thin rhombic crystals. Specific gravity may be very high (often greater than 1.050). History will reveal recent x-ray studies.
	Sulfa	Clear to brown sheaves of needles with eccentric, central constriction. History of sulfa medication.

* May be pathologic.

Miscellaneous: 450 ×

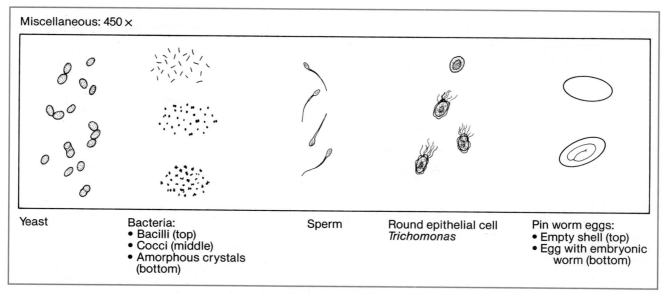

| Yeast | Bacteria:
• Bacilli (top)
• Cocci (middle)
• Amorphous crystals (bottom) | Sperm | Round epithelial cell
Trichomonas | Pin worm eggs:
• Empty shell (top)
• Egg with embryonic worm (bottom) |

FIGURE 32–10. Miscellaneous findings in urine.

PROCEDURE 32-6   ANALYZING URINE MICROSCOPICALLY

GOAL To perform a microscopic examination of urine to determine the presence of normal and abnormal elements.

EQUIPMENT AND SUPPLIES

Blood and body-fluid protection barriers (gloves, goggles, masks, and aprons or gowns)
Urine specimen
Centrifuge tube

Centrifuge
Disposable pipette
Microscope slide and coverslip
Microscope
Permanent marker

PROCEDURAL STEPS

1.   Wash and dry your hands. Follow the universal blood and body-fluid precautions. Glove yourself with nonsterile gloves.

2.   Gently mix the urine specimen.
     Purpose: If the urine is not well-mixed, elements that have settled to the bottom of the specimen container will be missed.

3.   Pour 10 ml of urine into a labeled centrifuge tube and cap tube (Fig. 32–11).

4.   Place the tube in the centrifuge (Fig. 32–12).

5.   Place another tube containing 10 ml of water in the opposite cup.
     Purpose: For proper operation, centrifuges must be carefully balanced. If not properly balanced, damage to the instrument can occur.

6.   Secure the lid, and centrifuge for 5 minutes or for the time specified for your instrument.
     Purpose: Timing varies based upon the speed and the size of the centrifuge head.

7.   Remove the tube from the centrifuge after the instrument has come to a full stop.

Continued

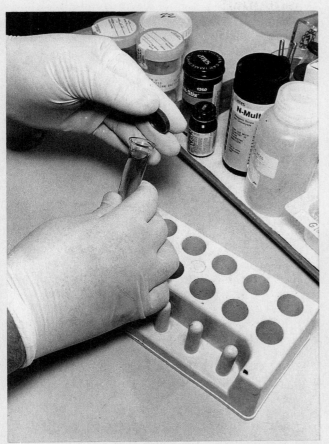

FIGURE 32–11.

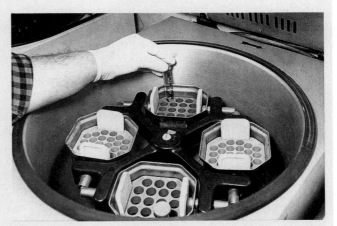

FIGURE 32–12.

   8. Pour off the clear supernatant from the top of the specimen by inverting the centrifuge tube over the sink drain (Fig. 32–13).

   9. Prevent the loss of sediment down the drain.
Purpose: The sediment is what you will examine under the microscope.

10. Thoroughly mix the sediment by grasping the tube near the top and rapidly flicking it with the fingers of the other hand until all sediment is thoroughly resuspended (Fig. 32–14).
Purpose: Elements centrifuge at different rates. Failure to completely mix the entire sediment will cause errors in quantification.

11. Using a disposable pipette, transfer one drop of sediment to a clean, labeled slide.

12. Place a clean coverslip over the drop, and place the slide on the microscope stage.

13. Focus under low power, and reduce the light.
Purpose: Mucus and casts are easily missed if reduced light is not used. Constant focusing helps locate them.

14. First, scan the entire coverslip for abnormal findings.
Purpose: Casts tend to migrate to the edges of the coverslip.

Continued

PROCEDURE 32-6 *Continued*

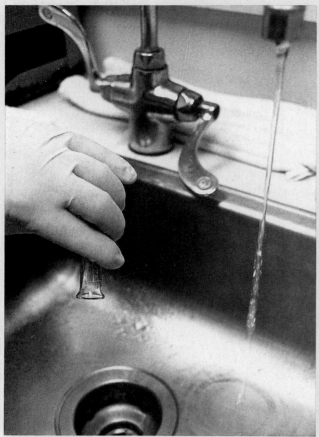

FIGURE 32-13.

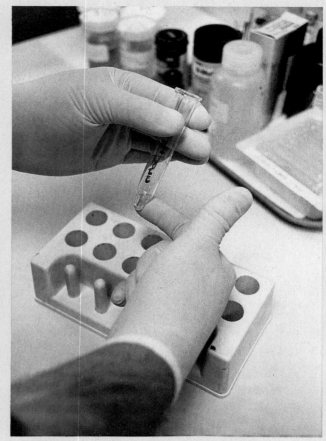

FIGURE 32-14.

15. Examine five low-power fields. Count and classify each type of cast seen, if any, and note mucus if present.
    Purpose: Choose five fields so that one is selected from each corner of the coverslip and the last one is chosen from the middle of the coverslip. If you move to an area and there is nothing there, record a zero.

16. Switch to high-power magnification, and adjust the light.
    Purpose: As magnification increases, more light is needed.

17. In five high-power fields, count the following elements: RBCs, WBCs, and round, transitional, and squamous epithelial cells.

18. In the same five fields, report the following as few, moderate, or many: crystals (identify and report each type seen separately), bacteria (identify as rods or cocci), sperm, yeast, and parasites.
    Purpose: These three terms are more easily and universally understood than are exact numbers.

19. Average the five fields, and report the results.

20. Clean up the work area.

21. Wash your hands.

putrid odor, numerous white blood cells, and bacteria are common in urinary tract infections. Bacteria may be rods or cocci and are identified under high-power magnification.

Sperm are often found in the urine specimens of both males and females. In the latter, their presence represents vaginal contamination of the specimen. Sperm usually have pointed, oval heads and long thread-like tails. They may be motile in fresh urine.

The most commonly encountered parasite in urine is *Trichomonas vaginalis*. It is usually a vaginal contaminant but may also be found in urine specimens from males. When urine is fresh and warm, the trichomonas may be motile. *Trichomonas* organisms are pear-shaped protozoa with four flagella. They are larger than round epithelial cells but smaller than squamous cells. *Trichomonas* organisms die when the specimen is cooled.

Mucous threads can be found in most urine specimens. They appear as pale, irregular, thready structures with tapered ends. Beginners often confuse hyaline casts and mucous threads. Increased numbers are seen in inflammation and when there has been contamination of the specimen with vaginal contents (see Fig. 32–6).

Reporting Findings of a Microscopic Examination

The slide is first examined under the low-power objective and low light to locate casts. Ten to 15 low-power fields are scanned, and the number of casts is counted and reported. The high-power objective and increased light is used to identify red and white blood cells, epithelial cells, yeasts, bacteria, and crystals. Ten to 15 high-power fields should be scanned, and the number counted, averaged, and reported. The method of counting varies considerably among laboratories. It is important that all workers in the same laboratory use the same counting and reporting systems. Report the results of the microscopic examination as follows (Table 32–6):

1. Separately total the numbers for each element counted, and then average. (Casts, WBCs, RBCs, and the three categories of epithelial cells are counted, totaled, and averaged.) Casts, WBCs, and RBCs are reported using numerical ranges based on the average:

0	10–20
0–1	20–30
1–2	30–40
2–5	40–50
5–10	>50

   Epithelial cells are reported as occasional, few, moderate, or many, according to the following:

0	
0–3	= occasional
3–6	= few
6–12	= moderate
>12	= many

2. Estimate the remaining elements as occasional, few, moderate, or many, according to the following:

   Occasional—Not seen in every field
   Few—Covers less than a quarter of the field

TABLE 32–6. CALCULATING A MICROSCOPIC URINALYSIS

Field	Per Low-Power Field — Casts	Mucus	WBC	RBC	Squamous Epithelial	Transitional Epithelial	Round Epithelial	Bacteria	Crystals	Other
1	0	Few	16	1	1	0	0	Moderate (rods)	Calcium oxalate—few Uric acid—few	—
2	1 hyaline	Few	32	0	3	0	0	Many	Calcium oxalate—few	Yeast
3	1 coarse granular	Moderate	21	2	3	0	0	Many	Calcium oxalate—few	Yeast
4	1 coarse granular	Few	12	1	5	0	1	Moderate	Uric acid—few	—
5	0	Few	25	0	4	0	0	Many	—	—
Total	1 hyaline 2 coarse granular	Few	106	4	16	0	1	Many	Calcium oxalate—few Uric acid—few	Yeast
Average	0.2 hyaline 0.4 coarse granular	Few	21.2	0.8	3.2	0	0.2	Many	Calcium oxalate—few Uric acid—few	Yeast
Report	0–1 hyaline 0–1 coarse granular	Few	20–30	0–1	Few	0	Occasionally	Many (rods)	Calcium oxalate—few Uric acid—few	Yeast

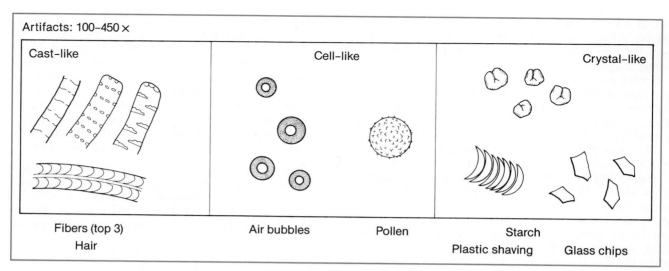

FIGURE 32–15. Urine artifacts.

Moderate—Covers approximately half of the field
Many—Covers the entire field
Do not report fibers, hair, talc granules, oil droplets, and other artifacts (Fig. 32–15).

Interpretation of Urine Cultures

Interpretation of urine cultures is performed by estimating the number of colonies and determining if one or more organisms are growing. The number of bacteria present in the urine can be estimated by counting the colonies that grow out after 24 hours of incubation (i.e., colony count) (Fig. 32–16). For example, if 30 colonies are counted on the medium and a 0.001-ml calibrated inoculating loop was used, the bacterial count is 30,000 per milliliter of urine. The number of colonies is multiplied by 1000, since only 1/1000 ml of urine was cultured. Usually, an infection is indicated when the *colony count* is over 100,000 bacteria per milliliter of urine.

After the organisms have been counted and isolated from the culture, they can then be identified by various means. Growth characteristics can be observed visually. Agglutination kits and biochemical strip tests are also available for identification of the isolated organisms.

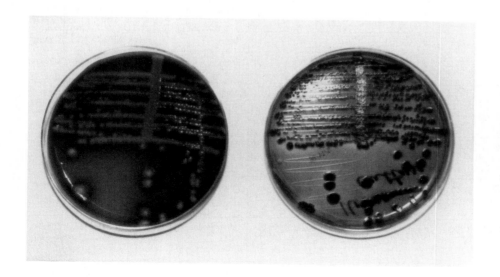

FIGURE 32–16. A culture showing between 75,000 and 100,000 CFU/ml (colony-forming units/ml). Growth is heavy in the original areas of inoculum and moderate in the third quadrant, and a few colonies are found in the fourth quadrant. The plate on the left is blood agar, and the one on the right is EMB agar (eosin-methylene blue agar). The organism growing is *Escherichia coli,* the most common cause of urinary tract infections.

PROCEDURE 32-7   COLLECTING A CLEAN-CATCH URINE SPECIMEN FOR CULTURE OR ANALYSIS

GOAL To collect a contaminant-free urine sample for culture or analysis using midstream clean-catch technique.

EQUIPMENT AND SUPPLIES

Sterile container with lid
Antiseptic towelettes

Set of written instructions

PROCEDURAL STEPS

1. Label the container and give the patient the supplies (Fig. 32–17).
    Purpose: Labeling the container avoids possible mixup of specimens.

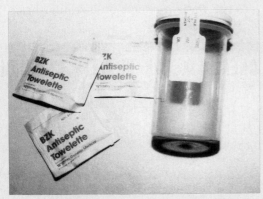

FIGURE 32–17.

2. Explain the instructions to adult patients or to the guardians of child patients.
    Purpose: Instructions must be understood if they are to be followed. By talking to the patient, you can determine if the patient understands.

    Female: Ask the patient to remove underclothing and to sit on the toilet, with one knee to the side as far as possible. Loosen the cap so that it can be removed from the container with one hand. Use fingers to spread the labia apart. Continue to hold the labia in this position throughout the entire procedure. Use three separate towelettes to clean the area from front to back three times—once down each side, and then once down the middle. Place the lid of the specimen cup, top side down, on a clean surface. Do not touch the rim or the inside of the lid or cup. Begin to urinate into the toilet, then hold the cup in the stream and collect a portion of the urine. Finish urinating into the toilet. Replace the lid on the container, and if needed, wipe the container with towels. For specimens collected at home, note the time on the container, and refrigerate until transporting to the laboratory. For specimens collected in the office, note the time on the container and process immediately or refrigerate.

Continued

Male: Loosen cap on the container. Retract the foreskin (if present), and use an antiseptic towelette to cleanse the glans and the urethral opening. Place the lid of the specimen cup, top side down, on a clean surface. Do not touch the rim or the inside of the lid or cup. Begin to urinate into the toilet, then hold the cup in the stream and collect a portion of the urine. Finish urinating into the toilet. Replace the lid on the container, and if needed, wipe the container with towels.

Infants: Obtain a sterile urine pouch. Using antiseptic towelettes, carefully cleanse the perineum and genital area. Tape the pouch in place over the penis or on the labia. Hold the infant so that the pouch is in position and urine flows into the pouch without touching the skin. Stimulate urination by placing the infant's feet in cold water, if necessary. Remove the pouch as soon as the specimen has been collected. Transfer the specimen to a sterile container.

QUALITY CONTROL

Quality control is a method of checking reagents, procedures, and personnel to ensure that results are accurate. Many commercially prepared products are available for use in both macroscopic and microscopic testing programs. Small laboratories using Ames products often use Chek-Stix for macroscopic quality control. Urintrol (Harleco) and Kovatrol (ICL Scientific) are intended for both macroscopic and microscopic quality control. It is good practice to use these products on a regular basis.

PROCEDURE 32–8   TESTING URINE WITH CHEK-STIX FOR QUALITY CONTROL

GOAL   To prepare, test, and record the results of Chek-Stix control product for macroscopic quality control.

EQUIPMENT AND SUPPLIES

Blood and body-fluid protection barriers
Chek-Stix
Distilled water
Centrifuge tube

Urinalysis reagent strips and tablets
Parafilm
Timer

PROCEDURAL STEPS

1. Wash and dry your hands. Follow the universal blood and body-fluid precautions. Glove yourself with nonsterile gloves.

2. Fill a graduated centrifuge tube with 12 ml of distilled water.
    Purpose: Tap water does not give accurate results because of pH differences.

3. Insert one Chek-Stix reagent strip, and cover the tube with Parafilm (Fig. 32–18). Invert the tube gently for 2 minutes.
    Purpose: Mixing is required for elution of chemicals from strip.

4. After 30 minutes have elapsed, mix again and discard the strip.

5. Test in the same manner as you would do a macroscopic urinalysis. The product may be used as a known, or it may be hidden in a batch of urine specimens and tested as an unknown.
    Purpose: "Blind" testing is often used to eliminate bias when the laboratory personnel know the results in advance.

Continued

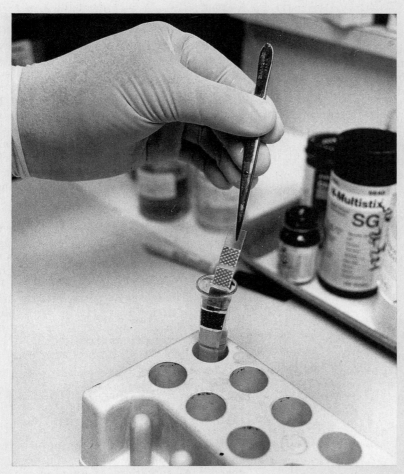

FIGURE 32-18.

6. Compare results with those given in the product insert.
   Purpose: Results should be within the range of given values for the procedure to be in control.

7. Record the results in the quality control log.
   Purpose: Values should be monitored over a period of time to check for trends that would indicate deterioration of reagents or problems with any one individual's test procedure. All laboratories must maintain quality control logs.

8. If test results show that the procedure is not in control, the following steps should be taken before you report any patient results:

   a. Retest the Chek-Stix with a new test strip, and be sure to time the procedure accurately.

   b. If the procedure is still not in control, prepare a new Chek-Stix and retest with a new reagent strip.

   c. If the procedure is still out of control, open a new bottle of reagent strips, and test with Chek-Stix.

   d. If still out of control, report your findings to your supervisor. Do not report out any patient results until the procedure is in control.

   Purpose: Test results should be an accurate indicator of the patient's condition.

9. Clean up the work area.

10. Wash your hands.

PREGNANCY TESTING

Medical assistants are often asked about the use of the home pregnancy tests now on the market. These tests are based on the same principles used in the kit methods most often used in laboratories. All the tests detect the presence of **human chorionic gonadotropin (HCG)** present in urine during pregnancy. The tests vary considerably in their sensitivity. Some of the home tests are able to detect HCG in urine as early as 9 days after a missed period. Other tests are more sensitive but are not available for home testing. The major drawback to the home test kits is their lack of positive and negative controls, which are supplied with the kits used in the laboratories. However, the home tests do show good agreement with the laboratory methods now in use.

A variety of home pregnancy tests are available in pharmacies. These urine assays for HCG are usually based on some type of enzyme assay procedure, which is usually simple. In spite of clearly written instructions, these tests have high false-positive and false-negative rates due to problems in technique and failure to use an adequate sample. The tests are somewhat expensive, and a physician will need to have the test repeated when the patient is first seen for a prenatal visit. The medical assistant should be familiar with these home tests, their techniques, and their shortcomings. You can be a great help in providing reliable consumer information and in encouraging patients to obtain proper testing and prenatal care (Fig. 32–19).

After pregnancy begins, the HCG levels in serum double every few days. This rapid rise occurs for approximately 7 weeks and then begins to slow. It is during this period that many women request a pregnancy test. The Wampole One-Step HCG is one such test that can be performed by using urine or serum. It is used routinely in many physicians' office laboratories. Procedure 31–9 is an example of a chromatographic immunoassay for the qualitative detection of HCG in serum and urine.

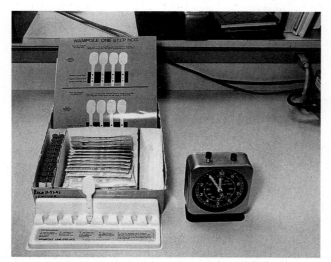

FIGURE 32–19. Pregnancy test, scrum, and urine one-step hCG manufactured by Wampole Laboratories. (Courtesy of Wampole Laboratories, a division of Carter-Wallace, Inc., Cranbury, NJ.)

GLOSSARY OF OTHER URINALYSIS-RELATED TERMS

diuresis Increase in the excretion of urine
dysuria Difficult or painful urination.
enuresis A condition of involuntary discharge of urine; *bedwetting.*
frequency Excessive urination.
incontinence The inability to control excretory functions.
nocturia Excessive urination during the night.
pyuria Presence of pus in the urine.
retention Accumulation of urine within the bladder because of the inability to urinate.
urgency The sudden, compelling desire to urinate.

PROCEDURE 32–9   PERFORMING A PREGNANCY DETECTION TEST

GOAL   To perform a pregnancy test on the specimen obtained.

EQUIPMENT AND SUPPLIES

Urine specimen
Pregnancy test kit
Clean test slide

Disposable mixing sticks
Reagents
Droppers

Continued

32

PROCEDURAL STEPS

1. Wash and dry hands. Follow the universal blood and body-fluid precautions. Glove yourself with nonsterile gloves.

2. Prepare the testing equipment.

3. Collect the needed specimen. If urine is to be used, collect approximately 0.250 ml in a clean container without preservatives. If serum is to be the testing agent, approximately 0.250 ml of serum is required to be collected by venipuncture into a clean tube without anticoagulants. Permit blood to form a clot for 20 to 30 minutes at room temperature. Centrifuge to obtain clear serum and transfer the serum into a clean glass or plastic tube.

4. Label the handle of the absorbent device or conjugate tube with the patient's name and control number.

5. Remove stopper from the conjugate tube. Discard the stopper (Fig. 32–20).
   Purpose: To prevent possible contamination.

6. With a disposable specimen dispenser, draw specimen to the 0.250 ml calibration line and expel specimen into the conjugate tube (Fig. 32–21).
   Purpose: To ensure accurate test results, specimen amount must be exact.

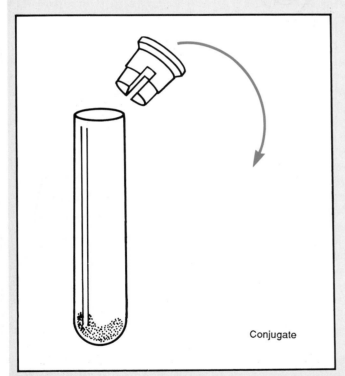

Conjugate

FIGURE 32–20.

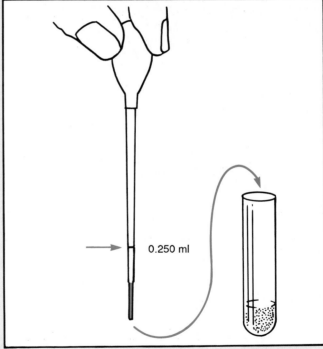

0.250 ml

FIGURE 32–21.

Continued

PROCEDURE 32–9 *Continued*

7. Mix briefly with a side-to-side motion to reconstitute the conjugate. Do not turn the tube upside down. Vortexing is not required or recommended. The mixture will appear cloudy (Fig. 32–22).

8. Place the conjugate tube into the work station (Fig. 32–23).

9. Place a labeled absorbent device into the conjugate tube.
   Purpose: To ensure proper identification of the test.

10. Read the reactions after 5 minutes for urine and 7 minutes for serum specimens. The absorbent device must be left in the conjugate tube when reading results.
    Purpose: Removing the device may alter the test results.

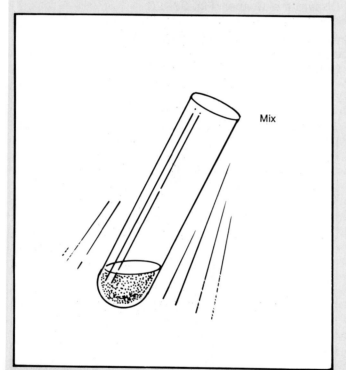

Mix

FIGURE 32–22.

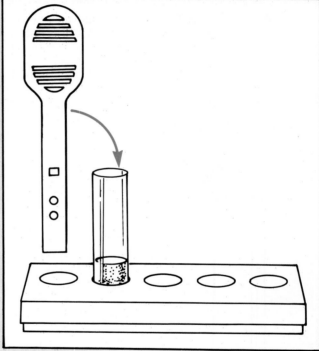

FIGURE 32–23.

Continued

11. To read the results, compare the color development in the three reaction zones (Fig. 32–24). If the pink-rose color in the sample reaction zone is darker than the negative control zone, the test result is *positive* (Fig. 32–25). If the pink-rose color in the sample reaction zone is equal to the color in the negative control zone, the test result is *negative* (Fig. 32–26).

12. Record test results.

13. Dispose of all used testing equipment in proper bio-waste container. Clean area. ***Purpose:*** Consider each component that comes in contact with specimen to be potentially infectious.

14. Remove gloves and wash hands.

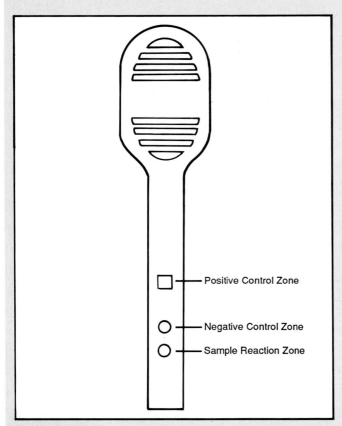

FIGURE 32–24.

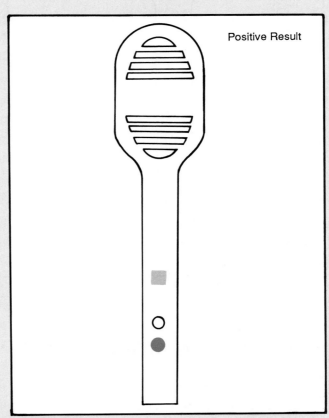

FIGURE 32–25.

Continued

PROCEDURE 32-9 *Continued*

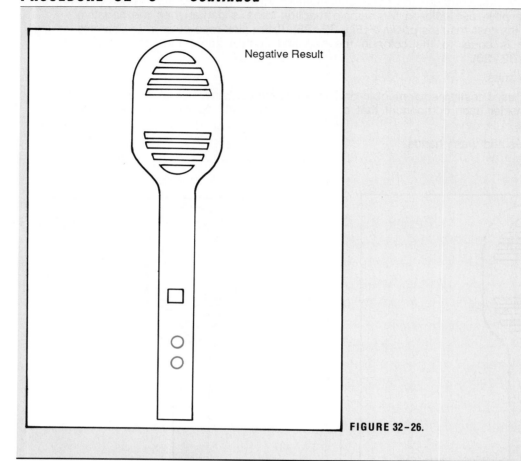

Negative Result

FIGURE 32-26.

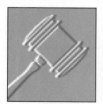

Like all other procedures, the test is only as valid as the specimen and the procedure performed on that specimen. You, as the physician's agent, are responsible for that validity when you instruct the patient and when you perform the test.

The medical assistant who is responsible for office laboratory testing must clearly understand the basic concepts of laboratory medicine. To do this, you must stay current with the rapid technologic advances in laboratory medicine and assist in the establishment of a protocol of the tests best suited to your physician/employer.

You have the responsibility for properly collecting specimens and accurately testing them. The office laboratory can provide a real challenge and the opportunity to work with the physician in promoting and improving the health of the patient.

▶ LEARNING ACHIEVEMENTS

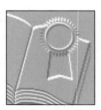

Upon successfully completing this chapter, can you in the time allowed by your evaluator:

1. Instruct a patient in the collection of a timed/24-hour urine specimen?
2. Instruct a patient in the collection of a clean catch midstream urine specimen?
3. Assess and record the color and turbidity of a urine specimen?
4. Perform calibration and testing for specific gravity to +0.002 of the actual specific gravity?
5. Perform chemical testing of a urine sample to a minimum performance level of 100% accuracy for negative reactions and within +1 color block of given results for positive reactions?

6. Perform the Clinitest procedure and record the results within +1 color block of the known value for that specimen?

7. Perform the acid precipitation test within +1 grade of the known results?

8. Perform a microscopic examination of urine within 20 minutes to a minimum performance level of +1 reporting range for casts, RBCs, WBCs, and epithelial cells and to a minimum performance range of 100% for the presence of mucus, crystals, yeast, and sperm?

9. Prepare and test the quality control product within 40 minutes, obtaining results that are within the range given by the product, and accurately record the results?

10. Demonstrate the proper use and care of:
    a. centrifuge?
    b. urinometer?
    c. microscope?
    d. other urinary testing equipment?

11. Perform a slide agglutination test for pregnancy to the minimum performance level of 100% accuracy for positive/negative controls and known specimens.

REFERENCES AND READINGS

Ames Company: *Modern Urinary Chemistry, A Guide to the Diagnosis of Urinary Tract Diseases and Metabolic Disorders,* revised reprint, Indiana, Elkhart, 1992.

Calbreath, D. F.: *Clinical Chemistry,* Philadelphia, W. B. Saunders Co., 1992.

Feingold, S. M., and Baron, E. J.: *Bailey and Scott's Diagnostic Microbiology,* St. Louis, C. V. Mosby Co., 1986.

Henry, J. B.: *Clinical Diagnosis and Management by Laboratory Methods,* 18th ed., Philadelphia, W. B. Saunders Co., 1991.

Wedding, M. E., and Toenjes, S. A.: *Medical Laboratory Procedures,* Philadelphia, F. A. Davis Co., 1992.

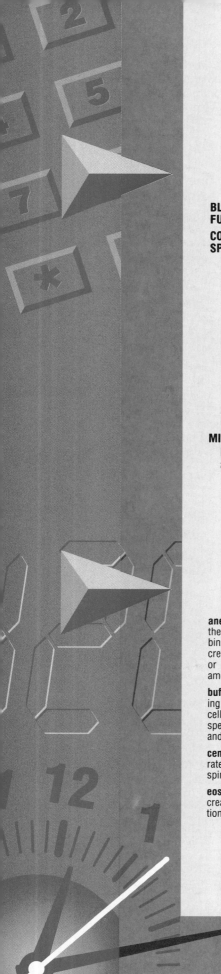

CHAPTER OUTLINE

VOCABULARY

anemia An abnormal decrease in the red blood cell count, hemoglobin, or hematocrit caused by increased red blood cell destruction or inability to produce sufficient amounts of normal red blood cells.

buffy coat The white layer separating the plasma and the red blood cell layers in a centrifuged blood specimen; contains the white cells and the platelets.

centrifuge An instrument that separates portions of samples by rapidly spinning them in a container.

eosin A granular leukocyte that increases in number in allergic conditions.

erythrocyte Red blood cell; contains the blood protein.

heparin A mixture of active principles capable of prolonging blood clotting time.

leukemia A malignant neoplasm of the blood-forming organs.

leukocyte White blood cell; primary function is fighting disease in the body.

morphology The study of the size, shape, and staining characteristics of a cell.

phagocytosis The engulfing of microorganisms and foreign particles by phagocytes.

plasma A straw-colored fluid that transports nutrients, hormones, and waste products; composed of 91% water.

polycythemia vera A condition that causes an overproduction of all formed elements of the blood.

serology A laboratory study of serum and the reactions between antigens and antibodies.

serum Plasma with the clotting proteins removed.

syncope A brief loss of consciousness; fainting.

thrombocyte Same as platelet; the smallest formed element of the blood.

tourniquet A device for the compression of an artery or a vein.

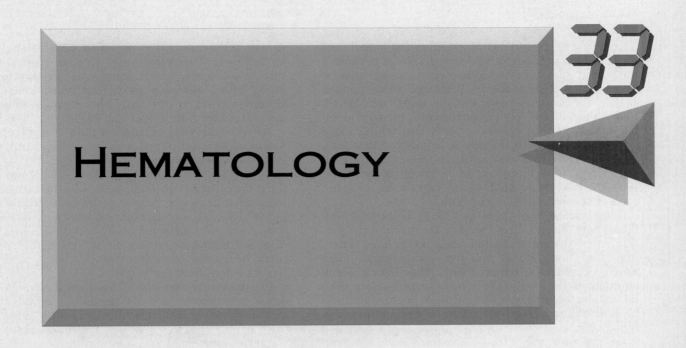

HEMATOLOGY

33

LEARNING OBJECTIVES

COGNITIVE

Upon successful completion of this chapter, you should be able to:

1. Define and spell the terms in the Vocabulary.

2. List the components of blood and the function of each.

3. Differentiate between plasma and serum.

4. List the blood tests that are performed for a complete blood count and the normal values of each.

5. List the sites used in obtaining capillary and venous blood for testing.

6. Explain the function of the Unopette.

7. Identify the parts of a hemacytometer.

8. Name the fluids used for red and white blood cell counts.

9. Discuss the normal cellular elements that may be observed in a blood smear.

10. State the normal values for the erythrocyte sedimentation rate.

PERFORMANCE

Upon successful completion of this chapter, you should be able to perform the following activities:

1. Demonstrate the correct procedure for obtaining a blood sample from a patient by venipuncture.

2. Demonstrate the correct procedure for obtaining a blood sample from a patient by capillary puncture.

3. Perform a microhematocrit on a sample of whole blood.

4. Perform a manual white cell count and calculate the results.

5. Perform a manual red cell count and calculate the results.

6. Demonstrate the proper use of a Unopette.

7. Prepare and stain a blood smear.

8. Perform a differential cell count on a properly stained blood smear.

9. Evaluate the morphology of red blood cells on a properly stained blood smear.

10. Estimate the number of platelets using a properly stained blood smear.

11. Determine an erythrocyte sedimentation rate.

Through the centuries, blood has fascinated and awed humans. Early myths about blood became a basis for sacrificial religious ceremonies, medical practices, and even poetry. Although these ancient beliefs about blood have, for the most part, disappeared, some still remain to frustrate modern medical procedures. In certain rural areas, taking blood samples is forbidden because it is believed that vital spirits needed to keep the body alive might be removed with the blood. Another primitive belief retained by some is that blood cannot be replaced once it is removed from the body.

The average body holds 10 to 12 pints of blood. The heart rotates this through the circulatory system more than a thousand times every day. There are more than 70,000 miles of passageways, most narrower than a human hair, that carry blood throughout the body. The blood contains more than 25 trillion cells; every second, the body replaces 8 million old red blood cells with 8 million new red blood cells.

Of the four major blood groups—A, B, O, and AB—about 85% are Rh positive and 15% are Rh negative.

- One person in three is O positive.
- One person in 15 is O negative.
- One person in three is A positive.
- One person in 16 is A negative.
- One person in 12 is B positive.
- One person in 67 is B negative.
- One person in 29 is AB positive.
- One person in 167 is AB negative.

Hematology is the study of blood. The modern hematology laboratory deals with the *counting* of red blood cells, white blood cells, and platelets; *differentiating* white blood cells on a stained smear; *measuring* the percentage of red blood cells in blood (hematocrit); and *determining* the oxygen-carrying capacity of the blood (hemoglobin).

The *complete blood count (CBC)* is the most frequent laboratory procedure ordered on blood. It gives a fairly complete look at the components of blood and can provide a wealth of information concerning a patient's condition. The CBC routinely includes the following:

- Red blood cell count
- White blood cell count
- Hemoglobin determination
- Hematocrit determination
- Differential white blood cell count
- Estimation of platelet numbers
- Red blood cell **morphology** (size and shape)

BLOOD COMPOSITION, FUNCTION, AND FORMATION

Whole blood is composed of formed elements suspended in a clear yellow liquid portion called **plasma.** Plasma makes up about 55% of the blood by volume. The remaining 45% consists of the formed elements, which are the **erythrocytes** (red blood cells), **leukocytes** (white blood cells), and **thrombocytes** (platelets). The average adult has approximately 5 to 6 quarts of blood.

Blood is the vital circulating fluid of the body and has at times been referred to as the "river of life." It is a transportation system bringing numerous substances of nourishment to all the cells of our body for growth, function, and repair and, in turn, carrying waste products away for disposal. In addition, blood functions to maintain the body at a uniform temperature; to keep the other body fluids in a state of equilibrium between alkalinity and acidity; and to carry hormones from the various glands to distant tissues where they are needed.

Plasma is the carrier for the formed elements and other substances such as proteins, carbohydrates, fats, hormones, enzymes, mineral salts, gases, and waste products. Plasma is composed of about 90% water, 9% protein, and 1% of various other chemical substances.

The cellular elements are produced and mature in the bone marrow, spleen, and lymph nodes. Then, they are released into the bloodstream. These cellular elements all have special functions.

The erythrocytes transport oxygen from the lungs to the body cells and carry carbon dioxide away from the cells, back to the lungs to be exhaled. They are disclike cells that have two concave sides and no nucleus. Their main constituent is the red pigment hemoglobin, which is composed of iron and protein. Hemoglobin actually carries the oxygen and carbon dioxide throughout the body. The life span of an erythrocyte is about 120 days. Then the cell is broken down, and the wastes are stored in the liver. The iron is reused for new red blood cell formation, and the protein is converted into a bile pigment.

The prime function of the leukocyte is to protect the body against infection and disease. The five types of leukocytes are classified into granular and agranular groups. The granular leukocytes are called *polymorphonuclear* leukocytes and include the neutrophils, eosinophils, and basophils. They are characterized by their heavily granulated cytoplasm and segmented nuclei. The *agranular* leukocytes are the lymphocytes and monocytes, which both have clear cytoplasm and a solid nucleus.

Thrombocytes play a vital role in initiating the clotting process of blood. When a small vessel is injured, thrombocytes adhere to each other and the edges of the injury, and form a plug that becomes a blood clot. This blood clot soon retracts and stops the loss of blood.

COLLECTION OF BLOOD SPECIMENS

For most hematology testing, an adequate blood sample can be obtained from capillaries by finger puncture. If a larger sample is required, blood can be obtained from a vein by venipuncture. To perform a CBC, venous blood is collected in a tube containing an *anticoagulant* that prevents clotting. Adding an anticoagulant results in a whole blood sample. When a blood specimen has had anticoagulant added, the liquid portion is called plasma. When a blood specimen is collected without an anticoagulant, it forms a clot and the liquid portion remaining is called **serum.**

Venipuncture

The most common method of obtaining blood for hematology testing is by venipuncture *(phlebotomy).* In a venipuncture, the blood is taken directly from a superficial vein. The vein is punctured with a needle, and the blood is collected in either a syringe or a tube. While a venipuncture is a safe procedure when performed by a trained professional, the procedure must be performed with care. You should routinely use appropriate barrier precautions when handling blood specimens. The good condition of the veins must also be preserved. Much practice is required to become skilled and confident in the art of venipuncture.

Generally, veins in the forearm or the elbow are used for venipunctures (Fig. 33–1). The puncture site should be carefully selected after inspecting both arms. The vein most frequently used is the median cephalic vein of the forearm. Alternative sites may be indicated if the area is cyanotic, scarred, bruised, edematous, or burned. You may use veins on the lower forearm, the back of the hand, or the wrist. Use foot or ankle veins only if the patient

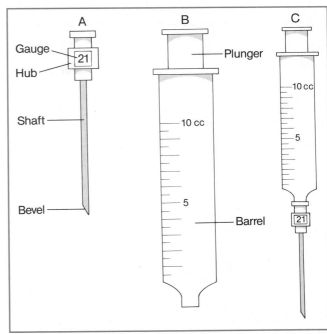

FIGURE 33–2. Materials for venipuncture. *A,* Hypodermic. *B,* Syringe. *C,* Syringe and needle assembled.

has good circulation of the legs and you have received permission from your supervisor or the physician.

Performing a venipuncture involves several important steps with which the medical assistant must be thoroughly familiar before attempting the procedure. The first step is to select the proper method for venipuncture (syringe or Vacutainer). Next, the patient must be prepared for the procedure. Patient preparation is followed by the actual venipuncture and specimen collection. The final step is care of the puncture site before discharging the patient.

Syringe Method

When veins are very small or fragile, the syringe method of venipuncture may be used. The equipment required includes a sterile syringe and hypodermic needle, tourniquet, 70% alcohol, sterile gauze, and a blood-collecting tube (Fig. 33–2). Most laboratories today use disposable needles and syringes. The needle and syringe must be assembled carefully to maintain sterility. Do not touch the tips of either needle or syringe, and do not uncap the needle until just prior to actual puncture. Needles of 20 to 22 gauge are used for venipunctures. The needle should be inspected to ascertain that it is sharp and smooth. The syringe plunger should be checked for free movement and should be left completely pushed into the barrel so that no air remains in the syringe.

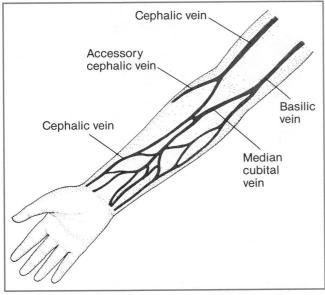

FIGURE 33–1. Veins of the arm commonly used for venipuncture.

TABLE 33-1. VACUTAINER TUBES, CONTENTS, AND THEIR USES

Stopper Color	Contents (Anticoagulant)	Uses*
Red	None	Serum for chemistry, serologic tests, typing, and crossmatching
Royal blue	Chemically clean	Trace metals (iron, lead); serum for chemistry
Black/red mottled (serum separation tube)†	Serum-separator gel	Serum for most chemistries, serologic tests
Black/yellow mottled (chlormerodrin accumulation test) (CAT)†	Clot activator, separator gel	Stat serum collections
Light blue†	Citrate	Coagulation studies, some hematology tests
Lavender†	EDTA	Hematology tests, some chemistries
Black†	Balanced oxalate	Coagulation
Green†	Heparin	Plasma for some chemistries, especially stats
Gray†	Fluoride	Stat glucose tests, alcohol levels, drug screening

*Specimen requirements vary, depending on the method used in testing. Always check the laboratory specimen requirements manual before collecting a specimen.
†Denotes tubes that must be thoroughly mixed by gentle inversion after the blood is collected.

Vacutainer Method

The Vacutainer system (Becton-Dickinson Company) is the most common collection system in use. It consists of evacuated tubes of various sizes with color-coded tops, indicating tube contents (Table 33–1); sterile disposable double-ended needles of different lengths and gauges; and a reusable plastic adapter that holds the needle and guides the tube (Fig. 33–3). Both pediatric- and adult-size adapters and tubes are available. The needle has two sharp ends. The short end is fitted into the adapter, and the long end is used to puncture the vein. After the vein is entered, the tube is pushed onto the needle in the adapter, and blood is drawn into the tube by vacuum. When the tube is full, it can be replaced by another tube.

Several tubes of blood can be collected using a variety of color-coded tubes with a single venipuncture. Tubes containing ethylenediamine-tetra-acetic acid (EDTA) anticoagulant additive are recommended for use when doing hematology studies. The white blood cells and platelets are best preserved in this type of tube, and better red blood cell morphology results will be obtained. This additive has no adverse effects on the blood sample when a sufficient quantity of blood is obtained. However, problems arise when too little blood is placed in the tube containing the additive. Misleading results and an incorrect diagnosis may occur.

Patient Preparation

Proper patient preparation begins with identification of the patient and a brief explanation of the procedure to minimize anxiety. The patient should be lying down or seated in a chair. Never have the patient standing or sitting on a high stool. Special venipuncture chairs are available with adjustable arm rests and a locking safety mechanism that prevents the patient from falling should fainting occur. (See Chapter 40 for the first-aid procedure for fainting.)

All necessary supplies should be within easy reach. When using the Vacutainer method, you should have extra tubes available in case you encounter a bad vacuum. **Tourniquets** should be flat, broad, and elastic. *Velcro* tourniquets are easy to apply and adjust; they come in several sizes. Blood pressure cuffs may be used. They can be easily inflated or deflated during the procedure, if necessary.

Alcohol from a dispenser or individual packets is used for most collections. For sterile or aseptic collections, individually packaged *povidone-iodine* swabs are used. Specimens for testing for blood alcohol levels are collected using *benzalkonium chloride* as the antiseptic. Alcohol may not be used for this collection, as it could interfere with the results of the test.

Needle disposal units should be available. Used needles should *not* be recapped, as this is the most

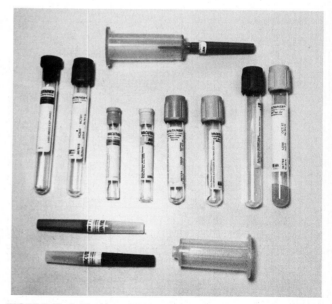

FIGURE 33-3. The Vacutainer system (Becton Dickinson Co.) consists of a reusable plastic adapter.

33

how to assemble

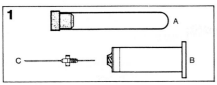

1

Description of parts:
A. Evacuated Glass Tube with Rubber Stopper
B. Plastic Holder with Guide Line
C. Double-Pointed Needle

A

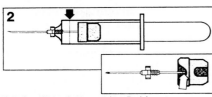

2

Thread needle into holder...tighten firmly!
Place tube in holder with needle touching stopper.

3

Push tube forward until top of stopper meets guide line. Let go.
Tube stopper will retract below guide line—leave it in that position.
At this stage, the full point of the needle is embedded in the stopper (see cross section) thus avoiding blood leakage upon venipuncture and preventing premature loss of vacuum.

Alternate Method
If needle and adapter are used, follow these instructions in place of steps 1 and 2.

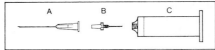

A   B   C

Description of parts:
A. Luer Hub Needle
B. VACUTAINER Adapter
C. Plastic Holder
Thread adapter into holder...tighten firmly!
Attach Luer Needle to Adapter slip as you would needle to a syringe. Place tube in holder with needle touching stopper, then proceed to step 3, above.

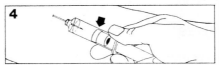

4

Where vein cannot be located — to conserve vacuum — remove tube from rear cannula (see arrow) before withdrawing needle from tissue.

how to use

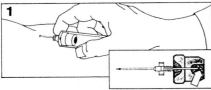

1

With rear point embedded in stopper, enter tissue—and immediately on tissue entry complete puncture of diaphragm.

B

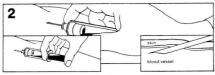

2

If in vein—blood flows immediately. Note: Technologist with small hands, proceed as you would with a hypodermic syringe. Holder provides finger grip and tube acts as plunger (see inset).

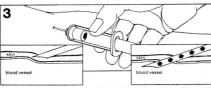

3

If in tissue instead of vein—blood will not be drawn. Proceed until venipuncture is signaled by intake of blood into VACUTAINER Tube, as shown.

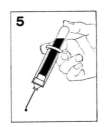

5

How to obtain blood drops for red and white cell counts, blood smears, etc. After tube is filled —grasp holder as illustrated and press firmly on bottom of tube. After each drop, release pressure and repeat for successive drops.

Additional Information
Incomplete Venipuncture, which may cause the tube to fill slowly or partially, may be corrected by deeper vein entry.
Transfixing of the vein may be corrected by pulling back slowly with needle until flow of blood indicates vein lumen re-entry.
Multiple Specimens (2, 3 or more) may be taken with one venipuncture and without loss of blood by releasing tourniquet while first tube is filling, and switching tubes while needle remains in vein.
Vein occlusion can be minimized by using VACUTAINER Adapter and smaller gauge needles (23, 24 or 25 gauge), thus slowing up flow of blood.
Proper degree of vacuum in each VACUTAINER Tube is doubly assured by the B-D Can Pack.

FIGURE 33–4. B-D Vacutainer method of making a venipuncture. *A,* How to assemble B-D Vacutainer. *B,* How to use B-D Vacutainer. (Courtesy of Becton Dickinson Co., Cockeysville, MD.)

probable cause of accidental needle sticks. Present guidelines for needle disposal recommend that the used needle be removed directly into the needle disposal unit, without cutting or recapping.

Keep your supplies clean and in order. The expiration dates of the evacuated tubes should be checked to be certain that outdated supplies are removed from use. Restock supplies as they are used.

Drawing the Blood

The patient's arm is fully extended and supported. A tourniquet is applied to the arm to make the veins more prominent by slowing blood flow.

The puncture site is located by gently pressing on the veins with your fingertips. This will determine the direction of the vein and the approximate size and depth. The area around the puncture site is cleansed with alcohol and sterile gauze. The site is then dried also using sterile gauze.

The syringe or assembled Vacutainer system (Fig. 33–4) is held in one hand, at a 15- to 30-degree angle to the arm. The needle is bevel up and pointing in the same direction as the vein. The skin and vein are entered with one smooth motion until the needle is in the lumen of the vein. The blood is obtained by gently pulling back on the plunger with the other hand while holding the syringe and needle motionless. When using the Vacutainer method, place two fingers at the end of the holder and, with your thumb, push the tube into the adapter. Release the tourniquet as soon as blood begins to fill the tube or to flow into the syringe. When you have obtained the required amount of blood, place a dry sterile gauze pad over the puncture site and remove the needle from the vein.

Care of the Puncture Site

Apply pressure for a few minutes. You may have the patient elevate the arm at this time to prevent oozing of blood. If you have used the syringe method, the blood must be transferred to a tube at this time. Gently insert the needle through the rubber stopper of a vacuum tube. The vacuum inside will draw the required amount of blood into the tube. For tubes that contain additives, gently invert eight to ten times to mix.

Check the puncture site and apply a Band-Aid, if desired. Discard the needle into the designated container, and clean the work area. Complete the laboratory requisition, and forward the blood specimen to the appropriate place. Wash your hands.

PROCEDURE 33-1   COLLECTING A VENOUS BLOOD SPECIMEN

GOAL   To collect a venous blood specimen.

EQUIPMENT AND SUPPLIES

Needle, syringe and tube or Vacutainer
   needle, adapter, and tube
70% alcohol

Sterile gauze pads
Tourniquet
Band-Aids

PROCEDURAL STEPS

1. Wash and dry your hands. Follow the universal blood and body-fluid precautions. Glove yourself with nonsterile gloves.
    Purpose: To prevent the spread of disease.

2. Check requisition for tests ordered and specimen requirements. Gather the materials needed (Fig. 33–5).
    Purpose: Allows for proper specimen collection.

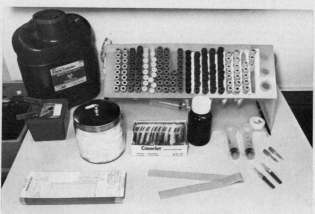

FIGURE 33-5.

Continued

3. Identify the patient and explain the procedure.
   Purpose: Ascertains patient identity, and explanations help gain the patient's cooperation.

4. Instruct the patient to sit with the arm well supported in a downward position.
   Purpose: Veins of the antecubital fossa are more easily located when the elbow is straight (Fig. 33–6).

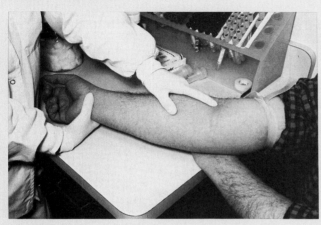

FIGURE 33–6.

5. Assemble equipment: Choice of syringe and needle sizes depends upon your inspection of the patient's veins. Attach the needle to the syringe or to the Vacutainer holder. Keep the cover on the needle.

6. Now, label tubes with the patient's name, the date, and time.

7. Apply the tourniquet around the patient's arm three to four inches above the elbow. The tourniquet should never be tied so tightly that it restricts blood flow in the artery (Fig. 33–7).
   Purpose: The tourniquet is used to make the veins more prominent.

8. Select the venipuncture site by palpating the antecubital space, and use your index finger to trace the path of the vein and to judge its depth. The vein most often used is the median cephalic, which lies in the middle of the elbow.
   Purpose: The index finger is most sensitive for palpating. Do not use the thumb, as it has a pulse of its own, which may confuse you (Fig. 33–8).

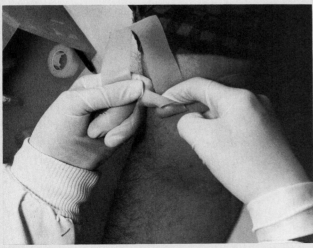

FIGURE 33–7.

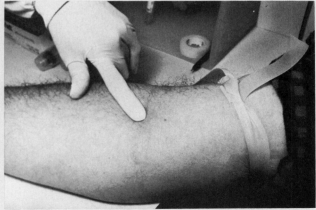

FIGURE 33–8.

Continued

PROCEDURE 33-1 *Continued*

9. Ask the patient to open and close his or her hand several times.
   Purpose: Clenching the fist produces engorgement of the vein.

10. Cleanse the site, starting in the center of the area and working outward in a circular pattern (Fig. 33-9).

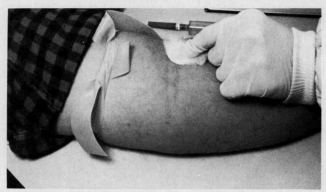

FIGURE 33-9.

11. Dry the site with a sterile gauze.
    Purpose: The circular pattern helps avoid recontamination of the area. Puncturing a wet area stings and can cause hemolysis of the sample.

12. Remove the needle sheath.

13. Hold the syringe or Vacutainer assembly in your dominant hand. Your thumb should be on top and your fingers underneath.

14. Grasp the patient's arm with the nondominant hand while using your thumb and forefinger to draw the skin taut over the site, to anchor the vein (Fig. 33-10).
    Purpose: Failure to anchor the vein makes puncturing more difficult and painful and may result in a missed vein.

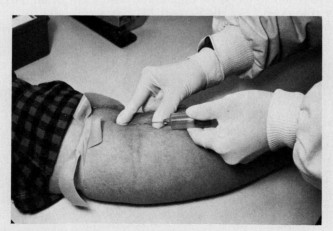

FIGURE 33-10.

Continued

15. Insert the needle through the skin and into the vein with the bevel of the needle up, aligned parallel to the vein, at a 15-degree angle, rapidly, and smoothly (Fig. 33–11). *Purpose:* The sharpest point of the needle is inserted first.

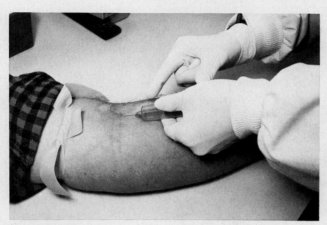

FIGURE 33–11.

16. Slowly pull back the plunger of the syringe with the nondominant hand *or* place two fingers on the flanges of the Vacutainer holder and, with the thumb, push the tube onto the needle inside the holder. Make sure that you do not move the needle after entering the vein. Allow the syringe or tube to fill to optimum capacity.

17. Remove the Vacutainer tube from the adapter prior to removing the needle from the vein. *Purpose:* A nontraumatic venipuncture produces the most reliable results. Proper tube filling ensures the correct ratio of blood to additive. Removal of the tube from the holder prior to removal from the vein prevents any excess blood from dripping from the tip of the needle onto the patient (Fig. 33–12).

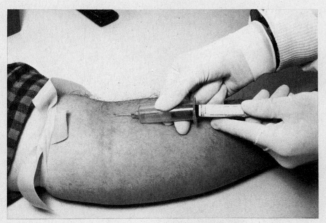

FIGURE 33–12.

18. Release the tourniquet when venipuncture is complete. It must be released before the needle is removed from the arm. *Purpose:* Removal of the tourniquet releases pressure on the vein and helps prevent blood from getting into adjacent tissues and causing a hematoma.

Continued

PROCEDURE 33 – 1   *Continued*

19. Place a sterile cotton ball over the puncture site at time of needle withdrawal (Fig. 33–13).

20. Instruct patient to apply direct pressure on puncture site with sterile cotton ball (Fig. 33–14). The patient may elevate the arm.
    Purpose: Direct pressure is the best method to stop bleeding. Elevating the arm above the heart also stops bleeding.

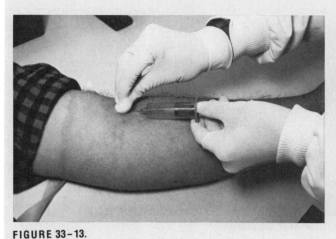

FIGURE 33–13.

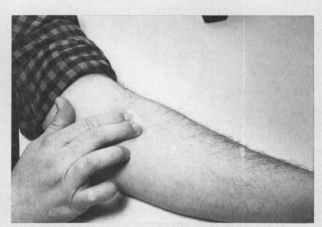

FIGURE 33–14.

21. Transfer the blood to a tube if using a syringe. Gently invert tubes to mix anticoagulants and blood. If tubes were not labeled prior to venipuncture, do so now (Fig. 33–15).
    Purpose: Prevents clotting of blood. Vigorous mixing may cause hemolysis.

22. Check the puncture site for bleeding.

23. Apply a Band-Aid (Fig. 33–16).

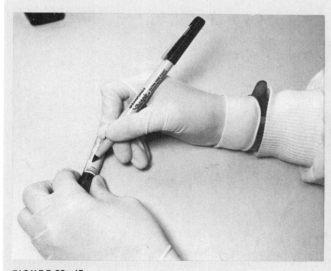

FIGURE 33–15.

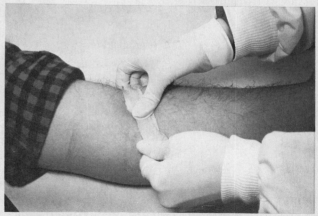

FIGURE 33–16.

Continued

24. Dispose of the needle safely. Allow it to drop directly into the disposal unit without touching it with your fingers. Do not recap used needles.
   Purpose: Most accidental needle sticks occur when a needle is being recapped. Report any accidents to your supervisor or the physician.

25. Clean the work area. Follow the recommendations for proper disposal of all materials.

26. Complete the laboratory requisition and route to the proper place.

27. Wash your hands.

Capillary Puncture

Capillaries are small blood vessels connecting the small arterioles to the small venules. The capillary puncture is an efficient means of collecting a blood specimen when only a small amount of blood is required or when a patient's condition makes venipuncture difficult.

Patient Preparation

In adults and children, the usual puncture site is the ring finger, but capillary blood can be obtained from the great finger, the earlobe, toe, or heel (Fig. 33–17). The puncture is made at the tip and slightly to the side of the finger.

The puncture site must be prepared by gentle massaging or placing the finger in warm water. This will increase blood circulation and allow a good flow of blood. The site is cleansed with 70% alcohol and wiped with a dry sterile gauze pad.

Obtaining the Blood

The patient's hand is held in a lateral position, with the skin near the puncture site pulled taut. A sharp-pointed blade called a *lancet* is used. Capillary punctures may also be performed using semiautomated devices such as the *Autolet*. The puncture is performed in one quick, smooth motion. The lancet should puncture the site to a depth of 3 to 4 mm. The first drop of blood is wiped away because it contains tissue liquid and would dilute any results. The second and following drops are used. The finger is massaged to increase blood flow. Squeezing the finger should be avoided, since this will force tissue fluid to dilute the blood. Samples must be collected quickly to avoid clotting. For this reason, it is important to assemble all equipment needed before performing the capillary puncture (Fig. 33–18).

Pipetting the Blood

Blood must be diluted before blood cells can be counted microscopically because the cellular elements of blood are so concentrated. Blood-diluting pipettes are used to dilute the blood with a diluting fluid, to manually perform leukocyte, erythrocyte, and thrombocyte counts. Blood is collected in glass blood-diluting pipettes, self-filling disposable pipettes, capillary tubes, or on glass slides.

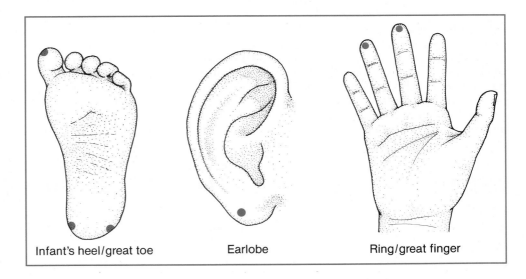

Infant's heel/great toe   Earlobe   Ring/great finger

FIGURE 33-17. Skin puncture sites.

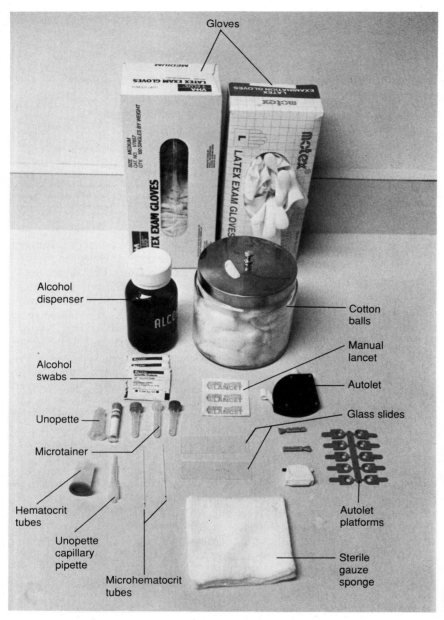

Gloves

Alcohol dispenser

Cotton balls

Manual lancet

Alcohol swabs

Autolet

Glass slides

Unopette

Microtainer

Hematocrit tubes

Autolet platforms

Unopette capillary pipette

Microhematocrit tubes

Sterile gauze sponge

FIGURE 33-18. Equipment needed for capillary puncture.

Self-filling and self-measuring disposable micropipette systems are also available for counting leukocytes, erythrocytes, and platelets. The *Unopette* system consists of a disposable self-filling diluting pipette and a plastic reservoir prefilled with a precise amount of diluting fluid.

Capillary tubes are available with and without the anticoagulant **heparin.** Tubes with a red ring around one end contain heparin, while those with a blue ring are nonheparinized. The microhematocrit specimen can be collected directly from the finger using the heparinized tubes.

The best specimen for a blood smear is capillary blood smeared directly onto a glass slide. The smear is stained, and the morphology of the cellular components can then be studied.

PROCEDURE 33-2   COLLECTING A CAPILLARY BLOOD SPECIMEN

GOAL   To collect a capillary blood specimen suitable for testing, using fingertip puncture technique.

Continued

EQUIPMENT AND SUPPLIES

Sterile disposable lancet
70% alcohol
Sterile gauze pads

Band-Aids
Supplies for requested test (e.g., Unopettes, slides, capillary tubes)

PROCEDURAL STEPS

1. Wash and dry your hands. Follow the universal blood and body-fluid precautions. Glove yourself with nonsterile gloves.

2. Greet and identify the patient.
   Purpose: Identifying the patient prior to the collection of the specimen is extremely important.

3. Explain the procedure.
   Purpose: Explanations help gain the patient's cooperation.

4. Assemble the needed materials, based upon the physician's requisition.
   Purpose: Once the skin has been punctured, the collection must proceed as rapidly as possible so the blood does not clot before the entire specimen has been collected.

5. Select a puncture site (side of middle finger of nondominant hand, outer edge of earlobe; medial or lateral curved surface of the heel or the great toe for an infant).
   Purpose: The nondominant hand may have fewer calluses. The side of the finger is less sensitive, and the skin is usually not as thick.

6. "Milk," or very gently rub, the finger along the sides.
   Purpose: This promotes circulation. If the finger is very cold, you may immerse it in warm water or moisten it with warm towels.

7. Clean the site with alcohol, and dry it with sterile gauze.
   Purpose: Puncturing wet skin is painful and can hemolyze the specimen.

8. Grasp the patient's finger on the sides near the puncture site, with your nondominant forefinger and thumb (Fig. 33–19).
   Purpose: Firmly holding the site allows control of the puncture.

9. Hold the lancet at a right angle to the patient's finger, and make a rapid, deep puncture on the patient's fingertip (Fig. 33–20).
   Purpose: Lancets are designed to puncture at a depth of 3 to 4 mm, which is sufficient to obtain the required drops of blood.

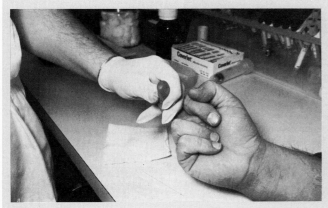

FIGURE 33–19.

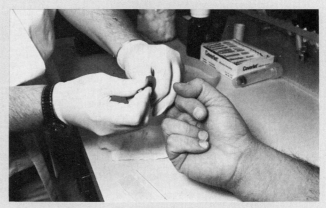

FIGURE 33–20.

Continued

PROCEDURE 33-2   *Continued*

10. Wipe away the first drop of blood (Fig. 33–21).
    Purpose: The first drop of blood contains tissue fluid.

11. Apply gentle pressure to cause the blood to flow freely (Fig. 33–22).
    Purpose: Squeezing liberates tissue that dilutes the blood and causes inaccurate results.

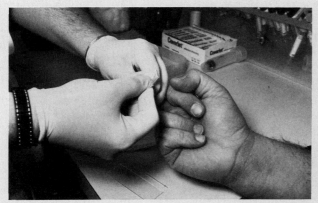

FIGURE 33-21.

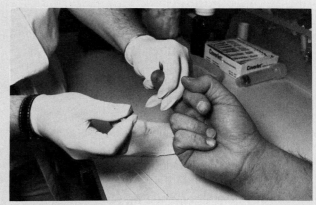

FIGURE 33-22.

12. Collect blood samples:
    a. Express a large, rounded drop of blood, and fill capillary tubes (Fig. 33–23).

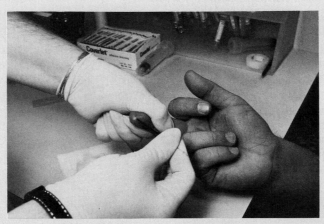

FIGURE 33-23.

    b. Wipe the finger with a clean sterile gauze pad, and place a fresh drop of blood on a slide for a smear (Figs. 33–24 and 33–25). Immediately make the smear, using the two-slide method (see Procedure 33–7).

13. Apply pressure to the site with clean sterile gauze.

14. Label all samples and requisitions correctly, and forward to laboratory for testing.

15. Check the patient for bleeding, and apply a Band-Aid if indicated.

16. Dismiss the patient.

Continued

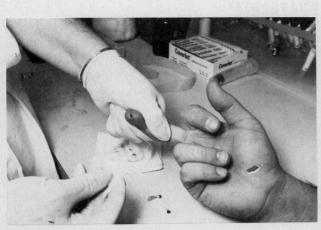

FIGURE 33-24.

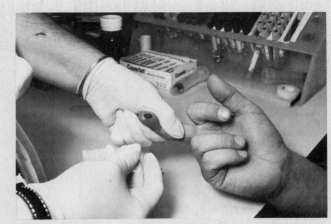

FIGURE 33-25.

17. Dispose of used materials in proper containers.

18. Clean the work area. Follow the recommendations for proper disposal of all materials.

19. Wash your hands.

MICROHEMATOCRIT

The microhematocrit (Hct) is a measurement of the percentage of packed red blood cells in a volume of blood. The test is based on the principle of separating the cellular elements from the plasma. The separation process is speeded up by centrifugation. Two or three drops of blood are collected in two capillary tubes and are placed in a specially designed microhematocrit **centrifuge.**

After centrifugation, the red blood cells will be at the bottom of the tube, the white blood cells and platelets in the center, and the plasma on top. From this separation, the microhematocrit is determined by comparing the concentration of red blood cells with the total volume of the whole blood sample.

The percentage is read by placing the tubes on a special microhematocrit reader. Some microhematocrit centrifuges have a built-in reading scale that reads calibrated capillary tubes. Microhematocrits should be performed in duplicate, and the average of the two results reported.

The microhematocrit is a commonly performed test requested by physicians separately or as part of the complete blood count. Since it is a simple procedure requiring only a small amount of blood, it is an ideal test for following the progress of patients.

The normal values vary with the sex and age of the patient (Table 33-2). The values range from a low of 36% in women to a high of 52% in men. Low microhematocrit readings can indicate **anemia** or the presence of bleeding in a patient; high readings may be caused by dehydration or a condition such as **polycythemia vera.** Values can be influenced by physiologic or pathologic factors, as well as by collection techniques.

TABLE 33-2. NORMAL HEMATOLOGY VALUES

Test	Men	Women
Microhematocrit	42-52%	36-48%
Hemoglobin	13.5-17.5 g/dl	12.5-15.5 g/dl
WBC	4500-11,000 cells/mm³	4500-11,000 cells/mm³
RBC	4.5-6.0 million cells/mm³	4.0-5.5 million cells/mm³
Platelets	150,000-400,000 cells/mm³ for both	

Differential for Both Men and Women	
Bands	0-7%
Segmented neutrophils	50-65%
Lymphocytes	25-40%
Monocytes	3-9%
Eosinophils	1-3%
Basophils	0-1%

PROCEDURE 33–3   PERFORMING A MICROHEMATOCRIT

GOAL   To perform a microhematocrit in duplicate.

EQUIPMENT AND SUPPLIES

Nonsterile gloves
EDTA anticoagulant blood
Capillary tubes

Sealing clay
Centrifuge

PROCEDURAL STEPS

1. Wash and dry your hands. Follow the universal blood and body-fluid precautions. Glove yourself with nonsterile gloves.

2. Assemble the materials needed.

3. Fill two plain (blue-tip) capillary tubes three-quarters full with well-mixed EDTA anticoagulant blood.
   Purpose: Duplicates should always be done as a means of quality control.

4. Plug the dry end of each tube with a sealing clay.
   Purpose: Sealing the wet end may result in loss of the plug and the sample during centrifugation.

5. Place the tubes opposite each other in the centrifuge, with sealed ends securely against the gasket (Fig. 33–26).
   Purpose: The centrifuge must always be balanced to avoid damage. If the clay ends of the capillary tubes are not outermost against the gasket, the sample will spin out of the tubes. Follow the universal blood and body-fluid precautions.

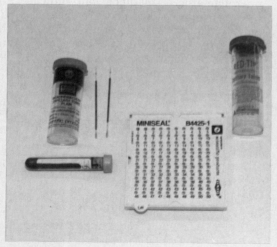
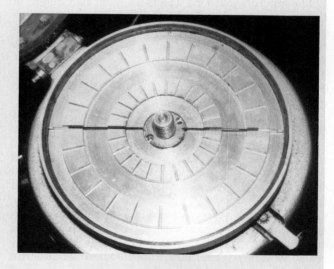

FIGURE 33–26.

6. Note the numbers on the centrifuge slots and record them.
   Purpose: The sample must be identified throughout the entire procedure.

Continued

33

7. Secure the locking top, fasten the lid down, and lock.
   Purpose: If the locking top is not firmly in place during the spinning cycle, the tubes will come out of their slots and break. The lid is always locked during centrifugation for safety purposes, to avoid aerosols or broken glass from being ejected.

8. Set the timer, and adjust the speed as needed.
   Purpose: The prescribed time is between 3 and 5 minutes. Check the manufacturer's instructions for time and speed.

9. Allow the centrifuge to come to a complete stop. Unlock the lids.

10. Remove the tubes immediately.
    Purpose: Tubes left in the centrifuge will show altered results, as the red blood cell layer spreads horizontally.

11. Determine the microhematocrit values, using one of the following methods:

    a. Centrifuge with built-in reader using calibrated capillary tubes.
       (1) Position the tubes as directed by manufacturer's instructions.
       (2) Read both tubes.
       (3) The average of the two results is reported.
       (4) The two values should not vary by more than ±2%.

    b. Centrifuge without built-in reader.
       (1) Carefully remove the tubes from the centrifuge.
       (2) Place a tube on the microhematocrit reader.
       (3) Align the clay–red blood cell junction with the zero line on the reader. Align the plasma meniscus with the 100% line. The value is read at the junction of the red cell layer and the **buffy coat** (Fig. 33–27).
       (4) Read both tubes.
       (5) The average of the two results is reported.
       (6) The two values should not vary by more than ±2%.

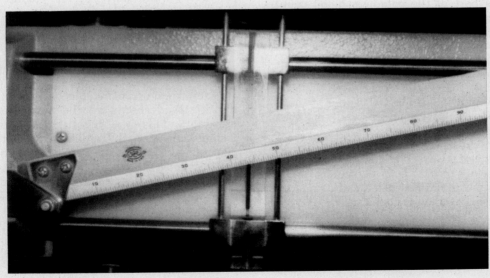

FIGURE 33–27.

12. Dispose of the capillary tubes in a biohazard container.

13. Clean the work area. Follow the recommendations for proper disposal of all materials.

14. Wash your hands.

HEMOGLOBIN

The hemoglobin (Hgb) determination is a rough measure of the oxygen-carrying capacity of the blood. Determining hemoglobin concentration can be performed as part of the complete blood count or as an individual test. Many methods of determining hemoglobin concentration have been used throughout the years. Today, the most widely used hemoglobin method is the *cyanmethemoglobin.* A sample of whole blood is diluted in *Drabkin reagent,* which breaks down (lyses) red cells, releasing the hemoglobin into the solution. The chemicals in the reagent react with the released hemoglobin to form the pigment cyanmethemoglobin, which can be measured by using a photometer.

The normal hemoglobin values vary throughout life. Values are normally quite high at birth, decline during childhood, then increase through the teens until the adult levels are reached (Table 33–2). Values range from a low of 12.5 g/dl in women to a high of 17.5 g/dl in men. The various factors that affect the hemoglobin level include age, sex, diet, altitude, and disease.

RED BLOOD CELL COUNT

The red blood cell count is a commonly performed procedure and is part of the complete blood count. The red blood cell count approximates the number of circulating red blood cells. The function of red blood cells is to transport oxygen to the tissues. The condition in which this oxygen-carrying capacity of the blood is below normal is called anemia. The red blood cell count is usually decreased in anemias. Increases are found in people with dehydration, polycythemia vera, or severe burns and in people who live at high altitudes, as an adaptation to the lower oxygen content of the air.

The normal values for red blood cell counts range from approximately 4 million cells per mm³ of blood to 6 million cells per mm³. Red blood cell counts are usually higher in males than females.

WHITE BLOOD CELL COUNT

The white blood cell count is one of the most frequently requested hematology tests. The white blood cell count gives an approximation of the total number of leukocytes in circulating blood. The count is performed to aid the physician in determining if an infection is present. It may also be used to follow the course of a disease and to determine if the patient is responding to treatment.

The normal white blood cell count varies with age. It is higher in newborns and decreases throughout life. The average adult range is between 4500 and 12,000 cells per mm³. Many factors affect the white blood cell count. Elevation in white blood cells is called *leukocytosis.* Physiologic increases in the white blood cell count are seen in pregnancy, stress, anesthesia, exercise, and exposure to temperature extremes and after treatment with steroids. Pathologic causes of leukocytosis include many bacterial infections, **leukemia,** appendicitis, and pneumonia. A decrease in the white blood cell count is called *leukopenia.* This condition may be caused by viral infections or by exposure to radiation, certain chemicals, and drugs.

METHODS OF COUNTING RED AND WHITE BLOOD CELLS

Manual Counts

Both the red blood cell count and the white blood cell count approximate the number of these circulating cells in the blood. These cellular elements are very concentrated in the blood. Therefore, the blood must be diluted for these cells to be counted microscopically. Blood-diluting pipettes and diluting fluids are used for this purpose. The counts are then performed using the diluted blood, a counting chamber called a *hemacytometer,* a hemacytometer coverslip, and a microscope.

Unopettes

Manual counts using blood-diluting pipettes and diluting fluid should not be performed by medical assistants. This type of testing is usually done in a formal laboratory by a licensed laboratory technician or technologist. A simpler and less error-prone method for performing manual counts is done by using a prefilled reservoir containing a premeasured diluting-fluid unit such as the Unopette (Becton-Dickinson, Cockeysville, MD.). This unit comes equipped with a capillary pipette and pipette shield. Unopettes are available for counting erythrocytes, leukocytes, and platelets (Fig. 33–28). Package inserts contain detailed instructions that, when correctly followed, result in a more accurate dilution than with the blood-diluting pipettes.

Hemacytometer

The hemacytometer is used to count the cellular elements of the blood. The hemacytometer is a heavy glass slide that, when viewed from the top, has two raised platforms surrounded by depressions on three sides. Each raised surface contains a ruled

PROCEDURE 33-4   FILLING A UNOPETTE

GOAL   To properly fill a Unopette pipette with blood and to transfer the sample to a Unopette reservoir.

EQUIPMENT AND SUPPLIES

 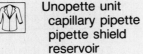

Unopette unit
  capillary pipette
  pipette shield
  reservoir

EDTA anticoagulant blood
Gauze pads
Test tube rack

PROCEDURAL STEPS

1.   Wash and dry your hands. Follow the universal blood and body-fluid precautions. Glove yourself with nonsterile gloves.

2.   Remove a Unopette reservoir from the storage container, and recap the container tightly.
     Purpose: The container is humidified. Loss of the humid conditions will allow evaporation, and the remaining Unopettes will give inaccurate results.

3.   Use the pipette shield to puncture the diaphragm of the Unopette reservoir. The hole must be large enough to allow the pipette to enter freely.
     Purpose: If the hole is too small, loss of a portion of the sample can occur when the pipette is inserted into the reservoir.

4.   Remove the pipette shield.

5.   Hold the pipette nearly horizontal.

6.   Place the tip of the pipette into a well-mixed tube of blood, and allow the pipette to fill by capillary action until blood reaches the end of the pipette. It will stop by itself.

7.   Place a finger over the hole in the end of the pipette to prevent loss of any sample, and carefully wipe the outside of the pipette with gauze to remove all traces of blood.
     Purpose: Blood on the outside of the pipette will enter the reservoir and give inaccurate results.

8.   Squeeze the reservoir gently with one hand.

9.   While holding your index finger over the hole in the top of the pipette, insert the pipette into the reservoir and seat it firmly in place with a twisting motion.
     Purpose: Squeezing the reservoir before inserting the pipette is necessary. It creates a vacuum, which will draw the sample into the reservoir.

10.   Release the pressure on the reservoir, and remove your finger from the top of the pipette. The sample will be drawn into the reservoir.

11.   Gently squeeze and release the reservoir several times to rinse all blood from the pipette into the reservoir. Liquid should rise to overflow chamber but should not be forced out of the top of the pipette.
      Purpose: The capillary pipette is calibrated to contain an amount of blood. It must be rinsed several times with the diluting fluid to ensure that all of the sample has been delivered into the reservoir.

12.   Mix the contents of the Unopette gently by inversion or by rolling between the palms of your hands.

13.   Identify the Unopette.
      Purpose: The sample must be identifiable at all times during the testing procedure.

14.   Allow the Unopette to sit for the specified amount of time, as stated in the directions.

15.   Place the shield on the top of the prepared Unopette to prevent evaporation.

16.   Clean the work area. Follow the recommendations for proper disposal of all materials.

17.   Wash your hands.

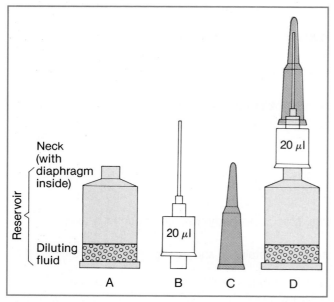

FIGURE 33-28. Parts of a disposable blood-diluting unit such as Unopette. *A*, Prefilled reservoir containing premeasured diluting fluid and sealed with diaphragm; *B*, capillary pipette with overflow chamber and capacity marking; *C*, pipette shield; and *D*, assembled unit.

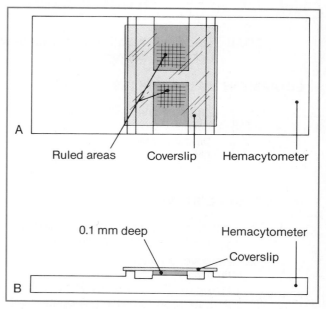

FIGURE 33-29. Top *(A)* and side *(B)* views of a hemacytometer. Sample should fill the shaded areas when the chamber is properly filled.

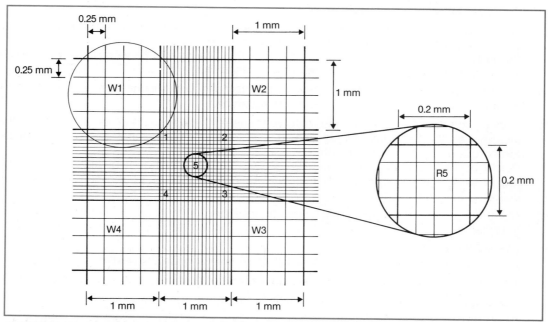

FIGURE 33-30. Neubauer ruling. The areas labeled "W" are used in counting white cells. Red cells are counted in the five areas in the center square. A blowup of the fifth red cell–counting area is shown as it would appear under the microscope's high-power magnification. Measurements of the ruled areas are shown.

counting area that is marked off by lines etched into the glass. The depressions surrounding these platforms are called "moats." The raised areas and depressions form an "H." A special hemacytometer coverslip of uniform thickness is used. The coverslip is positioned on the hemacytometer so that it covers the ruled areas, confines the fluid in the chamber, and regulates the depth of the fluid. The depth of the fluid in the most commonly used *Neubauer-type* hemacytometer is 0.1 mm with the coverslip in place (Fig. 33–29).

Each ruled area of the counting chamber consists of a large square, 3 mm × 3 mm. This area, in turn, is divided into nine equal squares, each of which is 1 mm². The white blood cell counting area consists of the four large corner squares labeled "W" (Fig. 33–30).

The center squares are used to count the red blood cells. Each center square is subdivided into 25 smaller squares. Only the four corner and center squares within the large center square are used to count red blood cells (see Fig. 33–30).

PROCEDURE 33-5 CHARGING (FILLING) A HEMACYTOMETER

GOAL To fill the hemacytometer for a manual cell count.

EQUIPMENT AND SUPPLIES

Nonsterile gloves
Neubauer ruled hemacytometer
Hemacytometer coverslip

Lint-free tissue
70% alcohol
Blood-diluting pipette or Unopette

PROCEDURAL STEPS

1. Wash and dry your hands. Follow the universal blood and body-fluid precautions. Glove yourself with nonsterile gloves.

2. Clean the hemacytometer and coverslip with 70% alcohol and lint-free tissue, and thoroughly dry.
 Purpose: Dirt, fingerprints, grease, or lint interferes with filling and counting.

3. Align the coverslip on the chamber.

4. Expel two drops from the well-mixed pipette or Unopette.
 Purpose: Diluent in the calibrated stem contains no cells and must be discarded before filling the chamber of the hemacytometer.

5. Touch the tip of the pipette to the edge of the coverslip in the loading area of the chamber.

6. Controlling the flow with the finger on the pipette or by gentle squeezing of the Unopette, fill the chamber in one smooth motion.
 Purpose: Chamber fills by capillary action. If the pipette is not touching the edge of the coverslip, the chamber will not fill properly.

7. Stop filling when the ruled area is full but do not overfill.

8. Fill both sides of the hemacytometer.

9. Allow the chamber to sit undisturbed for 1 or 2 minutes so that the cells settle, but do not allow the sample to dry.
 Purpose: Once the cells have settled in the chamber, the counting procedure is easier. Drying contracts the sample and elevates the count.

10. Clean the work area. Follow the recommendations for proper disposal of all materials.

11. Wash your hands.

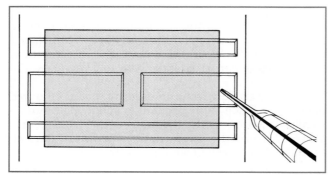

FIGURE 33–31. Charging the hemacytometer.

After the coverslip has been positioned, the hemacytometer is filled, or *charged*. This is accomplished by touching the tip of the diluting pipette or Unopette to the point where the coverslip and the raised platform meet (Fig. 33–31). The fluid will flow by capillary action into one side of the hemacytometer. The opposite side is also filled.

Counting

The hemacytometer is placed on the microscope. White blood cell counts are observed under ×10 objective, and red blood cells are counted under ×40 objective. A counting pattern of left to right and right to left is used to ensure that cells are counted only once. Counts should begin in the upper left corner square. All cells within the squares are counted. Only cells touching top and left boundary lines are counted (Fig. 33–32).

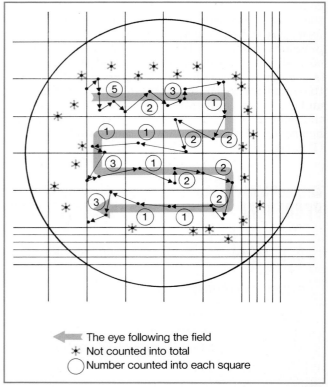

◀ The eye following the field
✳ Not counted into total
◯ Number counted into each square

FIGURE 33–32. Counting. (1) Begin counting cells in the upper left-hand corner. (2) Proceed across the top row, counting cells, including those that touch the top and left sides of each square. (3) Continue to count the remainder of cells in the same fashion. (4) Count in the direction of the arrows. The number of cells in each square is indicated by a circle.

PROCEDURE 33–6   COUNTING CELLS IN THE NEUBAUER RULED HEMACYTOMETER

GOAL To properly focus a hemacytometer, to locate the appropriate areas to count, and to direct your field of vision through the chamber in the proper manner while counting cells.

EQUIPMENT AND SUPPLIES

Properly filled hemacytometer (see Procedure 33–5)
Microscope
Hand tally counter (Fig. 33–33)

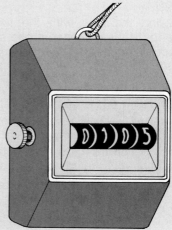

FIGURE 33–33.

Continued

33

PROCEDURAL STEPS

1. Wash and dry your hands. Follow the universal blood and body-fluid precautions. Glove yourself with nonsterile gloves.

2. Place the hemacytometer on the lowered microscope stage under low-power magnification.
   Purpose: The thick chamber will not fit under the objective unless the stage is lowered.

3. Center the ruled area over the opening in the stage.

4. Reduce the light intensity by closing the diaphragm and lowering the condenser.
   Purpose: The unstained cells require reduced light for counting.

5. Raise the stage carefully while watching from the side to be certain that the objective lens does not hit the coverslip.
   Purpose: The chamber or the microscope lens can easily be damaged by improper focusing techniques.

6. Focus and center the correct area (top left large "W" square for counting WBC), using the coarse adjustment and mechanical stage simultaneously.
   Purpose: You will be moving through several planes of focus. When you see the chamber moving through the ocular lens, you will know that you are in approximate focus and will be able to locate the lined area easily.

7. Adjust the light until the cells are easily visible.
   Purpose: Too much light will prevent you from visualizing the cells.

8. Count white cells under low power, by depressing the hand tally once for each cell seen.
   a. Begin in the top row, on the far left.
   b. Count the top row, moving visually from left to right.
   c. Count all cells within the boundaries of the square, and also cells touching the top and the left-hand lines of the square.
   d. Do not count cells touching the right-hand or the bottom lines of the square.
   e. When you come to the end of the top row, drop to the second row.
   f. Count the second row, moving visually from right to left.
   g. Continue counting in this zigzag pattern, ending at the bottom left small square.
      Purpose: Using the same sequence when counting helps you to count all cells that should be counted and to avoid counting cells twice or missing them entirely.

9. When you have finished counting a large square, record the number.

10. Return the tally to zero, move to the next large square, and begin to count.
    Purpose: You need to know the total cells counted in each square individually to determine if the chamber was filled correctly. An unevenly filled hemacytometer voids the count.

11. Switch to high power, and focus with the fine adjustment for counting red blood cells (top left "R" square).

12. Locate the remaining squares to be counted, and determine the number of cells in each. For WBC, the counts from each square should vary by no more than 10 cells. For RBC, the numbers should vary by no more than 20 cells. Greater variation indicates an unevenly filled hemacytometer. In such cases, the chamber should be cleaned and refilled.

Continued

PROCEDURE 33 - 6   *Continued*

13. Total the cells counted in all four squares for WBC and five squares for RBC.

14. Count the second side of the chamber in the same manner.

15. Average the counts from both sides.

16. Calculate the results:
    RBC — average times 10,000
    WBC — average times 50

17. Record the results.

18. Clean the work area. Follow the recommendations for proper disposal of all materials.

19. Wash your hands.

Calculations

Calculations for a red blood cell count are determined by counting both sides of the hemacytometer and obtaining an average. This number is then multiplied by 10,000. For white blood cell counts, the average of the two sides is multiplied by 50.

Automation

In the past, blood cell counts were usually performed manually in the physician's office. Automated counters were seen only in private laboratories and in hospitals. However, the current availability of many different types of instruments has made it possible for the physician's office to also be automated. The modern instruments range from relatively simple, inexpensive counters to the very complex and expensive machines. Many physicians are moving to the automated cell counters because they provide accurate results and do not require a technologist to operate.

Most of the automated cell counters operate by first diluting the cells in a fluid that conducts an electric current. Then, these diluted cells pass through a special narrow opening in the machine. The passing cells interrupt the flow of current, and each interruption is counted. Some machines use a laser beam instead of an electric current.

Automation has improved the accuracy of cell counting and has resulted in greater efficiency in the laboratory. In addition, automation reduces the frequency of handling the individual blood specimen and decreases the risk of exposure to blood-borne pathogens, such as the hepatitis B virus or HIV (AIDS viruses).

DIFFERENTIAL CELL COUNT

Preparation of Blood Smears

A blood smear enables you to view the cellular components of the blood in as natural a state as possible. The morphology of the leukocytes, erythrocytes, and platelets can be studied. Their size, shape, and maturity can be evaluated. Examining a blood smear is part of a complete blood cell count.

A blood smear is prepared by spreading a drop of blood on a clean glass slide. The slides must be free of dust and grease. The best specimen for a blood smear is capillary blood that has no anticoagulant added. EDTA anticoagulant blood can be used provided the smear is made within 2 hours of collection.

There are several methods of spreading the drop of blood on the slide that result in a good smear. One method is to place a small drop of blood one-half inch from the right end of a glass slide. The end of a second glass "spreader" slide is placed in front of the drop of blood at an angle of 30 to 35 degrees. The spreader slide is brought back into the drop until the blood spreads along the edge of the spreader slide. This is done with a quick but smooth gliding motion. The spreader slide is then pushed to the left with a quick, steady motion, spreading the blood across the slide.

A good smear should cover one half to three quarters of the slide. It should show a gradual transition from a thick to a thin end with a feathered edge. It should have a smooth appearance with no

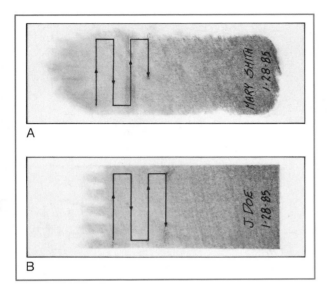

FIGURE 33-34. Shapes of blood smears. *A*, This smear is made by rapidly advancing the spreader slide before the drop of blood extends to the edge of the slide. *B*, This smear is made using a special spreader slide with ground edges and corners. Arrows show the pattern for performing a differential in this portion of the smear.

ridges, holes, lines, streaks, or clumps (Fig. 33-34). The cells should be distributed evenly, upon microscopic examination.

After the smear has been made, it should be allowed to dry. The slide should be propped up to dry with the thick end down. Do not blow on the slide to dry it. This can cause artifacts in the red blood cells from the moisture in your breath. Once dry, the slide is labeled in the thick portion of the smear by writing the patient's name in the dried blood film. If slides with frosted ends are used, the label can be written on the frosted end.

Following labeling, the slide is fixed in *methanol*, which preserves and prevents changes or deterioration of the cellular components. Many of the quick stains available on the market contain the fixative in the stain.

Staining of Blood Smears

The stains commonly used for examination of blood cells are called *polychromatic* because they contain dyes that will stain various cell components different colors. These stains usually contain *methylene blue,* a blue stain, and **eosin,** a red-orange stain. These stains are attracted to different parts of the cell. Thus, the cells and their structures are more easily visualized and differentiated. The most commonly used differential blood stain is *Wright stain.*

Wright stain is applied to the slide for approximately 1 to 3 minutes. A buffer is added on top of the stain and is mixed by gently blowing until a green metallic sheen appears. This usually takes 2

to 4 minutes. The slide is then gently rinsed and is allowed to air-dry. A properly stained smear should appear pinkish to the naked eye.

Identification of Normal Blood Cells

Much useful information can be gathered from the microscopic identification and evaluation of blood cells in a stained smear. A great deal more information can be acquired from the observation of these blood cells than from actual cell counts. Blood smears can impart more knowledge than any other laboratory test.

The features of blood cells that you will observe and evaluate are cell size, nuclear appearance, and cytoplasmic characteristics. The results of observing these three features will allow for cell identification, although much practice is required to be able to recognize and classify all the blood cells that may be seen in various disease states.

Cells are examined under the oil-immersion objective. The light should be bright to facilitate the visualization of colors and small structures. The slide is examined near the feathered end of the smear, where the cells are barely touching each other and are easiest to identify.

Red blood cells are the most numerous of the cellular elements. They are biconcave discs that have no nucleus. The red cells should appear pinkish-tan, as a result of the staining of the hemoglobin within the cells (Fig. 33-35).

Thrombocytes, or *platelets,* are the smallest of the cellular elements. They may be round or oval. No nucleus is present, since the platelet is just a fragment of cytoplasm from a large bone-marrow cell. They stain blue.

Leukocytes are the largest of the normal circulating blood cells. Each of the five types has a characteristic appearance. The granulocytes include neutrophils, eosinophils, and basophils. Granulocytes contain distinctive granules in their cytoplasm and may have segmented nuclei. The agranulocytes include lymphocytes and monocytes. They have few, if any, granules and nonsegmented nuclei. The nuclei of the leukocytes should appear purple, and their cytoplasm may vary from pink to blue or blue-gray.

Neutrophils are known by a variety of names, including *polymorphonuclear neutrophils, segmented neutrophils, polys,* and *segs.* They are the most numerous white blood cells in circulation in adults. They are produced in the bone marrow, are released into the circulation, and eventually enter tissue to fight off invading microorganisms by engulfing them **(phagocytosis).** Many types of bacterial infections stimulate increased production of neutrophils.

The *segmented neutrophil* nucleus is segmented into two to five lobes that are connected by a strand. The nucleus stains a dark purple. The cytoplasm is pale pink and contains fine pink or lilac granules.

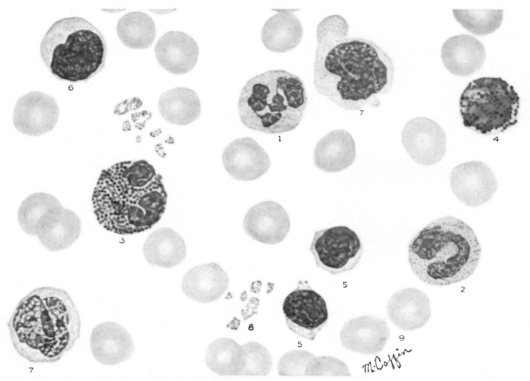

FIGURE 33-35. Normal cellular constituents of adult human blood. *1,* Segmented (polymorphonuclear) neutrophil; *2,* band (stab) neutrophil; *3,* segmented eosinophil; *4,* basophil; *5,* small lymphocyte; *6,* large lymphocyte; *7,* monocytes; *8,* thrombocytes; *9,* erythrocytes. (From Custer, R.P. [ed]: *An Atlas of the Blood and Bone Marrow,* 2nd ed., Philadelphia, W.B. Saunders Co., 1974.)

An immature form of the neutrophil is called a *band,* or *stab.* Instead of having a segmented nucleus, where the lobes are separated by a thin filament, the band has an unsegmented nucleus shaped like a horseshoe. The staining is the same as in the segmented neutrophil. An increase in bands is termed a "shift to the left" and is seen in infections such as bacterial meningitis, pneumonia, appendicitis, strep throat, and abscesses and in chronic granulocytic leukemia. The nucleus of the *eosinophil* is divided into two or three lobes that stain purple. The cytoplasm stains pink and contains large round or oval red-orange granules. Eosinophils are phagocytic and are associated closely with allergies such as hay fever and asthma, as well as certain parasitic infestations such as trichinosis, amebiasis, and schistosomiasis. The nucleus of the *basophil* is segmented and stains light purple. The large dark blue-black granules contain histamine, which is a part of the allergic response. Little is known about the function of basophils.

Lymphocytes are the second most numerous white cell in adults. In children, they are usually the most numerous. Their nucleus is usually oval or round and smooth. It stains purple. The cytoplasm stains blue. Lymphs, as they are commonly called, are responsible for the recognition of foreign antigens and the production of circulating antibodies for immunity to disease. Increased numbers of lymphocytes are found in most viral diseases; in some bacterial infections such as syphilis, brucellosis, tuberculosis, and typhoid and paratyphoid fevers; in leukemias; and in young children who are actively making antibodies. In many viral infections, stimulated or reactive lymphocytes, called *atypical lymphs,* are found. These are common in infectious mononucleosis.

Monocytes are the largest white blood cell in the circulation. The nucleus may be oval, indented, or horseshoe-shaped. The cytoplasm stains a dull gray-blue and may contain *vacuoles,* which appear as clear spaces in the cytoplasm filled with fluid or air. Monocytes are called macrophages and ingest bacteria and the debris of cellular breakdown. They are increased in certain viral infections such as hepatitis and mumps; rickettsial infections such as Rocky Mountain spotted fever; and bacterial infections such as brucellosis, tuberculosis, and typhoid (see Fig. 33–35).

Differential Examination

A specific area of the stained smear must be examined when doing the differential count. This area must be where the red blood cells are touching but are not clumped, when viewed microscopically. After

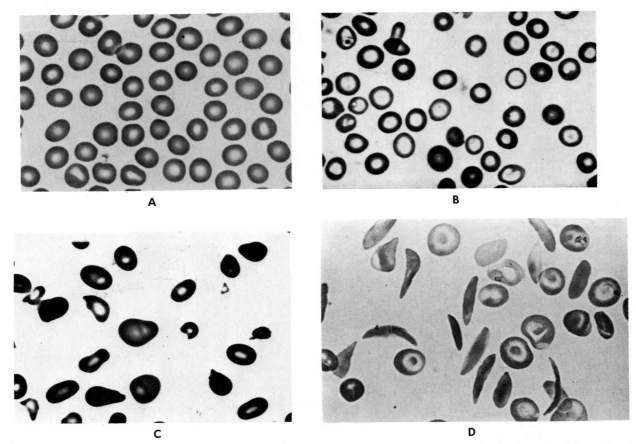

FIGURE 33-36. A comparison of red blood cells. *A,* Normal blood. *B,* Iron deficiency anemia. Note lack of color (hypochromia), smaller size (microcythemia), and elliptic cells. *C,* Megaloblastic anemia. Note varying size of cells (anisocytosis) and large cells (macrocytosis). (All from Henry, J.: *Clinical Diagnosis and Management by Laboratory Procedures,* 17th ed., Philadelphia, W.B. Saunders Co., 1984.) *D,* Sickle cell anemia, showing sickle-shaped cells and target cells. (From Raphael, S.S.: *Lynch's Medical Laboratory Technology,* 4th ed., Philadelphia, W.B. Saunders Co., 1983.)

you have located an appropriate area under low power, focus under oil immersion. The differential examination consists of counting and classifying 100 consecutive white blood cells while moving in a specific winding pattern through the smear. This pattern must be followed to avoid counting the same cells twice. A tally is kept of the cells observed on a *differential cell counter.*

Normal values vary with age (Table 33-2). Many disease states alter the ratios of the different types of leukocytes.

Red Blood Cell Morphology

After determining the differential cell count, the red blood cells are observed and evaluated. Normally, stained red blood cells are the same size and shape and are well filled with hemoglobin. Any variations from the normal state are reported.

Size

Normal-sized red blood cells are known as *normocytic.* If the cells are larger than normal, they are *macrocytic;* if smaller, *microcytic.* The condition in which different sizes of red blood cells are present is called *anisocytosis.*

Shape

Normal red blood cells are round or slightly oval. Cells may be shaped like sickles, targets, crescents, or burrs. *Poikilocytosis* is a significant variation in the shape of the red blood cells.

Content

A red blood cell with the normal amount of hemoglobin is called *normochromic.* Pale-staining cells are *hypochromic* and have less hemoglobin than normal (Fig. 33-36).

Platelet Observation

Platelets, or thrombocytes, are formed in the bone marrow by *megakaryocytes.* As megakaryocytes mature, platelets are shed from the cytoplasm and are released into the circulation, where they function in

PROCEDURE 33-7   PREPARING A SMEAR STAINED WITH WRIGHT STAIN

GOAL To prepare and stain a slide that meets the criteria for the performance of a differential examination.

EQUIPMENT AND SUPPLIES

Clean glass slides
Transfer pipette or capillary tube

Wright stain materials
EDTA anticoagulant blood specimen

PROCEDURAL STEPS

1. Wash and dry your hands. Follow the universal blood and body-fluid precautions. Glove yourself with nonsterile gloves.

2. Assemble the materials needed.

3. Mix the blood specimen.

4. Dispense a small drop of blood onto a slide, about one-half to three-fourths inch from the right end. Use a transfer pipette or capillary tube.

5. Hold the left side of this slide with your nondominant hand.

6. Place the spreader slide in front of the drop of blood at an angle of 30 to 35 degrees. Use your dominant hand.
   Purpose: An angle of 30 to 35 degrees makes a smear with a good feathered edge.

7. Pull back the spreader slide into the drop of blood, and allow the blood to spread to the edges of the slide.

8. Push the spreader slide forward with a quick smooth motion, maintaining the same angle throughout (Fig. 33-37).
   Purpose: If the motion is not smooth, ridges will occur in the smear.

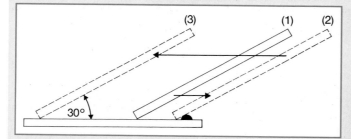 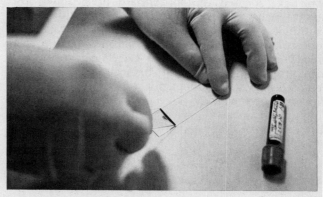

FIGURE 33-37.

9. Rapidly but gently wave the slide to accelerate the drying process.

10. Stand the slide with the thick end down, and allow the slide to complete drying.
    Purpose: If the thick end is up, the undried portion of the blood may run down into the dry thin area and ruin the smear.

11. Label the slide when it is dry. Use a pencil, and write the name in the thick end of the smear.
    Purpose: Pencil will scratch the name into the smear and will not wash off in the staining process.

Continued

33

12. Stain according to method used.
    Two-step method:
    a. Place the smear on a staining rack, with the blood side up.
    b. Flood the smear with Wright stain.
    c. Time for 1 to 3 minutes.
    d. Add an equal amount of buffer, drop by drop, on top of the Wright stain.
    e. Blow gently, and mix the two solutions until a green metallic sheen appears. This should appear within 2 to 4 minutes.
    f. Rinse thoroughly with distilled water.
    g. Drain water from the slide.
    h. Wipe the back of the smear with gauze.
    i. Stand the smear to dry.
    Quick stain:
    a. Place the smear into solutions according to the manufacturer's instructions.
    b. Proceed with steps f through i just listed.
13. Clean the work area. Follow the recommendations for proper disposal of all materials.
14. Wash your hands.

PROCEDURE 33-8   PERFORMING A DIFFERENTIAL EXAMINATION OF A SMEAR STAINED WITH WRIGHT STAIN

GOAL   To perform a differential cell count, evaluate the red blood cell morphology, and estimate the number of platelets.

EQUIPMENT AND SUPPLIES

Microscope
Immersion oil

Lens tissue
Lens cleaner

PROCEDURAL STEPS

1. Wash and dry your hands. Follow the universal blood and body-fluid precautions. Glove yourself with nonsterile gloves.
2. Assemble the materials needed.
3. Clean the microscope with lens tissue and lens cleaner.
   Purpose: Dirty optical surfaces interfere with viewing.

Continued

PROCEDURE 33 – 8   *Continued*

4. Place the slide on the stage, with the smear facing up.
   Purpose: If the slide is face down, you will not be able to focus under oil immersion.

5. Locate an area of the smear where the red blood cells barely touch each other or slightly overlap, using the low-power objective.
   Purpose: If the slide is too thick, the cells will be crowded, small, and difficult to evaluate. If the slide is too thin, the cells will be very far apart and will show the effects of excessive flattening.

6. Focus under oil immersion with the fine-adjustment knob and increased light.

7. Count 100 consecutive white blood cells in a winding pattern, identifying each cell encountered.

8. Record each white cell on the differential cell counter by depressing the appropriate key for each cell.
   Purpose: The differential examination must proceed systematically, to avoid missing cells or counting any cell twice.

9. Evaluate the red blood cells observed in 10 fields. Record any variations in:
   - Size — microcytosis, macrocytosis, anisocytosis
   - Shape — poikilocytosis, ovalocytosis, target cells, sickle cells, and so forth
   - Content — normochromic or hypochromic
   Purpose: The red blood cell evaluation gives the physician important information about the red blood cell population and is an important tool in the assessment of anemias and red blood cell diseases.

10. Count the platelets in 10 fields, obtain an average, and multiply that average by 15,000 to give an estimate of the platelet count. The normal platelet count is 150,000 to 400,000/mm^3. Report the count as normal, decreased, or increased.
    Purpose: Platelet numbers can be a clue to bleeding disorders.

11. Clean the microscope with lens tissue and lens cleaner.

12. Clean the work area. Follow the recommendations for proper disposal of all materials.

13. Wash your hands.

---

coagulation. When damage to a vessel occurs, platelets form a plug at the site, and eventually a fibrin clot seals the leak. On a stained smear, the morphology of the platelets is observed for any abnormalities. They are small and irregularly shaped and may vary considerably in size. The average number of platelets seen in 10 to 15 fields is reported. The normal platelet count is 150,000 to 400,000 per mm^3. An increase in platelets is called *thrombocytosis,* and a decrease is called *thrombocytopenia.*

ERYTHROCYTE SEDIMENTATION RATE

The erythrocyte sedimentation rate (ESR) is a laboratory test that measures the rate at which erythrocytes gradually separate from plasma and settle to the bottom of a specially calibrated tube. The number of these red blood cells that fall in one hour is the ESR. The test is not specific for a particular disease but is used as a general indication of inflammation. Increases are found in such conditions as acute and chronic infections, rheumatoid arthritis, tuberculosis, hepatitis, cancer, multiple myeloma, rheumatic fever, and lupus erythematosus.

Normal values vary slightly with age and sex (Table 33–2). Only increased ESR rates are significant.

Several methods of measuring the erythrocyte sedimentation rate are used, including *Wintrobe, Westergren,* and *Landau-Adams.* All these methods are based on the same principle and differ only in the amounts of blood needed and the tube size and calibration used.

The Wintrobe method is commonly used. It consists of a Wintrobe tube that is graduated from 0 to 100 mm and a specially designed Wintrobe rack, which holds the tube in a vertical position. A long-tipped *Pasteur pipette* is used to fill the Wintrobe tube with 100 ml of blood, to the zero mark on the tube (Fig. 33–38). The tube is placed in the Wintrobe rack for 1 hour. At the end of 1 hour, the level

33

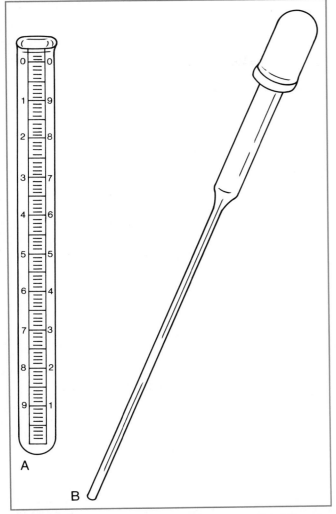

FIGURE 33-38. Materials for measuring erythrocyte sedimentation rate. *A*, Wintrobe sedimentation rate tube; *B*, long-stemmed Pasteur pipette.

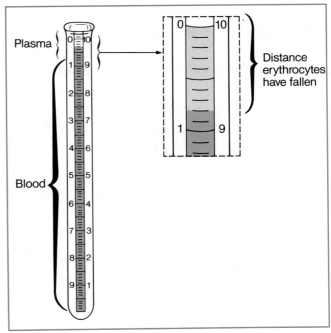

FIGURE 33-39. Sedimentation rate tube showing the settling of cells. Example shown illustrates a reading of 8 mm.

on the tube to which the erythrocytes have fallen is measured. The rate is recorded in mm/hour (Fig. 33-39).

Many factors can affect the sedimentation rate. The tube must be totally filled with blood and must not contain air bubbles. The tube must be allowed to sit in a vertical position undisturbed for a full hour. Minor degrees of tilting may increase the sedimentation rate; careful timing is important. Jarring or vibrations from nearby machinery will falsely increase the ESR. Testing must be performed within 2 hours after the blood has been collected.

PROCEDURE 33-9   DETERMINING A SEDIMENTATION RATE BY THE WINTROBE METHOD

GOAL   To properly fill a Wintrobe tube and observe and record the findings of an erythrocyte sedimentation rate, using the Wintrobe method.

EQUIPMENT AND SUPPLIES

EDTA anticoagulant blood specimen
Wintrobe tube
Wintrobe rack

Timer
Pasteur pipette
Bulb

Continued

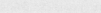

PROCEDURE 33 – 9 *Continued*

PROCEDURAL STEPS

1. Wash and dry your hands. Follow the universal blood and body-fluid precautions. Glove yourself with nonsterile gloves.

2. Assemble the materials needed.

3. Check the leveling bubble of the Wintrobe rack.
   Purpose: The rack must be horizontal to ensure that the tube is vertical.

4. Mix the blood well.
   Purpose: Cells settle when the specimen stands, and blood must always be well-mixed prior to sampling.

5. Fill the Pasteur pipette with blood, and insert the tip of the pipette to the bottom of the Wintrobe tube.

6. Fill the Wintrobe tube to the "0" mark, by squeezing the bulb of the pipette.

7. Slowly remove the pipette from the tube while keeping the tip of the pipette below the level of the blood.
   Purpose: If the tip of the pipette is above the level of the blood, bubbles will be trapped in the tube and will invalidate the test.

8. Place the tube in a numbered slot in the Wintrobe rack, and set the timer for 1 hour. The tube must be in a vertical position and free from all vibration.
   Purpose: Jarring will increase the sedimentation rate.

9. Measure the distance the erythrocytes have fallen after 1 hour. The ESR scale measures from 0 at the top to 100 at the bottom. Each line is 1 mm.

10. Record the findings.
    Purpose: The ESR is reported in mm/hour.

11. Clean the work area. Follow the recommendations for proper disposal of all materials.

12. Wash your hands.

LEGAL AND ETHICAL RESPONSIBILITIES

Phlebotomy is an *invasive* technique in which a sterile needle is inserted into a vein. The procedure is subject to the laws and regulations for surgical procedures because the skin is penetrated and body fluid removed. When performing venipuncture, regulations must be enforced, and deviations are not allowed. Be sure to follow the procedures established by your employer and the regulations of your state.

If the blood drawn is for drug level studies, **serology** evaluations, or HIV determinations, the procedure must be preformed *exactly* as the law dictates. Courts of law require absolute adherence to procedures and complete and exact documentation of the chain of events for collecting, handling, and analyzing the specimen. Skin preparation for a blood alcohol level test *must be* done with povidone-iodine (Betadine) rather than alcohol because the alcohol could falsely elevate the blood alcohol level. Many states have statutes that specify exactly how, when, and under what circumstances this testing can be done. You can find out the regulations for your state by requesting a copy of the legislation from the state hospital association, the state police headquarters, or a state congressman.

In 1991, many states adopted the Blood Safety Act, which requires physicians to provide patients with information concerning blood transfusion options. This information is given before surgery and before any medical procedure in which there is a possibility that blood transfusion may be necessary. Physicians also are required to note on each patient's medical record that a written summary was given to the patient. As the physician's agent, you share this responsibility. If this is needed for a particular patient, it is the responsibility of every member of the health care team to see to it that this information is supplied to the patient, noted on the chart, and initialed. The written summary has been formally prepared. Copies of it can be requested from the State Department of Health Services.

► PATIENT EDUCATION

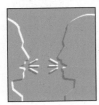

When working as a phlebotomist, the medical assistant must maintain a professional attitude and still be sympathetic to the fears and apprehensions of the patient. By establishing an environment that encourages the patient to relax, the amount of pain and discomfort experienced by the patient during the drawing procedure is kept to a minimum.

If the patient has a positive attitude, you need to provide little explanation about the procedure. Often, the patient can help you by telling from which site the last blood was successfully drawn. It is wise to follow the patient's suggested information in choosing the site for the removal of the blood specimen. When a patient is allowed to become an active participant in the procedure, he or she remains more relaxed, talkative, and confident in your expertise as a phlebotomist.

This atmosphere can change dramatically when the patient has had an unpleasant experience and associates pain and hurt with venipuncture. Such a patient usually is ill at ease, nervous, and apprehensive. When confronted with this scenario, you need to make every effort to perform the procedure quickly, efficiently, and effectively. Once the blood has been drawn and the patient has relaxed, you then will have an opportunity to help the patient develop a positive attitude.

If your patient has a history of **syncope** when blood is drawn, or if you suspect that this patient may faint during the procedure, have the patient lie down. Assemble your equipment and alert the physician before beginning the procedure. This type of professional care may help the patient get through the procedure without a traumatic effect.

Always remember to identify your patient and explain what you are going to do. Answer any questions the patient may have, and perform a skilled venipuncture before anxiety is allowed to set in.

► LEARNING ACHIEVEMENTS

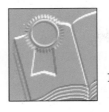

Upon successful completion of this chapter, can you in the time allowed by your evaluator:

1. Collect a blood specimen by venipuncture from a patient using either a syringe or Vacutainer method and complete the procedure in proper sequence?
2. Assemble the appropriate supplies; collect a capillary blood specimen suitable for testing, using fingertip puncture technique; and correctly complete each step of the procedure in proper order?
3. Perform a microhematocrit in duplicate to a minimum level of $\pm 1\%$?
4. Fill a Unopette capillary pipette and transfer to a Unopette reservoir, correctly completing each step in proper order?
5. Fill a hemacytometer chamber and correctly complete each step of the procedure in the proper sequence?
6. Using the filled hemacytometer, count and calculate a manual white or red blood cell count to a minimum performance level of ± 200 WBC/mm^3 and $\pm 50,000$ RBC/mm^3?
7. Prepare and stain a blood smear, using Wright stain, completing each step in proper sequence?
8. Perform a differential cell count, red blood cell examination, and platelet estimation to a minimum performance level of 90% accuracy?
9. Using an EDTA blood specimen, determine a sedimentation rate using the Wintrobe method to a minimum performance level of ± 1 mm?

REFERENCES AND READINGS

Bonewit, K.: *Clinical Procedures for Medical Assistants,* 3rd ed., Philadelphia, W.B. Saunders Co., 1990.

Calbreath, D. F.: *Clinical Chemistry,* Philadelphia, W.B. Saunders Co., 1992.

Feingold, S. M., and Baron, E. J.: *Bailey and Scott's Diagnostic Microbiology,* St. Louis, C.V. Mosby Co., 1986.

Garza, D., Becan-McBride, K.: *Phlebotomy Handbook,* 2nd ed., Norwalk, Connecticut, Appleton and Lange, 1989.

Henry, J. B.: *Clinical Diagnosis and Management by Laboratory Methods,* 18th ed., Philadelphia, W.B. Saunders Co., 1991.

Wedding, M. E., and Toenjes, S. A.: *Medical Laboratory Procedures,* Philadelphia, F.A. Davis Co., 1992.

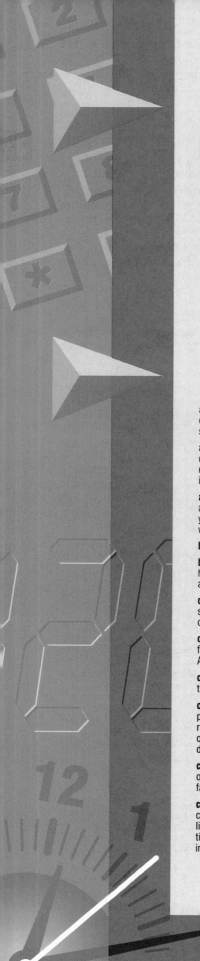

CHAPTER OUTLINE

VOCABULARY

amino acid One of the 20 organic compounds that form the chief constituents of protein.

anorexia nervosa An emotional disorder characterized by a refusal to eat and an altered physical self-image.

atherosclerosis A common type of arteriosclerosis in which deposits of yellow plaque form on the interior walls of the arteries.

biotin A type of B-complex vitamin.

bulimia An abnormal increase in hunger characterized by binge eating and self-induced vomiting.

calorie The amount of heat necessary to raise the temperature of 1 g of water 1°C, or a pint of water 4°F.

carotene The yellow-red pigment from food that converts to vitamin A.

cellulose A carbohydrate that forms the structure of most plants.

cholesterol A substance found in plant and animal fats, such as saturated oils, egg yolk, and milk; currently thought to produce fatty deposits in the blood vessels.

choline An essential part of the diet of mammals that helps to prevent fatty deposits in the liver.

cirrhosis A disease of the liver that causes impairment in the metabolism of nutrients and the detoxification of poisons absorbed from the intestines.

cretinism Congenital condition characterized by diminished development and dystrophy of the bones and soft tissues, as well as some mental retardation resulting from hypofunctioning of the thyroid gland.

deficiencies Conditions caused by a below-normal intake of a particular substance.

diabetes mellitus A disorder of carbohydrate metabolism caused by underproduction of insulin and characterized by excessive urinary output.

dietitian An individual with a bachelor's degree in foods and nutrition who is concerned with the maintenance and promotion of health and the treatment of diseases through diet.

digestion The process of converting food into chemical substances that can be used by the body.

endogenous Produced within or caused by factors within the organism.

exogenous Produced outside or caused by factors outside of the organism.

gliadin A protein from wheat that is soluble in alcohol.

glycogen A polysaccharide that is the principle form in which carbohydrates are stored in animal tissues.

goiter An enlargement of the thyroid gland.

hydrogenated Combined with, treated with, or exposed to hydrogen.

obesity An excessive accumulation of body fat (usually defined as more than 20% above the recommended body weight).

osteoporosis Loss of bone tissue occurring most frequently in small-boned, postmenopausal women.

pantothenic acid B-complex vitamin present in all living tissues.

phenylketonuria (PKU) A congenital disease resulting from a defect in protein metabolism that, when untreated, causes severe mental retardation.

protein A group of organic compounds occurring in plants and animals. It contains the major elements carbon, hydrogen, oxygen, and nitrogen and the amino acids essential for life maintenance.

scurvy A condition resulting from a deficiency in vitamin C (ascorbic acid). It is characterized by bleeding gums and ecchymosis.

tetany A continuous contraction or muscle spasm caused by inadequate blood calcium or accidental surgical removal of the parathyroid glands.

tryptophan Essential amino acid present in high concentration in animal and fish protein.

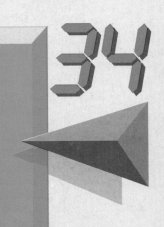

NUTRITION AND DIET MODIFICATION

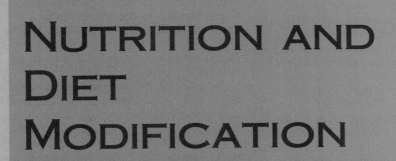

LEARNING OBJECTIVES

COGNITIVE

Upon successful completion of this chapter, you should be able to:

1. Define and spell the words listed in the Vocabulary.

2. Describe normal nutrition.

3. List the four major food groups.

4. Discuss the meaning of recommended dietary allowance.

5. Calculate the caloric value of carbohydrates, fats, and proteins.

6. Differentiate between fat-soluble and water-soluble vitamins.

7. Describe the role of carbohydrates in the daily diet.

8. Explain the need for minerals in the diet.

PERFORMANCE

Upon successful completion of this chapter, you should be able to perform the following activities:

1. Write a personal diet history for 2 weeks.

2. Calculate the total daily calories in your personal diet.

3. Determine whether your daily food intake includes the four basic food groups, in recommended servings.

4. Adjust your daily diet to meet the recommended daily allowances for nutrients.

5. Determine the daily calorie level needed to maintain your present weight.

NORMAL NUTRITION

Now more than ever, the public wants to know about the food it eats and how food affects health. Tremendous progress in the improvement of the general health of Americans has occurred over the past century, and an increase in longevity has resulted from the control of preventable disease through better nutrition. Factors that affect one's health include proper care and functioning of all body organs, good diet, and a sound mental attitude. It is generally agreed that good nutrition is one of the most important environmental factors that affect the health of an individual, a community, or a nation.

Good health is the state of emotional and physical well-being that is determined, to a large extent, by a person's diet. We are, quite literally, what we eat, since the food we consume is used to build and repair every part of our bodies. Consequently, it is important that the food choices we make are based on sound information and knowledge. A person who is well-nourished is usually more alert in every way and emotionally better balanced. The well-nourished person is also better able than the poorly nourished individual to ward off infections.

The physician, the medical assistant, and the dietitian all are closely involved in the nutritive care of the patient. The physician prescribes the diet, and, ideally, the dietitian instructs the patient in how to follow it. Frequently, however, such professional aid is not available. In this case, it is often necessary for the assistant to discuss the diet with the patient, answer questions, and explain certain aspects of the modifications involved. Many patients may hesitate to ask the physician details about the diet, or questions may arise after the patients leave the office. Such concerns typically include methods of preparation, sources of information, and interpretation of labels. The medical assistant is the one the patient turns to for answers. Consequently, the assistant should be able to answer basic questions on normal nutrition and should have a fundamental knowledge of the diets that physicians prescribe most often.

Nutrition and Dietetics

Nutrition refers to all the processes involved in the intake and utilization of nutrients. *Nutrients* are the organic and inorganic chemicals in food that supply the energy and raw materials for cellular activities. *Metabolism* refers to the cellular activities that occur inside and outside the cells. **Digestion** is a series of reactions occurring in the mouth, stomach, and small intestine that result in reducing large food molecules into simple absorbable forms. These absorbed nutrients are then carried by the bloodstream to all parts of the body, where they are metabolized.

The word *nutrition* is also used to indicate nutritional status, or the condition of the body resulting from the utilization of the essential nutrients available to the body. Public interest in nutrition has increased in recent years owing to the growing concern about physical fitness.

Dietetics is the practical application of nutritional science to individuals. It is "the combined science and art of feeding individuals or groups under different economic or health conditions according to the principles of nutrition and management." The **dietitian** is the individual who is concerned with this promotion of good health through proper diet and with the therapeutic use of diet in the treatment of disease.

Food

Food is defined as any material that meets the nutritive requirements of an organism for the maintenance of growth and physical well-being. To be classified as a food, a substance must perform one or more of three basic functions in the body: provide a source of fuel or energy; supply nutrients to build and repair tissues; and supply nutrients to regulate body processes (Fig. 34–1). Most foods supply both fuel and nutrients; however, no one food supplies all the nutrients required for proper metabolism. Consequently, a combination of different foods is necessary. With a little planning, a well-balanced diet supplying all the body's needs can be obtained. **Deficiencies** in a diet or an inadequate diet results in malnutrition and may lead to a variety of diseases. Good nutrition is particularly critical for pregnant women and young children, since malnutrition during development and growth may result in physical and mental retardation.

Energy

Every bodily action, whether voluntary or involuntary, requires energy. Even when asleep, the body still needs a source of energy to keep the heart beating, the lungs breathing, and other vital organs functioning. The involuntary activities of digestion and respiration also require energy even though they are not consciously controlled. *Basal metabolism* is the term used for this energy expenditure when the body is at rest.

There are basically two energy sources available to the body: **exogenous** and **endogenous.** When the quantities of food (exogenous) consumed are insufficient to furnish the required fuel, the body begins to break down its fat reserves (endogenous) in an attempt to supply the necessary energy. Generally, it is desirable for the daily food intake to

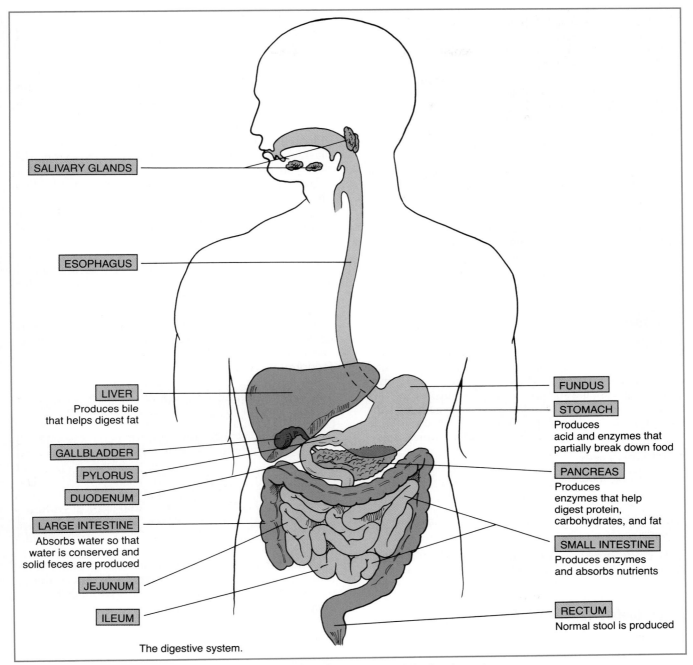

SALIVARY GLANDS

ESOPHAGUS

LIVER
Produces bile
that helps digest fat

GALLBLADDER

PYLORUS

DUODENUM

LARGE INTESTINE
Absorbs water so that
water is conserved and
solid feces are produced

JEJUNUM

ILEUM

FUNDUS

STOMACH
Produces
acid and enzymes that
partially break down food

PANCREAS
Produces
enzymes that help
digest protein,
carbohydrates, and fat

SMALL INTESTINE
Produces enzymes
and absorbs nutrients

RECTUM
Normal stool is produced

The digestive system.

FIGURE 34-1. The anatomy and physiology of the digestive system.

equal the total energy needs of the body (number of calories needed for both voluntary and involuntary activities).

Quantities of energy are expressed in units of heat energy called calories. A **calorie (cal)** is the amount of heat needed to raise the temperature of 1 g of water 1°C. Since this unit represents a relatively small amount of energy and metabolism involves much larger quantities of energy, the *large calorie (Cal),* or *kilocalorie (kcal),* is commonly used. A kilo-

calorie is defined as the amount of heat required to raise the temperature of 1 kg of water 1°C. Of the seven food constituents (carbohydrates, proteins, fats, water, minerals, vitamins, and fiber), only carbohydrates, proteins, and fats are capable of furnishing the body with energy. Carbohydrates and proteins yield 4 kcal/gm, whereas 1 gm of fat provides 9 kcal.

Determining energy needs can be done by using the Harris-Benedict formula:

Males: (5 × height) + (13.7 × weight + 660) − (6.8 × age) = Kcal/day
Females: (4.8 × height) + (9.6 × weight + 655) − (4.7 × age) = Kcal/day

Height should be expressed in inches, current weight in kilograms, and age in years.

Example: A 20-year-old woman weighs 110 pounds and is 5 feet 2 inches tall, thus:

(4.8 × 62) + (9.6 × 50 + 655) − (4.7 × 20) = 1338.6 Kcal/day

The amount of energy needed by a given individual varies considerably according to activity level and basal requirements; however, most adults require 1800 to 3300 kcal a day.

Dietary Evaluation

In 1940, the Food and Nutrition Board of the National Academy of Sciences was appointed to advise the government on food and nutritional matters. This board developed a scientific guide called *Recommended Dietary Allowances (RDA)* and published the first edition in 1943. The purpose of this guide was to provide standards to serve as a goal for good nutrition. The guide offers advice on a wide variety of nutritional problems, some of which are:

Nutritional needs

Establishing food standards

Designing nutrition education programs

Establishing guidelines for nutrition labeling of foods.

This guide is revised at regular intervals. The 10th edition was published in 1989 (Table 34–1).

Seven Dietary Guidelines for Americans

In 1985, the Public Health Service of the Department of Health and Human Services and the U.S. Department of Agriculture, revised and published the *Dietary Guidelines for Americans*. This report included seven recommendations that address the relationship between diseases and diet. The seven guidelines are:

- Eat a variety of foods.
- Maintain a healthy weight.
- Choose a diet low in fat, especially saturated fat, and cholesterol.
- Choose a diet with plenty of vegetables, fruits, and grain products.
- Use sugars only in moderation.
- Use salt and sodium only in moderation.
- If you drink alcoholic beverages, do so in moderation.

Even though a diet may be adequate in calories, it may not be adequate in nutrients. A *balanced diet* includes adequate amounts of all the essential food constituents. To meet the body's nutritional requirements, the U.S. Department of Agriculture developed a four food group system (Fig. 34–2). This guide divides commonly eaten foods into four groups according to the nutritional contributions of each group. A fifth group (fats, sweets, and alcohol) provides kilocalories but only a few nutrients. It is advisable to choose a wide variety of foods from the first four groups.

Individual eating styles must be considered when choosing foods from the four groups; however, if the suggested serving guide is followed, about 1200 kcal will be eaten. This will provide adequate protein and supply most of the daily vitamin and mineral needs for good health.

The four food group system is easy to follow and simple to remember. It provides a flexible guide for planning a general or *modified diet* restricted in kcal or in specific nutrients or fiber.

There are nine key nutrients that the body needs daily to maintain normal health. The following chart shows these nine important nutrients and the food groups that provide them:

- Meat, poultry, fish, dry beans, peas, eggs, and nuts group: iron, protein
- Fruit and vegetable group: calcium, vitamin C, vitamin A, iron
- Milk, yogurt, and cheese group: calcium, vitamin D, riboflavin
- Bread, cereal, rice, and pasta group: riboflavin, niacin, thiamine

Good nutrition is a balance between protein, vitamins, minerals, and fiber, with little fat, sodium, sugar, and alcohol. The energy intake must be balanced with the energy output.

Nutrients
Carbohydrates

Carbohydrates are chemical organic compounds composed of carbon, hydrogen, and oxygen and are mostly plant products in origin. They are divided into three groups based on the complexity of their molecules: simple sugars, complex carbohydrates (starch), and dietary fiber. Each has a function in health and consists of many variations.

When carbohydrates are small single units, they are called *molecules*. The molecules can combine to form double units, or they may form even larger structures and become complex units. Those that have a special significance in nutrition are the simple sugars—glucose, fructose, and galactose; the

TABLE 34–1. FOOD AND NUTRITION BOARD, NATIONAL ACADEMY OF SCIENCES—NATIONAL RESEARCH COUNCIL RECOMMENDED DIETARY ALLOWANCES* Revised 1989

Designed for the maintenance of good nutrition of practically all healthy people in the United States

Age (y) or Condition	Weight† (kg)	Weight† (lb)	Height† (cm)	Height† (in)	Protein (g)	Fat-Soluble Vitamins Vitamin A (µg RE)‡	Vitamin D (µg)§	Vitamin E (µg α-TE)‖	Vitamin K (µg)	Water-Soluble Vitamins Vitamin C (mg)	Thiamin (mg)	Riboflavin (mg)	Niacin (mg NE)¶	Vitamin B₆ (mg)	Folate (µg)	Vitamin B₁₂ (µg)	Minerals Calcium (mg)	Phosphorus (mg)	Magnesium (mg)	Iron (mg)	Zinc (mg)	Iodine (µg)	Selenium (µg)
INFANTS																							
0.0–0.5	6	13	60	24	13	375	7.5	3	5	30	0.3	0.4	5	0.3	25	0.3	400	300	40	6	5	40	10
0.5–1.0	9	20	71	28	14	375	10	4	10	35	0.4	0.5	6	0.6	35	0.5	600	500	60	10	5	50	15
CHILDREN																							
1–3	13	29	90	35	16	400	10	6	15	40	0.7	0.8	9	1.0	50	0.7	800	800	80	10	10	70	20
4–6	20	44	112	44	24	500	10	7	20	45	0.9	1.1	12	1.1	75	1.0	800	800	120	10	10	90	20
7–10	28	62	132	52	28	700	10	7	30	45	1.0	1.2	13	1.4	100	1.4	800	800	170	10	10	120	30
MALES																							
11–14	45	99	157	62	45	1000	10	10	45	50	1.3	1.5	17	1.7	150	2.0	1200	1200	270	12	15	150	40
15–18	66	145	176	69	59	1000	10	10	65	60	1.5	1.8	20	2.0	200	2.0	1200	1200	400	12	15	150	50
19–24	72	160	177	70	58	1000	10	10	70	60	1.5	1.7	19	2.0	200	2.0	1200	1200	350	10	15	150	70
25–50	79	174	176	70	63	1000	5	10	80	60	1.5	1.7	19	2.0	200	2.0	800	800	350	10	15	150	70
51+	77	170	173	68	63	1000	5	10	80	60	1.2	1.4	15	2.0	200	2.0	800	800	350	10	15	150	70
FEMALES																							
11–14	46	101	157	62	46	800	10	8	45	50	1.1	1.3	15	1.4	150	2.0	1200	1200	280	15	12	150	45
15–18	55	120	163	64	44	800	10	8	55	60	1.1	1.3	15	1.5	180	2.0	1200	1200	300	15	12	150	50
19–24	58	128	164	65	46	800	10	8	60	60	1.1	1.3	15	1.6	180	2.0	1200	1200	280	15	12	150	55
25–50	63	138	163	64	50	800	5	8	65	60	1.0	1.2	15	1.6	180	2.0	800	800	280	15	12	150	55
51+	65	143	160	63	50	800	5	8	65	60	1.0	1.2	13	1.6	180	2.0	800	800	280	10	12	150	55
PREGNANT					60	800	10	10	65	70	1.5	1.6	17	2.2	400	2.2	1200	1200	320	30	15	175	65
LACTATING																							
1st 6 mo					65	1300	10	12	65	95	1.6	1.8	20	2.1	280	2.6	1200	1200	355	15	19	200	75
2nd 6 mo					62	1200	10	11	65	90	1.6	1.7	20	2.1	260	2.6	1200	1200	340	15	16	200	75

(From Poleman, C. M. and Peckenpaugh, N. J.: *Nutrition Essentials and Diet Therapy*, 6th ed., Philadelphia, W. B. Saunders Co., 1991, inside cover.)

*The allowances, expressed as average daily intakes over time, are intended to provide for individual variations among most normal persons as they live in the United States under usual environmental stresses. Diets should be based on a variety of common foods to provide other nutrients for which human requirements have been less well-defined. See text for detailed discussion of allowances and of nutrients not tabulated.

†Weights and heights of reference adults are actual medians for the U.S. population of the designated age, as reported by NHANES II. The median weights and heights of those under 19 years of age were taken from Hamill et al. (1979) (see pages 16–17). The use of these figures does not imply that the height-to-weight ratios are ideal.

‡Retinol equivalents. 1 retinol equivalent = 1 µg retinol or 6 µg β-carotene. See text for calculation of vitamin A activity of diets as retinol equivalents.

§As cholecalciferol. 10 µg cholecalciferol = 400 IU of vitamin D.

‖α-Tocopherol equivalents. 1 mg d-α tocopherol = 1 α-TE. See text for variation in allowances and calculation of vitamin E activity of the diet as α-tocopherol equivalents.

¶1 NE (niacin equivalent) is equal to 1 mg of niacin or 60 mg of dietary tryptophan.

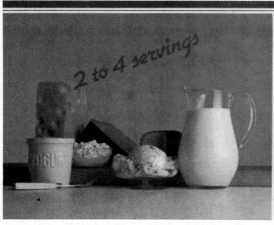

SERVINGS:
Adults 2
Children under 9 years old 2-3
Children 9 to 12 years old
and Pregnant Women 3
Teens and Nursing Mothers 4

1 SERVING IS:
1 CUP MILK OR YOGURT
1⅓ OUNCES CHEDDAR OR SWISS CHEESE
2 OUNCES PROCESSED CHEESE FOOD
1½ CUPS ICE CREAM OR ICE MILK
2 CUPS COTTAGE CHEESE

Skim, nonfat, and lowfat milk and milk products provide calcium and keep fat intake down.

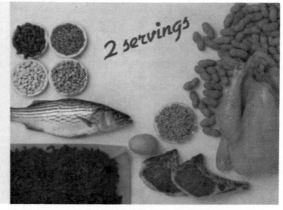

½ SERVING IS:
1 to 1½ OUNCES LEAN, BONELESS, COOKED MEAT, POULTRY, OR FISH
1 EGG
½ to ¾ CUP COOKED DRY BEANS, PEAS, LENTILS, OR SOYBEANS
2 TABLESPOONS PEANUT BUTTER
¼ to ½ CUP NUTS, SESAME OR SUNFLOWER SEEDS

Poultry and fish have less fat content than red meats.

FIGURE 34–2. The four food groups of the *Guide to a Better Diet.* (From the U.S. Department of Agriculture, Washington, DC, 1980.)

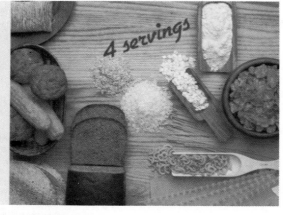

1 SERVING IS:
1 SLICE BREAD
½ to ¾ CUP COOKED CEREAL OR PASTA
1 OUNCE READY-TO-EAT CEREAL

Choose whole-grain products often.

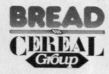

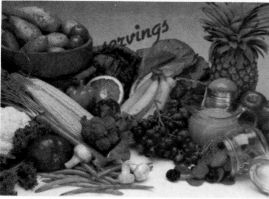

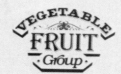

1 SERVING IS:
½ CUP   AN ORANGE
A SMALL SALAD   ½ CANTALOUPE
A MEDIUM-SIZED POTATO   ½ GRAPEFRUIT

Have citrus fruit, melon, berries, or tomatoes daily and a dark-green or dark-yellow vegetable frequently. For a good source of fiber, eat unpeeled fruits and vegetables and fruits with edible seeds — berries or grapes.

double units—sucrose, lactose, and maltose; and the complex units—starch, **glycogen,** and dietary fiber. Although there is no specific dietary requirement for carbohydrates, it is desirable to include them as a reasonable proportion of the caloric intake. They are the ideal energy source.

With the exception of fiber, carbohydrates are easily digested and absorbed into the body. Simple sugars are absorbed first; the complex sugars must be processed before they can be absorbed in the intestinal tract. Dietary fiber is indigestible and passes through the gastrointestinal tract unchanged.

Glucose is the sugar formed from all carbohydrates eaten. It is absorbed into the bloodstream, where it is metabolized into energy.

The primary function of carbohydrates is to supply the body's energy needs. Once these needs are met, the unused molecules are handled the same way as fats in maintenance action. Carbohydrates are easily converted to energy. One gram of carbohydrate yields 4 kcal.

Some of the common food sources of carbohydrates are:

- Cereal grains: rice, wheat, corn, oats, barley, and buckwheat
- Vegetables: green leafy vegetables, seeds, and dried peas and beans
- Sweets: table sugar, molasses, and maple and corn syrups

There are no animal sources that provide adequate carbohydrates.

Dietary fiber is commonly called *roughage* or *residue.* It is defined as the portion of the plant eaten that cannot be digested or absorbed. It is classified by its water solubility; it adds bulk to the intestinal tract; and it is beneficial for normal gastrointestinal functioning. The best way of adding fiber to the diet is to consume fruits, raw vegetables, legumes, and whole grains.

Fats

Fats, also composed of carbon, hydrogen, and oxygen, differ from carbohydrates in the proportions of each of these elements. Fats can be classified in several different ways: by their source, by their physical appearance, or by their chemical structure.

SOURCE: ANIMAL OR VEGETABLE. Animal fats are found in dairy products, meat, fish, and eggs. They are usually solid at room temperature. Vegetable fats are found in plants. Sources include corn, olives, cottonseed, nuts, and beans. They are generally liquid at room temperature and are called *oils.*

PHYSICAL APPEARANCE: VISIBLE OR INVISIBLE. Visible fats are those having a fatty appearance, such as butter or the fat around meat. Fats such as those in avocados or eggs are labeled invisible, since they are not discernible.

CHEMICAL STRUCTURE: SATURATED OR UNSATURATED. Saturated fats are those fatty acids that contain all the hydrogen possible. They are usually from animal sources and are solid at room temperature. Examples of saturated fats are lard, butter, meat fat, and **hydrogenated** fats. The main exceptions are coconut and palm oils, which are of plant origin but exceptionally high in saturated fat. Hydrogenated vegetable oils (shortening) are also saturated fats. Unsaturated fatty acids can take on more hydrogen under the proper conditions. They are found in plants and are usually liquid at room temperature. Examples are the oils from corn and safflower. Some fats, such as those of the soft-type margarines, are partially hydrogenated. That is, an unsaturated fat is treated so that it takes up a predetermined quantity of hydrogen, resulting in a product that exhibits properties of both a saturated and an unsaturated fat. These fats are usually soft at room temperature.

Cholesterol is a lipid commonly found in saturated fats. It is also manufactured within the body. The confusion between "good" and "bad" fats stems from the distinction between the fat in food and the fat in our bodies. The good fats in our diet are polyunsaturated and monounsaturated fats. The bad dietary fats are cholesterol and saturated fats. The fat in our bodies is divided into two categories. The good fat is high-density lipoprotein (HDL); the bad fats are low-density lipoprotein (LDL) and very low-density lipoprotein (VLDL). The HDL and the LDL levels can be successfully changed through diet. The American Heart Association offers specific guidelines for safe serum cholesterol and HDL and LDL levels (Table 34-2).

Fats make up about 35 to 40% of the total calories in the American diet. Since fats supply 9 kcal/gm, they are the most concentrated source of energy in our diet.

The major functions of fat in the body are to:

- Provide a source of energy.
- Carry fat-soluble vitamins A and D.
- Supply those fatty acids essential for growth and life.
- Slow down emptying time of the stomach, thus increasing the satiety value of the diet.

When fat is stored in the body as adipose tissue, it acts as a reserve energy supply and as insulation and padding for the body and its vital organs.

Some of the common food sources of fat are:

Animal sources: whole milk, butter, lard, meat fat, bacon, cheese, and egg yolk

Plant sources: vegetable oils, margarine, chocolate, peanut butter, salad dressings, olives, nuts, and avocados.

TABLE 34–2. PLASMA CHOLESTEROL CONCENTRATIONS ASSOCIATED WITH INCREASED RISK OF CARDIOVASCULAR DISEASE*

Age (y)	Total Cholesterol,* mg/dl		LDL† Cholesterol,* mg/dl		HDL† Cholesterol,* ‡mg/dl
	Moderate Risk	High Risk	Moderate Risk	High Risk	Increased Risk
MEN					
0–14	173	190	106	120	38
15–19	165	183	109	123	30
20–29	194	216	128	148	30
30–39	218	244	149	171	29
40–49	231	254	160	180	29
≥50	230	258	166	188	29
WOMEN					
0–14	170	174	113	126	36
15–19	173	195	115	135	35
20–29	184	208	127	148	35
30–39	202	220	143	163	35
40–49	223	246	155	177	34
≥50	252	281	170	195	36

(From Hoeg, J. M., et al.: An approach to the management of hyperlipoproteinemia. *JAMA* 1986;255:514–519. Copyright 1986, American Medical Association.)

*Values are adapted from the 75th percentile (moderate-risk) and 90th percentile (high-risk) values obtained by the Lipid Research Clinics.

†LDL: low-density lipoproteins; HDL: high-density lipoproteins.

‡The HDL cholesterol values for the lower fifth percentile were taken from the Lipid Research Clinics.

Proteins

The word **protein** comes from a Greek word meaning "to take first place," and rightly so, for protein is necessary to all living cells. Chemically, proteins are made of carbon, hydrogen, and oxygen, similar to the composition of carbohydrates and fats. However, they also contain nitrogen and several other elements, such as sulfur, phosphorus, and iron. It is the nitrogen that distinguishes proteins from other molecules.

Proteins are very large, complex molecules. They are composed of units known as **amino acids,** which are the materials that our bodies use to build and repair tissues. It is in the form of amino acids that proteins are absorbed into the system and metabolized. There are 23 amino acids, of which 10 are essential in the adult for normal growth and maintenance of tissues. These 10 essential amino acids must come from food.

Proteins are classified according to whether or not they contain all essential amino acids in good proportion to one another. A *complete protein* is one that contains a well-balanced mixture of all 10 essential amino acids. If it is the only source of protein in the diet, it will support life and normal growth. A *partially complete protein* is one that supplies an imbalanced mixture of essential amino acids. If it is the sole protein source, it will maintain life but will not support normal growth. An *incomplete protein* will support neither life nor normal growth. It must not be the sole protein source, for it is missing, or extremely low in, one or more of the essential amino acids. Food sources of these proteins are as follows:

Complete Proteins: meat, fish, poultry, eggs, and dairy products.

Partially Complete Proteins: grains and vegetables.

Incomplete Proteins: corn and gelatin.

Fortunately, most foods have a mixture of proteins that supplement each other. Since there is little, if any, storage of amino acids in the body, it is important that a source of protein be included at each meal. If incomplete or partially complete proteins are used, attempts should be made to balance them. That is, a protein deficient in one amino acid should be eaten with one that is high in the same amino acid.

Vegetarianism has become increasingly popular, and many different forms exist. Some vegetarians consume no red meats but will eat fish and poultry. Some include eggs and/or dairy products in their diets. Others (classified as vegans) consume no animal proteins at all, relying solely on vegetable foods for protein. Those who eat some animal protein in the form of fish, eggs, and milk are generally not at risk nutritionally. Vegetarians must include a variety of foods to ensure the nutritional adequacy of their diets. To supply sufficient protein, vegetables that complement each other must be eaten together. Vegetarians must compensate for the deficiencies in their diets by properly combining foods to get the correct proportion of amino acids. This is customarily done in the diets of different cultures. For example, in Mexico, beans are combined with rice, and in Middle Eastern countries, wheat bread is combined with cheese.

The recommended intake of proteins is 0.8 gm per kilogram of weight (Table 34–3). Of this, at least one third should be obtained from complete proteins. However, if the individual is a strict vegetarian, as already mentioned, care must be taken to balance the proteins consumed.

The average American diet is about 12 to 15% protein. Protein deficiency is the most common form of malnutrition and exists throughout the world. Almost one half of preschool-age children in developing countries are malnourished. A condition called *kwashiorkor* afflicts young children whose protein intake is deficient despite adequate caloric intake. Their diets are very poor in protein and consist mainly of carbohydrates and polished rice. The syndrome is characterized by edema, hypopigmentation, sparse and silky reddish hair, and a pathetic, fretful look. Another deficiency syndrome, called *marasmus,* results from a total decrease in both proteins and calories. It occurs in infants and young children and is characterized by emaciation, loose skin in folds, large sunken eyes, loss of flesh, and the general appearance of old age.

Of the numerous functions of protein in the body, the major ones are to:

- Build and repair body tissue (this cannot be accomplished with any other nutrient)
- Aid in the body's defense mechanisms against disease
- Regulate body secretions and fluids
- Provide energy

Vitamins

Vitamins are defined in the *Handbook of Diet Therapy* as organic substances "occurring in minute quantities in plant and animal tissues; essential for specific metabolic functions or reactions to proceed normally."

Vitamins are classified as body regulators because they:

- Regulate the synthesis of bones, skin, glands, nerves, brain, and blood
- Aid in the metabolism of protein, carbohydrates, and fats
- Prevent nutritional deficiency diseases
- Provide for good health at all ages

They do not supply calories in our diets. Rather, they function as catalysts and help or allow metabolic reactions to proceed. Originally, they were lettered or numbered as they were discovered. However, as they have been identified chemically, they have been given more specific names. In many cases, their chemical names are as well known as their letter designations.

Vitamins are divided into two groups: fat-soluble (A, D, E, and K) and water-soluble (C and the B complex). Deficiencies of a vitamin cause illness. However, there is no good evidence that large intakes of vitamins are useful in the healthy individual. Vitamins will not cure a disease or illness other than one caused by the lack of that nutrient. For example, vitamin C will not cure bleeding gums unless the condition is specifically caused by a lack of ascorbic acid, the chemical name for vitamin C. It should also be noted that toxic symptoms from excessive ingestion of vitamins A and D are proven clinical entities, and large intakes of some water-soluble vitamins may cause adverse effects.

FAT-SOLUBLE VITAMINS
Vitamin A, or Retinol. We can obtain vitamin A by two methods: as a vitamin or from a compound called **carotene,** which the body converts to vitamin A. Carotene is known as a precursor of vitamin A. It is probably a more important source of the vitamin than the preformed compound, since vitamin A, as such, is present in very few foods.

TABLE 34-3. RECOMMENDED DAILY ALLOWANCE FOR PROTEIN

	Age (y)	Weight (kg)	Weight (lb)	Height (cm)	Height (in)	Protein (g)
Infants	0.0-0.5	6	13	60	24	13
	0.5-1.0	9	20	71	28	14
Children	1-3	13	29	90	35	16
	4-6	20	44	112	44	24
	7-10	28	62	132	52	28
Males	11-14	45	99	157	62	45
	15-18	66	145	176	69	59
	19-24	72	160	177	70	58
	25-50	79	174	176	70	63
	51	77	170	173	68	63
Females	11-14	46	101	157	62	46
	15-18	55	120	163	64	44
	19-24	58	128	164	65	46
	25-50	63	138	163	64	50
	51	65	143	160	63	50
Pregnant women						60
Lactating women	first 6 mo					65
	second 6 mo					62

(From *Recommended Dietary Allowances,* 10th ed. Washington, DC, National Academy of Sciences—National Research Council, 1989.)

HUMAN REQUIREMENTS. The recommended daily dietary allowance for the adult is 800 to 1000 retinol equivalents (see Table 34–1). This can be supplied by many different foods; for example, one half an ounce of beef liver, one half a large potato, one third of a cup of cooked spinach, or three medium tomatoes (Table 34–4).

STABILITY. Vitamin A and carotene are not water-soluble and are resistant to heat if not in prolonged contact with it. Consequently, they are not lost through most cooking methods. However, fats will become rancid when in contact with warm air. Once this occurs, the major portion of vitamin A and carotene present is destroyed.

Vitamin D, or Cholecalciferol. Vitamin D may be obtained from a few foods, but the most significant source is produced in the body upon exposure to sunlight. The preformed vitamin is not widely distributed. However, through enrichment processes, it is added to a number of foods, mainly dairy products.

HUMAN REQUIREMENTS. The recommended daily dietary allowance for the adult is 5 μg, which should be readily supplied by exposure to sunlight (see Table 34–1). The level for children and pregnant or lactating women is 10 μg per day. This latter could be supplied by one half a teaspoon of cod-liver oil, three and one half ounces of tuna, or two cups of fortified milk (see Table 34–4).

TABLE 34–4. FAT-SOLUBLE VITAMINS

Functions	Good Sources	Symptoms of Deficiency	Symptoms of Toxicity
Vitamin A **(Nomenclature: Preformed—Retinol, retinal, retinoic acid** **Precursor—Carotene)**			

Maintenance of epithelial cells and mucous membranes
Constituent of visual purple—important for night vision
Necessary for normal growth, development, and reproduction
Necessary for adequate immune response
	Preformed vitamin A: liver
	Carotene (dark green, leafy):
	  spinach
	  broccoli
	  kale
	  Swiss chard
	  turnip greens
	  collard greens
	Carotene (deep orange):
	  carrots
	  sweet potatoes
	  orange winter squash
	  pumpkin
	  tomatoes
	  apricots
	  watermelon
	  cantaloupe
		Nyctalopia (night blindness)
		Keratinized skin (rough, dry skin)
		Dry mucous membranes
		Xerophthalmia (an eye disease)
			Appetite loss
			Hair loss
			Dry skin
			Bone and joint pain
			Enlarged liver and spleen
			Abnormal skin pigmentation
			Fetal malformations

Vitamin E **(Nomenclature: Tocopherol)**			
Prevents oxidative destruction of vitamin A in the intestine Protects red blood cells from rupture (hemolysis) Helps maintain normal cell membranes by reducing the oxidation of polyunsaturated fatty acids	Wheat germ Vegetable oils Legumes Nuts Whole grains Fish Green, leafy vegetables	Breakdown of red blood cells	Headache Nausea Inhibited blood clotting
Vitamin K **(Nomenclature: Menadione, Phylloquinone)**			
Necessary for formation of prothrombin and other factors necessary for blood clotting	Dark green, leafy vegetables Cauliflower Soybean oil Green tea Synthesis of intestinal bacteria	Hemorrhage	Hemolytic anemia Liver damage
Vitamin D **(Nomenclature: Ergocalciferol [vitamin D_2], cholecalciferol [vitamin D_3]** **Precursors: Ergosterol [plants], 7-dehydrocholesterol [in skin])**			
Aids in absorption of calcium and phosphorus Regulates blood levels of calcium Promotes bone and teeth mineralization	Fortified milk Fish with bones (salmon, sardines, and so on)	Rickets (children) Osteomalacia (adults)	Calcification of soft tissues Hypercalcemia Renal stones Appetite and weight loss Nausea and fatigue Growth failure

(From Poleman, C. M., and Peckenpaugh, N. J.: *Nutrition Essentials and Diet Therapy*, 6th ed., Philadelphia, W. B. Saunders Co., 1991, pp 100–101.
Data From Briggs, M. H.: *Vitamins in Human Biology and Medicine*, Boca Raton, FL, CRC Press, 1981; Briggs, M. H.: *Recent Vitamin Research*, Boca Raton, FL, CRC Press, 1984; Garrison, R. H., and Somer, E.: *The Nutrition Desk Reference*, New Canaan, CT, Keats Publishing, 1985; Griffeth, H. W.: *Complete Guide to Vitamins, Minerals and Supplements*, Tucson, AZ, Fisher Books, 1988; Pennington, J. A. T., and Church, H. N.: *Food Values of Portions Commonly Used*, 14th ed. New York, Harper & Row, 1985.)

STABILITY. Vitamin D is stable to heat and is not affected by most cooking methods.

Vitamin E, or Tocopherol. Vitamin E is the vitamin that is still looking for a disease. Over the years, there have been numerous attempts to link this vitamin with many illnesses in humans, but efforts largely have failed. However, it does have several very important functions that are linked with its ability to combine with oxygen and, thus, protect various substances that would otherwise be subject to oxidation.

HUMAN REQUIREMENTS. The recommended daily dietary allowance for the adult is 8 to 10 mg alpha tocopherol equivalents (see Table 34–1). This adult allowance could be met by one tablespoon of saf-flower, corn, or soybean oil, or 3 ounces of wheat germ (see Table 34–4).

Vitamin K. The major function of this vitamin in the body has to do with the formation of *prothrombin,* which is a clotting agent in the blood. Consequently, the vitamin is often used to treat certain types of hemorrhages. Deficiency is rare and is usually due to absorption problems rather than inadequate supply of the vitamin.

HUMAN REQUIREMENTS. There is no RDA for this vitamin. However, estimated safe and adequate daily intakes have been established (see Table 34–1) for adults at 70 to 140 μg day. Probably one half to two thirds of this is supplied by bacterial synthesis in the intestines. The remainder can be supplied by one half cup of broccoli, 3 ounces of beef liver, or one eighth of a head of lettuce (see Table 34–4).

WATER-SOLUBLE VITAMINS
Vitamin C, or Ascorbic Acid. Vitamin C was first used to treat **scurvy** in British sailors during the 18th century. Of course, at the time, the curative factor in the limes each sailor was required to consume daily while at sea was unknown. However, they did know that a lime daily seemed to prevent the dread disease. As a result, the British sailors were nicknamed "limeys," a term that is still used today.

HUMAN REQUIREMENTS. The recommended daily dietary allowance for adults is 60 mg (see Table 34–1). This amount of ascorbic acid would be supplied by 6 ounces of orange or grapefruit juice, 1 cup of strawberries, or three spears of fresh or frozen broccoli, cooked (Table 34–5).

STABILITY. Vitamin C is very easily destroyed by both heat and exposure to air. Since it is water-soluble, care must be used in cooking fruits and vegetables that contain vitamin C. Small amounts of water should be used and cooking times should be short. An alkaline medium will speed up the loss of vitamin C.

Vitamin B$_1$, or Thiamine
HUMAN REQUIREMENTS. Need for the vitamin depends on caloric intake; generally, 0.5 mg per 1000 calories is adequate. The level set by the National Research Council (NRC) is 1.0 to 1.4 mg per day, depending on sex (see Table 34–1). To obtain this amount of thiamine, an individual must eat 1 tablespoon of brewers' yeast, 4 ounces of lean pork, or 2 cups of 40% bran flakes (see Table 34–5).

STABILITY. Thiamine is destroyed by heat and alkaline mediums. Since it is water-soluble, small amounts of water should be used in cooking to preserve this nutrient.

Vitamin B$_2$, or Riboflavin
HUMAN REQUIREMENTS. The National Research Council established 1.2 to 1.6 mg per day (see Table 34–1). Foods supplying this would be 1½ ounces of calf liver, cooked; 3 cups of yogurt or milk; or 3 cups of 40% bran flakes (see Table 34–5).

STABILITY. Riboflavin is very unstable in light. Consequently, milk should be stored in either dark glass or plasticized paper containers. Riboflavin from foods other than milk can also be lost in cooking water or drippings since it is water-soluble.

Niacin. Niacin is obtained either from preformed niacin or from conversion of its precursor, **tryptophan,** in the body. Tryptophan is an essential amino acid, and the body converts it to niacin. About 1 mg of niacin is produced from approximately 60 mg of tryptophan.

HUMAN REQUIREMENTS. The recommended dietary allowance is 13 to 18 mg per day (see Table 34–1). This amount of niacin would be found in 6 ounces of round steak or 1½ cups of pinto beans (see Table 34–5).

Vitamin B$_6$, or Pyridoxine
HUMAN REQUIREMENTS. The National Research Council recommends 2 to 2.2 mg per day for adults (see Table 34–1). No single food is an outstanding source of vitamin B$_6$. However, it is widely distributed in foods, and eating a variety of foods easily supplies adequate amounts. The NRC allowance could be supplied by four bananas, two avocados, or 12 ounces of beef liver, fried (see Table 34–5).

Folic Acid, or Folacin
HUMAN REQUIREMENTS. The established allowance is 400 μg per day for adults (see Table 34–1).

STABILITY. Folacin is destroyed by heat and is frequently lost in cooking water. Storage and cooking losses are usually high irrespective of methods (see Table 34–5).

Vitamin B$_{12}$, or Cobalamin. Deficiency of this vitamin produces an anemia identical to that produced by a folic acid deficiency. However, if a deficiency of vitamin B$_{12}$ is allowed to continue untreated, serious neurologic symptoms will result. For this reason, folic acid cannot legally be added to multivitamin capsules except at very low levels. This is to prevent the folic acid from inadvertently masking the early symptoms of a vitamin B$_{12}$ deficiency.

HUMAN REQUIREMENTS. For adults, 3 μg per day is recommended (see Table 34–1). This is easily supplied by ¼ ounce of beef liver, fried; ¼ cup of frozen peas, cooked; or ¼ cup of canned pineapple (see Table 34–5).

TABLE 34–5. WATER-SOLUBLE VITAMINS

Functions	Good Sources	Symptoms of Deficiency	Symptoms of Toxicity
	Vitamin B₁ *(Nomenclature: Thiamine)*		
Plays a role in carbohydrate metabolism Helps the nervous system, heart, muscles and tissue to function properly Promotes a good appetite and good functioning of the digestive tract	Whole grains Wheat germ Enriched white flour products Organ meats Pork Legumes Brewer's yeast	Polyneuritis Beriberi Fatigue Depression Poor appetite Poor functioning of intestinal tract Nervous instability Edema Spastic muscle contractions Wernicke's encephalopathy Korsakoff's psychosis	Anaphylactic shock Lethargy Ataxia (loss of physical movement) Nausea Hypotension Possible electroencephalogram changes
	Vitamin B₂ *(Nomenclature: Riboflavin [formerly vitamin G])*		

Essential for certain enzyme systems that aid in the metabolism of carbohydrate, protein, and fat	Milk and milk products
	Eggs
	Green, leafy vegetables
	Organ meats
	   liver
	   kidney
	   heart
	Dry yeast
	Peanuts
	Peanut butter
	Whole grains
		Tongue inflammation
		Scaling and burning skin
		Sensitive eyes
		Angular stomatitis and cheilosis
		Cataracts
			No toxicity known in humans

	Vitamin B₃ *(Nomenclature: Niacin, nicotinic acid)*		
Part of two important enzymes that regulate energy metabolism Promotes good physical and mental health and helps maintain the health of the skin, tongue, and digestive system	Meats and organ meats Whole-grain flour products Enriched white flour products Legumes Brewer's yeast	Pellagra (rare) with skin and mouth manifestations Gastrointestinal disturbances Photosensitive dermatitis Depressive psychosis	Flushing caused by vasodilation Anorexia Nausea and vomiting Abnormal glucose metabolism Abnormal plasma uric acid levels Abnormal liver function tests Gastric ulceration Anaphylaxis (swelling, pain, fever, or asthmatic symptoms caused by physical sensitivity) Circulatory collapse
	Vitamin B₆ *(Nomenclature: Pyridoxine, pyridoxal, pyridoxamine)*		
Important in metabolism of protein and amino acids, carbohydrate, and fat Essential for proper growth and maintenance of body functions	Liver and red meats Whole grains Potatoes Green vegetables Corn	Not fully established but believed to lead to convulsions, peripheral neuropathy, secondary pellagra, possible depression, oral lesions	May inhibit prolactin secretion (a hormone necessary for adequate breast milk production) Sensory nerve damage Numbness of extremities Liver damage
	Vitamin B₁₂ *(Nomenclature: Cobalamin)*		
Aids in hemoglobin synthesis Essential for normal functioning of all cells, especially nervous system, bone marrow, and gastrointestinal tract Important in energy metabolism, especially folic acid metabolism	Foods of animal origin Meats Organ meats Dry milk and milk products Whole egg and egg yolk Not found in significant amounts in plant sources	Pernicious (megaloblastic) anemia Subacute combined degeneration of the spinal cord Various psychiatric disorders May cause anorexia	Inadequate evidence at this time

TABLE 34–5. WATER-SOLUBLE VITAMINS *Continued*

Functions	Good Sources	Symptoms of Deficiency	Symptoms of Toxicity
Folacin *(Nomenclature: Folic acid)*			
Functions in the formation of red blood cells and in normal functioning of gastrointestinal tract Aids in metabolism of protein	Glandular meats Yeast Dark green, leafy vegetables Legumes Whole grains	Impaired cell division Alterations of protein synthesis with possible neural tube defect Various psychiatric disorders Megaloblastic anemia Supplements mask the symptoms of pernicious anemia but not the neurologic manifestations	Possible hypersensitivity reactions
Choline			
A constituent of several compounds necessary for certain aspects of nerve function and lipid metabolism	Synthesized from methionine (an amino acid)	Occurs only when protein intake (methylamine) is low	None known in humans
Pantothenic Acid			
Essential part of complex enzymes involved in fatty acid metabolism	Animal products Liver Eggs Whole grains Legumes White potatoes Sweet potatoes	Nutritional melalgia (burning foot syndrome) Headache Fatigue Poor muscle coordination Nausea Cramps	None known
Biotin *(Nomenclature: Once known as vitamin H)*			
Essential for activity of many enzyme systems Plays a central role in fatty acid synthesis and in the metabolism of carbohydrates and protein	Liver Meats Milk Soy flour Brewer's yeast Egg yolk (raw egg white destroys biotin) Bacteria in the intestinal tract also produce biotin	Rare but includes certain types of anemia, depression, insomnia, muscle pain, dermatitis	None known in humans
Vitamin C *(Nomenclature: Ascorbic acid, dehydroascorbic acid)*			
Helps protect the body against infections and in wound healing and recovery from operations Is important for tooth dentin, bones, cartilage, connective tissue, and blood vessels	Citrus fruits Tomatoes Strawberries Cantaloupe Currants Green, leafy vegetables Green peppers Broccoli Cabbage Potatoes	Anemia Swollen and bleeding gums Loose teeth Ruptures of small blood vessels (bruises) Scurvy (rebound scurvy can occur when large doses, or megadoses, are suddenly stopped)	Urinary stones

(From Poleman, C. M., and Peckenpaugh, N. J.: *Nutrition Essentials and Diet Therapy,* 6th ed., Philadelphia, W. B. Saunders Co., 1991, pp 101–104. Data from Briggs, M. H.: *Vitamins in Human Biology and Medicine,* Boca Raton, FL, CRC Press, 1981; Briggs, M. H.: *Recent Vitamin Research,* Boca Raton, FL, CRC Press, 1984; Garrison, R. H., and Somer, E.: *The Nutrition Desk Reference,* New Canaan, CT, Keats Publishing, 1985; Griffeth, H. W.: *Complete Guide to Vitamins, Minerals and Supplements,* Tucson, AZ, Fisher Books, 1988; Pennington, J. A. T., and Church, H. N.: *Food Values of Portions Commonly Used,* 14th ed. New York, Harper & Row, 1985.)

STABILITY. Vitamin B_{12} is stable under most conditions, since it is attached to a protein in foods.

Other B Vitamins. Other vitamins that belong to the B complex, but for which no requirements have been established, are biotin, pantothenic acid, and choline. **Biotin** is synthesized by bacteria in the gastrointestinal tract and is important in several enzyme systems. Raw egg white contains a protein, avidin, which is capable of binding biotin, thus making it unavailable to the body. Avidin is changed by heating, so it will not function in this manner in cooked egg whites. The estimated safe and adequate intake of biotin is 100 to 200 μg, which could be supplied by 4 ounces of beef liver or 2 cups of cooked oatmeal. **Pantothenic acid** is involved in carbohydrate and fatty acid metabolism. It is present in almost all foods, and deficiency should not be seen if a mixed diet is consumed. The Food and Nutrition Board suggests an intake of 4 to 7 mg per day. An equivalent of this amount would be found in 3 ounces of beef liver, four to six eggs, or 1 quart of milk. **Choline** is important in the body mainly as a constituent of compounds known as phospholipids (primarily lecithin). Besides performing other functions, choline is involved in the transport and metabolism of fats. Choline is found in whole grains, meats, egg yolks, and legumes. No deficiency has been demonstrated in humans.

Minerals

Minerals are inorganic chemical elements that make up about 4% of body weight. Of the many that are used by the body, only 14 are felt to be essential. Of those, allowances have been established for only six. Most minerals are required in relatively small amounts, but even so, they are absolutely essential for life.

Minerals contribute to the body's water-electrolyte balance and acid-base balance, and some are cofactors for enzymes. The largest proportion of inorganic elements is found in the skeleton. Minerals present in the largest amount include sodium, potassium, chlorine, calcium, phosphorus, magnesium, and sulfur. Those present in very small amounts, the *trace elements,* include iron, zinc, copper, cobalt, manganese, iodine, and fluorine.

The minerals that are needed only in trace amounts seem either to behave as part of hormone or enzyme systems or to work with vitamins in various metabolic reactions throughout the body. For example, iodine is part of the thyroid hormone *thyroxine,* and another hormone, *insulin,* has zinc as part of its structure. Cobalt, on the other hand, is an essential part of the B_{12} molecule.

Like vitamins, these minerals can be obtained from common foods in a well-balanced diet. With the exception of iodine and iron, mineral deficiencies are rare in the average American diet.

MAJOR MINERALS

Calcium. In the American diet, calcium is the mineral that is the most likely to be deficient. The body requires calcium at all ages, but the highest requirements are during pregnancy, lactation, and childhood.

Osteoporosis is a condition in which the bones become increasingly porous and brittle because of a loss of calcium. This common condition of aging causes bones to fracture more easily. When the spine is involved, the vertebrae collapse, causing curvature and backache, as well as a decrease in stature. In women, osteoporosis is associated with the postmenopausal decrease in estrogen. Many physicians are recommending additional dietary supplements of calcium to forestall this condition (Table 34–6).

HUMAN REQUIREMENTS. The calcium requirement is 800 mg per day (see Table 34–1) and can be supplied by 2 to 3 cups of milk or yogurt, or 4 ounces of cheese.

Phosphorus. Phosphorus is a constituent of every living cell and, as such, has numerous functions in the body. In many cases, it works in the same manner as calcium. However, in addition, it is required for protein, fat, and carbohydrate metabolism, in energy metabolism, and in various buffering systems in the body. It is also involved in a number of vitamin and enzyme reactions. No specific disease is associated with a deficiency of this nutrient, but excessive and prolonged use of antacids containing aluminum hydroxide can produce symptoms of phosphorus deficiency (weakness, anorexia, and bone demineralization) (see Table 34–6).

HUMAN REQUIREMENTS. The phosphorus requirement is 800 mg per day (see Table 34–1) and can be supplied by 2 to 3 cups of milk or yogurt, or 4 ounces of cheese or tuna fish.

Magnesium. Most magnesium is found in combination with calcium and phosphorus in bone tissue. In addition to its role in bone metabolism, magnesium functions mainly in carbohydrate and amino acid reactions in the body. With other minerals, it is also important in nervous activity and muscle contractions. A deficiency of this element results in nervous irritability and, eventually, in convulsions similar to those seen in cases of **tetany** *(hypocalcemia).*

HUMAN REQUIREMENTS. The magnesium requirement is 300 to 350 mg per day for adults, depending on sex (see Table 34–1). No single food, eaten in normal amounts, is an outstanding source of magnesium, but a combination of ½ cup of peanuts and three bananas would supply the NRC allowance (see Table 34–6).

Sodium. This mineral is required mainly for control of fluid volume in the body; an increase in the level of sodium in the serum leads to water retention. One compartment expanded as a result of fluid retention is the vascular system. Sodium, then, is directly related to blood pressure. It functions in acid-base balance and is involved in both carbohydrate and protein metabolism. Deficiencies of sodium can result from inadequate production of adrenocortical hormone or from excessive perspiration. Symptoms of deficiency include nausea, vomiting, and muscle cramps. Extreme cases may lead to heart failure.

Excessive sodium may cause an effective increase in blood volume and, hence, an increase in blood pressure. Although many other factors besides sodium and water retention are involved in causing high blood pressure (hypertension), it appears reasonable to suggest that sodium intake be closely monitored. Estimates place sodium consumption at roughly 10 times the level actually required. Therefore, at least those persons who are predisposed to hypertension should try to use the salt shaker less frequently and should avoid obviously salty foods such as potato chips and broth. Salt substitutes, however, should not be used without medical supervision (see Table 34–6).

HUMAN REQUIREMENTS. The Food and Nutrition Board set the safe and adequate intake for this mineral at 1100 to 3300 mg daily. One teaspoon of table salt supplies 2000 mg of sodium, but 12 green olives or four ounces of ham could also supply over 1000 mg of sodium (see Table 34–1).

Potassium. This mineral functions in much the same way as sodium except that potassium is concentrated within the body cells. In addition to its involvement in fluid volume, potassium plays a multitude of roles in carbohydrate and protein metabolism. Deficiencies of potassium are rare and are usually related to either severe vomiting or diarrhea or to the use of diuretics (drugs that cause excretion of sodium and potassium, frequently used in treating hypertension). Symptoms of a potassium deficiency include nausea, vomiting, and muscle weakness. Severe losses of potassium result in rapid contractions of the heart and, eventually, death due to heart failure.

Too much potassium can also be dangerous. Usually, *hyperkalemia* (high potassium blood level) is due to kidney failure or to the combination of a reduced ability to excrete potassium along with overingestion of potassium, either from supplements or salt substitutes (see Table 34–6).

HUMAN REQUIREMENTS. The safe and adequate intake is set at 1875 to 5625 mg per day (see Table 34–1). No single food source can supply this amount. However, many fruits and vegetables supply 300 to 400 mg per serving, so a variety of foods from these groups should adequately supply potassium in the American diet.

Chlorine. As the ion chloride, this mineral acts as a companion to sodium. It is primarily involved in acid-base and fluid balance and is a component of hydrochloric acid in the stomach. Deficiencies are unusual and are generally related to sodium losses or to excessive vomiting and diarrhea. Toxicities of dietary chlorine are unknown, since it is readily excreted by the kidney. Chlorine in its gaseous form, however, is lethal (see Table 34–6).

HUMAN REQUIREMENTS. Safe and adequate intake of chlorine has been established to be 1700 to 5100 mg per day for adults (see Table 34–1). The amount of salt in the diet supplies more than enough of this nutrient.

Sulfur. Sulfur is used by the body in protein synthesis and in reactions in the liver. The amount of sulfur is normally adequate in diets in which the complete protein content is adequate (see Table 34–1). Deficiency of this mineral can result in dermatitis and imperfect development of hair and nails (see Table 34–6).

TRACE MINERALS
Iron. Although required in small amounts in comparison with such nutrients as phosphorus and calcium, iron is a vitally important element. It is an essential part of *hemoglobin* (the protein that is the oxygen-carrying substance in the blood) and is responsible for the color of red blood cells. The body is very conservative with iron; it reuses it again and again. However, deficiencies do occur, particularly in premenopausal women or during pregnancy or hemorrhagic conditions. A deficiency of iron results in a microcytic anemia (Table 34–7).

HUMAN REQUIREMENTS. The RDA allowance is 18 mg per day for adult women (see Table 34–1). Unless a woman eats liver and other rich sources of iron frequently, the ordinary diet may not supply a sufficient quantity of iron. In this case, an iron supplement may be desirable. For men, 10 mg per day is recommended. This lower amount for men can be supplied by one cup of 40% bran flakes or four ounces of beef liver.

Iodine. Iodine's only function in the body is as a part of the thyroid gland hormone *thyroxine*. Although the requirement for iodine is small, the thyroid gland fails to function properly without it, and the condition known as **goiter** occurs. Iodine deficiency in a pregnant woman can result in **cretinism** in the infant. This disease is characterized by dwarfing and retarded physical and mental growth (see Table 34–7).

TABLE 34–6. MAJOR MINERALS (MACRONUTRIENTS)

Functions	Sources	Deficiency Symptoms	Toxicity Symptoms
Mineral and Elemental Symbol: Calcium (Ca²⁺)			

Functions	Sources	Deficiency Symptoms	Toxicity Symptoms
Helps muscles to contract and relax, thereby helping to regulate heartbeat Plays a role in the normal functioning of the nervous system Aids in blood coagulation and the functioning of some enzymes Helps build strong bones and teeth May help prevent hypertension	Primarily found in milk and milk products; also found in dark green, leafy vegetables, tofu and other soy products, sardines, salmon with bones, and hard water	Poor bone growth and tooth development, leading to stunted growth and increased risk of dental caries, rickets (bowing of legs) in children, osteomalacia (soft bones) and osteoporosis (brittle bones) in adults, poor blood clotting, and possible hypertension	Kidney stones
Mineral and Elemental Symbol: Chloride (Cl⁻)			
Involved in the maintenance of fluid and acid-base balance Provides an acid medium, in the form of hydrochloric acid, for activation of gastric enzymes	Major source is table salt (sodium chloride); also found in fish and vegetables	Disturbances in acid-base balance, with possible growth retardation, psychomotor defects, and memory loss	Disturbances in acid-base balance
Mineral and Elemental Symbol: Magnesium (Mg²⁺)			
Helps build strong bones and teeth Activates many enzymes Participates in protein synthesis and lipid metabolism Helps regulate heartbeat	Raw, dark green vegetables, nuts and soybeans, whole grains and wheat bran, bananas and apricots, seafoods and coffee, tea, cocoa, and hard water	Rare but in disease states may lead to central nervous system problems (confusion, apathy, hallucinations, poor memory) and neuromuscular problems (muscle weakness, cramps, tremor, cardiac arrhythmia)	Drowsiness, weakness, and lethargy and in severe toxicity skeletal paralysis, central nervous system depression, respiratory depression, and ultimately coma and death
Mineral and Symbol: Phosphorus (PO₄)			
Helps build strong bones and teeth Present in the nuclei of all cells Helps in the oxidation of fats and carbohydrates (energy metabolism) Aids in maintaining the body's acid-base balance	Milk and milk products, eggs, meats, legumes, whole grains, soft drinks (used to make the "fizz")	Rare but with malabsorption can cause anorexia, weakness, stiff joints, and fragile bones	Hypocalcemic tetany (muscle spasms)
Mineral and Elemental Symbol: Potassium (K⁺)			
Plays a key role in fluid and acid-base balance Transmits nerve impulses and helps control muscle contractions and promotes regular heartbeat Needed for enzyme reactions	Apricots, bananas, oranges, grapefruit, raisins, green beans, broccoli, carrots, greens, potatoes, meats, milk and milk products, peanut butter and legumes, molasses, coffee, tea, cocoa	May cause impaired growth, hypertension, bone fragility, central nervous system changes, renal hypertrophy, diminished heart rate, and death	Hyperkalemia (excess potassium in the blood) with cardiac function disturbances

34

TABLE 34-6. MAJOR MINERALS (MACRONUTRIENTS) *Continued*

Functions	Sources	Deficiency Symptoms	Toxicity Symptoms
Mineral and Elemental Symbol: Sodium (Na⁺)			
Plays a key role in the maintenance of acid-base balance Transmits nerve impulses and helps control muscle contractions Regulates cell membrane permeability	Salt (sodium chloride) is the major dietary source; minor sources occur naturally in foods such as milk and milk products and several vegetables	Hyponatremia (too little sodium in the blood)	May cause hypertension, which can lead to cardiovascular diseases and renal (kidney) disease; in the form of salt tablets, can cause gastric irritation
Mineral and Symbol: Sulfur (SO₄)			
Part of three amino acids, and the B vitamins thiamine and biotin Plays a role in oxidation-reduction reactions	Protein-rich foods (meat, eggs, milk)	None documented in humans	Unlikely to cause significant symptoms

(From Poleman, C. M., and Peckenpaugh, N. J.: *Nutrition Essentials and Diet Therapy*, 6th ed., Philadelphia, W. B. Saunders Co., 1991, pp 126–127. Data from Garrison, R. H., and Somer, E.: *The Nutrition Desk Reference*, New Canaan, CT, Keats Publishing, 1985; Griffeth, H. W.: *Complete Guide to Vitamins, Minerals and Supplements*, Tucson, AZ, Fisher Books, 1988.)

TABLE 34-7. TRACE MINERALS (MICRONUTRIENTS)

Functions	Sources	Deficiency Symptoms	Toxicity Symptoms
Mineral and Elemental Symbol: Chromium (Cr³⁺)			
Activates several enzymes Enhances the removal of glucose from the blood	Liver and other meats, whole grains, cheese, legumes, and brewer's yeast	Weight loss, abnormalities of the central nervous system and possible aggravation of diabetes mellitus	Inhibited insulin activity
Mineral and Elemental Symbol: Cobalt (Co²⁺)			
An essential component of vitamin B₁₂ Activates enzymes	Figs, cabbage, beet greens, spinach, lettuce, watercress	Pernicious anemia	Polycythemia (excess number of red corpuscles in blood)
Mineral and Elemental Symbol: Copper (Cu²⁺)			
Aids in the production and survival of red blood cells Part of many enzymes involved in respiration Plays a role in normal lipid metabolism	Shellfish—especially oysters—liver, nuts and seeds, raisins, whole grains, and chocolate	Anemia, central nervous system problems, abnormal electrocardiograms, bone fragility, impaired immune response; may be a factor in failure to thrive in premature infants	In Wilson's disease and Huntington's chorea (both hereditary diseases), copper accumulation causes neuron and liver cell damage
Mineral and Elemental Symbol: Fluorine (F⁻)			
Helps the formation of solid bones and teeth, thereby reducing incidence of dental caries, and may help prevent osteoporosis	Fluoridated water (and foods cooked in fluoridated water), fish, tea, gelatin	Increased susceptibility to dental caries	Fluorosis and mottling of teeth
Mineral and Elemental Symbol: Iodine (I⁻)			
Helps regulate energy metabolism through being part of thyroid hormones Essential for normal cell functioning, helps to keep skin, hair, and nails healthy	Primarily from iodized salt, also found in saltwater fish, seaweed products, vegetables grown in iodine-rich soils	Goiter, cretinism in infants born to iodine-deficient mothers, with accompanying mental retardation and diffuse central nervous system abnormalities	Little toxic effect in individuals with normal thyroid gland functioning

Table continued on following page

TABLE 34–7. TRACE MINERALS (MICRONUTRIENTS) *Continued*

Functions	Sources	Deficiency Symptoms	Toxicity Symptoms
Mineral and Elemental Symbol: Iron (Fe³⁺)			
Essential to the formation of hemoglobin, which is important for tissue respiration and ultimately growth and development Part of several enzymes and proteins in the body	Heme sources: organ meats—especially liver, red meats, and other meats Nonheme sources: iron-fortified cereals, dark green, leafy vegetables, legumes, whole grains, blackstrap molasses, dried fruit, and foods cooked in iron pans	Iron-deficiency anemia and possible alterations that impair behavior	Idiopathic hemochromatosis, which can lead to cirrhosis, diabetes mellitus, skin pigmentation, arthralgias (joint pain), and cardiomyopathy
Mineral and Elemental Symbol: Manganese (Mn²⁺)			
Needed for normal bone structure, reproduction, normal functioning of cells and the central nervous system A component of some enzymes	Nuts, whole grains, vegetables and fruits, coffee, tea, cocoa, and egg yolks	None observed in humans	Iron-deficiency anemia through inhibiting effect on iron absorption; pulmonary changes, anorexia, apathy, impotence, headaches, leg cramps, and speech impairment; in advanced stages of toxicity resembles Parkinson's disease
Mineral and Elemental Symbol: Molybdenum (Mo)			
A component of three enzymes Important for normal cell function	Organ meats, legumes, whole grains, dark green vegetables	Vomiting, tachypnea (fast breathing), tachycardia, coma, hypermethioninemia in premature infants (methionine is an amino acid)	Growth retardation and weight loss reported in animals
Mineral and Elemental Symbol: Selenium (Se)			
Part of an enzyme system Acts as an antioxidant with vitamin E to protect the cell from oxygen	Protein-rich foods (meat, eggs, milk), whole grains, seafood, liver and other meats, egg yolks, and garlic	Keshan disease (a human cardiomyopathy) and Kashin-Beck disease (an endemic human osteoarthropathy)	Physical defects of the fingernails and toenails and hair loss
Mineral and Elemental Symbol: Zinc (Zn²⁺)			
Plays a role in protein synthesis Essential for normal growth and sexual development, wound healing, immune function, cell division and differentiation, and smell acuity	Whole grains, wheat germ, crabmeat, oyster, liver and other meats, Brewer's yeast	Depressed immune function, poor growth, dwarfism, impaired skeletal growth and delayed sexual maturation, acrodermatitis	Severe anemia, nausea, vomiting, abdominal cramps, diarrhea, fever, hypocupremia (low blood serum copper), malaise, fatigue

(From Poleman, C. M., and Peckenpaugh, N. J.: *Nutrition Essentials and Diet Therapy,* 6th ed., Philadelphia, W. B. Saunders Co., 1991, pp 128–129. Data from Garrison, R. H., and Somer, E.: *The Nutrition Desk Reference,* New Canaan, CT, Keats Publishing, 1985; Griffeth, H. W.: *Complete Guide to Vitamins, Minerals and Supplements,* Tucson, AZ, Fisher Books, 1988.)

HUMAN REQUIREMENTS. The iodine requirement is 150 μg per day for adults (see Table 34–1). One teaspoon of iodized salt supplies 420 μg of iodine, much more than the RDA. Three glasses of milk will supply 150 μg of iodine.

Zinc. Zinc is necessary for growth and *gonadal* development in humans. Zinc is part of the hormone insulin, which regulates carbohydrate metabolism. It is also a component of several enzyme systems in the body. A deficiency of this nutrient retards skeletal growth and sexual maturation. Additional symptoms include decreased ability to taste and delayed wound healing (see Table 34–7).

HUMAN REQUIREMENTS. Requirements are 15 mg per day for adults (see Table 34–1). This could be supplied by one oyster. One milligram of zinc is found in 1 ounce of most meats.

Fluoride. The major function of fluoride is in hardening bones and teeth. As a result, it is beneficial in reducing the amount of dental decay in infancy and childhood. Some evidence indicates that fluoride may also benefit adults who take it throughout life in protecting them against osteoporosis. In areas of the country where water is naturally fluoridated in excess of 6 to 8 ppm, *mottling* (brown staining) of the tooth enamel is observed.

However, at levels used in artificial fluoridation programs, no health hazard has been documented.

HUMAN REQUIREMENTS. The safe and adequate intake is set at 1.5 to 4 mg per day for adults. This would be supplied by 1.5 liters (L) of fluoridated water (see Table 34–7).

Copper. Copper contributes to iron absorption and metabolism and is involved in the formation of hemoglobin. Copper deficiencies are unusual and are generally linked to genetic defects. The safe and adequate intake is established at 2 to 3 mg per day for adults (see Table 34–7).

Water

Water is the most important nutrient, yet it is all too often overlooked when the average person considers nutritional status. It has a wide variety of functions in the body:

- Plays a key role in the maintenance of body temperature
- Acts as a solvent and a medium for most biochemical reactions
- Acts as a vehicle for transport of substances such as nutrients, hormones, antibodies, and metabolic wastes
- Acts as a lubricant for joints and mucous membranes

Approximately two thirds of the total body weight is water. It is lost daily from the body in urine, feces, and sweat and is expired in the air. Extensive water losses due to diarrhea, vomiting, burns, or perspiration can lead to electrolyte losses and resultant life-threatening imbalances. Drinking too much water (water intoxication) can also be dangerous.

Most of the daily requirements for water are satisfied by ingested fluids and foods and by water released by the metabolism of carbohydrates, fats, and proteins. All food contains some water. Most vegetables and fruits are more than 80% water, and meats are 40 to 60% water.

HUMAN REQUIREMENTS. None is set, but an adequate daily allowance for adults is 2 L (about eight glasses).

CLINICAL NUTRITION

Although the majority of patients a physician sees are treated medically without using a therapeutic diet, there are some illnesses and diseases that can be cured and patients whose recovery can be facilitated by the use of a special diet. In such cases, the normal (sometimes referred to as house or regular) diet is used as a basis of planning. The two major reasons for this are:

- The closer the special diet is to a normal one, the fewer changes the assistant will be asking the person to accept, and the easier it will be for the patient to adhere to the diet.
- It is easier to be certain that the patient's diet supplies adequate amounts of the essential nutrients if a regular diet pattern is used as a baseline.

Modifying a Diet

The normal diet can be modified with regard to the following features (or combination thereof) to create a therapeutic diet:

- Consistency
- Caloric level
- Levels of one or more nutrients
- Bulk
- Spiciness
- Levels of specific foods
- Feeding intervals

Consistency

Changes in consistency are sometimes ordered for individuals who have problems with their mouth, teeth, or esophagus. A texture restriction is also frequently called for in cases of illnesses of the gastrointestinal tract.

SOFT OR LIGHT DIET. Foods with roughage are eliminated (no raw fruits or vegetables). No strongly flavored or gas-forming vegetables are allowed (onions, beans, broccoli, and cauliflower). In many cases, spices are limited.

MECHANICAL SOFT DIET. A regular diet in which the food is either chopped, ground, or pureed, depending upon the degree of texture change required. No foods or spices are restricted.

LIQUID DIET. There are two types of liquid diets. The clear liquid diet includes only broth soups, tea, coffee, and gelatin. In some cases, apple juice and cranberry juice may be allowed. The full liquid diet includes all foods allowed on a clear liquid diet plus milk, custards, strained cream soups, refined cereals, eggnogs, milkshakes, and all juices.

The soft and mechanical diets should supply all the nutrients required by an individual. The clear liquid diet is not adequate and should be used for very brief periods of time. Full liquid diets can be made adequate, but they are usually not, and therefore they should also be used only for short periods.

Caloric Level

Calories may be either increased or decreased. Increased calories are ordered in cases of chronic underweight, as in the eating disorders **anorexia nervosa** and **bulimia;** following an illness; for malnutrition and hyperthyroidism; during times of growth, such as infancy and childhood; and during pregnancy and lactation. Under such circumstances, the total amounts of foods on the regular diet are increased, and the diet is usually higher in fats (since fat supplies more calories per gram than either carbohydrates or proteins). The number of meals eaten may also be increased from three to six or more.

Calories are restricted in cases of **obesity** and **diabetes mellitus.** The quantities of food consumed should be decreased, but no one food group should be eliminated. For diabetes, food containing carbohydrates, particularly the simple sugars, are controlled. Lists of foods that enable diabetics to plan their diets more easily have been prepared by the American Diabetic Association. (The lists are known as exchange lists, and various modifications of them are frequently used for calorie-restricted diets in general.)

High-calorie diets should be adequate in all nutrients. Low-calorie diets can usually be made adequate. However, diets supplying less than 1800 kcal will probably be inadequate.

Levels of One or More Nutrients

A large number of therapeutic diets modify the levels of one or more nutrients. This type of diet is used to treat specific deficiency diseases (for example, high-iron diet) or when a patient has had a toxic reaction to a specific vitamin or mineral (for example, low-vitamin A diet). Many inborn errors of metabolism are treated by eliminating or limiting the ingestion of a nutrient (for example, **phenylketonuria** is treated by limiting the quantities of the essential amino acid phenylalanine). In cases of hypertensive heart disease, sodium is restricted. For patients with **atherosclerosis,** a low-fat or low-cholesterol diet may be prescribed. Protein levels are changed for kidney and liver disease therapy. Fat is also restricted for gallbladder or liver disease.

In general, the normal diet is modified by restricting foods that are sources of the nutrient involved. Except for the nutrient in question, the RDA allowances can usually be met. However, if several restrictions are ordered for the same patient, a nutrient supplement may be necessary (Fig. 34–3).

Bulk

Bulk or residue is changed when treating problems of the colon or large bowel. In some cases,

high-residue diets are ordered; in others, low-residue diets. In either case, foods high in **cellulose** are considered to be high in residue because the body does not digest this carbohydrate well, and a residue is left in the colon. In some instances, a low-residue diet is distinguished from a low-fiber diet. In this case, a low-fiber diet eliminates those foods with a high cellulose content, and a low-residue diet restricts milk, in addition to fiber content. Either diet should supply all the nutrients needed; however, if milk is restricted drastically, the calcium level must be watched carefully.

Spiciness

A bland diet restricts those dietary components that are classified as gastrointestinal irritants. Such a diet limits any foods that are chemically (e.g., caffeine, pepper, chili, nutmeg, and alcohol) or mechanically (high-fiber) irritating. No fried foods or highly concentrated sweets are included. Gas-forming vegetables belonging to the onion and cabbage family are also eliminated. The diet is commonly used for problems occurring in the gastrointestinal tract (such as ulcers). The bland diet should supply sufficient nutrients for the individual to meet the RDA allowances, unless fruits and vegetables are eliminated (in which case, a supplement may be necessary).

Levels of Specific Foods

Diets that modify the levels of specific foods are most frequently used to treat allergies of various kinds. There are two basic elimination-type regimens. A simple elimination diet removes only one or two foods that are suspected of causing the allergy. The *Rowe* elimination diet involves a more extensive program. Using this method, the basic diet consists of a few hypoallergenic foods such as rice cereal, apples, pears, carrots, sweet potatoes, lamb, and milk substitutes. If no allergic reaction is observed, single food-family groups are added slowly in periods of about 10 days. In children, the most common allergies are to chocolate, wheat, eggs, and milk. *Celiac disease* (an intestinal malabsorption syndrome characterized by diarrhea, hypocalcemia, bleeding, and malnutrition) is treated by eliminating foods that contain a protein called **gliadin** (found in wheat). In some cases, it may be difficult to meet the RDA allowances for all nutrients. When this situation occurs, supplements should be ordered.

Feeding Intervals

Feeding intervals can be changed. Usually, more meals are ordered rather than fewer. Generally, the increase is from three meals to six or eight meals. Feeding intervals are shortened for treating prob-

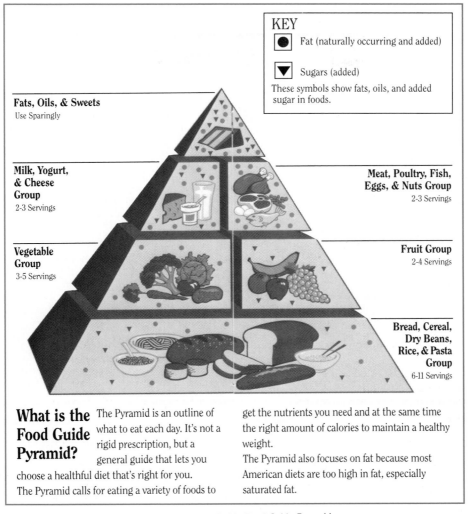

KEY

● Fat (naturally occurring and added)

▼ Sugars (added)

These symbols show fats, oils, and added sugar in foods.

Fats, Oils, & Sweets
Use Sparingly

Milk, Yogurt, & Cheese Group
2-3 Servings

Meat, Poultry, Fish, Eggs, & Nuts Group
2-3 Servings

Vegetable Group
3-5 Servings

Fruit Group
2-4 Servings

Bread, Cereal, Dry Beans, Rice, & Pasta Group
6-11 Servings

What is the Food Guide Pyramid? The Pyramid is an outline of what to eat each day. It's not a rigid prescription, but a general guide that lets you choose a healthful diet that's right for you. The Pyramid calls for eating a variety of foods to get the nutrients you need and at the same time the right amount of calories to maintain a healthy weight.

The Pyramid also focuses on fat because most American diets are too high in fat, especially saturated fat.

FIGURE 34-3. USDA's Food Guide Pyramid.

lems dealing with the gastrointestinal tract, malnutrition, or underweight. An individual who has had part or all of the stomach removed surgically (*surgical bypass of the intestine* or *gastric partitioning*) requires more meals. In some cases, the total food consumed per day is the same, but it is fed in smaller quantities at any given time. In other cases, more food is added at the extra meals. Unless the number of meals is reduced severely, the RDA allowances should be met.

Prescribing a Diet

Since there are so many different types of therapeutic diets, it is frequently impossible for the physician to stay abreast of all the restrictions and other considerations involved. For this reason, the physician will often rely on either a local dietitian or a nutritional consultant to plan the therapeutic diet and instruct patients on the modifications they should follow.

Basically, diet therapy involves a problem-solving process. First, data concerning the nutritional status of the patient must be collected (Table 34-8). This information is generally accumulated by a variety of health professionals (headed by the physician), including in some cases medical assistants, and is expanded and coordinated by the registered dietitian. The second step is the planning phase, during which the collected data are analyzed, the nutrition-related problems are delineated, and the possible solutions are outlined. The proposed dietary measures are then implemented as a planned dietary program. (Some of the most common nutrition-related problems and the dietary modifications used to treat them are shown in Table 34-9.) Last, the program, or diet, being used is evaluated in terms of the medical problem to determine whether the nutrition-related disorder is being or has been corrected. If necessary, the entire process is repeated. At all

TABLE 34-8. ACCEPTABLE WEIGHTS FOR MEN AND WOMEN

Height (Without Shoes)	Weight in Pounds (Without Clothes) 19-34 years old	35 years and older
5'0"	97-128	108-138
5'1"	101-132	111-143
5'2"	104-137	115-148
5'3"	107-141	119-152
5'4"	111-146	122-157
5'5"	114-150	126-162
5'6"	118-155	130-167
5'7"	121-160	134-172
5'8"	125-164	138-178
5'9"	129-169	142-183
5'10"	132-174	146-188
5'11"	136-179	151-194
6'0"	140-184	155-199
6'1"	144-189	159-205
6'2"	148-195	164-210
6'3"	152-200	168-216

(From U.S. Department of Agriculture, Human Nutrition Information Service: *1990 U.S. Dietary Guidelines for Americans.*)

TABLE 34-9. COMMON DIET-RELATED DISORDERS

Disorder	Major Dietary Components	Corrective Dietary Measures
Allergies	Wide variety of foods as possible allergens: wheat, milk, eggs, chocolate most common	Eliminate or restrict food sources of allergen
Anemia	Deficiency of iron, B_{12}, or folacin	Increase amount of deficient nutrient
Anorexia nervosa	Starvation; fear of becoming fat; altered body image	High-calorie diet, psychotherapy, behavior modification
Atherosclerosis	High cholesterol, high saturated fat, excessive calories	Control calories, decrease total fat in diet to 30 to 35% of calories, change to more unsaturated fats, lower cholesterol content of diet, stress complex carbohydrates rather than simple sugars
Bulimia	Binge eating, self-induced vomiting	Regular diet; behavior modification, psychotherapy
Cancer of the colon	Low fiber	Increase dietary fiber, increase fluids
Cirrhosis of the liver	Excessive ingestion of alcohol or nutrients such as iron, lead, vitamin A or D	Reduce dietary level of excessive nutrient or substance
Constipation/diverticulosis	Poor fiber intake, poor fluid intake	Increase dietary fiber and fluids
Diabetes mellitus	Obesity, excessive sugar consumption	Control calories and carbohydrates
Hypertension	Obesity, high salt intake	Control calories, decrease sodium intake
Obesity	Excessive calorie intake, inadequate physical activity	Decrease calories, increase activity; behavior modification, group therapy

times, it is preferable to involve the patient as much as possible to maximize results and maintain long-term dietary modifications.

If it is not feasible to use professional dietetic assistance, the physician may wish to use a service offered by some firms that develop diets, printed with the physician's name on them, that can be given to the patient. Numerous pharmaceutical or medical suppliers also supply diet lists, which usually are used as additional advertising for the products of the manufacturer. If such diets are employed, remember that one list is frequently used for more than one type of diet (for example, several different calorie levels may be listed in chart form), and it is left to the patient to decipher the information. Diets of this nature must be as clear and concise as possible so that the patient is not unduly confused or frightened.

It is important that the patient return home with written instructions after leaving the office. Many questions will arise after the diet has first been in-troduced in the office. A written list is the easiest method of answering these questions.

When a patient needs to follow a specific diet, it may be necessary to help him or her learn how to read labels for calorie, sodium, cholesterol, and fat content. To do this, it is necessary for the patient to become familiar with adjectival terms used in label-ing. The most frequently questioned terms are listed in the FDA Adjectival Terms and Definitions for Food/Shelf Labels for Calories, Sodium, Cholesterol, and Fat chart.

FDA ADJECTIVAL TERMS AND DEFINITIONS FOR FOOD/SHELF LABELS FOR CALORIES, SODIUM, CHOLESTEROL, AND FAT	
TERM	**DEFINITION AND REQUIREMENT**
Low calorie	Less than or equal to 40 calories per serving and less than or equal to 0.4 calories per gram
Reduced calorie	At least one third fewer calories, but otherwise nutritionally equiva-lent to the food it re-places; requires a statement of compari-son
Sodium free	Less than 5 mg sodium per serving
Very low sodium	Less than or equal to 35 mg sodium per serv-ing
Low sodium	Less than or equal to 140 mg sodium per serving
Reduced sodium	At least 75% reduction of sodium compared with the food it re-places; requires a statement of compari-son
Cholesterol free	Less than 2 mg choles-terol per serving
Low cholesterol	Less than or equal to 20 mg cholesterol per serving
Reduced choles-terol	At least 75% reduction of cholesterol com-pared with the food it replaces; requires a statement of compari-son
Low fat	Less than or equal to 2 g fat per serving and less than or equal to 10% fat on a dry weight basis
Reduced fat	At least 50% reduction of fat compared with the food it replaces; re-quires a statement of comparison

THE POLITICS AND ECONOMICS OF NUTRITIONAL RECOMMENDATIONS

Almost every American schoolchild is taught that a healthy diet is composed of a given number of daily servings from each of the four basic food groups. What the children (and even many adults) do not know is that dividing the American diet into four equal groups resulted more from political and economic pressures than from information relevant to health. According to Marion Nestle, professor of nutrition at New York University and an advisor to government nutrition agencies:

> "The standard four food groups are based on American agriculture lobbies. Why do we have a milk group? Because we have a National Dairy Council. Why do we have a meat group? Because we have an extremely powerful meat lobby."

In 1956, the four food groups were presented as equal segments of a food wheel with each food group (and its agricultural lobby) accorded equal weight in the graphic presentation. In 1991, to reflect the new dietary guidelines that called for more consumption of grains and less consumption of meat, sweets, and fats, the graphic design was changed from a wheel to a pyramid (Fig. 34–4). The grain group was placed at the bottom of the pyramid and the sweets and fats group was at the top to emphasize the difference in importance between the two groups in the diet. The USDA named the new design the "Eat Right Pyramid."

Just before the "Eat Right Pyramid" was to be introduced to the American public, the Secretary of Agriculture unexpectedly suspended its release. Rep-resentatives from the dairy and meat industries, fearing negative economic repercussions, objected to the placement of their food groups next to the sweets and fats group near the top of the pyramid. The message was quite clear—governmental nutri-tional advice is driven as much by political and eco-nomic considerations as by scientific recommenda-tions to improve public health; thus, each person has the responsibility to construct a healthy diet for himself or herself.

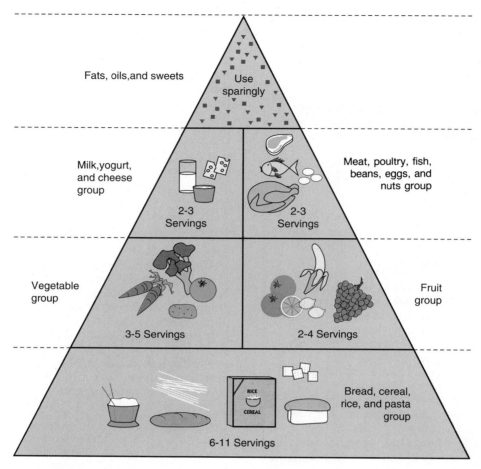

FIGURE 34-4. "Eat Right Pyramid" of the U.S. Department of Agriculture.

LEGAL AND ETHICAL RESPONSIBILITIES

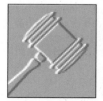

Always remember that you are not a doctor, nor are you a dietitian. Follow the doctor's instructions, and if the patient has questions that you are not sure of, *always* ask the physician for his or her advice in handling the question. If the office you work in employs a registered dietitian, refer questions involving meal patterns and food selection changes to him or her. When seeking advice in the field of nutrition, direct patients to someone who truly qualifies as an expert on nutrition.

▸ PATIENT EDUCATION

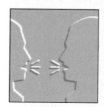

The medical assistant may be called upon to discuss the diet with the patient. It is extremely important to have a thorough knowledge of diet therapy in order to talk with the patient in a convincing manner. It is important that the patient understand the diet and the rationale behind its use. If the patient feels uneasy or has many unanswered questions, he or she will be less motivated to follow the diet. The medical assistant can be a very valuable asset to the physician, the dietitian, and the patient. A sound understanding of nutrition and diet therapy enables the assistant to function most effectively.

When talking to patients about a diet, the following may be helpful:

- Use charts and diagrams to illustrate diets.
- Consider the patient's dietary likes and dislikes.
- Remember ethnic and cultural foods are important.
- Allow the patient to play an active role in the learning process.
- Suggest local support groups that can help in diet maintenance.

► LEARNING ACHIEVEMENTS

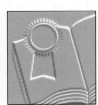

Upon completion of this chapter, can you in the time allowed by your evaluator:

1. List the major foods in each of the four major food groups?
2. Describe the seven dietary guidelines for Americans?
3. Explain the difference between "good" and "bad" cholesterol?
4. Calculate the total daily calories in your personal diet?
5. Adjust your daily diet to meet the recommended daily allowances for nutrients?

REFERENCES AND READINGS

Edlin, G., and Eric, G.: *Health and Wellness,* 4th ed., Boston, Jones & Bartlett Publishers, Inc., 1992.

Garrison, R. H., and Somer, E.: *The Nutrition Desk Reference,* New Canaan, CT, Keats Publishing, Inc., 1985.

National Academy of Sciences, National Research Council: *Recommended Dietary Allowances,* 10th ed., Washington, DC, 1989.

National Dairy Council: *Nutrition Source Book,* Rosemont, IL, 1980.

Poleman, C., and Peckenpaugh, N.: *Nutrition: Essentials and Diet Therapy,* 6th ed., Philadelphia, W. B. Saunders Co., 1991.

U.S. Department of Health and Human Services: *Facts About Blood Cholesterol,* Public Health Service, National Institutes of Health, Publication No. 85–2696, 1985.

U.S. Department of Health and Human Services: *Surgeon General's Report on Nutrition and Health,* DHHS Publication No. (PHS) 88–50210, 1988.

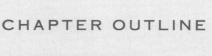

CHAPTER OUTLINE

VOCABULARY

abrasion Rubbing or scraping of the skin or mucous membrane (e.g., a skinned knee).

abscess A localized collection of pus that may be located under the skin or deep within the body. It causes tissue destruction.

approximation The act or process of drawing together skin or wound edges.

biopsy A small sample of tissue excised from the body for diagnostic or therapeutic purposes.

cannula A flexible tube that surrounds a sharp, pointed trocar inserted into the body. When the trocar is withdrawn, fluid escapes from the body through the cannula.

caustic A substance that burns or destroys organic tissue by chemical action.

curettage The act of scraping a body cavity with a surgical instrument, such as a curette.

cyst A sac of fluid or semisolid material located in or under the skin.

débridement Surgical removal of damaged, diseased, or contaminated tissue until healthy tissue is exposed.

dilatation Opening or widening the circumference of a body orifice with a dilating instrument.

diluent A substance, such as water, that renders a drug or a solution less potent.

dissect To cut or separate tissues with a cutting instrument or scissors.

fascia A sheet or band of fibrous tissue located deep in the skin that covers muscles and body organs.

fistula An abnormal, tubelike passage within the body tissues.

lesion A wound, sore, ulcer, tumor, or any traumatic tissue damage that causes a lack of tissue continuity or a loss of function.

lumen An open space, such as within a blood vessel, the intestine, or an examining instrument.

obturator A metal rod with a smooth rounded tip that is placed into hollow instruments to decrease destruction of the mucous membrane during insertion.

paroxysm Sudden return or amplification of symptoms such as a spasm or seizure.

patency The open condition of a body cavity or canal.

polyps Tumors on stems. They are frequently found on mucous membranes.

stylus A metal probe that is inserted or passed through a catheter, needle, or tube. It is used for clearing purposes or to facilitate passage into a body orifice.

suppuration Production of purulent material (pus) from a wound.

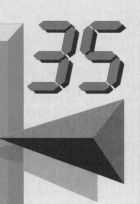

INTRODUCTION TO MINOR SURGERY

LEARNING OBJECTIVES

COGNITIVE

Upon successful completion of this chapter, you should be able to:

1. Define and spell the words in the Vocabulary.

2. Identify by name the instruments used in minor surgery procedures.

3. Identify types of suture strands and surgical needles.

4. State the rules for sterile technique.

5. Compare and contrast medical and sterile hand washing techniques.

6. Name five common fears that a patient may have when faced with either elective or emergency surgery.

7. List six preoperative procedures that need to be completed before the time of surgery.

PERFORMANCE

Upon successful completion of this chapter, you should be able to:

1. Prepare a surgical pack for the autoclave.

2. Perform the surgical hand wash without an error in technique.

Minor surgery is surgery that is restricted to the management of minor problems and injuries. Almost all medical assistants are expected to glove and assist with the preparation of the sterile field and the patient. A few are expected to assist with outpatient surgical procedures that were once performed in the hospital. Although these more difficult operations may involve complete gowning and gloving with surgical masks and caps, the next two chapters limit discussion and descriptions to the routines necessary to prepare for and assist in minor surgery only. This chapter includes surgical supplies, how to prepare for minor surgery, the difference between a circulating and scrubbed medical assistant, aseptic techniques, and the preoperative preparation of the patient. It prepares you for Chapter 36, in which specific minor surgical procedures and the postoperative care of the patient are presented.

A complete understanding of minor surgery procedures includes material presented in preceding chapters, specifically: Chapter 23, Basic Concepts of Asepsis, in which the principles of microbiology can be found; in Chapter 24, Sanitization, Disinfection, and Sterilization, in which the processes that do or do not achieve sterility are discussed; and Chapter 25, Acquired Immunodeficiency Syndrome, which covers the guidelines for pathogenic waste. You are urged to refer to these previous chapters frequently while reading these next two.

The following are composites of acceptable procedures and techniques for preparing for minor surgical procedures in the medical office, clinic, and urgent-care center. However, individual practices and preferences may modify some of these procedures as described.

SURGICAL SUPPLIES

When minor surgery is routinely performed, the medical office is usually designed to include a changing room and a minor surgery room that is separate from the other examining rooms. The larger surgery centers are frequently designed to include recovery rooms and family waiting areas. The minor surgery room should be near a workroom with a sink and an autoclave, if the room does not have its own. It should be easy to clean or decontaminate, and it should be uncluttered to allow easy movement and minimal dust collection. In addition to the operating table, equipment should include a clock with a second sweep, an operating light, sitting stools, and a Mayo stand. Cabinets with counter tops are necessary to serve as a side or back table during the surgery. All surgical supplies are stored in these cabinets. Supplies used in this room should not be used elsewhere; supplies used elsewhere should not be brought into this room.

Surgical Solutions and Medications

Treatment room supplies include standard solutions and medications that are used in minor surgery and dressing changes. Although the solutions and medications listed here are basic, every practice has preferred items and methods of applying them. Many of these items are used by the medical assistant. Others are used by the physician only, but the medical assistant is responsible for their care and supply.

Sterile distilled water is kept in two forms. Multiple-dose vials are used for injectable distilled water and as a **diluent** for medications. Larger containers of sterile distilled water are used for rinsing instruments that have been in a chemical disinfectant solution.

Sterile physiologic saline solution (0.85% sodium chloride) is also stocked in two sizes. The smaller multiple-dose vials are used for injection. The larger containers of physiologic saline are used for rinsing and irrigating wounds. Do not prepare these items in your office; purchase high-quality commercially prepared products.

Povidone-iodine (Betadine) is currently the preferred skin antiseptic. Isopropyl alcohol 70% was the antiseptic of choice in the past. Neither of these products is sporicidal. Betadine does not cause the problems of the earlier tincture of iodine and is used in several different ways: as a skin preparation for surgery, as a surgical hand scrub, for saturating dressings, and as a topical ointment.

Surgical soap, such as Betadine Scrub and Hibiclens, is used for hand washing, for the patient's skin preparation before surgery, and before the application of an antiseptic.

Hydrogen peroxide (H_2O_2) in a 3% solution is used as a mild antiseptic. It kills by its oxidizing power. The oxidizing action creates minute bubbles when applied to a skin **abrasion** or wound and has cleansing action. It is used in irrigations and **débridement** and is nonirritating.

Procaine and lidocaine (Xylocaine) are local anesthetics, and there are many others. They are usually purchased in multiple-dose vials of 30 to 50 cc (ml). When highly vascular areas are involved, anesthetics with epinephrine may be used. Epinephrine causes vasoconstriction at the site, which keeps the anesthetic in the tissues longer, prolonging its effect; it also minimizes local bleeding. Since epinephrine tends to maximize swelling at the site and to distort a close **approximation** of the wound edges, it is not generally used on the extremities. Epinephrine must be used with caution in patients with a history of heart disease.

Tincture of benzoin is applied as a protective coating over ulcers and abrasions. It is used under adhesive tape to increase holding power and to decrease skin sensitivity to the tape. Tincture of benzoin is supplied in spray cans as well as in solution for painting on the skin with an applicator.

Ethyl chloride is used as a skin anesthetic (topical). It is a highly volatile liquid that is sprayed on the skin. It evaporates so quickly that the tissue is immediately cooled and numbed. It has a very short duration and is sometimes called "freezing."

Epinephrine 1:1000 (Adrenalin) is a vasoconstrictor used to control hemorrhage, asthmatic **paroxysms,** and shock. It is also used to reverse allergic reactions. Administration can be topical, by inhalation, or parenteral.

Formalin, 10% solution, is used to preserve excised tissue for specimens, such as those taken in biopsy or for histologic studies.

Aromatic spirits of ammonia is supplied in bottles or in small glass ampules covered with cotton gauze to prevent injury when they are crushed to open. It is most commonly used for fainting, although recent studies have shown that its dangers may far outweigh any advantages for certain patients.

Vaseline (petroleum jelly, or petrolatum) is used to impregnate gauze squares or strips. It is packaged and sterilized by commercial manufacturers.

Iodoform gauze strips are slender strips of gauze, 1/4 to 1/2 in. wide, impregnated with iodoform (96% iodine). They are used to pack an abscess, acting as a wick to draw out the infection and as a local antibacterial (Fig. 35–1).

Silver nitrate ($AgNO_3$) is available in solution or coated on applicator sticks. It is a **caustic** and is applied topically. It must be kept in light-proof brown containers. The most commonly used solution is 20%, but 10% and 50% solutions are frequently employed. The applicator sticks are convenient for touching oral and nasal **lesions.** Silver nitrate may be used to promote the healing process after surgery.

Accessory Supplies

Certain pieces of equipment are frequently used in minor surgery.

An *electrosurgical unit* is used to cauterize blood vessels and incise tissue with an electric current.

Fiberoptic lights and headlights supply an intense light in a small area.

Wound drains are rubber drains introduced into a wound at the end of a surgical procedure, if the wound is filled with fluid or is oozing.

Surgical sponges are used to absorb blood and protect tissues during surgery. They also may be used to wipe blood or other debris from the instruments. The 4 × 4 gauze square is used in most minor surgery.

Syringes and needles are used to inject local anesthetics, to aspirate fluids from a wound, and to irrigate wounds.

Instruments are fundamental to the performance of diagnostic procedures and patient treatments. With the growth of urgent care centers and an increase in outpatient surgery, the medical assistant now must care for and use a greater variety of surgical instruments. The administrative medical assistant must properly spell the names of instruments when transcribing medical dictation as well as purchase and inventory them by name. The clinical medical assistant must know which instruments

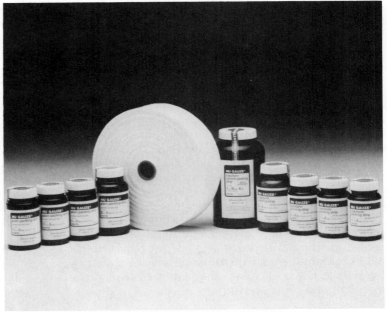

FIGURE 35–1. Commercially prepared Iodoform gauze (Nu Gauze Packing Strips) for packing an abscess and for facilitating drainage. (Courtesy of Johnson & Johnson Medical, Inc., Arlington, TX.)

are used for each procedure in order to package them for sterilization and setup and to assist the physician during surgery or an examination.

IDENTIFYING THE PARTS OF SURGICAL INSTRUMENTS

Instruments have clearly identifiable parts and can be visually differentiated from one another. The basic components are the handle, the closing mechanism, and the part that comes into contact with the patient, commonly called the *jaws.* Many instruments may be ordered straight (str) or curved (cvd), depending on the operator's preference.

Instruments have either ring handles (finger-rings) or spring handles (sometimes called thumb-handled or thumb grasp). Included in the instruments with a ring handle are scissors; tweezers are listed under spring-handled instruments. A ring-handled forceps is shown in Figure 35–2*A*; a spring-handled thumb forceps is pictured in Figure 35–2*B*.

Ratchets resemble gears and are located just below the ring handles. Ratchets are used to lock an instrument into position. Most ratchets can be closed at three or more positions, depending on the thickness of the material being grasped. An example of an instrument with a ratchet closing mechanism is shown in Figure 35–2*C*. Another type of locking mechanism is the box-lock (Fig. 35–2*D*).

The inner surfaces of the jaws on some instruments have sawlike teeth called *serrations,* and both ring-handled and thumb-type instruments may have them. These serrations may be crisscross, horizontal, or lengthwise (Fig. 35–2*E*). Serrations prevent small blood vessels and tissue from slipping out of the jaws of the instrument.

Jaws may be plain-tipped or mouse-toothed (Fig. 35–2*F*). If the tooth is large, the tip may be called *rat-toothed* rather than *mouse-toothed.* Toothed instruments are usually called *tissue forceps* and are identified by the number of intermeshing teeth (e.g., 1 × 2, 2 × 3, 3 × 4). Figure 35–2*G* shows part of an *Allis tissue forceps.* Because this forceps is used to grasp delicate soft tissues, the teeth are finer, shallow, and more rounded; others may be sharper and deeper. Still others have sharp hooklike single or double teeth, such as the *tenaculum* and *vulsellum.* Usually, the *tenaculum* has a single sharp hook on each jaw (see Fig. 35–10*D*). However, the *vulsellum* (Fig. 35–10*C*) has a double hook that resembles the fangs of a snake. Toothed instruments commonly have ratchets for locking into towels or human tissues.

An instrument is usually named for its use (e.g., *splinter forceps,* for removing splinters) or after the person(s) who developed it (e.g., *Mayo-Hegar needle holder*). Many general instruments are identified by the part of the body where they are used (e.g., *rectal speculum* and *nasal speculum*).

There are thousands of surgical instruments, and there are great variations in their names. The same instrument may carry two or three different names, depending on the physician or the part of the country. A physician may ask for a clamp or a forceps when a *Kelly hemostat* is wanted, and you will need to know what a clamp or forceps means in each case. As in building words from word parts, if you train yourself to recognize the distinctive parts of instruments and the reasons for each part, you will quickly build a working knowledge of hundreds of instruments.

CLASSIFICATIONS OF SURGICAL INSTRUMENTS

Surgical instruments are generally classified according to their use, and most belong to one of four groups:

- Cutting and dissecting
- Grasping and clamping
- Retracting
- Probing and dilating

Cutting and Dissecting Instruments

These are the cutting, incising, scraping, punching, and puncturing instruments. Included are scissors, scalpels, chisels, curettes, punches, drills, and needles. Instruments with a sharp blade or surface can cut, scrape, or **dissect.**

Scissors

Operating scissors (also called *surgical scissors;* Fig. 35–3*A* through *C*)

- Most frequently used length is 5¼ inches
- Used to cut tissue or fine sutures

Dissecting scissors (Fig. 35–3*D*)

- Narrow blunt blades
- May have inside and outside edges
- Used for dissecting or exposing growths and vessels

Bandage scissors (Fig. 35–3*E* and *F*)

- Probe tip is blunt
- Easily inserted under bandages with relative safety
- Used to remove bandages and dressings

Gauze shears (Fig. 35–3*G*)

- Has sharp blades and large ring handle
- Used to cut gauze, tubing, and adhesive

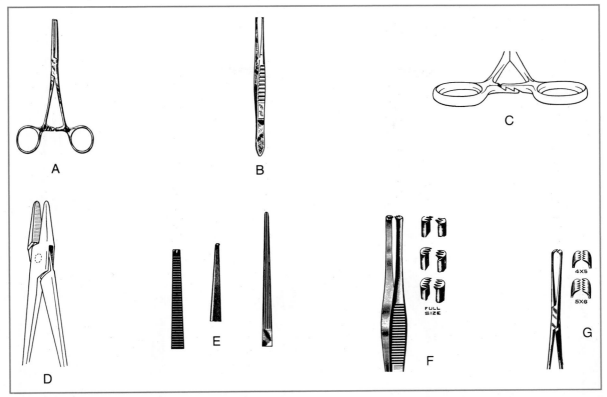

FIGURE 35-2. Identifying parts of an instrument. *A*, Ring handle. *B*, Thumb-type or spring-type handle. *C*, Ratchets. *D*, Box-lock. *E*, Serrations (horizontal, crosscross, longitudinal). *F*, Mouse-toothed (rat-toothed). *G*, Allis tissue forceps.

Littauer stitch or suture scissors (Fig. 35-3*H*)

- Blade has break or hook to get under sutures
- Used to remove sutures from healed incisional site

Iris scissors (Fig. 35-3*I*)

- Usual length is 4 inches
- Tips may vary as with operating scissors
- Used in suture removal (as per physician's preference)

Scalpels

Scalpel handles (Fig. 35-4*A*)

- Nos. 3, 3L, and 7 are the standard handles

Scalpel blades (Fig. 35-4*B*)

- No. 11 is commonly used
- Nos. 10, 12, and 15 are used for specialty incisions
- Blades with numbers from 10 to 15 fit into standard handles

Grasping and Clamping Instruments

Clamping instruments are used for many different tasks. Many have a sharp tooth or teeth and are used to retract, hold, and manipulate human **fascia**. The most common clamping instruments are the hemostats, which were originally designed to stop bleeding or to clamp severed blood vessels. Other clamping instruments are used to grasp other instruments or sterilized materials. Sometimes hemostats and the other clamping instruments are used interchangeably.

Forceps

Hemostatic forceps (Fig. 35-5*A* through *C*)

- Jaws may be fully or partially serrated, without teeth
- May be straight, curved, plain-tipped, or rat-toothed
- Used to clamp off small vessels or hold tissue

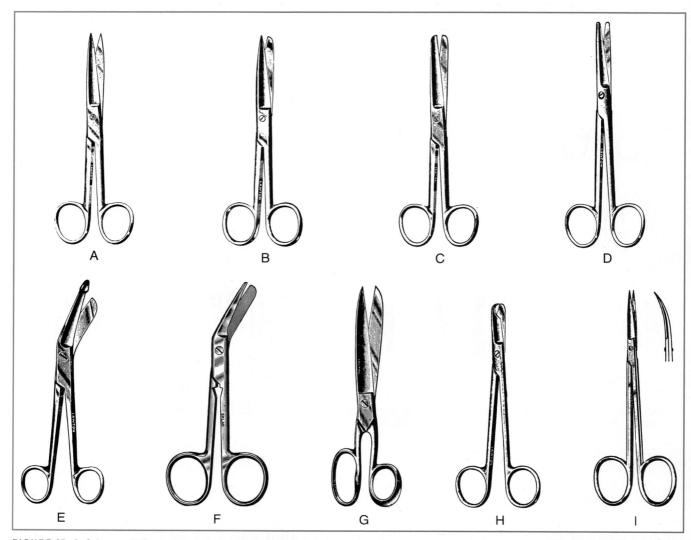

FIGURE 35–3. Scissors. *A*, Operating scissors, straight or curved, sharp-sharp. *B*, Operating scissors, blunt-sharp. *C*, Operating scissors, blunt-blunt. *D*, Mayo dissecting scissors, straight or curved, 6¾ in. *E*, Lister bandage scissors, 5½ in. *F*, Burnham finger bandage scissors. *G*, Gauze shears, army-type, 7½ in. *H*, Littauer stitch (suture) scissors, 5½ in. *I*, Iris (eye) scissors, straight or curved, 4⅛ in.

Needle holders (Fig. 35–5*D* through *F*)

- Jaws are shorter and look stronger than hemostat jaws
- Jaws are serrated and may have a groove in the center
- Used to firmly grasp a suture needle

Splinter forceps (Fig. 35–6*A* through *D*)

- Design and construction vary
- Fine tip for foreign object retrieval
- Used to grasp foreign bodies embedded in skin

Towel forceps (Fig. 35–6*E* and *F*)

- Have very sharp hooks
- Come in various lengths from 3 to 6½ inches
- Used to hold drapes in place during surgery

Sterilizer forceps (Fig. 35–7*A* and *B*)

- Have curved jaw surfaces
- Many types are available
- Used to retrieve sterilized items from the autoclave

Bard-Parker sterilizer forceps and container unit (Fig. 35–7*C*)

- A spring-operated metal float-basket rises as forceps is withdrawn; helps maintain sterile technique
- Attached lid provides a seal from the environment
- Used to retrieve and move items in a sterile field

35

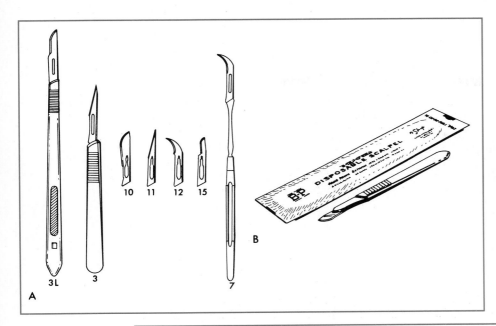

FIGURE 35-4. Scalpels and blades. *A*, Bard-Parker operating scalpels (handles with various disposable blades). *B*, Packaged, disposable sterile blade and reusable handle.

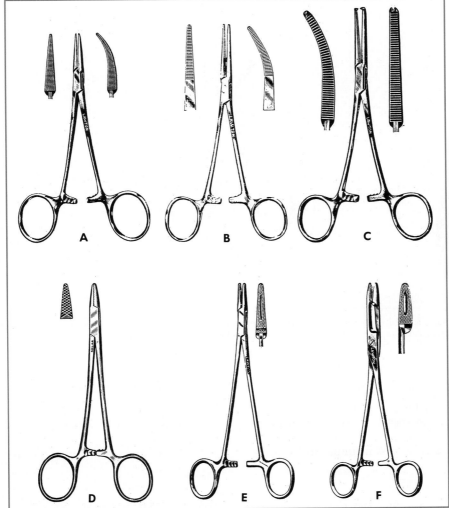

FIGURE 35-5. Hemostats and needle holders. *A*, Halsted mosquito hemostat, straight or curved, 5 in. *B*, Kelly hemostat, straight or curved, 5½ in. *C*, Rochester-Ochsner hemostat, straight or curved (toothed 1 × 2), 6½ in. *D*, Plain needle holder with grooved jar, 6, 7, or 8 in. *E*, Plain needle holder with grooved jaw, 6 in. *F*, Needle holder with grooved jaw and scissors, 5½ in.

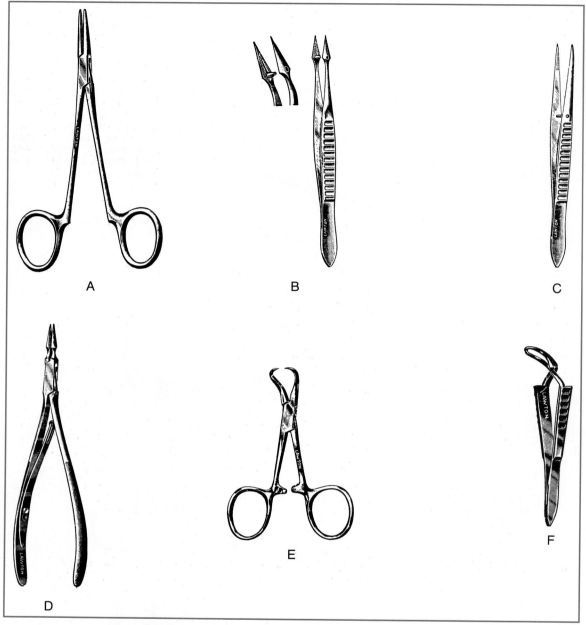

FIGURE 35–6. Splinter forceps and towel clamps. *A*, Physician's splinter forceps (ring handle). *B*, Hunter splinter forceps (thumb or spring handle). *C*, Plain splinter forceps. *D*, Virtus splinter forceps. *E*, Backhaus towel clamp. *F*, Jones towel clamp (spring handle).

Allis tissue forceps (Fig. 35–7*D*)

- Comes in different lengths and jaw widths
- Is less traumatic to tissue, as teeth are not as sharp
- Used to grasp muscle or skin flaps surrounding a wound

Plain tissue forceps (Fig. 35–7*E*)

- Pincher grip
- Same use as Allis tissue forceps

Plain thumb (dressing) forceps (Fig. 35–7*F*)

- Manufactured in lengths from 4 to 12 inches
- Has varying types of serrated jaws but no teeth
- Used to insert packing into or remove objects from the nose or ear

Retracting Instruments

Retracting instruments hold tissue away from the surgical wound (incision), so their use in minor sur-

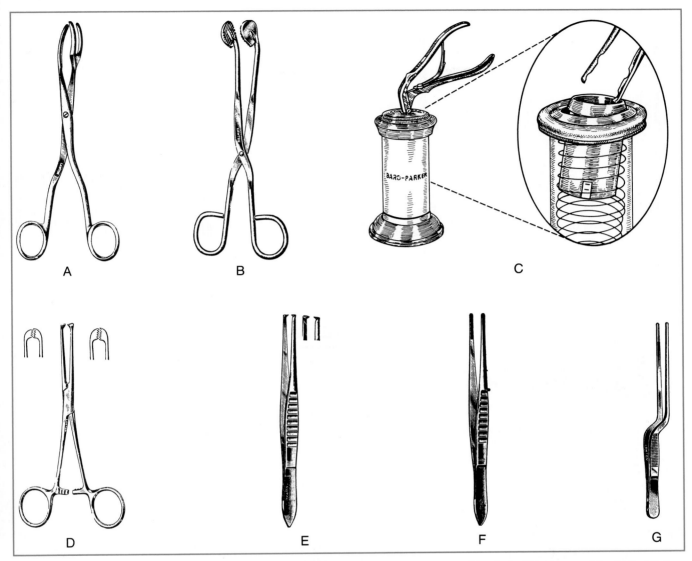

FIGURE 35-7. Sterilizer, tissue, and dressing forceps. *A,* Sterilizer forceps (tongs), three-pronged, 8 in. *B,* Sterilizer forceps, 8 in. *C,* Bard-Parker sterilizer forceps and container. *D,* Allis tissue forceps. *E,* Plain tissue forceps, 5½ in. *F,* Plain thumb forceps, 5½ in. *G,* Lucae bayonet dressing forceps, 5½ in.

gery is limited. By physician preference, the *Allis tissue forceps* and the *Kelly hemostat* are used to retract during most minor surgical procedures. A retractor may be hand-held (in which case an assistant is required to hold it in place) or self-retaining (holding itself in place by means of a ratchet).

Probing and Dilating Instruments

These instruments are used for both surgery and examinations. Probes may be used to search for a foreign body in a wound or to enter a **fistula.** Dilators are used to stretch a cavity or opening for examination or before inserting another instrument to obtain a tissue specimen.

Probes (Fig. 35–8*A* through *C*)

- Lengths range from 4 to 12 inches; available with or without bulbous tip
- May be smooth or have a director groove
- Used to find foreign bodies embedded in dermal tissue

Trocars and obturators (Fig. 35–8*D* and *E*)

- Consist of a sharply pointed **stylus (obturator)** contained in a **cannula** (outer tube)
- Come in various sizes
- Used to withdraw fluids from cavities or for draining and irrigating with a catheter

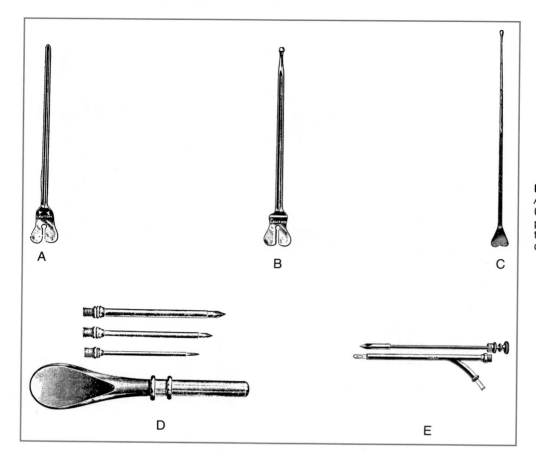

FIGURE 35-8. Probes and trocars. *A*, Grooved director, plain tip. *B*, Grooved director, probe tip. *C*, Larry probe, bulbous tip. *D*, Nested trocar, three sizes. *E*, Ochsner trocar with obturator and drain.

Specula (Fig. 35–9*A* through *F*)

- Most common dilator used
- Valves are spread apart, dilating the opening
- Used to open or distend a body orifice or cavity

Scopes (Fig. 35–9*G* and *H*)

- Do not have blades or bills that increase dilation
- Sizes range from 3½ to 10 inches in length
- Used to internally view the anus and colon

SPECIALTY INSTRUMENTS

Although all instruments fall under the same four categories as the surgical instruments just discussed, the remaining instruments are organized into specialty groupings. Presenting the instruments in this manner makes it easy to see how the instruments relate to particular examinations. In addition to recognizing the name and usage of each instrument, you must organize and set out the instruments needed for each particular examination on what is called a *tray setup.*

Instruments for Gynecology

Sims uterine curette (Fig. 35–10*A*)

- Six sizes are frequently used
- Spoon-shaped scraping instrument
- Used to remove minor **polyps,** secretions, and bits of afterbirth (placental tissue)

Bozeman uterine dressing forceps (Fig. 35–10*B*)

- Designed to hold sponges or dressings
- Capable of reaching the cervix and vagina easily
- Used to swab the area or apply medication

Schroeder uterine vulsellum forceps (Fig. 35–10*C*)

- Used to hold tissue (such as the cervix) while obtaining a tissue specimen, or to lift the cervix to view the fornix

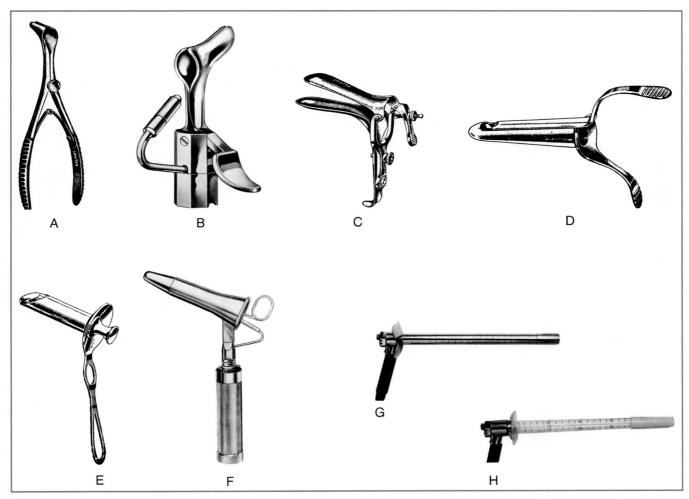

FIGURE 35–9. Specula and scopes. *A,* Vienna nasal speculum. *B,* Nasal speculum, bivalve, illuminated. *C,* Graves vaginal speculum. *D,* Brinkerhoff rectal speculum. *E,* Hirschman anoscope. *F,* Illuminated anoscope with removable obturator. *G,* Sigmoidoscope, reusable, illuminated, 25 cm (obturator not shown). *H,* Sigmoidoscope, disposable, fiberoptic.

Schroeder uterine tenaculum forceps (Fig. 35–10*D*)

- Has very sharp pointed tips
- Used in the same way as the vulsellum forceps

Foerster sponge forceps (Fig. 35–10*E*)

- Tips are round and serrated
- Used in the same way as the dressing forceps

Hegar uterine dilators (Fig. 35–10*F* and *G*)

- Come in sets of eight
- Are double-ended to produce 16 different sizes
- Used to dilate the cervix for **dilatation** and **curettage**

Sounds (Fig. 35–10*H* and *I*)

- Used to check the **patency** of the cervical os or the urethral meatus

Instruments for Ophthalmology and Otolaryngology

Nasal speculum (see Fig. 35–9*A* and *B*)

- Valves can be spread to facilitate viewing
- An applicator or snare can be introduced through the valves
- Used to spread the nostrils for examination

Krause nasal snare (Fig. 35–11*A*)

- Has a wire loop at the tip that can be tightened
- Used to remove polyps from the naris

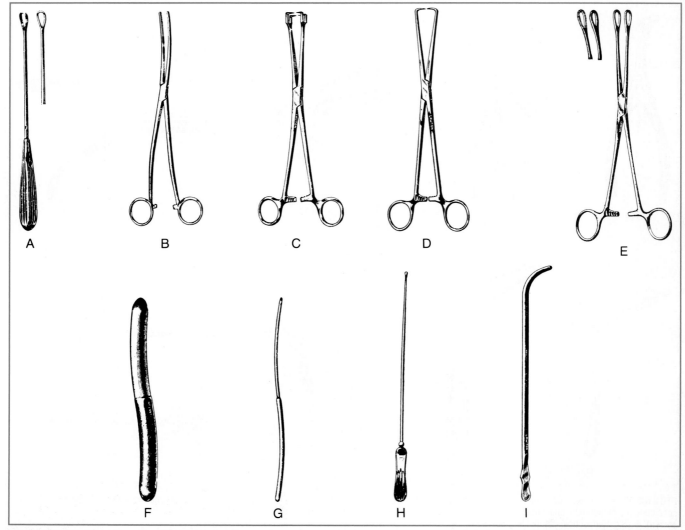

FIGURE 35-10. Instruments for gynecology. *A*, Sims uterine curette, sharp or blunt, 12 in. *B*, Bozeman uterine dressing forceps. *C*, Schroeder uterine vulsellum forceps, straight, 9 in. *D*, Schroeder uterine tenaculum forceps, 9 in. *E*, Foerster sponge forceps (uterine sponge forceps), straight or curved, 9½ in. *F*, Hegar uterine dilator, double-ended, largest. *G*, Hegar uterine dilator, double-ended, smallest. *H*, Sims uterine sound. *I*, Van Buren urethral sound.

Hartman "alligator" ear forceps (Fig. 35–11*B*)

- Has a 3½-inch shaft and is made in a variety of styles
- Action of the jaw is similar to that of an alligator's jaw
- Used to remove foreign bodies or polyps

Eye foreign body spud (Fig. 35–11*D* and *E*)

- Used to remove foreign bodies imbedded in the eye

Buck ear curettes (Fig. 35–11*F*)

- Made with sharp or blunt scraper ends
- Manufactured in various sizes
- Used to remove foreign matter from the ear canals

Reiner ear syringe (Fig. 35–11*H*)

- Fitted with a piston to forcibly inject fluid into the ear or a cavity
- A small splash shield collects the backwash into a basin
- Used for removal of cerumen and for irrigation

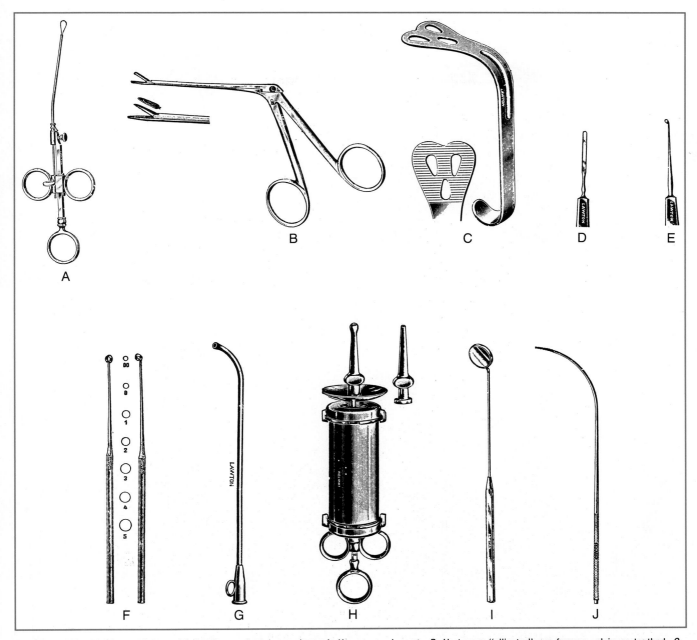

FIGURE 35–11. Instruments for ophthalmology and otolaryngology. *A*, Krause nasal snare. *B*, Hartmann "alligator" ear forceps, plain or toothed. *C*, Weider "metal" tongue depressor. *D*, Dix eye foreign body spud, flat end. *E*, Laforce eye foreign body spud ("golf-club" eye spud). *F*, Buck ear curette. *G*, Hartmann eustachian-tube catheter. *H*, Reiner ear syringe with shield and control handle, plain tip and bulbous tip. *I*, Laryngeal mirror. *J*, Ivan laryngeal metal applicator.

Laryngeal mirror (Fig. 35–11*I*)

- Made in various sizes
- May have a nonfogging surface
- Used for examination of the larynx and postnasal area

Ivan laryngeal metal applicator (Fig. 35–11*J*)

- Holds cotton in place with its roughened end
- Used to swab or sponge throat or postnasal tissue
- Is 9 in. long with curved end for use in throat or postnasal areas

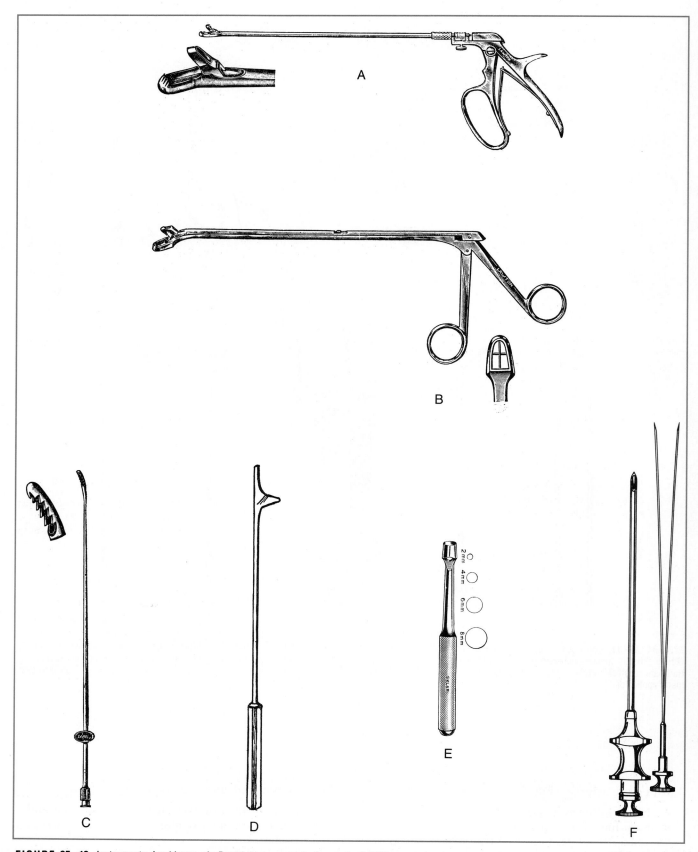

FIGURE 35–12. Instruments for biopsy. *A*, Rectal biopsy punch (forceps). *B*, Wittner uterine (cervical) biopsy forceps. *C*, Novak biopsy curette. *D*, Cervical spatula. *E*, Cutaneous punch (skin biopsy punch). *F*, Silverman biopsy needle with stylus (inserted) and biopsy cannula.

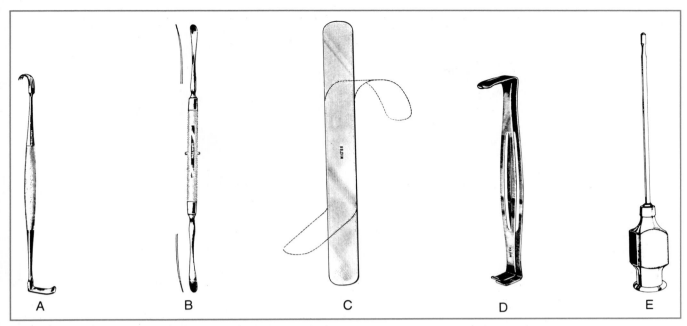

FIGURE 35–13. Instruments for wounds and wound drainage. *A,* Senn double-ended retractor and skin hook. *B,* Freer dissector and elevator. *C,* Crile Ribbon retractor. *D,* Langenbeck retractor. *E,* Abscess needle. (Courtesy of Becton-Dickinson & Co.)

Instruments for Biopsy

Rectal biopsy punch (Fig. 35–12*A*)

- Made with interchangeable stems
- Comes in different lengths and styles
- Used through a proctoscope or sigmoidoscope

Cervical biopsy forceps, curette, and spatula (Fig. 35–12*B* through *D*)

- Come in disposable kits
- Used to obtain specimens for diagnostic examination

Abscess needle (Fig. 35–12*E*)

- Attached to a syringe
- Used to withdraw fluids or suppuration (pus) from a cyst or abscess

Silverman biopsy needle (Fig. 35–12*F*)

- Works on the same principle as an obturator
- At biopsy site, stylus is removed, and a split cannula is inserted to retrieve specimen
- Needle biopsy can eliminate the need for surgical incision

Instruments for Wounds and Wound Drainage

Senn retractor and skin hook (Fig. 35–13*A*)

- A double-ended instrument; three-pronged end is a skin hook, and flat end is a retractor
- Used to hold open small incisions or to secure a skin edge for suturing

Freer dissector and elevator (Fig. 35–13*B*)

- Used to lift connective tissues from bone

Crile malleable (ribbon) (Fig. 35–13*C*)

- Used to hold open larger incisions or to hold connective tissue out of the surgical field

Langenbeck retractor (Fig. 35–13*D*)

- Used to hold open small incisions

Abscess needle (Fig. 35–13*E*)

- Used to withdraw fluids or **suppuration** (pus) from a **cyst** or **abscess.**
- Usually are disposable

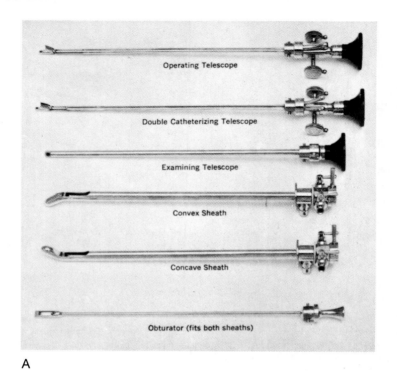

FIGURE 35-14. Instruments for urology. *A*, Brown-Buerger cystoscope. *B*, Robinson catheter. *C*, Foley catheter. *D*, Catheter guide.

Instruments for Urology

Brown-Buerger cystoscope (Fig. 35-14*A*)

- Used to visually examine the urethra and bladder

Robinson catheter (Fig. 35-14*B*)

- Soft rubber urethral catheter in sizes French 12 to 30
- The higher the number, the smaller the **lumen**
- Inserted into the bladder to obtain a sterile specimen

Foley catheter (Fig. 35-14*C*)

- Manufactured in sizes French 8 to 30
- Manufactured with a double rubber lining
- After insertion, sterile solution is injected into the inner lining, inflating a balloon

Catheter guide (Fig. 35-14*D*)

- Metal device
- To be used with extreme caution
- Used only when it is impossible to insert a catheter by normal means
- Used as an indwelling catheter

PROCEDURE 35-1   IDENTIFYING SURGICAL INSTRUMENTS

GOAL To identify, correctly spell the names of, and determine the use(s) of standard office instruments or those selected by your instructor.

EQUIPMENT AND SUPPLIES

Bard-Parker transfer forceps
Curved hemostat
Straight hemostat
Dressing forceps (thumb)
Allis tissue forceps
Towel clamp

Scalpel and blade
Vaginal speculum
Dissecting scissors
Bandage scissors
Ophthalmoscope
Paper and pencil

PROCEDURAL STEPS

1. Look for the following parts that determine usage: box-lock, serrations, finger rings, cutting edge, noncutting edge, thumb type, teeth, ratchets, and electric attachments.
   Purpose: To determine the combination of features and parts for each instrument.

2. Consider the general classification of the instrument: cutting and dissection, grasping and clamping, retracting, or probing and dilating.
   Purpose: The clue to the name of the instrument may be found by determining the classification.

3. Carefully examine its teeth and serrations.
   Purpose: The clue to the name of the instrument may be found by determining its distinctive parts.

4. Look at the length of the instrument to determine the area of the body for which it is used.
   Purpose: The clue to the name of the instrument may be found by determining where it can reach.

5. Try to remember whether the instrument was named for a famous physician, university, or clinic.
   Purpose: Many instruments are named for the inventor.

6. If the instrument is a pair of scissors, look at the points and determine whether they are sharp-sharp, sharp-blunt, or blunt-blunt.
   Purpose: The clue to the name of a pair of scissors may be found by determining the combination of points.

7. Carefully compare the instrument with similar instruments that you know, to determine whether it is in the same category or has the same name.
   Purpose: The clue to the name of an instrument may be found with the knowledge you already have.

8. Write, with correct spelling, the complete name of each instrument, including its category and usage.

CARE AND HANDLING OF INSTRUMENTS

Since instruments are expensive and the physician's skill is dependent on the quality of the instruments, the medical assistant must properly care for each instrument to maximize its life and ensure that every part is in safe, working order.

Most instruments are made of fine-grade stainless steel. The term "stainless" is usually taken too literally. Although stainless steel does resist rust and keeps a fine edge and tip longer, even the best stainless steel may develop water spots and stains, especially if water with a high mineral content is used. Proper hardness and flexibility are important. Inexpensive instruments may be too brittle or too soft. Mistreatment of chrome-plated instruments can cause minute breaks in the finish, which may become a source of contamination or may tear the surgeon's gloves.

Instruments should be carefully examined when they are purchased. Scissors should be tested to see if they shear the full length of the blades, completely to the tip. This can be checked by cutting a piece of cotton. If the scissors cut cleanly and do not chew at any point, even at the tip, they are functioning correctly. Teeth and serrations should be checked to see if they intermesh completely and if the jaws are even on the sides and tip. Each instrument should be felt over its entire surface for any rough areas that may tear or snag the surgeon's gloves. Box-locks and hinges must work freely but should not be too loose. Thumb- and spring-handled instruments must have the correct tension and meet evenly at the tips.

Under no circumstances should instruments be bunched together or allowed to become entangled. Avoid mixing stainless steel instruments with ones of aluminum, copper, or brass. This may cause electrolysis and may result in etching. Even mixing stainless steel with chrome-plated instruments is best avoided. If an instrument is accidentally dropped, it may be permanently damaged. If scissors are dropped with the blades partially open, there will be a nick at the point at which the blades cross. Do not leave ratchets closed. Do not leave an instrument clamped onto material such as a drape or gauze.

Reserve a special place during the surgical procedure to receive contaminated instruments. This is usually a basin of disinfectant solution placed in the sink or within reach of the assistant. If a metal basin is used, it is advisable to place a small towel on the bottom of the basin to prevent damage to the instruments as they are dropped into the solution. Never allow blood or other coagulable substances to dry on an instrument. If immediate cleaning is not possible, they should be rinsed well and placed in a cold water solution of a blood solvent and a mild detergent. The detergent increases the wetting ability of the water, allowing the instrument surfaces to be better exposed to the solution. It is best to use a detergent that has a neutral pH. It should be low-sudsing and easy to rinse off. Each manufacturer of the various disinfectants and blood solvents recommends the correct dilution and time of immersion for its product. Read the label.

Upon completion of the surgical procedure, the receiving basin for the instruments is transferred from the area to the cleaning and sterilization room. It is important to remove used instruments from the patient's view as soon as possible.

Separate the various types of instruments. Sharp instruments should be carefully handled to prevent damage to cutting edges or possible injury to the person sanitizing them. Rubber and plastic items are easily punctured and often discolor metals. Some plastic and rubber goods should not be soaked too long because they will discolor. Plastics may become porous and lose their glossy surface. Sanitize and sterilize surgical packs without delay. The instruments must be ready for the next scheduled procedure or any emergency. Surgical packs should be processed daily at a designated time.

Commercially prepared *disposable packs* are available for most minor surgical procedures. They are time-savers and convenient because they can eliminate linen laundering and supply autoclaving. Their disadvantages include high cost and their lack of custom-designed contents to suit regional practices and preferences. Available packs include towel packs, skin prep packs, irrigation sets, suture sets, suture removal sets, catheterization sets, biopsy sets, and shave prep packs.

Disposable Drapes

Disposable drapes are available in several different materials and sizes and may contain an opening (fenestration) for the operative site. A special incisional drape has an adhesive backing around the opening to prevent slippage (Fig. 35–15). This clear incisional drape adheres to the patient's cleansed skin and remains taped to the area throughout the procedure. The skin incision is made with the scalpel through the adhesive drape. In minor surgery in the medical office, disposable drapes are rapidly replacing the use of autoclaved linen towels and towel clamps.

Wounds

Types of Wounds

A wound is an interruption in the continuity of the internal or external body tissues. A wound may be *intentional* (such as in surgery) or *accidental,* and *open* or *closed* (Table 35–1). An open wound is one with an outward opening where the skin is broken, causing the underlying tissues to be exposed. A closed, or *nonpenetrating* wound does not have an outward opening, but the underlying tissues are damaged, as in a hematoma or contusion (bruise). Closed wounds are usually the result of a blow or a violent jar or shock (concussion) to the body. An aseptic (clean) wound is not infected with pathogens; septic wounds are infected with pathogens.

Open wounds may be classified according to the appearance of their openings. An *incised* wound has a clean edge and is made with a cutting instrument. An incised wound may be the result of intentional surgery or a criminal knife wound. A *lacerated* wound has torn or mangled tissues and is made by a dull or blunt instrument. The *penetrating,* or *puncture,* wound is caused by a sharp, slender object such as a needle or ice pick and passes through the

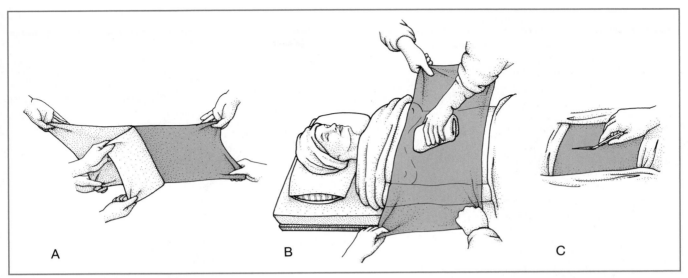

FIGURE 35–15. Application of the adhesive-backed incisional drape. *A,* Remove backing to expose sticky side of drape. *B,* Apply drape. Secure center, then work toward edge. *C,* Secure edges of drape.

skin into the underlying tissues. A *perforating* wound is a penetrating wound that passes through to a body organ or cavity.

Wound Healing

All wounds go through a healing, or repair, process that has three phases.

The *first phase* (lag) is the period when the blood vessels contract to control hemorrhage, and blood platelets form a network in the wound that acts like glue to plug the wound. Following a complex series of chemical reactions, a substance called *fibrin* is released into the wound that begins clotting. The fibrin continues to collect red blood cells, more platelets, and white blood cells, and the clot becomes a *scab*. About 12 hours later, special white blood cells arrive at the site to clear away debris and bacteria. Within 1 to 4 days, the fibrin threads contract and pull the edges of the wound together under the clot or scab.

The *second phase* (proliferation) is the wound healing and new growth period and lasts from 5 to 20 days. It is during this phase that the tissues repair themselves. New cells form, and the wound continues to contract and seal. If the wound is a clean surgical incision, complete contraction usually takes place during this phase, and there is no scarring or permanent fibrous tissue (cicatrix) formation.

The *third phase* (remodeling) occurs from the 21st day on. Whereas the clean, shallow wound may contract in the first two phases, large or mangled wounds require the time and cellular activity of this third phase to build a bridge of new tissue to close the gap of the wound. The cells produce a fibrous protein substance called *collagen* (connective tissue) that gives the wounded tissues strength and forms scar tissue. Scar tissue is not true skin; it is usually very strong, but it cannot stand the tension of the

normal skin because it lacks elasticity. Scar tissue is also devoid of normal blood supply and nerves.

Wounds are classified by the way they repair themselves. The clean, surgical wound that has been sutured closed and heals quickly without scarring does so by *first intention*. Tissues that are severely damaged, are purposely kept open, or fail to close are said to heal by granulation (healing from the bottom up), which is called *second intention*.

Several factors influence the healing process. People who are young and in good general health and have adequate nutrition heal more rapidly. Adequate protection and resting to the injured area also enhances the healing process. Destruction or reinjury during the second phase can delay healing and increase scarring.

Wounds are susceptible to infection because the normal skin barrier is broken. If there is debris in a wound as a result of the breakdown of the various cellular components, this dead (necrotic) tissue acts as a culture medium for bacterial growth. Suppuration (pus) is necrotic tissue with bacteria, dead leukocytes, and other products of tissue breakdown. Necrotic tissue must be removed. Removal of debris is called débridement, which may be natural or a surgical procedure.

OPEN WOUND HEALING. Sometimes the physician may prefer no dressing or bandage on small wounds. There are definite advantages to open wound healing:

- There are strong arguments for allowing air to freely circulate in the wound.
- The wound is not irritated or rubbed by a dressing or bandage.
- The wound stays dry, which inhibits bacterial growth, resulting in less chance of infection.
- Sutures stay dry and hold together better.
- In the patient who is shaved prior to surgery, dry shaving nicks heal faster than moist nicks.

TABLE 35–1. TYPES OF WOUNDS

Type	Description
Intentional (performed under surgical asepsis)	
1. Surgical incision	A neat, clean cut, performed with scalpel
2. Hypodermic puncture	Injection under the skin for the purpose of drug administration or fluid withdrawal

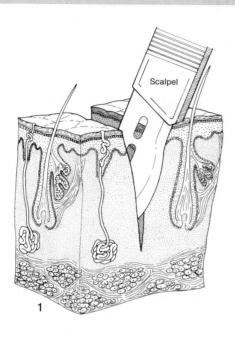

1

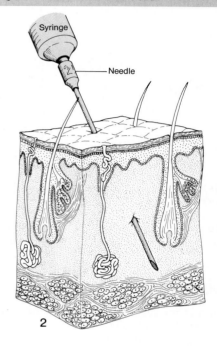

2

Type	Description
Accidental (septic, may cause infection)	
1. Contusion (hematoma)	Closed (nonpenetrating) wound in which blood from broken vessels accumulates in tissues
2. Incision	Neat, clean cut from sharp blade objects, such as glass, knives, or metal

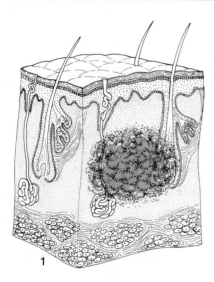

1

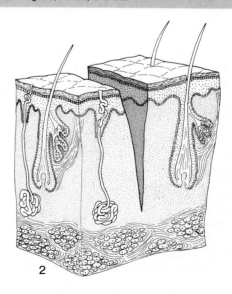

2

Continued

35

TABLE 35–1. TYPES OF WOUNDS *Continued*

Type	Description
3. Laceration	Jagged, irregular breaking or tearing of tissues, usually caused by a sharp blow to the body
4. Puncture	Skin is pierced by a pointed object, such as pin, nail, spllinter, or bullet

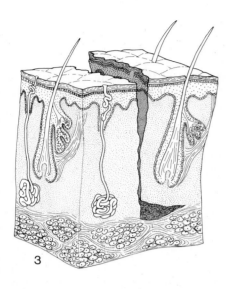

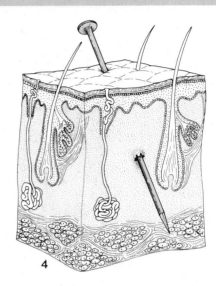

Type	Description
5. Abrasion	Superficial wound; scraping of the skin
6. Avulsion (sometimes amputation)	Tissue forcibly torn or separated from the body; may be jagged or mutilated; may be caused by automobile accidents, gunshot wounds, or animal bites

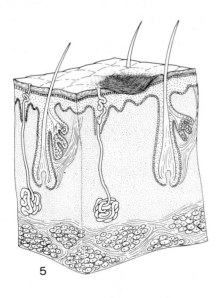

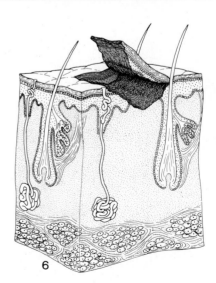

- Any pre-existing infection remains localized and is not spread by the dressing or bandage.

Sutures

The word *suture* is used as both a noun and a verb. As a noun, it refers to a surgical stitch or to the material used; as a verb, it refers to the act of stitching. Sutures were used as long ago as 2000 BC. History does not record the first surgical operations and the use of sutures, but ancient medical writings do make reference to using sinews and strings to tie off blood vessels and control bleeding.

Modern surgery and the use of sutures began in 1865, when Lister developed antisepsis and the disinfection of suture materials. Many kinds of materials have been used over the centuries, including precious metals, horsehair, animal tendons, and cotton and linen cord. Most of the improvements in suture materials and techniques have occurred in the last 50 years.

A suture may also be used as a *ligature*. This is a strand of suture material used to tie off a blood vessel or to strangulate tissue. A ligature may be tied around a skin growth and left there until the growth is strangulated and falls off. If a ligature is used to tie off an internal tubular structure, it must last permanently or long enough for the structure itself to disintegrate. To *ligate* means to apply a ligature.

Types of Suture

Sutures may be classified as either absorbable or nonabsorbable. Many different materials are available, each having its advantages and disadvantages. The following are commonly used suture materials in minor surgery procedures (Fig. 35–16).

ABSORBABLE SUTURE. The absorbable suture dissolves and is absorbed by the body's enzymes during the healing process; thus, it does not have to be removed.

- **Surgical catgut** is used in tissue that heals rapidly.
- **Plain catgut** is used in those tissues that heal most rapidly, such as mucous membrane and subcutaneous tissue.
- **Chromic catgut** is treated with chromic salts to slow its absorption rate to 20 to 40 days.

NONABSORBABLE SUTURE. Nonabsorbable suture is either left in the body (where it becomes imbedded in scar tissue) or is removed when healing is complete. It is frequently used in minor surgical procedures performed in the medical office because the majority of the suturing required is superficial and in areas where sutures can be removed after healing has taken place.

- **Silk** is widely used because it is strong and easy to tie. It is treated with Teflon or a similar coating to prevent tissue drag and flaking.
- **Surgical cotton** is not as strong as silk but has the same applications. Cotton can be strengthened by dipping the strands in sterile saline before use.
- **Polyester suture** is the strongest of all sutures except for surgical steel. It is usually multifilamented (braided) and may be coated with Teflon. It is used in facial, ophthalmic, and cardiovascular surgery.
- **Stainless steel** is the strongest suture and is well tolerated by the body. It is difficult to handle and is easily contaminated during a procedure. *Surgical staples* are made of stainless steel.
- **Nylon suture** is strong and has a high degree of elasticity. It is primarily used for skin closure. Owing to its elasticity and stiffness, many knots must be used, and these knots tend to untie if placed incorrectly.

Suture Sizing and Packaging

The diameter of the suture strand determines its size; for instance, size 2–0 is thinner than size 0, and size 0 is thinner than size 2. Suture as thin as

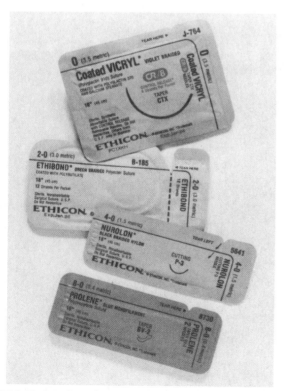

FIGURE 35–16. Suture packets labeled according to size, type, and length of suture material, type of needle point, and shape of the needle. Note: The second packet from the top contains sutures but no needle. (Courtesy of Ethicon, Inc.)

35

size 11-0 and as thick as size 7 is available. The sizes from 2-0 to 6-0 are the most frequently used in the medical office. The length of the suture is standardized. Strands are precut in 17-, 18-, 24-, 54-, or 60-inch lengths.

Suture is available in peel-apart packages for convenience. The sterile inner pack may be grasped by the physician or flipped onto the instrument tray by the medical assistant (see Fig. 35-16).

Needles

Surgical needles are chosen according to the area in which they are to be used and the depth and width of the desired stitch. They are classified according to shape and by the type of point, shaft, and eye (Fig. 35-17). The shape of a needle may be straight or curved. Straight needles are not easily manipulated and are restricted to use on the surface tissue. A curved needle allows the surgeon to swing the needle beneath the surface and then back up again on the other side. The sharper the curve of the needle, the deeper the surgeon can pass the needle. The point of a needle can be a taper or a cutting edge. A taper is used on delicate tissues; the cutting edge lacerates the skin as the needle is passed through, which is advantageous on the tougher tissues, such as the skin and connective tissue. The head of the needle can have an eye or can be eyeless. Eyeless needles are also called *atraumatic* because they cause the least amount of tissue trauma as the needle is pulled through. Manufacturers supply the suture strands with the suture needle attached in peel-apart packages, or separate needle packs and continuous reels of suture that will need to be autoclaved as used. The majority of suture materials used in the medical office are prepackaged, with the suture strand and needle attached. The most common needle type for minor skin repair is the curved, cutting-edged, atraumatic needle.

PREPARATION FOR SURGERY

Procedure File

Keep a card file for each procedure, listing the preferences of each physician in the office. This is particularly helpful for complicated procedures and procedures that are seldom performed. Color-code the 5 × 8 cards for each physician, and keep the information current. The cards usually contain information on the following:

- Preoperative instructions
- Preoperative and operative medications
- Universal blood and body-fluid precautions, listing specific protection barriers (goggles, masks, gowns, aprons, and gloves) to be worn

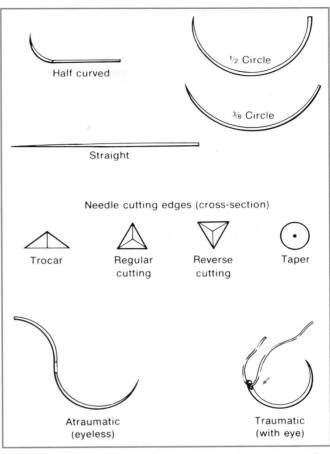

FIGURE 35-17. Needle shapes and the types of needle points and eyes. Most needles used in the medical office are of the atraumatic type.

by the surgeon and the assistants (see Chapter 25).

- Instruments used
- Syringe and needle sizes
- Glove sizes
- Postoperative instructions
- The number of days to the scheduled follow-up appointment

A more detailed procedures manual should be developed by you and the physicians. The procedures should be reviewed at regular intervals for revision and development. See Chapter 22 for directions on how to write a procedures manual.

Preparing Sterile Packs

Surgical packs must be prepared the day before the procedure or at least in enough time for the pack to be dry and cool for the procedure. (See Chapters 24 and 25.)

- Before closing the pack to be autoclaved, take a count, on at least two separate occasions, of the items required for the procedure. Use your procedure file card for guidance.

- If the items are numerous, label the pack with the name of the procedure rather than the individual contents.
- Sterilize transfer forceps in a separate pack. If you are not gloved, use the sterile transfer forceps to arrange the instruments on the sterile field in their sequence of use.
- If disposable sterile towels and drapes are not used, you may autoclave linen towels, one or two to a package. Fanfold the towels so they may be unfolded easily with the transfer forceps.
- In many cases, an entire setup may be autoclaved in one pack (instruments, sponges, dressings, suture materials, syringes, and needles), but you must be certain that the pack is not so thick that it prevents steam circulation to all the parts of the pack.
- Sterility indicators should be placed in the very middle of large packs to indicate whether proper sterilization has occurred throughout the pack.
- In case of contamination, it is always best to have more than one pack ready for every procedure.

PREOPERATIVE PREPARATION AND CARE OF THE PATIENT

Whether minor surgery is the result of an unforeseen accident or a planned, elective procedure, the patient needs psychologic care as well as physical care. The patient facing any surgical procedure suffers from fear of pain, disfigurement, and often the fear of cancer being discovered. An injured patient may feel anxious about the medical bills or loss of employment. Because surgery is a frightening and dehumanizing experience, you must take the time, both preoperatively and at the time of surgery, to help the patient through these fears and anxieties. The best method is to help the patient talk about the procedure or voice any concerns or misgivings. Questions should be answered directly, but answer only those questions that are within your scope of experience and the policies of the office. If you cannot answer a question, assure the patient that you will relay the question to the physician prior to the procedure. Don't forget to relay the message. What may seem to be a minor or unimportant question to you may be very frightening to the patient. A good technique is to write down the question in front of the patient, then give it to the physician. The minor surgery room can look very frightening to the patient, so, unless the patient is sedated, try to make conversation with the patient while you prepare for the physician's arrival.

The physical preparation may involve obtaining blood and urine for tests the day before surgery, completing forms and permissions, and gathering a current history concerning any recent illnesses or medications. Before the day of surgery, preoperative instructions may include a shave prep, cleansing enemas, food intake restrictions, special bathing, and a sedative medication.

On the day of surgery, the patient's vital signs are recorded, and the patient is assisted in undressing, if necessary, and then is asked to empty the bladder. Keep the patient on schedule but never appear to rush the process.

Preoperative Instructions

When planning office surgery, complete the following procedures before the time of the appointment:

- Have the necessary consent forms ready to sign.
- Give the patient all the necessary preoperative instructions, such as medications to be used and special skin cleansing.
- Instruct patients to bring a relative or friend to drive them home after the surgery.
- When appropriate, instruct the patient to wear special clothing that is easily removed and can be worn over bulky dressings or a cast.
- Instruct the patient to leave jewelry and other valuables at home.
- Call the patient the day before the surgery and confirm any special instructions.

Surgical Asepsis

Surgical asepsis is defined as the destruction of organisms *before they enter the body*. This technique is used for any procedure that invades the body's skin or tissues, such as surgery or injections. Any time the skin or mucous membrane is punctured, pierced, or incised (or will be during a procedure), surgical aseptic techniques are practiced. The surgical hand wash (scrub) must be used. Everything that comes into contact with the patient should be sterile, such as gowns, drapes, instruments, and the gloved hands of the surgical team. Minor surgery, urinary catheterizations, injections, and some specimen collections, such as blood and biopsies, are performed using surgical aseptic technique.

Because it is not possible to sterilize your hands, the goal of the hand scrub is to reduce skin bacteria by the use of mechanical friction, special surgical soaps, and running water. Normally, there are two types of bacteria on your skin:

TABLE 35–2. HOW TO DISTINGUISH BETWEEN MEDICAL AND SURGICAL ASEPSIS

	Medical Asepsis	Surgical Asepsis
Definition	Destruction of organisms *after* they leave the body	Destruction of organisms *before* they enter the body
Purpose	Prevent reinfection of the patient. Avoid cross-infection from one person to another	Care for open wounds. Use in surgery
Technique	Universal blood and body-fluid precautions Isolation techniques	Sterile technique
Procedure	Clean objects are kept from contamination Clean gloves and clean barriers used Objects disinfected as soon as possible after contact with the patient	Objects must be sterile Sterile gloves and articles used Objects must be sterilized before contact with the patient
When used	For examinations that do not involve open wounds or breaks in the skin or mucous membranes but do involve patient blood or body fluids. Isolating infected persons from others	Surgery, biopsy, wound treatment, insertion of instruments into sterile body cavities
Hand wash technique	Hands and wrists washed for 1–2 min; soap, water, and plenty of friction used to remove oil and microorganisms from fingers Hands held downward, running water allowed to drain off fingertips, hands dried with paper towels	Hand and forearms scrubbed for 3–10 min; surgical soap, running water, friction, and sterile brush used; fingernails must be cleaned Hands held up, under running water, to drain off elbows. Hands dried with sterile towels

35

- **Transient bacteria.** These are surface bacteria that are introduced by fomites and remain with you a short time.
- **Resident bacteria.** These are found under fingernails, in hair follicles, in the openings of the sebaceous glands, and in the deeper layers of the skin.

Resident bacteria in the deeper skin layers come to the surface with perspiration, which is why sterile gloves are used in addition to the surgical hand scrub. Some agencies recommend that you scrub for a specific number of minutes; others count the number of scrub strokes. Follow the guidelines of your employer and take periodic cultures from your scrubbed hands to determine whether or not your technique is effective.

Hand Washing

As stated in Chapter 23, there are two types of asepsis: medical and surgical. The purpose of both the medical and the surgical hand washes is infection control; however, there are differences between the two (Table 35–2).

The surgical hand wash is the same as the medical hand wash with the exception of several adaptations, which are described in Procedure 35–2.

PROCEDURE 35–2   HAND WASHING FOR ASSISTING WITH SURGICAL ASEPTIC PROCEDURES

GOAL   To wash your hands with surgical soap, using friction, running water, and a sterile (optional) brush to sanitize your skin before assisting with any procedure that requires surgical asepsis.

EQUIPMENT AND SUPPLIES

Sink with foot or arm control for running water
Nail file

Surgical soap in a dispenser
Sterile or nonsterile brush
Towels

Continued

PROCEDURE 35-2 *Continued*

PROCEDURAL STEPS

1. Remove all jewelry.
   Purpose: Jewelry harbors bacteria and is not permitted in surgical asepsis.

2. Inspect your fingernails for length and your hands for skin breaks.

3. Turn on the faucet and regulate the water to a comfortable temperature.

4. Keep your hands upright and held at or above waist level (Fig. 35-18).
   Purpose: Water running from the nonscrubbed area above the elbow down to the hands will drag bacteria back onto the hands. All areas below the waist are considered contaminated during all surgical procedures.

5. Allow water to run over your hands, apply acceptable solution, lather while holding your fingertips upward, and remember to rub between the fingers (Fig. 35-19).
   Purpose: The surfaces of the fingers have four sides.

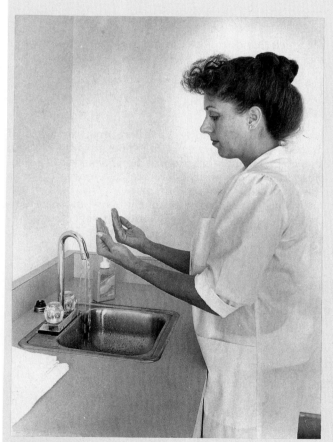

FIGURE 35-18.

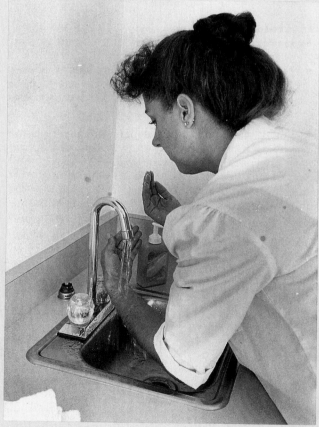

FIGURE 35-19.

Continued

35

6. Clean your fingernails with a file, discard it, and rinse your hands under the faucet without touching the faucet or the insides of the sink basin (Fig. 35–20).
   Purpose: The sink basin and fixtures are always considered contaminated.

7. Apply more solution and repeat the scrub, remembering to wash and use friction between each finger with a firm, circular motion.

8. Wash forearms and wrists while holding your hands above waist level (Fig. 35–21).

9. Scrub all surfaces with a brush, being careful not to abrade your skin. The second washing process should take at least 3 minutes.

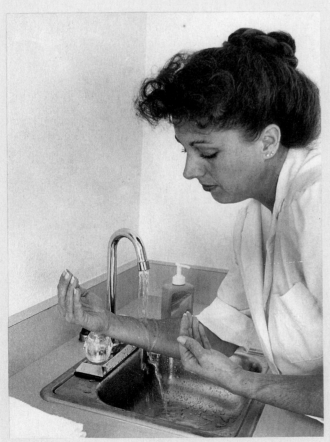

FIGURE 35–20.

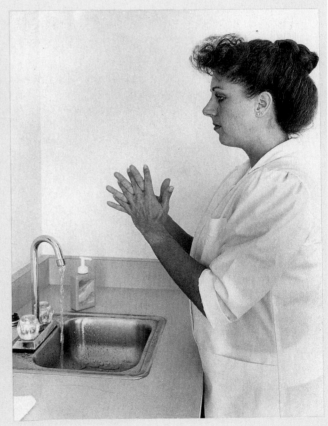

FIGURE 35–21.

Continued

PROCEDURE 35 – 2   *Continued*

10. Rinse thoroughly, keeping your hands up and above waist level (Fig. 35 – 22).

11. Dry your hands with a sterile towel or paper towel (Fig. 35 – 23).
    Purpose: To keep your clean hands from touching the part of the towel that comes into contact with your forearms, which are not as clean as your hands. If you are to gown and glove for a procedure, you will be required to use a sterile rather than a paper towel.

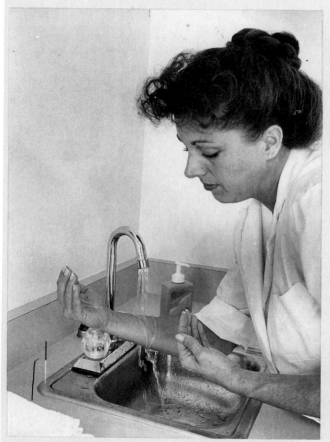

FIGURE 35 – 22.

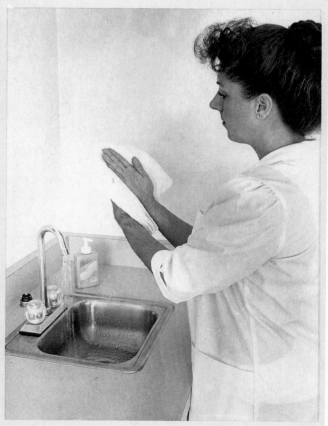

FIGURE 35 – 23.

Continued

12. Using a patting motion, continue to dry the forearms (Figs. 35–24 and 35–25).

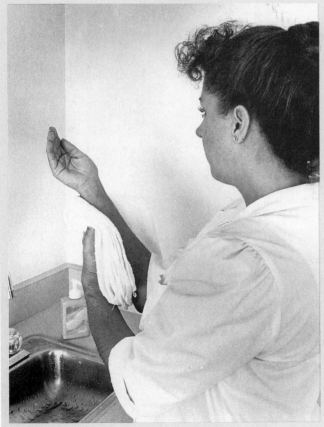

FIGURE 35–24.

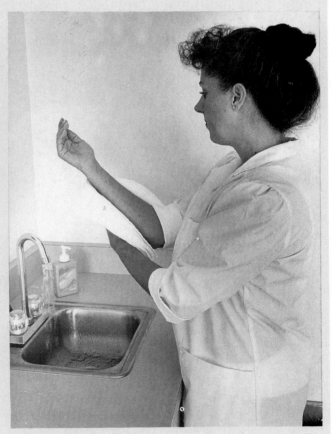

FIGURE 35–25.

Continued

PROCEDURE 35 – 2   *Continued*

13. Turn off the faucet with the foot or forearm lever, if available, or with the towel if it is a hand faucet (Fig. 35–26).
    Purpose: To separate the clean hand(s) from the contaminated faucet handle(s).

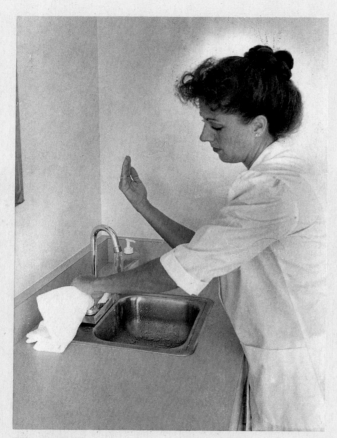

FIGURE 35–26.

35

LEGAL AND ETHICAL RESPONSIBILITIES

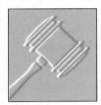

When surgical procedures are to be performed in the medical office, awareness of legal responsibilities is imperative. The medical assistant must know what procedure is to be performed and whether the patient has been informed regarding the procedure. It is your responsibility to obtain the patient's signature on the consent forms for all minor surgery procedures. Legal action primarily occurs when complications arise owing to failure to fill out procedure and consent forms correctly.

If the surgery to be done is a sterilization procedure for birth control, it is essential to follow the stipulated regulations of the state in which you are employed. A waiting period is usually required, and in some states, both the patient and the spouse must receive counseling and sign the consent for surgery forms.

► PATIENT EDUCATION

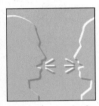

The medical assistant is often asked to have the patient sign a consent for surgery form. After obtaining the signature, there is still no guarantee that the patient understands the procedure to be done. If you know what the physician plans to do, then you can reinforce the physician's explanation. When this is done, you can help to reduce the risk of possible litigation. Increasing the patient's understanding ensures greater compliance with presurgical preparations and postsurgical care.

When giving the patient instructions, encourage him or her to ask questions if what has been said is not understood. This type of interaction makes the procedure easier to perform and encourages the patient to follow the advice given by the physician.

When the physical and psychologic needs of the patient are met, you can be assured that the patient has sufficient information to be comfortable before, during, and after a surgical procedure. Meeting such needs is one of the truly rewarding aspects of medical assisting.

► LEARNING ACHIEVEMENTS

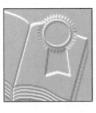

Upon completion of this chapter, can you in the time allowed by your evaluator:

1. Correctly identify and spell 90% of the instruments pictured, including each instrument's category and use?
2. Perform a 3-minute aseptic hand scrub without missing a step or incorrectly performing a step?
3. Give a patient instructions for a surgical procedure using words, diagrams, and pictures to be certain that the procedure is understood?
4. State the legal and ethical responsibilities of patient education?

REFERENCES AND READINGS

Anderson, R. M., and Romfh, R. F.: *Technique in the Use of Surgical Tools,* New York, Appleton-Century-Crofts, 1980.
Bonewit, K.: *Clinical Procedures for Medical Assistants,* 3rd ed., Philadelphia, W. B. Saunders Co., 1989.
Fuller, J. R.: *Surgical Technology: Principles and Practice,* 2nd ed., Philadelphia, W. B. Saunders Co., 1986.
Grewe, H. E., and Kremer, K.: *Atlas of Surgical Operations,* Philadelphia, W. B. Saunders Co., 1980.
Rice, M. R.: *Law, Liability, and Ethics,* Philadelphia, Delmar Publishers, 1988.
Sabiston, D. C. Jr.: *Textbook of Surgery,* 13th ed., Philadelphia, W. B. Saunders Co., 1986.

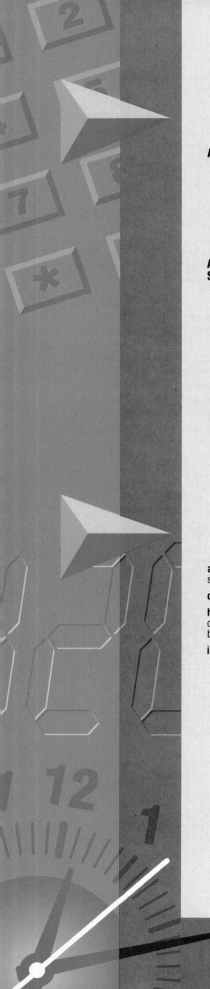

CHAPTER OUTLINE

VOCABULARY

approximate To bring wound or skin edges together.

coagulum A blood clot.

hematoma A localized collection of clotted blood caused by a broken blood vessel.

in situ Localized.

irrigation The flushing out of a cavity or wound with a solution.

microsurgery Surgery performed under a microscope using very small instruments.

pedunculated Having a stemlike connecting part.

photocoagulation Clotting of blood with light.

planing The rubbing away of a layer of tissue.

slough The shedding away of dead tissue cells.

untoward Hard to manage.

ASSISTING WITH MINOR SURGERY

LEARNING OBJECTIVES

COGNITIVE

Upon successful completion of this chapter, you should be able to:

1. Define and spell the terms in the Vocabulary.
2. Define the concepts of "aseptic technique."
3. List the routines of minor surgery in correct sequence.
4. Choose the correct type of bandage to use.
5. List postsurgical routines in proper sequence.
6. Instruct a patient in postoperative wound care.
7. List safety precautions necessary for electrosurgery.
8. List safety precautions necessary for laser surgery.

PERFORMANCE

Upon successful completion of this chapter, you should be able to:

1. Use transfer forceps.
2. Prepare a patient's skin for minor surgery.
3. Open a sterile linen pack.
4. Glove using the open-gloving method.
5. Open and add a sterile pack to a sterile field.
6. Add sterile items in a peel-back wrapper to a sterile field.
7. Assist with suturing.
8. Assist with a minor surgical procedure.
9. Bandage the injured site.
10. Assist with suture removal.

There are so many different minor surgical procedures and setups, and each physician–medical assistant team has individual preferences. We cannot cover all minor surgical procedures or even list all the specific items that may be used for a specific technique. The following procedures are merely composites of acceptable practices in minor surgical techniques. Once you know these basics, with a little bit of background information, you will be able to assist with any minor surgical procedure.

ASEPTIC TECHNIQUE

There is no mystery about aseptic technique. Handling sterile items requires a degree of dexterity and vigilance, but it is really a matter of concentration, with planned movements and steps.

Although the procedures outlined in this chapter and the next are for minor surgery, all the sterile techniques of major surgery must be observed. To have a sound knowledge of sterility and sterile technique, start with the analogy:

> Everything sterile is white, everything that is not sterile is black, and there is no gray.

Sterile surfaces must not come into contact with nonsterile surfaces. Honesty is important; an incomplete or incorrect step may lead to serious wound contamination and postoperative infection.

Personnel

Hands and hair are the two greatest sources of contamination. With practice, you will learn to know what may be touched with the hands and what must be touched only with sterile forceps or sterile gloved hands. Hair that is allowed to fall free over the shoulders and forward will give off a cloud of bacteria; it must be contained back and off the shoulders. In addition, the following rules are fundamental:

- Remember that air currents carry bacteria, so body motions and talking over a sterile field should be kept to a minimum.
- Sterile team members face each other.
- If you lose the sterile field from your line of vision, you can no longer assume the field is sterile; therefore, never turn your back on a sterile field or wander away from the sterile field.
- Nonsterile persons do not reach over a sterile field.

The Sterile Field

A sterile field is any sterile surface, usually containing sterile items. In surgery, a sterile field is created by draping sterile towels, prepackaged or from autoclaved packs, over a Mayo stand or table. A sterile field is also the draped surgical site after the patient's skin has been prepped and draped for surgery. The following rules demonstrate correct field techniques:

- Sterile field towels and sterile table drapes are fanfolded so that they may be unfolded easily by lifting one edge.
- If an entire setup is in a single package and is double-wrapped, the wrappings can be left underneath as the sterile table drape.
- Sterile tables are sterile only at table height.
- Any item below your waist level must be considered contaminated.
- A 1-inch edge around the entire sterile field is considered not sterile.
- The edges of all wrappers, packs, and towels are considered not sterile.
- The sides of containers are considered not sterile.
- Sterile goods must not be allowed to come into contact with the 1-inch edge around the sterile field, the edges of wrappers, or the sides of containers.
- If the sterility of an item is questionable, consider the item contaminated.

Moisture

Moisture carries bacteria from a nonsterile surface to a sterile surface; therefore:

- A sterile field placed on a drop of moisture results in the contamination of the field.
- Spills contaminate a sterile field.
- A sterile field remains sterile only as long as it is dry.

Handling Equipment

When two medical assistants work with the surgeon, one serves as the circulating assistant and the other serves as the scrub assistant. The scrub assistant washes with the surgical scrub, and gloves for the procedure. During the procedure, the scrubbed assistant receives only sterile items, cares for the open sterile field, and passes instruments and supplies to the surgeon. The circulating assistant wears nonsterile gloves, opens sterile supplies before and during the procedure, helps position the patient for the procedure, performs the scrub preparation on the patient, and handles all nonsterile equipment in the room during the procedure. Before every surgery, the team members review which universal blood and body-fluid precautions (goggles, masks, aprons, and special procedures) are necessary for the procedure.

If you are the single assistant, you must do all of these functions. The order in which you do things is

36

TABLE 36-1. PREPARATION FOR MINOR SURGERY: SINGLE-ASSISTANT PREPARATION

1. Wash your hands; gather all supplies.
   Sterile side (Mayo tray): two towel packs; skin-prep pack; patient drape pack; instrument pack; miscellaneous pack(s); three glove packs; masks; goggles; aprons or gowns
   Nonsterile side (side counter): syringes; suture material; anesthesia; solutions; additional sponges; dressings; bandages; transfer forceps; waste basin; waste receptacle; nonsterile gloves; masks; goggles; aprons or gowns
2. Escort patient into the room.
3. Greet and converse with patient.
4. Position patient on table.
5. Wash your hands.
6. Open first towel pack.
7. Open skin prep pack.
8. Pour soap and antiseptic solutions.
9. Expose the site to be prepped.
10. Scrub with the surgical hand wash.
11. Glove and arrange sterile field.
12. Place sterile towels at skin scrub boundaries.
13. Prep the patient's skin.
14. Discard skin prep materials.
15. Discard gloves; wash your hands.
16. Open table drape pack on Mayo stand to create sterile field.
17. Open instrument pack(s), and transfer instruments to sterile field. Add sterile syringe unit.
18. Add sterile items as requested.
19. Physician joins you and converses with the patient.
20. Open physician's glove pack (physician now gloves).
21. Open patient drape pack (physician now drapes the surgical site).
22. Cleanse and hold up anesthesia vial for physician to withdraw anesthesia with sterile syringe (physician will now administer the anesthesia).
23. Repeat surgical hand wash; reglove with a new glove pack.
24. Arrange sterile field instruments and other materials for safety and in sequence; check instrument condition.
25. Unwind suture materials, load the first suture into the needle holder.
26. Place two gauze sponges at the site.
27. Assist the procedure.*
    For physician—instrument pass; maintain field; anticipate needs; cut sutures.
    For patient—retract tissue; sponge blood from wound; specimen care.
28. Escort patient to recovery area.
29. Record and prepare specimens.
30. Clean the room; clear materials; discard gloves.
31. Chart the procedure on the medical record.
32. Help the patient to prepare to leave the office.
33. Disinfect and sterilize equipment at first available time.

*By law, the assistant may not clamp tissue, place sutures, or alter body tissues in any way.

vital. If you do not do things in the proper order, you might find yourself gloved and sterile with no packs open or with a nonsterile item to retrieve, or you may find that the surgeon is waiting and you cannot work because you do not have on your gloves. Not only is it important to learn aseptic technique, but it is important to learn, step-by-step, how to get from the beginning to the end. Table 36-1 outlines the chronologic steps for the assistant who must function as both the circulating and the scrub assistant.

Transfer Forceps

The first sterile procedure that you must master is the use of transfer forceps. If you are the circulating assistant and your hands are not gloved, you must use sterile transfer forceps to touch sterile items or to pass sterile items to the scrub assistant's or surgeon's hand. Even if you are not working with surgical patients, there is rarely a day that you will not need to transfer some sterile item from the autoclave or a sterile package. Sterile transfer forceps

PROCEDURE 36-1 USING TRANSFER FORCEPS

GOAL To move sterile items on a sterile field or to transfer sterile items to a gloved team member.

EQUIPMENT AND SUPPLIES

A sterile transfer forceps in a sterile forceps container or a Bard-Parker container
A sterile item to move or transfer

A Mayo stand set up with a sterile field and sterile instruments
A sterile gauze sponge in an individual wrapper

PROCEDURAL STEPS

1. Wash your hands, and dry them carefully.
   Purpose: Water on your hands could run down the forceps and contaminate the forceps and the sterile solution.

Continued

PROCEDURE 36-1   *Continued*

2. Peel open the sterile 4 × 4 or 3 × 3 gauze package, and set it down on the counter with the gauze sponge exposed and laying on the inside of the wrapper.

3. Remove the forceps by pulling it straight up and out of the solution, without touching the sides of the container.
Purpose: If you turn the tips upward, the solution will run onto the nonsterile area and then back down over the sterile end when you turn the tips down again, thus contaminating the forceps and the solution when you return the forceps to the container.

4. Dry the forceps by touching them, points down, to the piece of dry, sterile gauze.
Purpose: Wet forceps will contaminate a sterile field.

5. Grasp an item on the field with the forceps, points down, and move it to its proper position for the procedure (Fig. 36-1).

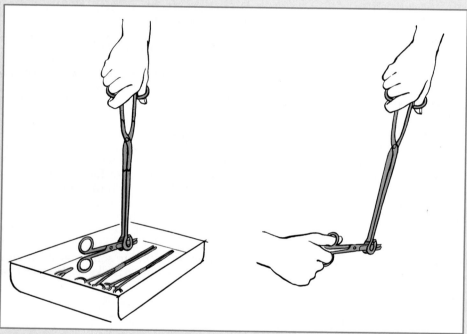

FIGURE 36-1.

6. Or, transfer an instrument to the surgeon's gloved hand.

7. Return the forceps, points down, into the forceps container, without touching the container sides.

---

may be autoclaved and kept dry in a pack or may be submersed in a sterile solution. The solution must be fresh and the container filled. At the time you change the solution, re-autoclave the transfer forceps and the container. The Bard-Parker transfer forceps, with its closed container system and spring-loaded inner lining, is sometimes preferred over the traditional open container. The closed system may prevent contamination from the air and dust, and the forceps are designed so that they cannot touch the sides of the container. This system must be changed, cleaned, and autoclaved as often as the open systems.

ASSISTING IN MINOR SURGICAL PROCEDURES

The physician is ultimately responsible for the surgical patient, but you are responsible for ensuring that everything you and the physician use in the care of the surgical patient is accounted for, ready for use, and prepared in a safe manner. A surgical conscience is the practice of good aseptic technique and demands that breaks in aseptic technique be reported immediately without regard to delays or embarrassment.

Every team has preferences regarding the sequence in which the team goes about the routines of minor surgery. Once a routine is established, it should be followed in every case. Sample setups for various types of minor surgery are provided in Table 36–2.

Positioning the Patient

Have the patient disrobe sufficiently to completely expose the surgical area. There is too much risk of contamination in doing the procedure while either you or the patient is holding back clothing that may slide into the area where the physician is working. Clothing may also act as a tourniquet or may make it difficult to apply a proper dressing or bandage. The patient's clothing may also be stained with the skin-disinfecting solution or may prevent a large area from being treated properly.

It is equally important to position the patient as comfortably as possible. An uncomfortable position can be held for only a limited time, and the patient will have to move, often in the middle of a procedure. If not comfortable, the patient's muscles may stiffen or ache after the surgery. If bandaging is applied to an area with the patient in an awkward position, the bandage may bind or improperly fit when the patient assumes a normal position. When

TABLE 36–2. SAMPLE MINOR SURGERY SETUPS

Procedure	Side Counter	Sterile Field	Comments	Postoperative Care
Suture repair	Local anesthetic; dressings and bandages; splints or guards; tape; drape; gloves; sterile physiologic saline	Syringe and needle; hemostats (3); scissors; sponges; suture material and needle; tissue forceps or skin hook; needle holder	If an emergency patient arrives in the office with a pressure dressing over a laceration, do not remove the pressure dressing until the physician is ready to suture. If the patient's pressure cloth *must* be removed, have ample sterile dressings ready to apply immediately. Ask the patient the possible length, depth, and exact location of the laceration. Usually there is limited cleansing of a wound because of the bleeding. If not, let the physician instruct you on the necessary cleansing.	Frequently, clean lacerations in a moderately protected area will not be dressed but left open. The patient will be instructed to keep the area clean and dry. Some lacerations may be closed with adhesive strips. These are becoming increasingly popular, since they reduce the chance of infection and do not leave suture scars.
Needle biopsy	Specimen bottle with sufficient fixative or preserving solution; laboratory form and label; local anesthetic; gloves	Biopsy needle; syringe and needle; sponges	A biopsy is the examination of tissue removed from the living body. Biopsies are usually done to determine whether a growth or swelling is malignant or benign; however, it may be done as a diagnostic aid in other diseases or infections. A needle biopsy may be done by aspiration with a needle and syringe or by a special biopsy needle. The specimen is then sent to a pathologist for either a cytologic or histologic examination.	Usually there is no special dressing required after a needle biopsy. A Band-Aid is often sufficient.
Cyst removal	Local anesthetic; disinfectant (skin prep); laboratory form; dressing, size depends on site; gloves; drape; specific bottle with sufficient fixative or preserving solution	Kelly hemostats; 2 str. and 2 cvd.; dressing forceps (2); suture and needle; scissors s/s or s/b; dissector (physician's choice); skin hook; syringe and needle; knife handle with blade #11 or #15; tissue forceps (2); Allis forceps; needle holder; sponges; coagulant gel	A sebaceous cyst is a benign retention cyst of a sebaceous gland containing fatty substance of the gland. It is also called a *wen*. They may occur any place on the body, with the exception of the palms of the hands and the soles of the feet. They are more common on the neck and shoulder, and because they are frequently the source of irritation, they are removed. Ordinarily, the cyst is attached only to the skin and moves freely over the underlying tissue. For cosmetic reasons, the physician will make the incision on the natural skin crease lines.	See suture repair above.

Table continued on following page

TABLE 36–2. SAMPLE MINOR SURGERY SETUPS *Continued*

Procedure	Side Counter	Sterile Field	Comments	Postoperative Care
Incision and Drainage (I & D)	Wax or plastic bag for contaminants; extra sponges; medications; skin antiseptic; bandages; ethyl chloride spray; extra applicators; gloves	Hemostats (2); probe; scissors; abscess needle; gauze stripping, iodoform; knife handle with blade #15; dressing forceps (2); sponges; dressing	An abscess is a localized collection of pus in a cavity formed by the disintegration of tissue. Abscesses may appear on any part of the body. Furuncle, boil, and carbuncle are names applied to different types of abscesses. In most abscesses, pyogenic cocci, usually staphylococci, are found, but it is not uncommon to find secondary organisms. The treatment for abscesses, other than those on the face, is usually incision and drainage. Because of the infectious organisms, extreme caution should be taken in handling the contaminated materials and instruments. The physician may choose to inject a local anesthetic if the abscess is deep rather than to use the ethyl chloride to "freeze" the area. The medical assistant may cut the length of gauze stripping for packing at the physician's request.	When dressing the area, several layers of gauze sponges should be placed over the abscess opening, especially if a drain has been inserted, and the gauze anchored with bandage. Frequently, a patient is instructed to apply warm moist packs for a couple of days. Daily dressing changes may also be indicated because of the copious drainage.
Cervical biopsy	Specimen bottle 10% formalin; laboratory form; skin antiseptic solution; gloves	Vaginal speculum; uterine dressing forceps (2); cervical biopsy punch; coagulant foam or gel; sponges; uterine tenaculum; vaginal tampon or packing	This is the examination of the tissue removed from the cervical area of the uterus. A biopsy is usually done to determine whether there is a malignancy present. It is also a diagnostic aid in diagnosing other diseases. If the Papanicolaou smear test is positive, it is usually confirmed by a cervical biopsy. The patient is placed in the lithotomy position, with a towel under the buttocks. Since the cervix is devoid of nerve endings that would respond to cutting and burning stimuli, there is very little discomfort. Postbiopsy bleeding may be controlled by the application of a coagulant gel or foam, or the physician may choose to lightly cauterize the area. The physician may also choose to remove a piece of tissue by means of electric conization.	Usually there are no special dressings or packing after a cervical biopsy. The patient is instructed to care for any discharge and to abstain from douching or sexual intercourse for a few days.
Nasal pack	Head mirror and light; emesis basin; medication; laryngeal mirror; tongue depressor; topical anesthetic; gloves	Nasal speculum; cotton applicators; scissors; metal applicator, str. and cvd.; nasal packing with string (4″); dressing forceps (bayonet); hemostatic forceps, str.; medicine glass; nasal pack, 1 inch, plain or iodoform	A nasal pack is inserted into the nasal cavity, usually for the purpose of stopping hemorrhage or for the application of medication. The patient is placed in a sitting position, with the back well-supported. Drape the front of the patient and give him or her some paper tissues.	The patient is instructed not to remove the pack, and a return visit is scheduled; or the patient is instructed how and when to remove the packing.

deciding on the correct patient position, consider where you and the physician will stand or sit, where the instruments will be placed, and the position of the light source. If the patient has an open wound, is bleeding, or has a wound that will need **irriga-** **tion**, wear nonsterile gloves to assist the patient into position for the procedure. If the bleeding is profuse, you should wear an apron or gown. If there is danger of blood or body-fluid contamination to your face, wear goggles and a mask.

Preparing the Patient's Skin

The human skin is a reservoir of bacteria (see Chapter 22). Resident organisms cannot be removed or completely destroyed; therefore, the skin cannot be sterilized. Transit bacteria, however, can be harmful, and all care must be given to cleanse the patient's skin of transit bacteria as much as possible. Cleansing the patient's skin prior to surgery is called a *skin prep.* A good skin prep eliminates, as much as possible, the transference of harmful organisms to the incision site. Sometimes the patient may be instructed to repeatedly cleanse the surgical area with bacteriostatic or antiseptic soap several days before the surgery. A patient may need to shave the surgical area immediately before coming to the office. Disposable skin prep trays are available. A patient skin prep is performed by a gloved assistant.

PROCEDURE 36-2   POURING A STERILE SOLUTION INTO A CONTAINER ON A STERILE FIELD

GOAL As a circulating assistant, pour a sterile solution into a stainless steel bowl or medicine glass that is sitting at the edge of a sterile field.

EQUIPMENT AND SUPPLIES

A sterile bottle of solution
A stainless steel bowl or medicine glass
A sterile field
A sink or waste receptacle

Note: A medicine glass or bowl on the sterile field should be near one edge of the field but inside the perimeter of the 1-inch barrier.

PROCEDURAL STEPS

1. Wash your hands, and dry them carefully.
   Purpose: Moisture on your hand may cause the bottle to slip from your hand.

2. Place your hand over the label, and lift the bottle. Note: If the container has a double cap, set the outer cap on the counter inside up, then proceed with Step 3.

3. Lift the lid of the bottle straight up, and then slightly to one side, and hold the lid in your minor hand facing downward.
   Purpose: Air currents carry contaminants that could settle on the inside of the lid.

4. Pour away from the label.
   Purpose: Spills down the side of the bottle stain or make the label unreadable.

5. If the container does not have a double cap, pour off a small amount of the solution into a waste receptacle.
   Purpose: To rinse any contaminants off the bottle lip.
   Note: If the container has a double cap, skip this step and proceed to Step 6.

6. Pour, away from the label, the desired amount into the glass or bowl, without allowing any part of the bottle to touch the glass or bowl (Fig. 36-2).
   Purpose: The bottle exterior is not sterile.

7. Tilt the bottle up to stop the pouring while it is still over the bowl or glass.
   Purpose: Solutions spilled on a sterile field contaminate the field.

Continued

PROCEDURE 36-2 *Continued*

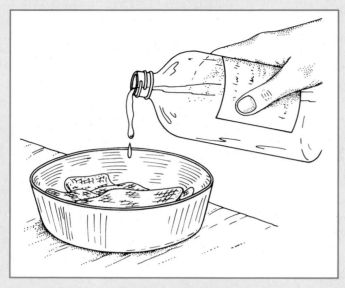

FIGURE 36-2.

8. Remove the bottle from over the sterile field.
   Purpose: Motion over a sterile field should be kept to a minimum.

9. Replace the cap(s) off to the side, away from the sterile field.

PROCEDURE 36-3 PREPARING A PATIENT'S SKIN FOR SURGERY

GOAL To prepare the patient's skin for a surgical procedure to reduce the risk of wound contamination.

EQUIPMENT AND SUPPLIES

Blood and body-fluid protection barriers
An autoclaved skin prep pack
   containing:
   12 to 24 4 × 4 gauze sponges
   Eight cotton-tipped applicators
   Two small stainless steel bowls

Antiseptic soap
Antiseptic
Waste receptacle on the side counter
Cotton balls, nail picks, and scrub
   brushes may also be needed

PROCEDURAL STEPS

1. Wash your hands, and dry them carefully. Follow universal blood and body-fluid precautions.
   Purpose: Moisture on your hands contaminates the pack.

2. Open your skin prep pack.

3. Arrange the items with the transfer forceps.
   Purpose: The skin prep field is a sterile field.

Continued

4. Add the soap and antiseptic solutions to the two bowls.

5. Expose the site. Use a light if necessary.

6. Glove yourself.
   Purpose: To protect the patient from your resident bacteria.

7. Place two sterile towels at the edges of the area to be scrubbed.
   Purpose: The area must be scrubbed up to the sterile towels, which will be beyond the opening of the surgical drape when the drape is applied.

8. Start at the incision site, and begin washing with the antiseptic soap on a gauze sponge in a circular motion, moving from the center to the edges of the area to be scrubbed (Fig. 36–3).
   Purpose: Circular motion from inside to outside drags contaminants away from the incision site.

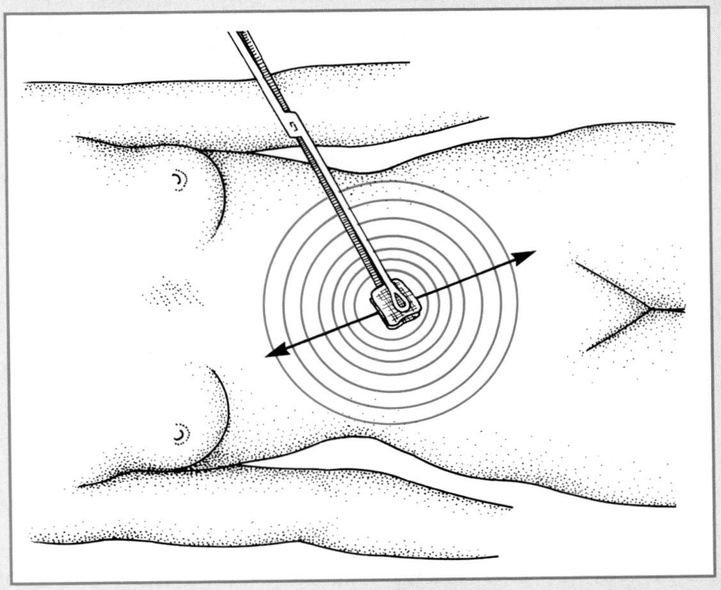

FIGURE 36–3.

9. After one wipe, discard the sponge, and begin again with a new sponge soaked in the antiseptic solution.
   Purpose: After one circular sweep, the sponge is now contaminated with skin bacteria and debris. When you return to the incision site for the next circular sweep, you must use sterile material.

10. Repeat the process, using sufficient friction for 5 minutes (or whatever is the policy for the length of time required for the skin prep).
    Purpose: Friction aids in the removal of *desquamated cells.*

11. Dry the area, using the same circular technique with dry sponges. The area may be dried by blotting with the third sterile towel.

12. Check that no solutions are pooling under the patient.
    Purpose: The solution will irritate or burn the skin.

13. Paint on the antiseptic with the cotton-tipped applicators, using the same circular technique and never returning to an area that has already been painted.

14. If the surgeon is not ready to begin the procedure, cover the site with the last sterile towel.

Surgery Routines

After receiving an assignment to assist in a minor surgical procedure, study the physician preference card to review the procedure and note the materials that are needed. Next, prepare the room and pull the supplies to be used. Supplies are opened just prior to the procedure; if there is a delay of longer than 1 hour, however, opened materials must be considered no longer sterile. Supplies should not be placed where they can be knocked over or dropped; wrapped supplies that fall to the floor must not be used. Once supplies are opened, a team member should stay in the room. The circulating assistant opens the packs, beginning with the pack that provides the sterile surface for the remaining sterile items.

The Mayo tray is usually prepared as soon as the scrub assistant is gloved and ready to manage the sterile field.

Drapes, towel packs, additional sponge packs, and other sterile packages are stacked on the side or back table. Items from this table may be added, if needed, during the procedure. A basin or trash bucket for waste is placed nearby during the surgery.

PROCEDURE 36-4   OPENING A STERILE LINEN PACK THAT WILL SERVE AS THE STERILE TABLE DRAPE

GOAL To open an autoclaved pack that contains a linen table drape, using correct aseptic technique.

EQUIPMENT AND SUPPLIES

An autoclaved pack that contains an inner linen towel that will serve as the sterile table drape

A Mayo stand
Disinfectant and gauze sponges

PROCEDURAL STEPS

1. Check that the Mayo stand is dust-free and clean. If it is not, clean it with 70% alcohol, or another disinfectant, and gauze sponges.
   Purpose: Although some areas cannot be sterile, steps must be taken to keep contamination to a minimum.

2. Wash your hands, and dry them carefully.
   Purpose: Moisture on your hands contaminates the pack.

3. Place the autoclaved pack on the Mayo stand, and read the label.
   Purpose: Most medical offices have a limited supply of surgical packs; to open a wrong package could mean not having enough instruments for a different procedure.

4. Check the expiration date (Fig. 36-4).
   Purpose: An expired pack is not considered sterile.

5. Position the package so that the outer envelope-flap is face up and at the top as you look at the package (Fig. 36-5).
   Purpose: This positions the pack for correct opening, using aseptic technique.

6. Open the first flap away from you (Fig. 36-6).
   Purpose: Otherwise, you will be reaching over a sterile field for the other three flaps.

7. Pull away the two side flaps. Be careful to lift each flap by reaching under the small folded-back tab and without touching the inner surface of the pack or its contents (Fig. 36-7).

Continued

36

Purpose: The tab and the outside surface are considered touchable and not sterile. Inside the 1-inch tab, the inner surface is considered sterile and not touchable.

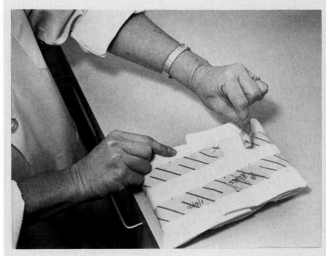

FIGURE 36–4.

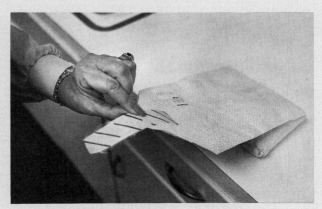

FIGURE 36–5.

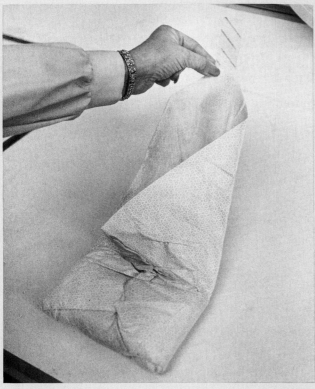

FIGURE 36–6.

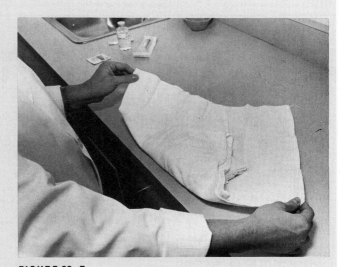

FIGURE 36–7.

Continued

PROCEDURE 36 – 4   *Continued*

8. Pull the last flap toward you by its tab, exposing the towel (Fig. 36–8).

9. Using sterile forceps (or a gloved hand) open the four-folded inside linen in the same manner as steps 6 through 8 previously listed.

10. You now have a sterile table drape as a sterile field to work from and for the distribution of additional sterile supplies and instruments.

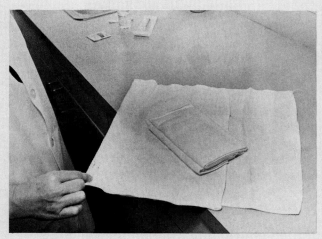

FIGURE 36–8.

PROCEDURE 36 – 5   GLOVING USING THE OPEN-GLOVING (WITHOUT A GOWN) METHOD

GOAL To apply your own sterile gloves before performing sterile procedures.

EQUIPMENT AND SUPPLIES

A pair of packaged surgical gloves in your size

PROCEDURAL STEPS

1. Perform the surgical hand scrub.

2. Dry your hands well.
   Purpose: Gloves do not slide easily over moist hands.

3. Open your glove pack. Remember, a 1-inch area around the perimeter of the glove pack is considered not sterile.
   Purpose: The open glove pack is a sterile field.

4. Glove your major hand first.
   Purpose: This will set up your major hand to do the more difficult step, which is to apply the second glove (Fig. 36–9, *left*).

Continued

5. With your minor hand, pick up the glove for your major hand, with your thumb and forefinger grabbing the top of the folded cuff, which is the inside of the glove (see Fig. 36–9, *left*).
   Purpose: The inside of the glove will be next to your skin and is considered not sterile.

6. Lift the glove up and away from the sterile pack.
   Purpose: Movement over a sterile field must be kept to a minimum.

7. Hold your hands away from you, and slide your major hand into the glove.

8. Leave the cuff folded (Fig. 36–9, *right*).
   Purpose: You will unfold the cuff later.

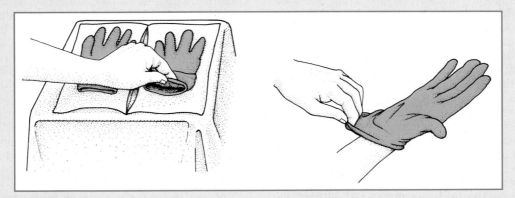

FIGURE 36–9.

9. With your gloved major hand, pick up the second glove by slipping your gloved fingers under the cuff so that your gloved hand only touches the outside of the second glove (Fig. 36–10, *left*).
   Purpose: Sterile surfaces must always touch sterile surfaces.

10. Slide your second hand into the glove, without touching the exterior of the glove or any part of your other hand (Fig. 36–10, *center*).

11. Still holding your hands away from you, unroll the cuff by slipping the fingers up and out. Stay away from your bare arm (Fig. 36–10, *right*).

12. Now, slip your gloved fingers up under the first cuff and unroll it, using the same technique.

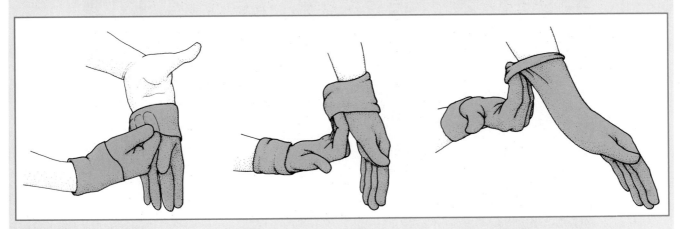

FIGURE 36–10.

The scrub assistant sorts and places the scalpels, hemostats, scissors, tissue forceps, and retractors on the field according to their sequence and frequency of use (Fig. 36–11). Scalpels and sharp instruments should be conspicuously placed so that they do not accidentally harm a team member. If the scrub assistant has not previously prepped the patient, the circulating assistant now performs the patient skin prep. The circulating assistant opens the drape pack. The physician enters the room, gloves, and begins draping the patient with towels or a fenestrated drape. The scrub assistant hands the drapes to the physician, one at a time. In many offices, the scrub assistant alone drapes the site. Once the site is draped, the Mayo stand is positioned below the site, and the scrub assistant stands opposite the physician, over the patient. The circulating assistant cleans the vial of anesthesia with alcohol and holds the vial (with the label up and visible to read) for the scrub assistant or the physician. The scrub assistant or physician lifts the syringe from the sterile field and withdraws the appropriate amount of anesthesia into the syringe. The physician administers the anesthesia, and the scrub assistant immediately places two sponges on the patient, next to the wound site, for sponging blood at the time of the first incision or to sponge an open injury as the first step of the procedure. Local anesthesia is administered either directly into the open wound or into the tissues surrounding the site to be incised. After the anesthesia has taken effect, the physician begins the procedure.

During the procedure, the scrub assistant must protect the sterile field from contamination, notify the physician if there is a break in sterile technique, dispose of soiled sponges into waste receptacles, and anticipate the surgeon's needs for instruments. The physician may verbally request instruments or may use hand signals (Fig. 36–12). As the team works together over time, the physician may not need to give any signals.

Instrumentation is logical: if the physician requests a suture, then scissors will be needed to cut the suture tie; if there is a sudden hemorrhage from a bleeder, the physician will need a hemostat. In gaining experience, the assistant watches, listens, and learns to judge what will be needed or performed next. Pass instruments with a firm and purposeful motion so that the physician will not have to look up. Wait until you feel the physician grasp the instrument, so it will not drop onto the patient or to the floor. Pass instruments so that the physician is protected from injury. Pass scalpels blade down. Hold all instruments by their tips, and pass the handle ends into the physician's palm or fingers. Avoid painful slapping of the instruments into the surgeon's hand. Correct passing produces a faint, gentle "snap" as it contacts the gloved hand.

If a specimen is collected during the procedure, it is placed in a sterile glass or basin. Do not remove the specimen from the sterile field until the physician gives the order. The physician may want to examine it again during the procedure.

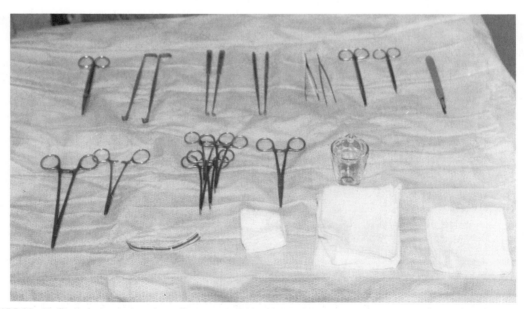

FIGURE 36–11. Sterile instruments and supplies on a sterile field in preparation for assisting with the minor surgical procedure.

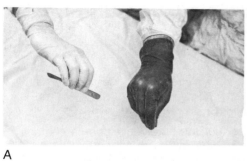

A

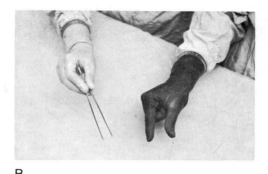

B

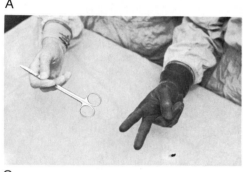

C

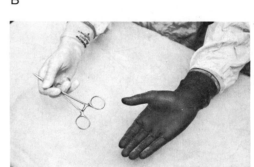

D

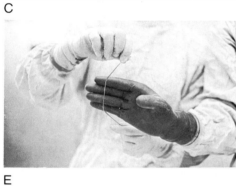

E

FIGURE 36-12. Passing instruments. *A,* Hand signal for scalpel. *B,* Hand signal for forceps. *C,* Hand signal for scissors. *D,* Hand signal for hemostat. *E,* Hand signal for suture strand without a needle (free tie). (From Nealon, T. F.: *Fundamental Skills in Surgery,* 3rd ed., Philadelphia, W.B. Saunders Co., 1979.)

PROCEDURE 36-6   OPENING A STERILE PACK TO ADD ITS CONTENTS TO A STERILE FIELD

GOAL   As a circulating assistant, add instruments from a sterile pack to a sterile field, using correct aseptic technique.

EQUIPMENT AND SUPPLIES

An autoclaved pack that contains at
   least three instruments or other
   sterile items
A Mayo stand set up with a sterile field

Continued

PROCEDURE 36 – 6 *Continued*

PROCEDURAL STEPS

1. Wash your hands, and dry them carefully.
   Purpose: Moisture on your hands contaminates the pack.

2. Position the pack on the palm of your minor hand so that the outer envelope-flap is face up and at the top as you look at the package (Fig. 36–13, *left*).
   Purpose: This positions the pack for correct opening, using aseptic technique.

3. Open the first flap away from you (Fig. 36–13, *right*).
   Purpose: Otherwise, you will be reaching over a sterile field for the other three flaps.

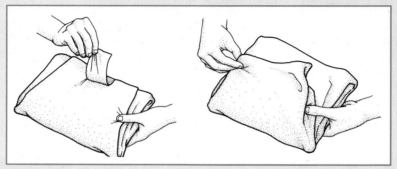

FIGURE 36–13.

4. Pull away the two side flaps. Be careful to lift each flap by reaching under the small folded-back tab and without touching the inner surface of the pack or its contents (Fig. 36–14, *left*).
   Purpose: The tab and the outside surface are considered touchable and not sterile. Inside the 1-inch tab, the inner surface is considered sterile and not touchable.

5. The last flap is pulled toward you by its tab, exposing the contents (Fig. 36–14, *center*).

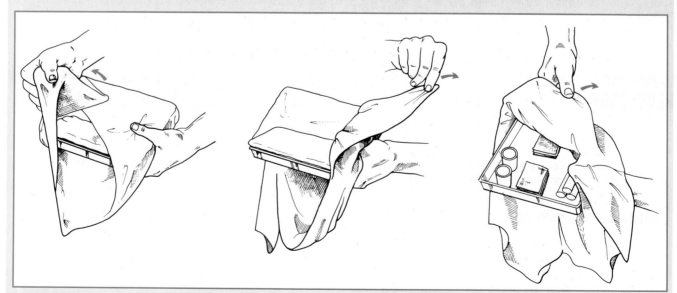

FIGURE 36–14.

Continued

6. By closing your open palm, grasp the items through the cloth at the tip ends (Fig. 36–14, *right*).
   Note: To make this possible, all items must be autoclaved in the same direction.

7. Hold the four flaps back around your wrist with your major hand (Fig. 36–13, *left*).
   Purpose: All parts of the four flaps are now considered not sterile, and you do not want them to touch any part of the instruments or the sterile field.

8. Slide the items, handles first, onto the field.
   Purpose: To avoid damaging the fine tips.

9. Do not reach over the field, yet place the instruments inside the perimeter of the 1-inch barrier.
   Purpose: The 1-inch perimeter around the sterile field is considered not sterile.

10. Or, hand the items to a gloved team member (Fig. 36–15, *right*).

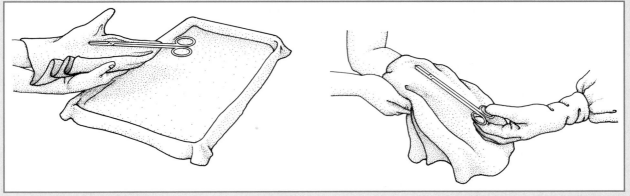

FIGURE 36–15.

PROCEDURE 36–7   ADDING STERILE ITEMS IN A PEEL-BACK WRAPPER TO A STERILE FIELD

GOAL To add the contents of a sterile pack, such as syringes, needles, and suture materials, to the sterile field, using correct sterile technique.

EQUIPMENT AND SUPPLIES

A package containing suture material
A package containing a disposable syringe and needle
A Mayo stand set up with a sterile field

Continued

PROCEDURE 36–7   *Continued*

PROCEDURAL STEPS

1. Wash your hands, and dry them carefully.
   Purpose: Moisture on your hands contaminates the pack.

2. Off to the side of the sterile field, hold the pack in your hand and read the label.
   Purpose: Most medical offices have a limited supply of items; to open a wrong package could mean not having enough supplies for a different procedure.

3. Hold the pack, and grab a peel-away edge in each hand.

4. Open by peeling the two flaps apart. Keep the flaps away from the sterile item by holding them outward. The item should be sticking straight out from between the peel-back sides (Fig. 36–16, *left*).
   Purpose: The edges of a sterile pack are considered not sterile.

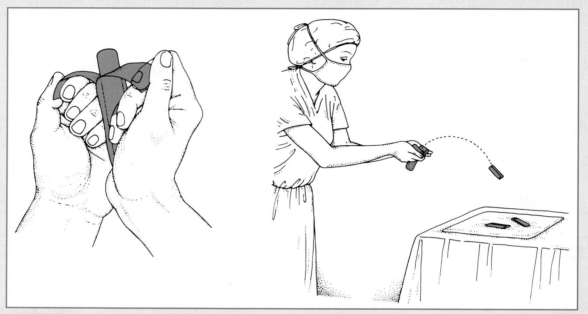

FIGURE 36–16.

5. Continue to peel with a snap of the hands to "pop" the items out of the package and onto the field from a distance of about 8 to 12 inches. Do not reach over the field, yet place the item inside the perimeter of the 1-inch barrier (Fig. 36–16, *right*).

Completion of the Surgical Procedure

At the conclusion of the procedure, the physician will begin the wound closure. The techniques and methods of tissue closure vary greatly, and it would be impossible to describe or illustrate all of them. There are two basic methods of suturing: the *continuous* (running) placement of a single strand; and the *interrupted* suture, in which each knot is placed and tied independently so that if one breaks, the others keep the wound closure intact (Fig. 36–17). The majority of skin closures in the medical office are limited to the interrupted technique.

The scrub assistant mounts the suture and needle in the needle holder and passes the unit to the physician. As the physician closes the wound, the scrub assistant assists by cutting the suture and sponging the site. The physician places the first interrupted suture at the midpoint of the incision. Then, each side of the first suture is mentally di-

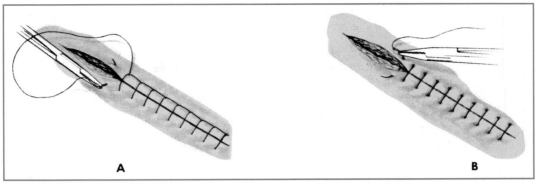

FIGURE 36–17. Types of skin closures. *A*, Continuous technique. *B*, Interrupted technique. (Courtesy of Ethicon, Inc.)

vided in half again, and the next two sutures are placed at each of these midpoints. The rest of the sutures are placed by the same technique of mentally dividing the remaining suture line in half until the length of the wound edge is totally **approximated.**

After skin closure, the wound site is cleaned with wet and dry sponges. This may be done by the surgeon or the scrub assistant. Care must be taken not to disturb the wound edges or the sutures. Next,

sterile dressings are placed over the incision, and the drapes are removed. Lift the drapes directly off the patient with minimum movement so as not to disturb the dressing or stir up the air currents. The circulating assistant or the surgeon then applies nonsterile bandage and tape to the dressing. Do not break down your Mayo stand until the patient has left the room. If there is an unexpected contamination of the wound site during the dressing, more materials will be needed from the sterile field.

PROCEDURE 36–8   ASSISTING WITH SUTURING

GOAL   To assist the physician in wound closure, without a break in sterile technique or injury to other team members.

EQUIPMENT AND SUPPLIES

A sterile field on a Mayo stand
Mayo-Hegar needle holder

Strands of atraumatic suture material
Surgical scissors
Gauze sponges

PROCEDURAL STEPS

1. Four to five inches over the sterile field, hold the curved needle point up in your minor hand (Fig. 36–18, *left*).
   Purpose: Keeping the suture material close to the surface prevents the strands from wandering onto a nonsterile area.

2. With the needle holder in your major hand, clamp the needle at the upper third of the total length (near the eyeless connection) with the needle holder (Fig. 36–18, *right*).
   Purpose: Clamping in the middle weakens or distorts the shape of the needle. Clamping too near the thread may cause the suture to detach from the needle. Clamping at the lower third of the needle damages the needle point.

3. With your major hand, hold the needle holder halfway down its shaft, at the box-lock, with the suture needle point up.
   Purpose: To prevent injury to the physician.

Continued

PROCEDURE 36-8 *Continued*

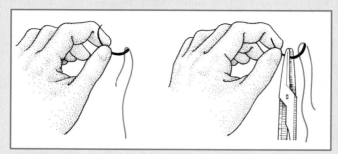

FIGURE 36-18.

4. With your minor hand, hold the suture strand, and pass the needle holder into the surgeon's hand (Fig. 36-19).
   Purpose: Holding the strand prevents it from touching anything else as it is being passed.

5. Pick up the surgical scissors with your major hand and a gauze sponge with your minor hand.

6. After the physician has placed a closure and holds the two strands taut, cut both suture strands in one motion, between the knot and the physician, at the length requested (about 1/8 inch) (Fig. 36-20).
   Purpose: Too long a suture may irritate the patient during recovery; too short a suture may untie during recovery.

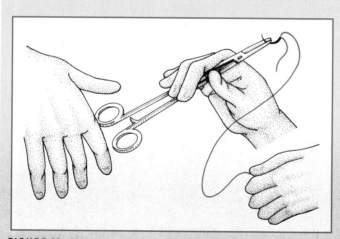

FIGURE 36-19.

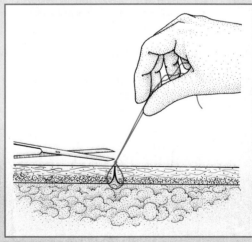

FIGURE 36-20.

7. Gently blot the closure once with the gauze sponge in your minor hand.
   Purpose: Rubbing or friction may damage the wound edges, and once a gauze sponge has been used, it must be discarded.

8. If additional strands of suture are needed, repeat the process.

PROCEDURE 36-9   ASSISTING DURING THE MINOR SURGICAL PROCEDURE

GOAL To maintain the sterile field and to pass instruments in a prescribed sequence during a surgical procedure that involves the making of a surgical incision and the removal of a growth.

EQUIPMENT AND SUPPLIES

An open patient drape pack on the side counter
A Mayo stand
A sterile field containing the following:
  A needle and syringe for the anesthesia
  A supply of gauze sponges

A scalpel handle and a no. 11 blade
One Allis tissue forceps
One skin retractor
Three hemostats
One medicine glass or bowl (specimen container)
A waste receptacle
A vial of anesthesia
Sterile gloves (at least two pairs)

PROCEDURAL STEPS

1. Scrub with the surgical hand wash; follow universal blood and body-fluid precautions.

2. Position the Mayo stand over the patient and below the site.

3. Invert the vial of anesthesia, and hold it for the gloved physician to withdraw the prescribed amount of anesthesia into the syringe.
   Purpose: The vial of anesthesia cannot be held after both team members are gloved.

4. Glove.

5. Grasp the patient drape in the open drape pack by holding one edge or corner in each hand.

6. Lift the drape from the pack without touching the drape to any of the pack edges.
   Purpose: A 1-inch barrier around any sterile field is considered not sterile.

7. Drape the surgical site without touching any part of the patient or the operating table with your gloved hands. The physician injects the local anesthesia.
   Note: The physician may drape the patient, while you glove.

8. Position yourself across from the physician. Arrange the sterile field. Check instrument condition.

9. Place two sponges on the patient, next to the wound site.

10. Grasp an Allis tissue forceps by the tips, and pass it to the physician to grasp a piece of tissue to be excised. Pass the handles into the surgeon's open palm with a firm and purposeful motion so that a gentle "snap" is heard as it contacts the surgeon's gloved hand.
    Purpose: The physician will not have to look up to receive the instrument.

11. Grasp the scalpel blade with a hemostat, and mount the scalpel blade onto the scalpel handle. Keep all sharp equipment conspicuously placed on the sterile field.
    Purpose: Sharp instruments that are not clearly visible may injure a team member.

12. Pass the scalpel, blade down, to the physician. The physician will take the scalpel with the thumb and forefinger in the position ready for use.
    Purpose: To protect the physician from injury.

13. Dispose of soiled sponges, using the waste receptacle.

14. Hold clean sponges in your minor hand, to pass as needed.

15. Hold out the specimen container to receive the specimen.

Continued

PROCEDURE 36–9 *Continued*

16. If there is a bleeder, or if a hemostat is requested, pass the hemostat in the manner described in Steps 9 and 10.
17. Receive instruments, and put them in the field.
18. Continue to sponge blood from the wound site.
19. Retract the wound edge with a skin retractor if so requested.

DRESSINGS AND BANDAGES

Dressings

A dressing is a sterile covering placed over a wound to:

- Protect the wound from injury and contamination
- Maintain a constant pressure
- Hold the wound edges together
- Control bleeding
- Absorb drainage and secretions
- Hide temporary disfigurement

A dressing usually consists of a strip of lubricated mesh or a nonstick Telfa pad placed over a sutured wound. It is important to use dressings that do not adhere to the wound itself. Gauze squares are usually placed over the nonadhering material. Body cavities or wounds that need to remain open for a time are dressed with long, thin packing material that is often impregnated with an antiseptic or lubricant. This is sometimes called *packing*. Regardless of the type of material, a good dressing must be effective and comfortable and must remain in place. If the dressing covers a hairless area, it may be anchored with tape only, but no tape may touch the wound.

Frequently, small, clean lacerations may be closed with special adhesive strips called Steri-Strips. These strips reduce the chance of infection and do not leave suture scars. Steri-Strips are used on areas of the body that are well protected from movement and stress; they are often used on the face. They should never be used on a knee or an elbow. Since Steri-Strips are a suture replacement, only the physician should place them. The physician places the strips onto the wound in the same sequence and at the same intervals as in interrupted sutures (Fig. 36–21).

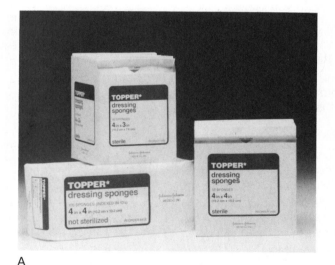

A

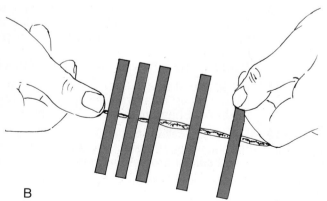

B

FIGURE 36–21. *A*, Probably the most commonly used dressing, this dressing sponge is manufactured in various sizes to accommodate wound sizes. It may be referred to as a sponge or a flat, but it is manufactured under the name "Topper Dressing Sponges." Each dressing is packaged individually in pull-apart sterile packages. (Courtesy of Johnson & Johnson Medical, Inc., Arlington, TX.) *B*, Sterile strip skin closures may be preferred for small lacerations. Sterile strips are applied in the same manner as sutures.

Bandages

Dressings are usually held in place by bandages, which further help to maintain even pressure, support the affected part, and keep the wound free from injury or contamination. Bandages can be gauze, cloth, or elastic cloth rolls and are bound by tape or tying. Dressings and bandages frequently appear easy and simple to apply, but special skill is required to apply a functional dressing that serves the purpose for which it is intended. Bandages that are too loose fall off. Bandages that are too tight may further harm the patient. Patients do not feel that good medical care has been given them if bandages are messy or uncomfortable. Swelling may occur after a dressing and bandage are applied, and the patient may need a dressing change sooner than scheduled.

Plain gauze roller bandage is almost a thing of the past. It is difficult to handle because it must be applied with reverse spiral turns if the area is uneven. Plain gauze roller bandage has no elasticity and tends to bind. Because it does not adhere to itself, it is also more likely to slip. *Wrinkled crepe-type bandages,* such as Kling, are preferred because they adhere to the various shapes of the body as well as to themselves (Fig. 36-22). Roller bandages are not applied without a dressing.

Plain elastic cloth bandage (Ace) or *elastic roller cloth with adhesive backing* makes a flexible and secure cover (Fig. 36-23). When applying Ace elastic roller bandage as a pressure bandage, especially to the lower limbs, it is absolutely essential to keep the bandage consistent in spacing and tension to ensure even pressure. Even and gentle pressure stimulates circulation and healing; uneven pressure causes constriction points that can create pressure sores or ulcers. All roller bandages are applied from the distal to the proximal part of the area. Bandaging can remain even and snug only if it is wrapped from a smaller to a larger circumference. Elevate the limb while you are bandaging, and work with the roller facing upward, close to the patient's skin. This technique is more likely to keep the tension consistent, and you will be less likely to drop the roll (Fig. 36-24A). Common bandaging techniques are shown in Figure 36-24B through H.

Adhesive bandages are commercially prepared elastic bandages, commonly called Band-Aids. They are available in various shapes to fit the various body parts. Small circular bandages are called "spots."

Seamless tubular gauze bandage, with or without elastic, is superior material for covering round surfaces, such as the arms, legs, fingers, and toes. It can be used as either a dressing or a bandage. Tubular bandage is applied with a cage-like applicator. Work with the cutting channel of the applicator facing toward the patient. You may start in the middle of the area to be dressed and anchor the dressing, if there is one, with a small piece of tape.

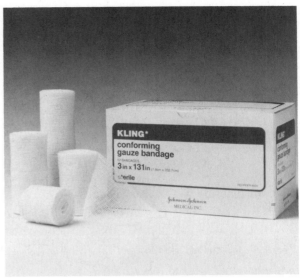

FIGURE 36-22. A wrinkled-crepe cotton bandage that adheres to itself and conforms to cover the body part. (Courtesy of Johnson & Johnson Medical, Inc., Arlington, TX.)

Hold the applicator in both hands, and control the tension flow with your fingers as the applicator is gradually rotated and the material slides off. Tubular dressings may be applied with or without slight pressure. Beyond the tip of the bandaged part, give the applicator a full half-turn, place the applicator again over the part, and repeat the process. Be very careful not to create a tourniquet effect when you reverse the applicator. When the desired thickness of the bandage is reached, cut the gauze, and anchor the final dressing with tape (Fig. 36-25). This lightweight gauze should not be used as a stockinette under a cast. Patients should be advised to call the physician's office if there is any problem with the dressing.

POSTSURGICAL ROUTINES

Cleaning the Operatory

While the circulating assistant escorts the patient from the room, the scrub assistant clears away the sterile field. Follow the universal blood and body-fluid precautions. The scrub assistant should not remove the gloves until all contaminated materials are removed and cared for. Sharp items are placed in separate basins and all instruments are taken to the work area; disposable items are properly placed in trash cans; and the linen is removed to the linen hamper. The room should be checked for any blood, spills, or other contamination. Decontaminate the room with soap and disinfectant as necessary. Label any specimens, and prepare them for transportation

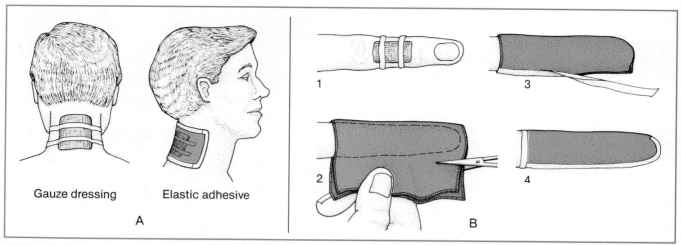

FIGURE 36–23. Elastic adhesive bandage used on *(A)* the neck and *(B)* the finger.

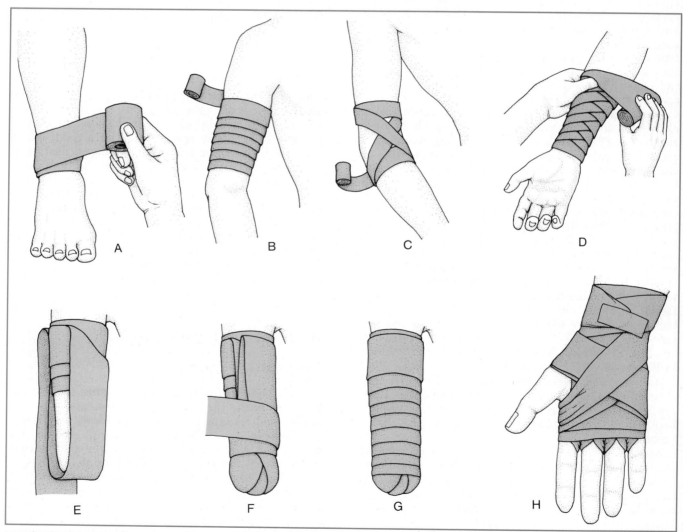

FIGURE 36–24. *A*, Applying a roller bandage. Start at the distal point. Keep the roll close to the patient and keep it upward. Maintain tension and spacing consistently even. *B*, Circular bandage. *C*, Figure-of-eight bandage. *D*, Reverse spiral bandage. *E*, Recurrent bandage for fingers. *F*, Circular turns for fingers. *G*, Reverse spiral for fingers. *H*, Combination recurrent and figure-of-eight turns for the hand.

to the laboratory. Chart the procedure on the patient's medical record, and place the chart on the physician's desk for any additional entries or comments. As soon as there is time, clean and reprocess the instruments and packs.

Postoperative Instructions and Care

Give the patient time to rest after the surgery. If a sedative was administered, make certain that the patient is sufficiently recovered to avoid injury during the journey home. If the patient has been given a topical or local anesthetic, explain to the patient that the anesthesia will soon be wearing off and that there may be discomfort at the site. Check with the physician if a pain medication has not been prescribed. If the physician has prescribed a pain medication, review with the patient the purpose of the medication and the directions for its use. Before the patient leaves the office, set the follow-up appointment.

Postoperative care extends for the total recovery period, not just for the time of immediate care before the patient leaves the office. Most medical assistants are responsible for teaching patients to care for themselves at home following the surgical experience. Since it is a known fact that the concentrative powers of the postoperative patient are diminished following the stress of surgery, instructions should be in writing that is simple in style and easily understood by the patient at home. These instructions can be preprinted forms for each type of surgery or a general form with boxes checked for whichever postoperative instructions apply to a particular patient. Printed instructions should include:

- How to apply a hot or a cold compress
- Whether or not to elevate a limb
- Whether or not to bathe
- Limitations of food intake or exercise
- When to return to work or school
- How to recognize and care for drainage if there is a wound drain in place
- What types of complications necessitate the patient calling the office
- Whether or not to change dressings
- The medications prescribed and their purposes
- The time the next day the patient should call to report in
- The date of the next appointment

Explain to the patient the importance of calling the office if there are any questions or **untoward** changes. If the patient does not call within the next 24 hours, you should call the patient. Many patients tend to "ride it out" or say they didn't want to bother you. Never allow the postoperative patient to

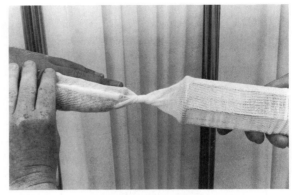

FIGURE 36-25. Tubegauz applied to a finger. (From Bonewit, K.: *Clinical Procedures for Medical Assistants*, 3rd ed., Philadelphia, W.B. Saunders Co., 1990, p. 214.)

leave the office without the physician's knowledge and approval.

Postoperative Return Visits

If the healing process is a long one or if the wound becomes infected, the patient may return for a dressing change. Check the patient's medical record, and follow the physician's instructions carefully. Follow the universal blood and body-fluid precautions. Glove, and wear other protection barriers as appropriate. Place the patient in a comfortable position, and adequately expose the area to be redressed. Try to obscure the wound site from the patient's vision, and do not reveal any unpleasant reactions, by either comment or facial expression. If at any time you determine that the wound may be infected, stop and notify the physician.

Reusable Ace bandage is rerolled in your hand as it is taken off the patient. Because microorganisms are carried by the air currents, keep the bandage close to the patient; do not let it fly around as you work.

Tape applied directly to the patient's skin is not the ideal dressing immobilizer. If tape has been used, it is hoped that it has been kept to a minimum. If there is tape holding a dressing in place, cut the tape next to the dressing. Always remove tape by pulling it toward the wound. If tape is adhering to a hairy area of the body, lift the outer tape edge with one hand and slowly and gently separate the underlying hair and skin from the tape with the thumb of your other hand. In other words, peel the skin from the bandage, not the bandage from the skin. Never rapidly "rip" tape from the body. If the tape is not irritating to the patient, it may be advisable to leave the tape on the skin until total healing has taken place.

After the physician examines the wound, you will either apply a new dressing or remove the patient's sutures.

PROCEDURE 36-10   REMOVING SUTURES

GOAL To remove sutures from a healed incision, using sterile technique and without injury to the closed wound.

EQUIPMENT AND SUPPLIES

Suture removal pack containing:
   One suture-removal scissors
   One thumb dressing forceps
   Gauze sponges

Skin antiseptic
Steri-Strips or Butterfly bandages
   (optional)

PROCEDURAL STEPS

1. Assemble necessary supplies.
2. Wash and dry your hands. Follow the universal blood and body-fluid precautions.
3. Open the suture-removal pack (Fig. 36-26).
4. Place dry toweling under the area.
   Purpose: To catch spills and to keep the patient dry.
5. Position and support the area.
6. If the area has not yet been cleaned, clean and blot dry with a sterile gauze sponge.
7. Place a gauze sponge next to the wound site.
   Purpose: To place the removed sutures.
8. Without pulling, grasp the knot of the suture with the dressing forceps.

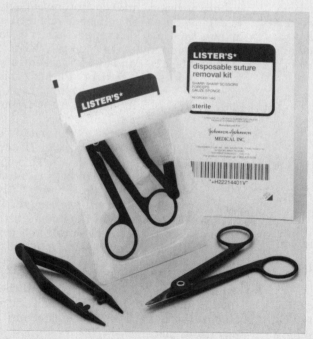

FIGURE 36-26. (Courtesy of Johnson & Johnson Medical, Inc., Arlington, TX.)

Continued

9. Cut the suture at skin level (Fig. 36–27).

10. Lift (do not pull) the suture toward the incision and out with the dressing forceps (Fig. 36–28).

11. Place the suture on the gauze sponge, and check that the entire suture strand has been removed.
    Purpose: Suture fragments left in a wound may cause infection and may prolong the healing process.

12. If there is any bleeding, blot the area with a new gauze sponge before continuing.

13. Continue in the same manner until all the other sutures have been removed.

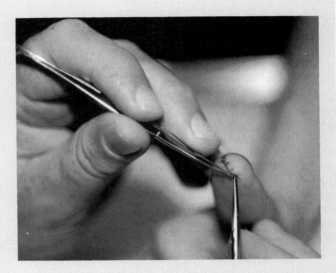

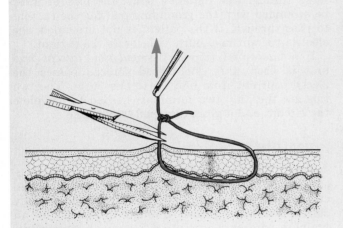

FIGURE 36–27.

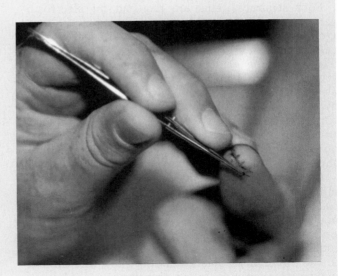

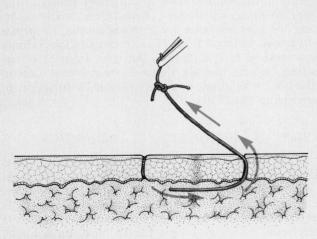

FIGURE 36–28.

Continued

PROCEDURE 36-10   *Continued*

14. Remove the gauze sponge with the sutures on it, and count the sutures.
   Purpose: To compare the count with the suture placement count on the patient's medical record, to ensure that all sutures are accounted for.

15. The physician may choose to apply Steri-Strips or Butterfly bandages for added support and strength.

16. Instruct the patient to keep the wound edges clean and dry and not to place excessive strain on the area.

ELECTROSURGERY

The electrosurgical unit incises, excises, or destroys tissue by using an electric current instead of a scalpel or curette. Electrosurgery is accomplished in minutes, and the shape and size of a surgical site can be well-controlled by the surgeon, making it advantageous to use in **microsurgery.** The electric current works on a minute scale, exploding the cells, which produces carbon and steam byproducts. This process also seals the cells and any blood vessels in the area, and cellular oozing and vascular bleeding can be kept to a minimum. In addition, the area is automatically sterilized by the heat generated by the current. Thus, electrosurgery is advantageous because:

- It is swift
- It controls bleeding by simultaneously cauterizing the surrounding blood vessels
- It is aseptic in technique

Four separate items are required for electrosurgery: the power unit, the patient grounding pad, the grounding cable (Fig. 36–29*A*), and the electrosurgical (electrocautery) needle or pencil (Fig. 36–29*B*). The grounding cable connects the machine to the grounding pad, which is placed on the patient as the electric ground. The pencil attaches to the machine by a long cord and is held by the surgeon. When the surgeon touches the tissue with the pencil, the electric current is activated by a foot pedal or a switch on the pencil, and proceeds from the machine through the cord and pencil into the tissues.

An electric current needs two terminals (biterminal, or bipolar) to complete a circuit. In the *monopolar unit,* the tip of the pencil is the first terminal and becomes the active electrode. The current continues through the patient's body, seeking an exit route that offers the least resistance to its flow back to the power unit. The grounding cable and grounding pad (sometimes called the dispersing plate, or indifferent plate) that is placed on the patient's body is the *ground* acting as the second terminal and provides the path back to the machine to complete the electric circuit. Because the electric current flows through the patient's body, the patient must be grounded with the grounding pad for the current to pass through. If the patient is not grounded, the electric current may burn or lacerate the patient.

If a *biterminal* (bipolar) *coagulation forceps* and unit is used, this dual-tipped forceps passes the electric current from one tip to the other. The two tips are the only two terminals needed to complete the circuit, and a grounding pad is not used.

Types of Current

Two types of current are generated by the electrosurgical unit: *undamped* and *damped.* Undamped current is a steady, unrestricted current and actually cuts tissue when guided through the tissue by an ordinary wire or the point of the pencil. An electrosurgical unit, when set in an undamped or "pure-cut" mode, produces a steady, uninterrupted high-frequency current, and the tissue is divided cleanly, with little or no bleeding.

Damped current is electricity that is restricted and diminished. It is used to coagulate tissue and to stop bleeding. In surgery, *coagulation* is the "clotting" of normal tissue, by physical means, to form a shapeless residual mass. Electrocoagulation is only one method of coagulation, but it is superior to the others, which include thermal coagulation, carbon dioxide coagulation, and coagulation by injection of sclerosing chemicals.

Types of Electrosurgical Techniques

There are four types of electrosurgical techniques: electrocoagulation, electrodesiccation, electrofulguration, and electrosection.

Electrocoagulation coagulates tissues and controls hemorrhage and **hematoma** formation. An active electrode, which may be a needle, disc, knife blade, or ball, is brought into contact with, or is inserted into, the lesion to be destroyed. A grounding pad may be placed in contact with or near the operative site. The amount of tissue destruction depends on

36

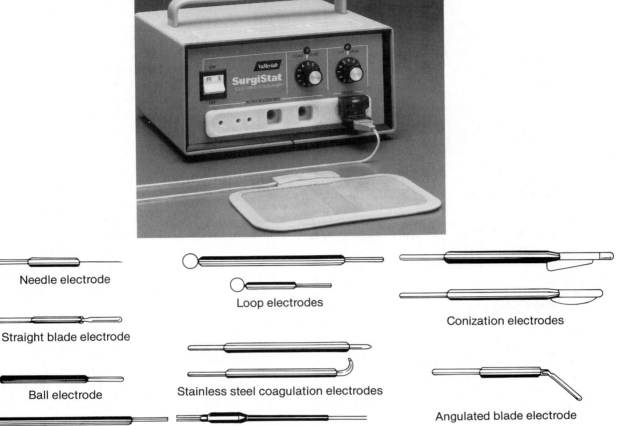

Needle electrode

Loop electrodes

Conization electrodes

Straight blade electrode

Ball electrode

Stainless steel coagulation electrodes

Angulated blade electrode

Disc electrode

Turbinate electrode

FIGURE 36–29. *A,* An electrosurgical power unit, which generates the electric currents necessary for electrosurgery. (Courtesy of Valleylab Inc., Boulder, CO.) *B,* Types of electrode pencils and tips used for electrosurgery.

the type of current and the length of time it is applied. This technique uses a moderately damped or modulated undamped current. This procedure may produce a great amount of necrosis, but it is advantageous in the treatment of larger or deeper growths. If bipolar coagulation forceps are used, coagulation takes place only between and immediately around the tips of the bipolar (biterminal) forceps. The destruction causes the tissue to turn grayish white. The tissue **sloughs** between 5 and 15 days, depending on the depth and the size of the area treated. When the slough has completely separated, healthy tissue appears underneath. Patients undergoing coagulation should be instructed that there will be a slight grayish discharge from the site. A topical antibiotic may be given, but it is usually not necessary because the electric current itself creates a sterile area.

Electrodesiccation destroys cells and tissues by means of a short electric spark gap that produces a highly or moderately damped current. The active electrode (usually a needle or ball) is inserted into or applied directly to the lesion. It produces coagulation of the tissue immediately surrounding the site

of application or insertion and usually results in less necrosis than does coagulation. Electrodesiccation may be used to destroy granulations and small polyps. It is sometimes used to destroy the stem of a **pedunculated** growth, after the growth has been removed by an instrument, to provide hemostasis and to minimize regrowth.

Electrofulguration is from the Latin "fulgur," meaning lightning or spark. Like electrodesiccation, it also destroys tissue by means of an electric spark, but the needle tip is not inserted into the tissue. It is held about 1 or 2 mm away from the surface of the site, allowing the current to produce a superficial desiccation. A grayish-white **coagulum** is formed on the surface and, depending on the mass, sloughs in a few hours to a few days. Small superficial growths carbonize when sparked and may be lifted off immediately, with no surface evidence.

Electrosection uses slightly damped, modulated undamped, or undamped currents. The active electrode is a knife blade, wire loop, or needle, and a large conductive metal plate is used as the grounding pad. This technique is used to incise or excise lesions and growths or for superficial **planing.**

Hazards of Electrosurgery

Safety precautions need to be taken with electrosurgery. If not, serious harm could come to the patient. Electric current should not be used around metal; therefore, the patient should be asked to remove all metal items and should be questioned whether or not there are any metal implants. Other implants that may pose a problem are those that may be disturbed by high-frequency voltage, such as pacemakers.

When a grounding pad is used, proper placement is important. The pad should be placed as close as possible to the wound site. Remember that all power concentrates and surges through the small tip of the active electrode and then seeks the grounding pad as the easiest exit pathway or ground. For the current to complete its circuit, there must be solid contact between the patient and the grounding pad. Therefore, the grounding pad should not be placed over hair, scar tissue, body protuberances, or highly irregular contours that would make it difficult to maintain an even contact between the pad and the body part. If the grounding pad is bent or wrinkled or has been applied unevenly, the current concentrates in the problem area, and "hot spots" or "cuts" can occur. A conductive medium (coupling gel) may be used to provide better contact between the patient and the grounding pad, but it must be applied uniformly to the pad and to the patient, covering the entire surface of each. Missed spots may cause burns, and areas coated too thinly may dry out during a lengthy procedure, resulting in hot spots. Pregelled electrodes make application easier, but care still must be taken in their application. Also, be careful that the patient is not placed in a position where contact may be made with metal of any type. The area to be treated must be dry and sufficiently exposed, and the patient should be in a comfortable position to limit movement during the procedure.

Anesthesia with Electrosurgery

Local anesthetics may or may not be used, depending on the method of the electrosurgery and the age and sensitivity of the patient. If a local anesthetic is injected into the patient, the surgeon may use a limited amount of anesthetic so as not to place too much liquid in the tissue that could heat with the passing current. Topical skin freezing with ethyl chloride is sometimes done, but care should be taken in using this flammable substance near an electric spark.

Postoperative Care

The crust resulting from electrosurgery is sterile. Thus, the postoperative application of an antiseptic solution is not necessary, nor is a dressing required if the treatment area is small and superficial. A small, dry gauze dressing or Band-Aid may be applied to protect the area from trauma or for cosmetic reasons. Dressings usually are not advisable, since the crust **in situ** should be kept dry, and a dressing may become moist. The patient should be instructed to keep the area dry, protected from trauma, and clean to prevent infection. A follow-up appointment should be scheduled for 3 to 5 days, so the area may be examined. Further treatment may be required in 2 to 6 weeks.

Care of Electrosurgical Equipment

If there is a break in an electric circuit, electricity will find another path back to the power unit. Breaks in the electric circuit can occur in damaged grounding cables or in the power unit. The grounding cable should be inspected after each surgical procedure. The power unit should be inspected regularly by a qualified engineer, and damaged parts must be replaced immediately. The electrode tips and needles sterilize themselves by means of the electric current, but you will need to keep them clean and polished. Fine steel wool or emery paper may be used for polishing them. The handles and cables may be wiped with alcohol or other germicide. As with all equipment that you must maintain, thoroughly read the manufacturer's instructions.

LASER SURGERY

LASER is the acronym for light amplification by stimulated emission of radiation. The first application of these light waves in medicine was in the treatment of diseases of the retina. Later, its application was expanded to **photocoagulation** therapy, and then to thermal vaporization and coagulation at a microscopic level. Today, laser surgery is used on the most delicate human tissues: the eyes, brain, spinal cord, gastrointestinal tract, and fallopian tubes.

Laser equipment is very expensive and therefore is mostly found in hospitals, but medical offices are beginning to purchase the equipment. There are many types of laser machines, but all are similar in design. They all have an optical tube, a laser medium, reflective mirrors, and an energy source. The principle behind the laser is that light waves stimulate molecules to generate more light waves until an intense beam of light is created that begins to act like matter. This light beam of "matter" exits from the machine and, when it reaches the human tissues, heats the cells to extremely high temperatures. The cells explode and change to carbon and steam. This coagulation and vaporization process can destroy tumors, abnormal cells, strictures, and ulcers.

Safety Precautions

The laser can be as dangerous as it is powerful. A special set of safety precautions is necessary for all personnel operating laser equipment.

- Safety glasses are required for the operators and the patient.
- Do not use flammable, alcohol-based products to prep the patient.
- Keep sterile saline solution available in case the beam accidentally ignites towels or linens.
- Post warning signs on entry doors.

The dangers of the laser include burns, the inhalation of carbon or steam when tissue is subjected to laser beams, and the electric hazards related to high-wattage equipment. Laser light destroys tissue and, improperly handled, can harm not only the patient but also you and the physician. A full laser safety program should be completed before assisting in laser procedures.

Assisting with Laser Surgery

Planning becomes very important when high technology tools are used in surgical procedures. You should have specific training regarding the type of laser to be used, accessory equipment for operating the laser, and safety intervention.

Carbon dioxide laser beams reflect off any shiny instrument surface. Protective supplies such as wet sponges should be available. Suction may be needed to eliminate smoke and debris that accumulate from the lasing process.

During the procedure, your primary function is to observe the field through safety goggles for possible contamination. Keep wet sponges ready. Remove any ignitable item out of the way of the carbon dioxide beam's path, and assist with the suctioning of smoke so the surgeon has a clear visual field. Always have a basin of sterile saline solution and a filled irrigating syringe ready. It may be necessary to cool thermally involved tissue or to extinguish any inadvertent heating of supplies. Watch each application of the beam and anticipate any need for protective supplies, special equipment, or instruments.

LEGAL AND ETHICAL RESPONSIBILITIES

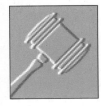

In the surgical setting, medical assistants realize the full extent of their role as the "patient's advocate" and the "physician's agent." Confirm the fact that the physician has explained the procedure to the patient and that the patient fully understands all aspects of the procedure that will be performed. This means that when the patient signs the consent form, he or she is truly informed. Breaks in technique invite legal action. The medical assistant must practice perfect aseptic technique, which protects both the patient and the surgeon.

Confidentiality of patient privacy plays a major role. Discussing a procedure with friends can have serious consequences for both the assistant and the surgeon.

▶ PATIENT EDUCATION

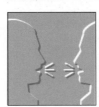

Many minor surgical procedures previously performed in the hospital are now being done in the medical office or clinic. As insurance companies continue to recognize the cost-effectiveness of performing minor surgical procedures in medical offices and clinics, the role of the medical assistant continues to increase.

With this shift comes the added responsibility of preparing the patient for the procedure and for postoperative self-care. The medical assistant must be well prepared to explain how the surgeon will perform the procedure. Listen while the surgeon explains the procedure to the patient; then, you should be able to answer any questions the patient may have. In this way, you can reinforce the physician's information and help the patient to feel confident about the care he or she receives.

If the patient wants members of the immediate family to be in the office while the procedure is being preformed, special allowances should be made.

▶ LEARNING ACHIEVEMENTS

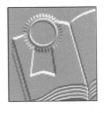

Upon completion of this chapter, can you in the time allowed by your evaluator:

1. Move a sterile item into proper position on the sterile field?
2. Transfer the sterile item to the surgeon's hand without a break in sterile technique?
3. Pour a sterile solution into a bowl or glass that is sitting at the outer perimeter of a sterile field without a break in sterile technique?
4. Drape and prep the skin for a surgical procedure, adhering to the principles of surgical asepsis, patient safety, and patient comfort?

5. Open a sterile linen pack without a break in sterile technique?

6. Put on a pair of sterile gloves without contaminating them?

7. Open a sterile pack and add its contents to a sterile field?

8. Add sterile prepackaged items to a sterile field without a break in technique?

9. Assist in the passing of suture materials and skin closure without delay to the surgeon?

10. Assist with a minor surgical procedure?

11. Remove sutures from a healed incision without injury to the patient?

REFERENCES AND READINGS

Anderson, R. M., and Romfh, R. F.: *Technique in the Use of Surgical Tools,* New York, Appleton-Century-Crofts, 1980.

Bonewit, K.: *Clinical Procedures for Medical Assistants,* 3rd ed., Philadelphia, W.B. Saunders Co., 1990.

Fuller, J.R.: *Surgical Technology: Principles and Practice,* 2nd ed., Philadelphia, W.B. Saunders Co., 1986.

Grewe, H.E., and Kremer, K.: *Atlas of Surgical Operations,* Philadelphia, W.B. Saunders Co., 1980.

Rice, M. R.: *Law, Liability, and Ethics,* Philadelphia, Delmar Publishers, 1988.

Sabiston, D. C., Jr.: *Textbook of Surgery,* 13th ed., Philadelphia, W.B. Saunders Co., 1986.

CHAPTER THIRTY-SEVEN

—

INTRODUCTION TO CLINICAL PHARMACOLOGY

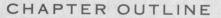

CHAPTER OUTLINE

VOCABULARY

angina pectoris Acute pain in the chest resulting from decreased blood supply to the heart muscles.

cardiotonic Increasing tonicity of the heart.

controlled substance Drugs that are regulated by the federal government (Drug Enforcement Agency).

ion An electrically charged particle.

nomogram Representation by graphs, diagrams, or charts of the relationships between numeric variables.

over-the-counter drugs Medications sold without a prescription.

permeability Ability to allow solutions to pass through a membrane.

synergism Joint action of agents that results in a combined effect that is greater than the effects of the individual components.

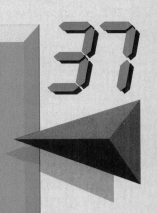

INTRODUCTION TO CLINICAL PHARMACOLOGY

LEARNING OBJECTIVES

COGNITIVE

Upon successful completion of this chapter, you should be able to:

1. Spell and define the words listed in the vocabulary.

2. Differentiate between a drug's generic name and trade name.

3. Cite the dangers of using over-the-counter drugs.

4. List the information needed in each part of a prescription.

5. Cite the Drug Enforcement Agency (DEA) regulations for the storage of guarded substances.

6. List the DEA regulations for prescription drugs under each of the five schedules of the Controlled Substance Act.

7. Define the major types of drug dependency.

8. Cite the clinical uses of drugs.

9. Recall the five steps that describe the fate of a drug in the human body.

10. Cite factors that influence the effect of a drug in the body.

11. Describe the use of the *Physicians' Desk Reference.*

PERFORMANCE

Upon successful completion of this chapter, you should be able to:

1. Calculate the correct dosage for drug administration using one system of measurement.

2. Calculate the correct dosage for drug administration using two systems of measurement.

3. Calculate the correct dosage for a child when only an adult medication is available.

4. Calculate the correct dosage for administration using body weight.

This chapter provides an overview and an introduction to the basic concepts of clinical pharmacology. *Pharmacology* is the broad science that deals with the origin, nature, chemistry, effects, and uses of drugs. *Clinical pharmacology* deals with the biologic effects a drug has on the patient when used as a medical treatment. It covers the actions of a drug in the body over a period of time, including the rate at which body tissues absorb a drug; where a drug is distributed or localizes in the tissues; the chemical changes of the drug that occur in the body; the specific effects a drug has on the body; the route by which a drug is excreted; and, finally, *toxicity,* which is a drug's poisonous effect.

As a result of the rapid, technical advances in drug therapy and biochemistry, the importance of how the body deals with a drug is now emphasized more than the specific effects that a drug has on the body. As a medical assistant, you should have a general understanding of the types of drugs that are available. For every drug that you administer, you should know the functional changes that particular drug brings about in the body. That is, you should know the drug's *effect* and how the body absorbs, uses, and eliminates the drug, which is the *fate* of a drug. With the advent of new drugs and with information on what happens to drugs once they are in the human body being discovered almost daily, you will continually need to update your knowledge of the specific drugs used in your particular practice. Your role as the person responsible for administering medications and instructing patients on drug administration may change from time to time, but you must always assist the physician, and sometimes the pharmacist, in providing safe drug therapy for the patients.

HISTORY AND BACKGROUND
Drug Sources

Some drugs have been with us since ancient times. Written recipes using opium, castor oil, alcohol, and iron have been found on Egyptian papyrus and Sumerian clay tablets dating back to 2000 BC. In medieval times, drugs derived from plants included belladonna (used to treat gastrointestinal disorders), ipecac (used to induce vomiting and now in many cough medicines), and digitalis (used in the treatment of cardiac disorders). The South American Indians have used quinine for reducing fevers and curare, a skeletal muscle relaxant, as an arrow poison for centuries.

Today, pharmacology has become a science, and the drug industry is able to isolate the chemical components of natural drugs and manufacture them synthetically, in a form purer than the plant counterpart. The development of pure drugs enables the administration of drugs to be exact, establishing dose-response relationships, that is, knowing exactly how much of a particular drug is needed to bring about a desired effect.

Natural Sources

Drugs can be obtained from the leaf, seed, sap, stem, or root of certain plants. For example, digitalis is an extract from the leaf of the purple foxglove *(Digitalis purpurea);* opium comes from the unripe capsules of the opium poppy *(Papaver somniferum);* ipecac, from roots of the *Cephaelis ipecacuanha;* and quinine, from the bark of the cinchona tree. As far back as the Stone Age, humans prepared extracts, fluid extracts, and tinctures from plants. *Alkaloids* are the nitrogenous chemicals extracted from plants and, in pure medicinal form, are quite potent. Although there are exceptions, drugs whose names end in "ine" are alkaloids. Morphine and atropine are examples. *Glycosides* are the sugars, such as glucose, extracted from plants, and their names usually end in "in" (for example, digoxin and digitoxin). Other products of plants include oils, such as castor oil; volatile oils, such as peppermint and clove; gums, used as soothing lotions or suspending agents; resins, such as pine; and tannins, used as protective coatings over burns.

Animals are another natural drug source and often supply replacement hormones for human therapy. Animal fats are used as bases for ointments. Insulin is a hormone extracted from the cells of the beef or sheep pancreas, and thyroid extract is obtained from the thyroid glands of some animals that are slaughtered for food. Some antibiotics come from substances that are excreted or secreted by bacteria, yeasts, and molds.

Minerals also supply a wide variety of natural drugs, such as sodium chloride and potassium, dietary replacements, and mineral oil.

Synthetic Sources

Early in the 19th century, chemists began isolating and extracting the pure principles from crude plant extracts. The first extraction of a pure form of a plant principle was morphine, discovered in 1805. This advance made dosage control possible. Further advances resulted in synthetic drugs, which are chemicals that duplicate the physical properties of natural substances. Synthetic drugs often can eliminate the many side effects that occur with natural substances and have increased *potency* (power). Oral insulin is one example of a synthetic replacement of a natural substance. Another is aspirin. In the late 19th century, a chemist experimenting with synthetic quinine accidentally discovered salicylates. Another chemist later discovered that coating salicylates with acetic acid made a safer form of salicylate. Thus, acetylsalicylic acid, or aspirin, was invented. Most drugs manufactured today are the controlled, more potent, synthesized substances that duplicate or replace the outdated, less reliable natural sources.

Drug Names

A single drug may have up to four different names:

- An organic name
- A chemical name
- A generic name
- A trade name

Some drugs have the same name in more than one of these categories. As an example, the various names of the **cardiotonic** drug digitalis follow.

Organic Name

This is the species name for a natural substance. *Digitalis purpurea* is a genus of herbs commonly called the purple foxglove whose leaves furnish digitalis.

Chemical Name

The chemical name of a drug represents its exact formula and is frequently difficult to understand. The chemical formula for digitalin, the digitalis glycoside extracted from the leaves, is $C_{36}H_{56}O_{14}$, with a hexose sugar name of 6-*desoxy*-D-allose, $CH_3(CHOH_3)CH$ (O-CH_3)-CHO. Chemical names are used by chemists and manufacturers. You will not need to know the formulas for drugs.

Generic Name

The generic name is the common name of the chemical or drug, and it is usually descriptive of a drug's chemical structure. This name is not owned by any particular company. It is nonproprietary, that is, not protected by a trademark. In this example, *digitalis* is the generic name.

Consumer group efforts have resulted in legislation in several states requiring pharmacists to fill prescriptions with generic forms of prescribed drugs rather than with the more expensive brand names, unless the physician specifically states a substitute is not acceptable. These groups claim that the less expensive generic products are the same as the more well-known brand names. Studies now show that generic substitutes may not always be chemically equivalent to certain name brands and that some generic drugs may not be as reliable as their name brand counterparts. Further testing and studies are being performed to resolve some of the controversy concerning equivalent formulations of products among various manufacturers and the high costs of name brand medications.

Trade (Brand) Name

The trade name is the name by which a particular manufacturer identifies the drug. A drug will have a different trade name with each pharmaceutical company that manufactures it. The trade names for digitalis include *Crystodigin* and *Purodigin*.

Drug Regulation

Drugs are regulated and controlled in their manufacture and distribution by the federal government. Basically, these regulations govern the following four areas of drug production:

- Drug development and evaluation before release for human use
- Drug quality and standardization
- Dispensing and administering drugs
- Drug use

Drug Development and Evaluation

The Food and Drug Administration (FDA) is an agency of the United States Department of Health and Human Services. It makes mandatory the testing of all drugs before release to the public. Testing includes toxicity tests in laboratory animals, then clinical studies in a controlled group of voluntary patients. A manufacturer must prove not only the safety of a drug but also its effectiveness. A drug that is safe but cannot be proved to have an advantageous effect on the human body will not be approved by the FDA. When all the phases of the preclinical and clinical studies pass investigation, the FDA will approve a new drug for marketing. Only one of ten new drugs ever reaches the clinical testing phase. Very few new drugs reach the consumer. After approval, a manufacturer must continue to demonstrate a drug's effectiveness and safety and must submit reports whenever unexpected adverse reactions are discovered. If there is evidence that an approved drug no longer appears safe or effective, the FDA may suspend or withdraw the drug from manufacture and distribution at any time.

Drug Quality and Standardization

Manufacturing standards are established by the FDA to ensure the proper identity, strength, purity, and quality of drugs shipped in interstate commerce, which includes nearly all the drugs that we encounter in the medical office. Every manufacturer must consistently do the following:

- Identify every drug by a particular color, form, shape, size, and label.
- Produce every dose at the same tested strength.
- Produce the exact formula approved by the FDA.
- Use ingredients that are free from contaminants and of the highest quality.

Dispensing and Administering Drugs

There are two methods of dispensing drugs: **over the counter** (OTC) and by prescription. Over-the-counter drugs are available to the public for self-medication. These drugs have been approved by the FDA and are considered safe for patients to use without the physician's advice.

OVER-THE-COUNTER DRUGS. As a health care worker who is directly involved in patient care, you should have an understanding of some basic facts regarding OTC drugs. Patients today are better informed about their personal health care and want to be active participants in health care decisions. They need facts to make informed choices when using OTC preparations. There is a trend toward making prescription drugs in controlled strengths available in OTC preparations. Most OTC preparations are safe if used as directed; however, the effectiveness of many OTC preparations has not been proved. It is not cost-effective for a woman with recurrent yeast infections to seek medical help for each recurrence when she herself is able to recognize the symptoms. Vaginal creams such as Monistat 7 are now available OTC for the treatment of such infections. OTC drugs also include drugs such as Benadryl, Motrin, and Dimetapp, which several years ago were available by prescription only. Facts that patients need to be familiar with are:

- OTC products provide safe minimal dosages that may have little therapeutic benefit.
- Many OTC products contain more than one active ingredient, which may not be desirable to the patient.
- Self-treatment with OTC products may mask symptoms and cause an aggravation of the problem.
- Patients may self-medicate and avoid professional medical care when it is needed.
- Multiple-drug interactions can lead to adverse reactions and even to toxicity.

PRESCRIPTION DRUGS. Federal law makes drugs that are dangerous, powerful, or habit-forming illegal to use except under a physician's order. A *prescription* is an order written by the physician for the compounding or dispensing and administration of drugs to a particular patient. Sometimes an order may be written for the medical assistant on the patient's medical record or to a nurse on the pa-

tient's chart. However, a prescription most often needs a written order on a prescription blank for the pharmacist to fill. A prescription must be given, and signed, by the physician, or the order cannot be carried out. There are four parts to a prescription, as follows:

- *Superscription:* Patient's name and address, the date, and the symbol ℞ (Latin for recipe, meaning "take").
- *Inscription:* Names and quantities of the ingredients.
- *Subscription:* Directions for compounding. Prescription writing is not as complicated for the physician as in earlier times because pharmaceutical manufacturers now prepare most medications ready for dispensing or administration. Rarely will a pharmacist have to compound or mix a medication.
- *Signature:* Directions for the patient. It is usually preceded by the symbol S (for the Latin *signa,* meaning "mark"). This is where the physician indicates what instructions are to be put on the label to tell the patient how, when, and in what quantities to use the medication.

Prescription directions may be in English or Latin. Set terms and abbreviations are used—a medical shorthand of sorts. It is easier to write "tab. 1 t.i.d. c. aq. p.c." than "one tablet three times each day with water after meals." A typical prescription is shown in Figure 37-1.

The medical assistant does not write prescriptions but must know prescription terms and abbreviations to communicate with the physician and the pharmacist and to administer medications by written order. The more common terms and abbreviations are listed in Table 37-1. Keep all prescription pads safe and out of view of the public.

Drug Use

Before the first law regulating the sale of foods and drugs in the United States was enacted in 1906, the consumer did not know the actual ingredients of foods and drugs. Cough medications contained excessive amounts of codeine. Vitamin and mineral supplements contained high levels of alcohol. A popular soft drink contained cocaine as its active ingredient. Over the years, more than 50 pieces of legislation have been enacted to control the dispensing and administration of drugs.

Today, narcotics and various other substances are controlled and regulated by the Drug Enforcement Agency (DEA), a branch of the Justice Department. The DEA regulates drugs under five schedules of controlled substances, known as Schedules I, II, III, IV, and V. Drugs are listed under a particular schedule, based on their abuse potential and medical usefulness. These schedules not only list the drugs regulated by each category, but also address regulations concerning the writing, telephoning, and refilling of prescriptions, and the storage and maintenance of drugs. Every medical practice should have a copy of the controlled substances regulations. The medical assistant may secure this list from a regional office of the DEA. It is also important to be on the DEA's mailing list to receive updates as drugs are added or deleted, or moved from one schedule to another.

SCHEDULE I. Schedule I includes substances that have no accepted medical use and a high potential for abuse. The possession of these drugs is illegal. Drugs included in this schedule are heroin, lysergic acid diethylamide (LSD), marijuana, mescaline, and peyote.

SCHEDULE II. Schedule II includes various narcotics such as opium, the opium derivatives (e.g., morphine), and the synthetic opium derivatives (e.g., synthetic morphine and methadone); stimulants, such as cocaine and amphetamines; and the commonly abused depressant barbiturates. To write these prescriptions, a physician must have a special license (DEA number). The prescription must be entirely handwritten by the physician on Federal Triplicate Order Forms imprinted with the DEA number or with the DEA number written in by the physician. These prescriptions must be filled within 72 hours and may not be refilled. In an emergency, a physician may telephone a Schedule II order to the pharmacist. However, the amount of the drug must be limited, and the physician must furnish to the pharmacy, within 72 hours, a written, signed prescription for the drug prescribed. If these drugs are kept in the medical office, they must be stored under lock and key and routinely counted and inventoried. The law requires that a dispensing record be kept on file for 2 years (or as otherwise specified by state law) and be subject to inspection by the DEA. The record must include the following:

- Full name and address of the patient
- Date of order
- Name, dosage form, and quantity of the drug
- Method (administered or dispensed)

SCHEDULE III. Schedule III includes the lesser abused combination drugs that contain limited quantities of codeine, narcotic substances, or amphetamine-like substances. The physician must handwrite the prescription, but a DEA number is not required. Refills, up to five in any 6-month period, are allowed, but they must be indicated on the original prescription order. When changes or additions are made by telephone, the physician must directly communicate with the pharmacist, and a written prescription order confirming the telephone request should be forwarded to the pharmacist as soon as possible.

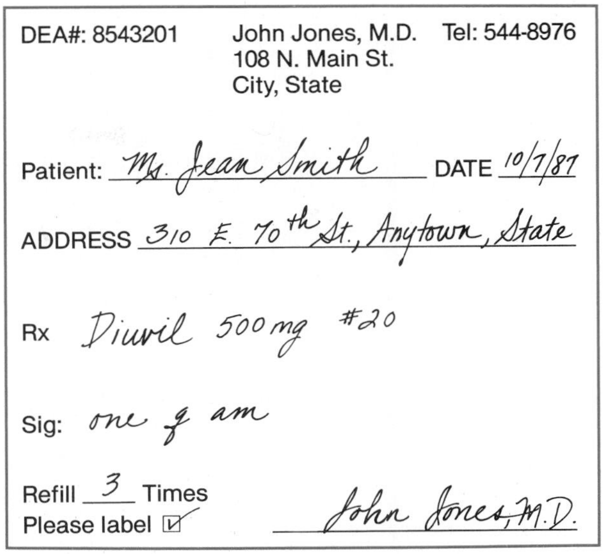

DEA#: 8543201   John Jones, M.D.   Tel: 544-8976
108 N. Main St.
City, State

Patient: *Ms. Jean Smith* _____ DATE *10/7/87*

ADDRESS *310 E. 70th St., Anytown, State*

Rx *Diuvil 500 mg #20*

Sig: *one g am*

Refill _*3*_ Times

Please label ☑   *John Jones, M.D.*

FIGURE 37–1. A sample prescription.

SCHEDULE IV. Schedule IV includes the minor tranquilizers and hypnotics that have a lesser potential for abuse. Prescriptions may be handwritten by the medical assistant under the physician's direction, but the physician must sign them. Up to five refills are allowed within a 6-month period. Requests for refills may be telephoned to the pharmacist by the medical assistant under order of the physician, but the physician should record the order on the patient's medical record. Schedule IV drugs include meprobamate (Equanil), chlordiazepoxide (Librium), diazepam (Valium), flurazepam (Dalmane), chloral hydrate, and the non-narcotic analgesic propoxyphene (Darvon).

SCHEDULE V. Schedule V includes miscellaneous mixtures containing limited amounts of narcotic drugs. Prescription orders and refills are the same as for Schedule IV drugs. Examples are most cough medications containing codeine and some drugs used for gastrointestinal disorders, such as Donnagel and diphenoxylate (Lomotil). In addition, all inventory records require the physician's name, address, DEA registration number, date of inventory, and the signature of the person taking the inventory.

All **controlled substances** must be stored in a safe or immovable locked cabinet. Prescription forms should be kept out of areas that are used by patients and preferably secured in an area that prohibits unauthorized or illegal use. The DEA Prescription Form 222 and the state triplicate forms also need to be kept in a locked area. Because of the increase in office thefts, many offices do not keep controlled substances in the office. If there is a loss of drugs, it must be reported to the regional DEA

TABLE 37-1. COMMON PRESCRIPTION ABBREVIATIONS

Abbreviation	Meaning	Abbreviation	Meaning	Abbreviation	Meaning
a.a.	of each	MS	morphine sulfate	SC	subcutaneous
a.c.	before meals	MTD	maximum tolerated dose	sub-q.	subcutaneous
ad lib.	as desired	NPO	nothing by mouth	s̄s̄	one-half
agit.	shake, stir	noct.	at night	stat.	immediately
a.m.	morning	N/S	normal saline	t.i.d.	three times a day
amp.	ampule	O₂	oxygen	tinct.	tincture
a.u.	each ear	OD	overdose	TO	telephone order
a.d.	right ear	OD	right eye	tus.	cough
a.s.	left ear	OS	left eye	U	unit
aq.	water	OU	both eyes	vag.	vagina
b.i.d.	twice a day	OTC	over-the-counter (drugs)	ves.	bladder
c̄.	with	p.c.	after meals	VO	verbal order
cap.	capsule	PL	placebo	W/O	water in oil
DC	discontinue	p.m.	afternoon	cm	centimeter
D.E.A.	Drug Enforcement Administration	PMI	patient medication instruction	mcg, μg	microgram
				mg	milligram
dil.	dilute	per os	by mouth	Gm, g	gram
disp.	dispense	p.r.	per rectum	kg	kilogram
ext.	extract	pulv.	powder	cc	cubic centimeter
F.D.A.	Food and Drug Administration	q.	every	ml	milliliter
fl.	fluid	q.d.	every day	L	liter
h	hour	q.h.	every hour	gr	grain
h.s.	at bedtime	q.2h	every 2 hours	dr	dram
inj.	injection	q.3h	every 3 hours	oz	ounce
IM	intramuscular	q.4h	every 4 hours	lb	pound
ID	intradermal	q.i.d.	four times a day	m	minim
IV	intravenous	q.m.	every morning	gtt	drops
med.	medicine	q.n.	every night	t, tsp	teaspoon
meq.	milliequivalent	q.o.d.	every other day	T, tbs	tablespoon
MLD	minimum lethal dose	q.s.	quantity sufficient	C	cup, Celsius
mn.	midnight	R	rectal	pt	pint
MO	mineral oil	℞	"take thou"	qt	quart
MOM	milk of magnesia	S, Sig	give the following directions	gal	gallon
MOPV	monovalent oral poliovirus vaccine	s̄	without	F	Fahrenheit

office and local law enforcement authorities immediately.

The expiration dates of medications must be checked on a regular basis, and a medication must be destroyed if its date has expired. *A drug cannot be given or dispensed to a patient after its expiration date.* Accepted methods for destroying different types of expired drugs are as follows:

- Liquids and ointments may be rinsed down the drain.
- Powders should be mixed with water and then flushed down the drain.
- Tablets and capsules should be flushed down the toilet.
- Vials and ampules should be opened and their contents poured down the drain.

As an added safety precaution, *two* employees should be present when drugs are destroyed, and both should sign and date the list of destroyed substances.

Drug Abuse

Any drug from aspirin to alcohol may be misused or abused. Today, there is a tremendous increase in the use of illegal and legal drugs. Nationally, treatment programs are available everywhere for people in all walks of life. Programs include detoxification, rehabilitation, and long-term rehabilitation maintenance. The American Medical Association (AMA) recognizes the problem of drug and alcohol abuse among physicians and other health professionals and has initiated therapy programs for its members. Medical assistants may frequently encounter patients who are misusing or abusing drugs. It is important for you to be alert to the symptoms of drug dependence and to notify the physician when you suspect a patient, or coworker, of having a problem with drug or alcohol dependency.

Drug misuse is the improper use of common drugs that can lead to dependence or toxicity. Examples of persons with chronic dependencies include people who cannot have a bowel movement unless they take a laxative; those who have used nasal decongestants for so long that they cannot breathe without the use of nasal sprays; or those who take so many antacids that they suffer systemic metabolic alkalosis. Alcoholic beverages are used by an estimated 75 million Americans. Even the controlled, social drinker can misuse alcohol and experience nausea, vomiting, a hangover, or dangerous accidents. *Drug abuse* is taking too much of a drug continually or periodically, in a manner that is considered not acceptable behavior by society. Drinking alcohol socially is acceptable. Drinking on the job is considered abusive. Cigarette smoking is an example of a once-accepted use of nicotine that is more and more being considered a form of drug abuse.

Drug dependency is the advanced stage of drug abuse. Dependency is the inability to function unless under the influence of a substance. *Psychologic dependency* is the compulsive craving for the effects of a substance. *Habituation* is a milder form of psychologic dependency. In this case, a person forms a habit of using a substance even to the detriment of physical health and well-being. Drinking coffee and soft drinks that contain caffeine and smoking cigarettes are common examples of habituation. *Physical dependency* is a person's need for a substance to avoid physical discomfort. This type of dependency occurs when abused substances produce biochemical changes, usually in the nervous system tissues. Discontinuing a substance that causes physical dependency creates the withdrawal syndrome. *Addiction* is a term that is now too broad to have any real meaning and is being replaced by the term *dependency.*

The following five types of drugs are the most commonly abused:

- The potent narcotic analgesics, such as heroin and morphine
- Depressant drugs, such as the barbiturates, sedatives, hypnotics, and anti-anxiety agents
- Psychomotor stimulants, such as cocaine and amphetamines
- Hallucinogens and psychosis-imitating drugs, such as LSD, mescaline, and peyote
- *Cannabis* derivatives, such as marijuana and hashish.

Regardless of the type of drug abused, it will have two effects on the person: acute and chronic. The acute effect is what the person feels when *intoxicated,* or directly under the influence of a particular substance. The chronic effects include the temporary or permanent physical and mental changes that result from long-term abuse.

The medical assistant often is called upon to answer patient questions concerning drug abuse and problems. You should read and keep up to date on the drug-related issues of our society. You should also have available for patients pamphlets and agency referral names for each of the five types of commonly abused drugs previously listed.

DRUG INTERACTIONS WITH THE BODY

The study of pharmacology used to focus on the *desired effect* a drug has on the human body, that is, the so-called end result. Now, knowledge of what happens to a drug while it is in the body (that is, the *fate* of the drug) is more important than the drug's effect, which we also know is often far from the drug's "end result." This shift has more value because we know that different patients react to the same dose of a drug in very different ways and that the same patient may react to the same dose of a drug differently at various times. Simply knowing the effect of a drug does not ensure the safety of the patient.

Uses of Drugs

Drugs may be called pharmaceuticals, medicines, or medications. As a form of therapy (that is, the treatment of disease by medicines), drugs occupy a prominent position. However, drugs also are used for other than therapeutic purposes. The uses of drugs include:

- **Therapeutic:** Used to cure a disease, such as antibiotics used to cure bacterial infections
- **Palliative:** Used to relieve the symptoms of a disease, such as pain relievers.
- **Preventive:** Used to prevent a condition, such as Dramamine for motion sickness
- **Replacement:** Used to replace or supplement what the body is not producing, such as insulin for the diabetic or vitamins and minerals.
- **Diagnostic:** Used to aid in the diagnosis of a disease or condition, such as dyes used in radiography examinations.

Generally, therapeutic drugs either eradicate foreign substances from the body, such as antibiotics destroying pathogens, or interfere with the functioning of the patient's own cells, tissues, or organs. This interference always has the potential to be poisonous to the body. However, the object of *rational drug therapy* is to control the degree of interference and to bring about the desired effect without any adverse, or *untoward*, effects.

Most drugs that affect the body tissues either bring about stimulation (increased activity) or depression (decreased activity). Some drug reactions are much more complicated: a drug may increase activity at the cellular level, which, in turn, decreases the activity of a particular organ, or vice versa. For example, a drug may decrease the nerve impulse transmission of certain cells in the heart, resulting in an increased heart rate. Some drugs stimulate one area of the body while depressing another. Morphine depresses the cough mechanism yet increases the mechanism that causes vomiting. Epinephrine (adrenalin) decreases (constricts) the openings of the blood vessels yet increases (dilates) the opening of the bronchial tubes.

Although most drugs can ultimately be classified as stimulants or depressants of some area of the body (especially the central nervous system), it is important to know how and where a drug affects the body, as well as what the drug does. Many drugs bring about the same effect, but in different ways from different parts of the body. For example, many drugs reduce blood pressure. Some act by depressing or stimulating central nervous system sites; some by relaxing the smooth muscle in the vessels in the heart; and others by decreasing the total fluid volume in the tissues. The end result, or effect, of all these methods is the same; a decreased blood pressure. However, each method is very different. Pain can be relieved by drugs acting in different ways at different sites. Some pain relievers act by relaxing smooth muscle spasms (antispasmodics); others block sensory nerve impulses to an area (local anesthesia); and still others dull the general senses of a patient so that an awareness of pain is lost (analgesics or general anesthesia).

People differ greatly in their reactions to drugs. Knowledge of how and where a drug produces its effect helps the physician to know which type of drug to use and when two or more drugs may be used for a more advantageous effect called **synergism** or synergistic effect. For example, treating a hypertensive patient with two drugs may be of more value than therapy with just one drug.

The Fate of Drugs

By knowing how the body handles a drug and what happens to the drug in the body, we can know the *onset* of a drug's activity (beginning), when its *intensity* is likely to peak, the *critical concentration* (the minimum amount of chemical necessary in the fluids that bathe the tissues for the tissues to respond to the drug), and the *duration* of a particular drug's activity. All these facts help to determine the dosage form, dosage amount, route, and frequency of administration of medications. The fate of a drug includes the following:

- **Absorption:** How a drug is absorbed into the body's circulating fluids, known as the *routes*
- **Distribution:** How a drug is transported from the site of administration to the various points in the body
- **Action:** What changes the drug causes once it has reached its destination
- **Biotransformation:** How the drug is inactivated, including the time it takes for a drug to be *detoxified* and broken down into byproducts
- **Excretion:** The route by which a drug is excreted, or eliminated, and the amount of time such a process requires

Drug Absorption

What happens to a drug from the time it is administered until it reaches the bloodstream is the first factor in determining the route of drug administration. An important point to remember is that no matter where a drug is absorbed, it can have one of two actions on the body: *local* (restricted to one spot or part; not general) or *systemic* (affecting the body as a whole). However, most drugs are used for their systemic effects. Even when drugs are used for local purposes, we know that none remains truly localized in the body. Any chemical that comes into contact with even the most superficial surface, such as the skin, has the potential to be absorbed into the bloodstream and to circulate to other tissues and organs. When we decide whether a drug is local or systemic, we should be thinking more of its intended use rather than its effect on the human organism.

ORAL ROUTE. Oral medications are convenient, safe, and inexpensive. However, drugs that can be destroyed in any way by the digestive tract must be given by injection. Injections are rapid but increase the danger of overdose or possible infection. The majority of oral medications are absorbed by the small intestine, but a few are absorbed more rapidly in the stomach. After absorption into the bloodstream from the small intestine, drugs are carried to the liver. In this organ, much of the drug's potency is inactivated before it circulates to the tissues. This inactivation by the liver often makes it necessary to administer higher dosages orally than when given by injection.

Food slows the absorption of drugs. Therefore, many medications are best prescribed 1 hour before or 2 hours after the ingestion of food. Food may also bind the drugs to them or in some other way destroy a drug. Tetracyclines, for example, are destroyed by milk products and antacids containing calcium salts. Patients on tetracycline should be advised not to eat dairy products or take liquid or solid forms of antacids.

The stomach acids present during digestion alone may destroy certain drugs. Because some drugs are destroyed by the components of the digestive tract or irritate the empty lining of the stomach, many oral drugs are *enteric-coated* to keep them intact for passage into the small intestine or to prevent gastric irritation or vomiting.

Some drugs are not affected by the digestive processes but cannot be absorbed through the intestinal walls into the bloodstream. For example, neomycin has no effect when taken orally (unless it is used to "sterilize" the bowel itself prior to bowel surgery). Other drugs may be unable to cross the bowel mucosa because of their poor solubility in lipids (fats), or they are inactivated by the pH of the gastrointestinal (GI) tract.

It is important to remember these absorption factors when administering medication by the oral route. If a patient has responded to a drug previously but is no longer responding, it may be important to question the patient's food-medication cycle. It could be that the patient is no longer taking the medication on an empty stomach as directed.

PARENTERAL ROUTE. Parenteral means "beside the digestive tract" and is the term for administering drugs by injection (hypodermically, under the skin). The parenteral route is the surest and fastest one, but there are several factors that determine its effectiveness.

The first is the amount of blood supply to the site of injection. The absorption of a drug in an aqueous (water) solution is faster in an area with more blood vessels. Therefore, drugs deposited in the muscle will be absorbed faster than drugs deposited in the upper layers of the subcutaneous tissues. The *intramuscular route* (IM) is chosen in an emergency for fast action or when larger amounts of the medication must be absorbed. The *subcutaneous route* (SC, or sub-cu) is chosen when a slower, prolonged effect is desired.

A second way that parenteral drug absorption may be controlled is physically. A drug's absorption may be quickened by hand massage after injection. Absorption may be slowed by injecting the drug in a physical form that slows absorption. One way of slowing the absorption of a drug and, therefore, increasing the duration of its effect is to suspend the drug in a solution that prolongs absorption, such as colloidal substances, fatty substances (oil), insoluble salts or esters, and epinephrine (adrenalin), which acts by constricting the blood vessels, thus retarding circulation and absorption. Insulin is suspended in protamine, which is a water-soluble protein extracted from the sperm of certain fish. Heparin is suspended in gelatin. Penicillin G is suspended with procaine (hydrochloride) salts. Aqueous drugs suspended in these substances slowly dissolve in the tissues over a long time, and the patient can be spared costly, frequent, and sometimes painful injections. Local anesthetics are sometimes mixed with epinephrine to keep the anesthetics and their effects in an area longer.

The third parenteral route is *intravenous* (IV), which is directly into the vein. This route is instantaneous and can be dangerously irreversible. Because of the dangers of intravenous administration, only those members of the medical team who are licensed to do so may inject medication intravenously. *The medical assistant is not licensed to perform the intravenous administration of medications to patients.* Because IV administration is so dangerous, medications given by IV are usually administered in small doses through an intravenous infusion (IV drip) to prevent toxic effects in the brain or the heart. Sometimes, an accidental overdose can be slowed by the application of a tourniquet between the injection site and the heart or the application of ice packs to the site. Both methods can constrict the blood vessels and retard the flow of the drug through the circulatory system.

Other forms of parenteral routes include the *intradermal* injection, which is below the skin but superficial to the subcutaneous tissues. This route is used mostly for allergy testing and skin testing (see Chapter 31). *Intrathecal,* or *intraspinal,* injections are used for spinal anesthesia and administering certain antibiotics into the spine for the treatment of meningitis. *Intra-articular* or *intralesional* injections are used for administering steroids into joints and lesions, or anticancer drugs into cancerous tumors.

MUCOUS MEMBRANE ABSORPTION. Drugs may be absorbed by the mucous membranes of the mouth, throat, nose, eyes, rectum, vagina, and the respiratory and urinary tracts. Some applications have a local effect, such as nasal sprays, eye drops, and a rectal suppository for constipation. Others have a systemic effect, such as a rectal suppository to control vomiting or a nitroglycerin tablet dissolved under the tongue (sublingual) to dilate the blood vessels and relieve the pain of **angina pectoris.** *Inhalation* is used to concentrate drugs locally in the lower respiratory passages or to produce systemic effects such as general anesthesia.

TOPICAL ABSORPTION. These routes include the application of medications to the skin, eyes, and ears. Most drugs are not absorbed by the outer layers of the skin. However, drugs in ointments, creams, lotions, and aerosols can be applied for the treatment of skin itching, inflammation, or other discomforts and for the treatment of skin infections with antibiotics. Nitroglycerin (for angina) and dimenhydrinate (Dramamine, for motion sickness) are two drugs that can be absorbed through the skin for systemic effects. *Dermal patches* containing these medications can be taped to the body for a slow, prolonged time-release of the drugs.

Drug Distribution

Once a drug is absorbed, it must be transported by the circulatory system to the area where it will have its effect. In the bloodstream, drugs can attach to plasma proteins and then be freed to pass from the blood into the site of action. Drugs are then carried through the fluids bathing the cells into the cells of the tissues and organs. The amount of blood supply to a part affects the speed with which drugs reach certain tissues. The high degree of blood circulating through the brain, heart, liver, and kidneys ensures that drugs will be concentrated in these areas rapidly. Drugs accumulate much more slowly in muscle, fat, and bone tissues.

The blood-brain barrier is a functional barrier between the brain cells and the capillaries circulating blood through the brain. This barrier determines which substances can cross. For the substances that can, it regulates the degree and rate of their absorption into the brain tissue. The general anesthetic thiopental sodium (Pentothal Sodium) is able to cross the blood-brain barrier immediately and produces sleep within seconds, whereas other sleep-producing drugs, such as the barbiturates, cross slowly and may take as long as 30 minutes to 1 hour to produce the same effect. While these drugs remain in the body, they may cross the blood-brain barrier several times, being redistributed to the rest of the body's tissues, then returning to the brain tissue. This is why some patients go back and forth between sleep and wakefulness.

Drugs can be distributed to the fetus of a pregnant woman by blood circulation exchange. Therefore, drugs of all types should be avoided during pregnancy. Some drugs may attach to and accumulate in bone tissue, which may interfere with normal growth and development. Tetracycline is an example. Distribution of this drug to the unborn fetus or a young infant may lead to its accumulation on the teeth and later discoloration of the tooth enamel. For the most part, this is a problem of the deciduous teeth (first set). However, administering tetracyclines to older children can cause a brownish discoloration of the permanent teeth.

Drug Action

No one theory explains why drugs act the way they do. The following is a general summary of the various theories of drug action:

- Drugs are believed to combine with body chemicals on the cell surface or within the cell itself. Correct cells are chosen because a particular drug has a *specific affinity* for a particular cell. The specific cell recipient is called a *receptor,* and the drug that has the affinity for it and produces a function change in the cell is called the *agonist.*
- Not all drugs that bind to specific cells cause a functional change in the cell. These drugs act as an *antagonist* to the natural process, and work by *blocking* a sequence of biochemical events.
- Some drugs are believed to act by affecting the enzyme functions of the body. Drugs attach to enzyme substances and rob the enzymes from cells. As a result, the enzyme products needed for normal cellular function are not supplied, and the cell fails to function properly.
- Certain anti-infective drugs have a *selected toxicity* for pathogens or parasites that have invaded the body. Penicillin and sulfonamides work because they poison, or interfere with the life processes of, bacteria without affecting the life processes of normal human cells. Research scientists continue to look for differences between cancer cells and normal cells to enable them to apply the principle of selected toxicity in cancer treatment. Most of the anticancer drugs in use today are not selectively toxic, and normal human cells are also poisoned by the cancer drugs.
- Both drugs that have a selective affinity for cells and those that bind with enzymes can be counteracted by administering large amounts of the natural substances with which the drugs

compete. This process is known as administering an *antidote* to a drug that may be acting as a poison.

- Some drugs alter the function of cells by affecting the physical properties of the cell membrane rather than altering the biochemical processes within the cell itself. This is especially true of drugs that affect nerve cells, such as anesthetics and alcohol. A change in the cell membrane changes the **permeability** of the membrane, which, in turn, changes the flow of **ions** in and out of the cells. This change in ion flow changes the polarity (opposite effects at two extremities, the two extremities being inside and outside the cell membrane) on which nerve pulses are conducted and produces general sleep or stupor.

Biotransformation of Drugs

This is the process by which drugs are converted into harmless byproducts. These byproducts are then more easily eliminated by the kidneys. Most drugs are broken down by the enzyme activity of the liver. The ability to break down the chemical components of a drug varies among individuals. Factors that determine this ability include age, the presence of other drugs, and liver disease. In some patients on long-term drug therapy, a drug may overstimulate the enzyme activity of the liver. This results in a too rapid destruction of the drug, and the patient has to take larger and larger doses for the drug to be effective. This situation is called *tolerance*.

Excretion of Drugs

The kidneys are the most important route for the elimination of drugs. Most drugs are filtered out of the circulation, broken down into harmless particles, and then excreted in the urine. Because the kidneys are so important in the elimination of drugs from the body, drug therapy must be carefully monitored in patients with kidney disease or malfunction. Drugs are also eliminated through the sweat glands and saliva and in bile. Exhalation, another mechanism for drug elimination, is the basis for measuring alcohol concentrations in the blood by the breathalyzer test. Drugs may be eliminated through the milk glands of the lactating mother, which means a woman breastfeeding a child has to be extremely careful about taking medications.

Factors That Influence the Effect of a Drug

As stated earlier, different people react to the same dose of medication in different ways, and the same patient can react to the same dose of the same drug differently on various occasions. The following factors are important in determining the correct medication for a patient.

Body Weight

A person's weight has a direct relationship with the effects of medication. Basically, the same dosage has a greater effect on a person who weighs less and a lesser effect on a patient who weighs more. Manufacturers of adult medications calculate dosages based on a normal adult weight (approximately 150 pounds). Sometimes, the physician will adjust the dosage to better suit the patient's body size. Pediatric medications are designed for the body weight or body surface area of children. If adult medications are used for children, the correct dosage must be calculated and adjusted for the child's body weight.

Age

In the newborn and the very elderly, age has its greatest effect on the body's response to a drug. This usually has to do with immature or deteriorating body systems. In addition, both groups are particularly sensitive to drugs that affect the central nervous system and to toxicity. Dosage calculations for these two groups must be carefully decided, and therapy usually begins with very small doses.

Sex

Drugs may affect men and women differently. As previously mentioned, the pregnant woman has to be extremely cautious, when taking medications, to avoid damage to the developing fetus. In addition, some drugs have side effects that can stimulate uterine contractions, causing premature labor and delivery. Intramuscular medications are absorbed faster by men. Because women have a higher body fat content and a musculature with less blood supply, intramuscular drugs remain in their tissues longer than in men's tissues. During certain times of the menstrual cycle, the immune response system is suppressed, and antibiotics given at this time may not be as effective as at other times.

Time of Day

Diurnal means "during the day" or "time of light." Diurnal body rhythms play an important part in the effects of some drugs. Sedatives given in the morning will not be as effective as when administered before bedtime, because the central nervous system is more stimulated and more resistant to the effects of the drug. Steroid administration is preferred in the morning because it best mimics the body's natural pattern of steroid production and elimination. Diuretics are best administered in the morning to reduce the need for the patient to get up during the night to void.

Pathologic Factors

Patients may adversely respond to drugs in the presence of liver or kidney disease because the body will not be able to detoxify and excrete chemicals properly. In patients with liver or kidney disease, some drugs may cause unconsciousness or death. Patients with other diseases or disorders may react quite differently than expected. Therefore, a thorough medical history is always required before administering medications. Even temporary pain and fever may alter the expected effect of a drug.

Immune Responses

The presence of a drug can stimulate a patient's immune response, and the patient will develop antibodies to a particular chemical. If the same drug is again administered, the patient will have an allergic reaction to the drug, ranging from a mild reaction to a serious respiratory and circulatory emergency.

Psychologic Factors

People may respond differently to a drug because of the way they feel about the drug. If a patient believes in the therapy, even a *placebo* (sugar pill or sterile water thought to be a drug) may help or bring about relief. A patient's personality can affect whether or not he or she will be cooperative in following the directions for a particular drug, and a patient's negative mind-set, or mental attitude, can reduce an expected response to a drug.

Tolerance

Tolerance is the phenomenon of reduced responsiveness to a drug. *Congenital tolerance* is an inborn resistance. *Acquired tolerance* occurs after taking a particular drug for a period of time. *Cross tolerance* occurs when a patient acquires a tolerance to one drug and becomes resistant to other similar drugs. *Physical dependence* often accompanies tolerance. The body becomes so adapted to the presence of the drug that it cannot function properly without it. To withdraw the drug is to throw the body out of its equilibrium, causing the well-known withdrawal syndrome.

Cumulation

When a drug is taken too frequently to allow for proper elimination, it accumulates in the tissues. The result is a more intense effect and a longer duration. Cumulation can cause overdose and toxicity. Proper dosage and timing of administration are the best prevention of drug accumulation.

Idiosyncrasy

Occasionally, a person reacts to a drug in a manner that is unexpected and peculiar to that individual only. An idiosyncrasy may manifest itself in many different ways, such as a hypnotic drug keeping a person awake, acting as a stimulant to this person rather than as a depressant. Usually, these reactions cannot be explained.

Classifications of Drug Actions

Clinical pharmacology is a complex subject. To make the subject easier, drugs are classified according to their actions on the body (for example, chemotherapeutics or emetics). Drugs also may be classified according to the body system that they affect (for example, drugs acting on the cardiovascular system). The following is a glossary of terms describing some basic drug actions. As you read some of the examples, remember that a drug classified as one type of agent may have other uses and actions on other systems of the body. For example, a drug classified as a diuretic may also be an antihypertensive drug, and a vasodilator may also be a respiratory antispasmodic. It takes time to understand not only the basic classification of a particular drug but also the many secondary uses and effects it has on the human body.

Adrenergic. A drug that acts like epinephrine, a hormone produced by the medulla of the adrenal glands (called adrenaline in Great Britain). It can be administered parenterally, topically, or by inhalation and acts as a vasoconstrictor, antispasmodic, or mimic of any of the effects that natural epinephrine has on the body. Adrenergics are used as emergency heart stimulants and to counteract allergic conditions such as hives and asthma. They are the most effective drug for counteracting the effects of anaphylactic shock. Adrenergic drugs are called *sympathomimetic* because their actions resemble the natural functions of the sympathetic nervous system.

Analgesic. A drug to relieve pain by lessening the sensory function of the brain. Analgesics vary greatly in their ability to relieve pain and range from aspirin to the opium derivatives. For narcotic analgesic examples, see Narcotic.

Analgesic — Antipyretic — Anti-inflammatory. A drug that relieves pain (usually originating in the joints, muscles, teeth, head, skin, and connective tissue), reduces fever (antipyretic), or acts as an anti-inflammatory or antirheumatic. Examples include acetaminophen (Tylenol), aspirin (acetylsalicylic acid), phenylbutazone (Butazolidin), ibuprofen (Advil, Motrin, Nuprin), naproxen (Naprosyn), piroxicam (Feldene), and indomethacin (Indocin).

Anesthetic. A drug used to produce insensibility to pain or the sensation of pain, local or general. *Topical anesthetics* are applied to the surfaces of the skin and mucous membranes and have a local action. *Local anesthetics* are infiltrated (injected into the tissues or nerves), intraspinal, or caudal (injected into the base of the spine). Their effects are local. *General anesthesia* is systemic and produces sleep.

Antibiotic. Agents that are produced both by living organisms and synthetically and are effective against bacterial infections. Some antibiotics are selective and have a *narrow spectrum*. Others have effects on a wide range of microorganisms and are called *broad-spectrum* antibiotics. There are four groups of antibiotics.

1. Those that result in the death of the bacterial cell (bacteriolytic). Examples include the penicillins (Pentids, Bicillin, Amoxil, and Ampicillin), cephalosporins (Keflin, Keflex), and bacitracin.
2. Those that interfere with the genetic production and reproduction of bacteria (bacteriostatic). Examples include the tetracyclines, streptomycin, gentamicin, erythromycin, chloramphenicol, and griseofulvin.
3. Those that dissolve the bacterial cell membranes (bacteriostatic or bacteriocidal). Examples include amphotericin and nystatin.
4. Those that interrupt the bacterial metabolic processes (bacteriostatic). Examples include the sulfonamides, para-aminosalicylic acid (PAS), and isoniazid (INH).

Antidepressant. Several drug groups are used to treat depression, including antidepressants, antipsychotics, antianxiety agents, psychomotor stimulants, and lithium. Antidepressants include amitriptyline HCl (Elavil) and imipramine pamoate (Tofranil).

Antiepileptic. Agent used to reduce the number or severity of epileptic attacks. These agents may be called anticonvulsants. However, convulsions do not occur in all types of seizures. Examples include sedatives and hypnotics (see following), phenytoin (Dilantin), methylphenidate HCl (Ritalin), and, sometimes, dextroamphetamine sulfate (Dexedrine).

Antifungal. Preparations to treat systemic or local fungal infections (mycoses), which include:

1. Those that treat the serious systemic fungal infections that spread to various vital organs via the bloodstream. One example is amphotericin B (Fungizone).
2. Those that are taken orally to treat ringworm-type infections of the skin, hair, and nails. An example is griseofulvin (Fulvicin U/F).
3. Those that are used to treat the yeast-like fungal infections, such as *Candida albicans (moniliasis)* of the vagina, mouth (thrush) or skin. Examples include miconazole (Monistat) and nystatin (Mycostatin).

Antihistamine — Histamine Blocker. An agent used to counteract the effects of histamine. Histamine is a natural substance in the body's tissues that aids in the body's inflammatory response to tissue injury and regulates the secretion of stomach acid. However, when histamine is released, it creates side effects that are the signs and symptoms of allergy, or even anaphylaxis, in certain hypersensitive persons. Antihistamines are used for the relief of allergic disorders, insect-sting reactions, and acute anaphylactic reactions. Because a side effect of antihistamines is drowsiness, they may also be used for sedation or motion sickness prevention. Examples include brompheniramine maleate (Dimetane), chlorpheniramine maleate (Chlor-Trimeton), diphenhydramine HCl (Benadryl, Benylin), and promethazine HCl (Phenergan)

Histamine blockers may be used to inhibit gastric acid secretions in the treatment of upper gastrointestinal problems and peptic ulcers. Examples are cimetidine (Tagamet) and ranitidine (Zantac).

Antihypertensive. A drug used to treat hypertension. There are many drugs for treating hypertension, including the following: diuretics (see following); sympathetic blocking agents (see following), such as atenolol (Tenormin), metoprolol tartrate (Lopressor), nadolol (Corgard); centrally acting agents, such as methyldopa (Aldomet); and vasodilators (see following).

Antispasmodic. An agent that relieves or prevents spasms from musculoskeletal injury or inflammation and from neurologic disorders resulting from central nervous system damage, or spasms of the smooth muscles such as the intestines or the uterus. Examples include methocarbamol (Robaxin) and carisoprodol (Soma), and levodopa (L-dopa).

Antitussive (Cough Suppressant). An agent that suppresses the cough reflex and dries up the secretion and normal discharge of a cough. Examples are dextromethorphan HBr (Romilar), codeine, and terpin hydrate with codeine.

Bronchodilator. An agent used to treat chronic bronchitis, bronchial asthma, and emphysema. Oral medications include aminophylline (Theophylline) and theophylline anhydrous (Theo-Dur). Parenteral medications include epinephrine (Adrenalin, Sus-Phrine). Aerosol inhalation medications include albuterol (Ventolin, Proventil) and isoproterenol HCl (Isuprel).

Carminative. A medication that relieves flatulence and aids in the expulsion of gas from the stomach and intestines. It usually contains a volatile oil or carbonated beverage.

Cathartic. An agent that increases and hastens bowel evacuation (defecation). Commonly called a laxative. The types range from mild laxatives to *purgatives,* which are severe cathartics. Some work by increasing the amount of bulk in the bowel. Others work by irritating the intestinal mucosa, which produces movement.

Chemotherapeutic. Now mostly refers to those chemical substances used to treat cancerous conditions and tumors. However, medically, it is the term for any drug that is used as an agent to treat infections.

Cholinergic. Drugs that act like the parasympathetic nervous system. They function to help restore energy and mimic the natural physiologic process that occurs when acteylcholine (a natural neurotransmitter) stimulates cholinergic nerves to transmit impulses to certain body structures and organs. Cholinergic drugs decrease the heart rate and act on smooth and skeletal muscle. However, because the site of action is so difficult to localize, or target, these drugs have limited clinical usefulness.

Decongestant. A drug that relieves local congestion in the tissues, usually the mucous membranes. The most popular are the nasal decongestants, such as ephedrine or phenylephrine (Neo-Synephrine). Decongestants are often combined with antihistamines.

Diaphoretic. A drug used to induce or increase perspiration.

Digestant. A drug that promotes the progress of digestion. Enzymes, antacids, and bile salts are included in this group.

Diuretic. A drug that increases the function of the kidneys and stimulates the flow of urine. It increases the water content of the blood through osmosis or salt action, freeing water from the tissues and reducing edema. Examples include hydrochlorothiazide (Dyazide, Esidrix, HydroDiuril) and furosemide (Lasix).

Emetic. A drug used to induce vomiting. Ipecac syrup is commonly used, and mild mustard and plain tepid water are home remedies used as emetics.

Expectorant. A drug used to increase the secretions and mucus from the bronchial tubes. It makes a cough more productive (expectoration) and breaks up congestion. Some expectorants are combined with antihistamines. An expectorant has an effect opposite that of a cough suppressant.

Hemostatic. A drug used to control bleeding; a blood coagulant. Absorbable hemostatics are applied directly to a wound, and an artificial clot is formed that is gradually absorbed. Gelfoam and Surgicel are examples.

Hypnotic. A drug that produces sleep and lessens the activity of the brain. A hypnotic has a sedative action when used in smaller doses. The barbiturates, both oral and injectable, are the most common hypnotics: pentobarbital (Nembutal), phenobarbital (Luminal), amobarbital (Amytal), secobarbital (Seconal), and secobarbital and amobarbital (Tuinal).

Hypoglycemic. Drugs used to compensate for a lack of effective insulin activity, such as the prompt-acting and long-acting insulins; or drugs that stimulate the pancreas to release insulin, such as chlorpropamide (Diabinese) and tolbutamide (Orinase).

Miotic. An agent that causes the pupil of the eye to contract.

Mydriatic. An agent used to dilate the pupil of the eye. Used by ophthalmologists in eye examinations.

Narcotic. Any of a group of drugs that depress the central nervous system and cause insensibility or stupor. Natural narcotics include the opium group. Synthetic narcotics include codeine phosphate (methylmorphine), meperidine HCl (Demerol), methadone (Dolophine), morphine sulfate, pentazocine (Talwin), and propoxyphene HCl (Darvon).

Opiate. The habit-forming drugs that are derived from or contain opium, such as morphine, codeine, heroin, papaverine, and tincture of opium (paregoric).

Parasympathetic Blocking Agent. Drugs that are called anticholingeric or cholinergic blocking agents because they block certain effects of acetylcholine (see Cholinergic). These agents include atropine sulfate, dicyclomine HCl (Bentyl), and methscopolamine (Scopolamine). Parasympathetic blocking agents are effective antidotes to cholinergic overdose and are used as gastrointestinal antispasmodics for the management of peptic ulcer, gastritis, and colitis. They are also used as heart rate stimulants, bronchial dilators, and pupil dilators for ophthalmic examinations.

Sedative. A drug that reduces excitement; a quieting agent that does not produce sleep as a hypnotic drug does. Antianxiety agents may also be classified as sedatives. Sedatives may be hypnotic drugs given in smaller doses or drugs such as the bromides, paraldehyde, chloral hydrate, or flurazepam (Dalmane). The newer antianxiety agents include alprazolam (Xanax), chlordiazepoxide HCl

(Librium), diazepam (Valium), and meprobamate (Equanil and Miltown).

Steroids. Drugs that mimic certain chemicals in the body such as the male and female hormones (testosterone, progesterone, and estrogen) and the hormones of the cortices of the adrenal glands. Agents affecting the female and male reproductive systems are used to treat reproductive system imbalances, for birth control, and in labor and delivery. The adrenocorticosteroids (commonly, cortisone) are widely used as anti-inflammatory, antiallergic, and antistress agents.

Sympathetic Blocking Agent. Drugs that are called adrenergic blocking agents (or *sympatholytic*) because they block certain functions of the adrenergic nerves (see Adrenergic). These agents are mainly useful in treating cardiovascular conditions such as hypertension, angina, and cardiac arrhythmias. Some examples are phenoxybenzamine HCl (Dibenzyline), phentolamine mesylate (Regitine), and propranolol HCl (Inderal).

Tranquilizer. A calming agent that reduces anxiety and tension without acting as a depressant. Tranquilizers are called psychotherapeutic drugs. In recent years, this group of drugs has greatly increased in number. The phenothiazine derivatives are often used. These include chlorpromazine (Thorazine), perphenazine (Trilafon), and thioridazine (Mellaril).

Vasoconstrictor. A drug that causes the blood vessels to constrict, narrows the lumen of a vessel, raises blood pressure, and causes the heart to beat more forcefully. Vasoconstrictors may be used to stop superficial bleeding, raise and sustain blood pressure, and relieve nasal congestion.

Vasodilator. The opposite of a vasoconstrictor. A drug that dilates blood vessels, lowers blood pressure by making the blood vessel lumen larger, and causes the heart to pump less forcefully. Used in the treatment of hypertension, angina pectoris, and peripheral vascular diseases. Nitroglycerin placed sublingually gives prompt vasodilation. Non-nitrate vasodilators include propranolol (Inderal) and nadolol (Corgard), both sympathetic blocking agents.

APPROACHES TO STUDYING PHARMACOLOGY

A pharmaceutical glossary could be endless. Many terms are combinations of the condition to be treated with the prefix "anti" (for example, antianginal, antianxiety, antiarrhythmic, anticoagulant, anticonvulsant, antidiarrheal).

Notice how these names emphasize the drug's effect (use) rather than its action in the body. More recent classifications, such as *parasympathomimetic*

and *cholinesterase inhibitors,* describe the pharmacologic action rather than the therapeutic use. However, both viewpoints are necessary for a more complete understanding of drugs and what they do once in the human body.

Of course no one can remember all there is to know about clinical pharmacology. Even if you did one day, there would be more to learn the next. The number of new drugs being introduced into use far exceeds the number of older drugs being replaced or discontinued. Thus, the number of drugs available for clinical use grows beyond the possible knowledge of one person. Therefore, numerous resources are necessary for study and review of the details concerning particular drugs. Remember, when in doubt, look it up before you use a drug.

Reference Materials

A good pharmacology textbook is handy for studying the principles and concepts of each drug classification. There are several comprehensive editions available in hospital and college bookstores. In addition, reference and cross-reference books that are updated annually or periodically should be available for easy reference. Most references list drug information in the following sequence:

1. *Action:* How the drug acts in the body.
2. *Indication:* The conditions for which the drug is used.
3. *Side Effects:* An effect on the body other than the one(s) for which the drug is given.
4. *Adverse Effects:* An effect on a tissue or organ system other than the one being sought by the administration of a medication.
5. *Precautions:* Actions necessary because of special conditions of the patient, drug, or environment that need to be considered for the drug to be successful or not harmful.
6. *Contraindications:* Conditions that make the administration of a drug improper or undesirable.
7. *Toxic Effects:* The poisonous effects and symptoms of toxicity.
8. *Dosage and Administration:* The usual route, dosage, and timing for administering the drug.

Package Inserts

Every drug package contains an insert describing all the significant aspects of using the drug, including information on the chemical formulation of the drug and clinical studies. The information on the inserts is controlled by the FDA.

Physicians' Desk Reference (PDR)

This reference book is published annually by the Medical Economics Company, Inc. (Oradell, NJ). For physicians who subscribe to *Medical Economics Magazine,* it is provided free. Copies can be purchased through the publisher or in local bookstores. Supplements are published throughout the year. This reference contains information on approximately 2500 drugs, and the product descriptions are identical to the package inserts. The drug manufacturers pay for this space, so the *PDR* could be called the "yellow pages of the drug industry."

The book's sections are color-coded and cross-referenced for easy use. The various sections allow you to begin searching for information concerning a drug from any starting point. You can start with the usage, classification, generic name, manufacturer's name, or trade name of a drug or what the drug looks like. There is a special photographic section for visual product identification. Once you know which drug you want to study, the product information section lists the actual package insert information alphabetically, first by the manufacturer, then by the brand name.

AMA Drug Evaluations

This reference is published by the American Medical Association (Chicago, IL) and replaces a former publication called *New Drugs*. The book provides information on over 1000 drugs, without the bias or endorsement of any particular brand or group of drugs.

The American Hospital Formulary

This reference is published by the American Society of Hospital Pharmacists (Bethesda, MD) and is available by subscription. The information is contained in a two-volume set, with four to six supplements added each year. Generic names are listed, and it is divided into sections based on drug actions.

The U.S. Pharmacopeia (USP)

This publication was first printed in 1820, and new editions are still published every 5 years. England and Canada each publish similar volumes. The *Pharmacopeia* is usually not an appropriate reference purchase for the medical office.

The U.S. Pharmacopeia/National Formulary (USP/NF)

This reference is the official source of drug standards for the United States. The *Pharmacopeia* was just recently combined with the *National Formulary*, which lists the chemical formulas for all accepted drugs. This new combined reference lists and describes all the approved medications that are considered useful and therapeutic in the practice of medicine. Single drugs rather than combined products (compound mixtures) are listed. If a drug name is the same as the official name in this volume, the drug will have the initials USP after it; for example, digitoxin, USP.

Learning About Drugs

The study of pharmacology is difficult, at best. However, there are a few ways you can make it easier.

First, take opportunities to observe the use of drugs in patient care. Studying about epinephrine (Adrenalin) becomes more meaningful when you see how its cardiovascular actions get a patient through an anaphylactic episode. This is more memorable than any textbook.

Second, concentrate on the most important drugs in each classification. For example, learn about digitalis (cardiovascular), morphine (narcotic analgesic), epinephrine (autonomic nervous system blocker), and atropine (autonomic nervous system mimetic). As you expand your knowledge to other drugs in each classification, you will easily understand new drugs by noting the similarities and differences between them and the basic, important drugs you studied first.

Third, learn about a drug's primary action and use, then expand your knowledge to its other actions and uses. Soon, you will be able to name the drug that is usually indicated for a particular condition. Then, by knowing a drug's secondary effects, you will be able to understand what side effects are likely to occur during the use of the drug. More important, you will be aware of the contraindications for the drug (conditions that make the use of the drug improper or undesirable). Knowledge of the drug's actions will also enable you to predict what toxic reactions could occur from overdose (Table 37–2).

It is hoped that pharmacology will always remain exciting and interesting to you as you work with patients and the other members of your team and that you will continue to assess and evaluate new drugs as their administration becomes your responsibility.

CALCULATING DRUG DOSAGES FOR ADMINISTRATION

The correct dosage of a medication may depend on the patient's age, weight, or state of health or on what other drugs the patient may be taking. Often, the physician will order a medication in a dosage that is different from that of the medications you stock. The difference may be in the system of measurement, the strength, or the form. There are formulas and mathematical tables of conversion for calculating the correct dosage of medication to be administered. Let's look at how you arrive at the correct calculation, one step at a time.

Mathematical Equivalents

You may need to review some basics of arithmetic before you begin to tackle drug calculations. You must thoroughly understand the addition, subtraction, multiplication, and division of fractions and decimals; the relationship of decimals and fractions; and how they are converted from one to the other. In addition, you need to review how decimals and percentages are converted back and forth. Table 37–3 provides some examples of these relationships.

The table shows that a fraction is, in another sense, a ratio. For example, ¼ (a fraction) is the same as the ratio 1:4 (one-to-four). If there is one apple and four oranges, then the number of apples that you have is ¼ the number of oranges, and the ratio of apples to oranges is 1:4. Now, divide the numerator 1 by the denominator 4 (a fraction is also an automatic division problem waiting to be solved):

$$4\overline{)1.00} \quad .25$$

The act of dividing a fraction results in a decimal number. Decimal numbers can then be converted to percentages by moving the decimal two (2) spaces to the right:

$$.25 = 25.0\%, \text{ commonly written } 25\%$$

Now, we can see all the relationships of Table 37–3. Using the example of apples and oranges, you can see that 1 is .25, or 25%, of 4. Therefore, the number of apples is .25, or 25%, of the number of oranges. If you need to review any of these concepts, please stop now and practice these steps of arithmetic. To go on without this background could be very frustrating as you attempt to understand problems in dosage calculations.

Ratio and Proportion

We have just reviewed that *ratio* is one way of expressing a fraction, or division problem, and shows the relationship of the numerator to the denominator. The comparison of *two* ratios is called a *proportion*. A proportion is written as follows:

$$\frac{4}{16} = \frac{1}{4} \text{ or } 4:16 :: 1:4$$

This is read as 4 divided by 16 equals 1 divided by 4, or four is to sixteen as one is to four. What we are saying here is that both ratios have the same proportions and are equal to one another even though the numbers are different. This is the key to calculating drug dosages. The physician's order for a medication may be a ratio different from that of the medication we stock. We will then compare the ordered ratio to the available ratio (what we have in stock) to find the correct proportion to administer. However, before going on, there is more background material that we need to know.

The preceding proportion example has all the answers in it; there is nothing to solve. In calculating

TABLE 37–2. PRESCRIPTION DRUGS DISPENSED IN U.S. COMMUNITY PHARMACIES, NEW AND REFILL PRESCRIPTIONS —ALL STRENGTHS

Ranking	Drug	Product Manufacturer
1	Amoxil	Beecham
2	Lanoxin	Burroughs Wellcome
3	Zantac	Glaxo
4	Xanax	Upjohn
5	Premarin	Wyeth-Ayerst
6	Cardizem	Marion
7	Ceclor	Lilly
8	Synthroid	Boots
9	Seldane	Merrell Dow
10	Tenormin ICI	Pharma
11	Vasotec	MSD
12	Tagamet	SKF
13	Naprosyn	Syntex
14	Capoten	Squibb
15	Ortho-Novum 7/7/7	Ortho
16	Dyazide	SKF
17	Ortho-Novum	Ortho
18	Proventil	Schering
19	Tylenol with/codeine	McNeil
20	Procardia	Pfizer
21	Calan	Searle
22	Ventolin	Allen & Hanburys
23	Inderal	Wyeth-Ayerst
24	Halcion	Upjohn
25	Theo-Dur	Schering
26	Lopressor	Geigy
27	Lasix	Hoechst
28	Voltaren	Geigy
29	Darvocet-N	Lilly
30	Dilantin	Parke-Davis
31	Monistat	Ortho
32	Augmentin	Beecham
33	Micronase	Upjohn
34	Feldene	Pfizer
35	Micro-K	Robins
36	Provera	Upjohn
37	Motrin	Upjohn
38	Mevacor	MSD
39	Triphasil	Wyeth-Ayerst
40	Prozac	Dista
41	Lo/Ovral	Wyeth-Ayerst
42	Valium	Roche
43	Retin-A	Ortho
44	Cipro	Miles
45	E-Mycin	Boots
46	Maxzide	Lederle
47	Coumadin	Du Pont
48	Carafate	Marion
49	Timoptic	MSD
50	Slow-K	Summit

(Extracted from *American Druggist*, New York, Hurst Publications, February 1992.)

dosages, we use mathematical proportions, but with one element unknown. We must solve for that unknown, or x. For example:

$$\frac{4}{16} = \frac{1}{x}$$

Always in a proportion, we solve the problem by *cross-multiplication*. Do not confuse this with plain

TABLE 37–3. MATHEMATICAL EQUIVALENTS

Percentage	Decimal	Fraction	Ratio
25%	.25	1/4	1:4
50%	.5	1/2	1:2
60%	.6	3/5 (6/10)	3:5
.5%	.005	1/200	1:200
.1%	.001	1/1000	1:1000
85%	.85	17/20	17:20
1%	.01	1/100	1:100

multiplication. If you see an equal sign (=) between two fractions, you know this is an *equation* to be *cross-multiplied.*

$$\frac{4}{16} = \frac{1}{x}$$

Now cross-multiply:

$$4 \times x = 16 \times 1$$

Therefore:

$$4x = 16$$

We know what 4x equals, but next we must find what 1x, or x, equals. To find the value of x, we must find a way to leave x (or 1x) alone on one side of the equation. We can change 4x to 1x by dividing the number 4 by itself:

$$4x \div 4 = 1x$$

But what we do on one side of an equation, we must do on the other side, or the equation will not be equal anymore. Therefore, we divide 16 by 4:

$$16 \div 4 = 4$$

The answer is x = 4. Let's put it all together now.

$$\frac{1}{x} = \frac{4}{16}$$

$$4 \times x = 16 \times 1$$

$$4x = 16$$

$$\frac{4x}{4} = \frac{16}{4}$$

$$1x = 4$$

We take the answer 4 and replace the x with it in the ratio. We have solved for x.

$$\frac{4}{16} = \frac{1}{4}$$

Calculating Dosages

When calculating dosages, a standard set of formulas is used. These formulas employ certain specific terms. Every drug has a *strength* (potency) and a *dosage unit (amount)*. The strength is the quantity of the drug held together in a particular form. The amount (volume) is what contains the drug. It may be a solid form, such as a tablet, or a liquid form, such as 1 cubic centimeter (cc) of injectable physiologic saline. In liquids, the drug strength is often called the *solute.* The solute is dissolved in an amount called the *solvent.* It is important to understand which measurements pertain to the strength (potency) of a drug and which pertain to the unit of dosage (form, volume, or amount). For example, a vial of injectable material may read "500 mg/cc." This means there are 500 mg (strength) of drug in every cc (amount) of liquid. When an oral medication reads "5 gr," it means that there are 5 grains (strength) in every tablet (amount). Let's use these two examples and the proportion formula previously reviewed to work out two problems: (1) filling a syringe and (2) administering tablets.

1. **Order:** Give 250 mg of a drug.
   Available: A vial marked 500 mg/cc.
   Standard Formula:

$$\frac{\text{available strength}}{\text{ordered strength}} = \frac{\text{available amount}}{\text{amount to give}}$$

Problem: Given the strength of the drug needed, the amount of fluid to be withdrawn must be determined.

We will set up a proportion with the three known quantities: the strength of the drug in the vial, the unit of fluid in which that strength is contained, and the strength of the drug the physician wishes to be administered to the patient.

Apply the problem to the standard formula:

$$\frac{500 \text{ mg}}{250 \text{ mg}} = \frac{1 \text{ cc}}{x \text{ cc}}$$

$$500 \times x = 250 \times 1$$

$$500x = 250$$

$$\frac{500x}{500} = \frac{250}{500}$$

$$1x = \frac{1}{2} \text{ cc} = 0.50 \text{ cc}$$

Solution: Administer 0.50 cc of the drug.

2. **Order:** Give 10 gr (grains) of a drug.
   Available: A bottle with tablets labeled 5 gr each.

Standard Formula:

$$\frac{\text{available strength}}{\text{ordered strength}} = \frac{\text{available amount}}{\text{amount to give}}$$

Problem: Given the strength of the drug needed, the number of tablets to be administered must be determined.

We will set up a proportion with the three known quantities: the strength of the drug in each tablet, the unit amount that is one tablet, and the strength of the drug the physician wishes to be administered to the patient.

Apply the problem to the standard formula:

$$\frac{5 \text{ gr}}{10 \text{ gr}} = \frac{1 \text{ tablet}}{\text{x (no. of tablets)}}$$

$$5 \times x = 10 \times 1$$

$$5x = 10$$

$$\frac{5x}{5} = \frac{10}{5}$$

$$1x = 2 \text{ tablets}$$

Solution: Administer 2 tablets.

Use the *standard formula* for any type of calculation. You may be using strengths that are measured in International Units (IU), as with insulin or penicillin; grams; milligrams; grains; or percentages. The forms in which drugs may be prepared include cubic centimeters (cc), or milliliters (ml); minims; drops; drams; ounces; pints; gallons (for making up diluted stock solutions from concentrated solutions, such as with alcohol and hydrogen peroxide); or spoonfuls. Follow the steps previously shown, and above all, discipline yourself to write down each step with complete calculations. This is the only way to ensure maximum accuracy and the safety of your patients. If you have difficulty with the calculation, or the answer does not seem quite right, ask the physician to check your calculation. A double check is always preferred.

Systems of Measurement

Sometimes, the physician will order a medication in a strength that is totally different from the one

---

PROCEDURE 37 – 1   CALCULATING THE CORRECT DOSAGE FOR ADMINISTRATION

GOAL To calculate the correct dosage amount and choose the correct equipment when the physician orders 2.4 million IU (International Units) of Bicillin (penicillin G benzathine) to be administered to a patient.

EQUIPMENT AND SUPPLIES

Premixed syringes of Bicillin in the following two strengths are available:

0.6 million IU/syringe
1.2 million IU/syringe

PROCEDURAL STEPS

1. Read the order in quiet surroundings to make sure that you fully understand it.
2. Using pencil and paper, write out the order.
3. Examine the drug labels to see what strengths and amounts are available.
4. Write down the standard formula.
   Purpose: To eliminate the chances of error, orders should never be carried out unless the calculations are completed in writing.
5. Rewrite the formula, replacing the unknown values with the known quantities. The unknown x will be the amount of the drug to give (amount to give).
6. Work the proportion problem by cross-multiplying to solve for x.
7. State your answer by filling in the blanks, as follows:
   To administer 2.4 million IU of Bicillin, I would select _____ of the premixed syringes labeled _____.

on the label of the vial or bottle. For example, the physician may order one grain of a drug, but the available dosage form is in milligrams. Before you can use the ratio and proportion formulas to arrive at the amount to administer, you first must convert to one system or the other. The best way is to convert to the measurement system that is on the label (what is available). After all, that is the system you will have to use. Dosage calculations would be easier if pharmacology dealt with just one system of measurement. Unfortunately, there are three: the metric system, the apothecary system, and the household system.

The *metric system* of weights and measures is now used throughout the world as the primary system for weight (mass), capacity (volume), and length (area). In the United States, it is used for scientific work, including most pharmaceuticals. However, some medication forms still use the older apothecary system, which necessitates learning the two systems and the relationships (conversions) between the two. A few hints about each system follow.

The metric system of weights and measures is a decimal system, which means that it uses the base ten (10). Each higher measure is 10 times the measure at hand; each lower, 1/10 the measure. The fraction is always written as a decimal, and the number precedes the letters designating the actual measure. Thus, one and a half liters would be written 1.5 L (Table 37–4). The *cubic centimeter* (cc) and the *milliliter* (ml) are interchangeable. In the metric system, 1 cc is a measurement of area, and an area this size holds exactly 1 ml (1/1000 of a liter) of fluid (volume). In fact, if you were to weigh 1 ml of water contained in 1 cc of area under certain conditions of temperature and barometric pressure, it would also weigh exactly 1 *gram* (g). In the metric system, these three basic units of measurement are convertible from one to the other.

With the *apothecary system,* the basic unit of weight is the *grain* (gr), and the basic unit of volume is the *minim* (M). As in the metric system, these two units are related: the grain is based on the weight of a single grain of wheat, and the minim is the volume of water that weighs one grain. Either Roman or Arabic numerals may be used, but it is not proper to use them together in the same prescription. Either symbols or abbreviations are used; for example, one and a half drams might be written ʒiss or d 1½. The number follows the symbol or abbreviation. Table 37–5 compares the units of weight and volume in the metric and the apothecary systems.

The *household system* is used in most American households. This system of measurement is important for the patient at home who has no knowledge of the metric or apothecary systems. The basic measure of weight is the *pound;* the basic measure of volume, the *drop.* The household drop is equal to the apothecary minim, so these two systems are sometimes easily interchangeable. Both the household and the apothecary systems use the terms dram and ounce as units of measurement, so always be sure of which system you are using. Medications are not measured in household weights, but many prescriptions contain directions using the household measurements of volume. Liquid oral medications are taken by the drop, teaspoon, or tablespoon, and are supplied in bottles labeled in ounces or pints. Tables 37–6 and 37–7 show the household system of measurement (note that there are some apothecary equivalents).

TABLE 37–4. ABBREVIATIONS AND SYMBOLS FOR SELECTED WEIGHTS AND MEASURES

	Apothecary System			Metric System	
	ℳ	Min. (M.)	minim	gm	gram
	℈	scr	scruple	L	liter
	ʒ	dr	dram	cc	cubic centimeter
fl	ʒ	f dr	fluid dram	ml	milliliter
	℥	oz	ounce		
fl	℥	fl oz	fluid ounce		
	O	pt	pint		
	C	gal	gallon		
		gr	grain		

TABLE 37–5. APPROXIMATE EQUIVALENTS FOR SOME COMMONLY USED MEASURES

| | | | Liquid Measure | | | |
			Apothecary		Metric	
Grains	Grams	Milligrams				
15	1.0	1000	1	quart	1000	ml (cc)
10	0.6	600	1	pint	500	ml
7½	0.5	500	8	fl oz	250	ml
5	0.3	300	7	fl oz	200	ml
4	0.25	250	3.5	fl oz	100	ml
3	0.2	200	1	fl oz	30	ml
2	0.12	120	4	fl d	15	ml
1½	0.1	100	2.5	fl d	10	ml
1	0.06	60	2	fl d	8	ml
¾	0.050	50	1	fl d	4	ml
½	0.030	30	45	M.	3	ml
⅜	0.025	25	30	M.	2	ml
¼	0.015	15	15	M.	1	ml
⅙	0.010	10	12	M.	0.75	ml
⅛	0.008	8	10	M.	0.6	ml
1/10	0.006	6	8	M.	0.5	ml
1/12	0.005	5	5	M.	0.3	ml
1/20	0.003	3	4	M.	0.25	ml
1/30	0.002	2	3	M.	0.2	ml
1/60	0.001	1	1.5	M.	0.1	ml
1/100	0.0006	0.6	1	M.	0.06	ml
1/120	0.0005	0.5	.75	M.	0.05	ml
1/150	0.0004	0.4	.5	M.	0.03	ml
1/200	0.0003	0.3				
1/250	0.00025	0.25				
1/300	0.0002	0.2				
1/400	0.00015	0.15				
1/500	0.00012	0.12				
1/600	0.0001	0.1				

Weight conversions; 1 lb = 0.45 kg; 1 kg = 2.2 lb; 10 lb = 4.5 kg; 10 kg = 22 lb; 30.0 g = 1 oz; 15.0 g = 4 d; 7.5 g = 2 d; 4 g = 1 d; 4 g = 60 grains; Domestic equivalents: 1 teaspoon = 5 ml (cc) = 1 fl d; 1 tablespoon = 15 ml = .5 fl oz; 1 measuring cup = 250 ml = 8 fl oz; 4 measuring cups = 1000 ml = 1 quart.

TABLE 37–6. HOUSEHOLD EQUIVALENTS

60 gtt	=	1 t or tsp		
3 t or tsp	=	1 T		
180 gtt	=	1 T	=	½ oz
2 T	=	1 oz	=	6 t or tsp
360 gtt	=	2 T		
1 oz	=	30 cc or 30 ml		
6 oz	=	1 tcp		
8 oz	=	1 C or 1 glass		
2 C	=	1 pt	=	16 oz
2 pt	=	1 qt	=	32 oz
4 C	=	1 qt	=	32 oz
4 qt	=	1 gal	=	128 oz

TABLE 37–7. COMMON HOUSEHOLD MEASURES

60 drops*	1 teaspoon
1 dash	Less than ⅛ teaspoon
3 teaspoons	1 tablespoon
2 tablespoons	1 ounce
4 ounces	1 juice glass
6 ounces	1 teacup
8 ounces	1 glass or cup
16 tablespoons or 8 ounces	1 measuring cup
2 cups	1 pint
2 pints	1 quart
4 quarts	1 gallon

* Drop (gtt) = approximate liquid measure depending on kind of liquid measured and the size of the opening from which it is dropped.

PROCEDURE 37-2 CALCULATING THE CORRECT DOSAGE FOR ADMINISTRATION USING TWO SYSTEMS OF MEASUREMENT

GOAL To choose the correct system of measurement and calculate the correct dosage amount when the physician orders 120 mg (milligrams) of a drug to be administered to a patient. (Tablet label reads 1 gr [grain] each.)

EQUIPMENT AND SUPPLIES

Tablets labeled 1 gr (grain) each
Standard mathematical formula:

$$\frac{\text{available strength}}{\text{ordered strength}} = \frac{\text{available amount}}{\text{amount to give}}$$

Conversion equivalent: 1 gr = 60 mg

PROCEDURAL STEPS

1. Read the order in quiet surroundings to make sure that you fully understand it.
2. Using pencil and paper, write out the order.
3. Examine the drug labels to see what strengths and amounts are available.
4. Convert the ordered system of measurement to the system of measurement on the label.
5. Write down the standard formula.
   Purpose: To eliminate the chances of error, orders should never be carried out unless the calculations are completed in writing.
6. Rewrite the formula, replacing the unknown values with the known quantities and using the system of measurement on the label. The unknown x will be the amount of the drug to give (amount to give).
7. Work the proportion problem by cross-multiplying to solve for x.
8. State your answer by filling in the blank, as follows:
   To administer 120 mg of a drug from tablets labeled 1 gr (grain) each, I would give _____ tablet(s).

Pediatric Dose Calculations

As noted earlier in the chapter, there is no perfect system for converting adult medications to proper pediatric dosages. In most cases, children are not able to tolerate adult medications, as a child's metabolism is very unstable compared with that of an adult. When it is necessary to administer an adult medication to a child, the following formulas are accepted. Calculating dosage in this manner is permitted only under the direct order and supervision of the physician.

Fried's Law

This calculation is for children under 1 year of age and is based on the age of the child in months compared with a child 12½ years old. The calculation assumes that an adult dose would be appropriate for a child aged 12½ years (150 mo).

$$\text{Pediatric dose} = \frac{\text{child's age in months}}{150 \text{ months}} \times \text{adult dose}$$

Young's Rule

Young's rule is for children over 1 year of age.

$$\text{Pediatric dose} = \frac{\text{child's age in years}}{\text{child's age in years} + 12} \times \text{adult dose}$$

Clark's Rule

This rule is based on the weight of the child. This system is much more accurate, since children of any age can vary greatly in size and body weight. Clark's rule uses 150 pounds (70 kg) as the average adult weight and assumes that the child's dose is proportionately less. The formula is:

$$\text{Pediatric dose} = \frac{\text{child's weight in pounds}}{150 \text{ pounds}} \times \text{adult dose}$$

West's Nomogram

West's nomogram calculates the body surface area of infants and young children. Many physicians use the **nomogram** because even a small miscalculation could be critical, especially when a child is ill, underweight, or overweight (Fig. 37–2).

$$\text{Pediatric dose} = \frac{\begin{array}{c}\text{basic surface area of child}\\ \text{(in square meters)}\end{array}}{1.73 \text{ square meters}} \times \text{adult dose}$$

You need complete mastery in calculating dosages, whether they be for children or adults. Until you master the arithmetic, the accurate placement of the decimal point, converting equivalents from one system to another, and the use of the ratio and proportion formula for every type of calculation, you must practice problems in dosages and solutions with someone who can check your work. Mastery of dosage calculations may take some time and much practice, but as with any other skill, you can achieve it if you take the time to understand the basics first, then advance to the concepts of ratio and proportion and, finally, the calculation of specific drugs and solutions.

37

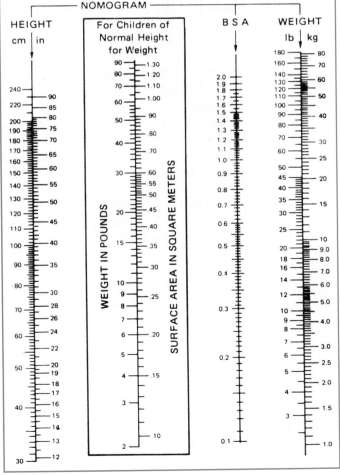

FIGURE 37–2. West's nomogram for estimation of body surface area. (From Behrman, R.E., and Vaughan, V.C. III: *Nelson Textbook of Pediatrics,* 13th ed., Philadelphia, W.B. Saunders Co., 1987.)

PROCEDURE 37-3 CALCULATING THE CORRECT DOSAGE FOR A CHILD WHEN ONLY AN ADULT MEDICATION IS AVAILABLE

GOAL To calculate the correct dosage amount for a 90-pound child using Clark's rule when the adult dosage is 250 mg.

EQUIPMENT AND SUPPLIES

Adult dosage 250 mg/cc
Clark's rule: Pediatric dose =

$$\frac{\text{child's weight in pounds}}{150 \text{ pounds}} \times \text{adult dose}$$

Standard mathematical formula:

$$\frac{\text{available strength}}{\text{ordered strength}} = \frac{\text{available amount}}{\text{amount to give}}$$

PROCEDURAL STEPS

1. Read the order in quiet surroundings to make sure that you fully understand it.
2. Using pencil and paper, write out the order.
3. Examine the drug labels to see what strengths and amounts are available.
4. Write down Clark's rule.
   Purpose: To eliminate the chances of error, orders should never be carried out unless the calculations are completed in writing.
5. Using Clark's rule, replace the unknown values with the known quantities. The unknown x will be the pediatric strength ordered (pediatric dose).
6. Write down the standard formula.
   Purpose: To eliminate the chances of error, orders should never be carried out unless the calculations are completed in writing.
7. Rewrite the formula, replacing the unknown values with the available quantities and the pediatric strength just determined. The unknown x will be the amount of the drug to give (amount to give).
8. Work the proportion problem by cross-multiplying to solve for x.
9. State your answer by filling in the blank, as follows:
   To administer an adult medication labeled 250 mg/cc to a 90-pound child, I will give _____ cc.

PROCEDURE 37-4 CALCULATING THE CORRECT DOSAGE FOR ADMINISTRATION USING BODY WEIGHT

GOAL To calculate correct dosage by using body weight method.
Ordered: Zovirax capsules 5 mg/kg every 8 hours times 7 days for a patient who has a diagnosis of herpes zoster. The patient weighs 132 pounds.
The capsules are labeled 50 mg = 1 capsule.
Weight: 2.2 lb = 1 kg

EQUIPMENT AND SUPPLIES

Capsules labeled 50 mg/kg
Balance scale
Formula for conversion of pounds to kilograms
Standard math formula: $\dfrac{\text{available strength}}{\text{ordered strength}} = \dfrac{\text{available amount}}{\text{amount to give}}$
Paper and pencil

PROCEDURAL STEPS

1. Read the order in quiet surroundings to make sure that you fully understand it.

2. Write out the order.

3. Examine the drug label to check the strength and amount.

4. Convert the patient's weight from pounds to kilograms.

5. Write down the standard formula.
   Purpose: To eliminate the chances of error.

6. Rewrite the formula, replacing the unknown values with the known quantities. The unknown x will be the amount of the drug to give.

7. Work the problem by cross-multiplying to solve for x.

8. State your answer by filling in the blank as follows:
   To administer 5 mg per kg of body weight of Zovirax from capsules labeled 50 mg each, I would give _____ capsule(s).

LEGAL AND ETHICAL RESPONSIBILITIES

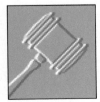

The medical assistant who prepares and administers medications is ethically and legally responsible for his or her own actions. Under the law, you are required to be licensed, registered, or authorized by a physician to administer medications. Laws vary from state to state. Therefore, it is essential that you become familiar with the laws in the state of your employment before giving medications. Legislation in some states gives physicians broad authority to delegate responsibility for giving medications. The medical assistant acts as the "agent" of the physician. The assistant is responsible and accountable for the acts performed and may be subject to penalty in case of default (see Chapter 5).

Regardless of the differences in state authorization laws, the courts will not permit the careless actions of health care workers to go unpunished, especially when such actions result in the harming or death of the patient. Under the law, those administering medications are expected to be familiar with the drugs administered and the effects that they might have on a patient. It is your responsibility to be aware of the drugs that your physician prescribes. Make it a habit to look up and check any drug that you are not familiar with. It is better to be safe than sorry.

Despite differences in the duties of drug administration assigned to you by your physician, the following considerations are your ultimate responsibility:

● To be informed about the drugs that you administer

- To ensure that a drug being used is correct in its order, dosage, route, time, and use
- To preassess the patient for any adverse effects, such as allergy or drug-to-drug or drug-to-food interactions
- To administer a drug appropriately
- To be aware of any adverse effects that might occur immediately following the administration of a medication
- To provide comfort, encouragement, and guidance to patients to ensure patient understanding, safety, and cooperation while the patient is on drug therapy

▸ LEARNING ACHIEVEMENTS

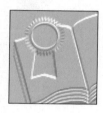

Upon completion of this chapter, can you in the time allowed by your evaluator:

1. Look up drugs in the *PDR* using the trade name index, the generic index, and the pharmaceutical index?

2. Given various medication orders and available medications packaged in different strengths, apply standard dosage calculation formulas to calculate correct dosages to be administered to patients?

3. Cite the dangers of using over-the-counter drugs?

4. Classify a given list of drugs by their actions on the body?

5. Cite 10 factors that influence the effect a drug may have on the body?

6. List six ethical and legal responsibilities in administering medications?

7. List, in order, the five steps that describe the fate of a drug in the human body?

Now that you have an introductory understanding of clinical pharmacology, and some guidelines for calculating drug dosages, you are ready to move on to Chapter 38, which covers the medical assisting process in drug administration and therapy.

Answers to Procedures 37–1 through 37–4

37–1. To administer 2.4 million IU of Bicillin, I would select two of the premixed syringes labeled 1.2 million IU per syringe.

37–2. To administer 120 mg of a drug from tablets labeled 1 gr each, I would give two tablets.

37–3. To administer an adult medication labeled 250 mg/cc to a 90-pound child, I would give 0.6 cc.

37–4. To administer Zovirax 5 mg/kg of body weight from capsules labeled 50 mg each, I would give a patient weighing 132 pounds two capsules (100 mg).

REFERENCES AND READINGS

Clark, J., Queener, S., and Karb, V.: *Pocket Guide to Drugs*, St. Louis, C. V. Mosby Co., 1986.

Physicians' Desk Reference, 44th ed. Oradell, NJ, Medical Economics, 1990.

Reynard, A., and Smith, C.: *Textbook of Pharmacology*, Philadelphia, W.B. Saunders Co., 1992.

Woodrow, R.: *Essentials of Pharmacology for Health Occupations*, 2nd ed., New York, Delmar Publishers, 1992.

CHAPTER THIRTY-EIGHT

—

ADMINISTRATION OF MEDICATIONS

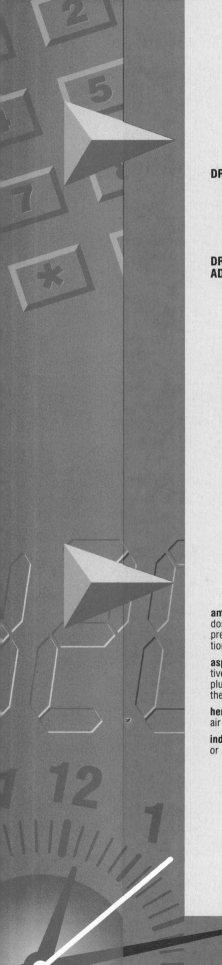

CHAPTER OUTLINE

VOCABULARY

ampule A small (usually a single-dose) glass container of medication prepared for parenteral administration.

aspirate To withdraw fluid by negative pressure; pulling up on the plunger of the syringe after inserting the needle to check for blood.

hermetically sealed Sealed so no air is allowed to enter.

induration An abnormally hard spot or place.

radical mastectomy The complete surgical removal of the breast, the surrounding muscles, and the lymph glands.

sublingual Under the tongue.

topical Applied to a certain area of the skin and affecting only that area.

vesiculation Formation of blister-like elevations on the skin.

vial A small bottle, usually glass.

viscosity The quality of being gluey and lacking the capability of easy movement.

volatile Referring to an explosive substance's capacity to vaporize at a low temperature.

wheal A localized area of edema on the body's surface.

ADMINISTRATION OF MEDICATIONS

38

LEARNING OBJECTIVES

COGNITIVE
Upon successful completion of this chapter, you should be able to:

1. Spell and define the words listed in the Vocabulary.

2. List six factors of patient assessment that may influence whether you should continue with an order to administer a drug.

3. State two situations in which it may be your responsibility to further assess an ordered drug before administering it.

4. State two environmental factors that would contraindicate the administration of a medication.

5. Recall the "three befores" and the "six rights."

6. List the basic solid and liquid oral dosage forms and give an example of each.

7. For each of the five mucous membrane sites, cite the methods for administering medications.

8. Differentiate among the nine types of topical medications.

9. For each parenteral method, list the preferred needle gauges and lengths and the usual syringe size.

10. State the risks of using reusable injection equipment and three advantages of disposable injection equipment.

11. List the contraindications for administering a parenteral drug in any particular site.

12. Locate the anatomic landmarks for each intramuscular injection site.

13. List the special considerations of anatomy when administering injectable medications to infants and small children.

14. Recall the Centers for Disease Control standards.

PERFORMANCE
Upon successful completion of this chapter, you should be able to:

1. Fill a syringe using sterile technique.

2. Demonstrate giving an intradermal injection.

3. Demonstrate giving a subcutaneous injection.

4. Demonstrate giving an intramuscular injection.

5. Demonstrate giving a Z-tract intramuscular injection.

6. Demonstrate using the transdermal patch.

Drug therapy has become one of the most significant aspects of patient care and one of the most significant responsibilities that a physician may delegate to a medical assistant. The medical assistant who is asked to administer medications must have a thorough understanding of the scientific principles of drug therapy and the confidence and assurance to follow through with the physician's request. Chapter 37 is an introduction to how drugs interact with the body, the basic routes of administration, and the standard formulas for dosage calculation. This chapter builds on the last, developing the specific skills of patient assessment and drug administration. Most of the drugs administered in the medical office will be by injection (parenterally). Most oral medications will be filled by prescription and will be started by the patient at home. Occasionally, you may be required to instill drops into a patient's eyes, ears, or nose, or you may be called upon to insert a rectal suppository into a pediatric patient.

No matter what type of medication you are to administer, the order must come from the physician. If the physician delegates drug administration to you as part of your job, it must be allowable under state laws. Every state has a medical practice act that will define whether or not a medical assistant can administer drugs under the supervision of a physician. Some states allow medical assistants to administer only certain types of medications, some prohibit medical assistants from giving injections. Information concerning the scope of practice for medical assistants in your particular state should be obtained from your local government or medical society. You should know what the law states and how your duties fit into that law.

DRUG THERAPY ASSESSMENT

Although medications may be given only under the direct order and supervision of the physician, you are a part of the assessment and problem solving processes in the care of the patient. In medicine, assessment never ends and never is the responsibility of just one person. A physician gives the order to administer medication to a patient based on a medical assessment, but you also must continue to assess the patient and the patient's environment as you follow through with the order. The physician depends on you to be alert to changes or new information that could result in a condition or consequence that would make the use of a drug improper or undesirable. Before giving any medication, you should assess the patient, the drug, and the environment.

Patient Assessment

Assessment of the patient includes the patient's history and current status. As you are about to act on a physician's order, you too should mentally review the following factors that may influence whether you continue with the order or return to the physician for further clarification:

- Are there any conditions that may contraindicate the use of the drug or the dosage ordered?
- Do you have special knowledge of any other drug use (a dependency, or the use of prescription or over-the-counter drugs) that may contraindicate the completion of the medication order?
- Does the patient have any allergies to drugs of this type or to certain foods or animals that may indicate that this drug will produce a similar allergic effect?
- Are the patient's age, height, and weight correct for the dosage ordered?
- Is there a reason that the route chosen for administration may not be desirable? For example, injections may be ordered for a particular site. However, you notice that at the site there is an injury, a swelling, or a recent change in texture or pigmentation, which would contraindicate the use of the site for injection.

Patient assessment does not end with the administration of the drug. Observe patients carefully for drug reactions that may follow injectable medications. Patients receiving penicillin (a drug with a high incidence of allergic response) or allergy immunotherapy (administering repeated injections of dilute extracts of the substance that causes the allergy; also called desensitization) must remain in the office for 20 to 30 minutes in case of acute anaphylactic reaction. Acute anaphylactic reaction can result in respiratory failure and circulatory collapse within minutes if not reversed with epinephrine. Lesser allergic reactions include hives, swelling, and itching. An antihistamine, such as Benadryl, may need to be administered (see Chapter 40).

Drug Assessment

Drug assessment includes evaluation of the dosage ordered and the drug itself. No medication should be administered without a written order. If you are to administer a medication by verbal order, be sure to have the physician sign or write the order on the patient's medical record as soon as possible. If there is doubt about a particular order, written or verbal, do not give the drug until you are sure that it is what the physician intends. If you still have doubts, confidentially and politely request that the physician personally administer the drug. Remember that you take the responsibility if you do not understand an order but administer the drug anyway.

You must also evaluate the drug's appropriateness. For example, you have a patient who is a diabetic, and the physician orders Ornade. You know that Ornade is a time-released antihistamine and that Orinase is an oral hypoglycemic. Never hesitate to question a misinterpretation or possible mistake on a drug order. So many drugs sound and are spelled alike that mistakes are possible. If you do not know the details of the drugs that you are administering, you will not be able to assess their appropriateness and, therefore, to support the physician and safeguard the patient.

Know the appropriate dosages. The standard abbreviations for dosages may not be clearly written, and you may need to know whether the order was for a minim (M.) or for a milliliter (ml). Since there are 15 to 16 minims in a milliliter, to guess or not to know the appropriate dosage, in this case, could result in a patient receiving 15 times the desired amount, or $\frac{1}{15}$ the necessary amount. Either way, harm may come to a patient from an irresponsible act on your part.

Environment Assessment

The patient's surroundings could determine an order's inappropriateness. The patient may become hysterical or uncooperative about receiving the medication, or the patient's family may protest the use of the drug. A patient may come to the office for a weekly drug treatment, but the physician may not be present. Drugs should not be administered to patients, even on order, if there is not someone present who can not only administer emergency first-aid but also reverse acute anaphylactic reactions with injectable epinephrine. The medical assistant cannot inject epinephrine without an order. In the absence of a physician, there would be no one to give that order in an emergency.

The environment must be safe for drug administration. Be sure that the patient is comfortable and protected from further injury. If a patient is to receive an injection, make sure to place the patient in a position that best exposes the site and protects the patient from injury in case he or she faints or has a drug reaction. If the patient is to take an oral medication with water, be sure that he or she is seated in a position that will prevent choking. Because any medication is potentially dangerous to a patient, there also must be emergency drugs, readily available, to counteract any adverse effects that might occur immediately following the administration of a medication. Emergency drugs should be in injectable form for rapid effect. Typically, emergency carts include adrenergics, such as epinephrine; anticholinergics, such as atropine; bronchodilators; and antihistamine-histamine blockers.

A note about your own environment. The entire process of administering medications should be completed in quiet surroundings and with concentration. When you are preparing and administering a medication, do not do anything else, including talking. The process requires organized and concise movements and involves "the three befores" and "the six rights."

The "Three Befores"

Before administering any drug, check the label for the correct drug choice and dosage three times:

1. *Before* removing the drug from the shelf. Make sure you start with the right medication and dosage.
2. *Before* pouring or preparing the drug. A double check while you work.
3. *Before* returning the drug to the shelf. A third check. Drugs are returned to the shelf before you leave the medication room to administer the medication to the patient.

The "Six Rights"

Before you leave the medication room, take the time to say yes to the following six questions.

Do I have the:

1. *Right patient?* Check the name on the patient's chart. (Before administering the drug, you will again check, by greeting the patient by name, to be sure that you have the right person.)
2. *Right drug?* Compare the written drug name with the label of the container that you are using. Does it seem appropriate? Know the medications that you are using. Never prepare medications from a bottle with a damaged label. READ THE LABEL THREE TIMES. Compare the written order with the strength labeled on the container. If the ordered strength is not available, you will have to give more or less, depending on the situation.
3. *Right dose?* Compare the written dosage order with the amount of drug that you prepare (number of tablets, quantity of solution). (Drug calculation formulas are located at the conclusion of Chapter 37.) READ THE LABEL THREE TIMES.
4. *Right time?* Should the medication be given now? Is it the correct time of day? Is it the correct time in a series of administrations? Is it the correct time in the body cycle?
5. *Right route?* Can the patient receive this medication by the route ordered? Is the particular drug available for the route ordered? Is the route an appropriate one?
6. *Right documentation?* Did I enter it on the patient's record? Was my entry precise and accurate? Did I initial the entry?

If you can say yes to all the preceding questions, then and only then are you ready to administer the drug.

DRUG FORMS AND ADMINISTRATION

As discussed in Chapter 37, the chosen route of drug administration determines whether or not the drug will have an effect and, often, the intensity of the effect. A drug prepared for one route but administered by another route may not have any effect at all or may potentially be dangerous. Each route requires different dosage forms.

Solid Oral Dosage Forms

The basic forms are tablets, capsules, powders, and lozenges (troches). Pills are rarely manufactured today, but many people mistakenly call tablets "pills."

Tablets and Caplets

Tablets are compressed powders or granules that, when wet, break apart in the stomach, or in the mouth if they are not swallowed quickly. Tablets may be *sugar* coated to taste better, or *enteric* coated to resist the acid action of the stomach. *Triturated* tablets are coated with a **volatile** liquid that dissolves in the mouth. An antacid tablet is an example.

Capsules

Capsules are gelatin coated and dissolve in the stomach, or they may be coated with substances that protect them from the acid action of the stomach. Timed- or sustained-release capsules are designed to dissolve at different rates, over a period of time, to reduce the number of times a patient has to take a medication.

Powders

Powders are no longer popular. Effervescent antacids and laxatives are now being manufactured in the form of a large tablet.

Lozenges (Troches)

Lozenges are flattened discs that are dissolved in the mouth for coating the throat.

Oral Administration

Make sure the patient has enough water to transport the drug to the stomach. Make sure that the patient is able to swallow the medication. It may be helpful to place the medication on the back part of the tongue, or the swallowing reflex can be stimulated by placing ice on the lips or tongue just prior to administering the drug. If a patient has difficulty in swallowing or is very young, you may crush and mix the solid form in a soft food, such as apple-sauce, provided that the food does not interact with the drug, or the drug is not enteric coated or a timed-release capsule. If your patient has been vomiting or is nauseated, an alternative route might be necessary.

Liquid and Oral Dosage Forms

Many types of liquid forms are available. They differ mainly in the type of substance used to dissolve the drug: water, oils, or alcohol.

Solutions: Drug substances contained in a homogeneous mixture with a liquid. Several types are:
Syrups: Solutions of sugar and water, usually containing flavoring and medicinal substances. Cough syrups are the most common.
Aromatic waters: Aqueous solutions containing volatile oils such as oil of spearmint, peppermint, or clove.
Liquors: Solutions that contain a nonvolatile material, such as alcohol, as the solute.

Suspensions: Insoluble drug substances contained in a liquid. Examples are:
Emulsions: Mixtures of oil and water that improve the taste of otherwise distasteful products such as cod liver oil.
Gels and magmas: Minerals suspended in water. Minerals settle; therefore, products containing minerals must be shaken before use. Milk of magnesia is an example.

Alcohol solutions: A drug substance mixed with alcohol to enhance the drug's properties. Examples are:
Fluidextracts: Combinations of alcohol and vegetable products that are more potent than tinctures. For example, belladonna fluidextract has a higher percentage of the powdered belladonna leaf than does tincture of belladonna.
Tinctures: An alcoholic preparation of a soluble drug or chemical substance, usually from plant sources. Examples are tinctures of belladonna and of opium. Less potent examples are camphorated tincture of opium (paregoric) and tincture of benzoin. One nonvegetable tincture is tincture of iodine.
Extracts: Very concentrated combinations of vegetable products and alcohol or ether that are evaporated until a syrupy liquid, solid mass, or powder is formed. Extracts are many times stronger than the crude drug itself.
Elixirs: Aromatic, alcoholic, sweetened preparations. Elixir of phenobarbital is one example; the alcoholic cough medicines, terpin hydrate with codeine and plain elixir of codeine, are two more. Elixirs differ from tinctures in that they are sweetened. They should be used with caution in patients with diabetes or in alcohol abusers.

Oral Administration

If the drug is not intended to coat the oral cavity or throat, liquid medications may be followed by a quantity of water. Use a straw for fluid iron preparations, acids, and certain other minerals to avoid staining the teeth. Then rinse the mouth with water. Liquid medications are not recommended for patients who are too weak to pour the liquid and to hold it steady in the spoon. Liquid medications are ideal for children. Solid drugs should not be administered to children until they reach the age when they can safely swallow a solid drug form without the danger of aspirating the drug. Always remain with the patient until you are certain that the medication has been totally swallowed.

Mucous Membrane Forms

Some mucous membranes are selected for their ability to absorb medication for a systemic effect. The most commonly used areas are the gums, cheeks (buccal), under the tongue (sublingual), rectum, and the respiratory mucosa (inhalation). Nasal, ophthalmic, rectal, and vaginal preparations may also be applied to these mucous membranes for their localized effects.

Rectal Administration

The rectal mucosa provides a rapid absorption even though the surface of the rectum is small. Drugs are absorbed directly into the bloodstream, without being altered as they would be by the digestive processes, and without irritation to the patient's gastric mucosa. Rectal medications are useful if the patient is nauseated, vomiting, or unconscious. Manufacturers supply rectal medications in the form of gelatin or cocoa butter–based suppositories, which melt in the warmth of the rectum and release the medication, or in the form of enemas. Suppositories and enemas are also used for their local effect, that is, to treat constipation. Rectal suppositories are used to soften the stool or stimulate evacuation of the bowel; enemas, to cleanse and evacuate.

The best time to administer a rectal drug intended for a systemic effect is following a bowel movement or enema. The patient should be cautioned to remain lying down for 20 to 30 minutes to prevent accidental evacuation of the drug by a bowel movement or elimination of the enema. Suppositories intended to treat constipation, of course, are administered to bring about bowel evacuation. The patient should be instructed to insert the suppository about two inches above the rectal sphincter muscles; a little mineral oil or vegetable oil may be used as lubrication. If suppositories are individually wrapped in foil, make sure the patient knows that the foil is the wrapper and is not part of the treatment.

Vaginal Administration

Vaginal suppositories, tablets, creams, and fluid solutions are used to treat local infections. Irrigating solutions (douches) may be used as anti-infectives or to acidify the area. Creams and foams are available as local contraceptives. Vaginal instillation is most effective if the patient remains lying down; many preparations are therefore prescribed at bedtime. The patient may need to wear a pad to absorb drainage. Liquid medications can be applied to tampons and inserted for a period of time; then a pad is usually not needed. Solid suppositories and tablets may be lubricated or moistened with water and inserted by hand or with an applicator. Creams are instilled with applicators. Prepackaged, disposable irrigation kits are available for douching.

In addition to prescription douches, many over-the-counter preparations are now marketed. Advise your patients that vaginal secretions have their own wash-effect that is antiseptic in nature. Frequent douching can remove the secretions and change the acidity of the vaginal canal, resulting in infection caused by either normal flora or invading bacteria. When instructing patients, confirm that the patient can differentiate the urinary meatus from the vaginal orifice and the rectum. Mistakes could result in vaginal infections or in damage or infection to the urinary tract. A simple drawing and explanation may be required.

Inhalation

Inhalation drugs are supplied in the form of droplets, vapors, or gas. Because of the large surface area and the rich blood supply of the respiratory membranes, the respiratory tract absorbs medications more rapidly than any other mucous membrane. Inhalation can be used to produce a local effect, such as with medications to liquefy bronchial secretions or to dilate the bronchi to bring relief to asthmatic or emphysemic patients. In addition, inhalation may be used for systemic effects, such as with oxygen and general anesthesia. Most inhalant substances do spill over into the bloodstream, however, and caution must be taken not to bring about cardiac irregularities and central nervous system side effects. Hand-held inhalers are very common today. Each brand is different, and the patient needs to carefully read the package insert for proper use of the inhaler.

Oral Administration

Mouth and throat agents come in the form of sprays, swabs, sublingual tablets, and buccal tablets. The mouth and throat membranes may be treated locally with antiseptics for oral hygiene and local infections; with anesthetics for relief of pain; and with astringents that form a protective film over the mucous membranes. The patient may have to gargle, or the area may be painted or sprayed. To paint or spray the throat, first look for the area of inflammation to be treated. Otherwise, the part needing treatment may be missed entirely. Avoid touching the posterior pharynx (back of the throat); this causes gagging and possibly vomiting.

Sublingual tablets are placed under the tongue, where they are rapidly absorbed into the bloodstream by the rich supply of capillaries. Sublingual absorption is systemic and bypasses the acids in the stomach, which inactivate many medications. Nitroglycerin, used for treating the chest pains of angina pectoris, is one of these medications. Used properly, it can bring relief within minutes. Instruct patients not to chew or swallow the medication, and tell them that a mild tingling will be felt under the tongue as the medication dissolves. The lack of the tingling feeling usually indicates that the medication has expired or, for some other reason, is inactive. The patient should be instructed not to smoke, eat, or drink during administration of the drug.

Buccal tablets are placed between the cheek and the upper molars. The same rules of sublingual administration apply to buccal administration.

Nasal Administration

Nose drops, nasal sprays, and tampons are used for their localized effect, but like the inhalation drugs, they may spill over into the bloodstream, causing a change in the heart rate, an increase in blood pressure, or central nervous system stimulation. Nasal medications are commonly used for blocked nasal passages (decongestants) and nosebleeds (hemostatics). Nose drops should be instilled with the patient's head tilted back. Then the patient should be instructed to tilt the head forward to distribute the medication properly. Short, quick breaths will help spread the solution. Any medication spilling down the throat should be expectorated; swallowing nasal preparations can result in systemic side effects.

Nasal sprays are designed for administration with the patient's head upright. Be sure that the spray tip is centered in the nostril and not against the side of the nasal cavity. Nasal decongestant sprays are often misused by patients. Be sure to teach the patient not to exceed the amount or frequency ordered by the physician. If too much is used, these drugs can dry the mucosa and make congestion worse.

Topical Forms

With a few exceptions, **topical** drugs are local in their effect. Most drugs applied to the skin cannot be absorbed into the bloodstream (unless there is a break in the skin). However, large amounts of a drug left on the skin for a long time can be absorbed and cause systemic poisoning. For example, the previous use of hexachlorophene soaps on hospitalized infants caused toxic reactions and even infant deaths. Now this drug is banned from use in nonprescription soaps and lotions. Oil-based substances have a better chance of being absorbed through the skin than do substances that are water based. One of the most common causes of poisoning in adults is the absorption of oil-based insecticides.

Skin medication forms include lotions, liniments, ointments, compresses, creams, and patches.

Lotions

Often used to control itching, lotions are applied by dabbing with a soft cloth, cotton ball, or tongue blade. Calamine is an example. Rubbing will increase the itching or irritation. If the condition is contagious, the medical assistant should wear gloves. Some lotions are used to relieve congestion and pain in muscles and joints. In these cases, the application is covered with a thick cloth to retain heat. It is said that these lotions and heat dilate the superficial blood vessels, thus drawing blood to the surface and away from the congested parts. However, this is controversial. Many believe that the effects of these lotions are limited to the skin surface where the medication is applied.

Liniments

Liniments (emulsions) have a higher portion of oil than do lotions, and volatile active ingredients may be added. Liniments are often used to protect dried, cracked, or fissured skin.

Ointments

Ointments are semisolid medications containing bases such as petrolatum and lanolin, or nongreasy bases. Ointments are applied to dry, scaly areas with little or no hair and can exert a prolonged effect. Ointments are used in small amounts and are applied with firm strokes to avoid increasing itchiness. Ointments that stain clothing should be covered. An ointment should be removed from a jar or tube with a tongue blade to prevent contamination of the remaining medication.

Soaks, Compresses, and Wet Dressings

These aqueous solutions of substances with mild astringent properties have a soothing, cooling, antipyretic effect when applied to blistered and oozing areas. Bandages may be soaked in the solution, then applied to the patient, or the patient's extremity may be immersed in the solution and then wrapped in cloth. Plastic wrap can be applied over the bandage or cloth, or the wet dressing can rest on a plastic-covered surface until the air dries the bandage. If the solution contains a dye, the patient should be advised that the treatment will stain clothing or bedding.

Hot Soaks and Compresses

Hot compresses are used to treat abscesses and cellulitis. Extreme care must be taken to avoid burning the patient. Hot soaks are applied for up to 20 minutes; after this amount of time, circulation to a part reaches maximum flow and dissipates heat as fast as the compress can create it.

Creams

Creams contain active ingredients incorporated into emulsions that vanish when they are rubbed into the skin.

The Transdermal Patch

Nitroglycerin hormones, and scopolamine (used to treat motion sickness) can be absorbed slowly through the skin to create a constant, timed-release systemic effect. The nitroglycerin patch is particularly useful for patients with frequent attacks of angina. Hormone patches, mainly estrogens, can also be absorbed slowly through the skin, providing the needed hormonal levels to women who are allergic to oral estrogen. The scopolamine patch is placed behind the ear, and additional amounts of the drug can be released with gentle pressure. With dermal patches, drugs can be administered in a timed-release manner for up to 3 days.

Ear Drops and Irrigations

Topical ear medications have a local effect and come in the form of drops and irrigations. Medications are instilled into the ear canal to treat infections, reduce inflammation, and bring about local anesthesia. Drops should be instilled with the patient lying down on the unaffected side. Ear drops are supplied in small bottles, with a dropper attached to the cork or cap. The bottle should be held in the hand for a few minutes to warm the solution to body temperature. Drops that are too cold or too warm can cause pain or dizziness. If the contents need mixing, roll the bottle between the palms; do not shake. The patient should lie still for 15 to 30 minutes to allow the medication to coat the ear canal and to be absorbed. Cotton ear plugs should not be used unless specifically ordered. In addition, ear irrigations are performed with the patient sitting; in infants, the patient should be supine.

Eye Drops, Ointments, and Irrigations

Drug forms for medicating the eye are sterile. Eye solutions come in dropper bottles; ointments are supplied in small tubes. Drops and ointments should not be applied to the sensitive cornea of the eye.

Tips of the dropper and the tube must not touch any portion of the eye or eyelid. Drugs instilled into the eye are generally absorbed slowly and affect only the area in contact. However, some medications can act systemically if improper administration techniques are used. If a medication is allowed to flow into the lacrimal system, it can travel down into the nasal cavity and can be absorbed into the circulatory system. To avoid this, you should apply pressure to the inner angle (inner canthus) of the eye with a tissue immediately following instillation of the medication onto the lower eyelid. Eye drops and ointments are placed between the eyeball and the lower lid. To teach the patient to self-administer eye drops, demonstrate how to hold back the head, open the eye wide, and let the drops fall into the lower portion of the eye. Tell the patient not to worry if the drops run onto the face; the solution is harmless.

Parenteral Medication Forms

Injectable medications must be sterile and in liquid form. The drug is usually in a solution that is minimally irritating to human tissues, such as physiologic saline or sterile water, and may contain a preservative or a small amount of antibiotic to prevent bacterial growth in the **vial**. All injectable medications are dated. Before use, check the expiration date, and examine the solution for possible deterioration. A parenteral medication is administered with a sterile syringe and needle.

Ampule

An **ampule** is a small **hermetically sealed** glass flask, usually containing a single dose of medication. Ampules have a neck with a weak point that is broken just before use. To open an ampule:

1. Gently tap the top of the ampule with your fingers to settle all the medication to the bottom portion of the flask (Fig. 38-1).
2. Wipe the neck of the ampule clean with alcohol.
3. It may be necessary to use a small file provided by the manufacturer to score an ampule at the breaking point to facilitate easier breaking.
4. Sharply tap the top so that the top breaks away from you.
5. If the top does not snap off easily, it may be necessary to "bend" it off. Hold each half of the ampule between your thumbs and fingers, in front of you and above waist level.
6. Snap your wrists toward your body to break the neck of the ampule in two. You will hear a pop because the ampule is vacuum sealed. The glass is designed not to shatter, and the medication will not spill out. Without touching the sides, a syringe and needle unit is inserted into the ampule, and the medication is withdrawn into the syringe.

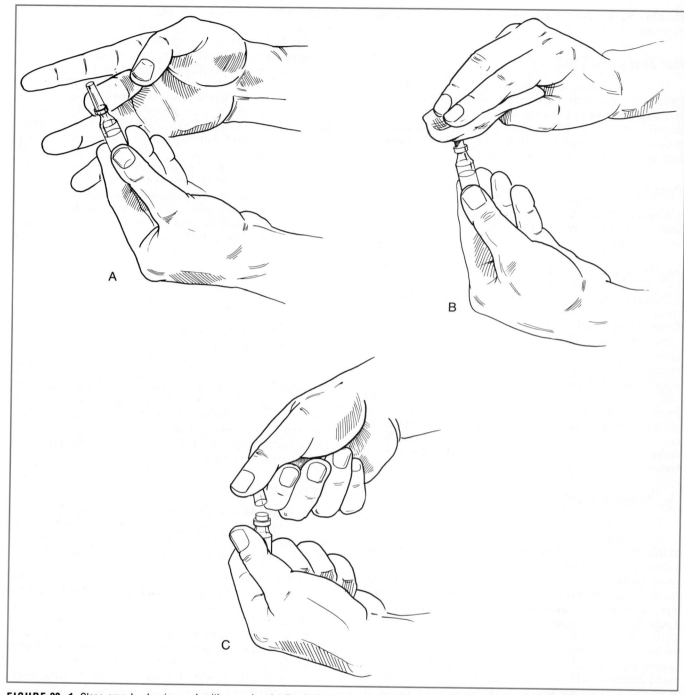

FIGURE 38–1. Glass ampule showing neck with a weak point line indicating breaking point. *A*, Tap neck of vial. *B*, Wipe neck of vial with alcohol prep. *C*, Snap off neck of vial.

Single-Dose Vial

A single-dose vial is a small bottle with a rubber stopper through which you insert a sterile needle to withdraw the single dose of medication inside. Before a sterile syringe and needle unit can be introduced into the solution, the rubber stopper must be wiped in a circular motion with alcohol or another suitable disinfectant.

Multi-Dose Vial

A multi-dose vial is a bottle with a rubber stopper that contains enough medication for multiple injections (Fig. 38–2). A vial may contain 30 cc of a drug. If the usual dosage is 0.5 cc, the bottle contains enough medication for 60 injections. Vials vary greatly in size, from 2 cc to 100 or more doses. Because multi-dose vials are entered more than once, extreme caution must be taken every time a needle is inserted into the medication. Contamination could cause very serious infections in future patients. If at any time, you feel that an error has been made or you suspect possible contamination, discard the vial. Never return unused medication to the vial. Learn to withdraw fluids to the correct mark. If you have more medication than you need in the syringe, eject the excess after you remove the unit from the vial. However, remember, your employer will not tolerate excessive waste of drugs due to imprecise withdrawing of medications for injection.

Vials are vacuum sealed. Each time you withdraw medication from a vial, you must first replace the portion of withdrawn medication with the same portion of air. Not enough replaced air will make it difficult to withdraw the medication; too much replaced air will force the medication into the syringe without your pulling on the plunger to withdraw it.

Prefilled Syringe

A prefilled syringe is a sterile disposable syringe and needle unit packaged by the manufacturer with a single dose of medication inside and ready to administer.

Cartridge Injection System

A cartridge injection system is a prefilled syringe and needle that is loaded into a metal cartridge for administration. The prefilled syringes are purchased by the box, and you use the same cartridge-loader over and over (Fig. 38–3).

Parenteral Medication Equipment

Both syringes and needles are manufactured in countless varieties for specific purposes and, sometimes, for specific medications. For example, there is a special syringe for insulin. Also, there is a special syringe unit for diabetics to use for self-injecting.

Hypodermic needles are manufactured in many lengths and widths, depending on the depth needed and the **viscosity** of the medication to be injected. Needles may be purchased separately or as part of a needle-syringe unit. Figure 38–4 shows the construction of a needle and the three common types of needle points. There are some facts to remember about the construction of a hypodermic needle. The following statement was prepared by the Becton Dickinson Company:

The size of the needle is governed by four factors: safety, rate of flow, comfort of the patient, and depth of penetration. There are three standard dimensions: length, outside diameter of the cannula, and wall thickness. Regular needles are measured for length from where the cannula joins the hub to the tip of the (needle) point.

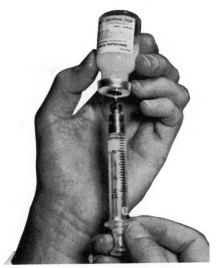

FIGURE 38–2. Filling a syringe from a multiple-dose vial. Keep the syringe at eye level.

Needle Gauge

The width of a needle is called its *gauge,* and needle gauges range in size from 14 (the largest) to 28 (the smallest). The smallest gauges (27 to 28) are used for intradermal injections when a very small opening is desired. These fine needle widths leave a small amount of medication just below the surface of the skin, with a minimum amount of injury. Gauges 25 and 26 are commonly used for subcutaneous injections. With a medication that is in an aqueous solution and is easily injected through a small opening, these two gauges cause minimal tissue damage, and the patient experiences less pain. Larger needles (gauges 20 to 23) are usually necessary for intramuscular injections when the medication is thick, such as penicillin, or the length of the needle requires the extra support of a thicker gauge. A patient cannot feel the difference between a 20- and a 22-gauge needle. In fact, the medication is not forced as strongly into the tissues with the larger 20-gauge needle as with the 22-gauge one, and the patient actually experiences less pain. Needles larger than 20 gauge are not used for drug therapy. They are mostly used for venipuncture, blood donations, and blood transfusions.

Needle Length

The choices of needle lengths vary from ⅜ inch to 4 inch, depending on the area of the body to be injected and the route (depth) used. Intradermal injections require only the short ⅜-inch needle. Needles that are ½ or ⅝ inch long are used for subcutaneous injections. Longer needles are necessary for depositing drugs intramuscularly. The choice of a 1-inch, 1½-inch, 2-inch, 2½-inch, or 3-inch length depends on both the muscle being used and the size of the patient.

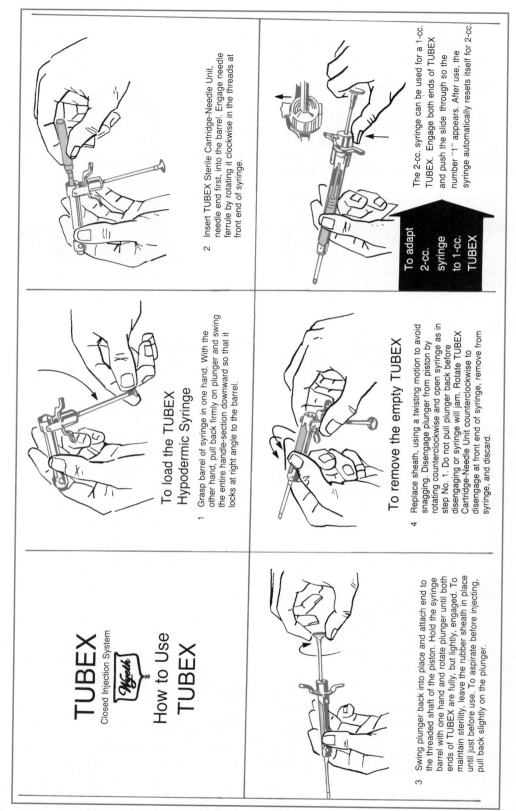

TUBEX
Closed Injection System

Wyeth

How to Use
TUBEX

1 Grasp barrel of syringe in one hand. With the other hand, pull back firmly on plunger and swing the entire handle-section downward so that it locks at right angle to the barrel.

To load the TUBEX Hypodermic Syringe

2 Insert TUBEX Sterile Cartridge-Needle Unit, needle end first, into the barrel. Engage needle ferrule by rotating it clockwise in the threads at front end of syringe.

3 Swing plunger back into place and attach end to the threaded shaft of the piston. Hold the syringe barrel with one hand and rotate plunger until both ends of TUBEX are fully, but lightly, engaged. To maintain sterility, leave the rubber sheath in place until just before use. To aspirate before injecting, pull back slightly on the plunger.

4 Replace sheath, using a twisting motion to avoid snagging. Disengage plunger from piston by rotating counterclockwise and open syringe as in step No. 1. Do not pull plunger back before disengaging or syringe will jam. Rotate TUBEX Cartridge-Needle Unit counterclockwise to disengage at front end of syringe, remove from syringe, and discard.

To remove the empty TUBEX

To adapt 2-cc. syringe to 1-cc. TUBEX

The 2-cc. syringe can be used for a 1-cc. TUBEX. Engage both ends of TUBEX and push the slide through so the number "1" appears. After use, the syringe automatically resets itself for 2-cc.

FIGURE 38–3. Procedure for administering an injection using a Tubex closed injection system. The method of administration is the same as with a conventional syringe. Remove the rubber sheath, introduce the needle into the patient, aspirate, and inject. (From Bonewit, K.: *Clinical Procedures for Medical Assistants,* 3rd ed., Philadelphia, W. B. Saunders Co., 1990, p 240.)

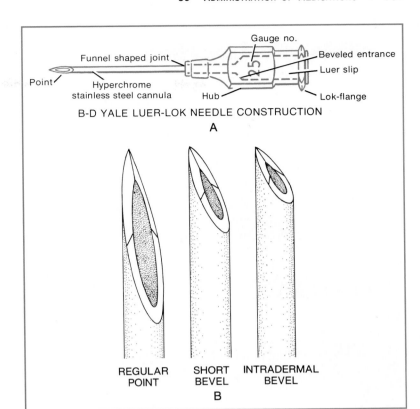

FIGURE 38-4. *A*, The construction of a hypodermic needle. *B*, Needle points.

Syringes

Figure 38-5 illustrates the construction of a 2.0-cc and a 10.0-cc syringe. The parts of a syringe are its barrel, calibrated scale(s), plunger, and tip. *Regular* syringes that hold up to 3.0 cc (ml) are usually calibrated with two scales: cc (ml) and minims. Larger *regular* syringes are calibrated in cc (ml) only. The *tuberculin* syringe is used for small quantities of drug, as it holds only up to 1.0 cc of injectable material (Fig. 38-6). The *insulin* syringe is calibrated in units specifically for diabetic use (Fig. 38-7).

Most syringes and needles are disposable—the advantages being the prevention of cross-infection, equipment that has not been damaged by use, and freedom from the duties of autoclaving and sterilization. Disposable needles are siliconized and are extremely smooth and sharp. Disposable units are packaged in sealed, rigid plastic containers (Fig. 38-8*A*) or in peel-apart paper wrappers (Fig. 38-8*B*). Both have an internal, rigid plastic sheath protecting the needle. Both individual needles and syringe-needle units are color coded for easy identification. Do not attempt to cut expenses by purchasing inferior or unknown brands of needles or

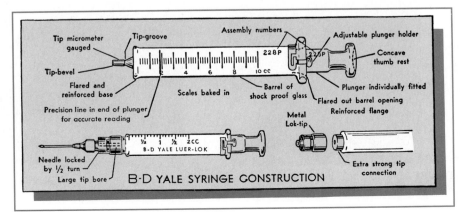

FIGURE 38-5. The basic construction of syringes, showing the 10-cc syringe and the 2-cc syringe. (Courtesy of Becton Dickinson Co.)

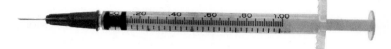

FIGURE 38-6. The disposable 1.0-cc tuberculin syringe with a detachable needle. This type of syringe is generally used for intradermal injections, such as allergy test, and for administering minute amounts of medication subcutaneously.

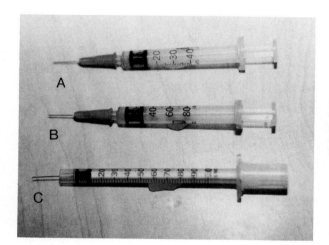

FIGURE 38-7. Insulin syringes have special calibrations to accommodate the various strengths of insulin that are manufactured. The drug is administered by concentration, which is measured in Units (U) and not in cubic centimeters (cc) or milliliters (ml). The U 100 syringe is becoming the "standard." *A,* Insulin syringe U 40. *B,* Insulin syringe U 80. *C,* Insulin syringe U 100.

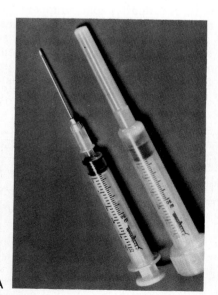

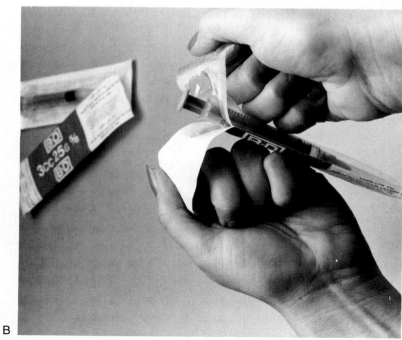

FIGURE 38-8. *A,* A rigid, disposable plastic package containing a syringe and needle unit. (Courtesy of Sherwood Medical Co., St. Louis, MO.) *B,* Sterile paper packaging containing a syringe and needle unit. (Courtesy of Becton Dickinson Co.)

syringes. Table 38–1 summarizes the needle and syringe sizes used for injections.

Biojector

The *Biojector* is a high-speed, pneumatically powered jet injector that uses compressed gas acting against a piston to eject medication through a small orifice at approximately the speed of sound. This jet action effectively causes medications to penetrate the skin, delivering them subcutaneously and intramuscularly. There is no needle, and thus, the risk of the accidental puncture of a nerve sheath or of the injection of the drug into a vein or artery is eliminated. This system also eliminates the possibility of an accidental needlestick to the health care worker. The Biojector is loaded and cared for similarly to the tubex injection equipment (Fig. 38–9).

PARENTERAL ADMINISTRATION

With practice, giving medications by injection will become easy and even automatic, but as stated before and stressed often, always follow the physician's orders, the "three befores," and the "six rights." Develop techniques that provide maximum safety and comfort for the patient. Injections are least painful when the needle is inserted swiftly and the medication injected slowly. Remember that the same aseptic conditions necessary for minor surgery are necessary whenever you penetrate the protective skin barrier.

Injections are not given near bones or blood vessels. Injections should never be given in an area where there is scar tissue, a change in skin pigmentation or texture, or excess tissue growth such as a mole or a wart. The point of injection should be as far as possible from any major nerve, and the site selected should be capable of holding the amount of medication that is injected. Never inject into an arm from which the lymph nodes have been removed (as after a **radical mastectomy**), as the medication cannot be absorbed into the bloodstream.

Make certain that all materials are ready for use. Many offices have a central room where medications are prepared. The medication is then taken to the waiting patient in another room. Handling medication administration in this way has many advantages, but care must be taken that the syringe and needle unit are transported with sterile technique. After a syringe is filled, the cap is replaced for transport to the patient. Never wrap a needle in gauze or cotton.

When carrying a syringe and needle, hold it horizontally and parallel to your body. Never transport more than one injection at a time, unless two or more are for the same patient or unless you have a

TABLE 38–1. NEEDLE AND SYRINGE SIZES FOR INJECTIONS

Route	Gauge	Length	Syringe
Intradermal	27–28	⅜ in	Tuberculin
Subcutaneous	25–26	½, ⅝ in	2 cc; tuberculin; insulin
Intramuscular	20–23	1–3 in	2–5 cc

special medication tray that has a named position for each syringe. Never combine two medications in a single syringe unless specifically ordered by the physician. If you are preparing a medication for the physician to give, place the vial or empty ampule beside the filled syringe. This shows what medication is in the syringe and offers a double check.

Use a professional approach and tell the patient what you are going to do. Small talk can keep the patient's mind off the procedure. Never tell a patient that it will not hurt; you may destroy your credibility. Make the patient as comfortable as possible, and allow for privacy. Never allow the patient to stand during the procedure. Keep the equipment out of the patient's sight as much as possible. Wear gloves and other blood and body-fluid protection barriers.

Destruction of Used Syringes and Needles

Follow guidelines in Chapter 25. After giving an injection, dispose of the syringe, needle, and gloves by placing them into a closed container immediately (Fig. 38–10). The cap should not be replaced on the needle, and the needle should not be cut or broken.

Reusable Syringes

Reusable syringes are not recommended; however, there are some medications that must be administered in glass syringes. If you must use reusable syringes, the Centers for Disease Control state, "Needles should be discarded in a puncture-resistant rigid container immediately. Reusable glass syringes should be thoroughly rinsed in cold water after use and soaked in a 10% bleach solution or commercial recommended soak." Syringes should be wrapped and sterilized (see Chapter 24).

Intramuscular Injections

Intramuscular injections are given into the muscle when (1) drugs will irritate the subcutaneous tissues, (2) a more rapid absorption is desired, or (3) the volume of the medication to be injected is large. The

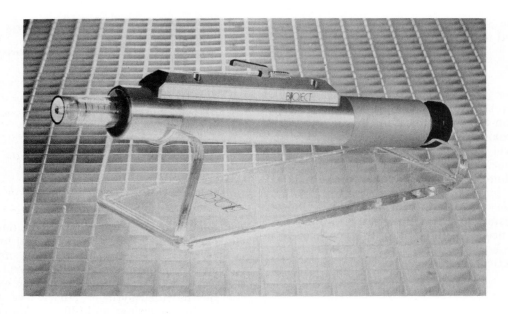

Biojector® Jet Injection System
Easy to use.

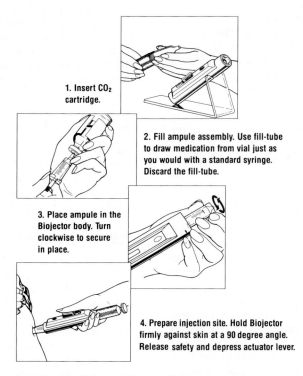

1. Insert CO_2 cartridge.

2. Fill ampule assembly. Use fill-tube to draw medication from vial just as you would with a standard syringe. Discard the fill-tube.

3. Place ampule in the Biojector body. Turn clockwise to secure in place.

4. Prepare injection site. Hold Biojector firmly against skin at a 90 degree angle. Release safety and depress actuator lever.

Biojector® is a registered trademark of Bioject Medical Systems Ltd. and its subsidiary, Bioject Inc.
©1990 Bioject Inc.
171-0108-00, 11/90

FIGURE 38–9. Biojector Jet Injection System. (Courtesy of Bioject Medical Systems Ltd. and its subsidiary, Bioject Inc.)

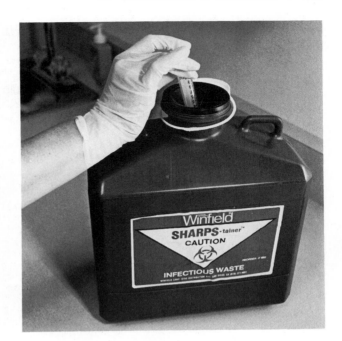

FIGURE 38-10. A rigid, puncture-resistant, disposable container into which needle-syringe units are placed immediately after use.

PROCEDURE 38-1   FILLING A SYRINGE

GOAL To fill a syringe with 1.5 cc of sterile water from a multipurpose vial, using sterile technique.

EQUIPMENT AND SUPPLIES

A vial or ampule containing the material
   to be injected
Antiseptic sponges

A sterile needle and syringe unit
A written order, including the drug
   name, strength, and route

PROCEDURAL STEPS

1. Read the order and choose a correct vial of medication (Fig. 38-11).
    Purpose: To check the medication the first of three times.

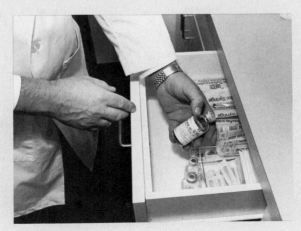

FIGURE 38-11.

Continued

PROCEDURE 38-1 *Continued*

2. Choose the correct syringe and needle size, depending on the site and the quantity of medication to be injected (Fig. 38-12).

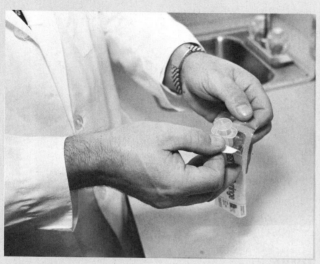

FIGURE 38-12.

3. Wash your hands.

4. Compare the order to both the name of the drug on the vial of medication and the amount to be withdrawn in the syringe.
   Purpose: To check the medication the second of three times.

5. Gently agitate the medication by rolling the vial between your palms (Fig. 38-13).
   Purpose: To mix any medication that may have settled.

6. Check the quality of the medication and the expiration date.
   Purpose: Medications may become contaminated or outdated.

7. Cleanse the rubber stopper of the vial with the antiseptic sponge, using a circular motion (Fig. 38-14).

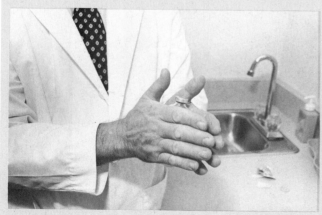

FIGURE 38-13.

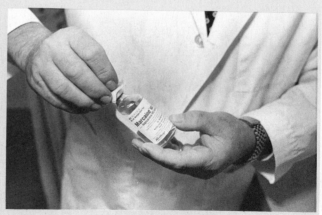

FIGURE 38-14.

Continued

8. Set down the vial. (You may hold the vial in the palm of your minor hand while you continue, if you do not contaminate the rubber stopper.)

9. Take the needle-syringe unit and remove the cap from the plastic protective case, or peel away the protective wrapper.

10. Remove the syringe.

11. Grasp the plunger and draw up an amount of air equal to the amount of medication ordered.
    Purpose: Not enough replaced air will make it difficult to withdraw the medication; too much replaced air will force the medication into the syringe without your pulling on the plunger to withdraw it.

12. Grasp the plastic sheath covering the needle between two fingers on the posterior side of your minor hand, and pull the syringe out of the sheath with your major hand.
    Purpose: To keep the sheath sterile for replacing it on the needle for transportation to the patient. The sheath may not be placed on a nonsterile surface or touched near its opening.

13. If you are not already holding the vial with the sheath in your minor hand, pick up the vial with the same hand that is holding the empty sheath, being careful not to touch the sheath to any nonsterile surface.

14. Turn the vial upside down without touching the rubber stopper.

15. Fully insert the needle into the center of the rubber stopper with your major hand.

16. Inject the air in the syringe into the vial.

17. Slowly pull back on the plunger until the proper amount of medication is withdrawn.
    Purpose: Withdrawing medication rapidly will cause air bubbles to form in the syringe (Fig. 38–15).

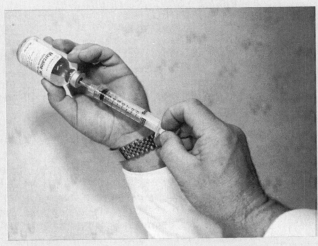

FIGURE 38–15.

Continued

PROCEDURE 38-1 *Continued*

18. While the needle is still in the vial, check that there are no air bubbles in the syringe.
    Purpose: Air bubbles displace medication, and the patient will not receive the proper amount of medication.

19. If there are air bubbles, slip the fingers holding the vial down to grasp the vial and syringe as a single unit.
    Purpose: This frees your major hand.

20. With your free hand, tap the syringe until the air bubbles dislodge and float into the tip of the syringe.

21. Gently expel these tiny air bubbles through the needle, then continue withdrawing the medication.

22. Withdraw the needle from the vial, and replace the sheath over the needle without the needle touching the sides of the sheath.

23. Return the medication to the shelf or the refrigerator, checking that you have the correct drug and dosage.
    Purpose: This is the third of the "three befores" of drug checking.

24. Clean the area.

---

angle of insertion is 90 degrees (Fig. 38–16), and the preferred sites are the *gluteus medius, vastus lateralis, deltoid, and ventrogluteal muscles* of the adult (Fig. 38–17). It is believed that some intramuscular injections are not given with a long enough needle, and medications may, therefore, be deposited into the upper adipose (fatty) tissue by

error. Fatty tissue does not absorb medications well, and the medication may remain at the site of the injection. Be certain to select needles that are long enough, especially for obese patients.

When locating a site for an intramuscular injection, expose the site so that you are able to visualize and palpate the landmarks correctly. Table 38–2 lists the sites as well as the criteria for choosing one site over another.

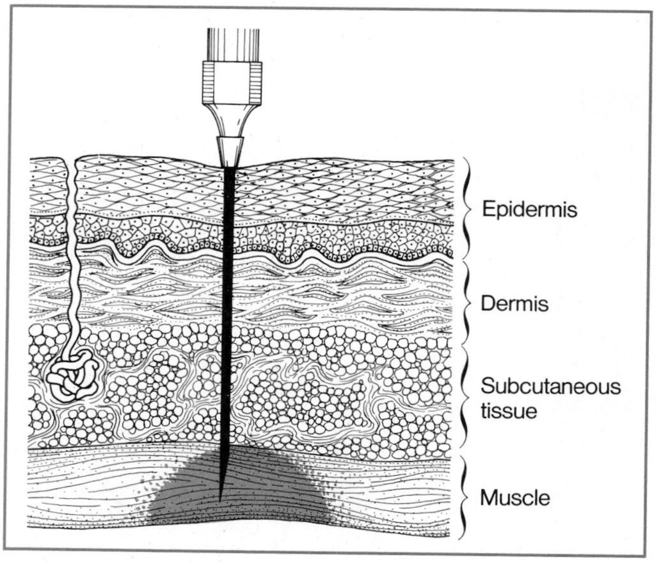

FIGURE 38-16. An anatomic illustration of the intramuscular injection. Note that the needle is inserted at a 90-degree angle and deposits the medication into the large central part of the muscle.

Labels in figure: Epidermis, Dermis, Subcutaneous tissue, Muscle

Vastus Lateralis (Thigh) Site

This muscle is part of the *quadriceps group* of the thigh. It is one of the body's largest muscles, and because it is developed at birth, it is considered the safest for infants. Many experts feel that as a site for adult intramuscular (IM) injections, the vastus lateralis is better than either the deltoid or the dorsogluteal sites because there are fewer major nerves and blood vessels in the vastus lateralis. The vastus lateralis muscle fills the midportion of the upper, outer thigh. In the adult, it can be located from one hand's width below the proximal end of the *greater trochanter* to one hand's width above the top of the *patella* (knee cap). Wyeth Laboratories states, "For infants and children, the acceptable position of this region lies below the greater trochanter of the femur and within the upper lateral quadrant of the thigh" (Fig. 38–18). The adult patient may sit or lie supine, but it is easier to locate the vastus lateralis with the patient lying down.

38

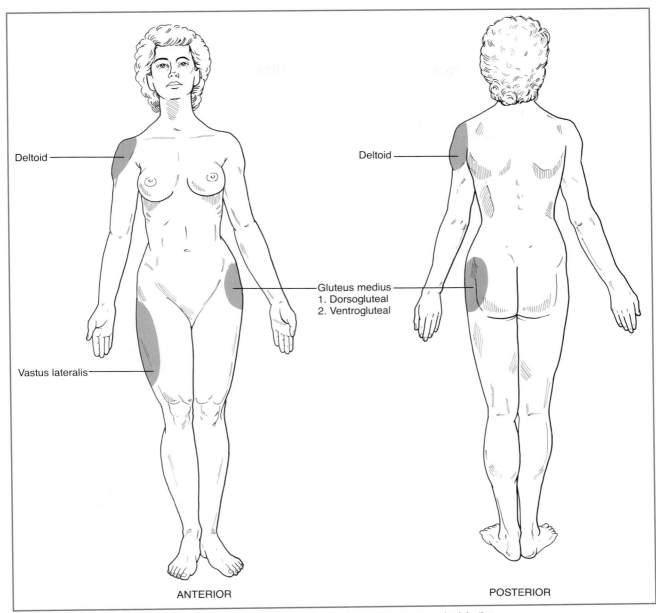

Deltoid

Vastus lateralis

Deltoid

Gluteus medius
1. Dorsogluteal
2. Ventrogluteal

ANTERIOR

POSTERIOR

FIGURE 38-17. The muscles commonly used for intramuscular injection.

Dorsogluteal (Gluteus Medius) Site

This is the traditional site for deep IM injections. However, complications due to sciatic nerve injury are frequent enough that experts are suggesting that this site be abandoned and replaced with the vastus lateralis and ventrogluteal sites. The dorsogluteal site continues to be popular, and it is still acceptable for adults if care is taken to locate the exact site. It is recommended that this site *not* be used for infants. The patient must lie in the prone position. To relax the muscles, the toes should be pointing inward. To locate the site, draw an imaginary diagonal line starting at the *greater trochanter* of the femur, across the buttocks, to the *posterior spine of the ilium*. Palpate these bony prominences to make

certain that you are at the correct site. The injection is made into the gluteus medius muscle several inches below the *iliac crest* (Fig. 38–19).

Ventrogluteal (Gluteus Medius) Site

Although considered safe, this site is not used as frequently as the others. This technique uses a larger mass of the gluteus medius muscle than when using the dorsogluteal site. The area is free of major nerves and blood vessels, and it is considered safe for both infants and adults (Fig. 38–20). All types of IM medications can be injected here, including the thick oily preparations. To locate the site, place your right palm on the patient's *greater trochanter,*

TABLE 38-2. TYPES OF INJECTIONS

Method	Drug Amount	Sites	Examples
IM	Adult, 1–2 cc	Deltoid	Adrenalin (epinephrine)
	Adult, 2–5 cc	Vastus lateralis	Penicillin
		Dorsogluteal, ventrogluteal	Demerol (meperidine)
	Child, 1–2 cc	Vastus lateralis, ventrogluteal	Penicillin
IM, Z	As above	Dorsogluteal, ventrogluteal	Irritating drugs
SC	Adult, 0.1–2.0 cc	Deltoid	Insulin
		Thigh	Vaccines
		Abdomen	Toxoids
	Child, 0.5 cc	Deltoid	Vaccines
		Thigh, abdomen	Toxoids
ID	Adult and child, 0.1–0.5 cc	Forearm	Tuberculin test, skin tests

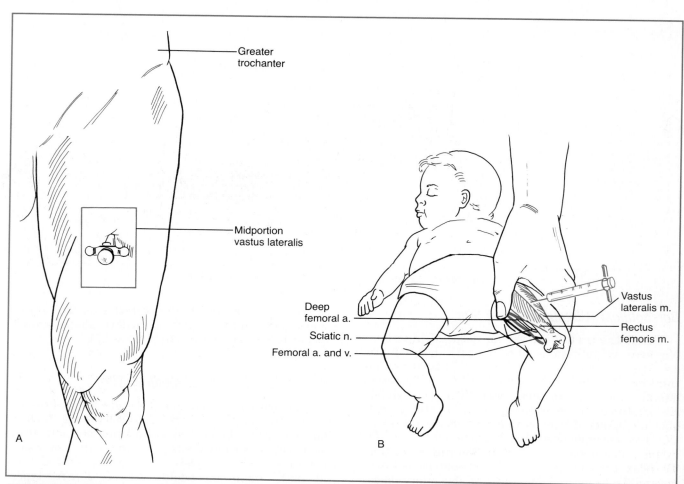

FIGURE 38-18. The vastus lateralis muscle is the preferred site for intramuscular injections in infants and children. *A,* Site selection for adults. *B,* Site selection for infants and children.

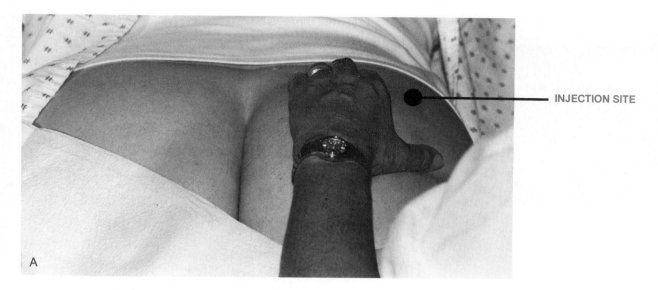

A

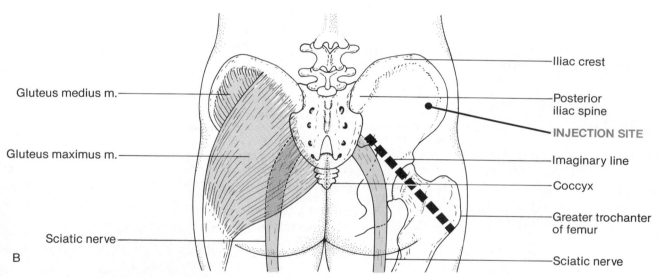

B

FIGURE 38-19. The dorsogluteal (gluteus medius) site is still preferred by many physicians.

then put your index finger on the *anterior iliac spine,* and spread your middle finger back as far as possible from your index finger, trying to touch the *crest of the ilium.* The center of the triangle formed by your index and middle fingers is the site for the injection. Choose the hand that is the opposite of the patient's side, that is, use your left hand to palpate the patient's right ventrogluteal site, and your right hand to palpate the patient's left side. For a child, you will need a 1-inch needle, whereas in an obese adult patient, you may need a 2½-inch needle to reach the depth of the muscle.

Deltoid Site

The deltoid muscle, the muscular cap of the shoulder, is located at the top of the upper, outer arm. The muscle mass is somewhat limited, so it cannot hold a large volume of medication. This triangular muscle is located between the *acromion* and *deltoid tuberosities* and fills an area approximately two fingerbreadths below the *acromion process* (Fig. 38-21). The major nerves and blood vessels located in the posterior portion of the arm must be avoided. Aqueous medications are most appropriate here, for

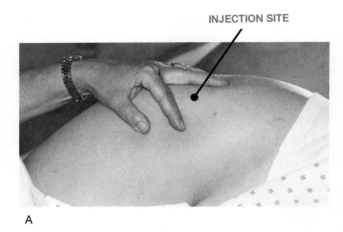

A

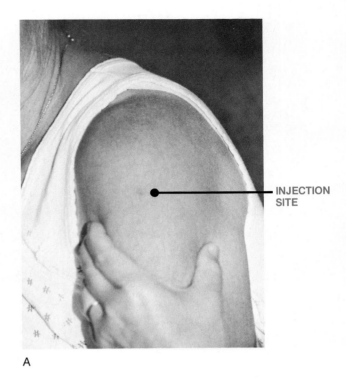

A

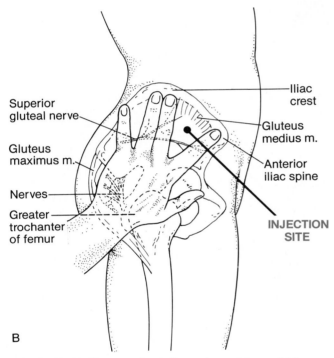

B

FIGURE 38-20. The ventrogluteal site can be used for most intramuscular injections.

example, vitamin B_{12}. If frequent injections are ordered, rotate the site and alternate the right and left arm. The deltoid site is acceptable for adults and older children, but it should not be used when the muscle is small or underdeveloped. For a small arm, you may need only a 25-gauge ⅝-inch needle; the 23-gauge 1-inch needle is most often used for the average-sized arm. When injecting, expose the entire shoulder rather than rolling up the sleeve. Grasp the muscle, and stretch the skin before injecting the medication. The patient may be seated or lying down.

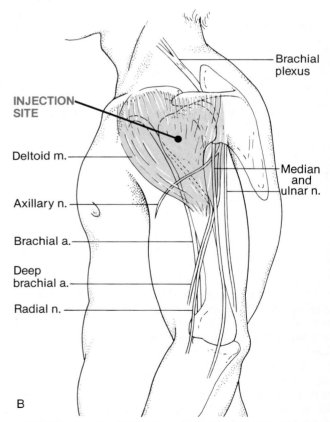

B

FIGURE 38-21. The deltoid muscle site is used for both intramuscular and subcutaneous injections. It is not recommended for infants because the muscle is not developed until later in childhood.

GOAL To inject 2 cc of medication into the muscle, using a needle and syringe of the correct size, as directed by the physician.

EQUIPMENT AND SUPPLIES

A vial or ampule containing the material to be injected
Antiseptic sponges
A sterile needle and syringe unit

A written order, including the patient's name, when to give the drug, the route of administration, and the name and strength of the drug

PROCEDURAL STEPS

1. Wash your hands. Follow universal blood and body-fluid precautions. Glove yourself with nonsterile gloves.

2. Select the correct medication from the shelf or the refrigerator.
   Purpose: Some medications must be refrigerated.

3. Read the label to be sure that you have the right drug and the right strength.
   Purpose: One medication may be manufactured and prepackaged in different strengths; for instance, a particular drug may be available in vials of both 250 mg/cc and 500 mg/cc.

4. Warm refrigerated medications by gently rolling between your palms.

5. Prepare the syringe, calculating the right dose.

6. Transport the medication to the patient.

7. Greet and identify the patient by name.
   Purpose: To be sure that you have the right patient.

8. Position the patient comfortably.

9. Expose the site.

10. Cleanse the patient's skin with the antiseptic sponge, using a circular motion, moving outward from the center (Fig. 38-22).

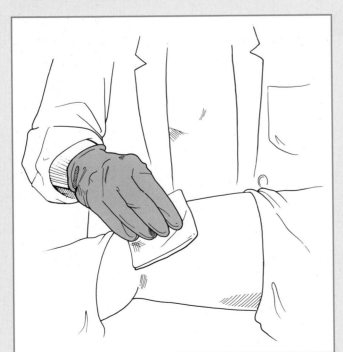

FIGURE 38-22.

Continued

PROCEDURE 38-2 *Continued*

11. Compare the order with the prepared medication, and the patient to the name on the order, to make sure that this is the right time to administer the drug.
    Purpose: This is the last of the six checks to be made before administering a medication. If there is any doubt, do not proceed. Check first with the physician.

12. Remove the sheath from the needle.

13. With the thumb and first two fingers of your minor hand, spread the skin tightly at the site to be injected, or pinch a large portion of the muscle at the site to be injected (Fig. 38–23).
    Purpose: Smoothing the skin by stretching or pinching facilitates the insertion of the needle.

14. Grasp the syringe as you would a dart, and with one swift movement, insert the entire needle up to the hub, at a 90-degree angle into the muscle (Fig. 38–24).
    Purpose: The depth of the injection is determined by the choice of needle length, not by how far you insert the needle. Once the needle is at the tissue layer, do not move the needle while injecting the medication. Being in as far as the hub helps to keep the needle in one place.

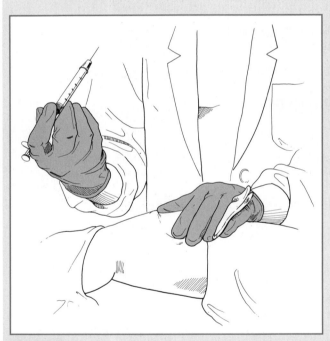

FIGURE 38-23.

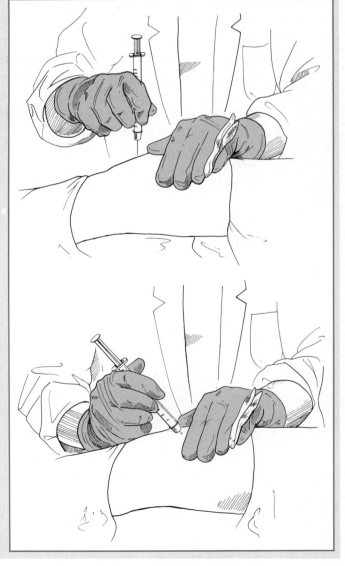

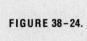

FIGURE 38-24.

Continued

15. Aspirate: Withdraw the plunger slightly to be sure that no blood enters the syringe (Fig. 38–25).
   Purpose: Blood in the syringe means that the needle is in a blood vessel and is not in the muscle tissue. You may *not* administer an intramuscular medication by the intravenous route.

16. If blood appears, immediately withdraw the syringe, and compress the injection site with the sponge.

17. Begin again with step 1.
   Purpose: Blood is now mixed with the medication, and the medication is considered contaminated. Blood may interact with the drug and may be irritating to the intramuscular tissues.

18. If no blood appears in the syringe, push in the plunger slowly and steadily until all medication has been administered (Fig. 38–26).
   Purpose: A rapid injection may tear the muscle tissue.

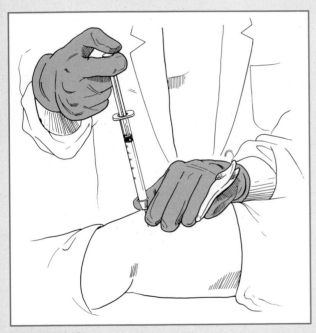

FIGURE 38–25.

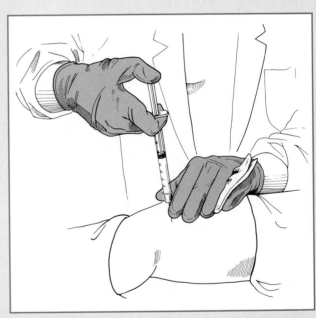

FIGURE 38–26.

19. Cover the area with the sponge, and withdraw the needle at the same angle of insertion (Fig. 38–27).

20. Gently massage the site with the antiseptic sponge.
   Purpose: Massage helps to increase absorption and to decrease pain (Fig. 38–28).

21. Make sure that your patient is comfortable and safe.

22. Dispose of the needle and syringe.

23. Observe the patient for any adverse reaction. You may need to keep the patient under observation for 20 to 30 minutes.

Continued

PROCEDURE 38-2 *Continued*

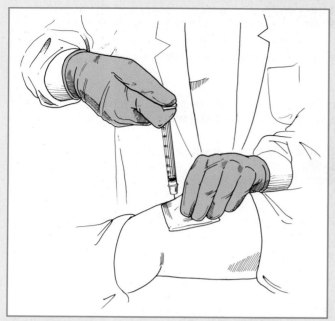

FIGURE 38-27.

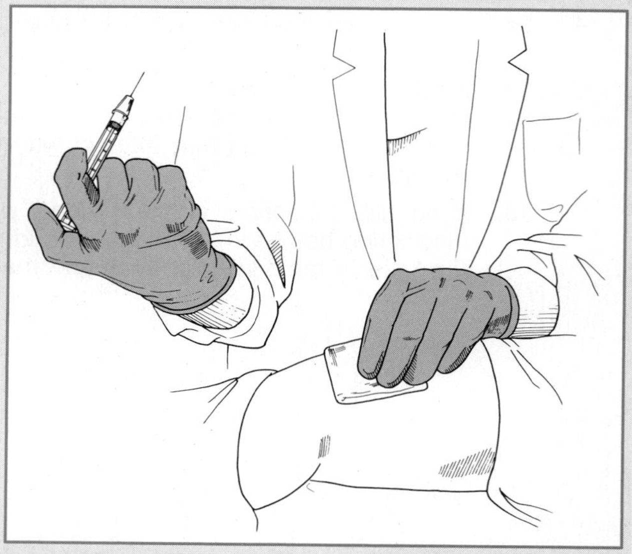

FIGURE 38-28.

24. Wash your hands.

25. Record the drug administration on the patient's medical record, and on the required DEA record if the medication is a controlled substance.

Z-Tract Intramuscular Injection

Some intramuscular medications are irritating to the skin and subcutaneous tissues. The injection must be given in such a way as to prevent any leakage back from the deep muscle into the upper subcutaneous layers. The Z-tract method displaces the upper tissue laterally before the needle is inserted (Fig. 38-29). The skin is pulled to one side before the tissue is grasped for the injection. After the needle is withdrawn, the tissue is released, with the needle tract to one side of where the medication is deposited in the muscle. The medication cannot leak out. These medications are always injected into the gluteus medius muscle of the buttocks. Because the medication is so irritating to the tissues, the needle should be changed after

withdrawing the medication from the vial.

Some medications require the injection of 0.5 cc of air following an injection. This air will clear the needle of the medication and will prevent the medication from flowing back along the tract of the injection. This air can be pulled into the syringe after the medication has been drawn in. Because the syringe is pointed downward during the injection, the air will float to the other end of the syringe and will be the last to enter the tissue. Wait a few seconds before withdrawing the needle. Wait 10 seconds before releasing the skin.

Many medications that require the Z-tract method should not be massaged after injection; just hold a sponge over the area for a few seconds. Walking will help the medication absorb. Use alternate sides for multiple or frequent injections.

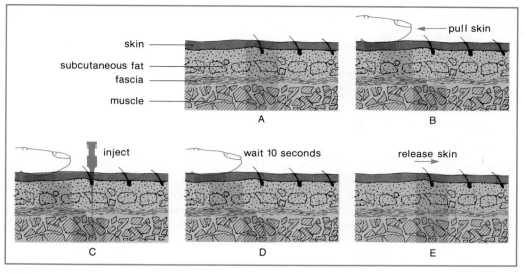

FIGURE 38-29. The Z-tract method of intramuscular injection is used when medications are irritating to subcutaneous tissues. This technique helps prevent the medication from leaking into the subcutaneous tissues.

PROCEDURE 38-3   GIVING A Z-TRACT INTRAMUSCULAR INJECTION

GOAL   To inject 1 cc of medication into the muscle using a needle and syringe of correct size and the Z-tract method, as directed by the physician.

EQUIPMENT AND SUPPLIES

A vial or ampule containing the material to be injected
Antiseptic sponges
A sterile needle and syringe unit

A written order, including the patient's name, when to give the drug, the route of administration, and the name and strength of the drug

PROCEDURAL STEPS

1. Wash your hands. Follow universal blood and body-fluid precautions. Glove yourself with nonsterile gloves.

2. Select the correct medication from the shelf or the refrigerator.
   Purpose: Some medications must be refrigerated.

3. Read the label to be sure that you have the right drug and the right strength.
   Purpose: One medication may be manufactured and prepackaged in different strengths; for instance, a particular drug may be available in vials of both 250 mg/cc and 500 mg/cc.

4. Warm refrigerated medications by gently rolling the container between your palms.

5. Prepare the syringe, calculating the right dose.

6. If the manufacturer so directs, draw 0.5 cc of air into the syringe.

7. Replace the sheath on the needle, and give a slight turn to loosen the needle. Secure a new needle, still in its sheath, to the tip of the syringe. Discard the contaminated needle.
   Purpose: The needle that was used to withdraw the medication is covered with a substance irritating to the skin and subcutaneous tissues.

Continued

PROCEDURE 38-3 *Continued*

8. Transport the medication to the patient.

9. Greet and identify the patient by name.
   Purpose: To be sure that you have the right patient.

10. Position the patient comfortably.

11. Expose the site.

12. Cleanse the patient's skin with the antiseptic sponge, using a circular motion, moving outward from the center.

13. Compare the order with the prepared medication, and the patient with the name on the order, to make sure that this is the right time to administer the drug.
    Purpose: This is the last of the six checks to be made before administering a medication. If there is any doubt, do not proceed. Check first with the physician.

14. Remove the sheath from the needle.

15. Pull the skin to one side and hold it firmly in place. If the skin is slippery, use a dry gauze sponge to hold the skin in place.
    Purpose: Displacing the skin prevents irritating medications from leaking back to the surface.

16. Grasp the syringe as you would a dart, and with one swift movement, insert the entire needle up to the hub, at a 90-degree angle into the muscle.
    Purpose: The depth of the injection is determined by the choice of needle length, not by how far you insert the needle. Once the needle is at the tissue layer, do not move the needle while injecting the medication. Being in as far as the hub helps to keep the needle in one place.

17. Aspirate: Withdraw the plunger slightly to be sure that no blood enters the syringe.
    Purpose: Blood in the syringe means that the needle is in a blood vessel and not in the muscle tissue. You may *not* administer an intramuscular medication by the intravenous route.

18. If blood appears, immediately withdraw the syringe, and compress the injection site with the sponge.
    Purpose: To minimize bleeding and bruising.

19. Begin again with step 1.
    Purpose: Blood is now mixed with the medication, and the medication is considered contaminated. Blood may interact with the drug and may be irritating to the intramuscular tissues.

20. If no blood appears in the syringe, push in the plunger slowly and steadily until all medication has been administered.
    Purpose: A rapid injection may tear the muscle tissue.

21. Wait a few seconds, then cover the area with the sponge, and withdraw the needle at the same angle of insertion. Wait 10 seconds, then release the skin.

22. If the manufacturer recommends it, gently massage the site with the antiseptic sponge.
    Purpose: Massage helps to increase absorption and to decrease pain.

23. Make sure your patient is comfortable and safe.

24. Dispose of the needle and syringe.

25. Observe the patient for any adverse reaction. You may need to keep the patient under observation for 20 to 30 minutes.

26. Wash your hands.

27. Record the drug administration on the patient's medical record, and on the required DEA record if the medication is a controlled substance.

Subcutaneous Injections

Subcutaneous injections are given just under the skin, into the fatty areolar layer called *adipose tissue* (Fig. 38–30). Smaller doses of less irritating drugs are given by this method. The angle of insertion is 45 degrees; however, heparin and insulin are usually administered at a 90-degree angle. The deltoid area is an injection site; however, the abdomen, thigh, and upper back may be used (Fig. 38–31). When multiple or frequent injections are ordered, the sites must be rotated. It is best to keep a rotation record. Most analgesics and immunizations are administered by subcutaneous injection.

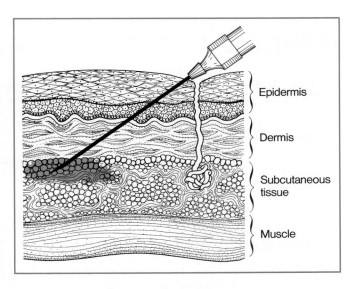

FIGURE 38–30. The subcutaneous injection is administered with a needle smaller and shorter than that used for the intramuscular injection. This method is used for small amounts of nonirritating medications in aqueous solution. It is injected at a 45-degree angle (at a 90-degree angle for insulin and heparin). The most common site is the deltoid region of the upper arm.

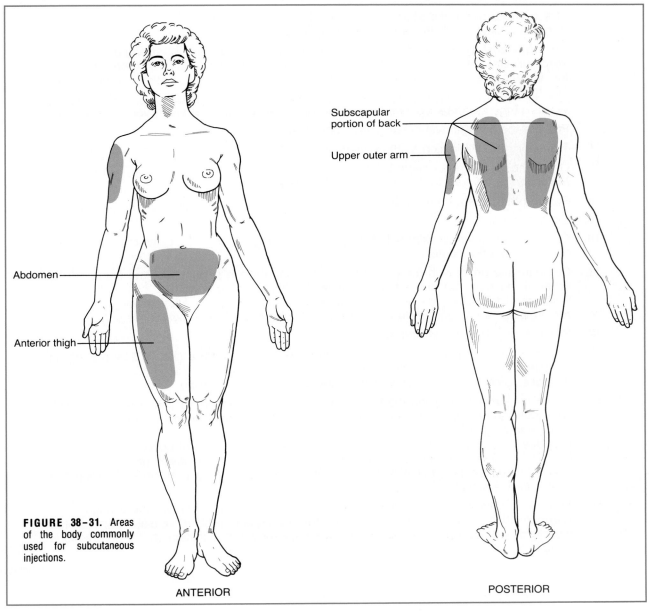

FIGURE 38–31. Areas of the body commonly used for subcutaneous injections.

ANTERIOR

POSTERIOR

PROCEDURE 38-4   GIVING A SUBCUTANEOUS INJECTION

GOAL   To inject 0.5 cc of medication into the subcutaneous tissue using a needle and syringe of correct size, as directed by the physician.

EQUIPMENT AND SUPPLIES

A vial or ampule containing the material to be injected
Antiseptic sponges
A sterile needle and syringe unit

A written order, including the patient's name, when to give the drug, the route of administration, and the name and strength of the drug

PROCEDURAL STEPS

1. Wash your hands. Follow universal blood and body-fluid precautions. Glove yourself with nonsterile gloves.

2. Select the correct medication from the shelf or the refrigerator.
   Purpose: Some medications must be refrigerated.

3. Read the label to be sure that you have the right drug and the right strength.
   Purpose: One medication may be manufactured and prepackaged in different strengths; for instance, a particular drug may be available in vials of both 250 mg/cc and 500 mg/cc.

4. Warm refrigerated medications by gently rolling the container between your palms.

5. Prepare the syringe, withdrawing the right dose.

6. Transport the medication to the patient.

7. Greet and identify the patient by name.
   Purpose: To be sure that you have the right patient.

8. Position the patient comfortably.

9. Expose the site.

10. Cleanse the patient's skin with the antiseptic sponge, using a circular motion, moving outward from the center.

11. Compare the order with the prepared medication, and the patient with the name on the order, to be sure that this is the right time to administer the drug.
    Purpose: This is the last of the six checks to be made before administering a medication. If there is any doubt, do not proceed. Check first with the physician.

12. Remove the sheath from the needle.

13. With the thumb and first two fingers of your minor hand, form a skin fold by picking up the tissue or by pulling the skin taut.
    Purpose: Smoothing the skin facilitates the insertion of the needle.

14. Grasp the syringe between the thumb and the first two fingers of your major hand with your palm up, and with one swift movement, insert the entire needle up to the hub at a 45-degree angle (Fig. 38-32).
    Purpose: The depth of the injection is determined by the choice of needle length, not by how far you insert the needle. Once the needle is at the tissue layer, do not move the needle while injecting the medication. Being in as far as the hub helps to keep the needle in one place.

15. Aspirate: Withdraw the plunger slightly to be sure that no blood enters the syringe.
    Purpose: Blood in the syringe means that the needle is in a blood vessel and not in the muscle tissue. You may *not* administer a subcutaneous medication by the intravenous route.

Continued

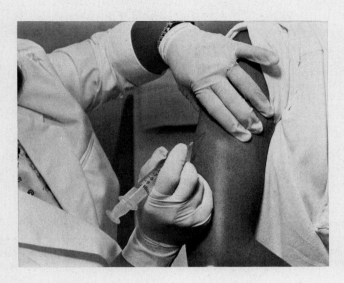

FIGURE 38-32.

16. If blood appears, immediately withdraw the syringe, and compress the injection site with the sponge.
    Purpose: To minimize bleeding and bruising.

17. Begin again with step 1.
    Purpose: Blood is now mixed with the medication, and the medication is considered contaminated. Blood may interact with the drug and may be irritating to the subcutaneous tissues.

18. If no blood appears in the syringe, push in the plunger slowly and steadily until all medication has been administered.
    Purpose: A rapid injection may damage the tissues.

19. Cover the area with the sponge, and withdraw the needle at the same angle of insertion.

20. Gently massage the site with the antiseptic sponge.
    Purpose: Massage helps to increase absorption and to decrease pain.

21. Make sure that your patient is comfortable and safe.

22. Dispose of the needle and syringe.

23. Observe the patient for any adverse reaction. You may need to keep the patient under observation for 20 to 30 minutes.

24. Wash your hands.

25. Record the drug administration on the patient's medical record, and on the required DEA record if the medication is a controlled substance.

Intradermal Injections

Intradermal injections differ from subcutaneous injections in that they are given *within the skin,* not under the skin layer (Fig. 38–33). When correctly administered, a small **wheal** (elevation) is raised on the skin. A very short needle and a small gauge are used. The angle of insertion is 15 degrees, almost parallel to the skin surface. The best site of injection is the center of the forearm, but the upper chest and back areas are also used (Fig. 38–34). An area with minimum hair is preferred. Most intradermal injections are skin tests for allergies. When intradermal injections are given properly, **vesiculation** forms immediately at the site of the injection. **Induration** will follow if there is an allergic reaction.

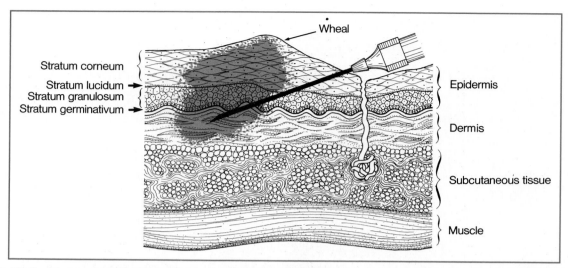

FIGURE 38-33. The intradermal injection is administered just under the epidermis. The drug is dispersed into an area where many nerves are present, thus it causes momentary burning or stinging. Minute amounts of medication are injected. This method is used to test for allergies, drug sensitivities, and susceptibility to some diseases.

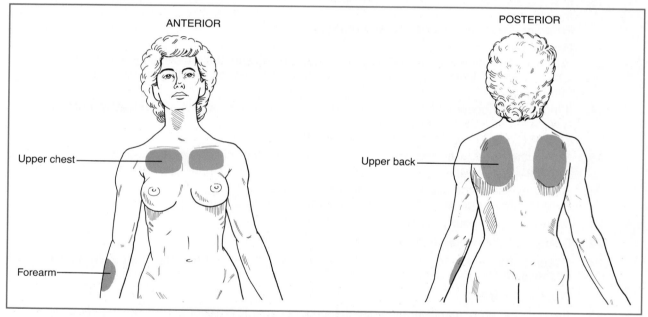

FIGURE 38-34. Sites recommended for intradermal injections.

Infants and Children

Administering injections to infants and small children requires some special considerations. The choice of a site is based upon muscular development, as well as the absence of major nerves and blood vessels. The most popular site for intramuscular injection is the vastus lateralis muscle (lateral thigh). Other sites are avoided for the following reasons:

- Babies do not have well-developed deltoid muscles.
- The sciatic nerve is proportionately larger in the infant.
- The gluteus medius is not well developed until the child is walking.

The best policy is to ask the physician to show you just where to inject. Any site selected for infants and children has a greater margin for error

PROCEDURE 38-5 GIVING AN INTRADERMAL INJECTION

GOAL To inject 0.1 cc of medication into the skin using a needle and syringe of correct size, as directed by the physician.

EQUIPMENT AND SUPPLIES

A vial or ampule containing the material to be injected
Antiseptic sponges
A sterile needle and syringe unit

A written order, including the patient's name, when to give the drug, the route of administration, and the name and strength of the drug

PROCEDURAL STEPS

1. Wash your hands. Follow universal blood and body-fluid precautions. Glove yourself with nonsterile gloves.

2. Select the correct medication from the shelf or the refrigerator.
   Purpose: Some medications must be refrigerated.

3. Read the label to be sure that you have the right drug and the right strength.
   Purpose: One medication may be manufactured and prepackaged in different strengths; for instance, an allergen may be available in 1:1000, 1:100, or 1:10 dilutions.

4. Warm refrigerated medications by gently rolling the container between your palms.

5. Prepare the syringe, withdrawing the right dose.

6. Transport the medication to the patient.

7. Greet and identify the patient by name.
   Purpose: To be sure that you have the right patient.

8. Position the patient comfortably.

9. Locate the antecubital space, then find a site several fingerwidths down the forearm.

10. Cleanse the patient's skin with the antiseptic sponge, using a circular motion, moving outward from the center.

11. Allow the antiseptic to dry.
    Purpose: Because the injected drug is deposited so near the skin surface, the antiseptic could interact with the drug.

12. Compare the order with the prepared medication, and the patient with the name on the order to be sure that this is the right time to administer the drug.
    Purpose: This is the last of the six checks to be made before administering a medication. If there is any doubt, do not proceed. Check first with the physician.

13. Remove the sheath from the needle.

14. With the thumb and first two fingers of your minor hand, stretch the skin taut.
    Purpose: Stretching the skin facilitates the insertion of the needle.

15. Grasp the syringe between the thumb and first two fingers of your major hand, palm down, with the needle bevel upward.

16. At a 15-degree angle, carefully insert the needle through the skin about ⅛ inch, keeping the needle visible through the skin (Fig. 38-35).

17. Turn the syringe 180 degrees to turn the bevel downward.
    Purpose: To prevent the medication from breaking through the skin by the force of the injection.

Continued

PROCEDURE 38-5 *Continued*

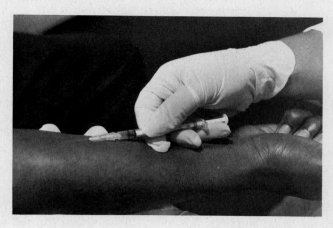

FIGURE 38-35.

18. Slowly and steadily inject the medication.
   Purpose: A rapid injection may force the substance through to the surface.

19. When a wheal appears, stop, and withdraw the needle.

20. Do not massage.
   Purpose: Massaging will interfere with the intended results.

21. Make sure that your patient is comfortable and safe.

22. Dispose of the needle and syringe.

23. Observe the patient for any adverse reaction. You may need to keep the patient under observation for 20 to 30 minutes.

24. Wash your hands.

25. Record the drug administration and any reactions that occurred at the site of the injection on the patient's medical record.

---

because the muscles are smaller than the muscles of the adult.

Babies have to be restrained by another assistant or the parent to avoid injury. If the child is old enough to understand, be honest and explain that the injection may "sting" for a minute, but that it is important to hold very still. Obtain assistance when giving an injection to an uncooperative child. You may keep the fact that the child is to receive an injection from the child until the last minute, but always let the child know. After the injection, praise the child for being helpful; show appreciation and assurance. If you do this, the child will remember more than just the "hurt" of the needle and will trust in you and the process of health care in general. Many children like to have an adhesive bandage applied after the injection as a badge of bravery. Do not give a used syringe to a child for play. It is contaminated and must be disposed of properly.

LEGAL AND ETHICAL RESPONSIBILITIES

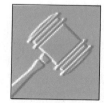

The medical assistant must be extremely knowledgeable when given the responsibility of administering medications in the physician's office. When the physician has written an order for the medication, follow it exactly. If you have a question about the order, ask for clarification before you proceed with the order. It is advisable to give a medication only after the order is written in the patient's chart. This helps eliminate errors and possible omissions in the medication therapy. Legal responsibilities include the prevention of error by carefully following safe practice procedures in pouring and administering drugs. Memorize the "six rights." Any person administering a drug must know the possible serious complications related to the drug and watch for side effects of the medication. The assistant must demonstrate compliance with the laws governing medications and their administration. Precise charting of the administration of medications cannot be overemphasized.

The administration of drugs also involves ethical principles. The patient always comes first, and with that foremost in mind, you cannot risk giving an incorrect medication. There is no chance for a "slight" error because any such error may result in a patient's death. If an error is made, it must be reported immediately to the physician so that measures can be taken to help the patient. It is difficult to admit that a mistake has been made, but it is *absolutely* necessary. For that reason, be sure to double-check your calculations with a coworker or the physician. Errors in medication administration can cause serious problems for the patient.

PATIENT EDUCATION

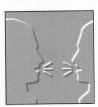

It is extremely important that a patient be instructed about how to take a medication and why he or she is taking it. Ideally, the patient is informed by the physician, but the medical assistant should be prepared to reinforce the physician's information to the patient or explain parts of the information that the patient did not understand. When the patient does not understand the need for the medication or the directions regarding how to take it, there is a greater risk of the medication being taken incorrectly. As a result, the physician's orders will not be carried out. The patient should fully understand the type of medication, its route of administration, its desired effect, and the side effects that need to be reported if they occur.

If a patient is given a diuretic in the office, he or she needs to know what the immediate effect is going to be; this helps the patient understand the urgency and polyuria that he or she will experience within a relatively brief period of time. When a pain medication that may inhibit vision or cause drowsiness is given, the patient should have full knowledge so that the possibility of personal injury can be avoided.

Emphasis should be placed on instructing the patient to take all of the medication prescribed. Many times, if a prescription is not completed, the treatment objectives are altered. Patients should also be instructed to take their medication in the time sequence prescribed. This keeps the optimum level of the drug circulating in the bloodstream.

When sample medications are dispensed in the office to the patient, the package contains inserts that can be helpful in educating the patient. If there are certain parts of the inserts that the patient is especially to remember, highlight this information for quick reference. If the physician has specific written instructions for the patient to follow, read over the form with the patient before giving it to him or her.

Always remember that the more the patient knows and understands about how to take the medication and why it is prescribed, the greater the chances are that the drug treatment will be successful.

► LEARNING ACHIEVEMENTS

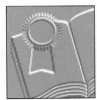

Upon completion of this chapter, can you in the time allowed by your evaluator:

1. Fill a syringe with the correct amount of medication, using sterile technique?
2. Inject a medication into the subcutaneous tissue using a needle and syringe of correct size, as directed?
3. Prepare and administer an intradermal injection using a needle and syringe of correct size, as directed?
4. Inject medication into muscle using a needle and syringe of the correct size, as directed?
5. Inject a medication into the muscle using a needle and syringe of correct size by the Z-tract method, as directed?
6. Apply a transdermal drug to the skin surface safely and securely?
7. Instruct the patient in the use of an oral medication?
8. Instruct the patient in the use of a rectal medication?
9. Instruct the patient in the use of a vaginal medication?
10. Instruct the patient in the use of an inhaler?

REFERENCES AND READINGS

Clark, J., Queener, S., and Karb, V.: *Pocket Guide to Drugs,* St. Louis, C. V. Mosby Co., 1986.
Physicians' Desk Reference, 44th ed., Oradell, NJ, Medical Economics, 1990.
Reynard, A., and Smith, C.: *Textbook of Pharmacology,* Philadelphia, W. B. Saunders Co., 1992.
Rice, J.: *Pharmacology for Medical Assisting,* Philadelphia, Delmar Publishers Inc., 1989.
Woodrow, R.: *Essentials of Pharmacology for Health Occupations,* 2nd ed., New York, Delmar Publishers, 1992.

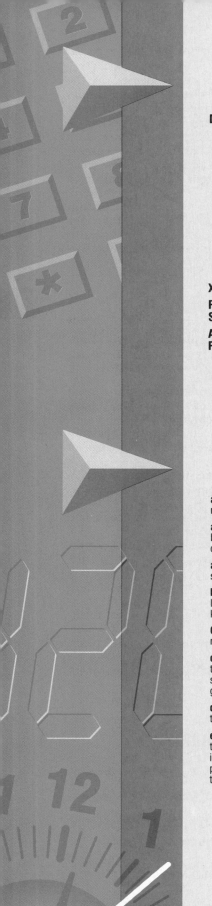

CHAPTER OUTLINE

VOCABULARY

arthritis Inflammation of a joint or many joints.

asthma Panting and wheezing caused by the swelling and spasm of bronchial tubes.

atrophy Wasting away; decrease in size and substance.

bursitis Inflammation of the bursae located in the shoulder and the knee.

COPD Chronic obstructive pulmonary disease.

cystic fibrosis A generalized hereditary disorder associated with widespread dysfunction of the endocrine glands.

denervation A condition in which the nerve supply has been blocked.

emphysema A pathologic accumulation of air in the tissues or organs in which the bronchioles become plugged with mucus and lose elasticity.

erythema A red color to the skin due to capillary congestion resulting from injury, infection, or inflammation.

expiration The act of breathing out or expelling air from the lungs.

extravasation Bleeding into the tissues.

inspiration The act of breathing in or inhaling air into the lungs.

maneuver A physical procedure.

osteoarthritis The most common type of arthritis, which causes the joints to degenerate.

osteoporosis A disorder characterized by loss of bone tissue.

quackery Pretense of possessing medical skill.

rad A measurement of the actual absorbed dose of radiation.

radiation The transfer through space of any form of energy, such as light, heat, or x-rays.

rem Method of measuring the amount of radiation absorbed by a patient exposed to x-rays; similar to **rad.**

roentgen Unit used to measure x-ray dosage.

sprain A traumatic injury without separation of muscle, tendon, or ligament surrounding a bone.

strain A muscular injury resulting from excessive physical exertion.

tone A normal state of balance in muscle tissue; when the muscles are at rest.

vital capacity The maximum volume of air inspired with a maximally forced effort from a position of maximum expiration.

volume capacity The maximum volume of air expired with a maximally forced effort from a position of maximum inspiration.

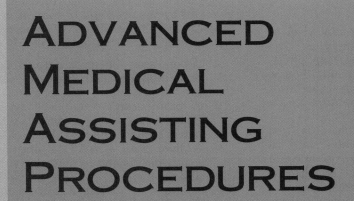

ADVANCED
MEDICAL
ASSISTING
PROCEDURES

LEARNING OBJECTIVES

COGNITIVE

Upon successful completion of this chapter, you should be able to:

1. Define and spell the words in the Vocabulary.

2. Explain your role in relation to diagnostic procedures.

3. Identify safety and precautionary measures pertinent to x-ray equipment.

4. State the purpose of contrast media in x-ray procedures.

5. Discuss the various special x-ray diagnostic procedures.

6. Identify the steps in preparing a patient for spirometric testing.

7. State the five characteristics of an acceptable spirometric maneuver.

8. State the recommendations for infection control when using spirometric equipment.

9. Recall the effects of heat on the body and why heat is an important treatment modality.

10. Recall the effects of cold on the body and why cold is an important treatment modality.

11. Explain the importance of physical therapy in the treatment of physical disabilities.

12. State the importance of range-of-motion exercises.

13. Recall three theories of pain control.

14. Discuss patient teaching activities for x-ray, spirometry, and therapeutic modalities.

DIAGNOSTIC RADIOLOGY

Diagnostic x-ray procedures allow radiologists to view internal body structures and function. The findings obtained by these procedures help physicians in disease diagnosis and treatment. Today, there are many special diagnostic x-ray procedures available that allow for greater observation inside the body.

A contrast medium is a *radiopaque* substance used in diagnostic radiology. It is sometimes used to allow for a more accurate visualization of internal body structures and tissues in contrast to adjacent structures. Contrast media may be gases (air, oxygen, carbon dioxide), heavy metals (barium sulfate, bismuth carbonate), or organic iodines. These can be administered orally, parenterally, or through an enema. Each contrast medium is specific for the examination of a particular organ, body cavity, or passage. The contrast medium makes the area opaque, allowing for both structural and functional visualization as in Figure 39–1. The following is a list of x-ray procedures using a contrast medium and the areas that are visualized:

- angiocardiography — heart and large vessels
- angiography — blood vessels
- arteriography — arteries
- arthrography — joints
- barium enema — lower intestinal tract
- barium meal — upper intestinal tract
- bronchography — bronchial tree and lungs
- cholecystography — gallbladder
- hysterosalpingography — uterus and fallopian tubes
- intravenous cholangiography — bile ducts
- intravenous pyelography — renal pelvis, ureters, and bladder
- lymphangiography — lymphatic vessels
- myelography — spinal cord

Nuclear Medicine

Nuclear medicine, also known as radionuclide imaging, is the branch of radiology that uses radioactive elements and compounds for diagnosis and treatment. In conventional x-ray imaging, radiation passes through the body from an outside source. Nuclear medicine involves detecting radiation from a radioactive chemical placed within the body or mixed with a sample of blood or urine for laboratory analysis.

Nuclear scans provide images that give information about the function and structure of organs and systems. Scans can visualize some organs that cannot be seen on conventional x-ray films. A patient undergoing a scan is given a drug or chemical that contains a radionuclide designed to concentrate in a particular part of the body. It is usually administered by injection.

A gamma camera is used to detect the radiation given off by the drug and to convert it into an image that can be photographed or displayed on a television screen. Scans that are frequently ordered are:

- A bone scan — helps to detect fractures, tumors, and inflammation; used to determine bone growth
- A brain scan — often used together with an image of the brain produced by tomography to detect tumors and vascular problems
- A liver scan — useful in diagnosing cirrhosis and hepatitis and in detecting tumors and liver abscesses
- A lung scan — often done to detect blood clots that have traveled through the bloodstream to the lungs
- A thyroid scan — uses radioactive iodine because iodine accumulates in the thyroid, and the rate of uptake is an indicator of thyroid function

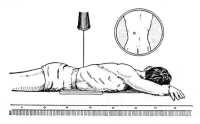

A

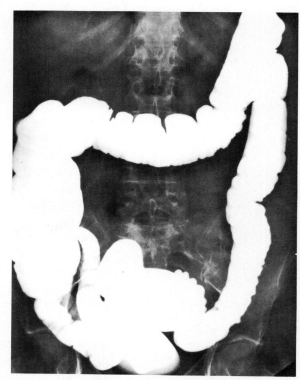

B

FIGURE 39–1. *A,* Positioning the patient for colon x-rays. *B,* The radiograph shows the colon distended with barium. (From Meschan, I.: *Radiographic Positioning and Related Anatomy,* 2nd ed., Philadelphia, W. B. Saunders Co., 1978.)

Computed Tomography (CT Scan)

Computed tomography was introduced in 1972 as another diagnostic x-ray tool. The machine, known as a scanner, examines the body site by rotating a full circle and taking a series of cross-sectional x-ray films. Films are made of the structure from all sides. The rates at which the x-rays are absorbed are detected, and a computer calculates the densities into a picture of the body site on a visual screen. The pictures obtained are very detailed and simulate a three-dimensional appearance (Fig. 39–2).

Magnetic Resonance Imaging

Magnetic resonance imaging uses a combination of radio waves and a strong magnetic field to produce images of the soft tissues. It is extremely useful in diagnosing cancer and other tumors and masses of the soft tissues.

Fluoroscopy

Fluoroscopy, also called *radioscopy*, is an x-ray examination that permits both structural and functional visualization of internal body structures. Through the use of a contrast medium, motion of a body part can be viewed. Thus, a physician can observe the action of the esophagus and stomach after a patient swallows a barium mixture. The patient is placed between the x-ray tube and the screen. X-rays pass through the body and project the structures as shadowy images on the screen. The image on the fluoroscope can be recorded on film to produce a permanent record called a *photofluorogram*.

Mammography

With the advent of new films and exposure techniques, it is now possible to make an x-ray visualization of breast tissue to detect tumors and to determine the presence of a malignancy. Lesions too tiny to produce symptoms can also be detected. Mammography is performed without the use of a contrast medium. Mammography should not be considered a substitute for breast biopsy, but it is an effective device for differential diagnosis in fibrocystic disease (Fig. 39–3).

Stereoscopy

This technique, also called *stereoscopic radiography* or *stereoradiography*, uses a special instrument to view films that have been taken at different angles. This produces a three-dimensional image having depth as well as height and width. Stereoscopy is used primarily for x-ray studies of the skull.

Thermography

This is a technique that reveals internal structures without the use of x-rays but is usually performed by radiographers. Thermography is a heat-sensing technique used primarily in the detection of breast tumors. Using an infrared camera, a photograph is taken that records the variations in skin temperatures. Cool areas appear dark, warm areas light, and intermediate temperatures as various shades of gray. Since inflammatory or malignant areas produce more heat than does surrounding normal tissue, these areas are clearly visible.

Ultrasonography

This procedure is not a radiologic procedure, but it permits visualization of internal structures by the use of high-frequency sound waves that echo off the body. An instrument called a *transducer*, similar to a microphone, is passed over the body part to be examined. It picks up the echoes, which are then displayed on an oscilloscope. The echoes are produced by the sound waves passing through the skin, striking the body part, and bouncing back to the transducer. Since sound waves do not expose the patient to radiation, ultrasound examination is ideal for observing the developing fetus and detecting the presence of multiple fetuses. It is also particularly useful for producing images of soft tissue tumors or lesions in the brain, eyes, abdomen, reproductive organs, and breasts.

Xeroradiography

In xeroradiography, the x-ray studies are processed on specially treated Xerox paper instead of x-ray film. The process takes only 90 seconds and permits visualization of soft tissues. For this reason, it is most often used to detect lesions or calcifications in the soft tissue of the breast.

Flat Plates

X-ray films can also be taken of various body parts without the use of special techniques or the use of a contrast medium. Flat plates are also called *plain films*. Several x-ray views are usually taken for review by the radiologist. Examples of these diagnostic x-ray films include skull, sinuses, chest, abdomen, and bone.

39

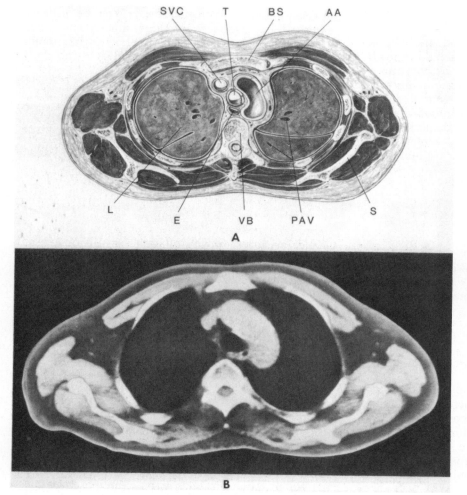

FIGURE 39–2. A computed tomograph through the aortic arch level. Lungs, bone, spine, and blood vessels can be visualized and compared with anatomic drawings. (*T*: Trachea; *SVC*: superior vena cava; *L*: lungs; *E*: esophagus; *BS*: body of sternum; *AA*: aortic arch; *S*: scapula; *PAV*: pulmonary arteries and veins; *VB*: vertebral body.) (From Meschan, I.: *Synopsis of Radiologic Anatomy with Computed Tomography*, Philadelphia, W. B. Saunders Co., 1980.)

X-RAY MACHINE

The x-ray machine consists of tube, table, and control panel (Fig. 39–4). The tube is the part in which the x-rays are produced and then are directed out as an x-ray beam. The entire tube is surrounded by a protective material (lead), except at the point where the rays are emitted. The lead absorbs the radiation like a sponge. The tube is designed to move the entire length of the table. The table is where the patient is positioned for the x-ray study. It is designed to rotate into different positions, as necessary for specific x-ray films. The control panel contains the knobs for operating the tube and the table. It is located behind a lead-lined wall, in another area away from the table and the tube.

RADIATION HAZARDS AND SAFEGUARDS

Excessive exposure to radiation can cause both tissue destruction and a variety of ill effects. Harmful effects include temporary or permanent damage to the skin, eyes, and reproductive and blood-forming organs. X-rays may produce harmful effects on the developing embryo and the fetus, causing malformations or death. Overexposure to x-rays produces a variety of symptoms. These include nausea, fatigue, diarrhea, constipation, bleeding, and loss of appetite.

All radiation exposure is cumulative and adds up to a total radiation dosage that is measured in **rads, rems,** or **roentgens.** Monitoring devices called *dosimeters* are worn by persons working near sources of x-rays. These monitors contain special photographic film that is sensitive to radiation and serve as a guide to the amount of radiation to which a person has been exposed. Monitors are submitted periodically for evaluation, and a report of any radiation exposure is maintained on all x-ray personnel.

Radiation exposure can come directly from the x-ray beam or from what is known as scattered radiation. Scattered radiation is the diffusion or deviation of the x-rays that is produced when they pass through a patient or anything in the patient's path. Even though the entire x-ray tube is enclosed in lead, scattered radiation may result from leakage through the tube. To prevent this from happening, all machines must be checked on a regular basis by licensed physicists.

Shielding is of special importance to both patients and personnel. Patients should be protected from unnecessary radiation by using lead aprons to cover the reproductive organs, especially for pregnant patients and all children. Personnel can obtain additional protection by wearing lead aprons and gloves when assisting. The walls of x-ray rooms are also lined with lead, which absorbs the scattered radiation, protecting all others in the area.

In addition to monitors and shielding, all x-ray personnel should have routine periodic blood counts performed to detect the presence of any abnormal or pathologic condition that may result from excessive radiation exposure.

ASSISTING WITH RADIOLOGIC PROCEDURES

As previously stated, there may be occasions when the medical assistant will be called upon to assist in the performance of basic x-ray procedures under the physician's supervision. The medical assistant's x-ray responsibilities may include scheduling examinations; instructing and positioning patients; processing film; and filing and storing films and written reports.

Preparing the Patient

The medical assistant is responsible for preparing the patient for the x-ray procedure. Preparation requires a thorough knowledge of the procedure and the ability to communicate all instructions, both written and oral, to the patient to ensure that these instructions are understood. Written instructions are essential, since oral instructions can be easily forgotten. Most physicians use their own printed material or use product literature provided by pharmaceutical companies detailing step-by-step instructions (Fig. 39–5).

The medical assistant should briefly explain the procedure using proper terminology but should avoid complex descriptions. Encourage the patient to ask questions and discuss any apprehensions. Reinforce the rationale for the x-ray procedure.

Many diagnostic x-ray examinations require special preparation by the patient the night before or the morning of the test. Patients may be instructed to eat a low-fat evening meal, not to eat after midnight, to drink plenty of fluids, or take special tablets, laxatives, or enemas.

Positioning the Patient

An important responsibility of the medical assistant is the proper positioning of the patient for spe-

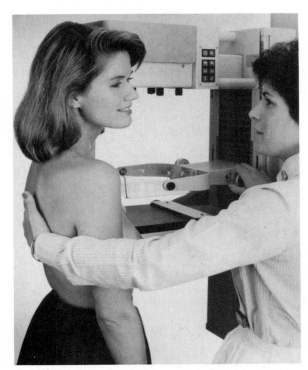

FIGURE 39–3. The patient is being assisted with the placement of her breast on the film holder in order to get a good image for the mammogram. (Courtesy of Lorad Medical System, Inc., Danbury, CT.)

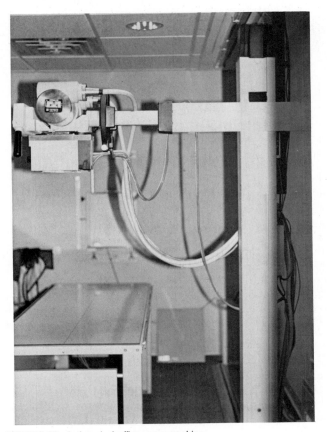

FIGURE 39–4. A typical office x-ray machine.

THE COLON X-RAY
(BARIUM ENEMA)

Your doctor has requested an x-ray examination of your colon (lower bowel). This is a thorough examination of the colon. A special enema (barium) is given, which allows the colon to be visible on x-rays.

****Please Note: This preparation is a laxative. It will empty your colon. Expect to have several loose or liquid bowel movements during the night. Do not be alarmed if you experience cramping and feel some weakness.

The following preparation is necessary to insure a satisfactory examination of the colon.

BEGIN DAY PRIOR TO EXAM DAY

1) Lunch should be a light diet. 1-2 cups soup, 4 Saltines or 1-2 slices bread or toast (butter and jelly ok), 1 serving fruit. May also have: 1 serving cake or up to 3 cookies. Beverage: Any juice, coffee or tea (no milk).

2) Please drink at least one full glass or more of water or clear liquids every 1-2 hours between noon and bedtime. (At least six 8 oz. glasses).

3) 1/2 hr. before evening meal take Fleet Phospho Soda. Pour contents (1 1/2 oz.) into one-half glass cool water. Drink, following immediately with one full glass of water.

4) Eat a liquid evening meal (bouillon, strained fruit juice and plain jello). No solid foods. No dairy products (milk, cream or cheese). No carbonated beverages.

5) At 8 P.M., take four yellow Fleet Bisacodyl tablets, swallowing tablets whole with a full glass of water. Do not chew or dissolve tablets.

6) Drink nothing after taking the tablets.

7) Eat nothing after the evening meal. **(NO BREAKFAST).**

ON THE MORNING OF THE EXAMINATION

1) At least one hour before leaving for your exam use Fleet Bisacodyl Suppository. Remove foil wrap from suppository. Lie on side, insert rounded end of suppository as high as possible in rectum. Wait 15 minutes before evacuating even if urge is strong.

2) On the x-ray table you will be given a barium enema. You will experience a sensation similar to a cleansing enema. It will be only a matter of minutes before you have to go to the bathroom and expel the enema.

3) The radiologist (an x-ray physician specialist) will examine your abdomen by pressing it with his hands and observing the colon with the fluoroscope (television) and x-ray films.

4) When the radiologist has completed his portion of the examination, an x-ray technologist will take some additional films and immediately take you to the bathroom. After you feel you have expelled all of the enema, please have a seat in the hallway and the technologist will take an additional film of your abdomen to visualize your empty bowel.

5) The colon exam will usually require approximately 1/2 hour.

Report to your doctor's receptionist the morning of your examination and you will be given a request slip for your x-rays.

We appreciate your cooperation.

FIGURE 39–5. Patient instruction sheet for barium enema. (Courtesy of Jackson Clinic, Madison, WI.)

cific x-ray films. Radiographs are made by directing the x-rays produced by the x-ray tube toward a specific body part. The body part must be positioned correctly between the x-ray film and the x-ray tube (Fig. 39–6). The patient's position is determined by the type of examination required and the specific body part to be visualized. Usually, several views are taken in an attempt to achieve a three-dimensional picture for better diagnosis by the radiologist. The basic x-ray views are:

- *Anteroposterior (AP) view:* The anterior aspect of the body faces the x-ray tube, and the posterior aspect faces the film. The x-ray beam is directed from front to back (see Fig. 39–6).
- *Posteroanterior (PA) view:* The posterior aspect of the body faces the x-ray tube, and the anterior aspect faces the film. The x-ray beam is directed from back to front (see Fig. 39–6).
- *Lateral view:* The body part is placed on its side. The x-ray beam is directed from one side (see Fig. 39–6).
- *Right lateral (RL) view:* The right side of the body faces the film.
- *Left lateral (LL) view:* The left side of the body faces the film.
- *Oblique view:* The body is placed on an angle. The x-ray beam is directed at an angle (see Fig. 39–6).

The basic x-ray positions are:

- *Supine position:* The patient lies on his or her back.
- *Prone position:* The patient lies on his or her abdomen.

Terms to describe the direction of the x-ray beam are:

- *Axillary:* The beam is directed toward the axilla (underarm).
- *Craniocaudal:* The x-ray beam is directed downward from head to toe.
- *Mediolateral:* The x-ray beam is directed from the midline toward the side of the body part of which a film is being made.

Exposing X-Ray Film

X-rays, which can be produced by high-velocity electrons in a vacuum tube, expose (turn black) a sheet of x-ray film. X-rays can also be absorbed by substances, to a degree relative to the density of that substance. Thus, if part of the body is positioned on a *cassette* (film holder) and x-rays are directed through it, the rays will be absorbed or scattered by the various substances in the body and will expose the film to varying degrees. The resulting image will show the pattern of substances inside the body. Air, for instance, is least dense and appears as black areas, whereas water, fat, and metal appear increasingly white. Since the human body is made of different materials and is of varying thicknesses, the final image is composed of various degrees of black and white.

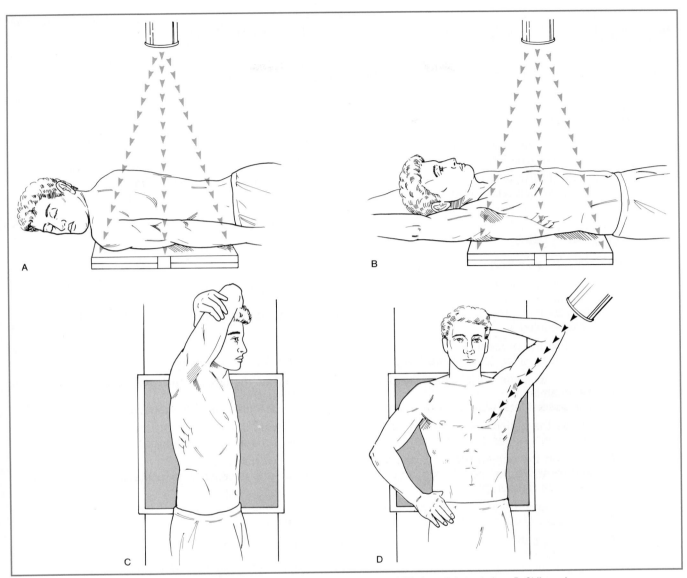

FIGURE 39-6. *A,* Posteroanterior (PA) view. *B,* Anteroposterior (AP) view. *C,* Lateral view. *D,* Oblique view.

Processing X-Ray Film

Film development takes place in a darkroom. No natural light is permitted in this area. The only artificial light used is a specially designed low-wattage bulb that will not expose the film. For x-ray film processing, most modern medical offices use automatic developers, which produce images quickly and automatically.

Filing X-Ray Films and Reports

X-ray films are permanent records that must be preserved many years for both medical and legal reasons. Medical assistants are often responsible for storing the patient's films after processing is completed and after the physician has read them. The films are placed in large envelopes, with the patient's name, the patient's number (if used), and the date clearly marked on the outside. These films should be stored in a dry, cool place. In a general practice office, the films are usually kept in a readily accessible area for viewing.

X-ray films are the property of the medical office where the films are taken. They do not belong to the patient. Written x-ray reports may be sent out, but the actual films must remain as part of the patient's file.

PROCEDURE 39–1   ASSISTING WITH AN X-RAY EXAMINATION

GOAL   To assist with an x-ray examination under the supervision of a physician.

EQUIPMENT AND SUPPLIES

Physician's order for an x-ray
  examination
X-ray machine
X-ray film and holder

X-ray darkroom
X-ray automatic developer or manual
  processing solutions

PROCEDURAL STEPS

1. Check order and equipment needed.

2. Introduce yourself, and confirm the identity of the patient. Ascertain if any special preparations were employed.
   Purpose: If special preparations were not followed, the examination may need to be rescheduled.

3. Explain the procedure.
   Purpose: Helps to reassure the patient and alleviates fear and anxiety.

4. Check to make certain that the patient has removed all metal objects from the area to be examined.
   Purpose: Metal objects appear on the film and may obscure the final image.

5. Drape the patient as necessary, and shield the abdominal area.
   Purpose: Drapes provide warmth, and shields protect the reproductive areas.

6. Position the patient properly, and immobilize the part, if necessary.
   Purpose: Proper positioning and complete stillness are necessary to achieve a clear, readable radiograph.

7. Stand behind a lead shield during the exposure.
   Purpose: Lead shields provide protection from scattered radiation.

8. Ask the patient to assume a comfortable position after the examination is completed, and wait until the films are processed.
   Purpose: In the event that it is necessary to retake an x-ray film, the patient will be readily accessible.

9. Develop the film, using automatic or manual film processing.

10. Dismiss the patient if all films are satisfactory.

11. Place the dry, finished x-ray film in a properly labeled envelope, and file it according to the policies of the office.

12. Record the x-ray examination on the patient's chart, along with the final written x-ray findings.

SPIROMETRY

Spirometry is regarded as an essential component of the medical evaluation of patients who complain of shortness of breath. It is also widely used in patients with allergy problems, asthma, COPD, cystic fibrosis and emphysema and in occupational therapy.

Although cardiopulmonary technologists have been the mainstays of pulmonary function testing, today, because of the increased awareness of lung disease resulting from smoking and environmental and occupational exposures, we find respiratory therapists, nurses, industrial hygienists, and medical assistants measuring and assessing pulmonary function.

Physiology of Spirometry

Although the lung is sometimes regarded as a sort of bellows system that moves air in and out of the body, it is a complex organ involved in many physiologic processes. Breathing is divided into two phases: **inspiration** and **expiration.** Inspiration is caused by the contraction of the respiratory muscles; expiration occurs with the relaxation of the respiratory muscles. Thus, during inspiration, the chest expands, the lungs fill with air, and the gases within the lungs are exchanged. Upon expiration, the gases that the body cannot use escape from the lungs.

Diagnostic Spirometry

During spirometry, the forced expiratory maneuver consists of a maximum inspiration and then a rapid, forceful, and complete expiration. A comparison is made of the **vital capacity,** amount of air inhaled, with the **volume capacity,** amount of air exhaled. In addition to checking the vital and **volume capacity,** the time it takes to complete each phase is also calculated. When these two factors are measured and compared, it is possible to determine the ability of the lung to provide the gas exchange needed for good health.

Instrumentation

The volume displacement spirometer shown in Figure 39–7 is the model most frequently used in the physician's office. Such spirometers are small, lightweight, and simple to use. Machines can be purchased with or without a microprocessor and programmed to measure exhaled volumes only. The patient breathing tube connects to the bottom of the unit. A rubber diaphragm fits snugly into the lower housing. As the patient's exhaled air enters the lower housing, it pushes the bottom side of the diaphragm upward. As the diaphragm moves upward, it pushes a pusher plate upward and the volume is measured. The exhaled air escapes back out of the patient breathing tube when the patient's mouth is removed. A volume–time tracing can be obtained if the instrument is equipped with a microprocessor.

SPIROMETRIC TECHNIQUE

Successful spirometry requires the application of a consistent technique for preparing the patient, explaining and performing the procedure, and inspecting the results.

Patient preparation really begins when the patient is scheduled. At that time, the patient should be instructed on such things as which medications should be withheld (if any), whether he or she should stop smoking for a specific time period, and

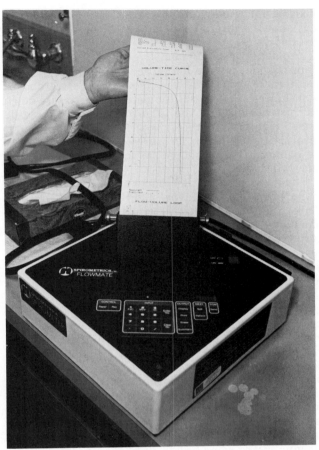

FIGURE 39–7. The diaphragm-type spirometer, which collects exhaled air beneath a diaphragm that pushes upward on a pusher-plate and writing mechanism.

possibly other factors. It is necessary that you have written orders from the physician regarding precisely what each patient should do to prepare for this test.

Patient Preparation

When the patient arrives for testing, the assistant should explain the purpose of the test, determine if there are any contraindications to performing the test, obtain the patient's height and weight, position the patient, and explain the actual maneuver. Explain spirometry in simple terms, and be brief. One statement that works well is "I am going to have you blow into a machine to see how big your lungs are and how fast the air comes out. It doesn't hurt, but it does require your cooperation and lots of effort."

The next step is to get the patient comfortable and in the proper position. Have the patient loosen any tight clothing such as neckties, belts, or bras. There is no significant difference between the sitting and standing positions, so have the patient do what is most comfortable. If sitting, the patient's legs should be uncrossed and both feet should be on the floor.

Explain the actual maneuver next. Show the patient the mouthpiece and noseclips. Explain how the mouthpiece fits into the mouth. If a cardboard mouthpiece is used, tell the patient not to bite down as this will obstruct the tubing hole. Lips should be sealed tightly, and the tongue should not stick out into the mouthpiece. Dentures that fit poorly may be a nuisance and should be removed if you think they will interfere.

Show the patient the proper chin and neck position. The chin should be slightly elevated and the neck slightly extended (Fig. 39–8). This position should be maintained throughout the forced expiratory procedure. Don't let the patient bend the chin to the chest. Bending at the waist is common and acceptable, but discourage the patient from bending all the way over.

Give specific instructions in simple, direct terms. For example, "I want you to take the deepest breath possible, put the mouthpiece in your mouth and seal your lips tightly, and then blast all your air into the tube as hard and as fast as you can in one long, complete breath." For spirometers that allow the patient to already be breathing on the mouthpiece, the instructions are simpler. One analogy that is sometimes helpful to further explain the maneuver is "It's like blowing out the candles on a birthday cake and they all don't go out, so you need to keep blowing in the same breath until they do."

Next, demonstrate the maneuver. Many patients will forget some or all of the instructions they just received, so the demonstration reinforces exactly what they are to do. Show the patient proper chin and neck position, how to get the mouthpiece in at the right time, and how to blast the air out and continue to blow.

When the demonstration is done, remind the patient of the following points:

- Take as deep a breath as possible.
- Blast air out hard.
- Don't stop blowing until you are told to stop.

Use good active and forceful coaching while the patient is performing the maneuver (Fig. 39–9). You may need to raise your voice with some urgency, using such phrases as "blow, blow, blow!" "Keep blowing, keep blowing!" and "Don't stop blowing!" Coaching improves the performance of most effort-dependent activities, which include spirometry. After the maneuver, give the patient some feedback on the quality of the test and describe what improvements could be made. Continue to repeat efforts until *three acceptable maneuvers* are obtained. If after eight trials no acceptable curves are obtained, stop and report this to the physician.

ACCEPTABLE MANEUVERS

Acceptability consists of five characteristics (Fig. 39–10):

- No coughing
- Good start of test
- No early termination
- No variable flows
- Consistency

INFECTION CONTROL

After a spirometric test is completed, the medical assistant must clean the equipment thoroughly. Microorganisms reportedly have been collected from pulmonary function devices. The transmission of the microorganisms to other patients has also been reported. There is a risk of cross-contamination when using pulmonary function equipment. It would also seem safe to speculate that this risk is in proportion to the frequency of cleaning or changing equipment parts. The use of filters to trap microorganisms might reduce this risk; however, these filters are costly and may interfere with the accuracy of the test. The National Association of Respiratory Care Therapists recommends the following:

1. Use disposable mouthpieces and discard after patient use. If rubber mouthpieces are used, clean with high-level disinfection between every patient.
2. Change external spirometer tubing between patients. Give the contaminated tubing high-level disinfection; dry the tubing before reuse.
3. Change noseclips between patients, and discard or clean with high-level disinfection.
4. Change water in water-sealed spirometers monthly.
5. Don't spend a great amount of time and effort cleaning the surfaces inside the spirometers.
6. Wash hands thoroughly, using good handwashing technique, before and after performing testing maneuvers whether or not gloves are worn.

TEST RESULTS

Place the results of the **maneuvers** with the patient's chart on the physician's desk when the tests are completed. Many physicians rely on the assistant to include comments pertinent to the testing with these results. If there are any questions regarding the quality of the results, you should ask the patient to wait while you check with the physician. Never allow the patient to leave the office before the physician gives you approval to do so. If the patient has delayed taking medication, check with the physician as to when the patient should resume taking it.

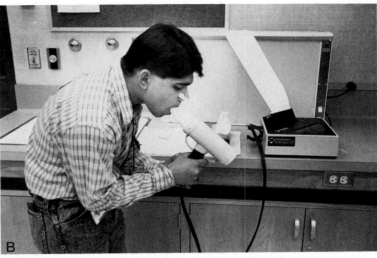

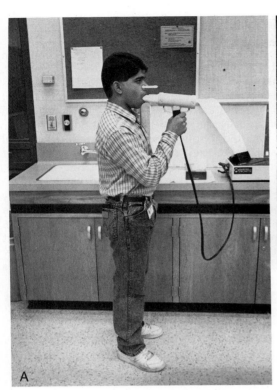

FIGURE 39–8. *A*, Good posture. *B*, Incorrect posture (too much bending of neck and chin).

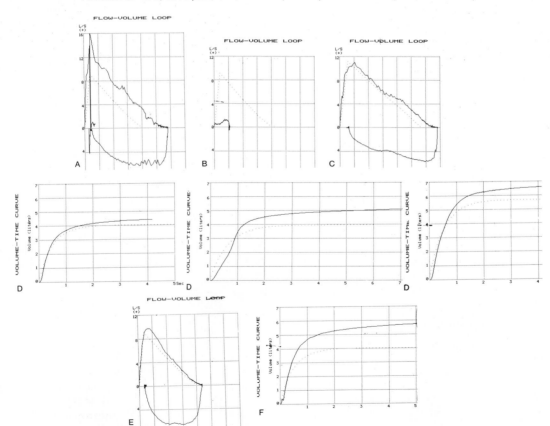

FIGURE 39–9. *A*, Significant coughing. *B*, Poor start. *C*, Abrupt end to flow. *D*, Inconsistency—three maneuvers. *E*, No change in volume. *F*, Good start. (*Solid line*, measured; *dotted line*, predicted).

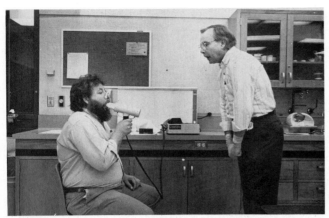

FIGURE 39-10. It is important to use good coaching during forced spirometry.

THERAPEUTIC MODALITIES

This section describes some of the more common applications of physical agents used in therapy. These physical agents are called *modalities* and include heat and cold therapy with water, the use of electric currents as a form of physical therapy, and therapeutic exercise.

Heat or cold applications to injured or painful body parts have been used throughout history. Heat and cold therapies are two well-practiced, common-sense home treatments easily applied with or without the direction of a physician. It is most likely that you have had the occasion to apply heat to a swollen, sore body part or ice to a burn or bruise. You have been applying the principles we are about to discuss, even though you may not have understood the underlying reasons that these therapies

PROCEDURE 39-2   PERFORMING VOLUME CAPACITY SPIROMETRIC TEST

GOAL   To perform volume capacity testing (Fig. 39-11).

EQUIPMENT AND SUPPLIES

Balance scale with measuring device
Volume capacity spirometer with
    recording paper in place
External spirometric tubing
Disposable mouth piece
Nose clip

PROCEDURAL STEPS

1. Introduce yourself and confirm the identity of the patient. Ascertain if any special preparation was needed by this patient and if it was followed.
   Purpose: If special procedures were not followed, the test may have to be rescheduled.

2. Explain the purpose of the test (Fig. 39-12).
   Purpose: To help reassure the patient.

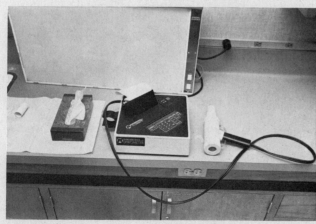

FIGURE 39-11.

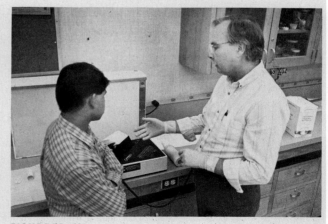

FIGURE 39-12.

Continued

3. Obtain the patient's height and weight.

4. Explain the actual maneuver.
   Purpose: The patient needs to understand the maneuver so he or she can cooperate fully to obtain best testing results.

5. Be certain the patient is comfortable and in proper sitting or standing position.
   Purpose: Proper positioning is necessary to ensure accurate test results.

6. Loosen any tight clothing such as neckties, belts, or bras.
   Purpose: Tight clothing may restrict breathing capacity.

7. Show the patient the proper chin and neck position (Fig. 39–13).

8. Practice the maneuver with the patient (Fig. 39–14).
   Purpose: To relieve apprehension and enhance understanding.

39

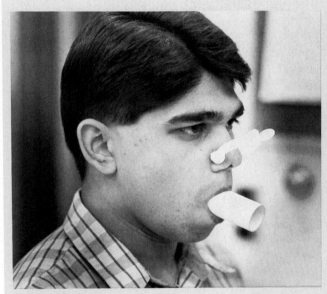

FIGURE 39–13.

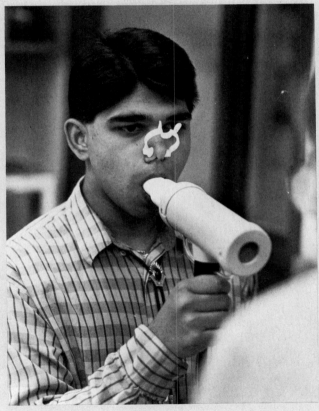

FIGURE 39–14.

Continued

PROCEDURE 39-2   *Continued*

9. Use active, forceful coaching during testing (Figs. 39-15 through 39-17).
   Purpose: Coaching improves performance.

10. Give the patient feedback after the maneuver is completed.
    Purpose: Compliments and explanations of mistakes in the maneuver will help improve patient compliance.

11. Continue testing until three acceptable maneuvers have been obtained (Fig. 39-18).

12. Dismiss the patient only if results are satisfactory.

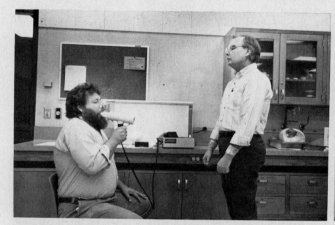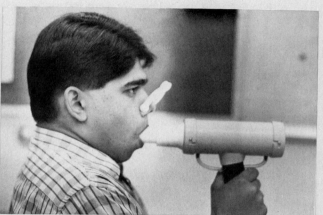

FIGURE 39-15. Maneuver performed with patient sitting *(left)* or standing *(right)*.

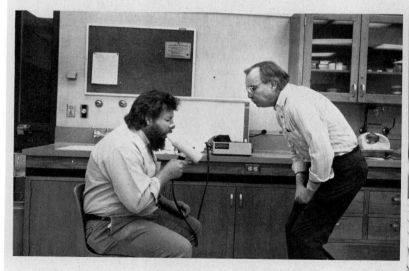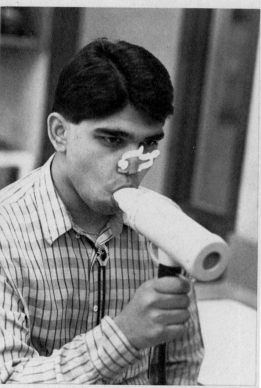

FIGURE 39-16. In sitting position *(above)* or in standing position *(right)*.

Continued

13. Clean and disinfect the equipment. Discard waste in a biologic waste container.

14. Remove gloves and wash hands.

15. Record testing information on the patient's chart and place the chart with the test results on the physician's desk for interpretation.

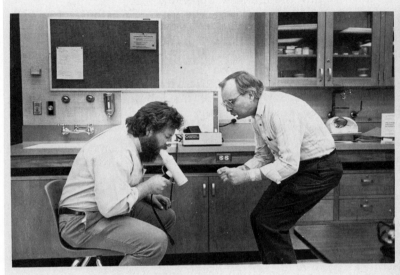

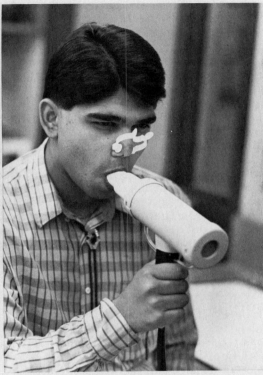

FIGURE 39–17. In sitting position *(above)* or in standing position *(right).*

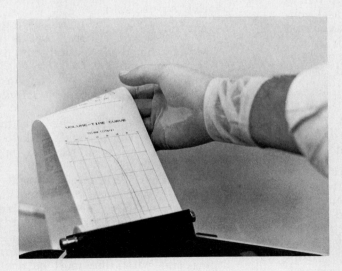

FIGURE 39–18. An acceptable tracing.

are so useful. These two physical measures, along with some other of the more complicated devices we will discuss in this chapter, are used primarily to improve circulation, minimize pain, and correct or alleviate muscular and joint malfunction.

Physical therapy and therapeutic exercise involve the scientific use of physical measures, devices, and body movement to restore normal function to injured tissues. Physical therapy is a separate allied health profession practiced by physical therapists and physical therapy assistants and aides. The Association of Physical Therapists states that "physical therapy treatments should be administered by a trained physical therapist or the treatment should be supervised by a registered physical therapist." Registered physical therapists work mainly in hospitals or in specialized private practices.

Your role may be limited to referring the patient to a physical therapist and explaining pre-appointment instructions, or, if it is permitted in your area of the United States, you may be able to administer limited physical therapy under the supervision of a physician or a registered physical therapist. Before participating in the physical treatment of patients, it is important for you to know which procedures are permitted by state law to be performed by someone other than a licensed physical therapist.

GENERAL PRINCIPLES OF HEAT APPLICATION

Heat produces local vasodilation and increases circulation. It speeds up the inflammatory process, promotes local drainage, relaxes muscles, and repairs tissue cells. Heat can be applied to relax and relieve pain in a **strained** muscle; to promote drainage from an abscess or infected area; to relieve tissue congestion and swelling, such as nasal congestion or a localized collection of **extravasated** blood in the tissues; or to improve the repair time of a **sprained** joint (Fig. 39–19). However, the effects of external heat applications also depend on the following conditions:

- The type of heat used
- The length of time the heat is applied
- The general condition of the patient
- The size of the area needing treatment

Heat can be harmful. Prolonged application of heat increases the secretions of the skin, softening it and lowering its resistance to injury. Extreme heat works adversely by constricting the blood vessels and causing burns. Heat applied too often may increase a patient's tolerance to heat so that the patient may be burned without knowing it. Infants and the elderly are particularly susceptible to burns, so extreme caution must be used when treating them. Infants and patients who cannot report a burning sensation should be evaluated and watched carefully, as should persons with diseases of the cardiovascular, renal, sensorineural, and respiratory system, and those with **osteoporosis.** In addition, special precautions must be taken with patients with impaired circulation, such as those with diabetes. Because heat can increase the inflammatory process, it should never be applied to the abdomen if appendicitis is suspected. In this instance, heat can rupture the inflamed appendix.

When deciding whether or not to treat a body part with heat, the following conditions all are generally contraindications. Of course, there may be special conditions, or directions given by the physician, to treat with heat even though one or more of these conditions exist. However, *do not* treat a patient having any of the following conditions until you have specifically discussed the condition with the physician:

- Acute inflammatory conditions: heat should not be used in most acute inflammatory processes for the first 48 hours.
- Severe circulatory problems, such as blockage and bleeding: heat can increase the blockage and cause hemorrhaging.
- The lack of sensation in a body part: there is danger that the patient cannot report burning. A lack of sensation may indicate a lack of circulation in the body part.
- Pregnancy or menstruation: heat can cause uterine contractions and increase menstrual flow.
- Areas containing encapsulated pus and having no drainage: heat increases the inflammatory process, and the encapsulated area could rupture.
- Blisters from hot water bottles, heating pads, skin ointments, or salves previously applied by the patient: heat should not be applied over newly burned skin.
- Scar tissue does not have a normal supply of blood vessels; therefore, heat is not carried away by blood circulation, and burns could occur.
- Body areas that may contain malignant tumors: Malignant tumor activity may be stimulated by heat.
- **Erythema,** redness of the skin, may indicate a blood clot, which could break loose with an increase in circulation caused by application of heat.
- Metal materials: Heat concentrates in metal materials, such as metal implants, prostheses, and certain IUDs. Therefore, patients with internal metal devices should not have those areas treated. To avoid burns, metal objects such as jewelry, watches, hearing aids, hairpins, and metal clips must be removed before treatment. Treatment must be administered on nonmetal tables and chairs.

Body parts may be heated to 110°F (44°C) without damage to the tissues. Redness appears because

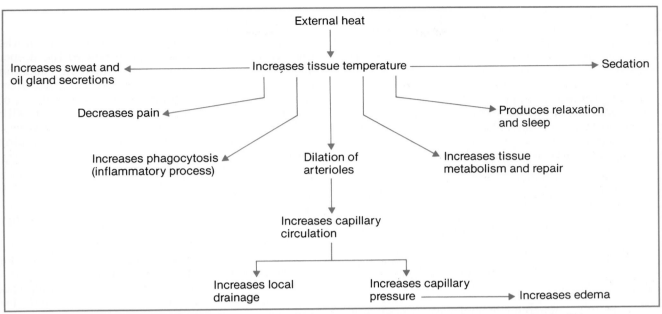

FIGURE 39-19. Body responses to local heat application. (Adapted from St. Mary's Hospital, Inc., Russelville, AR.)

the capillaries become congested with blood at the skin's surface. Continuous heat for more than 20 minutes usually results in the increased circulation carrying away the heat as rapidly as it is applied, and the therapy may lose its effectiveness. Heat applied for more than 1 hour causes the blood vessels to constrict, thereby decreasing the blood supply to the area and adversely affecting the effectiveness of the treatment.

Moist heat penetrates better than dry heat. Moist heat (heat hydrotherapy) may be applied with hot packs and compresses, soaks, or baths. Dry heat may be applied in the form of hot water bottles or electric heating pads and lamps, or by the use of electric current when the treatment of the deeper tissues is necessary. Let's look at some of the more common methods of treatment by heat.

Heat Hydrotherapy

Soaks

With heat hydrotherapy, a body part is immersed gradually into medicated or plain water for approximately 15 minutes at a temperature no greater than 110°F (44°C). The extremities are often treated by this method. Patients can take their own soaks at home, but special instructions in aseptic techniques must be given to the patient if the area being treated is an open wound.

Whirlpool Treatment

This method uses a tank with special equipment that agitates the water to provide gentle massage. It is useful for exercise or to cleanse wounds. The temperature is the same as for any method of heat hydrotherapy.

Paraffin Bath

This is especially useful in treating chronic joint disease. A mixture of seven parts paraffin and one part mineral oil is heated to melting at about 127°F. The patient's body part is dipped into the warm paraffin mixture and removed, and then this is repeated until a thick coat is formed on the body part. The paraffin is left on for about 30 minutes and then is peeled off. It leaves the skin soft, warm, and pliable, with a slight erythema.

Hot Moist Compresses

These are used to increase blood flow to small areas of the body, such as the hands. Compresses may be made at home with soft cloths or a clean washcloth. If hot moist compresses are applied to an open wound in the office, use sterile gauze sponges, a sterile solution, and surgically aseptic conditions. Follow the universal blood and body-fluid precautions. Dispose of used materials in a closed container so that personnel and other patients are not in danger of contact with the contaminated materials.

Often, you will be asked to instruct patients on how to apply hot moist compresses at home. Patient instructions for home care should be explicit and simple. The patient should remove all jewelry and should be instructed *not* to apply a hot moist compress if a rash appears or the skin is broken. A plastic covering will help keep in the moisture. A hot water bottle may be used to keep the compress hot. If you are speaking to the patient over the telephone, be sure that the patient writes down the instructions as you read each step. Never assume that the patient knows the correct method. When instructing patients in person, it is best to have preprinted instructions for you to review and give to the patient to take home. The following list of steps may be used in preparing patient instructions for applying hot compresses at home:

1. Moisten a clean hand towel with warm water.
2. Wring it out.
3. The compress should be warm, not hot.
4. Place the towel directly onto the skin.
5. Cover the towel with plastic to keep in the moist heat.
6. Continue the therapy for the prescribed length of time and the prescribed number of times each day.

Commercially prepared hot moist compresses are packs made of canvas containing a silicon gel, which retains heat (Fig. 39–20). They may be purchased for home use and may be heated in warm water.

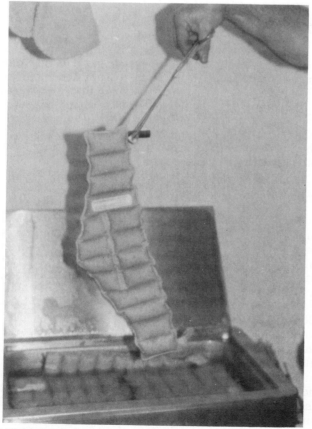

FIGURE 39–20. Commercially prepared hot moist pack made of canvas that contains a silicon gel.

Dry Heat

Methods of dry heat can produce heat on the superficial skin surfaces or penetrate to the deeper muscle tissues. Heating pads, infrared radiation (heat lamps and hot water bottles), and ultraviolet rays generate heat that can penetrate to a depth of 10 mm. Deeper penetration of heat, produced with high-frequency electric current, is called *diathermy*. Diathermy is derived from the Greek words meaning "heating through."

Heating Pads

The least complicated method of applying dry heat, heating pads are often used by the patient at home. When giving instructions for use at home, caution the patient that heating pads must not be used near moisture. Instruct the patient to turn the heat control to low or medium (never the high setting) and to keep the pad on the body part only for a prescribed length of time. Heating pads with automatic thermostats are preferred over the older models that do not control the temperature evenly.

Infrared Radiation Lamps

These generate heat within a metal coil element or a special heat-producing electric bulb. This source of energy produces very shallow heat penetration. The penetration is about 3 to 5 mm, or 0.1 to 0.2 inch, and depends on the principle of conduction to warm the deeper tissues (Fig. 39–21). This treatment produces an approximate 1°F temperature increase at the site being treated.

Before treatment, the skin is cleansed to remove any ointments and skin oils. The treatment extends for usually 20 to 45 minutes, according to the physician's instructions. During the course of the treatment, the patient's skin becomes flushed, but a "sunburn" does not occur. However, if used improperly, the infrared lamp is capable of producing skin burns in exactly the same manner as touching a hot stove or oven. In addition to dry heat treatments, the infrared lamp can be placed above a moist dressing to extend the time of a moist heat treatment.

Maintenance of the infrared lamp is simple. The heating element should be kept in a down position when not in use, to prevent dust from accumulating on the element. The electric connections should be checked and kept in good working condition.

Ultraviolet Radiation

Ultraviolet radiation is produced by the sun or by lamps, sometimes called sun lamps. Ultraviolet radiation is more penetrating than infrared radiation and can cause skin burns or pigmentation changes resulting in tanning. Ultraviolet rays are also capa-

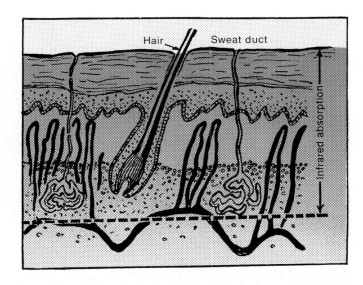

FIGURE 39-21. The broken line indicates the depth of penetration of the infrared rays into the skin.

39

ble of killing bacteria. It is this bactericidal action that makes ultraviolet radiation so useful in therapy. It is effective in treating skin diseases caused by bacteria, such as acne, psoriasis, and ulcerations.

Ultraviolet rays are generated by different types of lamps. One type discharges a current of electricity through certain gases in a quartz tube. The process produces ultraviolet rays with very little heat generation. This lamp is called the *cold quartz lamp* and is most frequently used in the physician's office.

There are two types of cold quartz ultraviolet lamps. One type is used for general body radiation. This energy is very potent, and precautions must be taken to avoid tissue damage from overexposure. The physician must give an exact order in seconds or minutes for the length of exposure and the exact distance between the patient and the lamp. At a distance of 36 inches from the unit to the patient, a first-degree burn can be produced in 30 seconds to 1 minute, a second-degree burn in 1 to 2 minutes, and a third-degree burn in 2 to 4 minutes.

Test the lamp on the patient's forearm for a few seconds before you begin treatment to determine the presence of skin sensitivity. Some patients cannot tolerate any ultraviolet radiation. A history of sun exposure may help you determine this. Ultraviolet rays are considered carcinogenic if their use is prolonged. Certain drugs, especially the sulfonamides, increase the sensitivity of the skin to ultraviolet rays, and treatments should be postponed or the dosage reduced accordingly. Additional precautions include using a towel to cover the genitalia and other areas of the patient's body not being treated. Both the operator and the patient should wear ultraviolet-filtered glasses.

The size of the dose is usually governed by the erythematous response of the patient's skin. Treatments are generally given every other day because 24 hours is not enough time to evaluate the maximum erythematous response of the skin. The penetration of the rays is less than 0.1 mm, and there may be some tanning of the skin. The intensity of the radiation is greatest when the rays strike the skin at right angles (90 degrees). At an angle of 30 degrees, the intensity decreases to 80% (Lambert's Cosine Law). If the distance from the patient to the lamp is decreased by one half, the strength of the radiation is increased four times (inverse square law). Because of these two factors, it is important that the distance and the angle of the ultraviolet rays are correct and the same for each treatment.

The *portable Spot-Quartz lamp* is useful when treating small areas (Fig. 39-22). The portable lamp is placed near or in contact with the area to be treated. Practically no heat is generated in the lamp coils, thus skin burns do not occur. The treatment time extends from a few seconds to minutes, depending on the skin condition and the distance between the patient and the lamp. A masking adapter for small areas attaches to the face of the lamp, and a filter (Wood's filter) eliminates the visible light. The glass coils of the lamp must be protected from breakage and must be kept free of dust and soil. They may be cleaned with alcohol.

Hot Water Bottles

These are often used at home without any thought to correct technique. When teaching patients how to use this method at home, caution them to keep the water temperature at or below 125°F (52°C). If the patient is a child, keep the temperature below 115°F (46°C) to prevent burns. A hot water bottle that is less than one half full conforms better to the body and is more comfortable.

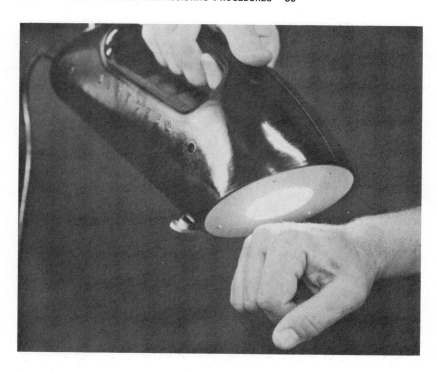

FIGURE 39–22. The Spot-Quartz is a portable, cold quartz lamp. (Courtesy of the Bircher Corporation.)

Heat Application to Deeper Tissues

Three methods of heat application to the deeper tissues are short-wave, microwave, and ultrasound diathermy. All three forms are applied to increase blood flow and speed up metabolism and electrolyte flow across the cell membranes. Treatment is used to stretch and repair tendons, joint capsules, and scars. Treatments usually relieve stiffness of joints, relax muscles, and decrease muscle spasm.

Short-Wave Diathermy

This method produces energy similar to that emitted by a radio station transmission. This energy penetrates deep into the body tissues and creates heat. The use of short-wave diathermy may be indicated for all types of inflammatory processes (acute, subacute, and chronic). Many patients report pain relief within 36 to 48 hours. Treatments may be prescribed as often as three times a week for 20 to 30 minutes.

Two condenser plates are placed on either side of the body part to be treated. As these high-frequency waves are transmitted through the body from one plate to the other, heat is generated in the tissues. Most short-wave diathermy plates are placed 1 inch from the skin. The dosage panel should be adjusted until a mild heat is felt by the patient. Some patients may believe that if a little warmth produces good results, more heat will be even better. This is not true with short-wave diathermy. Do not increase the volume of energy above the amount ordered by the physician, and carefully explain to the patient that only a gentle warmth is appropriate for effective treatment. Conversely, notify the physician that you need to lower the volume of energy if the amount ordered is too much for the patient. Position the machine so that the patient cannot adjust the controls. If necessary, place a towel on the patient to collect perspiration.

The short-wave diathermy machine must be wiped down after use on each patient. Do not permit the electric cords to tangle. Do not move the machine in any position that will pull the electric cord at any of the connections. The cables leading to the patient electrode plates should not cross one another or touch the patient. Electricity follows the path of least resistance and may flow from one cord to another, thus rerouting the energy away from the area being treated. Almost all machines have "spacers" on the cables to prevent this. Some machines may require a warm-up period before they can be used in treatment.

Microwave Diathermy

This method uses radar waves. It works on the same principle as microwave ovens used for cooking. Microwaves have a higher frequency and shorter wavelength than radio waves. This mode is the easiest to use (one electrode is placed above the body part to be treated), but it has less penetration than does short-wave diathermy. Microwaves cannot be used over moist dressings or near persons with implanted electronic cardiac pacemakers.

Ultrasound Diathermy

Ultrasound energy is sound energy. The basic principle of ultrasonography is the same as that of sonar, used in oceanography. Ultrasonic waves are concentrated into a narrow beam and are transmitted through a medium in the form of vibrations. The customary sounds that we hear are produced by sound waves vibrating at a rate of 100 to 12,000 cycles per second (hertz). Ultrasound waves vibrate at the rate of one million times per second. In therapeutic ultrasound machines, this frequency is created by an electric current passing through an applicator (transducer). In the applicator is a quartz crystal. The current passes through the quartz, causing the quartz to vibrate at an extremely high frequency. When the applicator containing the quartz is brought into contact with the body, the vibrations are transferred and continue through the tissues.

Though the frequency of this vibration is high, the total energy transmitted to the patient is very low. It is normally indicated on an output meter on the machine, in total watts or watts per square centimeter of the applicator element area (Fig. 39–23). Ultrahigh-frequency sound waves do not travel through air. The applicator must be held in contact with the body surface and aided with a *coupling agent*. A coupling agent may be either water or a gel. If the area of the body to be treated can be immersed in a basin or tank, treatment may be administered under water. For areas of the body that cannot be immersed, gel is applied to the applicator and to the body part to be treated. The gel should be water-soluble and nonstaining to clothing or skin.

Ultrahigh-frequency sound waves cause the tissues to vibrate, which, in turn, vibrates the circulatory system and speeds up circulation. The increased blood flow creates a chemical action in the tissues that has a favorable effect on the body's healing process. All this takes place with little or no heat, and the patient feels no sensation except a little warmth. Because ultrasound waves travel best through water, they penetrate the deep body tissues that have a high water content, such as the muscles. However, because ultrasound waves cannot penetrate and "move" along tissues that have a low water content, such as bone, the waves are capable of concentrating and "bombarding" bone and causing damage. Ultrasound treatment must be used very carefully where bones are near the surface of the skin.

Most acute ailments, such as strains, sprains, and torn muscles and tendons, are treated with ultrasound power as low as 0.5 to 1.0 watt per square centimeter. Ultrasound treatment is not recommended within the first 48 hours for these acute conditions. During this first 48-hour period, the best treatment is application of cold compresses. Chronic conditions, such as **arthritis** and **osteoarthritis,** may be treated at a higher power, 1.5 to 2.5 watts per square centimeter. The duration of any treatment varies from 5 to 15 minutes, depending on the physician's instructions.

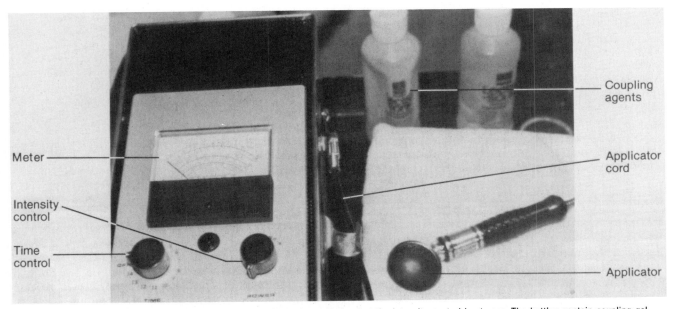

FIGURE 39–23. The ultrasound machine and its parts are shown here. Notice that the intensity control is at zero. The bottles contain coupling gel.

PROCEDURE 39-3   ASSISTING WITH ULTRASOUND THERAPY

Note: The medical assistant should perform ultrasound therapy only under the supervision of the physician or a registered physical therapist.

GOAL   To apply ultrahigh-frequency sound waves to the patient's deep tissues for therapy.

EQUIPMENT AND SUPPLIES

Ultrasound machine
Coupling agent

PROCEDURAL STEPS

1. Wash your hands.
2. Confirm the patient's identity.
3. Explain the procedure, and ask the patient to indicate if there is any discomfort.
   Purpose: To ensure that the patient does not experience any pain or injury.
4. Question the patient for the presence of any internal or external metal objects.
5. Position the patient comfortably, with the area to be treated exposed.
6. Apply a warmed coupling agent liberally over the area to be treated and to the applicator.
   Purpose: To transmit the sound waves through water or a water-soluble substance.
7. Begin treatment with the intensity control at the lowest setting.
8. Set the timer on the machine.
   Purpose: The timer starts the machine.
9. Increase the intensity control to the ordered amount.
10. Hold the applicator at a 90-degree angle against the patient's skin.
    Purpose: To ensure close contact.
11. Work the applicator over the area to be treated in a circular fashion, within a radius of 2 inches per second.
    Purpose: Constant motion prevents "hot spots" from occurring from excessive ultrasonic waves to one area.
12. If the alternative method of "stroking" is ordered, move the applicator in short 1-inch strokes so that each stroke overlaps the last stroke about ½ inch.
13. Keep the applicator moving until the timer sounds. The timer shuts off the machine automatically.
14. Return the intensity control to zero.
15. Remove the coupling agent from the patient and from the applicator with a paper wipe.
16. Assist the patient to the dressing room.
17. Record on the patient's medical record the treatment date, area treated, intensity, duration, and any unusual occurrences or reaction(s) that may have occurred during the treatment.

GENERAL PRINCIPLES OF COLD APPLICATION

Cold applications such as ice packs and cold compresses act as vasoconstrictors and cause contraction of the involuntary muscles of the skin. These two actions cause a reduced blood supply to the skin and numbing of the sensory nerve endings. Cold applications are used to control bleeding or to slow down inflammatory reactions. Cold reduces swelling and relieves pain. Occasionally, it is used to slow down the activity of living cells, thereby controlling infection. It is important to understand that while cold applications prevent further swelling, they do not reverse any swelling that is already present in the tissues. Such swelling is later treated with heat.

Cold applications may be used in an emergency to treat burns and to control internal bleeding and edema. Cool sponge baths, using cool water and alcohol, are employed to reduce fevers. A generalized lowering of the body's temperature depresses the activity of the body, slowing the heart and the pulse rate and decreasing cellular activity.

Cold Compresses

Cold compresses are applied to small areas such as the face and the head. Gauze sponges or washcloths are most often used. The first cloth should be applied gently so that the patient gets used to the cold. Compresses should be changed every 3 minutes, and the total treatment is ordered usually for 20 minutes at a time. Advise patients to check the skin for signs of redness and swelling at the application site. Applications should be stopped if the cold causes pain.

PROCEDURE 39-4 APPLYING AN ICE BAG

39

GOAL To instruct a patient on how to apply dry cold to a body area to prevent swelling.

EQUIPMENT AND SUPPLIES

Ice bag
Small cubes or chips of ice
Towel

PROCEDURAL STEPS

1. Wash your hands.
2. Identify the patient.
3. Explain the procedure, and answer any questions that the patient may ask about home care.
4. Specifically ask the patient if he or she has any questions about how to perform the treatment.
5. If the patient is not sure how to do the procedure, demonstrate the following steps.
6. Check the bag for possible leaks.
7. Fill the bag with small cubes or chips of ice until it is about two thirds full.
   Purpose: Small chips conform better to the body part.
8. Push down on the top of the bag to expel excess air, and apply the cap.
   Purpose: To remove air, which is a poor conductor of cold.
9. Dry and cover the bag.
10. Help the patient position the ice bag on the affected area.
11. Advise the patient that the damaged tissues will benefit from the cold even though the treatment may feel uncomfortable.
12. Advise the patient to leave the ice bag in place for about 30 minutes or until the area feels numb.
13. Check the skin for color, feeling, and pain.
    Purpose: If the area being treated becomes very painful, remains numb, or is pale or blue, the ice bag should be removed and the physician notified.
14. Clean the ice bag by emptying the water, rinsing it, and allowing it to dry in the air without the cap on.
15. Chart the procedure and the patient teaching session.

Ice Packs

Ice packs can be applied to the head to treat headache, fever, delirium, and minor head injuries; to the abdomen to slow down inflammation within the abdominal or pelvic cavity; or to the eyes to control swelling and inflammation. Ice packs may be prescribed following some surgical procedures to control swelling and bleeding and may be used to relieve the symptoms of hemorrhoids.

Usually, an ice pack is applied up to 1 hour or until the patient complains of pain from the cold or numbness, whichever occurs first. Ice packs should be covered with a cloth or towel to keep the patient dry. Ice packs without a covering may be too cold for the patient to tolerate.

Do not assume that a patient knows the correct technique of applying an ice pack. Instruct the patient on how to care for and apply ice packs at home. Ice packs may be made from items found in the home such as plastic bags and towels. Commercially prepared dry ice packs may be purchased, but they are effective only for a few minutes. Commercially available ice bags are the most effective.

THERAPEUTIC EXERCISE

A therapeutic exercise program is designed to correct specific disabilities of the patient. An exercise program may restore mobility, coordination, and strength to a part or may result in relaxation and relief of tension or pain. Extensive evaluation of the patient's actual physical condition is necessary when exercise therapy is prescribed. This is also a time when a great amount of patient education and encouragement is required. The physical therapist and the physician work together in evaluating the best type of treatment. Often, therapeutic exercise is combined with the heat and heat hydrotherapy treatments already mentioned in this chapter.

Joint Mobility

If motion is restricted even for a short time, the joint tissues become dense, hard, and shortened. These changes occur even in normal joints in as short a time as 4 days. It is important to institute joint exercise as soon as possible during therapy. Treatment of joint immobility or disability is accomplished either actively or passively by exercising a joint to its highest degree of possible motion.

Active Exercise

Active exercise is body movement voluntarily initiated and controlled by the patient, although the patient may be assisted by the physical therapist or physical therapist assistant. Active exercise may require specialized equipment, similar to gymnasium equipment. Some devices that are prescribed are stationary bicycles and free weights.

Passive Exercise

Passive exercise is moving a body part without the voluntary action of the patient. The movement is performed by someone other than the patient or by the force of a machine.

Range-of-Motion (ROM) Exercises

ROM exercises are specially designed exercises that move each joint of the body through its full range of motion (Fig. 39–24). After an injury to a joint, it is recommended that the patient exercise the injured part to its full range of motion three times, at least twice daily. If the patient cannot exercise actively, another individual can exercise the part passively. Range-of-motion exercises should be done slowly and gently, and only after the patient has been specifically instructed in correct techniques by a physical therapist. If the exercises are done too early or improperly, pain and even fracture or bleeding within the joint can occur.

Muscle Training and Strength

Muscle training is used to teach patients to gain or regain use of their muscles. This training can involve rehabilitation of muscle control lost as a result of physical trauma or diseases, such as poliomyelitis or cerebral palsy, or learning to use crutches or a wheelchair. Endurance exercises are used in the rehabilitation of the patient whose goal is to return to an active life after a long and debilitating illness or injury.

Electromuscle Stimulators

These are low-voltage machines that create a controlled electric current similar to that coming from an ordinary wall outlet. These low-voltage currents are useful for stimulating the motor and sensory nerves supplying the muscles. Such stimulation provides a passive means of exercising a muscle when a patient cannot activate the muscle voluntarily because of nerve damage. The purpose of the treatment is to revitalize a muscle or prevent **atrophy** of normal muscle.

Small electrode pads are moistened with tap water to increase their contact with the patient's skin. The pads are held by the technician until they are strapped into place. The machine is then operated by passing electric currents into the patient's muscles. The path of the electric current varies, depending on the exact placement of the two pads. As the current is applied to the muscles, the various waves act like the body's own nerves, causing the muscles to contract and relax.

One type of therapeutic current can stimulate and exercise **denervated** muscles and, if applied often enough, maintain a nearly normal muscle **tone.** Stimulation is also beneficial in retraining a patient to use injured muscles. The current artificially contracts and relaxes the muscles, and the patient is able to remember the feel of moving the body part. This often produces spectacular results and demonstrates to the patient that a muscle is not "dead" but can be revitalized.

Crutches

Crutches are used for mobility in cases of leg injury. You may be asked to help the patient select and adjust the proper size of crutches. Have the patient stand tall, with the head and back straight. If extra support is needed to maintain posture while measuring the crutches, have the patient stand straight against a wall. Adhere to the following steps to ensure a comfortable fit:

1. Crutch tips should be placed about 6 inches away from and parallel to the toes. (A thin person should move the tips slightly forward; a heavy person, with wide hips, should allow more space between the crutches and the toes.)
2. Adjust the length of the crutches so that two or three fingers fit between the armpit and the crutch top (about 2 inches). You may measure from the anterior axillary fold to the heel and then add 2 inches more.
3. Have the patient bend the elbow about 20 to 30 degrees when holding the hand grip.
4. Ask the patient to push down on the crutches and lift the body slightly. Now the arms should be nearly straight.
5. The hands and the arms should hold all the body weight with each stride. (Remember that weight borne by the axillary region may cause permanent nerve damage.)
6. Ask the patient to walk a few steps to be sure that the weight is distributed properly (Fig. 39–25).
7. As crutch-walking skills improve, so will posture. Instruct the patient to make adjustments at regular intervals. Young children outgrow crutches rapidly; check for fit frequently.

Tips for Patients Using Crutches

- Check that all wing nuts are tight.
- Check your crutch tips for wear. Crutch tips may be purchased at any drugstore or hardware store.
- Foam pads at the armpits and around the hand grips are more comfortable.
- Wear a sturdy low-heeled shoe on your unaffected foot.
- Keep the injured leg as relaxed as possible, and bend the knee to ensure that the leg clears the floor.
- Avoid scatter rugs, spills on the floor, extension cords, pets, and walking in the dark.
- Special safety equipment for the kitchen and bathroom is available for purchase or rental.

Wheelchairs

Wheelchairs use arm muscles rather than leg muscles for mobility. The folding wheelchair is very popular because it is lightweight and folds easily for travel.

Tips for Patients Using a Wheelchair

- Lock the chair so that it cannot move.
- Fold back the foot rests.
- Back into the chair, and support yourself on the arm rests as you lower your body into the seat.
- To leave the chair, first lock the chair and then fold back the foot rests.
- Lift your body, supporting yourself on the arm rests.
- Place your unaffected foot flat on the floor, just slightly under the seat.
- Push into an upright position, using your thigh muscles along with your arm and shoulder muscles.

Relief of Tension and Pain

A growing branch of medicine and physical therapy employs exercise to relax the muscles and to provide relief from tension and pain resulting from stress or a wide variety of physical disorders.

Pain Control

This includes such techniques as relaxation, massage, the application of heat and liniments, mechanical electric stimulation, acupuncture, and hypnosis. Mechanical electric stimulation was introduced 100 years ago as an analgesic. It was regarded as **quackery** at that time, even though some patients reported pain relief. Acupuncture, adapted from ancient Chinese techniques, has received wide acceptance during the last few decades. Along with acupuncture, hypnosis has proved helpful in pain relief for many patients. During the past 15 years, the effectiveness of relaxation exercises, heat, and massage for pain relief has been explained scientifically.

There are several theories about pain and its control. The "gate theory" offers one possible explanation. In 1937, Ronald Melzack and Patrick Wall hypothesized that pain signals can be modified by a hypothetic gate in the spinal cord that opens and closes. Gentle stimulation causes impulses to travel so fast that they rush ahead and close the gate, which keeps the pain signals from reaching the brain.

Since this theory was first proposed, we have learned that our bodies contain morphine-like substances called *cephalins* and *endorphins*. These two analgesic substances are found naturally in the

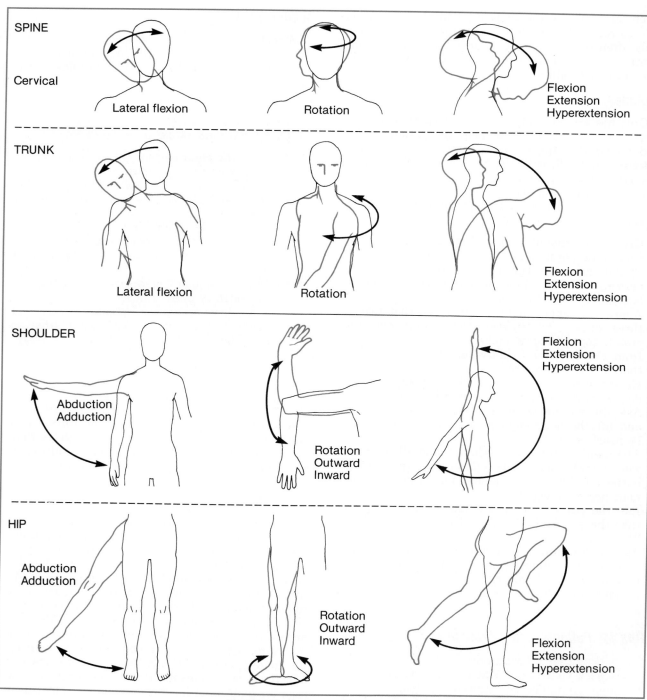

FIGURE 39–24. Range-of-motion exercises.

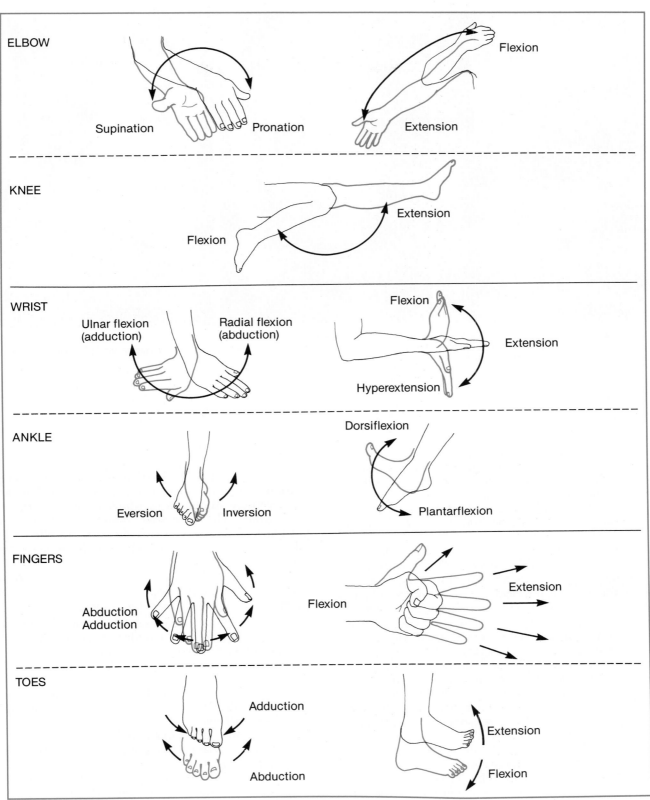

FIGURE 39-24. *Continued*

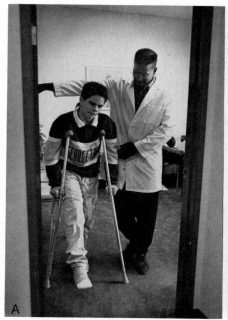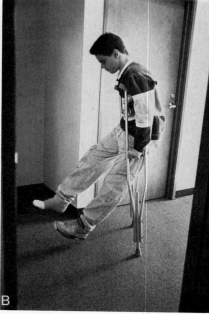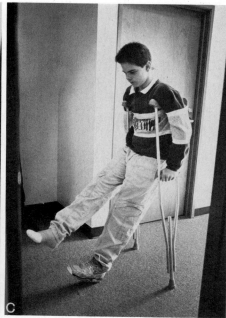

FIGURE 39–25. *A,* One type of crutch walking, the swing through gait, is shown here. It is used when the affected foot can bear no weight. *A,* The unaffected foot bears the body weight, and both crutches advance together. *B,* The arm muscles bear the body weight as the body swings through. *C,* Completion of the step with weight returning to the unaffected foot.

brain and spinal cord and appear to block the transmission of pain signals upward along the spinal cord to the brain. Another discovery is that certain thick sensory fibers extending from tactile receptors in the skin can compete with and suppress the transmission of pain to the brain from the thinner nerve fibers.

The most significant number of chronic pain sufferers seen in the medical office are those with muscle or joint pain such as arthritis, **bursitis,** and low back pain. All the physical pain control techniques previously mentioned have been useful in treating these conditions. *Intractable pain* is defined as that which cannot be relieved except through the use of addicting drugs or incapacitating sedation. The patient with chronic, prolonged, unrelenting pain becomes a slave to the torment. Indeed, pain may destroy a person's personality or life productivity. Until the last decade, intractable pain was managed by surgical excision of the sensory nerve pathways (pain receptors) to the brain.

For the patient with intractable pain, the electric muscle stimulator can increase blood flow through the area and relieve pain. The TENS-PAC is one type that transmits electric stimulation to the patient's nerves by touching the skin (Fig. 39–26) and is called a "transcutaneous electric nerve stimulator." Patients can be taught to use this device at home.

Massage

Massage is a form of passive exercise that relieves tension and pain. Massage activates the thicker tactile receptors in the skin, which compete with the pain signals. The systematic, therapeutic stroking or kneading of the body or a body part can effectively relieve localized pain, as well as pain at a distant site.

The medical assistant is usually not asked to apply therapeutic massages to patients, but you should be familiar with the terminology used:

- *Effleurage* is a stroking movement. In natural childbirth, a light circular stroke of the lower abdomen is done in a rhythm with controlled breathing to aid in the relaxation of the abdominal muscles.
- *Friction* is deep stroking or rubbing that involves deeper tissues. The traditional back rub uses friction.
- *Pétrissage* is a kneading or rolling type of massage with pressing of the muscles. It is also called *foulage.*
- *Tapotement* is a rapidly repeated, light percussion or tapping done with the sides of the hands. It may be called vibratory if it is done with a vibratory instrument or a sound.

The emphasis of this chapter has been on the basic physical techniques that are used to treat and

39

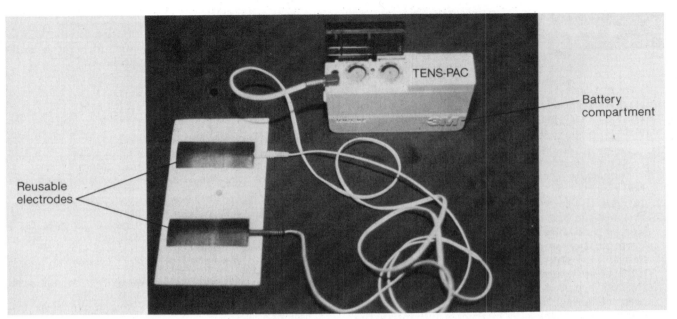

FIGURE 39-26. The small, portable TENS-PAC is prescribed by physicians to help control acute pain.

promote the repair of diseased or injured tissues and to relieve pain. Many of these treatments will be performed by you under the supervision of the physician or the physical therapist. If you are interested in the numerous other therapies that are performed in hospitals or physical therapy practices, you should consider visiting one of these institutions to observe firsthand how these modalities are further integrated into the restoration and rehabilitation of the patient to normal health and functioning.

LEGAL AND ETHICAL RESPONSIBILITIES

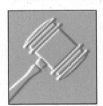
The procedures described in this chapter are not the basic procedures that the medical assistant will be required to perform when first securing a position in a medical facility. These techniques all involve additional training and practice. Before performing any of the described procedures, it is strongly recommended that you check with your local or state medical assistant organization regarding the laws in your state. Whenever you perform the techniques described in this chapter, you are responsible for the procedures. Remember the following:

- You must have a written order before doing the procedure.

- You must follow the procedure as it is ordered.
- Never advise the patient without permission.
- Reinforce the instructions given to the patient by the physician or therapist.
- If you have a concern about the procedure, discuss it with the physician or therapist privately before proceeding with the test.

Always remember, you are *assisting* with this procedure. If you keep this foremost in your mind, you will stay within the law and ethics of your state and your association.

▶ PATIENT EDUCATION

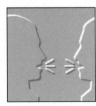
Throughout this chapter, you have read about the importance of teaching the patient. The reasons for patient education can be divided into two categories: to assist you in performing the procedure, and to obtain the best possible results. In addition, the informed patient is better prepared to continue with the intervention at home when this is needed. When you work with the physician and the therapist in helping the patient, you become an integral part of the health care team. This type of involvement leads to patient satisfaction and personal achievement.

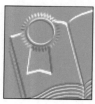

▶ LEARNING ACHIEVEMENTS

Upon completion of this chapter, can you in the time allowed by your evaluator:

1. Explain proper preparation of selected radiologic examinations to patients?
2. Assist with the positioning of patients for selected radiologic examinations?
3. Demonstrate the proper filing of x-ray studies and reports?
4. Prepare the spirometer for testing?
5. Instruct the patient in the spirometric maneuver testing procedure?
6. Perform the spirometric volume capacity maneuver and obtain three satisfactory tests with ±3% of deviation?
7. Instruct a patient in applying a hot, moist compress at home?
8. Apply an ice pack and instruct a patient in the application of an ice pack?
9. Assist with the administration of ultrasound therapy?
10. Demonstrate range-of-motion exercises?
11. Create patient education activities for the various applications of heat and cold, for crutch walking, and for the use of a wheelchair?

REFERENCES AND READINGS

American Thoracic Society Statement: Standardization of Spirometry, *Am Rev Respir Dis* 1987; 136:1030–1050

Bartrum, R.J., and Crow, H.C.: *Real-Time Ultrasound,* 2nd ed., Philadelphia, W.B. Saunders Co., 1983

Meschan, I., and Ott, D.J.: *Introduction to Diagnostic Imaging,* Philadelphia, W.B. Saunders Co., 1984

Miller, B.F., and Keane, C.B.: *Encyclopedia and Dictionary of Medicine, Nursing and Allied Health,* 4th ed., Philadelphia, W.B. Saunders Co., 1987

Nelson, S.B.: *Performance Evaluation of Contemporary Spirometers, Chest* 1990; 97:288–297

Snopek, A.: *Fundamentals of Special Radiographic Procedures,* 3rd ed., Philadelphia, W.B. Saunders Co., 1992

Swanson, M.A.: *Crutches on the Go,* Issaquah, WA, Medic Publishing Co., 1987

Taylor, R.: *Physical Therapy: Improving Movement and Function,* Daly City, CA, Krames Communications, 1984

Wanger, J.: *Pulmonary Function Testing, A Practical Approach,* Baltimore, Williams & Wilkins, 1992

CHAPTER FORTY

——

MEDICAL EMERGENCIES

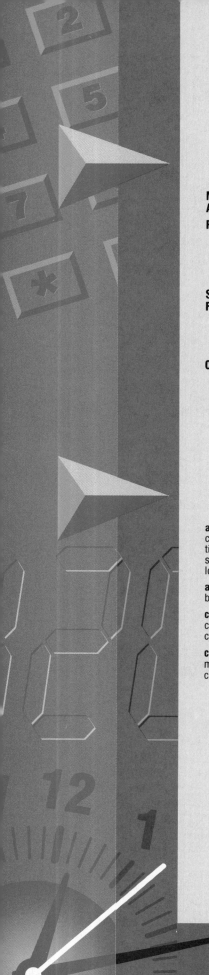

CHAPTER OUTLINE

VOCABULARY

anaphylaxis An allergic condition caused by an antigen/antibody reaction. May cause shock, bronchoconstriction, airway obstruction, and loss of consciousness.

apical pulse Pulse felt over the base (apex) of the heart.

convulsion A series of involuntary contractions of the voluntary muscles.

cyanosis Blue color of the mucous membranes and body extremities caused by lack of oxygen.

diaphragmatic Pertaining to the primary muscle of respiration; separates the thoracic and the abdominal cavities.

epistaxis Nosebleed.

insulin shock Shock brought about by too much insulin, too little food, or excessive exercise; when untreated, it can result in death.

Ipecac (syrup of ipecac) A syrup given to induce vomiting.

mediastinum The space in the center of the chest under the sternum, containing the heart, great vessels, esophagus, and trachea.

paroxysm The sudden onset of symptoms, such as a spasm or seizure.

syncope Loss of consciousness; fainting.

traumatic Pertaining to, resulting from, or causing physical injury or shock.

triage To sort or to choose; to determine the priority of need for treatment.

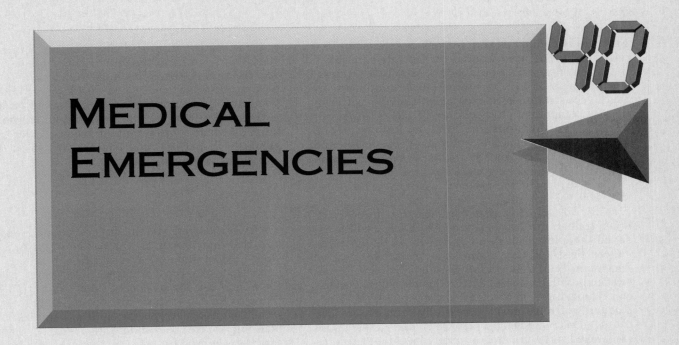

MEDICAL EMERGENCIES

40

LEARNING OBJECTIVES

COGNITIVE
Upon successful completion of this chapter, you should be able to:

1. Define and spell the words in the Vocabulary.

2. Describe the medical assistant's legal and ethical responsibilities in an emergency.

3. Recall two resources that can help to make your medical office accident-proof.

4. List the basic items that must be included on a crash tray.

5. Explain how and why a defibrillator is used in an emergency.

6. Recognize a choking victim.

7. Recall the conditions that necessitate the implementation of cardiopulmonary resuscitation.

8. Identify the major symptoms associated with heart attack.

9. List four medications that are indicated for a victim experiencing a severe cardiac disorder.

10. Describe the emergency medical care that is usually given to victims of asthma, anaphylactic shock, convulsions, and hemorrhagic shock.

11. State the functions of a Poison Control Center.

PERFORMANCE
Upon successful completion of this chapter, you should be able to perform the following activities:

1. Demonstrate cardiopulmonary resuscitation on an approved manikin.

2. Demonstrate the Heimlich maneuver.

3. Demonstrate fracture immobilization and proper technique in moving the injured.

4. Demonstrate triage technique in simulated emergency situation.

First aid is defined as the immediate care given to a person who has been injured or has suddenly taken ill. It includes well-chosen words of encouragement, a willingness to help, a promotion of confidence by the demonstration of competence, and the performance of temporary physical care to alleviate pain or a life-threatening situation. First-aid knowledge and skill can often mean the difference between life and death, temporary and permanent disability, and rapid recovery and long-term hospitalization.

It is frequently the medical assistant who is responsible for initiating first aid in the office and continuing to administer first aid until the physician or other trained medical teams arrive. Each medical assistant should enroll in an American Red Cross Advanced First-Aid Course and American Red Cross or American Heart Association Cardiopulmonary Resuscitation (CPR) Course. All graduates of the American Association of Medical Assistants (AAMA) accredited programs must successfully complete a CPR course. Basic knowledge of CPR and life-support skills need to be updated annually because of recommended changes for procedures as new techniques are developed. It is strongly recommended that medical assistants encourage their local chapters of the AAMA to offer workshops conducted by physicians and emergency personnel from the community.

There are many acceptable approaches to emergency care. All offices should establish written policies concerning the handling of medical emergencies. The medical assistant should consult with the physician-employer for his or her preferences in handling emergencies in that particular practice. Medical assistants should perform only emergency procedures that they have been trained to handle, and while in the office, only those designated by the physician. If an emergency occurs in the office, the medical assistant should notify the physician or any other available physician. If a physician is not located, then the assistant should contact the local emergency medical services team.

Medical assistants do not assume the responsibility of diagnosing but are expected to make decisions based on their medical knowledge. A major goal in emergency care of the injured is to cause no further harm.

In a true emergency, the law permits anyone to do whatever is reasonably necessary, provided that the care given is within the scope of competence of the person administering first aid. The law holds persons giving emergency care to be responsible for any injury that they cause as a result of their negligence or failure to exercise reasonable care. You, the medical assistant, are limited to the standards of your state laws, and your physician-employer is legally responsible for your mistakes.

MAKING THE OFFICE ACCIDENT-PROOF

Usually, it is the medical assistant's responsibility to make the office as accident-proof as possible. Do not use scatter rugs or delicate chairs, and be sure that floors are not slippery. Keep cupboard doors and drawers closed. Wipe up spills immediately, and pick up dropped objects. All medications should be kept out of sight; dangerous drugs should be kept in locked cupboards. If there are children in the office, keep all sharp objects out of reach. Never leave a seriously ill patient or a restless, depressed, or unconscious patient unattended.

PLANNING AHEAD

The office staff should discuss possible emergencies that may occur in that office or area. For instance, local industries may present unique problems that call for very specialized care. Plan for these, and ask the physician's advice on what procedures to follow. If there are several employees, each should be assigned specific duties. Organization and planning make the difference between organized care for the patient and complete chaos. Some offices have set up the "buddy system." This system allows one person to take immediate charge of the patient while another obtains needed materials and calls for assistance. They can also relieve each other in more strenuous work such as resuscitation and external heart massage.

Using Community Emergency Services

Many communities have established an emergency medical services (EMS) system. This system includes an efficient communications network, such as the emergency telephone number 911; well-trained rescue personnel; properly equipped vehicles; an emergency facility that is open 24 hours a day to provide advanced life-support; and hospital intensive care for the victims.

There are over 300 poison control centers in the United States ready to provide emergency information for treating victims of poisonings. Many of the centers have toll-free lines. Some have systems for communicating with deaf persons.

Every office should post a list of local emergency numbers. This list should be in plain sight and should be known to all office personnel. Include on the list the local EMS system, poison control center, ambulance, fire, rescue squad, and police department numbers.

Preventing Children's Accidents

Accidents are the leading cause of death among children under 15 years of age. Even more common are home accidents that cause injuries that do not kill but require hospitalization. More than one-half million of such accidents occur each year. The Children's Bureau of the Department of Health, Education, and Welfare has published pamphlets containing helpful tips on preventing accidents.

Child-resistant bottle caps, safer toys, better-educated parents, more responsible toy manufacturers, and government regulations have helped to cut dramatically the number of childhood deaths and injuries. Parents should be encouraged to use car safety seats, make their homes accident-proof, purchase safe toys, become familiar with basic first-aid procedures, and know the local emergency numbers. Medical assistants in both pediatrics and family practice specialties may be called upon to educate families in these matters.

SUPPLIES AND EQUIPMENT FOR EMERGENCIES

Crash Tray

The emergency, or crash, tray is a properly equipped tray of first-aid items needed for a variety of emergencies. Contents of the tray vary to some degree, according to the type of emergencies each office encounters (see Basic Crash Tray Items). The tray should be kept in an easily accessible place known to all personnel in the office. A firm rule must be made that no one borrows any items from the tray. Medication expiration dates should be checked and the tray replenished with fresh supplies after use.

BASIC CRASH TRAY ITEMS

Activated charcoal, bottle of 30 to 50 g
Adhesive tape
Airways in assorted sizes
Amobarbital sodium (Amytal Sodium)
Antihistamine, injectable and oral
Apomorphine hydrochloride
Atropine
Dextrose
Diazepam (Valium)
Digoxin (Lanoxin)
Disposable syringe and needle units
Epinephrine (Adrenalin), injectable
Furosemide (Lasix)
Glucagon
Hot and cold packs (instant type)
Ipecac syrup
Isoproterenol hydrochloride aerosol spray (Isuprel)
Lidocaine (Xylocaine)
Metaraminol (Aramine)
Muslin sling or cravat bandage to be used as a tourniquet
Orange juice
Sterile dressings (miscellaneous sizes, including two abdominal pads)

Epinephrine is a vasoconstrictor used to check hemorrhage. It relaxes the bronchioles, is used to relieve asthmatic **paroxysm,** and is an emergency heart stimulant used to treat shock. Epinephrine should be in a ready-to-use cartridge syringe and needle unit. These are supplied in 1.0-cc cartridges.

Other drugs used are atropine, digoxin (Lanoxin), and lidocaine (Xylocaine). Atropine decreases secretions, increases respiration and heart rates, and is a smooth muscle relaxant. It dilates the pupil of the eye and is a general cerebral stimulant. Atropine relieves gastrointestinal cramps and hypermotility and may also be used to relieve pain locally. Digoxin is a cardiotonic. It is used to treat congestive heart failure and is good for emergency use because it has a relatively rapid action. Lidocaine is used as both a local and a topical anesthetic.

Apomorphine hydrochloride is a prompt and effective emetic and is used in cases of poisoning when a stomach pump cannot be employed. **Syrup of ipecac** is also an emetic and one that many physicians are recommending be kept on hand in the home for use in emergencies.

Antihistamines are used to counteract the effect of histamine and are used in the treatment of allergic reactions and **anaphylaxis.**

Isoproterenol, an antispasmodic, is used in bronchial spasm and is also a cardiac stimulant. Some trademarks for this product are Isuprel (Winthrop-Breon), Medihaler-Iso (Riker), and Norisodrine (Abbott).

Other medications that may be found on a crash tray are metaraminol (Aramine) (50%, in a prefilled syringe), for severe shock; amobarbital sodium (Amytal) and diazepam (Valium), for convulsions and as sedatives; dextrose and insulin, to treat diabetic patients; and furosemide (Lasix), for congestive heart failure. Glucagon is primarily used to counteract severe hypoglycemic reactions in diabetic patients taking insulin.

Small cans, with pull-tab openers, of orange juice are handy for quick sugar administration in cases of diabetic patients experiencing **insulin shock.**

Most physicians and others involved in emergency care do not recommend a tourniquet because of the danger that may result from incorrect usage. A tourniquet that completely stops blood flow to the point of no measurable pulse is potentially hazardous and should be used very cautiously. It is much better to apply pressure directly over the bleeding area. Today, rather than a tourniquet, a constricting band is employed for the purpose of decreasing lymphatic and superficial venous blood flow for bites by insects and snakes. In these cases, the constricting band is applied just above the bite area.

Crash Cart

As more patients come to clinics and physicians' offices to seek emergency care, the medical assistant will need to become even more familiar with specialized equipment on the emergency, or "crash," cart to help save lives. This cart contains many more items than the smaller crash tray commonly found in most physicians' offices. Figure 40–1

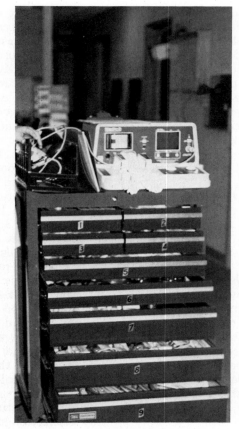

A

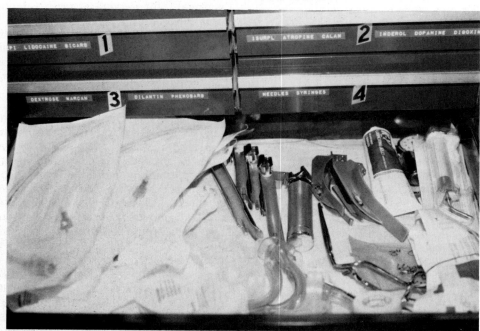

B

FIGURE 40–1. *A,* A typical crash cart in clinics and urgent care centers. It is on wheels, and the top is large enough to hold a defibrillator. *B,* The interior of the crash cart drawer reveals a good supply of airways, a laryngoscope with extra batteries, and some sterile wrapped supplies that are readily available in an emergency situation. (Courtesy of Dean West Urgent Care, Madison, WI.)

shows the outside and the inside of a typical crash cart. The cart contains numerous locking drawers in which supplies and medicines are kept.

Defibrillators

The medical assistant who works in a large clinic or in an urgent-care center may be required to assist the team with defibrillation of emergency patients. Defibrillators are instruments that send a massive jolt of electricity into the heart muscle by means of plates or paddles applied to the chest to re-establish the proper rhythm of the heartbeat. One paddle is placed to the right of the upper sternum and the other is placed just to the left of the nipple, at the apex of the heart.

The office defibrillator is portable and is powered by batteries. The monitor has a nonfading display, and it is possible to freeze the monitor for prolonged viewing. If a permanent record of the victim's heart rate is desired, the machine can make a printed copy.

COMMON EMERGENCIES

The general rules to follow in an emergency are few but very important (see General Rules for Emergencies chart).

GENERAL RULES FOR EMERGENCIES

- The first and most important rule is to keep calm. Reassure the patient and make him or her as comfortable as possible.

- Survey the situation to determine the nature of the emergency. A decision must be made as to whether the need is immediate. This decision requires calm judgment and may call for some medical knowledge.

- Take immediate steps to remedy the situation. Calmly but firmly give specific instructions to the patient and to other office personnel. Never say, "Will someone call the doctor?" Say, "YOU call the doctor," "YOU get a blanket," and "YOU get the emergency tray."

- After the emergency is under control, make certain that all the events and the medications used are recorded accurately. Be precise when recording. Have statements of how the accident happened or what events just preceded the emergency.

- Follow the universal blood and body-fluid precautions.

The basic principles and procedures for the following emergencies are covered thoroughly in the manuals published by the American Red Cross,

which are listed at the end of this chapter. Wound care, dressings and bandages, burns, and poisonings are among the topics included in the American Red Cross Standard First-Aid course, which is the minimum requirement for accredited programs of medical assisting as defined by the Committee on Allied Health Education of the American Medical Association. These manuals are readily available at modest cost everywhere in the United States. The following sections of this chapter serve as a review and reference source for administering first aid in common emergencies.

Fainting (Syncope)

One of the most common emergency problems to confront the medical assistant is fainting. **Syncope** is usually caused by lack of oxygen in the blood, with a consequent lack of oxygen to the brain. Prior to fainting, a person may appear pale, may feel cold, weak, dizzy, or nauseated, and may have numbness of the extremities. Immediately lay the patient flat, with the head lower than the heart. Loosen all tight clothing, and maintain an open airway. Apply a cold washcloth to the forehead. Pass aromatic spirits of ammonia back and forth under the patient's nostrils. Be careful not to hold the ammonia too close to the nose. Obtain the patient's pulse, respiration rate, and blood pressure; and then report the findings to the physician. Keep the patient in a supine position for at least 10 minutes after consciousness has been regained.

If recovery is not prompt, summon the physician or emergency medical rescue team for transportation to the hospital. This might be a brief episode in the development of a serious underlying illness.

Emergency Respiratory Resuscitation

Breathing may suddenly cease for a variety of reasons, including shock, disease, and trauma. The most obvious sign that breathing has stopped is when the chest is no longer moving. Artificial respiration must be begun immediately, since death may follow within 4 to 6 minutes.

Resuscitation techniques should be studied and practiced in courses directed toward this purpose. The basics are presented here as an introduction or a reference. First, the airway must be opened by positioning the patient on the back and relieving possible obstruction of the air passage by the tongue. Extreme caution must be used if there is any chance that the patient has suffered a cervical neck injury, as should be assumed in any accident. If neck injury is not suspected, the head is tilted by downward pressure on the forehead and upward pressure under the chin. If neck injury may be present, grasp the angle of the victim's lower jaw without extending the neck.

Mouth-to-mouth resuscitation is begun if breathing does not follow opening of the airway. Position yourself on the side of the patient's head. One hand should continue pressing on the forehead and should also be turned so that the fingers can hold the nose shut. The other hand should continue lifting the chin upward. Place your mouth over the mouth of the victim and give two full breaths. Check for the carotid pulse. If the pulse is present, continue ventilating the lungs every 5 seconds. If the pulse is absent, you must provide artificial circulation in addition to artificial respiration (see Cardiopulmonary Resuscitation section later in this chapter).

There is a mouth-to-nose and a mouth-to-stoma method for resuscitation of victims with tracheotomies. Please refer to the American Red Cross *Standard First Aid Manual* for specific procedures and precautions.

Artificial airways may be inserted by trained personnel to establish or maintain breathing. Airways of various types and sizes should be kept ready on the emergency tray and cart (Fig. 40–2).

Cardiopulmonary Resuscitation

Cessation of breathing may be accompanied by a cessation of the heartbeat (cardiac arrest), which is identified by the lack of a pulse. Artificial respiration must then be accompanied by external (closed) cardiac massage. This is called cardiopulmonary resuscitation (CPR), which is the combination of artificial circulation and artificial breathing.

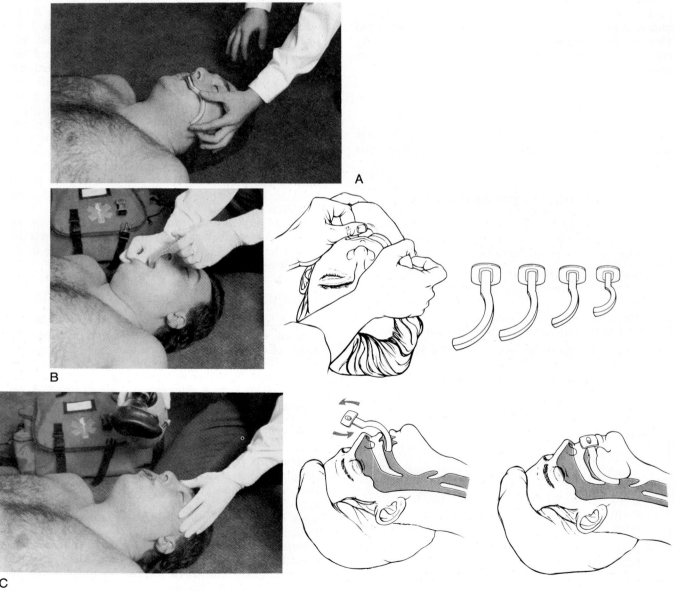

FIGURE 40–2. *A,* Measure the airway from the center of the patient's mouth to the angle of the jaw. *B,* To open the mouth, place your index finger on the top teeth and the thumb on the lower teeth and apply pressure in opposite directions. Insert the oropharyngeal airway in the mouth with the tip pointing toward the roof of the mouth. *C,* Rotate the airway 180 degrees into position at the base of the oropharynx. Once fully inserted, the flange of the airway should rest against the lips. If the patient gags during the insertion, quickly remove the airway and do not attempt reinsertion. Have suction on standby in case of vomiting. (From Henry, M., and Stapleton, E. R.: *EMT: Prehospital Care,* Philadelphia, W. B. Saunders Co., 1991, p 101.)

The basic ABC steps of CPR include:

A—airway

B—breathing

C—circulation

When both breathing and pulse stop, the victim has suffered sudden death. There are many causes of sudden death, including choking, drowning, poisoning, suffocation, electrocution, and smoke inhalation. CPR must be started immediately in an attempt to prevent death or permanent damage to body organs, especially the brain.

Since CPR may cause injuries to the ribs, heart, liver, lungs, and blood vessels, it should be performed only by individuals properly trained in the techniques and only if cardiac arrest has occurred.

In CPR, the heart is compressed by downward pressure on the sternum, which should cause the blood to circulate. The proper position is for the heel of the one hand to be placed on the sternum, two fingerwidths above the lower notch where the ribs join. The other hand is placed on top, and the rescuer presses straight down. The sternum will be depressed one and one-half to two inches with sufficient pressure.

Compressions should be given at a rate of 80 to 100 compressions per minute (15 compressions should take 9 to 11 seconds). Compress down and up smoothly, keeping hand contact with the victim's chest at all times. After every 15 compressions, move back to the mouth, open the airway with the head-tilt/chin-lift, and breathe two full breaths into the victim. After three cycles have been completed, locate and check the carotid pulse, feeling for 5 seconds. Continue CPR until a qualified person can relieve you or until advanced life support is available.

CPR for infants and small children is similar to that for adults, but a few important differences must be remembered. When handling an infant be careful that you do not overextend the head when tilting it back (Fig. 40–3A). The infant's neck is so pliable that forceful backward tilting might block breathing

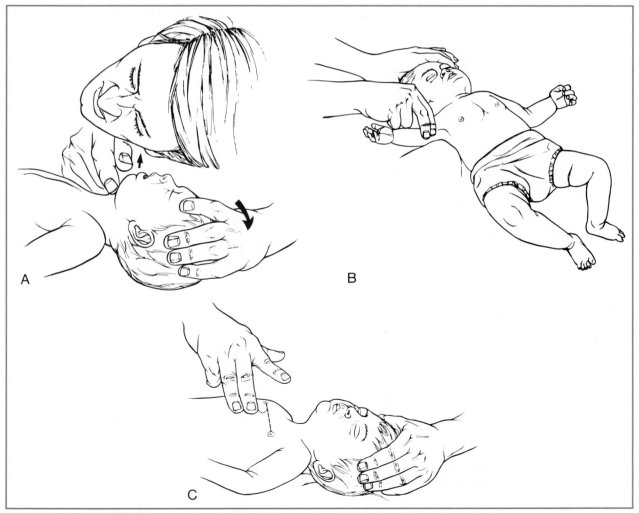

FIGURE 40–3. Modifications necessary for the CPR procedure when the victim is an unresponsive infant. *A,* Gently tilt the head backward but do not hyperextend it. *B,* Locate the brachial pulse between the elbow and the shoulder. *C,* Place the fingers one finger's width below the nipple line. (From Henry, M., and Stapleton, E. R.: *EMT: Prehospital Care,* Philadelphia, W. B. Saunders Co., 1991, pp 249–250.)

passages instead of opening them. With an infant who is not breathing, be certain to cover both the mouth and the nose with your mouth and deliver two slow "puffs" that are just strong enough to make the chest rise. With a small child, pinch the nose, cover the mouth, and breathe as for an infant. In an infant, check the brachial pulse (Fig. 40–3*B*) between the elbow and the shoulder. Use only the fingertips at the center of the sternum for compressions on the infant (Fig. 40–3*C*). Compress the sternum between ½ and 1 inch, at a rate of at least 100 times per minute. Only the heel of one hand is used for compressions on a small child. Depress the sternum 1 to 1½ inches, at a rate of 80 to 100 times per minute. CPR for children over 8 years of age is the same as that for adults.

PROCEDURE 40–1   PERFORMING CARDIOPULMONARY RESUSCITATION

GOAL   To restore a victim's breathing and blood circulation when respiration and pulse stop.

EQUIPMENT AND SUPPLIES

Nonsterile gloves (sterile gloves may be preferred)

An American Heart Association– approved manikin equipped with a printout for demonstration of the proper technique for your instructor.

PROCEDURAL STEPS

(To be performed on an approved manikin ONLY.)

1. Begin a primary survey. Tap the victim and ask, "Are you OK?" Wait for victim to respond.
   Purpose: To determine whether the victim is conscious.

2. Shout for help. Put on gloves.
   Purpose: To alert other rescue personnel to the problem.

3. Tilt the victim's head and lift the chin. Look, listen, and feel for signs of breathing. Place your ear over the mouth and listen for breathing. Watch the rising and falling of the chest for evidence of breathing (Fig. 40–4).
   Purpose: To determine whether the victim is breathing and to open the airway.

4. Begin rescue breathing by pinching the nose tightly with your thumb and forefinger if none of the signs of breathing are present (Fig. 40–5).
   Purpose: An airtight seal must be present so that air cannot escape through the nose when you perform mouth-to-mouth resuscitation.

5. Maintain an airtight seal with your mouth on the victim's mouth (Fig. 40–6).

6. Give two full breaths.
   Purpose: May be sufficient stimulus to initiate breathing by the victim.

7. Check the carotid pulse (Fig. 40–7).
   Purpose: The pulse is easier to feel in this area.

8. Continue mouth-to-mouth resuscitation at the rate of approximately one full breath every 5 seconds *if the pulse is present.*

9. Initiate CPR *if there is no pulse.*

10. Kneel at the victim's side opposite the chest. Move your fingers up the ribs to the point where the sternum and the ribs join. Your middle fingers should fit into the area and your index finger should be next to it across the sternum.

Continued

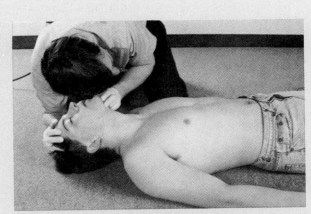

FIGURE 40–4. Establishing breathlessness. (From Henry, M., and Stapleton, E. R.: *EMT: Prehospital Care*, Philadelphia, W. B. Saunders Co., 1991, p 244.)

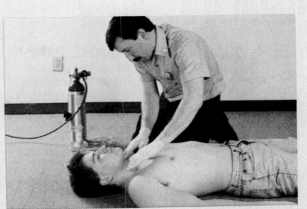

FIGURE 40–5. Checking for responsiveness. (From Henry, M., and Stapleton, E. R.: *EMT: Prehospital Care*, Philadelphia, W. B. Saunders Co., 1991, p 244.)

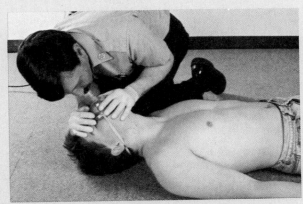

FIGURE 40–6. Mouth-to-mask ventilation. (From Henry, M., and Stapleton, E. R.: *EMT: Prehospital Care*, Philadelphia, W. B. Saunders Co., 1991, p 245.)

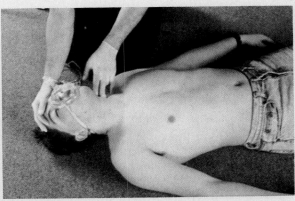

FIGURE 40–7. Check for carotid pulse. (From Henry, M., and Stapleton, E. R.: *EMT: Prehospital Care*, Philadelphia, W. B. Saunders Co., 1991, p 245.)

11. Place the heel of your hand on the chest midline over the sternum, just above your index finger (Fig. 40–8).
12. Place your other hand on top of your first hand and lift your fingers upward off of the chest (Fig. 40–9).
    Purpose: This position gives you the most control, allowing you to avoid injuring the victim's ribs as you compress the chest.
13. Bring your shoulders directly over the victim's sternum as you compress downward, and keep your arms straight.

Continued

PROCEDURE 40-1 *Continued*

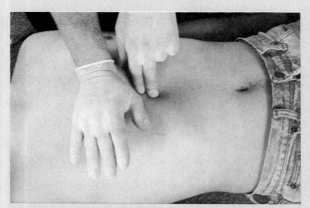

FIGURE 40-8. Place the heel of the hand closest to the patient's head next to your fingers. (From Henry, M., and Stapleton, E. R.: *EMT: Prehospital Care*, Philadelphia, W. B. Saunders Co., 1991, p 245.)

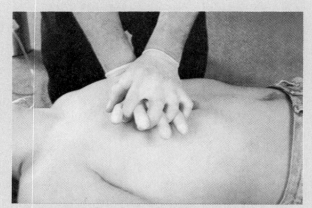

FIGURE 40-9. Place the heel of the other hand directly over the hand on the sternum and interlock your fingers to avoid pressure in the area of the ribs. (From Henry, M., and Stapleton, E. R.: *EMT: Prehospital Care*, Philadelphia, W. B. Saunders Co., 1991, p 245.)

14. Depress the sternum 1½ to 2 inches for an adult victim. Relax the pressure on the sternum after each compression but *do not remove your hands* from the victim's sternum.
   Purpose: The depth of compression is needed to circulate blood through the heart. Movement of the hands may cause injury to the victim.

15. After performing 15 compressions, open the airway and give two full breaths.

16. Complete three cycles of compressions and breaths, ending with breaths. Check the carotid pulse for 5 seconds. If there is no pulse, resume CPR at the rate of 15 compressions to 2 breaths. Always start and end each cycle with two full breaths.

Choking

Choking is caused by a foreign object, usually food, lodged in the upper airway. Often, exhalation can take place, but inhalation is blocked. Thus, the lungs quickly empty. The choking victim who has food or a foreign object lodged in the throat cannot speak, breathe, or cough. The victim may clutch the neck between the thumb and index finger. This universal distress signal should be viewed as a sign that the victim needs help (Fig. 40-10). The face pales and turns blue. Eventually, there is loss of consciousness and cardiopulmonary arrest. If the object is not removed, the victim may die within 4 to 6 minutes.

If the victim has good air exchange or only partial obstruction, and can speak, cough, or breathe, do not interfere. If the victim cannot speak, cough, or breathe, use the Heimlich maneuver. Give sub-**diaphragmatic** abdominal thrusts until the foreign body is expelled or the victim becomes unconscious

(Fig. 40-11). If the victim becomes unconscious, position the victim on his or her back, and call out for help. Sweep your finger in the victim's throat in an attempt to remove the foreign body. Open the airway, and attempt rescue breathing. If you are still unsuccessful in removing the foreign body, use the Heimlich maneuver and give six to ten subdiaphragmatic abdominal thrusts (Fig. 40-12). Repeat the sequence until you are successful. After the obstruction is removed, begin the ABCs of CPR, if necessary.

It is possible to perform the abdominal thrust maneuver on yourself if you are choking and there is no one nearby to help you. Press your fist into your upper abdomen with quick upward thrusts or lean forward and press the abdomen quickly against a firm object such as the back of a chair (Fig. 40-13).

To dislodge a foreign object from an infant, place the victim face down, over your forearm and across your thigh. The head should be lower than the

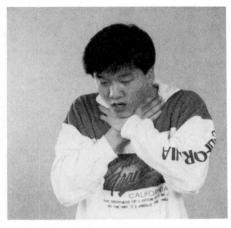

FIGURE 40-10. The choking sign. The distress of the choking victim must be distinguished from that of the coronary victim. In both cases, the face develops a blue color owing to the lack of oxygen. The choking sign consists of the victim grasping at the throat. The immediate use of the Heimlich maneuver is indicated. (From Henry, M., and Stapleton, E. R.: *EMT: Prehospital Care*, Philadelphia, W. B. Saunders Co., 1991, p 128.)

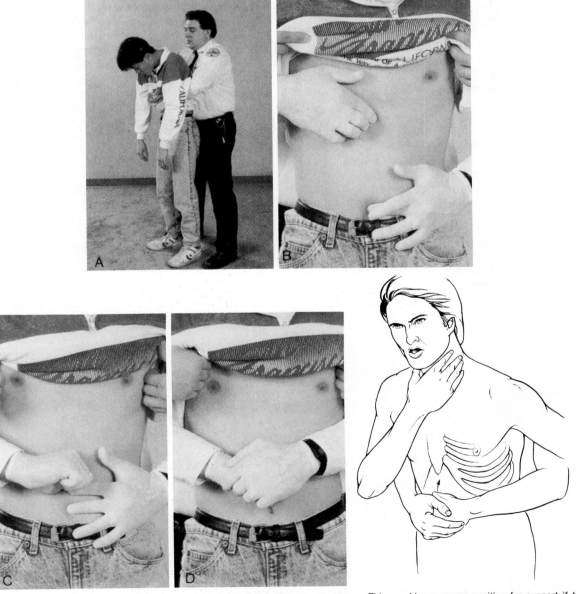

FIGURE 40-11. *A*, The rescuer should stand directly behind the victim with an open stance. This provides a secure position for support if the victim becomes unconscious. (From Henry, M., and Stapleton, E. R.: *EMT: Prehospital Care*, Philadelphia, W. B. Saunders Co., 1991, p 129.) *B*, Locate the victim's xiphoid and umbilicus. *C*, Place your fist just above the umbilicus with the thumb side in. *D*, Grab the fist with the other hand and apply an inward and upward thrust to the abdominal wall.

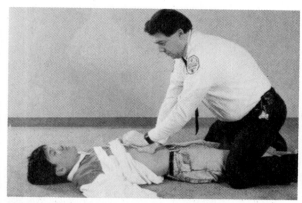

FIGURE 40–12. Straddle the victim at the level of the thighs and place the heel of one hand just above the umbilicus. (From Henry, M., and Stapleton, E. R.: *EMT: Prehospital Care*, Philadelphia, W. B. Saunders Co., 1991, p 130.)

trunk. Next, support the head and neck of the victim with one hand. Using the heel of the other hand, deliver four blows to the back, between the infant's shoulder blades (Fig. 40–14). Place the infant on his or her back, with the head lower than the trunk. Using two or three fingers, deliver four thrusts in the sternum area. Repeat the sequence until the foreign body is expelled or the infant becomes unconscious (Fig. 40–15).

If the infant becomes unconscious, position the infant on his or her back and call out for help. Sweep your finger in the throat in an attempt to remove the foreign body (Fig. 40–16). Open the airway, and attempt rescue breathing. If you are still unsuccessful in removing the foreign body, perform the sequence of back blows and chest thrusts until you are successful. After the obstruction is removed, begin the ABCs of CPR, if necessary (Fig. 40–17).

Chest Pain

Chest pain can be associated with both heart and lung disease, as well as a few other conditions. It can be quite serious; all patients with chest pain are treated as cardiac emergencies until a physician has ruled out this diagnosis. The patient is usually sweating and has a gray, ashen appearance. The lips and fingernails may be blue (a sign of **cyanosis**). Frequently, the patient is clutching the chest in pain. This pain may radiate from the **mediastinum** down the left arm and up the left side of the neck. The pulse may be rapid and weak. Frequently, there is nausea.

Do not have the patient walk any distance. A wheelchair or a chair with rollers is an excellent method of moving this patient to a quiet room. The patient will probably prefer to have his or her head slightly elevated or even to be in a semisitting position. Keep the patient quiet and warm. Loosen all tight clothing. Record **apical pulse** and radial pulse. Remember, you must use a stethoscope when obtaining an apical pulse. Administer oxygen if the physician has previously given these instructions. *Absolutely no smoking should be allowed by the patient or by anyone within the vicinity.* Prepare the medication that the physician is most likely to use. This may be epinephrine (Adrenalin), atropine, digitalis, calcium chloride 10%, or morphine. Determine whether the conscious patient is carrying any medication. Ask about the medication. Usually, this medication is nitroglycerin tablets that are administered sublingually. You may give them to the patient with the patient's consent. Do not give the patient alcohol, food, or water by mouth without the physician's permission. Do not give spirits of ammonia.

If the physician is in the office or is on the way, connect the patient to the electrocardiograph, and

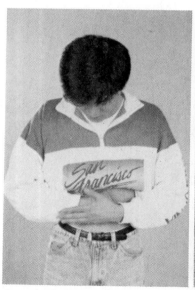

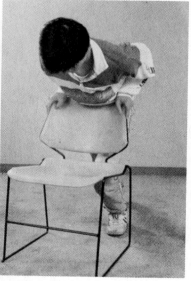

FIGURE 40–13. *A,* Self-administered abdominal thrusts using fist. *B,* Self-administered abdominal thrusts using back of chair. (From Henry, M., and Stapleton, E. R.: *EMT: Prehospital Care,* Philadelphia, W. B. Saunders Co., 1991, p 130.)

A

B

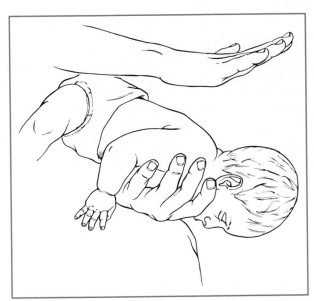

FIGURE 40–14. When back blows are being administered, the infant should be supported on your arm and thigh. The infant's head can rest across your palm to give further support to the head. (From Henry, M., and Stapleton, E. R.: *EMT: Prehospital Care*, Philadelphia, W. B. Saunders Co., 1991, p 657.)

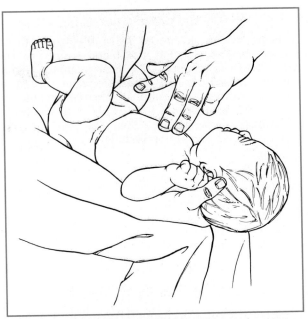

FIGURE 40–15. Chest thrusts are administered in the same position as are cardiac compressions. The infant should be placed on a firm surface in order to deliver the most effective thrust. (From Henry, M., and Stapleton, E. R.: *EMT: Prehospital Care*, Philadelphia, W. B. Saunders Co., 1991, p 658.)

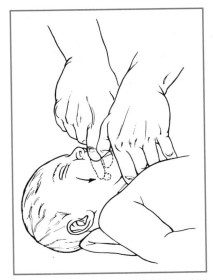

FIGURE 40–16. The finger sweep in the infant should be done while maintaining a jaw lift. The finger sweep is performed only after visualizing the foreign body. (From Henry, M., and Stapleton, E. R.: *EMT: Prehospital Care*, Philadelphia, W. B. Saunders Co., 1991, p 658.)

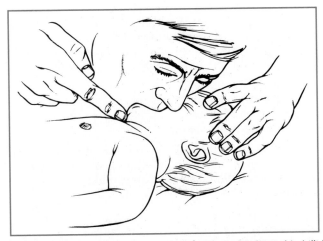

FIGURE 40–17. The infant is ventilated after performing a head-tilt/chin-lift procedure. The head is placed in the "sniffing" or neutral position. At times, a folded sheet or towel placed under the shoulder blades helps maintain this position. This is particularly important when performing cardiopulmonary resuscitation. Mouth-to-mouth and mouth-to-nose ventilation methods are used in infants. (From Henry, M., and Stapleton, E. R.: *EMT: Prehospital Care*, Philadelphia, W. B. Saunders Co., 1991, p 659.)

record a few tracings. Lead II is usually considered to be the monitoring lead. If the physician cannot be reached, call the emergency rescue team. It may be necessary to start mouth-to-mouth resuscitation if the patient is unconscious and there is no evi-dence of breathing. If chest pain progresses to car-diac arrest, CPR must be performed.

The office staff must remain calm and offer emo-tional support and reassurance, since all heart pa-tients are extremely frightened and anxious.

Signals of Heart Attack

A heart attack is caused by a blockage of the coronary arteries, so that the blood supply to the heart muscles is stopped. The most common signal of heart attack is an uncomfortable pressure, squeezing, fullness, or pain in the center of the chest, in the mediastinal area. This may spread to the shoulder, neck, jaw, or arms. The pain may not be severe. Other symptoms include:

- Sweating
- Nausea
- Indigestion
- Shortness of breath
- Cold and clammy skin
- A feeling of weakness
- Extreme apprehension

Cerebrovascular Accident (Stroke)

A cerebrovascular accident (CVA) is a disorder of the blood vessels serving the cerebrum that results in an impairment of the blood supply to a part of the brain. The term *stroke* is often applied to this problem. This interruption in the normal circulation of blood through the brain leads to a sudden loss of consciousness and some degree of paralysis, which may be temporary or permanent depending on the severity of the oxygen deprivation of the brain cells.

Usually, minor strokes do not produce unconsciousness, and the symptoms depend on the location of the hemorrhage and the amount of brain damage. Symptoms of a minor stroke include:

- Headache
- Confusion
- Slight dizziness
- Ringing in the ears

This may be followed by minor difficulties in speech, memory changes, weakness of the extremities, and some disturbance of personality.

Symptoms of a major stroke include:

- Unconsciousness
- Paralysis on one side of the body
- Difficulty in breathing and swallowing
- Loss of bladder and bowel control
- Unequal pupil size
- Slurring of speech

Treatment

The patient should be protected against any further injury or physical exertion. Keep the patient lying down and covered lightly. Maintain an open airway. Position the head so that any secretions will drain from the side of the mouth to prevent choking. Do not give the patient anything to eat or drink. Vital signs should be taken at regular intervals and recorded for the physician. Have an ambu-

lance take the patient to the hospital as soon as possible.

Poisonings

All poisonings are considered medical emergencies. Poisoning can occur by mouth, absorption, inhalation, and injection. Aspirin poisoning is by far the most common type of poisoning seen in young children. Other typical household poisons include medicines, detergents, cleaners, disinfectants, bleaches, insecticides, ammonia, glues, cosmetics, and poisonous plants. Symptoms of poisoning vary greatly. Important signs of poisoning include:

- Open bottles of medicines or chemicals
- Stains on clothing
- Burns on hands and mouth
- Changes in skin color
- Nausea
- Shallow breathing
- Convulsions
- Stomach cramps
- Heavy perspiration
- Dizziness
- Drowsiness
- Unconsciousness

When a person calls to report a poisoning, ask for

- The location and the phone number
- The name of the poison taken
- How much was taken
- How long ago the poison was taken
- Whether or not vomiting has occurred
- The name, weight, and age of the victim
- Any first aid being given

Instruct the caller not to hang up and not to leave the victim unattended. Call the local poison control center. Quickly forward all directions to the caller. Tell the caller to bring the container of poison or of vomitus to the office or hospital.

Treatment

Speed is essential in administering first aid in poisonings. In all cases, it is most important to dilute the poison, to induce vomiting (except when the person has swallowed a corrosive poison), and to seek medical attention. Generally, it is safe to try to dilute the poison with 1 or 2 cups of water or milk. It is important to dilute the poison before vomiting is induced. Do not induce vomiting if the victim is unconscious or having a **convulsion.** Do not attempt to induce vomiting when the victim has swallowed a strong corrosive or petroleum product. Give 1 tablespoon of syrup of ipecac and one cup of water. If vomiting does not occur after 20 minutes, repeat the procedure. It may be necessary to make the victim gag to start vomiting. The gag reflex is started by touching the back of the tongue lightly.

Encourage the victim to drink fluids until the emesis is reasonably clear. When vomiting has stopped, administer 30 to 50 g of activated charcoal, which absorbs any residual toxic substance and inhibits the absorption of poisons.

Insect Stings

Treatment

Remove the stinger, if there is one, by gently brushing it off or by using forceps or tweezers. Be careful not to squeeze the stinger. This injects more venom into the skin. Place the forceps as close to the skin as possible, not over the stinger sac, and gently remove the stinger. Apply ice in a towel or a plastic bag around the area, to relieve the pain and slow the absorption of the venom. Calamine lotion or a paste of baking soda may be applied to relieve itching. Keep the patient's activities to a minimum to slow down circulation and, thus, the spread of the venom.

If the patient gives a history of allergies, especially to insect venom, the patient should be transported to the nearest hospital for immediate care. This patient may experience dyspnea and a decrease in blood pressure. A wet, itchy, swollen rash may occur. The victim may complain of shortness of breath or difficulty in breathing. Sometimes, there is edema of the lips and the face. Difficulty in talking is a sign of edema in the throat. In this situation, there is the possibility of complete airway obstruction. These are signs of a true emergency. Epinephrine and oxygen should be ready for immediate administration on the physician's orders. Antihistamines may be used, as well as cortisone, but the action of these are considerably slower than that of epinephrine. If the patient experiences acute **anaphylactic shock,** death may occur within 1 hour without the intervention of a physician.

Shock

Shock is a condition that produces a depressed state of many vital body functions. It is a physiologic reaction resulting from a **traumatic** condition to the body. Shock is often caused by an injury, accident, hemorrhage, illness, surgical operation, or overdose of drugs or by burns, pain, fear, or emotional stress. Shock may be immediate or delayed, mild or severe, and even fatal.

Signs of shock may include:

- Paleness
- Clamminess
- Dilated pupils
- Weak and rapid pulse
- Low blood pressure
- Thirst
- Lethargy
- Faint feeling
- Labored breathing

Treatment

Ensure an open airway, and check for breathing and circulation. Place the patient on his or her back, with the legs elevated. Loosen all tight clothing. Cover the patient with a blanket for warmth. Do not move the patient unnecessarily. Fluids may be given by mouth if not contraindicated or if medical care will be delayed for more than 60 minutes. Because there are so many different causes of shock, it is advisable to administer only basic first-aid care and to have the patient transported to the hospital.

Asthmatic Attack

Asthma is a condition characterized by wheezing, coughing, choking, and shortness of breath resulting from spasmodic constriction of the bronchi in the lungs. Attacks vary greatly. Severe attacks rarely last for more than a few hours, but milder symptoms may persist much longer.

Some asthmatic patients carry respiratory inhalators with them. You may assist them with using their inhalators. A bronchodilator such as epinephrine or aminophylline may be ordered by the physician. Other medications are used to thin the mucus in the air passages so that the patient can clear the lungs more easily.

The patient should be warned of the hazards of overstimulation of the body, such as exercise and emotional upsets causing laughing or crying. Explain the importance of relaxation to the patient with asthma.

Seizures

Seizures are frightening to witness, but usually the patient is not suffering, nor is there great danger. Establishing a tranquil environment is usually an essential component of caring for patients experiencing seizures.

Treatment

Loosen clothing but do not attempt to restrain the patient's movements, except to prevent injury. Remove anything that might be in the way that could cause harm. Always protect the head. Give neither fluids nor medication by mouth. If the patient remains unconscious after the jerking has subsided, position the patient in a semiprone position to maintain an open airway and to allow drainage of excess saliva. Do not attempt to place anything between the teeth during the convulsion because forcing an object through a tightly clenched mouth may damage the teeth. After the seizure is over, let the patient rest or sleep in a quiet room. If the patient has not regained consciousness within 10 to 15 minutes, it may be advisable to contact the physician.

Abdominal Pain

Abdominal pain is any pain or discomfort in the abdomen. Causes of abdominal pain include:

- Stress
- Inflammation
- Hemorrhage
- Obstruction
- Ulcers
- Tumors
- Excessive eating, drinking, or smoking

All abdominal pain should be investigated. Severe and persistent abdominal pain, especially when accompanied by fever, should receive medical attention as soon as possible.

Treatment

Treatment varies with the cause of the pain. Keep the patient warm and quiet. Have an emesis basin available. Administer nothing by mouth. Do not apply heat to the abdomen unless so instructed by the physician. Check and record the patient's vital signs.

Obstetric Emergencies

The types of problems found in an obstetric office are unique to this specialty. Every medical assistant employed in an office where the physician delivers babies should be trained to handle emergencies. The majority of these problems will be presented to you over the telephone. If there are physicians in the office, those calls should be transferred to them immediately.

If a pregnant patient calls in to report vaginal bleeding, you must ask some specific questions. Is the bleeding like a menstrual flow or is it a gushing type of hemorrhage? Is it painful or without any pain? If the bleeding is gushing, the patient must be told to lie down immediately while you send for an ambulance. In such a situation, the mother and baby could bleed to death in a matter of a few minutes as the result of a ruptured uterus. If the bleeding is like a normal menstrual flow, have the patient go to bed, with the foot of the bed elevated. Tell her that you will report this to the physician immediately. If the tissue passed is liver-like, it may be a blood clot; white tissue may be fetus. No matter what the appearance of the tissue, have the patient take it with her to the hospital.

Sprains

A sprain is an injury to a ligamentous structure surrounding a joint and is frequently due to twisting or wrenching of that part.

Treatment

Today, the most accepted first aid is elevation, mild compression, and immediate application of ice. There is considerable advantage if the ice is applied within 20 to 30 minutes after the injury has occurred. The ice should remain on the part for 24 hours, with the injured area elevated. After 24 to 36 hours, application of mild heat is usually indicated. The patient may be advised to immobilize the part.

Fractures

A fracture is a break or crack in a bone and can result from trauma or disease (Fig. 40–18). Fractures in which the bone penetrates the skin, causing an open wound, are called *open* or *compound* fractures. Fractures in which there is no break in the skin are called *closed* or *simple* fractures.

Treatment

When a patient with a fracture is brought into the office, the medical assistant should make the patient as comfortable as possible. Have the patient lie down in a position that does not place strain on the area. First aid includes preventing movement of the injured part; elevation of the affected extremity; application of ice; and control of bleeding, if present. Do not apply too much pressure on the bleeding area if there is a fracture beneath. Be gentle. Do not attempt to straighten the fracture or move it in any way. If the patient must be moved, give support to the fractured area before moving. If possible, an x-ray film of the area should be ready when the physician arrives.

Burns

Burns are the most frequent cause of all injuries and the leading cause of accidental death in the United States. Burn injuries can result from heat, chemicals, or radiation. Burns are classified as first-degree, second-degree, or third-degree, depending on the depth of the wound (Fig. 40–19).

First-Degree Burn

A first-degree burn shows erythema of the epidermis only. The tissue destruction is superficial, without blistering. The use of cold packs on a first-degree burn until the pain stops may prevent it from becoming a second-degree burn.

Second-Degree Burn

A second-degree burn includes the entire epidermal layer and varying depths of the dermis. Blisters are usually formed and there is some pain. There is also danger of infection in the blistered area. If the burn is deep enough, there may be some destruction of the hair follicles and the sebaceous glands.

Third-Degree Burn

A third-degree burn is the destruction of all the epithelium and may involve underlying muscle tissue. Destroyed skin sloughs leaving a raw area. There is danger of infection. Third-degree burns themselves do not cause pain, as the nerve endings are destroyed.

Burns are also classified according to the percentage of body surface involved (Fig. 40–20). A method called the *Rule of Nines* has been developed to determine burn surface involvement.

In adults, the body surface area is divided into areas of 9% and 18%. Areas involving 9% of the body surface are the head, neck, and each arm. Areas involving 18% of the body surface are the front torso, the back torso, and each leg. The genitalia and each palm represent 1% each. The sum of all body percentages is 100%. In children, an adjustment is made because a child's head is relatively large compared with the body. The head is given 18%, and each lower limb is considered 14%.

Treatment

First aid for burns includes relief of the pain, prevention of infection, and treatment of shock. Burns are extremely painful and dangerous. Recommended first aid for a first-degree burn is to immerse it immediately in cool water. This gives fast relief from the pain. If immersion in water is not possible, then apply sterile, wet compresses to the area. There is always the danger of infection from contamination because the burned tissue acts as a culture medium for bacteria and there is poor circulation through this tissue to carry medications such as antibiotics. Apply a sterile, dry dressing over the wet compress. If the burn is over a large area, wrap a sterile towel over the area, and get the patient to the hospital as soon as possible.

Second-degree burns are immersed in cold water for 1 to 2 hours. Do not open blisters. Do not apply any medications or ointments unless instructed to do so by the physician. Apply a dry, sterile protective bandage.

For third-degree burns, do not remove adhered particles or charred clothing. Cover the burns with thick, sterile dressings. Keep the patient warm and quiet, and provide him or her with emotional support. Chemical burns should be thoroughly rinsed with plenty of running water and should be covered with a sterile dressing.

Fourth-degree burns involve deep tissue damage, even bone. Electric and chemical burns can cause damage to deeper underlying structures as the current or chemical travels through and penetrates the tissue.

The most serious effect of extensive burns is shock. Observe the patient for any signs and symptoms of shock, and begin first aid immediately.

Lacerations

Lacerations are a common presentation in general practice and pediatrics. A lacerated wound displays a jagged or irregular tearing of the tissues. Bleeding may be profuse. Since there is much tissue destruction, the possibility of contamination exists.

Treatment

Have the patient lie down. Keep the patient quiet. Cover the injured area with a sterile dressing; use a dressing that is thick enough to absorb the bleeding. If bleeding persists or is profuse, apply direct pressure to the dressing and also to the area just above the wound. The injured part of the body should be elevated above the level of the victim's heart.

Wounds that are not bleeding severely and that do not involve deep tissues should be cleansed. Wash in and around the wound with soap and water to remove bacteria and other foreign matter. If the laceration is extremely dirty, it may be irrigated with sterile normal saline solution. Hydrogen peroxide is not generally recommended for fresh wounds as it may damage tissue. Rinse the wound thoroughly with clean water, and blot dry. Then cover the injured area with a sterile dressing.

A butterfly closure strip may be used over small lacerations, to hold the edges together. If the wound is superficial and has straight edges, it may be closed with a microporous tape, which eliminates the discomfort of suturing and suture removal as well as some of the potential risks of infected sutures. The tape (available in ¼- or ½-inch widths) is placed at approximately ¼-inch intervals until the wound is closed. Generally, closure is started near one end. However, a longer wound could be brought together in quarters, and then the intervening spaces closed next. Figure 40–21 shows an excellent method of informing patients as to the nature of their injury and of both the office and the home treatment required. If you work in a multicultural community, forms should be printed in different languages for non-English–speaking patients.

Animal Bites

Any animal bite that breaks the skin should be seen by a physician and reported to the authorities. The animal must be identified and confined for quarantine. The animal should not be killed because a positive rabies identification is almost impossible to make if the animal has been dead for a while. Many pet owners will not admit that their pet has bitten a person because they fear that the animal will be killed. Assure them that the Health Depart-

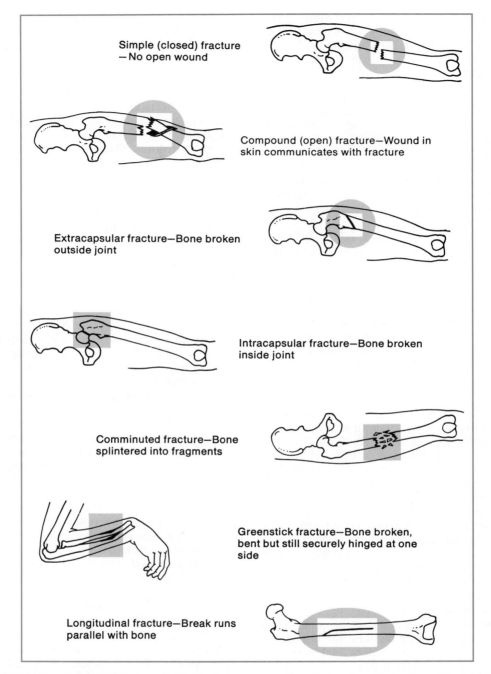

Simple (closed) fracture
— No open wound

Compound (open) fracture—Wound in
skin communicates with fracture

Extracapsular fracture—Bone broken
outside joint

Intracapsular fracture—Bone broken
inside joint

Comminuted fracture—Bone
splintered into fragments

Greenstick fracture—Bone broken,
bent but still securely hinged at one
side

Longitudinal fracture—Break runs
parallel with bone

FIGURE 40-18. Various types of fractures encountered in emergency care. (From Ethicon, Inc.: *Nursing Care of the Patient in the O.R.*)

ment authorities only want to confine the animal for observation.

Treatment

The bite should be washed thoroughly with soap and water and should be treated as any other wound would be. The victim should be seen by a physician.

Nosebleeds (Epistaxis)

Nosebleed, or **epistaxis,** is a hemorrhage from the nose usually resulting from the rupture of small vessels within the nose. Nosebleeds can result from injury, disease, strenuous activity, high altitudes, and exposure to cold.

40

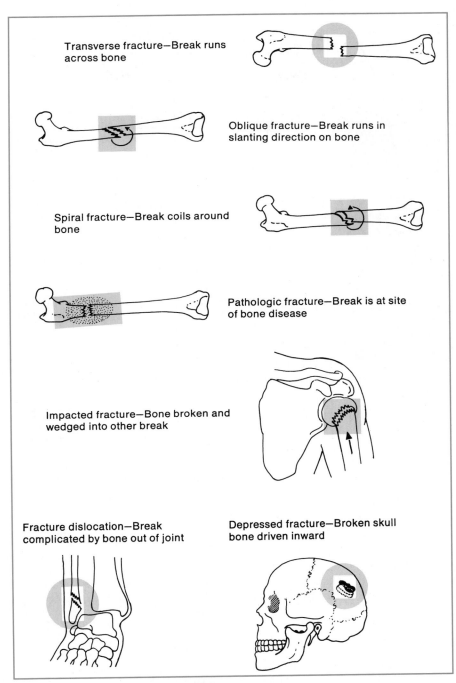

Transverse fracture—Break runs across bone

Oblique fracture—Break runs in slanting direction on bone

Spiral fracture—Break coils around bone

Pathologic fracture—Break is at site of bone disease

Impacted fracture—Bone broken and wedged into other break

Fracture dislocation—Break complicated by bone out of joint

Depressed fracture—Broken skull bone driven inward

FIGURE 40–18. *Continued*

Treatment

Keep the patient quiet and in a sitting position. Apply external pressure to the affected nostril. Cold compresses to the nose and face may also be of value. If bleeding cannot be controlled, insert a clean pad of gauze into the nostril.

Hemorrhages

Bleeding may be external or internal. Those administering first aid can do little about internal bleeding, except to keep the patient quiet and warm to minimize shock. Get medical help immediately.

External bleeding is not as complex as internal

		APPEARANCE	SENSATION	COURSE
EPIDERMIS	SUPERFICIAL BURN	Mild to severe erythema; skin blanches with pressure	Painful	Discomfort lasts about 48 hours
Sweat duct			Hyperesthetic	
Capillary		Skin dry	Tingling	Desquamation in 3–7days
		Small, thin-walled blisters	Pain eased by cooling	
Sebaceous gland	PARTIAL-THICKNESS BURN	Large thick-walled blisters covering extensive area (vesiculation)	Painful	Superficial partial-thickness burn heals in 10–14 days
Nerve endings			Hyperesthetic	Deep partial-thickness burn requires 21–28 days for healing
DERMIS		Edema; mottled red base; broken epidermis; wet, shiny, weeping surface	Sensitive to cold air	
Hair follicle				Healing rate varies with burn depth and presence or absence of infection
Sweat gland	FULL-THICKNESS BURN	Variable, e.g., deep red, black, white, brown	Little pain	Full-thickness dead skin suppurates and liquefies after 2–3 weeks
		Dry surface		Spontaneous healing impossible
Fat		Edema	Anesthetic	Requires removal of eschar and skin grafting
Blood vessels		Fat exposed		Scarring deformities and function loss
SUBCUTANEOUS TISSUE		Tissue disrupted		Beneath eschar capillary tufts and fibroblasts organize into granulating tissue

FIGURE 40–19. Classification of burn depth in relation to the skin. First-degree (superficial), second-degree (partial thickness), and third-degree (full thickness). (From Luckmann, J., and Sorensen, K. C.: *Medical-Surgical Nursing: A Psychophysiologic Approach*, 3rd ed., Philadelphia, W. B. Saunders Co., 1987, p 1616.)

bleeding in that you can frequently see the source of the bleeding. Shock and loss of consciousness may occur from a rapid loss of blood in a short time. There are four practical ways of controlling severe bleeding.

Methods of Controlling Bleeding

The first technique is to use direct pressure over the area by applying a sterile dressing. If blood soaks through the entire pad, do not remove the pad, but add additional pads of thick cloth and continue direct pressure. The second method is elevation of the injured part. Elevation uses the forces of gravity to control blood flow. The third method is to apply pressure over the nearest pressure point between the bleeding area and the heart. This compresses the main artery supplying the affected limb. The last resort is the application of a tourniquet. The use of a tourniquet is dangerous and should be used only for a life-threatening hemorrhage. By deciding to use a tourniquet, you have made a decision that the patient will bleed to death without it.

TOURNIQUET. The types of wounds that would most probably require a tourniquet involve deep lacerations into an artery of the midupper arm, or amputation of the arm at the same level, and deep lacerations into an artery of the thigh, or amputation of the leg at the thigh level.

A tourniquet must be at least 2 inches wide. Less width may cause tissue damage under the tourniquet and, thus, the possibility of amputation at a higher level on the extremity. A broad, flat tourniquet is best, and a pad should be used under the area of the tie. Wrap it twice around the extremity, about 1 to 2 inches above the wound. Tie a halfknot, and place a short stick on this knot. Tie a full knot over this stick. Twist the stick to tighten the tourniquet until you can no longer feel a pulse. Gently tighten the tourniquet until the bleeding is stopped. Do not make it any tighter, since the tissues beyond the tourniquet can die without blood circulation. Do not release the tourniquet but seek medical help immediately. If possible, avoid covering the tourniquet, so that emergency medical personnel will see it immediately. Also, write the time of the application on

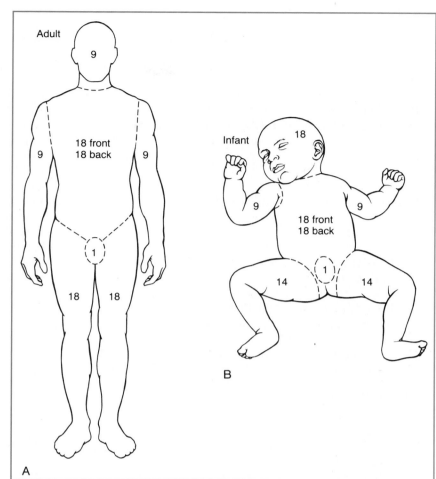

FIGURE 40–20. Body surface chart of the "Rules of Nines." *A*, Adult. *B*, Child. (From Henry, M., and Stapleton, E. R.: *EMT: Prehospital Care*, Philadelphia, W. B. Saunders Co., 1991, p 503.)

the victim's forehead, or pin a note on his or her clothing.

Because a tourniquet completely obstructs the flow of blood to an extremity, the victim may lose the injured extremity. In other words, the extremity may be sacrificed to save the victim's life.

Head Injuries

The severity of a head injury can vary greatly. With a head injury, the patient may appear normal, may experience dizziness, severe headache, or memory loss, or may even be unconscious. The loss of consciousness may be brief or prolonged; it may appear immediately or may be delayed. The victim may experience vomiting, loss of bladder and bowel control, and bleeding from the nose, mouth, or ears. The pupils of the eyes may be of unequal diameters.

Treatment

All head injuries must be considered serious. Seek medical attention immediately. Have the victim lie flat unless there is difficulty in breathing. In such a case, raise the head and shoulders slightly unless there is evidence of neck injury. Control any hemorrhage. Do not administer anything by mouth. Keep the patient warm and quiet. Watch the pupils of the eyes, and record any changes. Obtain the vital signs. Record the extent and duration of any unconsciousness.

Foreign Bodies in the Eye

This kind of emergency is most uncomfortable, and it is often extremely difficult to keep the patient from rubbing the eye. Tell the patient not to touch the eye in any way. If the doctor has given you prior permission, you may put a few drops of ophthalmic topical anesthetic in the eye. The patient will greatly appreciate this and will experience almost immediate relief. The eye may be rinsed with tepid tap water in an attempt to remove the object. Unless the foreign object is clearly visible, do not attempt to search for it or to remove it.

LACERATIONS

What you need to know . . .

It is important to prevent infection and to allow your cut to heal. Call your doctor or return to him or her immediately if any of the "danger signs" occur.

Return for recheck in _____ days
Return for suture removal in _____ days

Danger signs to watch for . . .

1. Increasing pain, swelling, redness, and warmth in the injured area.
2. Pus in or around the cut.
3. Fever greater than 100°F (38°C).
4. Blood soaking through the dressing.

If any of these signs occur, contact your doctor or return to the Emergency Department.

What to do at home . . .

1. Take all medicines exactly as directed.
2. Raise the injured area above your heart level for 1 to 2 days.
3. Keep the wound and bandage clean and dry. For cuts on the face, a bandage is often not necessary. All finger dressings must be changed within 24 hours.
4. Remove the bandage/dressing in 24 hours.
5. After 24 hours, you may shower or bathe. Begin cleaning the wound with clear water twice each day to remove crusting and scabbing. Then apply ointment (Polysporin).
6. Prevent sunburn. Use a sunscreen for 6 months (e.g., Pre-Sun or Eclipse).
7. If you have a private doctor or are a member of an HMO (e.g., Kaiser), you should call for an appointment for your recheck and suture removal. If you can't get an appointment, you are welcome to return here to complete your care.

Please remember . . .

1. The exam and treatment you have just received are not intended to provide complete medical care. You need to call your doctor to schedule a follow-up visit.

2. The X-rays or E.C.G. taken today will be reviewed by a specialist. If there is any change in your diagnosis, we will contact you.

FIGURE 40-21. Typical educational and informational literature given to the patient to assist in his or her home care of a wound. (Courtesy of Community Emergency Medical Group, Fresno, CA.)

Treatment

The medical assistant should never attempt to remove a foreign body from the cornea. The patient should be placed in a darkened room to wait. Have plenty of tissues available. If there is a contusion and swelling, cold wet compresses will help. If you have been trained to turn an upper eyelid out, then do so gently and search for the foreign body. Be very careful not to place any pressure on the eye. If the foreign body cannot be found, then ask the patient to close the eyes. Cover both eyes with eye pads and hold them in place with a strip of tape until the physician arrives.

LEGAL AND ETHICAL RESPONSIBILITIES

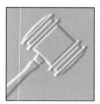

Most states have enacted Good Samaritan laws to encourage health care professionals to provide medical assistance at the scene of an accident without fear of being sued for negligence. These statutes vary greatly, but all seem to have the intent of protecting the caregiver. It is helpful for the medical assistant to understand the legal responsibilities and the rights of the caregiver. A physician or other health care professional is not legally obligated to give emergency care, regardless of the ethical and moral considerations. Legal liability is limited to gross neglect of the victim or willfully causing further injury to the victim. As a caregiver, you are required to act as a reasonable person and cannot be held liable for personal injury resulting from an act of omission. The Good Samaritan statutes provide for the evaluation of the caregiver's judgment.

If you have never been trained in CPR, you cannot be expected to perform the procedure. However, in many states, a health care provider with CPR training and skills who is present at the scene can be declared negligent if cardiac arrest occurs and he or she does not administer CPR to the victim.

Remember, if the victim is conscious or if a member of his or her immediate family is present, obtain a verbal consent for the emergency care procedure before you begin. Consent is implied if the patient is unconscious and no family member is present.

▶ PATIENT EDUCATION

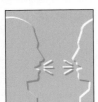 Emergencies can occur in the home, while on vacation, or in the physician's office. Patients need to be instructed in handling an emergency, both by example and through actual instruction. The medical assistant must remain calm, **triage** the situation, call for help, and be prepared to administer appropriate first-aid intervention. This attitude helps the patient learn how to report and handle an emergency. You can give patients brochures that instruct them in home safety. These are of particular importance when there are young children in the house. Remember to keep your American Red Cross and American Heart Association cards current. Take advantage of community workshops to maintain and extend your skills. Post a list of community safety workshops in an area where it can be seen by patients, and encourage them to attend. Your participation in emergency care workshops and your encouragement to have others participate may help to save lives.

▶ LEARNING ACHIEVEMENTS

 Upon completion of this chapter, can you in the time allowed by your evaluator:

1. Assess an accident, telephone the emergency operator, and correctly report the accident?
2. Demonstrate how and why the defibrillator is used?
3. Recognize the major symptoms of a heart attack?
4. Successfully perform the Heimlich maneuver?
5. Obtain pertinent information from the local poison control center?
6. Advise a patient in ways to control accidents at home?
7. Perform CPR on an approved manikin, following the correct sequence and not omitting a step in the procedure?
8. Immobilize the injured area and move a patient with a fractured limb?
9. Triage a simulated emergency situation?

REFERENCES AND READINGS

American National Red Cross: *Advanced First Aid and Emergency Care,* 3rd ed., 1988.

American National Red Cross: *Cardiopulmonary Resuscitation,* 1988.

American National Red Cross: *Community CPR,* 1988.

American National Red Cross: *Standard First Aid and Personal Safety,* 3rd ed., 1988.

Henry, M., Stapleton, E.: *EMT—Prehospital Care,* Philadelphia, W. B. Saunders Co., 1992.

Ignatavicius, D. D., and Bayne, M. V.: *Medical and Surgical Nursing,* Philadelphia, W. B. Saunders Co., 1991.

Roberts, J. R.: *Clinical Procedures in Emergency Medicine,* 2nd ed., Philadelphia, W. B. Saunders Co., 1990.

Safar, P., and Bircher, N.: *Cardiopulmonary Cerebral Resuscitation,* 3rd ed., Philadelphia, W. B. Saunders Co., 1990.

40

GLOSSARY

abet To encourage or support. **(4)**

abrasion Rubbing or scraping of the skin or mucous membrane (e.g., a skinned knee). **(35)**

abscess A localized collection of pus which may be located under the skin or deep within the body. It causes tissue destruction. **(35)**

abstract A written summary of the key points of a book, paper, or case history. **(20)**

academic degree A title conferred by a college, university, or professional school on completion of a program of study. **(12)**

accelerating Causing to act or move faster. **(3)**

account A single financial record. **(16)**

account balance The debit or credit balance remaining in the account. **(16)**

accounting equation Assets = Liabilities + Proprietorship. **(16)**

accounts payable Amounts charged and not paid. **(16)**

accounts receivable Amounts owed to the doctor. **(16)**

accounts receivable control A summary of unpaid accounts. **(16)**

accounts receivable ledger The combined record of all the patient accounts. **(16)**

accounts receivable ratio A formula for measuring how fast outstanding accounts are being paid. **(18)**

accounts receivable trial balance A method of determining that the journal and the ledger are in balance. **(16)**

accrual basis of accounting Income is recorded when earned; expenses are recorded when incurred. **(16)**

acidosis Chemical imbalance caused by a decrease in the alkaline content of body fluids. **(27)**

acknowledgment Recognition given to a patient for contribution to the conversation. **(6)**

Acquired Immunodeficiency Syndrome (AIDS) Disease involving the total collapse of the human immune system. Its cause is still unknown. **(25)**

acrotism The absence of a pulse. **(26)**

adjustment column An account column used for entering discounts. It is sometimes included to the left of the balance column. **(16)**

administer To instill a drug into the body of a patient. **(5)**

administrative Having to do with management duties. In medical assisting, refers to all "front office" activities. **(1)**

administrative law Regulations set forth by government agencies. **(5)**

aerophagia Swallowing or gulping air, which produces rapid and/or irregular breathing. **(26)**

afebrile Without fever. **(23), (26)**

age analysis A procedure for classifying accounts receivable by age from the first date of billing. **(18)**

agenda A list of the specific items under each division of the order of business to be presented at a business meeting. **(20)**

agglutination The clumping together of particles (antigens and antibodies) resulting from their interaction with specific antibodies (or antigens); used in laboratory tests for blood typing and many other pathologic tests. **(31)**

alignment The state of being in the correct relative position. **(13)**

aliquot A portion of a well-mixed sample that is removed for testing. **(31)**

allergic reaction Bodily response brought about by a hypersensitivity to certain irritating substances. **(9)**

alphabetic filing Any system that arranges names or topics according to the sequence of letters in the alphabet. **(14)**

alphanumeric Systems made up of combinations of letters and numbers. **(14)**

amenorrhea Absence of the menstrual period. **(29)**

amino acid One of the 20 organic compounds that form the chief constituents of protein. **(34)**

ampule A small (usually single-dose) glass container of medication prepared for parenteral administration. **(38)**

anaphylaxis An allergic condition caused by an antigen/antibody reaction; may cause shock, bronchoconstriction, airway obstruction, and loss of consciousness. **(40)**

ancillary Subordinate; auxiliary. **(22)**

anemia An abnormal decrease in the red blood cell count, hemoglobin, or hematocrit caused by increased red blood cell destruction or the inability to produce sufficient amounts of normal red blood cells. **(33)**

anesthesia Natural or artificially induced absence or loss of feeling or sensation. **(2)**

angina pectoris Acute pain in the chest, resulting from decreased blood supply to the heart muscles. **(37)**

ankylosis Immobility of a joint due to disease or injury. **(29)**

annotate To furnish with notes, which are usually critical or explanatory. **(12)**

anorexia nervosa An emotional disorder characterized by a refusal to eat and an altered physical image. **(34)**

anoscope Instrument used to examine the anus. **(29)**

anthrax An acute infectious disease caused by a bacillus. Humans contract the disease from contact with animal hair, hides, or waste matter. **(2)**

antibody An immunoglobulin produced by lymphoid tissue in response to substances interpreted as foreign invaders gaining entry into the body. **(31)**

anticoagulant A substance added to a blood sample that prevents coagulation. **(31)**

antisepsis The process of applying substances that render microorganisms harmless. **(24)**

anuria Complete suppression of urine formation by the kidney. **(32)**

anxiety A feeling of uneasiness, apprehension, or dread; fear of the unknown. **(6)**

aphonia Loss of the ability to speak. **(2)**

aphrodisiacs Drugs that arouse the sexual instinct. **(2)**

apical pulse Pulse felt over the base (apex) of the heart. **(40)**

apnea Absence or cessation of breathing. **(26)**

appraisal Setting a value on or judging as to quality. **(22)**

approximate To bring wound or skin edges together. **(36)**

approximation The act or process of drawing together skin or wound edges. **(35)**

arbitration The hearing and determination of a cause in controversy by a person or person either chosen by the parties involved or appointed under statutory authority. **(5)**

arbitrator A neutral person chosen to settle differences between two parties in controversy. **(5)**

arrhythmia Irregular pulse rhythm. An abnormality or irregularity in heart rhythm. **(26)**, **(29)**, **(30)**

arthritis Inflammation of a joint or many joints. **(39)**

artificial insemination The introduction of semen into the vagina or cervix by artificial means. **(4)**

asepsis Free from infection or infectious materials. **(24)**

aspirate To withdraw fluid by negative pressure. Pulling up on the plunger of the syringe after inserting the needle to check for blood. **(38)**

assault An intentional, unlawful *attempt* of bodily injury to another by force. **(5)**

assignment of benefits A statement authorizing an insurance company to pay benefits directly to a physician. **(15)**, **(19)**

asthma Spasmodic constriction of the bronchi; panting and wheezing caused by bronchial tube swelling and spasm. **(29)**, **(39)**

atherosclerosis A common type of arteriosclerosis in which deposits of yellow plaques form on the interior walls of the arteries. **(34)**

atrioventricular node (AV node) Part of the conductive system located between the atria and the ventricles near the septum. It receives the impulses from the SA node and sends them down the bundle of His and the bundle branches. **(30)**

atria The upper chambers of the heart. **(30)**

atrophy Wasting away; decrease in size from normal. **(27)**, **(39)**

attenuated Made thin or weaker. **(2)**

auscultation The act of listening for sounds within the body. **(2)**

avocational Pertaining to a subordinate occupation or a hobby. **(7)**

bacteria Single-celled microscopic organisms. **(2)**

balance column The account column on the far right that is used for recording the difference between the debit and credit columns. **(16)**

balance sheet A financial statement for a specific date that shows the total assets, liabilities, and capital of a business. **(16)**

bariatrics The field of medicine dealing with obesity. **(29)**

batch A collection of similar work that can be processed in one operation. **(8)**

battery A willful and unlawful use of force or violence upon the person of another. **(5)**

beneficiary The person receiving the benefits of an insurance policy. **(19)**

benign Noncancerous (as when describing a mass or tumor). **(29)**

benign hypertension Hypertension of slow onset, usually without symptoms. **(26)**

bibliography A list of the works referred to

in a text or that were consulted by the author in producing a text. **(20)**

bigeminal pulse Two regular beats followed by a pause. **(26)**

bilirubin The orange-yellow pigment that is formed from the breakdown of hemoglobin in old red blood cells. **(27)**

biopsy Excision of a small sample of tissue from the body for diagnostic or therapeutic purposes. **(35)**

biotin A type of B-complex vitamin. **(34)**

body fluids External and internal fluids, secretions and excretions of the human body, including blood, semen, vaginal secretions, saliva, tears, breast milk, cerebrospinal fluid, amniotic fluid, and urine. **(25)**

bookkeeping The recording part of the accounting process. **(16)**

bounding pulse A pulse characterized by high tension. **(27)**

bradycardia Slow heart beat; a pulse that is below 60 beats per minute. **(26)**, **(30)**

bradypnea Respirations that are regular in rhythm but slower than normal in rate. **(27)**

bruit An abnormal sound or murmur heard on auscultation of an organ, vessel, or gland. **(27)**

buffy coat The white layer separating the plasma and the red blood cell layers in a centrifuged blood specimen; contains the white cells and the platelets. **(33)**

bulimia An abnormal increase in hunger characterized by binge eating and self-induced vomiting. **(34)**

bundle of His Atrioventricular bundle of impulse-conducting fibers in the myocardium. **(30)**

bursitis Inflammation of the bursae located in the shoulder and the knee. **(39)**

calorie The amount of heat necessary to raise the temperature of 1 kilogram of water 1 degree Celsius or of a pint of water 4 degrees Fahrenheit. **(34)**

cancer Any malignant cellular tumor or neoplastic disease in which there is a transformation of normal body cells into malignant cells. **(29)**

candid Frank; straightforward. **(22)**

cannula A flexible tube that surrounds a sharp pointed trocar that is to be inserted into the body. The trocar is withdrawn, and fluid escapes from the body through the cannula. **(35)**

capital purchase Purchase of a major item of furniture or equipment. **(21)**

caption A heading, title, or subtitle under which records are filed. **(14)**

cardiac arrest Total cessation of a functional heartbeat. **(30)**

cardiotonic Increasing tonicity of the heart. **(37)**

carotene The yellow-red pigment from food that converts to vitamin A. **(34)**

cash basis of accounting Income is recorded when received; expenses are recorded when paid. **(16)**

cash flow statement A financial summary for a specific period that shows the beginning cash on hand, the cash income and disbursements during the period, and the amount of cash on hand at the end of the period. **(16)**

cash payment journal A record of all cash paid out. **(16)**

cassette A magnetic tape wound on two reels and encased in a plastic or metal container. *Microcassette* A very small cassette tape that may be used in a hand-held dictating unit. **(13)**

casts Fibrous or protein materials that are thrown off into the urine in kidney disease. **(32)**

categorically Pertaining to a division in any classification system. **(21)**

catheterization The insertion of a tube through the urethra and into the urinary bladder to withdraw urine from the bladder. **(32)**

causative The organism or agent that is responsible for an effect or condition. **(24)**

caustics Substances that corrode or eat away tissues; a substance that burns or destroys organic tissue by chemical action. **(21)**, **(35)**

cellulose A carbohydrate that forms the structure of most plants. **(34)**

censure The act of blaming or condemning sternly. **(4)**

Centers for Disease Control (CDC) National agency located in Atlanta, Georgia, responsible for the reporting of statistics for communicable diseases. **(25)**

centrifuge An instrument that rapidly separates portions of samples by rapidly spinning them in a container. **(33)**

cerebrospinal fluid A fluid within the subarachnoid space, the central canal of the spinal cord, and the four ventricles of the brain. **(31)**

cervical vertebra The upper seven bones of the spinal column; the skeleton of the neck. **(2)**

cervix The narrow lower end of the uterus. Sometimes called the *neck* of the uterus. **(28)**

chancre The primary lesion of syphilis that occurs at the site of entry of the infection. **(28)**

chemotherapy The treatment of disease using chemical agents. **(2)**

cholera An acute, infectious, bacillus-caused disease involving the entire small bowel. **(2)**

cholesterol A substance found in plant and animal fats, such as saturated oils, egg yolk, and milk, that is currently thought to produce fatty deposits in the blood vessels. **(34)**

choline An essential part of the diet of mammals that helps to prevent fatty deposits in the liver. **(34)**

chronologic In the order of time. **(7)**

chronologic order Same as *chronologic*. **(14)**

circumvention Going around; avoidance. **(22)**

cirrhosis A disease of the liver that causes impairment in the metabolism of nutrients and the detoxification of poisons absorbed from the intestines. **(34)**

claim A demand to an insurer by an insured

person for the payment of benefits under a policy. **(19)**

clarity The state of being clear or lucid. **(11), (12)**

clinical Pertaining to actual observation and treatment of patients. **(1)**

coagulable Capable of being formed into clots. **(24)**

coagulum A blood clot. **(36)**

coding Converting verbal descriptions of diseases, injuries, and procedures into numeric and alphanumeric designations. **(19)**

coinsurance/copayment A policy provision by which both the insured person and the insurer share in a specified ratio the expenses resulting from an illness or injury. **(19)**

colitis Inflammation of the colon. **(29)**

collection ratio A formula for measuring the effectiveness of the billing system. **(18)**

colloquialism An expression that is acceptable and correct in ordinary conversation or informal speeches but unsuited for formal speech or writing. **(20)**

colony The visible growth on a culture plate usually resulting from a single bacterium. **(31)**

command An instruction telling the computer to do something with a program. **(8)**

communicable Capable of being transmitted from one person to another. **(5)**

compensatory damages General or special damages without specific monetary value. **(5)**

compulsory Obligatory; enforced. **(4)**

computer A machine that is designed to accept, store, process, and give out information. **(8)**

concise Expressing much in brief form. **(12)**

concurrent Operating or occurring at the same time. **(3)**

condylomata Soft and moist pink or red swellings that grow rapidly and have a cauliflower appearance. When sexually transmitted, they are known as *genital warts*. **(36)**

congenital Present at or existing from the time of birth. **(28)**

consultation report A report of the findings of the consulting physician to be sent to the referring physician. **(13)**

contagious Transmitted readily from one person to another by direct or indirect contact. **(5)**

contamination The act of soiling, staining, or polluting, especially the introduction of infectious materials or germs that produce disease; a surface that has become soiled through contact with nonsterile material. **(2), (24)**

continuation page The second and following pages of a letter. **(12)**

continuity The quality or state of being continuous. **(14)**

continuous fever Temperature is elevated and remains at the elevated level with little or no fluctuation within a 24-hour period. **(23), (26)**

contract law Enforceable promises. **(5)**

contraindication A condition that renders a treatment improper or undesirable. **(29)**

controlled substance Drugs that are regulated by the federal government (Drug Enforcement Agency). **(37)**

convulsion A series of involuntary contractions of the voluntary muscles. **(40)**

coordination of benefits The provision in an insurance contract that limits benefits to 100% of the cost. **(19)**

COPD Chronic obstructive pulmonary disease. **(39)**

correlation The act or process of correlating; mutual relation. **(14)**

CPU Central Processing Unit; the part of a computer system that processes information. **(8)**

credit balance The amount of advance payment or overpayment on an account. **(16)**

credit column The account column to the right of the debit column that is used for entering funds received. **(16)**

cretinism Congenital condition characterized by diminished development and dystrophy of the bones and soft tissues as well as by some mental retardation resulting from hypofunctioning of the thyroid gland. **(34)**

crisis Sudden drop of high temperature to normal or subnormal that generally occurs within 24 hours. **(23), (26)**

cross-reference A notation in a file that indicates that a record is stored elsewhere and that gives the reference. **(14)**

crossover claim A claim for benefits under both Medicare and Medicaid. **(19)**

culminate To reach a decisive point; to bring to a head. **(4)**

curettage The act of scraping a body cavity with a surgical instrument such as a curette. **(35)**

cursor A symbol appearing on the monitor of a computer that shows where the next character to be typed will appear. **(8)**

cyanosis A bluish discoloration of the skin, extremities, and mucous membranes caused by a decreased level of oxygen transported to cells. **(2), (27)**

cyst A sac of fluid or semisolid material located in or under the skin. **(35)**

cystic fibrosis A generalized hereditary disorder associated with widespread dysfunction of the endocrine glands. **(39)**

daily journal The book in which all transactions are first recorded; the book of original entry or general journal. **(16)**

daisy wheel A plastic or metal printing element of an electric typewriter or impact printer that consists of a disk with spokes bearing type. It derives its name from its shape, which is like that of a daisy. **(8), (13)**

database A collection of related files that serves as a foundation for retrieving information. **(8)**

debit column The account column on the left that is used for entering charges. **(16)**

débridement Surgical removal of damaged, diseased, or contaminated tissue until healthy tissue is exposed. **(35)**

deceptive Misleading; having the power to deceive. **(4)**

deductible A statement in an insurance policy that the insuring company will pay the expenses incurred after the insured person has paid a specified amount. **(19)**

defibrillator An apparatus used to produce electroshock to the heart via electrodes placed on the chest wall. **(30)**

deficiencies Conditions caused by a below-normal intake of a particular required substance. **(34)**

demographic Relating to the statistical characteristics of populations, such as births, marriages, mortality, health, and so forth. **(8)**, **(14)**

denervation A condition in which the nerve supply has been blocked. **(39)**

dessication Drying. **(24)**

deviation A noticeable or marked departure from accepted norms of behavior. **(10)**

diabetes mellitus A disorder of carbohydrate metabolism caused by underproduction of insulin and characterized by excessive urinary output. **(34)**

dialysis Separating out from the blood the harmful waste products of the body that are normally excreted in the urine. **(2)**

diaphragmatic Pertaining to the primary muscle of respiration, the diaphragm, which separates the thoracic and abdominal cavities. **(40)**

dictation The process of recording the spoken word onto a storage medium from which a printed copy will be produced. **(13)**

diction Choice of words to express ideas, especially with regard to correctness, clearness, or effectiveness. **(11)**

dietitian An individual with a bachelor's degree in foods and nutrition who is concerned with maintenance and promotion of health and the treatment of diseases through diet. **(34)**

digestion The process of converting food into chemical substances that can be used by the body. **(34)**

dilation Opening or widening the circumference of a body orifice with a dilating instrument. **(35)**

dilemma A situation involving choice between equally unsatisfactory alternatives. **(4)**

diluent A substance, such as water, that renders a drug or a solution less potent. **(35)**

diplopia Double vision. **(29)**

direct filing system A filing system in which materials can be located without consulting an intermediary source of reference. **(14)**

directory A logical area on a disk within which programs and data are stored. Each directory functions similarly to a single floppy disk. **(8)**

disability The condition resulting from illness or injury that makes an individual unable to be employed. **(19)**

disbursements Funds paid out. **(17)**

disbursements journal Record of every amount paid out, the date paid, the check number, and the purpose of payment. **(16)**

discharge summary The final progress note for a hospital patient that contains the patient's admitting and discharge diagnoses, any surgeries performed, the patient's course while hospitalized, and his or her condition upon discharge. **(13)**

discount A subtraction from the patient's balance. **(16)**

discretion Quality of being discreet, tactful, or prudent. **(1)**

discrimination A distinction based on race, religion, sex, or some other factor, especially one resulting in unfair or injurious treatment of an individual belonging to a particular group. **(22)**

disinfection Destruction of pathogenic organisms by chemical or physical means. **(24)**

disk A flat, circular plate with a magnetic surface that is capable of storing computer programs. Some disks are flexible *(floppy disks)* and some are hard *(hard disks)*. **(8)**

disk drive A device that loads a program or data stored on a disk into a computer. **(8)**

dispense The giving of drugs, in some type of bottle, box, or other container, to the patient. (Under the Controlled Substances Act of 1970, the definition of "dispense" includes the administering of Controlled Substances). **(5)**

disruption A breaking down or upset. **(10)**

dissect To cut or separate tissues with a cutting instrument or a scissors. **(35)**

dissection The process of cutting apart or separating tissues for anatomic study. **(2)**

dissemination The act of broadcasting or spreading over a considerable area. **(3)**, **(22)**

diuresis Increase in the excretion of urine. **(32)**

dot matrix printer An impact printer that forms characters using patterns of dots. **(8)**

draft A preliminary outline or writing that the author expects to amend or revise. **(20)**

ductus deferens The testicular duct that carries sperm from the epididymis to the ejaculatory duct. **(28)**

dysplasia Abnormal development of cells and tissues. **(29)**

dyspnea Difficult or painful breathing. **(26)**, **(30)**

dysuria Difficult or painful urination. **(32)**

eczema A common allergic reaction in children; atopic dermatitis. **(29)**

editing The process of examining text to determine accuracy and clarity. **(13)**

ejaculation Ejection of the seminal fluid from the male urethra. **(28)**

elastic pulse A pulse with regular alterations of weak and strong beats without changes in cycle. **(27)**

electronic mail Communications transmitted via computer using a telephone modem. **(8)**

emancipated minor A person under legal age who is self-supporting and living apart from parents or a guardian. **(5)**

embryology The science or study of the development of living organisms during the embryonic stage. **(2)**

empathy Intellectual and emotional awareness of another person's thoughts, feelings, and behavior. **(6)**

emphysema A pathologic accumulation of air in the tissues or organs in which the bronchioles become plugged with mucus and lose elasticity. **(27), (39)**

endogenous Produced or caused by factors from within the body. **(27), (34)**

endorsement Sanction or approval. **(3)**

endorser Person who signs his or her name on the back of a check for the purpose of transferring title to another person. **(17)**

endotoxin A poisonous substance found in certain bacteria that is released after the death of the bacteria. It causes fever, chills, and other symptoms. **(31)**

enunciation The act of pronouncing words distinctly. **(11)**

enuresis A condition of involuntary discharge of urine; bedwetting. **(32)**

enzymatic reaction A chemical reaction controlled by an enzyme. **(32)**

eosin A granular leukocyte that increases in number in allergic conditions. **(33)**

epididymis Oblong coiled body on top of the testis that stores the sperm cells. **(28)**

epistaxis Nose bleed. **(40)**

erythema Redness or inflammation of the skin caused by congestion of the capillaries in the skin layers. Results from injury, infection, or inflammation. **(29), (30), (39)**

erythrocyte Red blood cell; contains the blood protein. **(33)**

essential hypertension Sometimes called *primary* or *essential hypertension;* It develops for no apparent reason, and its cause is unknown. **(26)**

established patient A patient who has received care from the physician within the last 3 years. **(19)**

establishing guidelines Making statements regarding roles, purpose, and limitations for a particular interaction. **(6)**

eupnea Normal breathing. **(26)**

eustachian tube A narrow tube leading from the middle ear to the pharynx. **(29)**

exemplary Serving as a warning. **(5)**

exogenous Produced outside or caused by factors outside the body. **(27), (34)**

exophthalmos An abnormal protrusion of the eyes. **(27)**

expendable Describing supplies or equipment that are normally used up or consumed in service. **(21)**

expiration The act of breathing out or of expelling air from the lungs. **(39)**

expulsion Act of expelling or forcing out. **(4)**

externship The practice of receiving employment experience in qualified health care facilities under the cooperative supervision of the medical staff and the program instructor as part of the educational curriculum. **(1), (7)**

extracurricular Relating to those activities that form part of the life of students but are not part of the courses of study. **(7)**

extravasation Bleeding into the tissues. **(39)**

fallopian tubes The tubes that carry the ovum from the ovary to the uterus; the oviducts. The location where fertilization usually takes place. **(2), (28)**

fascia A sheet or band of fibrous tissue, deep in the skin, that covers muscles and body organs. **(35)**

fasting To go without solid food for a specified period of time. **(31)**

febrile Refers to a fever and is used descriptively. *Fever:* elevation of body temperature above normal. It is sometimes classified as follows: low—99° to 101° F (37.2° to 38.3° C); moderate—101° to 103° F (38.3° to 39.5° C); high—103° to 105° F (39.5° to 40.6° C). **(23), (26)**

fee profile A compilation of a physician's fees over a given period of time. **(15)**

fee schedule A list of services or procedures indemnified by the insurance company and of the specific dollars that will be paid for each service. **(19)**

fee splitting Sharing a fee with another physician, laboratory, or drug company not based on services performed. **(4)**

felony A crime of a graver nature than one designated as a misdemeanor. Generally, an offense punishable by imprisonment in a penitentiary. **(5)**

file An orderly, self-contained collection of data that is stored on a permanent storage device such as a disk. **(8)**

filing system A plan for organizing records so that they can be found when needed. **(14)**

fiscal agent A financial representative. **(15)**

flatus Gas expelled through the anus. **(29)**

floppy disk (diskette) A thin disk (diskette) of magnetic material capable of storing a large amount of information. The floppy disk was developed to provide users of small computer systems with an inexpensive and convenient way of storing information. **(8)**

focusing Questions and statements used to help the patient develop an idea. **(6)**

font A set of printing type that is one size and style. **(13)**

footnote A comment placed at the bottom of a page that would be distracting if placed within the main text. **(20)**

foreskin Loose skin covering the end of the penis. **(28)**

format Shape, size, and general make-up of a publication such as a resume **(7)**; To magnetically create tracks on a disk where information will be stored; to initialize. **(8)**

freestanding emergency center An emergency facility not associated with a hospital. **(1)**

frequency Excessive urination. **(32)**

fringe benefit A benefit granted by an employer that involves a money cost without affecting basic wage rates. **(19)**

fumigation Using a gaseous agent to destroy organisms such as insects and vectors. **(24)**

fungicide An agent that destroys fungi. **(24)**

galley proof A printer's proof taken from composed type before page makeup. **(20)**

general journal The book of original entry in accounting. **(16)**

genetics The branch of biology dealing with heredity and variation among related organisms. **(4)**

germicide/bactericide Destroys pathogenic organisms. **(24)**

ghost surgery A situation in which a patient has consented to have surgery done by one surgeon, but without the patient's knowledge or consent, the surgery is actually performed by another surgeon. **(4)**

glans penis The cone-shaped glans at the end of the penis covered by the foreskin in the uncircumcised male. **(28)**

gliadin A protein from wheat that is soluble in alcohol. **(34)**

glycogen A polysaccharide that is the principal form in which carbohydrate is stored in animal tissues. **(34)**

glycosuria The presence of glucose in the urine. **(32)**

goiter An enlargement of the thyroid gland. **(34)**

group policy A policy that covers a group, such as all employees of one company, under a master contract. **(19)**

group practice The provision of services by a group of at least three practitioners. **(1)**

hard copy The readable paper copy or printout of information from a computer. **(8)**

hardware Computer machinery. **(8)**

HCFA Health Care Financing Administration; the authority that administers Medicare. **(13)**

HCPCS HCFA's Common Procedure Coding System, used in determining Medicare fees. **(13)**

health maintenance organization (HMO) An organization that provides comprehensive health care to an enrolled group for a fixed periodic payment. **(1)**

hemangioma A benign tumor of dilated blood vessels. **(36)**

hematoma A localized collection of clotted blood caused by a broken blood vessel. **(31), (36)**

hematuria The presence of blood in the urine. **(32)**

hemiplegia Paralysis of one side of the body. **(2)**

hemoccult Hidden blood; a test for occult blood in the stool. **(29)**

hemolysis The destruction of red blood cells. **(31)**

hemolyzed Describing a blood sample in which the red cells have been ruptured. **(31)**

heparin A mixture of active principles capable of prolonging blood clotting time. **(33)**

hermetically sealed Sealed so that no air is allowed to enter. **(38)**

high-level disinfection A chemical procedure that kills vegetative organisms and viruses but not large numbers of bacterial spores. **(25)**

histologic Pertaining to the study of tissue cells. **(25)**

histologist One who specializes in the study of the minute structure, composition, and function of the tissues. **(2)**

history and physical The record of a patient's present illness, past medical and surgical history, and family history, and a review of the patient's present condition by body systems. **(13)**

human chorionic gonadotropin (hCG) A hormone secreted in large amounts by the placenta during gestation to stimulate the formation of interstitial cells. **(32)**

Human Immunodeficiency Virus (HIV) The virus that causes AIDS. It is transmitted through sexual contact or exposure to infected blood or blood components, and from an infected mother to her fetus. **(25)**

hydrocele A painless swelling in the scrotum caused by fluid in the testis. **(28)**

hydrocephaly An enlargement of the cranium caused by abnormal accumulation of cerebrospinal fluid within the cerebral system. **(28)**

hydrogenated Combined with, treated with, or exposed to hydrogen. **(34)**

hyperplasia An increase in the number of cells. **(29)**

hyperpnea Increased rate of respiration. **(26)**

hypertension High blood pressure in which systolic pressure is consistently above 160 mm Hg and diastolic pressure is above 90 mm Hg. **(26)**

hyperthermia Synonym for fever. **(23)**

hyperventilation Abnormally prolonged and deep breathing that is usually associated with acute anxiety or emotional tension. **(27)**

hypotension Blood pressure that is below normal in which systolic pressure is below 90 and diastolic pressure is below 50 mm Hg. **(26)**

hypoxia Reduction in the amount of oxygen that is transported to body tissues. **(26)**

ICD-9-CM International Classification of Diseases, 9th Revision, Clinical Modification. **(13)**

immunology A science that deals with the phenomena and causes of immunity and immune responses. **(2)**

in balance Total ending balances of patient ledgers equal the total of the accounts receivable control. **(16)**

in situ Localized. **(36)**

in vitro In glass; in a test tube or other artificial environment. **(4)**

incontinence Inability to control excretory functions. **(29), (32)**

indemnity A benefit paid by an insurer for a loss insured under a policy. **(19)**

indicator strip A charted strip that is inserted into the dictation unit and on which the dictator marks the beginning and end point of each document and any corrections to be made. **(13)**

individual policy A policy usually held by a person who does not qualify for a group policy. **(19)**

induration An abnormally hard spot or place. **(29), (38)**

infarction An area of tissue that has died because of lack of blood supply. **(30)**

infectious Capable of causing infection. **(5)**

informed consent A consent in which there is understanding of what treatment is to be undertaken and of the risks involved, why it should be done, and alternative methods of treatment available and their attendant risks. The alternatives include the failure to treat and the attendant risk. **(5)**

infraction Breaking the law. **(5)**

innovation Act of introducing something new or novel. **(2)**

inoculate To place a specimen in a culture medium to allow it to grow so that it can be identified. **(31)**

I/O (input/output) *Input* is any information that is entered into and used by a computer; *output* is any information that is processed by a computer and transmitted to a monitor, printer, or other device. **(8)**

ion An electrically charged particle. **(37)**

inspiration The act of breathing in or inhaling air into the lungs. **(39)**

insubordination Refusing to submit to authority. **(22)**

insulin shock Shock brought about by too much insulin, too little food, or excessive exercise. When untreated, it can result in death. **(40)**

integral Essential; being an indispensable part of a whole. **(10)**

interaction A two-way communication. **(10)**

intercom An intercommunication system; in a telephone system, a direct line from one station to another. **(9)**

intermittent Coming and going at intervals; not continuous. **(10)**

intermittent fever Body temperature is elevated at certain times within a 24-hour period but falls to a normal or even subnormal level during the same period of time. **(23)**, **(26)**

intermittent pulse A pulse in which occasional beats are skipped. **(26)**

intrinsic Inward; indwelling. **(12)**

invasion of privacy Unauthorized disclosure of a person's private affairs. **(18)**

invasive procedure A surgical entry into tissues, cavities, or organs. **(25)**

inventory A list of articles with the description and quantity of each. **(21)**

invoice A paper describing a purchase and the amount due. **(16)**

invulnerable Incapable of being injured or harmed. **(2)**

ionizing Process in which a neutral atom or molecule gains or loses electrons and then acquires a negative or positive electric charge. **(39)**

Ipecac (syrup of ipecac) A syrup given to induce vomiting. **(40)**

irregular pulse A pulse that varies in force and frequency. **(26)**

irrigation The flushing out of a cavity or wound with a solution. **(36)**

ischemia Temporary deficiency of blood supply to a tissue or organ; decreased blood flow to a body part or organ that is caused by constriction or plugging of the supplying artery. **(30)**, **(32)**

isolation The act of placing alone, apart from others. **(3)**

jargon The technical vocabulary of a special group. **(1)**

jaundice Yellow color of the skin, sclera, mucous membranes, and secretions resulting from increased levels of bilirubin. **(27)**, **(29)**

Kaposi's sarcoma A tumor of the walls of the blood vessels. It usually appears as pink to purple spots on the skin. **(25)**

keratosis Any horny growth, such as warts. **(36)**

keyboarding The process of entering characters into the memory of a word processor. **(13)**

labia majora Two folds of adipose tissue that extend from the mons pubis to the perineum. **(28)**

labia minora Two thin folds of epithelial tissue between the labia and the opening of the vagina. **(28)**

laissez faire Management style of "hands off" when dealing with employees. **(6)**

legend The heading or title of a figure. **(20)**

lesion A wound, sore, ulcer, tumor, or any traumatic tissue damage that causes a lack of tissue continuity or a loss of function. **(35)**

lethargic Describing a condition of drowsiness or indifference. **(40)**

leukemia A malignant neoplasm of the blood-forming organs. **(33)**

leukocyte White blood cell. Its primary function is to fight disease in the body. **(33)**

leukoderma White patches on the skin. **(29)**

lexicographic Pertaining to the definition of words and the compilation of dictionaries. **(20)**

liability State or quality of being liable; that for which one is liable, such as debts. **(3)**

ligation The process of tying up something to close it, usually a blood vessel, during surgery. The ties are called *ligatures*. **(2)**

listening An active process of receiving information and examining one's reaction to the messages received. **(6)**

litigation Contest in a court of justice for the purpose of enforcing a right. **(5)**, **(14)**

lumen An open space, such as within a blood vessel, the intestine, or an examining instrument. **(35)**

lymphoma A group of cancers that usually affect the lymph nodes, but in HIV infections, they often affect other tissue. **(25)**

main memory The section of a computer where information and instructions are stored. **(8)**

maker (of a check) Any individual, corporation, or legal party who signs a check or any type of negotiable instrument. **(17)**

malfeasance The doing of an act that is wholly wrongful and unlawful. **(5)**

malignant Having properties of metastasis; resulting in death. **(29)**

malignant hypertension High blood pressure that develops rapidly and may be fatal if not treated immediately. **(26)**

malpractice Professional misconduct, improper discharge of professional duties, or failure to meet the standard of care by a professional that results in harm to another. **(5)**

mammary glands The breasts. **(28)**

mandatory In the nature of a mandate or command; obligatory. **(1)**

maneuver A physical procedure. **(39)**

manuscript A written or typewritten document, as distinguished from a printed copy. **(20)**

matrix Something in which something else originates, develops, takes shape, or is contained; a base upon which to build. **(10)**

mediastinum The space in the center of the chest under the sternum, containing the heart, great vessels, esophagus, and trachea. **(40)**

medical indigent One who is able to take care of ordinary living expenses but who cannot afford medical care. **(15)**, **(19)**

melanosis Unusual deposits of black pigment on the skin. **(29)**

member physician A physician who has agreed to accept the contracts of an insurer; this usually includes accepting the insurance benefits as payment in full. **(19)**

menarche The onset of the menstrual cycle. **(28)**

meningitis An acute inflammation of the membranes of the spinal cord and the brain. **(25)**

meniscus The concave surface of a column of a liquid in a tube or cylindrical container. **(27)**

menopause The biologic end of the reproductive cycle of the female; also called *climacteric*. **(28)**

menstruation The cyclic shedding of the lining (endometrium) of the uterus. **(28)**

meticulous Extremely careful of small details. **(22)**

microcephaly A small size of the head in relation to the rest of the body. **(28)**

microcomputer Desk-top computer, originally designed as a personal computer. **(8)**

microfilming Photographing records in reduced size on film. **(14)**

microorganism An organism of microscopic or ultramicroscopic size. **(2)**

microsurgery Surgery performed under a microscope using very small instruments. **(36)**

millennia Thousands of years (*mille* = thousand). **(2)**

minicomputer Medium-size computer that has larger storage capacity than a microcomputer and that can accommodate multilocation terminals. **(8)**

misdemeanor A crime less serious than a felony. **(5)**

misfeasance The improper performance of a lawful act. **(5)**

modem An acronym for MOdulator DEModulator; a device that enables data to be transmitted over telephone lines. **(8)**

monitor A device used to display computer-generated information; a video screen; a CRT **(8)**; to listen to a matter transmitted by telephone as a third party. **(11)**

monograph A learned treatise on a small area of knowledge; a written account of a single thing or class of things. **(20)**

mons pubis The fat pad that covers the symphysis pubis. **(28)**

mons veneris The rounded, elevated area overlying the symphysis pubis that is covered with hair after puberty. **(2)**

mordant A chemical (Gram's iodine) used to make a primary stain adhere to the cells it stains. **(31)**

morphology The study of the size, shape, and staining characteristics of a cell. **(33)**

motivation Process of inciting a person to some action or behavior. **(22)**

multiparous Describing a woman who has had two or more pregnancies. **(28)**

myocardium The middle layer of the walls of the heart muscle. **(30)**

myoglobinuria Abnormal presence of a hemoglobin-like chemical of muscle tissue in urine that results in muscle deterioration. **(32)**

myringotomy Incision of the tympanic membrane. **(29)**

mysticism The experience of seeming to have direct communication with God or ultimate reality. **(2)**

mythology A branch of knowledge that deals with the interpretation of myths. **(2)**

myxedema A condition resulting from advanced hypothyroidism. **(27)**

negotiable Legally transferable to another party. **(17)**

neophyte A beginner. **(2)**

neoplasia New growth of cells. Used interchangeably with the term *cancer*. **(29)**

nevi Round moles or birthmarks varying in color from yellow-brown to black. **(27)**

new patient A patient who has not received any professional services from the physician in the past 3 years. **(19)**

nocturia Excessive urination during the night. **(32)**

nomogram Representation by graphs, diagrams, or charts of the relationships between numeric variables. **(37)**

nominal Existing in name only. **(5)**

noncommittal Not revealing any specific attitude or opinion. **(11)**

nonfeasance The failure to do something that should have been done. **(5)**

nonparticipating provider A physician who does not accept assignment under Medicare or the Blue Plans. **(19)**

no-show A person who fails to keep an appointment without giving advance notice of such failure. **(10)**

nosocomial Pertaining to or originating in a hospital. **(32)**

numerical filing Filing records, correspondence, or cards by number. **(14)**

obesity An excessive accumulation of body fat, usually defined as more than 20% above the recommended body weight. **(34)**

objective Something toward which effort is directed; an aim or end of action. **(7)**

obturator A metal rod with a smooth rounded tip, placed in hollow instruments to decrease destruction of the mucous membrane during insertion. **(35)**

occult Hidden; not visible with the eye alone. **(31)**

onset Beginning of a fever. **(23)**, **(26)**

open-ended questions General questions that ask the patient to determine the direction the communication should take. **(6)**

operation record A report dictated immediately following surgery that contains the preoperative and postoperative diagnoses, the procedure performed, the anesthesia administered, the names of the patient, surgeon, assistant surgeon (if any), and the anesthetist, the beginning and ending time of the surgery, and the patient's condition on leaving the operating room. This report becomes a permanent part of the patient's chart. **(13)**

oral hygiene Proper care of the mouth and teeth for the maintenance of health and prevention of disease, characterized by clean teeth and absence of unpleasant breath. **(9)**

order of business A list of the different divisions of business in the order in which each will be called for at business meetings. **(20)**

orientation The determination or adjustment of one's intellectual or emotional position with reference to circumstances. **(22)**

orthopnea Breathing in an upright or straight position. **(26)**

orthostatic blood pressure Blood pressure measurement taken with the patient in a standing, erect position. **(26)**

osteoporosis Loss of bone tissue occurring most frequently in small-boned, postmenopausal women. **(34)**, **(39)**

otitis Inflammation of the ear canal. **(29)**

OUTfolder A folder used to provide space for the temporary filing of materials. **(14)**

OUTguide A heavy guide that is used to replace a folder that has been temporarily removed from the filing space. **(14)**

ovaries A pair of almond-shaped organs located at the distal end of the fallopian tubes. Responsible for the development and release of the ova and the production of a large percentage of the female hormones. **(28)**

over-the-counter Describing medications sold without a prescription. **(37)**

oviducts The pair of tubes in the female that carry the egg from the ovary to the uterus; fallopian tubes. **(2)**

packing slip An itemized list of objects in a package. **(16)**

pallor The absence of color to the skin and mucous membranes. **(27)**

pandemic Affecting the majority of the people in a country or a number of countries. **(2)**

pantothenic acid B complex vitamin present in all living tissues. **(34)**

paroxysmal Describing the sudden onset of symptoms such as a spasm or seizure. **(35)**, **(40)**

participating provider A physician who accepts assignment under Medicare or the Blue Plans. **(19)**

passive Describing the movement or exercising of a body part by an externally applied force. **(27)**

patency The open condition of a body cavity or canal. **(35)**

pathologic Altered or caused by disease. **(2)**

pathology report The report dictated by the pathologist following any surgery that involves removal of tissue in the hospital. The report contains a description of the tissue removed (gross and microscopic) as well as the diagnosis; it is signed by the pathologist. It becomes a permanent part of the patient's chart. **(13)**

payables Amounts owed to others. **(16)**

payee The person named on a draft or check as the recipient of the amount shown. **(17)**

payer Person who writes a check in favor of the payee. **(17)**

pedunculated Having a stem-like connecting part. **(36)**

pejorative Having negative connotations; a depreciatory word. **(14)**

penis The male organ of copulation. **(28)**

percussion The act of striking a part of the body with short, sharp blows as an aid in diagnosing the condition of the underlying parts by the sound obtained. **(2)**

perfusion The passing of a fluid through spaces. **(2)**

pericardium The sac that surrounds the heart. **(30)**

periodical A journal published with a fixed interval (of greater than 1 day) between the issues or numbers. **(20)**

peripheral A device—such as a printer, disk drive, or mouse—that can be attached to a computer for input, output, or storage purposes. **(8)**

perjured testimony Telling what is false when sworn to tell the truth. **(5)**

permeability Ability of solutions to pass through a membrane. **(24)**, **(37)**

personal inventory A *complete* summary of pertinent information about oneself. **(7)**

phagocytosis The engulfing of microorganisms, other cells, and foreign particles by phagocytes. **(2)**, **(33)**

phenylalanine An essential amino acid found in milk, eggs, and other common foods. **(32)**

phenylketonuria (PKU) A congenital disease resulting from a defect in protein metabolism that, when untreated, causes severe mental retardation. **(34)**

philosophy The general laws that furnish the rational explanation of anything. **(22)**

phonetic Pertaining to the voice or its use. **(9)**

photocoagulation Clotting of blood with light. **(36)**

photometer An instrument that measures the intensity of a beam of light passing through it; the intensity of a beam is directly related to the concentration of the substance the beam passes through. **(31)**

pitch The vibratory frequency of a tone or sound. **(11)**

placenta The vascular structure that develops

within the uterus during pregnancy and through which a fetus receives nourishment. **(2)**

planing The rubbing away of a layer of tissue. **(36)**

plasma A straw-colored fluid that transports nutrients, hormones, and waste products. It is 91% water. **(33)**

pneumocystis carinii **pneumonia (PCP)** A lung infection usually occurring in immunocompromised people. Caused by a protozoan that is present almost everywhere but is normally destroyed by healthy immune systems. **(25)**

polycythemia vera A condition that causes an overproduction of all formed elements of the blood. **(33)**

polyps Tumors on stems frequently found on mucous membranes. **(35)**

POMR Problem Oriented Medical Record. **(14)**

portfolio A set of documents either bound in book form or loose in a folder. **(12)**

posting The act of transferring information from one record to another. **(16)**

power of attorney A legal statement in which a person authorizes another person to act as his or her attorney or agent. The statement may be limited to the handling of certain procedures. The person authorized to act as agent is known as an *attorney in fact.* **(17)**

preamble An introductory portion; a preface. **(4)**

precept A practical rule guiding behavior or technique. **(4)**

pre-existing condition A physical condition of an insured person that existed prior to the issuance of the insurance policy. **(19)**

premium The periodic payment required to keep a policy in force. **(19)**

prepaid plan A prepaid plan that provides all covered services to a policyholder for payment of a monthly fee. **(19)**

prerogative An exclusive and unquestionable right belonging to a person or body of persons. **(10)**

presbyopia Diminution of accommodation of the lens of the eye occurring normally with aging; results in farsightedness. **(29)**

prescribe To issue a prescription for the patient; to direct, designate, or order use of a remedy. **(5)**

preservative A substance added to a specimen that prevents deterioration of cells or chemicals in the specimen. **(31)**

primary tumor Tumor at the site of origin. **(29)**

printout The output from a printer; also called *hard copy.* **(8)**

probationary Pertaining to a trial or a period of trial to ascertain fitness for a job. **(22)**

professional courtesy Reduction or absence of fee to professional associates. **(15)**

Professional Standards Review Organization (PSRO) A group of physicians working with the government to review cases for hospital admission and discharge under gov-ernment guidelines; sometimes referred to as *Peer Review.* **(19)**

proficient Competent as a result of training and practice. **(10)**

prognosis Forecast of the course of a disease. **(20)**

progress notes Records of patient visits, telephone calls, progress, and treatment that are inserted into the patient's medical chart. **(13)**

prompt A symbol used by some computers to indicate when the computer is ready to accept input. **(8)**

pronunciation The act or manner of pronouncing words. **(11)**

proofreading Checking a document for spelling, sentence structure, punctuation, capitalization, style, and format. **(13)**

prostate A fluid-secreting gland that surrounds the neck of the urethra in the male. **(28)**

protein A group of organic compounds occurring in plants and animals; contains the major element nitrogen and the amino acids essential for life maintenance. **(34)**

proteinuria An excess of serum protein in the urine. **(32)**

protozoa Primitive animal organisms, each of which consists of a single cell. **(2)**

protozoal Pertaining to a pathogenic organism that can be ingested and transmitted through contaminated feces. Handwashing and the taking of precautions when handling stools are highly recommended. **(25)**

prudent Capable of directing or conducting oneself wisely and judiciously. **(3)**

pruritus Itching. **(29)**

ptosis Drooping of the upper eyelid. **(29)**

public domain The realm embracing property rights that belong to the community at large and that are subject to appropriation by anyone. **(4)**

puerperal fever The fever that accompanies an infection of the birth canal following delivery of a child; childbed fever. **(2)**

pulse deficit Difference between the apical pulse and the radial pulse. **(26)**

pulse pressure Difference between the systolic and the diastolic blood pressures; fewer than 30 points or more than 50 points is considered normal. **(26)**

punitive Inflicting punishment. **(5)**

purulent Consisting of or containing pus. **(2)**

pustule Raised pus-filled area or sac. **(2)**

putrefaction Decomposition of animal matter that results in a foul smell. **(2)**

pyrexia Synonym for fever. **(23)**, **(26)**

pyuria Presence of pus in the urine. **(32)**

quackery Pretense of medical skill. **(3)**, **(39)**

quality assurance A law-enforced program that guarantees quality patient care. **(31)**

quality control The operational procedures used to implement the quality assurance program. **(31)**

rabies An acute infectious disease of the nervous system caused by a virus, usually communicated to humans through animal bite. **(2)**

rad A measurement of the actual absorbed dose of radiation. **(39)**

radiation The transfer through space of any form of energy, such as light, heat, or x-ray. **(39)**

radical mastectomy The complete surgical removal of the breast, the surrounding muscles, and the lymph glands. **(38)**

radiology reports Radiology reports are dictated in the radiology department of a hospital or imaging center and include reports of x-rays and other imaging procedures. **(13)**

rales Abnormal or crackling chest sounds that occur during breathing; abnormal respiratory sounds heard on inspiration. **(26), (29)**

random access memory (RAM) The computer's temporary memory; it stores data and programs that are input. **(8)**

rapport A relationship of harmony and accord between the patient and the health care worker. **(6)**

read-only memory (ROM) Memory that can be altered only by changing the physical structure of the chip. ROM chips are usually used to store information that is essential to the operation of a computer. **(8)**

receipts cash received. **(16)**

receivables Amounts that are owed by others. **(16)**

reciprocity An obligation under which something is done or given by each of two to the other. **(3)**

reconciliation (of bank statement) The process of proving that the bank statement and the checkbook balance are in agreement. **(17)**

recruitment The supplying of new members or help. **(22)**

reducing distance Diminishing the physical space between the medical assistant and the patient. **(6)**

re-entry student One who has been away from formal education or employment for several years and who is now preparing to re-enter the workplace. **(7)**

reference laboratory A large laboratory that accepts specimens from smaller laboratories to perform tests not done by the smaller laboratories. **(31)**

reference values The listings of accepted ranges for normal values for routine hematology tests. **(31)**

reflecting Directing back to the patient his or her ideas, feelings, questions, or concerns. **(6)**

regional Pertaining to a region or territory; local. **(1)**

rem Method of measuring the amount of radiation absorbed by a patient while exposed to x-ray. Similar to *rad*. **(39)**

remittent fever A fever in which temperature fluctuates greatly but never falls to the normal level. **(23), (26)**

reprint A reproduction of printed matter. **(20)**

reputable Honorable; having a good reputation. **(21)**

requisition A formal written request from the physician authorizing a laboratory procedure. **(31)**

resident A graduate and licensed physician receiving training in a specialty in a hospital. **(4)**

residual Refers to urine left in the bladder after urination. **(32)**

resonance Sound or echo produced by percussion of a body part or cavity. **(27)**

restating Repeating to the patient what you believe is the main thought or idea expressed. **(6)**

resumé A *selective* summary of one's education and employment record tailored to the position being sought. **(7)**

rete mucosum The innermost layer of the epidermis (*rete* = network of nerves or vessels). **(2)**

retention Accumulation of urine within the bladder because of inability to urinate. **(32)**

retention schedule A listing of dates until which records are to be kept, based on statutes of limitations, tax regulations, and other factors. **(14)**

revocation The act of annulling by recalling or taking back. **(4), (5)**

rhinitis Inflammation of the nasal membranes. **(29)**

rhonchi Rattling noises in the throat that may resemble snoring. **(26)**

rhonchus Abnormal sounds heard when the airway is obstructed; also called a *wheeze*. **(29)**

rider A legal document that modifies the protection of a policy. **(19)**

roentgen Unit used to measure x-ray dosage. **(39)**

rural Pertaining to the country, as distinguished from a city or town. **(1)**

sanitization Reducing the number of microorganisms to a level that is relatively safe. **(24)**

scanner An input device that converts printed matter into a computer-readable format. **(8)**

screen The act of determining to whom a telephone call is to be directed. **(11)**

screening test A laboratory test done on large numbers of people for the purpose of detecting occult diseases. **(31)**

scrotum The double pouch that contains the testicles and epididymis. **(28)**

scurvy A condition resulting from a deficiency in vitamin C (ascorbic acid). It is characterized by bleeding gums and ecchymosis. **(34)**

secondary hypertension Elevated blood pressure due to another condition. For example, *prenatal hypertension* is elevated blood pressure that returns to normal when the pregnancy terminates. **(27)**

seeking clarification Asking for additional inputs to understand the message received. **(6)**

seeking consensual validation Attempts to reach a mutual meaning for a specific word used in the conversation. **(6)**

semen Thick, whitish secretion containing the spermatozoa. **(28)**

seminar A group of students meeting regularly and informally with a professor to discuss ideas and problems. **(7)**

senile Pertaining to old age. **(36)**

sensitivity disk An antibiotic-impregnated paper that is placed on a specially inoculated culture plate to determine whether an organism is sensitive or resistant to that antibiotic. **(31)**

sequential Succeeding or following in order or as a result. **(14)**

serology A laboratory study of serum and the reactions between antigens and antibodies. **(33)**

serum Plasma with the clotting proteins removed. **(33)**

service benefit plan A plan that agrees to pay for certain surgical and medical services and that is not restricted to a fee schedule. **(19)**

shelf filing A system that uses open shelves (rather than cabinets) for storing records. **(14)**

sigmoidoscope An instrument used to examine the sigmoid colon; may be rigid or flexible. **(29)**

silence Periods of no verbal communication. **(6)**

sinoatrial node (SA node) Pacemaker of the heart located in the right atrium. **(30)**

slough The shedding of dead tissue cells. **(36)**

slow pulse A pulse rate between 40 and 60 beats per minute. It may be noted in athletes and the aged during rest. **(26)**

socioeconomic Relating to a combination of social and economic factors. **(10)**

software The programming necessary to direct the hardware of a computer system; computer programs. **(8)**

solo private practice One physician practicing alone. **(1)**

specimen A sample of body fluid, waste product, or tissue that is collected for analysis. **(31)**

spermatozoa Mature male sex cells or germ cells. **(2), (28)**

sprain A traumatic injury without separation of muscle, tendon, or ligament surrounding a bone. **(39)**

staging Used to describe the extent of cancer spread. **(29)**

stand-alone system Any complete computer system located within an office. **(8)**

stat Do immediately. **(31)**

stat report An immediate report (from the Latin *statim*, meaning "at once"). **(10)**

statement A request for payment. **(16)**

statement of income and expense A summary of all income and expenses for a given period. **(16)**

statute of limitations The time limit within which an action may legally be brought upon a contract. **(14), (18)**

statutory body A part of the legislative branch of a government. **(3)**

sterilization Complete destruction of all forms of microbial life. **(24)**

stertorous Describing a deep snoring sound that occurs with each inspiration. **(26)**

stethoscope An instrument for listening to sounds within the body. **(2)**

strain A muscular injury resulting from excessive physical exertion. **(39)**

stridor High-pitched, harsh sound heard when the larynx is obstructed. **(29)**

stylus A metal probe that is inserted or passed through a catheter, needle, or tube for clearing purposes or to facilitate passage into a body orifice. **(35)**

subject filing Arranging records alphabetically by names of topics or things rather than by names of individuals. **(14)**

sublingual Under the tongue. **(38)**

subscriber A person named as principal in an insurance contract. **(19)**

subscript A symbol or number written immediately below another character. **(13)**

subsidize To aid or promote something (such as a private enterprise) with public money. **(18)**

substantiated Having been established as true by proof or competent evidence; verified. **(3)**

summary A synopsis of the main points of a longer text. **(20)**

superbill A combination charge slip, statement, and insurance reporting form. **(18)**

superscript A symbol or number written immediately above another character. **(13)**

suppuration Production of purulent material (pus) by a wound. **(37)**

surrogate A substitute; someone appointed to act in the place of another. **(4)**

suspension The act of interrupting or discontinuing temporarily, but with an expectation or purpose of resumption. **(4)**

swine erysipelas A contagious disease affecting young swine in Europe. **(2)**

symmetry Relative proportion of the opposite sides of the body and their parts to each other. **(27)**

syncope A brief loss of consciousness; fainting. **(33), (40)**

synergism Joint action of agents so that their combined effect is greater than the actions of the individual components. **(37)**

syntax error A computer system response to a mistake in instructions, such as a transposition of characters or an omission of a character or word. **(8)**

syphilitic chancre The primary sore of syphilis. **(2)**

T-cells (T-lymphocytes) Small circulating lymphocytes that are produced in the bone marrow. Their primary function is to indirectly aid cellular immune responses (i.e., to facilitate the destruction of virus-infected cells and cancer cells). **(25)**

tab The projection on a file folder or guide on which the caption is written. **(14)**

tachycardia Fast heart rate; pulse greater than 100 beats per minute. **(26), (30)**

tachypnea Respirations that are regular in rhythm but faster than normal in rate. **(27)**

technical Pertaining to the practical or procedural details of a trade or profession. **(1)**

technologic Relating to the application of scientific knowledge or methods. **(4)**

telecommunications The science and technology of communications by transmission of information from one location to another via telephone, television, or telegraph. **(8)**

teller A bank employee who is assigned the duty of serving the bank's customers. **(17)**

testicle The male gonad. **(28)**

tetany A continuous contraction or muscle spasm caused by an inadequate blood calcium level or accidental surgical removal of the parathyroid glands. **(34)**

third-party check A check written to the order of the person offering payment and unknown to the payee, who is a third party in the process. **(17)**

third-party payor Someone other than the patient, spouse, or parent who is responsible for paying all or part of the patient's medical costs. **(15)**

thready pulse A pulse that is very faint and scarcely perceptible. **(26)**

thrombocyte A platelet; the smallest formed element of the blood. **(33)**

thrush *Candida albicans;* a yeast infection usually seen on the mucous membranes of the mouth and nose. **(25)**

tickler (file) A chronologic file used as a reminder that something must be taken care of on a certain date. **(10)**, **(14)**

tinnitus Ringing in the ears. It is a symptom of labyrinthitis, eighth cranial nerve damage, or cerebral arteriosclerosis. **(27)**, **(29)**

tone A normal state of balance in muscle tissue; when the muscles are at rest. **(39)**

topical Applied to a certain area of the skin and affecting only that area. **(38)**

tort An act that brings harm to a person or damage to property, caused negligently or intentionally. **(5)**

tourniquet A device for the compression of an artery or a vein. **(33)**

toxin A poisonous protein substance produced by some plants, animals, and pathogenic bacteria that builds up in the body as the microorganisms multiply. **(31)**

transaction The occurrence of a financial event or condition that must be recorded. **(16)**

transcription The process of transcribing from notes or a recording to the printed page; listening to recorded dictation and transcribing it into written form. **(12)**, **(13)**

transfer Removing inactive records from the active files. **(14)**

transmitter The part of a telephone into which one speaks. **(11)**

traumatic Pertaining to, resulting from, or causing physical injury or shock. **(40)**

treason A crime against the United States. **(5)**

treatise A systematic exposition or argument in writing. **(20)**

trespass To exceed the bounds of what is lawful, right, or just. **(5)**

triage To sort or to choose; to determine the priority of need for treatment. **(40)**

tryptophan Essential amino acid that is present in high concentration in animal and fish protein. **(34)**

tutorial Instruction on paper or disk intended to give practical information about using a specific computer program. **(8)**

unequal pulse Difference between right and left radial and/or femoral pulse counts. **(27)**

unit Each part of a name that is used in indexing. **(14)**

universal precautions A set of guidelines based on the assumption that every medical patient has a blood-borne infection that can be transmitted by blood, bloody fluids, and genital secretions. **(25)**

untoward Hard to manage. **(36)**

urban Characteristic of or pertaining to a city or town. **(1)**

uremia A toxic renal condition characterized by the lack of excretion of waste nitrogenous substances in the blood. **(27)**

urethra The canal through which urine and sperm are discharged. **(28)**

urgency The sudden compelling desire to urinate. **(32)**

usual, customary, and reasonable (UCR) A formula for determining medical insurance benefits payable. **(15)**

uterus A pearshaped organ located in the pelvic cavity between the bladder and the rectum and attached to the cervix. Holds the fetus during pregnancy. **(28)**

vagina The canal in the female that extends from the vulva to the cervix. **(2)**, **(28)**

vas deferens Ductus deferens. **(28)**

vasectomy Sterilization procedure for the male. **(28)**

venereal Due to or propagated by sexual intercourse. **(5)**

ventricle One of the lower chambers of the heart. **(30)**

vermicide Agent that destroys parasitic worms or intestinal parasites. **(24)**

vertigo Sensation of rotation or movement; dizziness. **(27)**, **(29)**, **(30)**

vesiculation Formation of blister-like sacs or elevations on the skin. **(29)**, **(38)**

vial A small bottle, usually glass. **(38)**

virulent Exceedingly pathogenic, noxious, or deadly. **(2)**

viscosity The quality of being a gluey substance lacking easy movement. **(38)**

vital capacity The maximum volume of air inspired with a maximally forced effort from a position of maximum expiration. **(39)**

vitiligo White patches on the skin caused by loss of melanin. **(27)**, **(29)**

vivisection Operation or cutting on a living animal for research purposes. **(2)**

void To urinate. **(28)**, **(32)**

volatile Referring to an explosive substance's capacity to vaporize at a low temperature. (38)

volume capacity The maximum volume of air expired with a maximally forced effort from a position of maximum inspiration. (39)

vulva The external female genitalia; an area beginning at the mons pubis and terminating at the anus. (28)

wasting syndrome A decrease of total body mass seen in the infected patient, usually caused by lack of appetite and persistent watery stools. (25)

WATS Wide Area Telephone Service. (11)

wheal A localized area of edema on the skin that is usually accompanied by itching. (29), (38)

word processing (WP) A system used to process written communications through the use of modern equipment, greater employee specialization, and an increase in the application of standardized procedures. (8)

xeroderma Dry skin. (29)

INDEX

Note: Page numbers in *italics* indicate illustrations; those followed by (t) refer to tables and procedures.

A

Abandonment, of patient, avoiding charges of, 388
Abbreviations, apothecary system, 778(t)
  in drug prescriptions, 764(t)
  in manuscript preparation, 343(t)
  in medical transcription, 195, 203
  in patient history and physical exam, 209(t)
  metric system, 778(t)
Abdomen, acute vs. chronic, 525
  division of, into quadrants, 485, *486*
    into regions, 485, *486*
  physical examination of, 485–486, *486*, 488, 492
Abdominal pain, causes of, 870
  treatment of, 870
Abdominal thrusts, self-administered, 864, *866*
  subdiaphragmatic, 864, *865–866*
Abduction, 536
Abortion, ethics of, Judicial Council opinions on, 42
  incomplete, 493
  spontaneous, 493
Abrasion, skin, hydrogen peroxide for, 694
Abridged Index Medicus, 339
Abscess, characteristics of, 399(t)
Abscess needle, 707, *707*
Abstracts, 336
  preparation of, 337
Abuse, ethics of, Judicial Council opinions on, 42
Academies, early medical education and, 28
Accidents, in children, prevention of, 856–857
Account balance, 248
Account cards, 248, *249–250*
Accounting, cash and accrual bases for, 246
  software for, 103
  terminology of, *247*, 247–248
Accounting equation, 254
Accounting systems, 245–265
  adjustments in, 256
  advantages and disadvantages of, 251(t)
  checkbook in, 248, *251*
  collection agency payments in, 259
  credit balances in, 256–257
  disbursements journal in, 248
  double-entry, 252, 254
  general (daily) journal in, 248
  ledger in, 248, *249–250*

Accounting systems *(Continued)*
  nonsufficient funds checks in, 257, *257*
  one-entry cash transactions in, 257, 259
  open book, statutes of limitations regarding, 305
  payroll records in, 265. See also *Payroll records.*
  pegboard (write-it-once), 254
    end-of-day summarizing in, 256
    entering and posting in, *255*, 255–256
    ledger cards in, 255
    materials required for, 254
    posting service charges and payments in, 258(t)
    preparation of, 255
    recording payments and charges in, 256
    use of, 254–256
  periodic summaries in, 263–264
  petty cash record in, 248, 251
  refunds in, 257
  single-entry, 251–252, *252–253*
    statutes of limitations regarding, 305–306
  software for, 264–265
  special entries in, 256–259
  vocabulary for, 244
Accounts payable, 260–264
  for petty cash, 262–263, *262–263*
  invoice and statements in, 260
  paying for purchases in, 260, 262
  recording disbursements in, *261*, 262
  recording personal expenditures in, 262
Accounts receivable, *259*, 259–260
  aging, 297, 299, *299*
  insurance protection for, 308
  ledger for, 248, *249–250*
    account card/statement from, 252, *253*
  locating and preventing errors in, 260
  trial balance of, 260, 264
Accounts receivable ratio, 296–297, *297*
Accrediting Bureau of Health Education Schools (ABHES), Registered Medical Assistant (RMA) examination and, 10
Ace bandage, 747, *748*
Acetest, urinary ketone measurement with, 608
Acetylsalicylic acid, invention of, 760–761
Achilles tendon, etymology of, 16
Acid precipitation test, of urinary protein, 612
Acidosis, breath odors in, 482
Acids, disinfection with, 411
Acknowledgment, in communication, 71
Acne vulgaris, 523

Acquired immunodeficiency syndrome (AIDS), 403, 427–437, 583. See also *Human immunodeficiency virus (HIV) infection.*
  AIDS-related complex in, 430
  annual deaths from, 428, *429*
  cause of, 428, 430
  Centers for Disease Control criteria for, 430
  characteristics of, 401(t)
  clinical manifestations of, 431–432
    bacterial infections in, 432
    candidiasis in, 431–432
    Cryptosporidium infection in, 431
    cytomegalovirus infection in, 432
    Kaposi's sarcoma in, 430–431
    lymphoma in, 431
    opportunistic infection in, 431
    Pneumocystis carinii pneumonia in, 431
    viral infection in, 432
    wasting syndrome in, 431
  geographic distribution of, 430, *430*
  impact of, 428
  incidence of, 428, *429*
  information on, organizations for, 437
  legal and ethical responsibilities in, 437
  population affected by, 431
  progression from HIV infection of, 430
  transmission of, 431
    portals of entry in, 431, 431(t)
  tuberculosis with, 582–583
  vocabularly for, 426
Acrotism, definition of, 466
Acuity testing, of color vision, 528, *529*, *531*, 531(t)
  of distance vision, 527, *527*
  of near vision, 527–528, *528*
Acupuncture, pain control with, 847
Addiction, drug, 765
Adduction, 536
Administration, terminology in, glossary of, 879–893
Administration area, utilization and care of, 352–353
Administrative law, 52
Adolescent, examination of, 505
Adrenergics, definition and uses of, 770
Adrenocorticosteroids, definition of, 772
Adults, incompetent, informed consent for, 58
Advertisements, classified, 86, *88*
  response to, by letter, 87, 87(t)
Advertising, ethics of, Judicial Council opinions on, 44

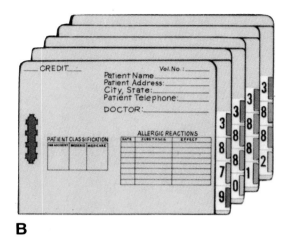

B

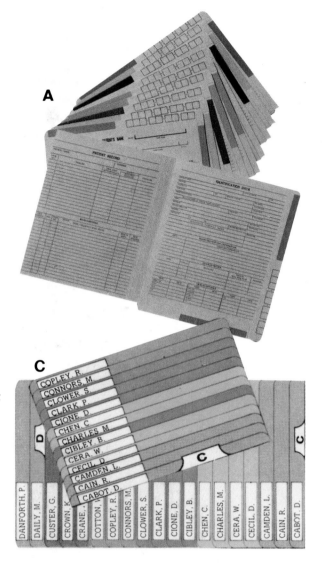

A

C

A good filing system for the efficient medical practitioner's office will often use a color-coded system for patient records.

A) Patient record folders are available with colored tabs, which can be used for either an alphabetical or numeric system. Use of a color-coded system will significantly minimize misfiling. (Courtesy of Ames Color-File, Division of Ames Safety Envelope Company, Somerville, Massachusetts.)

B) A numeric system is appropriate for large or multiple-physician offices. (Courtesy of Bibbero Systems, Inc.)

C) For alphabetical color coding, the second letter of each patient's name determines the color used. Misfiled folders are easily detected. (Courtesy Bibbero Systems, Inc.)

D) Working examples of alphabetical (left) and numeric (right) systems.

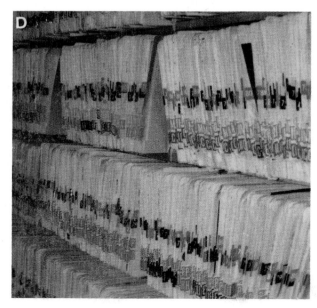

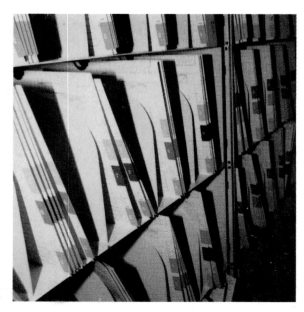